Advanced Nutrition and Human Metabolism

FOURTH EDITION

Sareen S. Gropper
Auburn University

Jack L. Smith
University of Delaware

James L. Groff

THOMSON
WADSWORTH

Australia • Canada • Mexico • Singapore • Spain
United Kingdom • United States

THOMSON
WADSWORTH

Publisher: Peter Marshall
Development Editor: Elizabeth Howe
Assistant Editor: Elesha Feldman
Editorial Assistant: Lisa Michel
Technology Project Manager: Travis Metz
Marketing Manager: Jennifer Somerville
Marketing Assistant: Melanie Banfield
Advertising Project Manager: Shemika Britt
Project Manager, Editorial Production: Sandra Craig
Creative Director: Rob Hugel
Print/Media Buyer: Judy Inouye
Permissions Editor: Sarah Harkrader
Production: Mary Douglas, Rogue Valley Publications
Text Designer: Susan Schmidler
Photo Researcher: Myrna Engler
Copy Editor: Mary Roybal
Cover Designer: Ross Carron
Cover Image: Sulforaphane, found in broccoli and one of the best-studied phytochemicals, is a small molecule that expedites the excretion of carcinogens from cells. *Photo:* Michael W. Davidson at Florida State University
Cover Printer: Phoenix Color Corp
Compositor: Progressive Information Technologies
Printer: Quebecor World/Versailles

Printed in the United States of America
1 2 3 4 5 6 7 08 07 06 05 04

For more information about our products, contact us at:
Thomson Learning Academic Resource Center
1-800-423-0563

For permission to use material from this text or product, submit a request online at **http://www.thomsonrights.com.**

Any additional questions about permissions can be submitted by email to **thomsonrights@thomson.com.**

Library of Congress Control Number: 2004101648

Student Edition: ISBN 0-534-55986-7

International Student Edition: ISBN 0-534-56013-X (Not for sale in the United States)

THIS BOOK IS PRINTED ON ACID-FREE RECYCLED PAPER

Thomson Wadsworth
10 Davis Drive
Belmont, CA 94002-3098
USA

Asia
Thomson Learning
5 Shenton Way #01-01
UIC Building
Singapore 068808

Australia/New Zealand
Thomson Learning
102 Dodds Street
Southbank, Victoria 3006
Australia

Canada
Nelson
1120 Birchmount Road
Toronto, Ontario M1K 5G4
Canada

Europe/Middle East/Africa
Thomson Learning
High Holborn House
50/51 Bedford Row
London WC1R 4LR
United Kingdom

Latin America
Thomson Learning
Seneca, 53
Colonia Polanco
11560 Mexico D.F.
Mexico

Spain/Portugal
Paraninfo
Calle Magallanes, 25
28015 Madrid, Spain

*To my parents for their love, support, and encouragement.
To Michael and Michelle who keep my life balanced and give me such joy. To my husband Daniel for his ongoing encouragement, support, faith, and love. And finally, to quote my husband, who told me to whom the book really needed to be dedicated, that is "To the carbon atom."*

Sareen Gropper

To my wife Carol, for her support for my coauthoring this new edition and for her assistance in the book's preparation. She has been very understanding of the changes in my career and our anticipated new directions.

Jack Smith

Brief Contents

Contents

Preface

Since the first edition was published in 1990, much has changed in the science of nutrition. But the purpose of the text—to provide thorough coverage of normal metabolism for upper-division nutrition students—remains the same. We continue to strive for a level of detail and scope of material that satisfy the needs of both instructors and students. With each succeeding edition, we have responded to suggestions from instructors, content reviewers, and students that have improved the text by enhancing the clarity of the material and by assuring accuracy. In addition, we have included the latest and most pertinent nutrition science available in order to provide future nutrition professionals with the fundamental information vital to their careers.

Just as the body of information on nutrition science has increased, so has the team of authors working on this text. Dr. James Groff and Dr. Sara Hunt coauthored the first edition. In subsequent editions, Dr. Sareen Gropper became a coauthor as Dr. Sara Hunt entered retirement. In this fourth edition, Dr. Jack L. Smith has joined the author team of Gropper and Groff.

NEW TO THIS EDITION

In this edition, we introduce a two-color design to visually emphasize important concepts in the chapters. The second color is also used in the figures to highlight reactants, products, and movement through the biochemical pathways. We hope this use of color will improve student learning.

Several new perspectives at the end of the chapters reflect the current thrust of nutrition research. While the chapter text concentrates on normal nutrition and physiological function, the perspectives deal with clinical, pathological, and applied aspects germane to the subject of each corresponding chapter. Many of the perspectives from the previous edition remain. New perspectives include "Phytochemicals and Herbal Supplements in Health and Disease" (Chap. 5), "Nutrigenomics: The Foundation for Individualized Nutrition" (Chap. 6), "Nutrient Usage during Strenuous Exercise" (Chap. 8), "Genetics and Nutrition: Human Folate Needs and Chronic Disease Risk" (Chap. 9), and "Nutrient–Drug Interactions" (Chap. 12).

In addition to a second color and new perspectives, this edition incorporates a thorough integration of the latest Dietary Reference Intakes, including new information on energy calculations and recommendations for carbohydrates, fiber, fat, fatty acids, cholesterol, protein, amino acids, vitamins, and minerals. We have also added a glossary to provide students with easy access to terminology used throughout the text. Cross-references have been retained to facilitate locating associated topics.

To our consideration of regulators of metabolism we have added a discussion of glycemic index and glycemic load and their proposed role in influencing metabolism. The information in Chapter 16, "Nutrition and the Central Nervous System," in the third edition has been incorporated into appropriate chapters throughout the text. The topics of other chapters remain the same as in the third edition.

PRESENTATION

The presentation of the fourth edition is designed to make the book easier for the reader to use. The second color, and cross-references draw attention to important elements in the text, tables, and figures and help generate reader interest. The perspectives provide applications of the information in the chapter text and have been well received by reviewers and users.

Because this book focuses on normal human nutrition and physiological function, it is an effective resource for students majoring in either nutrition science or dietetics. Intended for a course in advanced nutrition, the text presumes a sound background in the biological sciences. At the same time, however, it provides a review of the basic sciences—particularly biochemistry and physiology, which are important to understanding the material. This text applies biochemistry to nutrient use from consumption through digestion, absorption, distribution, and cellular metabolism, making it a valuable reference for health care workers. Health practitioners may use it as a resource to refresh their memories with regard to metabolic and physiological interrelationships and to obtain a concise update on current concepts related to human nutrition.

We continue to present nutrition as the science that integrates life processes from the molecular to the cellular level and on through the multisystem operation of the whole organism. Our primary goal is to give a comprehensive picture of cell reactions at the tissue, organ, and system levels. Subject matter has been selected for its relevance to meeting this goal.

ORGANIZATION

Each of the 16 chapters begins with a topical outline followed by a brief introduction to the chapter's subject matter. These are followed in order by the chapter text, a brief summary that ties together the ideas presented in the chapter, a reference list, and one or more perspectives with their own reference lists.

The text is divided into five sections. Section I (Chaps. 1–3) focuses on cell structure, gastrointestinal tract anatomy and function with respect to digestion and absorption, and energy transformation. Section II (Chaps. 4–8) discusses the metabolism of the macronutrients. This section reviews primary metabolic pathways for carbohydrates, lipids, and proteins, emphasizing those reactions particularly relevant to issues of health. We include a chapter on fiber as well as a chapter on the interrelationships among the metabolic pathways. Also included in Section II (Chap. 8) is a description of the metabolic dynamics of the fed-fast cycle, along with a presentation of exercise and sports nutrition and the impact of physical exertion on the body's metabolic pathways. Section III (Chaps. 9–13) concerns those nutrients considered regulatory in nature: the water- and fat-soluble vitamins and the minerals, including the macrominerals, microminerals, and ultratrace minerals. These chapters cover nutrient features such as digestion, absorption, transport, function, metabolism, excretion, deficiency, toxicity, and assessment of nutriture, as well as the latest recommended dietary allowances (RDAs) or adequate intakes (AIs) for each nutrient. Section IV (Chaps. 14 and 15) covers the maintenance of the body's homeostatic environment. It includes discussion of body fluids and electrolyte balance, pH maintenance, body composition, and energy expenditure. The final chapter (Chap. 16), "Experimental Design and Critical Interpretation of Research," constitutes Section V and is supplementary to the rest of the book. This chapter discusses the types of research and the methodologies by which research can be conducted. It is designed to familiarize students with research organization and implementation, to point out problems and pitfalls inherent in research, and to help students critically evaluate scientific literature.

SUPPLEMENTARY MATERIAL

To enhance the teaching and learning of the textbook, a Multimedia Manager CD-ROM is available. This multimedia collection of visual resources provides instructors with the complete collection of figures from the textbook. Instructors may use illustrations to create custom classroom presentations, visually-based tests and quizzes, or classroom support materials. In addition, a robust test bank is available both electronically on the Multimedia Manager CD-ROM and in printed form. Students will find online practice tests for each chapter at www.nutrition.wadsworth.com.

ACKNOWLEDGMENTS

While this textbook represents countless hours of work by the authors, it is also the work of many other hard-working individuals. We cannot possibly list everyone who has helped, but we would like to call attention to a few individuals who have played particularly important roles. We thank Michelle Gropper for her assistance in formatting the text to begin the revision process. We thank our undergraduate and graduate nutrition students for their ongoing feedback. We thank our publisher, Pete Marshall; our developmental editor, Elizabeth Howe; our marketing manager, Jennifer Somerville; our Project Manager for Editorial Production, Sandra Craig; and our permissions editor, Sarah Harkrader. We extend special thanks to our production team, especially Mary Douglas and our copy editor, Mary Roybal.

We also thank two contributors to the fourth edition of the text, Ruth M. DeBusk, Ph.D., R.D. for writing the perspective, "Nutrigenomics: The Foundation for Individualized Nutrition" and Rita M. Johnson, Ph.D., R.D., F.A.D.A. for the perspective, "Genetics and Nutrition: Human Folate needs and Chronic Disease Risk."

In addition, we thank Richard Morel for his careful examination of page proofs and thoughtful feedback. We are indebted to the efforts of Carole A. Conn (University of New Mexico), who prepared the test bank and a set of student practice quizzes for the book's web site.

We owe special thanks to the reviewers whose thoughtful comments, criticisms, and suggestions were indispensable in shaping this text.

Fourth Edition Reviewers

Victoria Castellanos, Florida International University
Prithiva Chanmugam, Louisiana State University
Kate J. Claycombe, Michigan State University
Richard Fang, University of Delaware
Leonard Gerber, University of Rhode Island
V. Bruce Grossie, Jr., Texas Woman's University
Cindy Heiss, California State University, Northridge
Jessica Hodge, Framingham State University
Satya S. Jonnalagadda, Georgia State University
Jay Keller, Idaho State University
Mark Kern, San Diego State University
M. Elizabeth Kunkel, Clemson University
Margery L. Lawrence, Saint Joseph College
Jaimette McCulley, Fontbonne University
Anahita Mistry, Florida State University
Kevin Schalinske, Iowa State University
Jean T. Snook, Ohio State University
Therese S. Waterhous, Oregon State University
M. K. (Suzy) Weems, Stephen F. Austin State University

Third Edition Reviewers

Eldon Wayne Askew, Utah State University
Janine T. Baer, University of Dayton
Irene Berman-Levine, University of Pennsylvania
Patricia Brevard, James Madison University
Lou Ann Carden, University of Tennessee at Martin
Richard A. Cook, University of Maine
Jamie Erskine, University of Northern Colorado–Greeley
Coni C. Francis, University of Colorado, School of Medicine
Howard P. Glauert, University of Kentucky
Jessica Hodge, Framingham State College
Rita M. Johnson, Indiana University of Pennsylvania
Mary F. Locniskar, University of Texas at Austin
Barbara Lohse Knous, University of Wisconsin–Stout
Mark Kern, San Diego State University
M. E. Kunkel, Clemson University
Phylis B. Moser-Veillon, University of Maryland
Carol P. Ries, Eastern Illinois University
Neil Shay, University of Illinois
Joanne Slavin, University of Minnesota
May-Choo Wang, San Jose State University
M. K. (Suzy) Weems, Stephen F. Austin State University

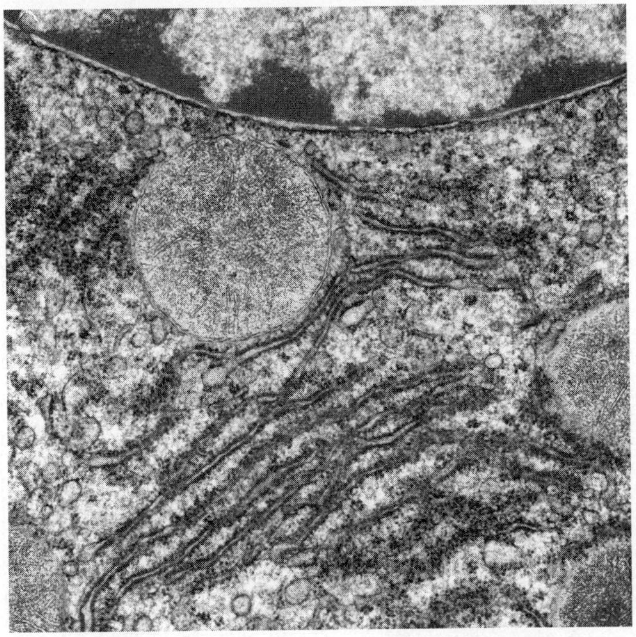
© Dr. Gopal Murti/Visuals Unlimited

A human liver cell

Components of Typical Cells
Plasma Membrane
Cytoplasmic Matrix
Mitochondrion
Nucleus
Endoplasmic Reticulum and Golgi Apparatus
Lysosomes and Peroxisomes
Cellular Proteins
Receptors and Intracellular Signaling
Transport Proteins
Catalytic Proteins (Enzymes)
Apoptosis
perspective
Cellular Enzymes on the Loose: Indicators of Disease

chapter 1 The Cell: A Microcosm of Life

CELLS ARE THE VERY ESSENCE OF LIFE. Cells may be defined as the basic living, structural, and functional units of the human body. They vary greatly in size, chemical composition, and function, but each one is a remarkable miniaturization of human life. Cells move, grow, ingest food and excrete wastes, react to their environment, and even reproduce.

Cells of all multicellular organisms are called **eukaryotic cells** (from the Greek *eu,* meaning "true," and *karyon,* "nucleus"). Eukaryotic cells are known to have evolved from simpler, more primitive cells called **prokaryotic cells.** The major distinguishing feature between the two cell types is that eukaryotic cells possess a defined nucleus, whereas prokaryotic cells do not. Also, eukaryotic cells are larger and much more complex structurally and functionally than their ancestors. Because this text addresses human metabolism and nutrition, all discussions of cellular structure and function in this and subsequent chapters pertain to eukaryotic cells.

Specialization among cells is a necessity for the living, breathing human, but cells in general have certain basic similarities. All human cells

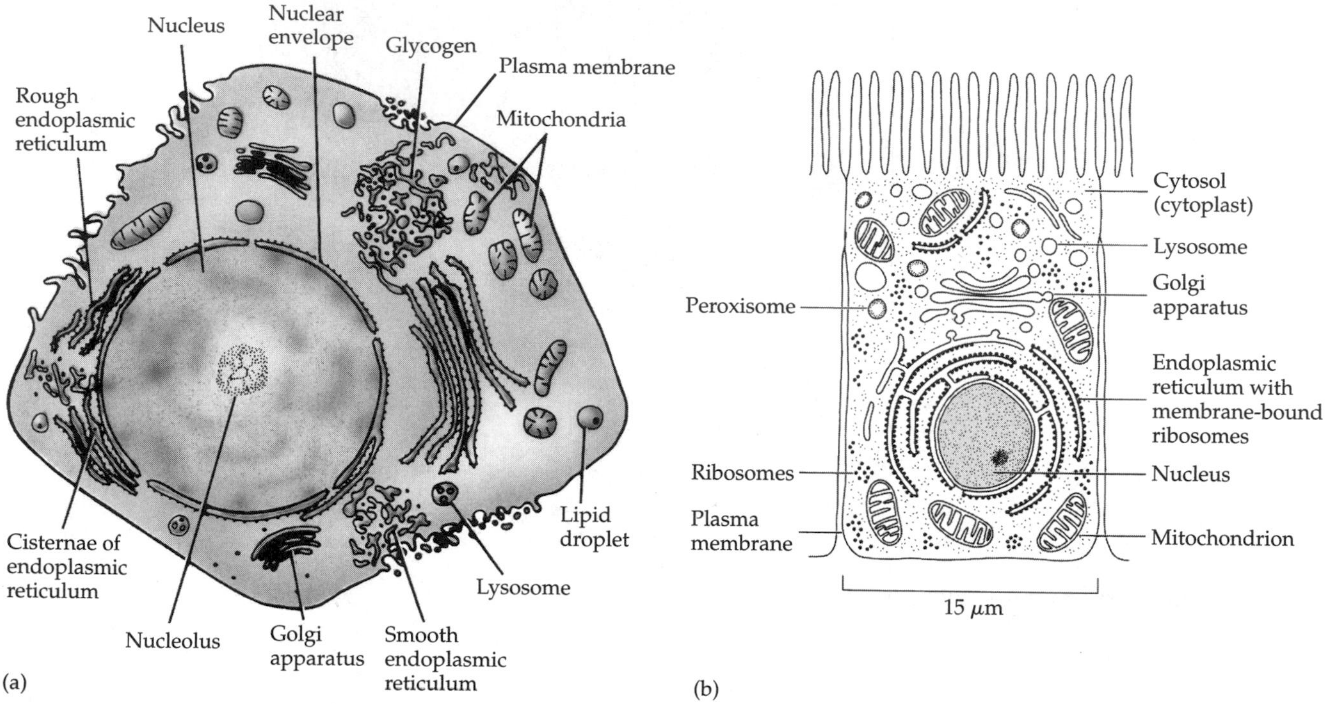

Figure 1.1 The fine structure of a typical animal cell (hepatocyte) is shown in (a), while (b) depicts a typical animal absorptive cell.

have a plasma membrane and a nucleus (or have had a nucleus), and most contain an endoplasmic reticulum, Golgi apparatus, and mitochondria. For convenience of discussion, a so-called "typical cell" is considered to allow us to identify the various organelles and their functions, which characterize cellular life. Considering the relationship between the normal functioning of a typical cell and the health of the total organism—the human being—brings to mind the old rule: "A chain is only as strong as its weakest link."

Figure 1.1a shows the fine structure of a mammalian liver cell (hepatocyte) to represent a typical animal cell, while Figure 1.1b gives a schematic view of a typical animal absorptive cell (such as an intestinal epithelial cell), showing its major components or organelles.

Our discussion begins with consideration of the plasma membrane, which forms the outer boundary of the cell, and then moves inward to examine the organelles held within this membrane.

COMPONENTS OF TYPICAL CELLS

Plasma Membrane

The **plasma membrane** is the membrane encapsulating the cell. By surrounding the cell, it lets the cell become a unit by itself. The plasma membrane, like other membranes found within the cell, has distinct functions and structural characteristics. Nevertheless, all membranes share some common attributes:

- Membranes are sheetlike structures composed primarily of lipids and proteins held together by noncovalent interactions.
- Membrane lipids consist primarily of phospholipids, which have both a hydrophobic and a hydrophilic moiety. Because of this structural property of phospholipids, they spontaneously form bimolecular sheets in water, called lipid bilayers, as shown in Figure 1.2. Because of their hydrophobic core, these bilayer sheets retard the passage of many water-soluble compounds into and out of the cell. Although such an arrangement requires transport systems across the membrane, it allows retention of essential water-soluble substances within the cell.
- Phosphoglycerides and phosphingolipids (phosphate-containing sphingolipids) comprise most of the membrane phospholipids. Of the phosphoglycerides, phosphatidylcholine and phosphatidylethanolamine are particularly abundant in higher animals. Another important membrane lipid is cholesterol, but its amount varies considerably from membrane to membrane. Molecular structures of these lipids are detailed in Chapter 6.
- Membrane proteins confer on biological membranes their functionality: they serve as pumps, gates, receptors, energy transducers, and enzymes.

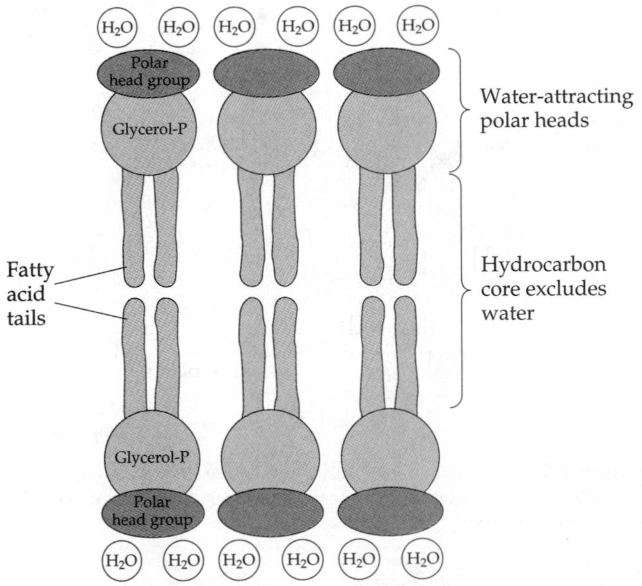

Figure 1.2 Lipid bilayer structure of biological membranes. Structures are schematic representations of phosphoglycerides (glycerophosphatides), which consist of fatty acid tails attached to polar "heads." Contained within the polar heads are glycerol, phosphate (P), and a polar head group, which can be choline, ethanolamine, serine, or inositol.

Figure 1.3 schematically illustrates the functions and positioning of some membrane proteins.

- Membranes are asymmetrical. The inside and outside faces of the membrane are different.
- Membranes are fluid structures in which lipid and protein molecules can move laterally with ease and rapidity.

Membranes can no longer be considered entities that are structurally distinct from the aqueous compartments they surround. For example, the **cytoplasm,** which is the cell's aqueous ground substance, affords a connection among the various membranes of the cell. Such an interconnection creates a structure that makes it possible for a signal generated at one part of the cell to be transmitted quickly and efficiently to other regions of the unit.

The plasma membrane provides protection to the cellular components while at the same time allowing them sufficient exposure to their environment for stimulation, nourishment, and removal of wastes. Chemical differences that distinguish the plasma membrane from other membranes in the cell follow:

- It has greater carbohydrate content owing to the presence of glycolipids and glycoproteins. Although some carbohydrate is found in all membranes, most of the glycolipids and glycoproteins are associated with the plasma membrane.
- It has a higher cholesterol content. Cholesterol enhances the mechanical stability of the membrane and regulates its fluidity.

Figure 1.4 illustrates the positioning of a cholesterol molecule between two phospholipid molecules. The orientation is such that the hydrocarbon side chain of the cholesterol molecule associates with the hydrocarbon fatty acid tails of the phospholipids, creating a hydrophobic region. The hydroxyl groups of the cholesterol are positioned close to the polar head groups of the phospholipid molecules, resulting in a more hydrophilic region [1]. It is this layering of polar and nonpolar regions that has led to the lipid bilayer notation to describe the plasma membrane structure. The rigid planar steroid rings of cholesterol are positioned so as to interact with and stabilize those regions of the hydrocarbon chains closest to the polar head groups. The rest of the hydrocarbon chain remains flexible and fluid. Cholesterol, by regulating fluidity of the membrane, regulates membrane permeability, thereby exercising some control over what may pass into and out of the cell. Fluidity of the membrane also appears to affect the structure and function of the proteins embedded in the lipid membrane.

The carbohydrate moiety of the glycoproteins and the glycolipids in membranes helps maintain the asymmetry of the membrane, because the oligosaccharide side chains are located exclusively on the membrane layer facing away from the cytoplasmic matrix. In plasma membranes, therefore, the sugar residues are all exposed to the outside of the cell, forming what is called the **glycocalyx,** the layer of carbohydrate on the cell's outer surface. On the membranes of the organelles, however, the oligosaccharides are directed inward into the lumen of the membrane-bound compartment. Figure 1.5 illustrates the glycocalyx and the location of oligosaccharide side chains in the plasma membrane.

Although the exact function of the sugar residues is unknown, it is believed that they act as specificity markers for the cell and as "antennae" to pick up

Figure 1.3 Schematic representation of various functions performed by cell membrane proteins.

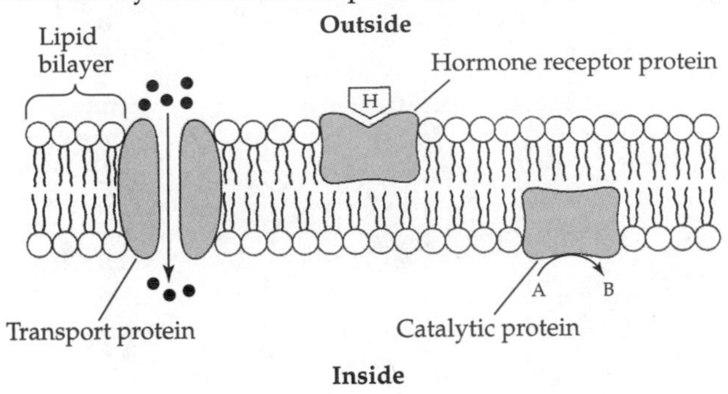

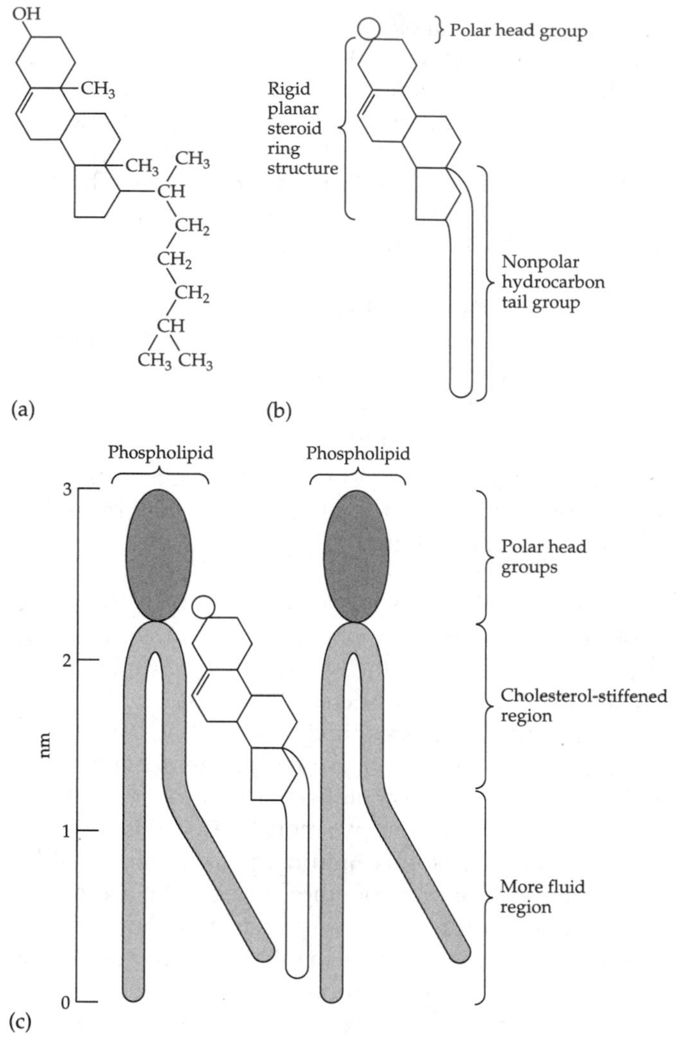

Figure 1.4 The structural role of cholesterol in the cell membrane is represented by a formula (a), by a schematic drawing (b), and as it interacts with two phospholipid molecules in a monolayer (c).

signals for transmission of substances in the cell. The membrane glycoproteins are crucial to the life of the cell, very possibly serving as the receptors for hormones, certain nutrients, and various other substances that influence cellular function. Glycoproteins also may help regulate the intracellular communication necessary for cell growth and tissue formation. Intracellular communication refers to pathways that convert information from one part of a cell to another in response to external stimuli. Generally, it involves the passage of chemical messengers from organelle to organelle or within the lipid bilayers of membranes. Intracellular communication is looked at more closely in the section "Receptors and Intracellular Signaling."

Whereas the lipid bilayer determines the structure of the plasma membrane, proteins are primarily responsible

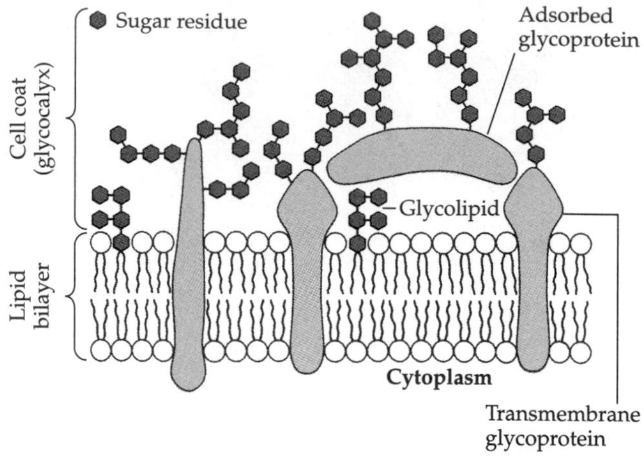

Figure 1.5 Diagram of the cell membrane glycocalyx, illustrating that all carbohydrate is located on the outside of the membrane.

for the many membrane functions. The membrane proteins are interspersed within the lipid bilayers, where they mediate information transfer (e.g., receptors), transport ions and molecules (channels, carriers, and pumps), and speed up metabolic activities (enzymes). Figure 1.6 illustrates the functions of these proteins in the transport of molecules into and out of the cell.

Membrane proteins are classified as either integral or peripheral. The integral proteins are attached to the

Figure 1.6 Schematic illustration of the role of proteins in transport, showing four ways in which molecules (•) may cross cellular membranes: (a) simple diffusion through the lipid bilayer; (b) diffusion through the membrane pores created by channel proteins; (c) facilitated diffusion or transport, necessitating a carrier protein specific for the molecule; and (d) active transport, a mechanism that, like facilitated transport, requires a specific transporter but that also requires the expenditure of energy in the form of ATP hydrolysis. Molecules crossing membranes by simple or facilitated diffusion are moved only from a region of higher concentration on one side of the membrane to a region of lower concentration on the other. Actively transported molecules, in contrast, can be moved against a concentration gradient.

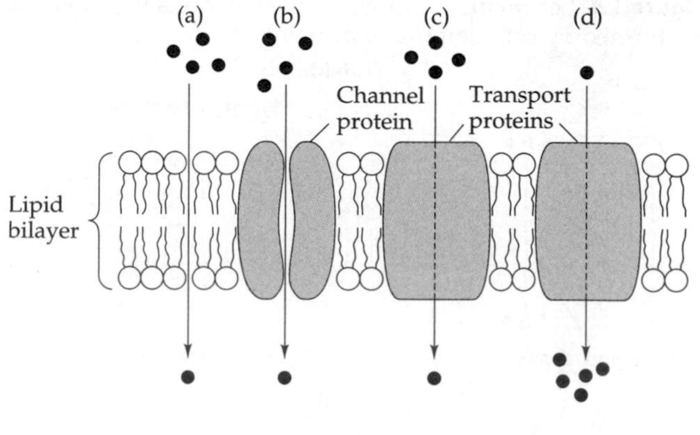

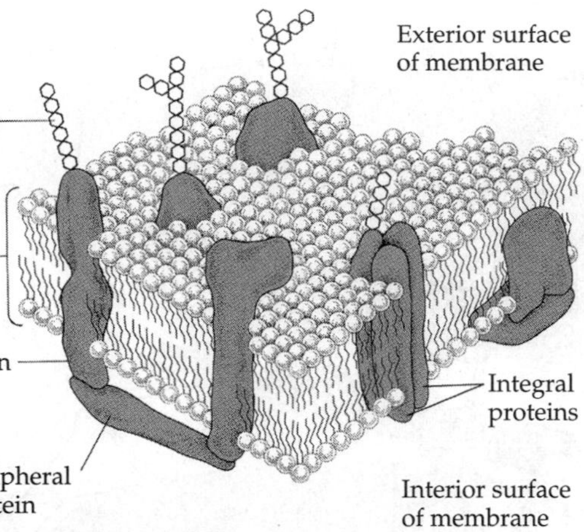

Figure 1.7 Positioning of proteins in the plasma membrane. Proteins that penetrate into the interior of the lipid bilayer are called integral proteins. Proteins that lie on the surface and do not penetrate the lipid bilayer are called peripheral proteins. Polysaccharides are frequently attached to membrane proteins and membrane lipids on the exterior side of the membrane.

membrane through hydrophobic interactions and are embedded in the membrane. Peripheral proteins, in contrast, are associated with membranes via ionic interactions and are located on or near the membrane surface (Fig. 1.7). Peripheral proteins are believed to be attached to integral membrane proteins either directly or through intermediate proteins [1].

Most receptor and carrier proteins are integral proteins, whereas the glycoproteins of the cell recognition complex are peripheral proteins [1]. Functions of membrane proteins, as well as functions of proteins located intracellularly, are discussed later in the chapter.

Cytoplasmic Matrix

A new frontier in the study of cell structure and cell physiology was made possible with the advent of the electron microscope. This microscope was able to identify the microtrabecular lattice, a fibrous cord of connective tissue that supports and controls the movement of cell organelles. The microtrabecular lattice is actually an intercommunication system of proteins and other macromolecules held in some state of aggregation. A model of this lattice, as shown in Figure 1.8, shows the microtrabeculae as being continuous with the proteins underlying the plasma membrane, the surface of the endoplasmic reticulum, the microtubules, and the filaments of the stress fibers. The lattice also appears to support certain extracellular extensions emanating from the cell surface. For example, the **microvilli,** which are extensions of intestinal epithelial cells, are associated with the microtrabeculae. Microvilli are designed to present a large surface area for the absorption of dietary nutrients. Microtubules, together with a network of filaments that interconnect them, form what is called the **cytoskeleton.** The cellular matrix, of which the cytoskeleton is a part, is most commonly called the cytoplasm. An alternative term that may be more appropriate is the **cytoplast,** because it suggests the structural and functional unity that is such an important feature of the matrix.

Like the microtrabecular lattice, microfilaments and microtubules apparently are complex polymers of many different proteins, including actin, myosin, and tubulin, the last a protein necessary for the formation of microtubules. These structures provide mechanical support for the cell and also serve as binding surfaces for soluble macromolecules such as proteins and nucleic acids that are present in the aqueous portion of the cytoplasmic matrix. In fact, evidence suggests that the nonfilamentous aqueous phase of the cell contains very few macromolecules and that many proteins in the cytoplasmic matrix are bound to the filaments for a large portion of their lives. Filling the intertrabecular spaces is the fluid phase of the cytoplasmic matrix, which contains small molecules such as glucose, amino acids, oxygen, and carbon dioxide. This arrangement of the polymeric and fluid phases apparently gives the cytoplasm (cytoplast) its gel-like consistency.

The spatial arrangement of the lattice or polymeric phase with the aqueous phase improves the efficiency of the many enzyme-catalyzed reactions that take place in the cytoplast. Because the aqueous phase contacts the polymeric phase over a very broad surface area, enzymes that are associated with the polymeric phase are brought into close proximity to their substrate molecules in the aqueous phase, thereby facilitating the reaction (see the discussion of enzymes, p. 17). Furthermore, if enzymes catalyzing the reactions of a metabolic pathway were oriented sequentially so that the product of one reaction was released in very close proximity to the next enzyme for which it is a substrate, the velocity of the overall pathway would be greatly enhanced. Evidence indicates that such an arrangement of the enzymes participating in glycolysis does in fact exist.

Possibly all metabolic pathways occurring in the cytoplasmic matrix may be influenced by its structural arrangement. Metabolic pathways of particular significance that occur in the cytoplasmic matrix and that might be affected by the structure include

- glycolysis,
- hexose monophosphate shunt (pentose phosphate pathway),
- glycogenesis and glycogenolysis, and
- fatty acid synthesis, including the production of nonessential, unsaturated fatty acids.

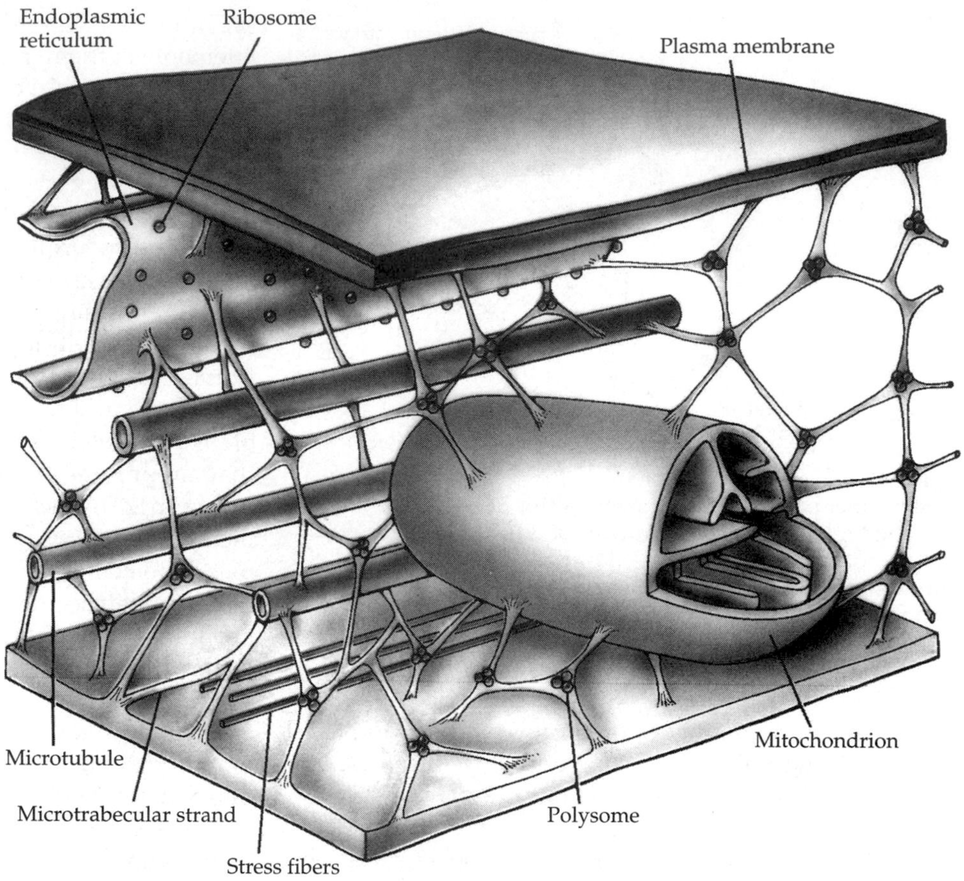

Figure 1.8 A model of the cytoplast (microtrabecular lattice). The cytoplast is shown at about 300,000 times its actual size and was derived from hundreds of images of cultured cells viewed in a high-voltage electron microscope. The model illustrates how the microtrabecular filaments are related to other components of the cell cytoplasm—the substance of the cell outside the cell nucleus. In the model the microtrabeculae suspend the elongated structures of the endoplasmic reticulum, the mitochondria, and the microtubules. At junctions of the microtrabecular lattice are polysomes, or organized clusters of ribosomes. (Adapted from Porter and Tucker, "The Ground Substance of the Cell." Copyright © 1981 by Scientific American, Inc. All rights reserved.)

Normal intracellular communication among all cellular components is vital for cell activation and survival. The importance of the microtrabecular network is evidenced by its function to support and interconnect cellular components.

Mitochondrion

The **mitochondria** are the primary sites of oxygen use in the cell and are responsible for most of the metabolic energy (adenosine triphosphate, or ATP) produced in cells. The size and shape of the mitochondria in different tissues vary according to the function(s) of the tissue. In muscle tissue, for example, the mitochondria are held tightly among the fibers of the contractile system. In the liver, however, the mitochondria have fewer restraints, appear spherical in shape, and move freely through the cytoplasmic matrix.

The mitochondrion consists of a matrix or interior space surrounded by a double membrane (Fig. 1.9). The mitochondrial outer membrane is relatively porous, whereas the inner membrane is only selectively permeable, thereby serving as a permeability barrier between the cytoplasmic matrix and the mitochondrial matrix. The inner membrane has many invaginations, called the cristae, that serve to increase the surface area of the inner membrane in which all the components of the electron transport (respiratory) chain are embedded.

The electron transport chain is central to the process of **oxidative phosphorylation,** the mechanism by which most cellular ATP is produced. Its components act as carriers of electrons in the catalytic oxidation of nutrient molecules by enzymes functioning in the mitochondrial

Figure 1.9 The mitochondrion.

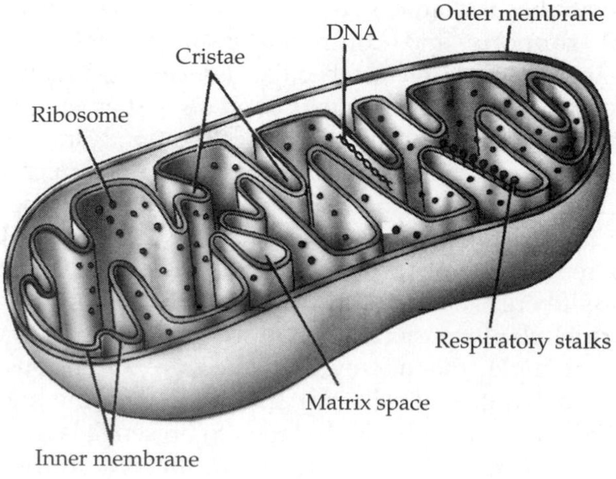

matrix. Flow of electrons through the electron transport chain is strongly exothermic, and the energy released is used in part for the synthesis of ATP, an endothermic process. Molecular oxygen is ultimately, but indirectly, the oxidizing agent in these reactions. The function of the **electron transport chain** is to couple the energy released by nutrient oxidation to the formation of ATP. The precise positioning of the chain components within the inner membrane is fortuitous, because it brings them into close proximity to both the oxidizable products released in the matrix and molecular oxygen. Figure 1.10 shows the flow of major reactants into and out of the mitochondrion.

Among the metabolic enzyme systems functioning in the mitochondrial matrix are those catalyzing the reactions of the Krebs cycle and fatty acid oxidation. Other enzymes are involved in the oxidative decarboxylation and carboxylation of pyruvate (Chap. 4) and in certain reactions of amino acid metabolism.

While the nucleus contains most of the cell's deoxyribonucleic acid (DNA), the mitochondrial matrix contains a small amount of DNA and a few ribosomes, so limited protein synthesis occurs within the mitochondrion. Of interest is that the genes contained in mitochondrial DNA, unlike those in the nucleus, are inherited only from the mother. The primary function of mitochondrial genes is to code for proteins vital to the production of ATP [2]. Most of the enzymes operating in the mitochondrion, however, are coded by nuclear DNA and synthesized on the rough endoplasmic reticulum (RER) in the cytoplasm. They are then incorporated into existing mitochondria.

All cells in the body, with the exception of the erythrocyte, possess mitochondria. The erythrocyte disposes of its mitochondria in the process of maturing and then must depend solely on the energy produced through anaerobic mechanisms, primarily glycolysis.

Nucleus

The nucleus of the cell is the largest of the organelles and because of its DNA content initiates and regulates most cellular activities. Surrounding the nucleus is the **nuclear envelope,** composed of two membranes (an inner and an outer membrane) that appear to be dynamic structures. The dynamic nature of these membranes makes possible communication between the nucleus and the cytoplasmic matrix and allows a continuous channel between the nucleus and the endoplasmic reticulum. At various intervals the two membranes of the nuclear envelope fuse, creating pores in the envelope (Fig. 1.11). The nucleus and the microtubules of the cytoskeleton appear to be interdependent. The polymerization and the intracellular distribution of the microtubules are controlled by nucleus-based activities. Clusters of proteins on the outer nuclear membrane are centers of these activities. These clusters, called microtubule organization centers (MTOCs), begin their polymerization and organization of the microtubules during mitosis. A review of MTOC activity has been published [3].

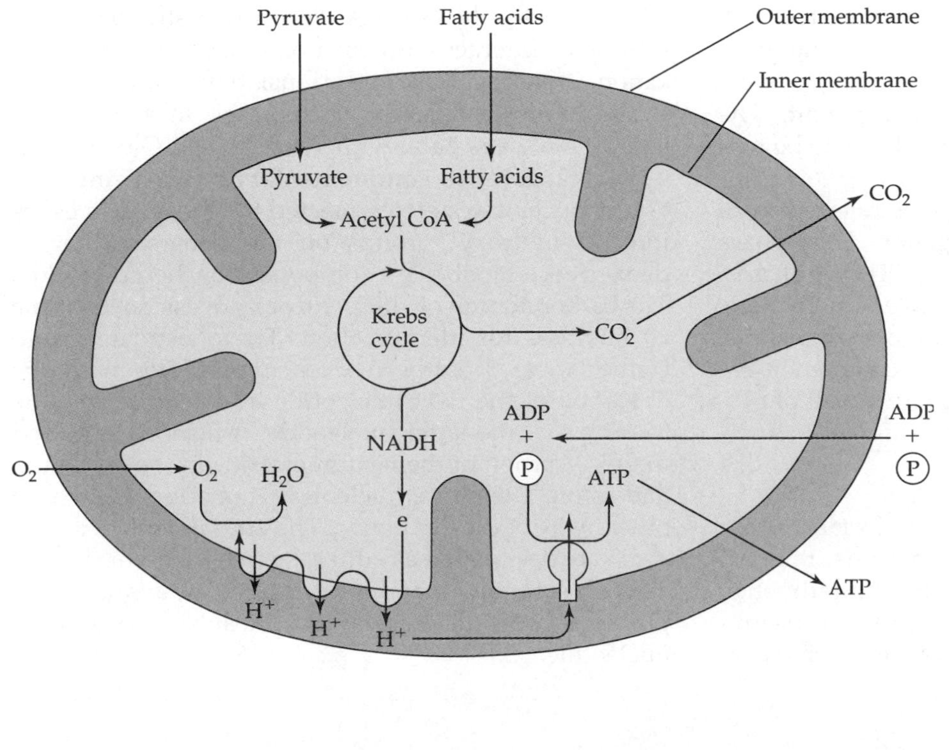

Figure 1.10 The flow of major reactants into and out of the mitochondrion.

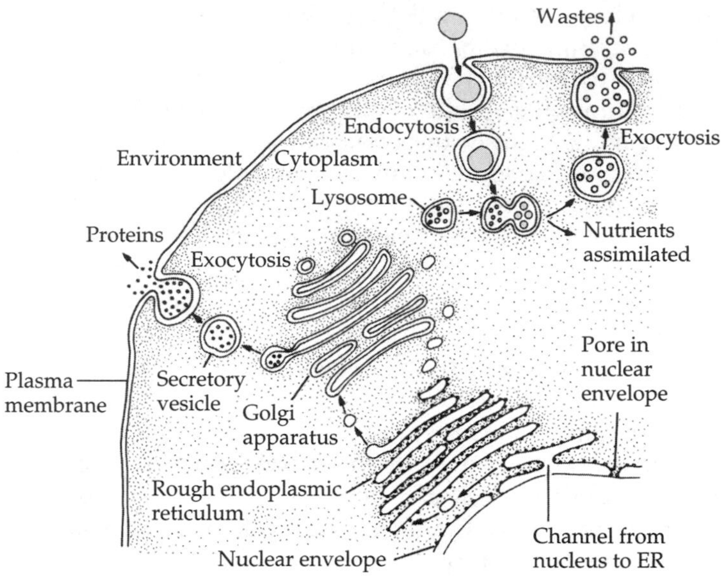

Figure 1.11 Communication between the nucleus and other cell components. Membrane material in the nuclear envelope, the endoplasmic reticulum, the Golgi apparatus, and the plasma membrane are cycled continuously, as illustrated.

The matrix held within the nuclear envelope is composed of chromatin plus all the enzymes and minerals necessary for the activity of the nucleus. Condensed regions of the chromatin called **nucleoli** contain not only DNA and its associated alkaline proteins (histones) but also considerable amounts of RNA (ribonucleic acid). This particular RNA is believed to give rise to the microsomal RNA (i.e., RNA associated with the endoplasmic reticulum).

Encoded within the nuclear DNA of the cell are thousands of genes that direct the synthesis of proteins, with each gene encoding a single specific protein. The cell **genome** is the entire genetic DNA within the cell. Barring mutations that may arise in the DNA, daughter cells, produced from a parent cell by mitosis, possess the identical genomic makeup of the parent. The process of DNA replication enables the DNA to be precisely copied at the time of mitosis.

Protein biosynthesis occurs in phases referred to as transcription, translation, and elongation. Each phase requires DNA and/or RNA activity. These phases, together with replication, will be reviewed briefly here, but the reader is reminded of the large scope of this subject and should consult a current, comprehensive biochemistry text for a more thorough treatment of protein biosynthesis.

Nucleic Acids

Nucleic acids (DNA and RNA) are formed from repeating units called **nucleotides,** sometimes referred to as nucleotide bases or just bases. Structurally, they consist of a nitrogenous core (either purine or pyrimidine), a pentose sugar (ribose in RNA, deoxyribose in DNA), and phosphate. Five different nucleotides are contained in the structures of the nucleic acids: adenylic acid, guanylic acid, cytidylic acid, uridylic acid, and thymidylic acid. The nucleotides are more commonly referred to by their nitrogenous base core only—namely, adenine, guanine, cytosine, uracil, and thymine, respectively. For convenience, particularly in describing the sequence of the polymeric nucleotides in a nucleic acid, the single-letter abbreviations A, G, C, U, and T are most often used. Adenine (A), guanine (G), and cytosine (C) are common to both DNA and RNA, while uracil (U) is unique to RNA and thymine (T) is found only in DNA. When two strands of nucleic acids interact with each other, as occurs in replication, transcription, and translation, bases in one strand pair specifically with bases in the second strand: A always pairs with T (or U), and G pairs with C, in what is called **complementary base pairing.**

The nucleotides are connected by phosphates esterified to hydroxyl groups on the pentose—that is, deoxyribose or ribose—component of the nucleotide. The carbon atoms of the pentoses are assigned prime (′) numbers for identification. The phosphate group connects the 3′ carbon of one nucleotide with the 5′ carbon of the next nucleotide in the sequence. The 3′ carbon of the latter nucleotide in turn is connected to the 5′ carbon of the next nucleotide in the sequence, and so on. Therefore, nucleotides are attached to each other by 3′, 5′ diester bonds. The ends of a nucleic acid chain are designated as either the free 3′ end or the free 5′ end, meaning that the hydroxyl groups at those positions are not attached by phosphate to another nucleotide.

Cell Replication

Replication: Synthesis of a daughter duplex DNA molecule identical to the parental duplex DNA.

At cell division the chromatin is condensed into chromosomes, with each chromosome containing a single molecule of DNA. The DNA exists as two large strands of nucleic acid that are intertwined to form a double helix (duplex DNA). During cell division the two unravel at one end, with each forming a template for the synthesis of a new strand via complementary base pairing. Incoming nucleotide bases first pair with their complementary bases in the template and then are connected through phosphate diester bonds by the enzyme DNA polymerase. The end result of the **replication** process is two new DNA chains that, together with their parent chains, permit the production of two duplex DNA molecules from the single parent molecule. Each new duplex DNA is therefore identical in base sequence to the parent, and each new cell of a tissue consequently carries within its nucleus identical information to direct its functioning.

The two strands of double helical DNA are antiparallel, which means that the free 5′ end of one strand is connected to the free 3′ end of the other. Base-paired DNA strands may be represented as follows:

free 3′ A–G–T–C–C–A–T— — —G–G–C–T–A–C–G free 5′ end

free 5′ T–C–A–G–G–T–A— — —C–C–G–A–T–G–C free 3′ end

The broken line in this simplified example represents a very large number of additional base pairs. Although only 14 base pairs at the chain termini are shown, the reader is reminded that millions of base pairs actually exist in eukaryotic cell DNA molecules.

Cell Transcription

Transcription: The process by which the genetic information (base sequence) in a single strand of DNA is used to specify a complementary sequence of bases in an mRNA chain.

Transcription proceeds continuously throughout the entire life cycle of the cell. In the process, various sections of the duplex DNA molecule unravel, and one strand—designated the **sense strand**—serves as the template for the synthesis of messenger RNA (mRNA). The genetic code of the DNA is transcribed into mRNA via complementary base pairing, as in DNA replication, except that the purine adenine (A) pairs with the pyrimidine uracil (U) instead of with thymine (T). **Genes** are composed of critically sequenced base pairs along the entire length of the DNA strand that is being transcribed. A gene, on average, is just over 1,000 base pairs in length, compared with the nearly 5×10^6 base pair length of typical chromosomal DNA chains. Although these figures provide a rough estimate of the number of genes per transcribed DNA chain, not all the base pairs of a gene are transcribed into functional mRNA.

A puzzling feature of eukaryotic genes is that certain regions of nucleotide sequences get transcribed into complementary mRNA sequences but do not code for the ultimate protein product. These segments, called **introns** (intervening sequences), have to be removed from the mRNA prior to its translation into protein (discussion of the translation process follows). The introns are enzymatically excised from the newly formed mRNA, and the ends of the functional, active segments are spliced together in what is called posttranscriptional processing of the mRNA. The gene segments that get both transcribed and translated into the protein product, called **exons** (expressed sequences), require no posttranscriptional processing.

Protein Biosynthesis

Following processing, the mRNA is exported into the cytoplasmic matrix, where it is attached to the ribosomes of the RER or to the freestanding polysomes. On the ribosomes, the transcribed genetic code becomes translated so as to bring amino acids into a specific sequence to produce a protein with a clearly delineated function. This process is called **translation.**

Translation: The process by which genetic information in an mRNA molecule specifies the sequence of amino acids in the protein product.

The genetic code for specifying the amino acid sequence of a protein resides in the mRNA in the form of three-base sequences called **codons.** A given codon codes for a single amino acid. For example, any of the codons—CUU, CUC, CUA, or CUG—codes for the amino acid leucine. Although a given amino acid may therefore have several codons, a given codon can code for only one amino acid. The transition from nucleic acid base sequence to protein synthesis lies in the translation of the mRNA codons by **anticodons,** which are three-base sequences of nucleotides on molecules of a different RNA called transfer RNA (tRNA). The anticodons attach to the codons by, once again, complementary base pairing.

Amino acids are first activated by ATP at their carboxyl end and then transferred to their specific tRNAs that bear the anticodon complementary to each amino acid's codon. For example, because codons that code for leucine are sequenced CUU, CUC, CUA, or CUG, the only tRNAs to which an activated leucine can be attached would need to have the anticodon sequence GAA, GAG, GAU, or GAC. The tRNAs then bring the code-designated amino acids to the mRNA situated at the protein synthesis site on the ribosomes. After the amino acids are positioned according to codon-anticodon association, peptide bonds are formed between the aligned amino acids in a process called **elongation.**

Elongation: Extension of the polypeptide chain of the protein product.

Each incoming amino acid is connected to the C-terminal end of the growing polypeptide chain by peptide bond formation. New amino acids are incorporated until all the codons (corresponding to one gene) of the mRNA have been translated. At this point, the process stops abruptly, signaled by a "nonsense" codon that does not code for any amino acid. The completed protein dissociates from the mRNA and some post-translational chemical modification may be required for it to attain its active form.

To summarize, it can be seen that information for protein biosynthesis flows from chromosomal DNA to ribosomal mRNA to protein. Figure 1.12 provides a schematic overview of the process.

Endoplasmic Reticulum and Golgi Apparatus

The **endoplasmic reticulum** (**ER**) is a network of membranous channels pervading the cytoplast and providing continuity between the nuclear envelope, the Golgi apparatus, and the plasma membrane. This structure, therefore, is a mechanism for communication from the innermost part of the cell to its exterior (Fig. 1.11).

The ER cannot be separated from the cell as an entity by laboratory preparation. During mechanical homogenization, the structure of the ER is disrupted and re-forms into small spherical particles called microsomes. The ER is classified as either rough (granular) or smooth (agranular). The granularity or lack of granularity is determined by the presence or absence of ribosomes. Rough endoplasmic reticulum (RER), so named because it is studded with ribosomes, abounds in cells where protein synthesis is a primary function. Smooth endoplasmic reticulum (SER) is found in most cells; however, because it is the site of synthesis for a variety of lipids, it is more abundant in cells that synthesize steroid hormones (e.g., the adrenal cortex and gonads) and in liver cells, which synthesize fat transport molecules (the lipoproteins). In skeletal muscle, SER is called **sarcoplasmic reticulum** and is the site of the calcium ion pump, a necessity for the contractile process.

Ribosomes associated with RER are composed of ribosomal RNA (rRNA) and structural protein. They are the primary site for protein synthesis. All proteins to be secreted (or excreted) from the cell or destined for incorporation within an organelle membrane in the cell more than likely are synthesized on the RER. The clusters of ribosomes (i.e., polyribosomes or polysomes) that are freestanding in the cytoplast are also the synthesis site for some proteins, but all proteins synthesized here are believed to remain within the cytoplasmic matrix.

Figure 1.12 A schematic representation of protein biosynthesis in the cell. Information flows in the direction DNA ⟶ RNA ⟶ protein. (a) Transcription of the sense strand of DNA to produce progenitor mRNA. Introns (see text) are shown as colored segments in the DNA and transcribed RNA strands. (b) Processing of progenitor mRNA by the excision of introns and the splicing of translatable (exon) regions. (c) Processed, nuclear mRNA prior to transportation to the cytoplast. (d) mRNA associated with ribosomes of the rough endoplasmic reticulum. Translation of the mRNA as amino acid–bearing tRNA molecules bring code-designated amino acids to mRNA codons via a ribosome. Following each incorporation of a new amino acid, ribosomes translocate to the next codon on the mRNA strand, exposing a new site for the next amino acid to be added. (e) Elongation of the polypeptide chain as peptide bonds are formed between amino acids and ribosomes continue their process of translocation and elongation.

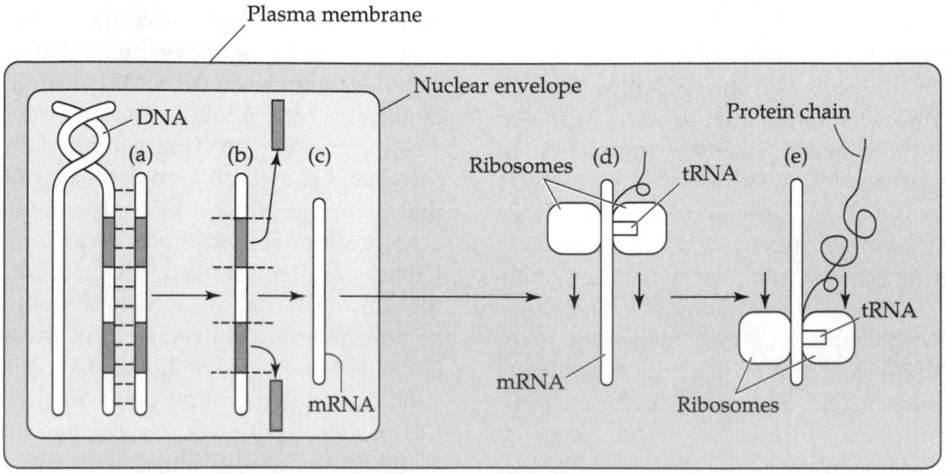

Located on the SER of liver cells is a system of enzymes very important in the detoxification and metabolism of many different drugs. This enzyme complex consists of a family of cytochromes, designated the P450 system, that functions along with other enzymes. The P450 system is particularly active in the oxidation of drugs, but because its action results in the simultaneous oxidation of other compounds as well, the system is collectively referred to as the mixed-function oxidase system. Lipophilic substances—for example, the steroid hormones and numerous drugs—can be made hydrophilic by oxidation, reduction, or hydrolysis, thereby enabling them to be excreted easily via the bile or urine.

The **Golgi apparatus** functions closely with the ER in the trafficking and sorting of proteins synthesized in the cell. It is particularly prominent in neurons and secretory cells. The Golgi apparatus consists of four to eight membrane-enclosed, flattened cisternae that are stacked in parallel (Fig. 1.11). The Golgi cisternae are often referred to as "stacks" because of this arrangement. Tubular networks at either end of the Golgi stacks have been identified:

- The cis-Golgi network acts as an acceptor compartment of newly synthesized proteins coming from the ER.
- The trans-Golgi network is the exit site of the Golgi apparatus. It is responsible for sorting proteins for delivery to their next destination [4].

Cisternae positioned between the cis- and trans-Golgi networks are designated as medial cisternae (Fig. 1.13).

The Golgi apparatus is the site for membrane differentiation and the development of surface specificity. For example, the polysaccharide moieties of mucopolysaccharides and of the membrane glycoproteins are synthesized and attached to the polypeptide during its passage through the Golgi apparatus. Such an arrangement allows for the continual replacement of cellular membranes, including the plasma membrane.

Sorting and trafficking of proteins in the secretory pathway between the ER and the Golgi stacks are not thoroughly understood. We do know, however, that the ER is a quality-control organelle in that it prevents proteins that have not achieved normal tertiary or quaternary structure from reaching the cell surface. The ER can retrieve or retain proteins destined for residency within the ER, or it can target proteins for delivery to the cis-Golgi compartment. Retrieved or exported protein "cargo" is coated with protein complexes called coatomers, abbreviated COPs (coat proteins). Some coatomers are structurally similar to the clathrin coat of endocytic vesicles. The choice of what is retrieved/retained by the ER and what is

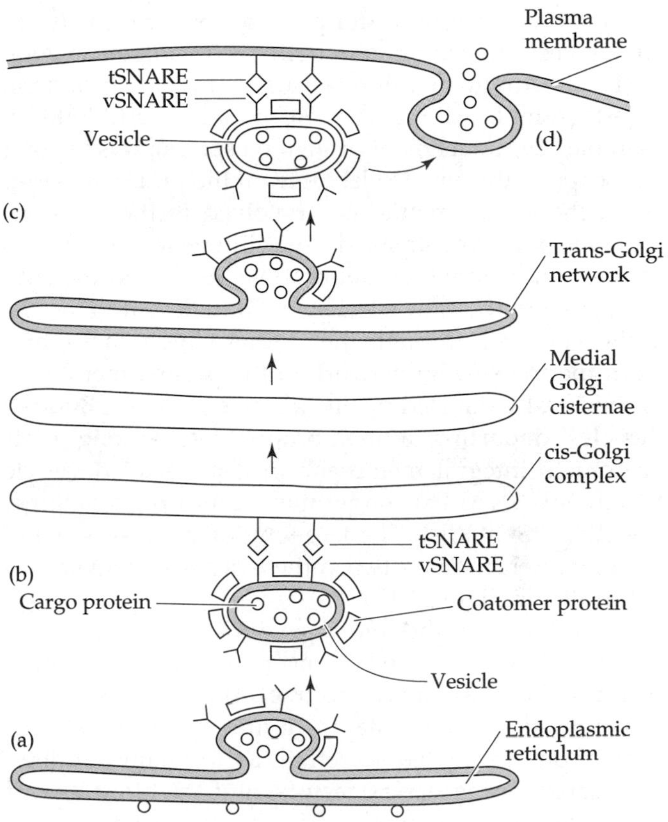

Figure 1.13 Proposed secretory pathway for cellular proteins, illustrating the delivery of ER-synthesized (cargo) proteins to the plasma membrane and secretion from the cell. Cargo proteins are depicted as small circles. (a) Budding and pinching off of cargo protein–containing vesicle from the ER. (b) Docking of vesicle with cis-Golgi complex. The specificity of the transport is postulated to reside in vSNARE (vesicle snare) and tSNARE (target snare) interaction (see text). (c) Vesicle formation following budding from the trans-Golgi network and vSNARE-tSNARE interaction at the plasma membrane. Sorting among proteins to determine those to be secreted and those to be retained occurs on the trans-Golgi network. (d) Vesicle fusion with the plasma membrane and release of cargo proteins into the extracellular environment.

exported to the Golgi apparatus is probably mediated by signals that are inherent in the terminal amino acid sequences of the proteins in question. Certain amino acid sequences of cargo proteins are thought to interact specifically with certain coatomers [5].

The membrane-bound compartments of the ER and the Golgi apparatus are interconnected by transport vesicles, through which cargo proteins are moved from compartment to compartment. The vesicles leaving a compartment are formed by a budding and pinching off of the compartment membrane, and the vesicles then fuse with the membrane of the target compartment. The specificity of vesicle-membrane interactions has been the focus of considerable research [5]. The current literature abounds with acronyms for proteins that are reactive in the process, according to hypothesis. Examples include NSF (N-ethylmaleimide-sensitive fusion proteins), SNAP (soluble NSF attachment proteins), and SNARE (soluble NSF attachment protein receptors). It is beyond the scope of this text to elaborate on the proposed series of reactions and interactions involved in the secretory protein pathway. Instead, the interested reader is referred to informative publications related to the subject [5,6]. Briefly, vesicle transport from the ER to the cis-Golgi complex, through the medial Golgi stacks, and from the trans-Golgi network to the plasma membrane is specifically directed by SNAPs and SNAREs. Budded vesicles departing a membrane have among their coatomers integral membrane proteins called vesicle SNAREs (vSNAREs). Target membranes possess target SNAREs (tSNAREs). The targeting of vesicles is mediated by interactions between these types of proteins, as illustrated in Figure 1.13.

Secretion from the cell of products such as proteins can be either constitutive or regulated. If secretion follows a constitutive course, the secretion rate remains relatively constant, uninfluenced by external regulation. Regulated secretion, as the name implies, is affected by regulatory factors, and therefore its rate is changeable.

Lysosomes and Peroxisomes

Lysosomes and **peroxisomes** are cell organelles packed with enzymes. Whereas the lysosomes serve as the cell's digestive system, the peroxisomes perform some specific oxidative catabolic reactions.

Lysosomes are particularly large and abundant in cells that perform digestive functions—for example, the macrophages and leukocytes. Approximately 36 powerful enzymes capable of splitting complex substances such as proteins, polysaccharides, nucleic acids, and phospholipids are held within the confines of a single thick membrane. The lysosome, just like a protein synthesized for excretion, is believed to develop through the combined activities of the ER and the Golgi apparatus. The result is a very carefully packaged group of lytic enzymes (Fig. 1.11).

The membrane surrounding these catabolic enzymes has the capacity for very selective fusion with other vesicles so that **catabolism** (or digestion) may occur as necessary. Wastes produced by this process can be removed from the cells by exocytosis, as indicated in Figure 1.11. Important catabolic activities performed by the lysosomes include participation in **phagocytosis,** in which foreign substances taken up by the cell may be digested or rendered harmless. An example of digestion by lysosomes is their action in the proximal tubules of the kidney. Lysosomes of the proximal tubule cells are believed to digest the albumin absorbed via endocytosis from the glomerular filtrate. Lysosomal phagocytosis serves as protection against invading bacteria, becoming part of the normal repair process following a wound or an infection.

A second catabolic activity of lysosomes is **autolysis**, in which intracellular components, including organelles, are digested as a result of degeneration or cellular injury. Autolysis also can serve as a survival mechanism for the cell as a whole. Digestion of dispensable intracellular components can provide the nutrients necessary to fuel functions essential to the life of the cell. The mitochondrion is an example of an organelle whose degeneration requires autolysis. It is estimated that the mitochondria of liver cells must be renewed approximately every 10 days.

Another catabolic activity of the lysosomes is bone resorption, an essential process in the normal modeling of bone. Lysosomes of the osteoclasts promote the dissolution of mineral and the digestion of collagen, both of which are necessary actions in bone resorption and regulation of calcium and phosphorus homeostasis.

Lysosomes, with their special membrane and numerous catabolic enzymes, also function in hormone secretion and regulation. Of particular significance is their role in the secretion of the thyroid hormones (Chap. 12).

In the early 1960s the peroxisomes were first recognized as separate intracellular organelles. These small bodies are believed to originate via "budding" from the SER. The peroxisomes are similar to the lysosomes in that they are bundles of enzymes surrounded by a single membrane. Rather than having digestive action, however, the enzymes within the peroxisomes are catabolic oxidative enzymes. Although the mitochondrial matrix is the major site of fatty acid oxidation to acetyl coenzyme A (acetyl CoA), the peroxisomes can carry out a similar series of reactions. Acetyl CoA produced in peroxisomes, however, cannot be further oxidized for energy at that site and must be transported to the mitochondria for oxidation via the Krebs cycle.

Peroxisomes are also the site for certain reactions of amino acid catabolism. Some of the oxidative enzymes involved in these pathways catalyze the release of hydrogen peroxide (H_2O_2) as an oxidation product. Because H_2O_2 is a very reactive chemical that could cause cellular damage if not promptly removed or converted, H_2O_2-releasing reactions are segregated within these organelles. Present in large quantities in the peroxisomes is the enzyme catalase, which degrades the potentially harmful H_2O_2 into water and molecular oxygen. Other enzymes in the peroxisomes are important in detoxifying reactions. Particularly important is the oxidation of ethanol to acetaldehyde.

CELLULAR PROTEINS

Proteins synthesized on the cell's ribosomes may be destined for secretion, or they may remain within the cell to perform their specific structural, digestive, regulatory, or other functions. Among the more interesting areas of biomolecular research has been the attempt to understand how newly synthesized protein that is to remain in the cell finds its way from the ribosomes to its intended destination. The answer lies in leader sequences within the proteins. Leader, or signaling, sequences are amino acid sequences attached to the amino end of the newly synthesized protein to direct it to its ultimate destination. Leader sequences are required for

- proteins destined for secretion from the cell,
- proteins to be retained in the cell's lysosomes and peroxisomes, and
- proteins intended for incorporation into various membranes of the cell.

Interaction between the leader sequences and specific receptors located on the various membranes permits the protein to enter its designated membrane. As the proteins move into their site of localization, the leader sequence is cleaved. Figure 1.14 illustrates the principle of a leader (or signal) sequence for the movement of a secretory protein into the ER from membrane-free ribosomes.

A long list of metabolic diseases is attributed to a deficiency of, or the inactivity of, certain enzymes. Tay-Sachs disease, phenylketonuria, maple syrup urine disease, and the lipid and glycogen storage diseases are a few well-known examples. As a result of research on certain mitochondrial proteins, it is believed that in at least some cases the enzymes are not necessarily inactive or deficient but rather fail to reach their correct destination [7,8].

Cellular proteins of particular interest to the health science student are

- **receptors,** proteins that modify the cell's response to its environment;
- **transport proteins,** proteins that regulate the flow of nutrients into and out of the cell; and
- **enzymes,** the catalysts for the hundreds of biochemical reactions taking place in the cell.

Receptors and Intracellular Signaling

Receptors are highly specific proteins located in the plasma membrane facing the exterior of the cell. Bound to the outer surface of these specific proteins are oligosaccharide chains, which are believed to act as

Figure 1.14 The signal (leader) peptide hypothesis. A membrane-free ribosome begins the synthesis of protein on an mRNA specific for the particular protein to be secreted. The signal peptide (consisting of ~80 amino acids) emerges first from the ribosome (A) and is recognized (B, C) by a complex of several proteins called the *signal recognition particle (SRP)*. Translation stops (C) until the ribosome-SRP complex binds to the rough endoplasmic reticulum (RER) membrane via a specific receptor for the SRP called the *docking protein (DP)*. Translation then resumes following the dissociation of the SRP between (C) and (D). The binding of the SRP to the DP creates a channel in the RER membrane through which the *signal peptide (SP)* travels, emerging in the RER cisterna, where it is eventually removed from the rest of the protein by a proteolytic enzyme, the membrane-bound signal peptidase, SPase (E). Protein synthesis continues, with the completed protein folding within the RER (G). (N indicates the end of the protein strand.)

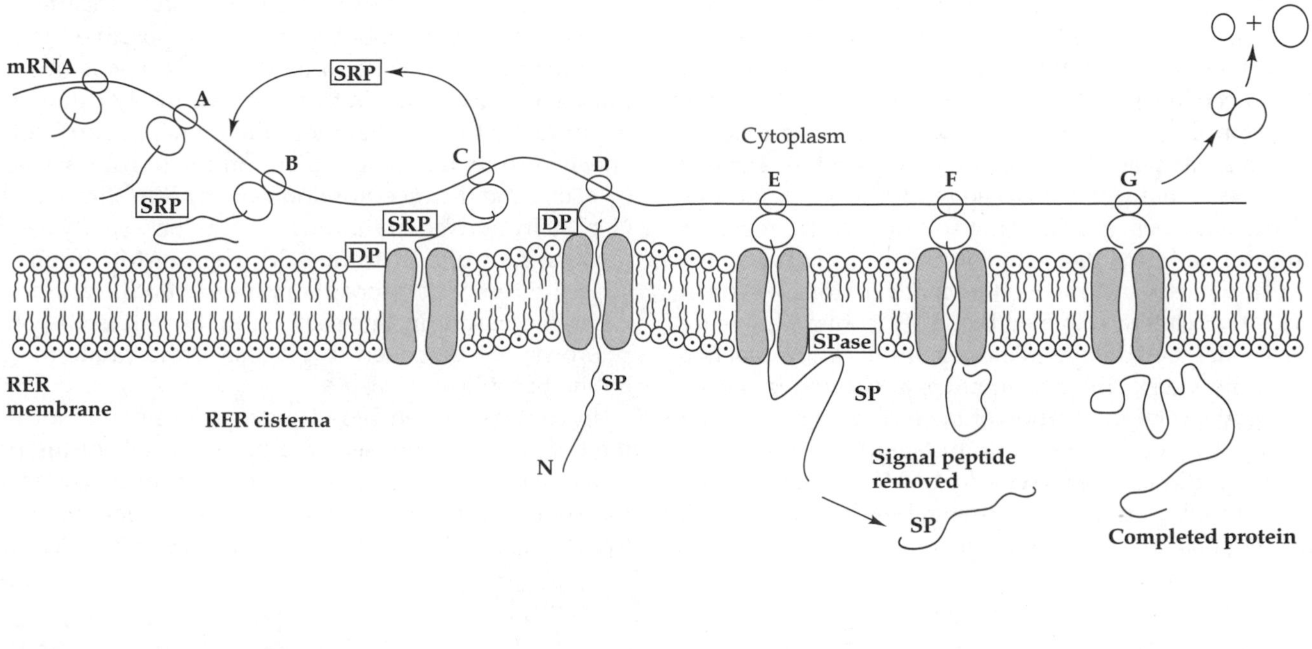

recognition markers. Membrane receptors act as attachment sites for specific external stimuli such as hormones, growth factors, antibodies, lipoproteins, and certain nutrients. These molecular stimuli, which bind specifically to receptors, are called **ligands.** There are also receptors located on the membrane of cell organelles; less is known about them, but they appear to be glycoproteins necessary for the correct positioning of newly synthesized cellular proteins.

Although most receptor proteins are probably integral membrane proteins, some may be peripheral. In addition, receptor proteins can vary widely in their composition and mechanism of action. Although the composition and mechanism of action of many receptors have not yet been determined, at least three distinct types of receptors are known to exist:

1. those that bind the ligand stimulus and convert it into an internal signal that alters behavior of the affected cell,
2. those that function as ion channels, and
3. those that internalize their stimulus intact.

Examples of these three types of receptors follow.

Internal Chemical Signal

The internal chemical signal most often produced by a stimulus-receptor interaction is 3′,5′-cyclic adenosine monophosphate (cyclic AMP, or cAMP). It is formed from adenosine triphosphate (ATP) by the enzyme adenylate cyclase. Cyclic AMP is frequently referred to as the second messenger in the stimulation of target cells by hormones. Figure 1.15 presents a proposed model for the ligand-binding action of receptors, which leads to production of the internal signal cAMP. As shown in the figure, the stimulated receptor reacts with the guanosine triphosphate (GTP)-binding protein (G protein), which is responsible for the activation of adenylate cyclase and the production of cAMP from ATP.

The mechanism of action of cAMP signaling within the cell is complex, but it can be viewed briefly as follows: cAMP is an activator of protein kinases. **Protein kinases** are enzymes that phosphorylate (add phosphate groups to) other enzymes and, in doing so, convert the enzymes from inactive forms into active forms. In some cases, the phosphorylated enzyme is the inactive form. Protein kinases that can be activated by cAMP contain two subunits, a catalytic and a regulatory subunit. In the inactive form of the kinase, the two subunits are bound in such a way that the catalytic portion of the molecule is inhibited sterically by the presence of the regulatory subunit. Phosphorylation of the enzyme by cAMP causes dissociation of the subunits, thereby freeing the catalytic subunit, which regains its full catalytic capacity.

Ion Channel

Receptors can also act as ion channels in stimulating a cell. In some cases, the binding of the ligand to its receptor causes a voltage change, which then becomes the signal for an appropriate cellular response. Such is the case when the neurotransmitter acetylcholine is the stimulus. The receptor for acetylcholine appears to function as an ion channel in response to voltage change. Stimulation by acetylcholine becomes a signal for the channels to open, allowing sodium (Na) ions to pass through an otherwise impermeable membrane [9].

Internalization Stimulus

The internalization of a stimulus into a fibroblast via its receptor is illustrated in Figure 1.16. Receptors that perform in such a manner exist for a variety of biologically active molecules, including the hormones insulin and triiodothyronine. Low-density lipoproteins (LDLs) are internalized in much the same fashion (see Chapter 6), except that their receptors, rather than being mobile, are already clustered in coated pits. These coated pits, vesicles formed from the plasma membrane, are coated with several proteins, among which clathrin is primary. A coated pit containing the receptor with its ligand soon loses the clathrin coating and forms a smooth-walled vesicle. This vesicle delivers the ligand into the depths of the cell and then is recycled along with the receptor into the plasma membrane. If the endocytotic process is for scavenging, the ligand (perhaps a protein) is not used by the cell but instead undergoes lysosomal degradation, as shown in Figure 1.16 and exemplified by the endocytosis of LDL.

The reaction of a fibroblast to changes in blood glucose levels is a good example of cellular adjustment to the existing environment that is made possible through receptor proteins. When blood glucose levels are low, muscular activity leads to release of the hormone epinephrine by the adrenal medulla. Epinephrine becomes attached to its receptor protein on the fibroblast, thereby activating the receptor and causing it to stimulate the G protein and adenylate cyclase, which catalyzes the formation of cAMP from ATP. Then cAMP initiates a series of enzyme phosphorylation modifications, as described earlier in this section, that result in the phosphorolysis of glycogen to glucose 1-phosphate for use by the fibroblast.

In contrast, when blood glucose levels are elevated, the hormone insulin, secreted by the β-cells of the pancreas, reacts with its receptors on the fibroblast and is transported into the cell via receptor-mediated endocytosis (Fig. 1.16). The action of insulin is to allow diffusion

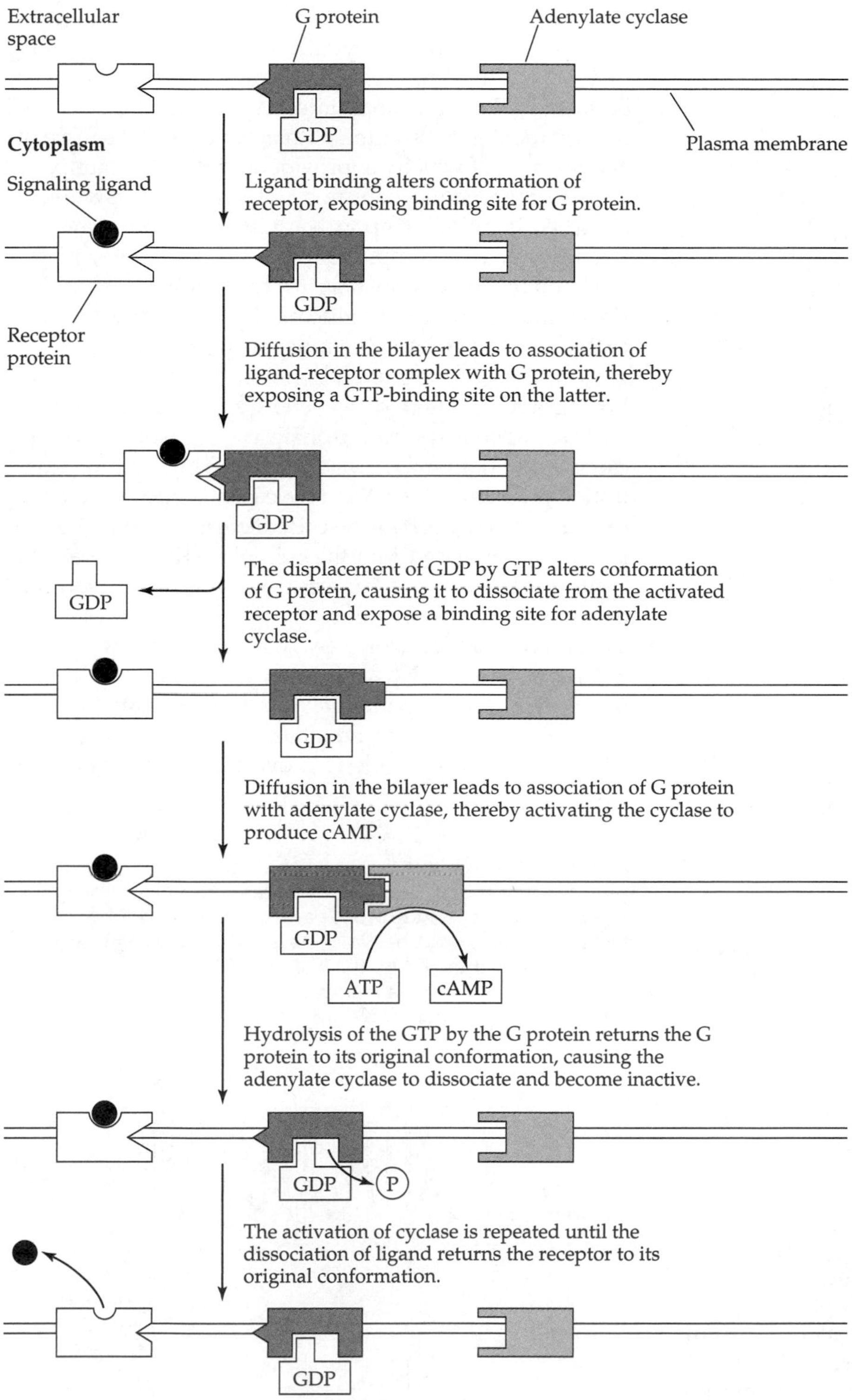

Figure 1.15 A proposed model for production of the internal signal cAMP. The response to an activated receptor protein is much greater than shown in this model because each activated receptor protein activates many molecules of G protein. Also, rather than diffusing independently through the plasma membrane and interacting only after the ligand binds to the receptor protein, the G protein and adenylate cyclase may be permanently associated. (Alberts B, Bray D, Lewis J. *Molecular Biology of the Cell.* New York: Garland, 1983, p. 385.)

of glucose into the cell, but the mechanism of action is not fully understood. It is postulated that insulin increases the number of glucose receptors in the cell membrane and that these in turn promote diffusion of glucose via its transport protein. Glucose transporters will be discussed in Chapter 4. The hormone itself is degraded within the cell [1].

Many intracellular chemical messengers other than those cited as examples in this section are known [10]. Listed here, along with cAMP, are several additional

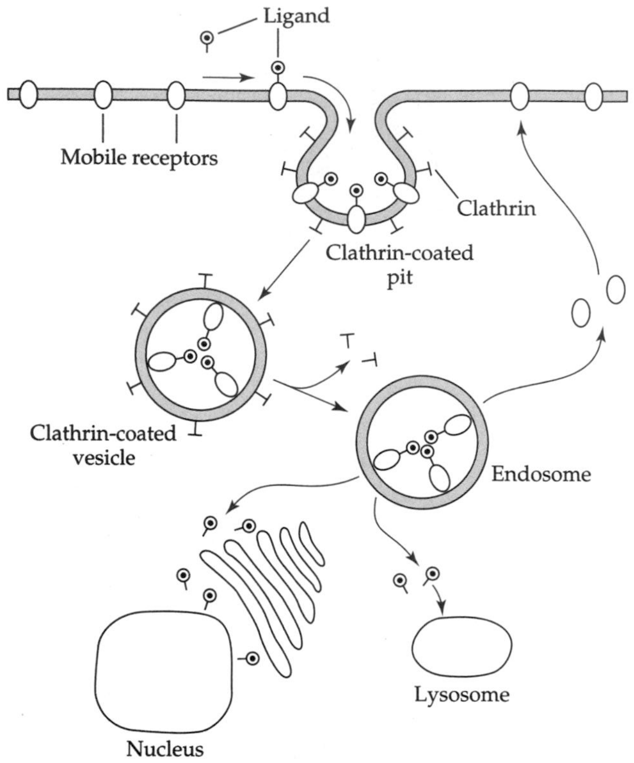

Figure 1.16 Receptor-mediated endocytosis, summarizing the steps involved in the binding, clustering, and entry of a typical ligand into a fibroblast. In this example, the receptor is recycled to the plasma membrane, and the ligand can either be used by the cell or undergo lysosomal degradation.

examples of intracellular messengers. Page numbers are included for those that are discussed in more detail in subsequent chapters.

- cyclic AMP
- cyclic GMP
- Ca^{+2}
- inositol triphosphate
- diacyl glycerol
- fructose 2,6-bisphosphate

Transport Proteins

Transport proteins are responsible for regulating the flow of nutrients and other substances into and out of the cell. They may function by acting as carriers (or pumps) for the substances, or they may provide protein-lined passages (pores) through which water-soluble materials of small molecular weight may diffuse. Figure 1.6 is an illustration of these various transport proteins.

The active transport protein that has been studied most is the sodium (Na^+) pump. Not only is the Na^+ pump essential for the maintenance of ionic and electrical balance, but it also is necessary for the intestinal and renal absorption of certain key nutrients (e.g., glucose and certain amino acids). These nutrients move into the epithelial cell of the small intestine against a concentration gradient, necessitating both a carrier and a source of energy, both of which are provided by the Na^+ pump.

The proposed mechanism by which glucose is actively absorbed is called symport because it is a simultaneous transport of two compounds (Na^+ and glucose) in the same direction. A transport protein with two binding sites binds both Na^+ and glucose. The attachment of Na^+ to the carrier increases the transport protein's affinity for glucose. Sodium, because it is moving down a concentration gradient created by energy released through Na^+/K^+ adenosine triphosphatase (ATPase), is able to carry along with it glucose that is moving up a concentration gradient. When Na^+ is released inside the cell, the carrier's affinity for glucose is decreased, and glucose also can be released into the cell. Na^+/K^+-ATPase then "pumps" the Na ions back out of the cell. The sodium pump is illustrated in Figure 1.17.

Na^+/K^+-ATPase works by first combining with ATP in the presence of Na^+ on the inner surface of the cell membrane. The enzyme then is phosphorylated by the breakdown of ATP to adenosine diphosphate (ADP) and consequently is able to move three Na ions out of

Figure 1.17 The active transport of glucose. Glucose is pumped into the cell's apical membrane by a Na^+-powered glucose symport, and glucose passes out of the cell by facilitated diffusion. The Na^+ gradient driving the glucose symport is maintained by the Na^+/K^+-ATPase in the basal and lateral plasma membrane, which keeps the internal concentration of Na^+ low.

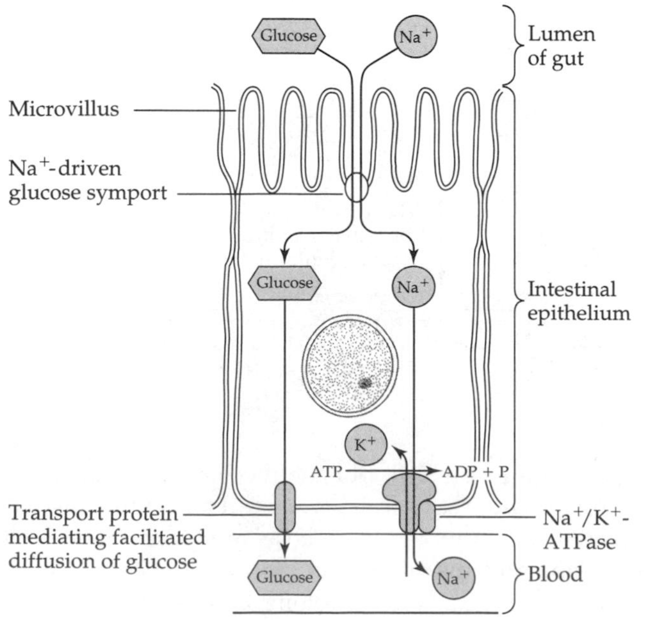

the cell. On the outer surface of the cell membrane, ATPase becomes dephosphorylated by hydrolysis in the presence of K ions and then is able to return two K ions to the cell. The term *pump* is used because the Na and K ions are both transported across the membrane against their concentration gradients. This pump is responsible for most of the active transport in the body.

Transport of glucose and amino acids into the epithelial cells of the intestinal tract is active in that the carriers needed for their transport are dependent on the concentration gradients achieved by the action of Na^+/K^+-ATPase at the basolateral membrane. The activity of Na^+/K^+-ATPase is the major energy demand of the body at rest. The process of facilitated (non-energy-dependent) transport is also a very important mechanism for regulating the flow of nutrients into the cell. It is used broadly across a wide range of cell types. Proteins involved in this function are often called transporters; probably the most thoroughly studied of these are the glucose transporters, discussed in Chapter 4.

Catalytic Proteins (Enzymes)

Enzymes are distributed throughout all cellular compartments. Those that are components of the cellular membranes are usually found on the inner surface of the membranes. Exceptions are the digestive enzymes: isomaltase, the disaccharidases (lactase, sucrase, and maltase), and certain peptidases located on the brush border of the epithelial cells lining the small intestine. Membrane-associated enzymes are found distributed throughout the cell organelles, with the greatest concentration found in the mitochondria. As mentioned earlier, the enzymes of the electron transport chain, where energy transformation occurs, are located within the inner membrane of the mitochondria.

Metabolic processes occurring in the cells are governed by enzymes that, for the most part, have been synthesized on the cell's RER under the direction of nuclear DNA. The functional activity of most enzymes, however, depends not only on the protein portion of the molecule but also on a nonprotein prosthetic group or coenzyme. If the nonprotein group is an organic compound, it usually contains a chemically modified B-complex vitamin. Commonly, however, the prosthetic group may be inorganic (i.e., metal ions such as Mg, Zn, Cu, Mn, Fe).

Enzymes have an active center that possesses a high specificity. This means that a substrate must fit perfectly into the specific contours of the active center. The velocity of an enzyme-catalyzed reaction increases as the concentration of the substrate that is available to the enzyme increases. However, this relationship applies only to a concentration of substrate that is less than the concentration that "saturates" the enzyme. At saturation levels of substrate, the enzyme molecule functions at its maximum velocity (V_{max}), and the occurrence of a still higher concentration of substrate cannot increase the velocity further.

K_m, or the Michaelis constant, is a useful parameter that aids in establishing how enzymes will react in the living cell. K_m represents the concentration of a substrate that will be found in an occurring reaction when the reaction is at one-half its maximum velocity. If an enzyme has a high K_m value, then an abundance of substrate must be present to raise the rate of reaction to half its maximum; in other words, the enzyme has a low affinity for its substrate. An example of an enzyme with a high K_m is glucokinase, an enzyme operating in the liver cells. Because glucose can diffuse freely into the liver, the fact that glucokinase has a high K_m is very important to the regulation of blood glucose. The low affinity of glucokinase for glucose prevents the removal of too much glucose from the blood during periods of fasting. Conversely, when the glucose load is high—for example, following a high-carbohydrate meal—excess glucose will still be able to be converted by glucokinase, which does not function at its maximum velocity when glucose levels are in the normal range. The enzyme therefore can be thought of as a protection against high cellular concentrations of glucose.

The nature of enzyme catalysis can be described by the following reactions:

$$\text{Enzyme (E)} + \text{substrate (S)} \longleftrightarrow \text{E-S complex}$$

(reversible reaction)

$$\text{E-S} \longleftrightarrow \text{E-P}$$

The substrate activated by combination with the enzyme is converted into an enzyme-product complex through rearrangement of the substrate's ions and atoms:

$$\text{E-P} \longrightarrow \text{E} + \text{P}$$

The product is released, and the enzyme is free to react with more of the substrate.

Most biochemical reactions are reversible, meaning that the same enzyme can catalyze a reaction in both directions. The extent to which a reaction can proceed in a reverse direction depends on several factors, the most important of which are the relative concentrations of substrate (reactant) and product and the differences in energy content between reactant and product. In instances when a very large disparity in energy content or concentration exists between reactant and product, the reaction can proceed in only one direction. Such a reaction is unidirectional as opposed to reversible. In unidirectional reactions, the same enzyme cannot catalyze in both directions. Instead, a different enzyme is required to catalyze the reverse direction of the reaction (see Chapter 3). Comparing glycolysis with gluconeogenesis allows us to see how unidirectional reactions may be reversed by the introduction of a different enzyme.

Simultaneous reactions, catalyzed by various multienzyme systems or pathways, constitute cellular metabolism. Enzymes are compartmentalized within the cell and function in sequential chains. A good example of a multienzyme system is the Krebs cycle located in the mitochondrial matrix. Each sequential reaction is catalyzed by a different enzyme, and some reactions are reversible while others are unidirectional. Although some reactions in almost any pathway are reversible, it is important to understand that the removal of one of the products drives the reaction toward formation of more of that product. Removal (or use) of the product, then, becomes the driving force that causes reactions to proceed primarily in the desired direction.

A very important aspect of nutritional biochemistry is the regulation of metabolic pathways. Anabolic and catabolic reactions must be kept in a balance appropriate for life (and perhaps growth) of the organism. Regulation involves primarily the adjustment of the catalytic activity of certain participating enzymes. There are three major mechanisms for this regulation:

1. covalent modification of enzymes via hormone stimulation,
2. modulation of allosteric enzymes, and
3. increase in enzyme concentration by induction.

The first of these mechanisms, *covalent modification of enzymes,* is usually achieved by the addition of or hydrolytic removal of phosphate groups to or from the enzyme. This is the mechanism involving cAMP and protein kinase activation previously discussed (p. 14). An example of covalent modification of enzymes is the regulation of glycogenesis and glycogenolysis.

The second important regulatory mechanism is that exerted by certain unique enzymes called *allosteric enzymes.* The term *allosteric* refers to the fact that these enzymes possess an allosteric or specific "other" site besides the catalytic site. Specific compounds, called modulators, can bind to these allosteric sites and profoundly influence the activity of these regulatory enzymes. Modulators may be positive (i.e., causing an increase in enzyme activity), or they may exert a negative effect (i.e., inhibit activity). Modulating substances are believed to alter the activity of the allosteric enzymes by changing the conformation of the polypeptide chain or chains of the enzyme, thereby altering the binding of its catalytic site with the intended substrate. Negative modulators are often the end products of a sequence of reactions. As an end product accumulates above a certain critical concentration, it can inhibit, through an allosteric enzyme, its own further production.

An excellent example of an allosteric enzyme is phosphofructokinase in the glycolytic pathway. Glycolysis gives rise to pyruvate, which is decarboxylated and oxidized to acetyl CoA and enters the Krebs cycle by combination with oxaloacetate to form citrate. Citrate is a negative modulator of phosphofructokinase. Therefore, an accumulation of citrate causes an inhibition of glycolysis through its regulation of phosphofructokinase. In contrast, an accumulation of AMP or ADP, which indicates a depletion of ATP, signals the need for additional energy in the cell in the form of ATP. AMP or ADP therefore acts to modulate phosphofructokinase positively. The result is an active glycolytic pathway that ultimately leads to the formation of more ATP through the Krebs cycle/electron transport chain connection.

The third mechanism of enzyme regulation, *enzyme induction,* creates changes in the concentration of certain inducible enzymes. Inducible enzymes are adaptive, meaning that they are synthesized at rates dictated by cellular circumstances. In contrast, constitutive enzymes, which are synthesized at a relatively constant rate, are uninfluenced by external stimuli. Induction usually occurs through the action of certain hormones such as the steroid hormones and the thyroid hormones and is exerted through changes in the expression of genes encoding the enzymes. Dietary changes can elicit the induction of enzymes necessary to cope with the changing nutrient load. This regulatory mechanism is relatively slow, however, compared to the first two mechanisms discussed, which exert effects in terms of seconds or minutes.

Specific examples of enzyme regulation will be cited in subsequent chapters dealing with metabolism of the major nutrients. It should be noted at this point, however, that *enzymes targeted for regulation catalyze essentially unidirectional reactions.* In every metabolic pathway, at least one reaction is essentially irreversible, exergonic, and enzyme limited. That is, the rate of the reaction is limited only by the activity of the enzyme catalyzing it. Such enzymes are frequently the regulatory enzymes, capable of being stimulated or suppressed by one of the mechanisms described. It is logical that an enzyme catalyzing a reaction reversibly at near equilibrium in the cell cannot be regulatory, because its up or down regulation would affect its forward and reverse activities equally. This, in turn, would not accomplish the purpose of regulation, which is the stimulation of the rate of the metabolic pathway in one direction compared with the rate of the pathway in the reverse direction.

Enzymes participating in cellular reactions are located throughout the cell in both the cytoplasmic matrix (cytoplast) and the various organelles. The location of specific enzymes depends on the site of the metabolic pathways or metabolic reactions in which those enzymes participate. Enzyme classification, therefore, is based on the type of reaction catalyzed by the various enzymes. Enzymes fall within six general classifications:

1. **Oxidoreductases** (dehydrogenases, reductases, oxidases, peroxidases, hydroxylases, oxygenases) are enzymes that catalyze all reactions in which one compound is oxidized and another is reduced. Examples of oxidoreductases are the enzymes found in the electron transport chain located on the inner membrane of the mitochondria. Other examples are the cytochrome P450 enzymes located on the ER of liver cells.

2. **Transferases** are enzymes that catalyze reactions not involving oxidation and reduction in which a functional group is transferred from one substrate to another. Included in this group of enzymes are transketolase, transaldolase, transmethylase, and the transaminases. The transaminases (α-amino transferases), which figure so prominently in protein metabolism, fall under this classification and are located primarily in the mitochondrial matrix.

3. **Hydrolases** (esterases, amidases, peptidases, phosphatases, glycosidases) are enzymes that catalyze cleavage of bonds between carbon atoms and some other kind of atom by the addition of water. Digestive enzymes fall within this classification, as do those enzymes contained within the lysosome of the cell.

4. **Lyases** (decarboxylases, aldolases, synthetases, cleavage enzymes, deaminases, nucleotide cyclases, hydrases or hydratases, dehydratases) are enzymes that catalyze cleavage of carbon-carbon, carbon-sulfur, and certain carbon-nitrogen bonds (peptide bonds excluded) without hydrolysis or oxidation-reduction. Citrate lyase, which frees acetyl CoA for fatty acid synthesis in the cytoplast, is a good example of an enzyme belonging to this classification.

5. **Isomerases** (isomerases, racemases, epimerases, mutases) are enzymes that catalyze the interconversion of optical or geometric isomers. Phosphohexose isomerase, which converts glucose 6-phosphate to fructose 6-phosphate in glycolysis (occurring in the cytoplast), exemplifies this particular class of enzyme.

6. **Ligases** are enzymes that catalyze the formation of bonds between carbon and a variety of other atoms, including oxygen, sulfur, and nitrogen. Formation of bonds catalyzed by ligases requires energy that usually is provided by hydrolysis of ATP. A good example of a ligase is acetyl CoA carboxylase, which is necessary to initiate fatty acid synthesis in the cytoplast. Through the action of acetyl CoA carboxylase, a bicarbonate ion (HCO_3^-) is attached to acetyl CoA to form malonyl CoA, the initial compound in de novo fatty acid synthesis.

APOPTOSIS

It is said that dying is a normal part of living. So it is with the cell. Like every living thing, a cell has a well-defined life span, after which its structural and functional integrity diminishes and it is removed by other cells through phagocytosis.

As cells die, they are replaced by new cells that are continuously being formed by cell mitosis. However, both daughter cells formed in the mitotic process do not always enjoy the full life span of the parent. If they did, the number of cells, and consequently tissue mass, could increase inordinately. Therefore, one of the two cells produced by mitosis generally is programmed to die before its sister. In fact, most dying cells are already doomed at the time of their formation. Those targeted for death are usually smaller than their surviving sisters, and their phagocytosis begins even before the mitosis generating them is complete [11]. The processes of cell division and cell death must be carefully regulated in order to generate the proper number of cells during development. Later, in the mature state, it is important that the desired number of cells be maintained. The mechanism by which naturally occurring cell death arises has been subjected to intense research in recent years.

Many terms have been used to describe naturally occurring cell death. It is now most commonly referred to as *programmed cell death,* to distinguish it from pathological cell death, which is not part of any normal physiological process. The emergent term describing programmed cell death is **apoptosis,** a word borrowed from the Greek meaning to "fall out."

Apoptotic cells are recognizable morphologically. They contract, the chromatin condenses, and the cytoplasmic organelles initially remain intact. Apoptosis also involves activation of a Ca^{+2}-dependent endonuclease that cleaves the genome of the cell into fragments of approximately 180 base pairs. Dead cells are removed by phagocytosis. Although the process of apoptosis has been extensively studied [11], how many distinct mechanisms are involved in causing cell death remains unclear.

Cell death appears to be activated by specific genes in dying cells. Genes designated ced-3 and ced-4 must be expressed within dying cells for cell death to occur. The ced-3 and ced-4 genes encode products (proteins) that activate cytotoxic activity, and they therefore must be tightly controlled to avoid damage to the wrong cells. A major control factor is a third gene, ced-9, which negatively regulates the ced-3 and ced-4 genes.

Mutations to ced-9, which inactivate the gene, have been shown to kill an animal under study by causing the death of cells otherwise intended to survive [11].

There is also interest in the possible involvement in the apoptotic process of the gene designated p53. The gene has been garnering a great deal of attention in the cancer field because of the tumor suppressor properties of some of its protein products. The connection of p53 to apoptosis is that it is believed to regulate the reduction/oxidation state of the cell and is able to increase concentrations of reactive oxygen species (ROS). ROS may, in turn, signal the beginning of apoptosis. The mechanisms underlying p53-dependent apoptosis are largely unknown, but a documented property of p53—its ability to activate gene transcription—may be a factor. Following is a proposed sequence of events by which p53 results in apoptosis:

1. The transcription induction of redox-related genes
2. Formation of ROS
3. Oxidative degradation of mitochondrial components, resulting in cell death [12]

Recently, the release of cytochrome c from the mitochondrion into the cytoplasmic matrix has been investigated as one factor that promotes apoptosis. Once cytochrome c has translocated to the cytoplasmic matrix, it activates certain proteolytic enzymes that are products of the ced-3 genes and therefore are associated with apoptosis [13]. A cytochrome c–apoptosis connection is supported by the discovery of a protein designated Bcl-2 (B-cell lymphoma gene product) that appears to block the release of mitochondrial cytochrome c. By blocking the release of mitochondrial cytochrome c, Bcl-2 interferes with the apoptotic process. Bcl-2 is an integral membrane protein on the outer membrane of the mitochondrion. Two observations are relevant:

- Bcl-2 prevents the efflux of cytochrome c from the mitochondrion to the cytoplasmic matrix.
- Genetic overexpression of Bcl-2 prevents cells from undergoing apoptosis in response to various stimuli.

Therefore, a possible role of Bcl-2 in preventing apoptosis is to block release of cytochrome c from the mitochondrion [14].

Much remains to be learned about the mechanisms underlying apoptosis. What is obvious is the intense interest in the mechanism. Once the apoptotic process is understood, can scientific intervention designed to slow the rate of programmed cell death be far behind?

summary

This brief walk through the cell—beginning with its outer surface, the plasma membrane, and moving into its innermost part, where the nucleus is located—has provided a view of how this living entity functions.

Characteristics of the cell that seem particularly notable are these:

- The flexibility of the plasma membrane in adjusting or reacting to its environment while protecting the rest of the cell as it monitors what may pass into or out of the cell. Prominent in the membrane's reaction to its environment are the receptor proteins, which are believed to have been synthesized on the rough endoplasmic reticulum and to have moved through the Golgi apparatus to their intended site on the plasma membrane.
- The communication among the various components of the cell made possible through the cytoplast, with its microtrabecular network, and also through the endoplasmic reticulum and Golgi apparatus. The networking is such that communications flow not only among components within the cell but also between the nucleus and the plasma membrane.
- The efficient division of labor among the cell components (organelles). Each component has its own specific functions to perform, with little overlap. Furthermore, much evidence is accumulating to support the concept of an "assembly line" not only in oxidative phosphorylation on the inner membrane of the mitochondrion but also in almost all operations, wherever they occur.
- The superb management exercised by the nucleus to ensure that all the proteins needed for a smooth operation are synthesized. Proteins needed as recognition markers, receptors, transport vehicles, and catalysts are available as needed.
- The fact that, like all living things, cells must die a natural death. This programmed process is called apoptosis, a particularly attractive focus of current research.

Despite the efficiency of the cell, it is still not a totally self-sufficient unit. Its continued operation is contingent on receiving appropriate and sufficient nutrients. Nutrients needed include not only those that can be used for production of immediate metabolic energy (ATP) or for storage as chemical energy, but also those required as building blocks for structural macromolecules. In addition, the cell must have an adequate supply of the so-called regulatory nutrients (i.e., vitamins, minerals, and water).

With a view of the structure of the "typical cell," the division of labor among its component parts, and the location within the cell where many of the key metabolic reactions necessary for the continuation of life take place, we can now turn to consideration of how the cell receives its nourishment so that life can continue.

References Cited

1. Berdanier CD. Role of membrane lipids in metabolic regulation. Nutr Rev 1988;46:145–49.

2. Young P. Mom's mitochondria may hold mutation. Sci News 1988;134:70.

3. Baluska F, Volkmann D, Barlow P. Nuclear components with microtubule-organizing properties in multicellular eukaryotes: functional and evolutionary considerations. In: Kwang W. Jeon, ed. International Review of Cytology 1997;175:91–135.

4. Griffiths G, Simons K. The trans Golgi network: sorting at the exit site of the Golgi complex. Science 1986;234:438–43.

5. Teasdale R, Jackson M. Signal-mediated sorting of membrane proteins between the endoplasmic reticulum and the Golgi apparatus. In: Annu Rev Cell Dev Biol 1996;12:27–54.

6. Rothman J. Mechanisms of intracellular protein transport. Nature 1994;372:55–63.

7. How do proteins find mitochondria? Science 1985;228:1517–18.

8. Wickner WT, Lodish JT. Multiple mechanisms of protein insertion into and across membranes. Science 1985;230:400–07.

9. A potpourri of membrane receptors. Science 1985;230:649–51.

10. Barritt GJ. Networks of extracellular and intracellular signals. In: Communication within Animal Cells. Oxford, England: Oxford University Press, 1992, pp. 1–19.

11. Ellis R, Yuan J, Horvitz H. Mechanisms and functions of cell death. In: Annu Rev Cell Biol 1991;7:663–98.

12. Polyak K, Xia Y, Zweler J, Kinzler K, Vogelstein B. A model for p53-induced apoptosis. Nature 1997;389:300–05.

13. Kluck R, Bossy-Wetzel E, Green D, Newmeyer D. The release of cytochrome c from mitochondria: a primary site for Bcl-2 regulation of apoptosis. Science 1997;275:1132–36.

14. Yang J, Liu X, Bhalla K, et al. Prevention of apoptosis by Bcl-2: release of cytochrome c from mitochondria blocked. Science 1997;275:1129–32.

Suggested Reading

Alberts B, Johnson A, Lewis J, Raff M, Roberts K, Walter P. Molecular Biology of the Cell, 4th ed. New York: Garland, 2002.

Barritt GJ. Networks of extracellular and intracellular signals. In: Communication within Animal Cells. Oxford, England: Oxford University Press, 1992, pp. 1–19.

Garrett RH, Grisham CM. Biochemistry, 2nd ed. New York: Harcourt College Publishers, 1999.

Masters C, Crane D. The Peroxisome: A Vital Organelle Cambridge, England: Cambridge University Press, 1995. This is a clearly written overview of the multifaceted functions of this important organelle.

Rhoades R, Pflanzer R. Human Physiology, 4th ed. Pacific Grove, CA: Thomson, 2003.

Web Sites

www.nlm.nih.gov
National Library of Medicine: MEDLINE

www.chid.nih.gov/welcome/welcome.html
National Institutes of Health: Combined Health Information Database

perspective

Cellular Enzymes on the Loose: Indicators of Disease

All of the hundreds of enzymes present in the human body are synthesized intracellularly, and most of them function within the cell in which they were formed. These are the enzymes responsible for catalyzing the myriad of metabolic reactions occurring in the cell. As explained in the section "Cellular Proteins" in this chapter, they are directed to specific locations within the cell following their synthesis on the ribosomes. Some enzymes, on the other hand, are secreted from the cell, usually in an inactive form, and are rendered active in the extracellular fluids where they function. Examples of secreted enzymes are the digestive proteases and other hydrolases formed in the cells of the pancreas and then secreted into the lumen of the small intestine. Other secreted enzymes, called plasma-specific enzymes, function in the bloodstream. Examples include the enzymes involved in the blood-clotting mechanism.

Diagnostic enzymology focuses on intracellular enzymes, which, because of a perturbation of the cell structure, egress from the cell and ultimately express their activity in the serum. By measuring the serum activity of the released enzymes, both the site and the extent of the cellular damage can be determined. If the site of the damage is to be determined with reasonable accuracy, the enzyme being measured must exhibit a relatively high degree of organ or tissue specificity. For example, an enzyme having an intrahepatocyte concentration many times greater than its concentration in other tissues could potentially be a marker for liver damage should its serum activity increase. The rate at which intracellular enzymes enter the bloodstream is based on two factors:

1. Those that affect rates at which enzymes leak from cells
2. Those that affect rates of production either by increased synthesis or by accelerated proliferation of enzyme-producing cells

Leakage Factors

Intracellular enzymes normally are retained within the cell by the plasma membrane. The plasma membrane is metabolically active, and its integrity depends on the cell's energy consumption and therefore its nutritive status. Any process that impairs the cell's use of nutrients can compromise the structural integrity of the plasma membrane. Membrane failure can also arise from its mechanical disruption, such as would occur due to a viral attack on the cell. Damage to the plasma membrane is manifested as leakiness and eventual cell death, allowing unimpeded passage of substances, including enzymes, from intracellular to extracellular compartments.

Factors contributing to cellular damage and resulting in abnormal egress of cellular enzymes include the following:

- tissue ischemia, (**ischemia** refers to an impairment of blood flow to a tissue or part of a tissue; it deprives affected cells of oxygen and oxidizable nutrients),
- tissue necrosis,
- viral attack on specific cells,
- damage from organic chemicals such as alcohol and organophosphorus pesticides, and
- hypoxia (inadequate intake of oxygen).

Increases in blood serum concentrations of cellular enzymes can be good indicators of even minor cellular damage because the intracellular concentration of enzymes is hundreds or thousands of times greater than in blood and also because enzyme assays are extremely sensitive.

Not all intracellular enzymes are valuable in diagnosing damage to the cells in which they are contained. Several conditions must be met for the enzyme to be suitably diagnostic:

- *There must be a sufficiently high degree of organ or tissue specificity of the enzyme.* Suppose an enzyme is widely distributed among organ or tissue systems. Although an abnormal increase of its activity in serum does indicate a pathological process with cellular damage, it cannot precisely identify the site of the damage. An example is lactate dehydrogenase (LDH). LDH activity is widely distributed among cells of the heart, liver, skeletal muscle, erythrocytes, platelets, and lymph nodes. Therefore, elevated serum activity of LDH can hardly be a specific marker for tissue pathology. In practice, however, LDH does have diagnostic value if it is first separated into its five different isoenzyme forms and these are quantified individually. LDH isoenzyme forms are designated LDH1, LDH2, LDH3, LDH4, and LDH5. Each isoform is more organ-specific than total LDH, with LDH1 being associated primarily with heart muscle and LDH5 with liver cells.
- *There must be a steep concentration gradient of enzyme activity between the interior and exterior of the cells under normal conditions.* If this were not true, small increases in serum activity would not be detectable. Examples of enzymes that are in compliance with this requirement and that have been useful over the years as disease markers are prostatic acid phosphatase, with a prostate cell/serum concentration ratio of $10^3:1$, and alanine aminotransferase, with a hepatocyte/serum ratio of $10^4:1$. These enzymes have been useful in the diagnosis of prostatic disease (primarily carcinoma) and viral hepatitis, respectively.
- *The enzyme must function in the cytoplasmic compartment of the cell.* If the enzyme is compartmentalized within an organelle such as the nucleus or mitochondrion, its leakage from the cell is impeded even in the event of significant damage to the plasma membrane. An example of an enzyme not in compliance with this condition is the mitochondrial enzyme ornithine carbamoyl transferase, which functions within the urea cycle. Although the enzyme adheres rigidly to the two previous conditions (i.e., it is strictly liver specific, and its cell/serum concentration is as high as $10^5:1$), it provides little value in the diagnosis of hepatic disease.
- *The enzyme must be stable for a reasonable period of time in the vascular compartment.* Isocitrate dehydrogenase has an extremely high activity in heart muscle. Yet, following the resultant damage of a myocardial infarction, the released enzyme is rapidly inactivated upon entering the bloodstream, thereby becoming indeterminable.

Increased Production Factors

The most common cause of increased production of an enzyme, resulting in a spike in its serum concentration, is malignant disease. Substances that occur in body fluids as a result of malignant disease are called tumor markers. A tumor marker

- may be produced by the tumor itself or
- may be produced by the host in response to a tumor.

In addition to enzymes and isoenzymes, other forms of tumor markers include hormones, oncofetal protein antigens such as carcinoembryonic antigen (CEA), and products of oncogenes. **Oncogenes** are mutated genes that encode abnormal, mitosis-signaling proteins that cause unchecked cell division.

Products of malignant cells, such as intracellular enzymes, exhibit a predictably increased rate of synthesis because of the nature of the disease process. Should the proliferating cells of the tumor retain their capacity to synthesize the enzyme, the gross output of the enzyme will be markedly elevated. Furthermore, the enzyme can be released into the systemic circulation as a result of tumor necrosis or the change in permeability of the plasma membrane of the malignant cells.

While tumor markers are present In higher quantities in cancer tissue or blood from cancer patients than in benign tissue or the blood of normal subjects, few markers are specific for the organ in which the tumor is located, because most enzymes are not unique to a specific organ. A possible exception is prostate specific antigen (PSA).

PSA is a proteolytic enzyme produced almost exclusively by the prostate gland. Its value as a tumor marker is further enhanced by the fact that metastasized malignant prostate cells produce nearly 10 times as much PSA as do normal prostate cells. A significant rise in serum PSA concentration therefore may signal that a tumor has metastasized to other sites in the body, suggesting a different therapeutic approach. Though other causes exist for an increase in PSA levels besides cancer, PSA has become a valuable screening and diagnostic tool. Prostate cancer is the leading cause of death among older men.

Table 1 offers a list of enzymes that have been used successfully as indicators of organ or tissue pathology. The principal sources of the enzymes and the clinical significance of their serum determination are also included.

Table 1 Diagnostically Important Enzymes

Enzyme	Principal Sources	Principal Clinical Significance
Acid phosphatase	Prostate, erythrocytes	Carcinoma of prostate
Alanine amino transferase	Liver, skeletal muscle, heart	Hepatic parenchymal cell disease
Aldolase	Skeletal muscle, heart	Muscle diseases
Amylase	Pancreas, salivary glands	Pancreatitis, carcinoma of pancreas
Cholinesterase	Liver	Organophosphorus insecticide poisoning, hepatic parenchymal cell disease
Creatine kinase (CK-2 isoform)	Heart, skeletal muscle	Myocardial infarction
Gamma glutamyl transferase	Liver, kidney	Alcoholism, hepatobiliary disease
Prostate specific antigen (PSA)	Prostate	Carcinoma of prostate

Suggested Reading

Moss DW, Henderson AR. Enzymes (Chap. 19); and Chan DW, Sell S. Tumor markers (Chap. 21). In: Tietz, Fundamentals of Clinical Chemistry, 4th ed., Burtis C and Ashwood E, eds. Philadelphia: Saunders, 1996;297–350.

Web Site

www.clinchem.org
Clinical Chemistry; Journal of the American Association for Clinical Chemistry

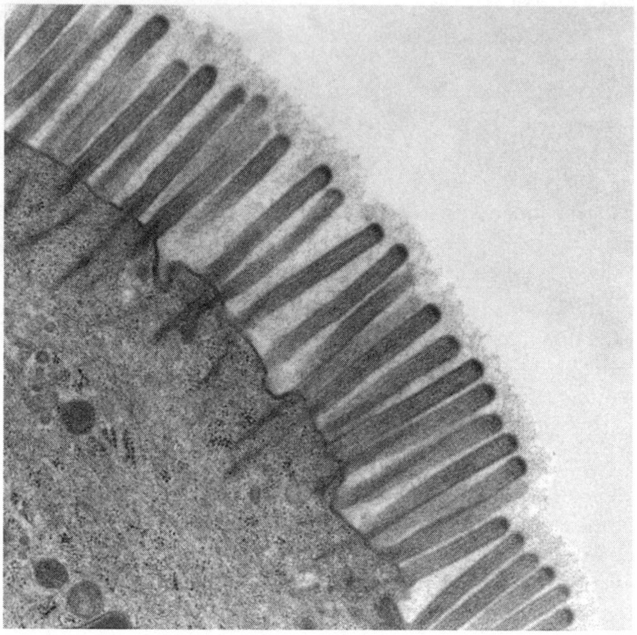

Intestinal microvilli

chapter 2 The Digestive System: Mechanism for Nourishing the Body

NUTRITION IS THE SCIENCE OF NOURISHMENT. Ingestion of foods and beverages provides the body with at least one, if not more, of the nutrients needed to nourish the body. There are six classes of nutrients that the body needs: carbohydrate, lipid, protein, vitamins, minerals, and water. For the body to use the carbohydrate, lipid, protein, and some minerals found in foods, the food must be digested first. In other words, the food first must be broken down mechanically and chemically. This process of digestion occurs in the digestive tract and on its completion yields nutrients ready for absorption and use by the body.

AN OVERVIEW OF THE STRUCTURE OF THE DIGESTIVE TRACT

The digestive tract, approximately 16 ft in length, includes organs that comprise the alimentary canal (also called the gastrointestinal tract) as well as certain accessory organs. The main structures of the digestive tract include the oral cavity, esophagus, stomach, and small and large intestines. The accessory organs include the pancreas, liver, and gallbladder. The accessory organs provide or store secretions that ultimately are delivered to the lumen of the digestive tract and aid in the digestive process. Figure 2.1

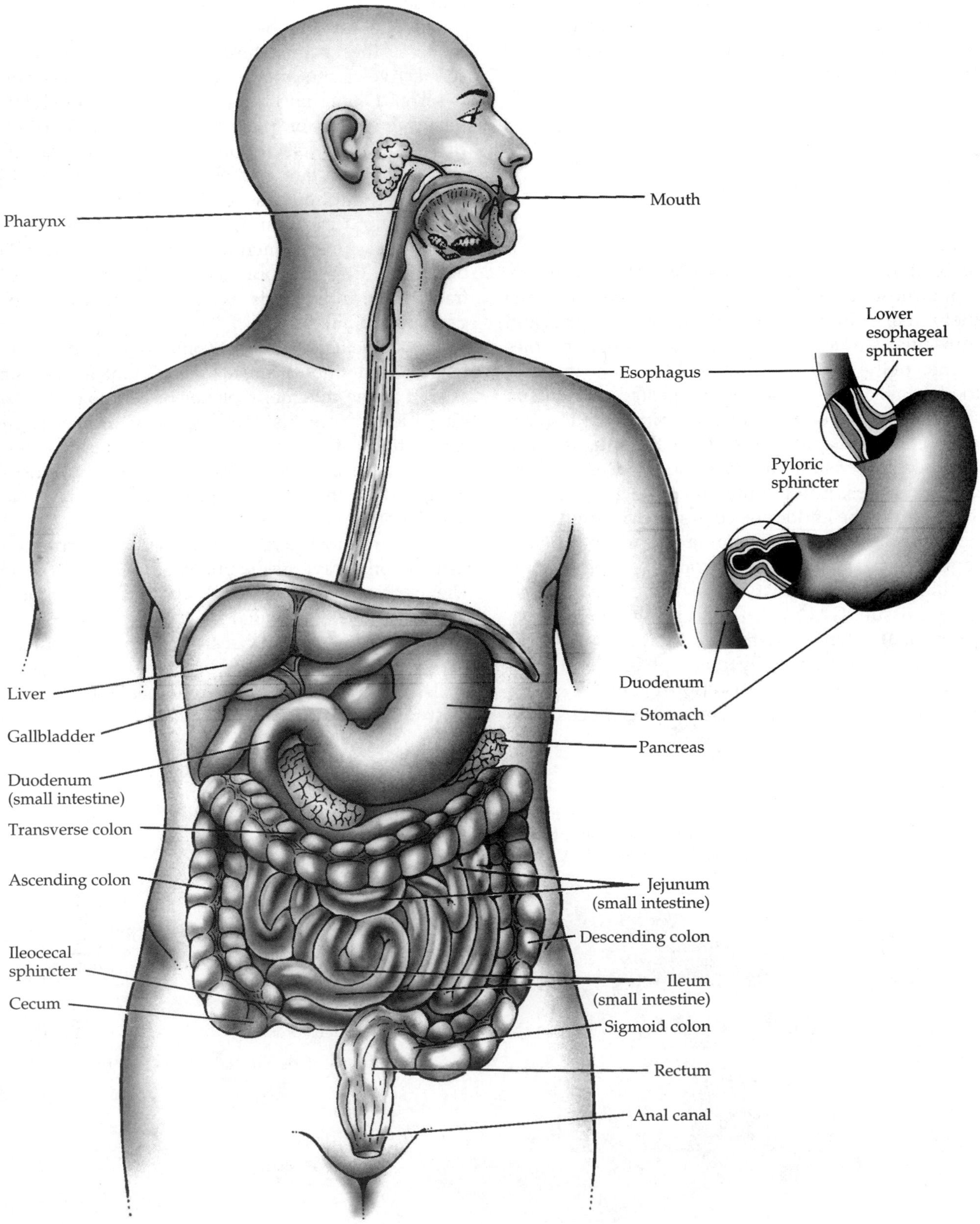

Figure 2.1 The digestive tract and its accessory organs.

illustrates the digestive tract and accessory organs. Figure 2.2 provides a cross-sectional view of the gastrointestinal tract showing the lumen (interior passageway) and the four main tunics, or layers, of the gastrointestinal tract:

- the mucosa,
- the submucosa,
- the muscularis externa, and
- the serosa or adventitia.

Some of these layers contain sublayers. The mucosa, the innermost layer, is made of three sections: the epithelium or epithelial lining, the lamina propria, and the muscularis mucosa. The mucosal epithelium lines the lumen of the gastrointestinal tract. It is the mucosal epithelium that is in contact with ingested nutrients in the food we eat. Exocrine and endocrine cells also are found among the epithelial cells of the mucosa. The exocrine cells secrete a variety of substances, such as mucus and juices, into the lumen of the gastrointestinal tract, while the endocrine cells secrete various hormones into the blood. The lamina propria lies below the epithelium and consists of connective tissue and small blood and lymphatic vessels. Gut-associated lymphoid tissue (GALT) also is found within the lamina propria. This lymphoid tissue contains a number of white blood cells, especially macrophages and lymphocytes, which provide protection against ingested microorganisms. The third sublayer of the mucosa, the muscularis mucosa, consists of a thin layer of smooth muscle.

Next to the mucosa is the submucosa. The submucosa, the second tunic or layer, is made up of connective tissue and more gut-associated lymphoid tissue and contains a network of nerves called the submucosal plexus or plexus of Meissner. This plexus controls, in part, secretions from the mucosal glands and helps regulate mucosal movements and blood flow. The lymphoid tissue in the submucosa is similar to that found in the mucosa and functions to protect the body against foreign substances. The submucosa binds the first mucosa layer of the gastrointestinal tract to the muscularis externa, or third layer of the gastrointestinal tract.

The muscularis externa contains both circular and longitudinal smooth muscle, important for peristalsis, as well as the myenteric plexus or plexus of Auerbach. This plexus controls the frequency and strength of contractions of the muscularis to affect gastrointestinal motility. The myenteric and submucosal plexuses are discussed in more detail on page 32 under "Neural Regulation."

The outermost layer, the serosa or adventitia, consists of connective tissue and the visceral peritoneum. The peritoneum is a membrane that surrounds the organs of the abdominal and pelvic cavities. In the abdominal cavity, the visceral peritoneum surrounds the organs, and the parietal peritoneum lines the cavity walls. Between the two peritoneums is the peritoneal cavity.

Figure 2.2 Cross section of a digestive tract segment showing the four layers: the mucosa, submucosa, muscularis externa, and serosa. (Adapted from Stalheim-Smith and Fitch, *Understanding Human Anatomy and Physiology*, St. Paul: West, 1993, p. 793.)

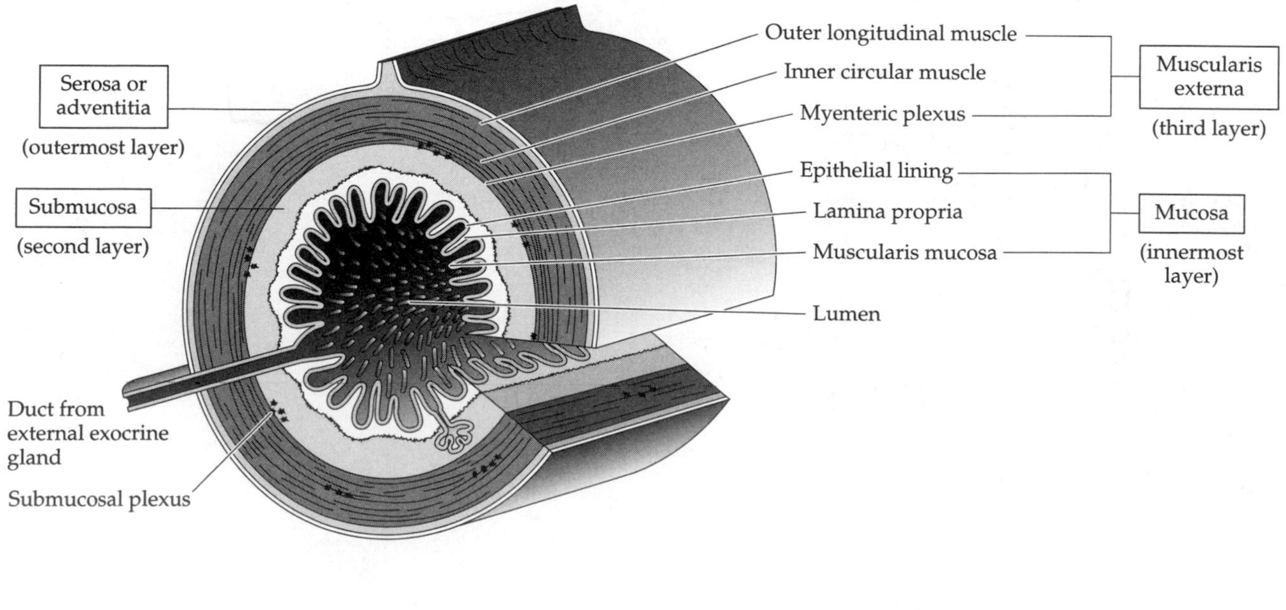

The Structures of the Upper Gastrointestinal Tract

The upper gastrointestinal tract consists of the oral cavity, esophagus, and stomach. The mouth and pharynx constitute the oral cavity and provide the entryway to the digestive tract. Food is passed from the mouth through the pharynx and into the esophagus. The esophagus is about 10 in. long and contains both striated and smooth muscles. Sphincters or valves, which are circular muscles, also are located throughout the digestive tract and allow for the passage of food from one section of the gastrointestinal tract to another. For example, an area of the esophagus referred to as the lower esophageal sphincter (LES) lies just above the juncture of the esophagus and stomach. Relaxation of this sphincter permits the passage of food from the esophagus into the stomach. The stomach is a J-shaped organ located on the left side of the abdomen under the diaphragm, extending from the LES to the duodenum, the upper or proximal section of the small intestine. The stomach mixes the food with digestive juices and enzymes and then holds the partially digested food before releasing it in small quantities at regular intervals into the lower gastrointestinal tract. The volume of the stomach when empty (resting) is about 50 mL (~2 oz), but on being filled it can expand to accommodate from 1 L to approximately 1.5 L (~37–52 oz). The pyloric sphincter, located at the distal end of the stomach, controls the release of **chyme** (partially digested food existing as a thick semiliquid mass) from the stomach into the duodenum.

The Structures of the Lower Gastrointestinal Tract and Accessory Organs

The lower gastrointestinal tract consists of the small and large intestines. The small intestine is composed of the duodenum (slightly less than 1 ft long) and the jejunum and ileum (which together are approximately 9 ft long). Microscopy is needed to identify where one of these sections of the small intestine ends and the other begins. The lumen of the jejunum is generally larger than that of the ileum. The small intestine represents the main site for nutrient digestion and absorption. The duodenum receives secretions from the liver, gallbladder, and pancreas, which are accessory organs. These secretions are necessary for the digestion of nutrients.

The liver, pictured in Figures 2.1, 2.3, and 2.4, is the largest single internal organ of the body. The liver is made up of two lobes called the right and left lobes. These lobes in turn contain functional units called lobules. The lobules are made up of liver cells called hepatocytes. Blood passes through the liver via sinusoids from branches of the portal vein and hepatic artery. Hepatocytes synthesize bile, which is necessary for fat digestion. Bile is then released into bile canaliculi, which lie between the hepatocytes in the hepatic plates. Bile drains from the plates into bile ducts. As shown in Figure 2.4a, the right and left hepatic bile ducts join to form the common hepatic duct. The common hepatic duct unites with the cystic duct, which leads into and out of the gallbladder, to form the common hepatic bile duct.

The gallbladder, a small organ with a capacity of approximately 40 to 50 mL (1.4–1.8 oz), is located on the surface of the liver (Fig. 2.1) and is also considered an accessory organ necessary for digestion. The gallbladder functions to concentrate and store the bile made in the liver until it is needed for fat digestion in the small intestine. Bile flow into the duodenum is regulated by the intraduodenal segment of the common hepatic bile duct and the sphincter of Oddi, located at the junction of the common hepatic bile duct and the duodenum (Fig. 2.4a).

The pancreas, the third accessory organ, is a slender, elongated organ ranging in length from about 6 to 9 in. The pancreas is found behind the greater curvature of the stomach, lying between the stomach and the duodenum (Figs. 2.1 and 2.4). Two types of active tissue are found in the pancreas (Fig. 2.4b):

- the ductless endocrine tissue that secretes hormones, primarily insulin and glucagon, into the blood, and
- the acini or ducted exocrine tissue that produces the digestive enzymes as well as pancreatic juice.

Figure 2.3 Structure of a liver lobule.

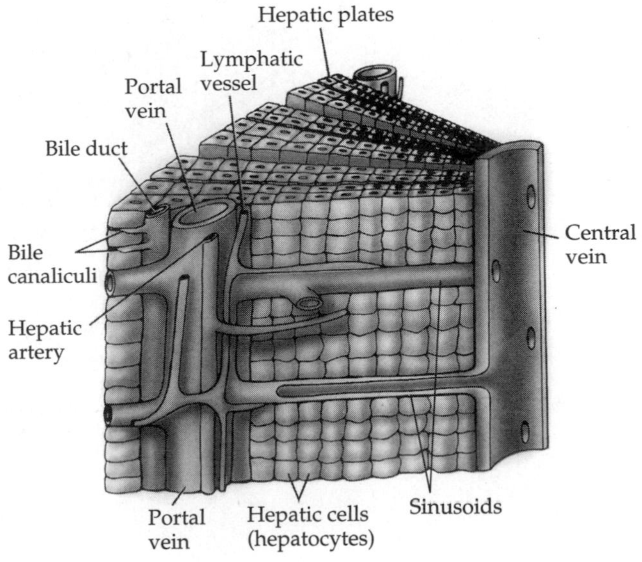

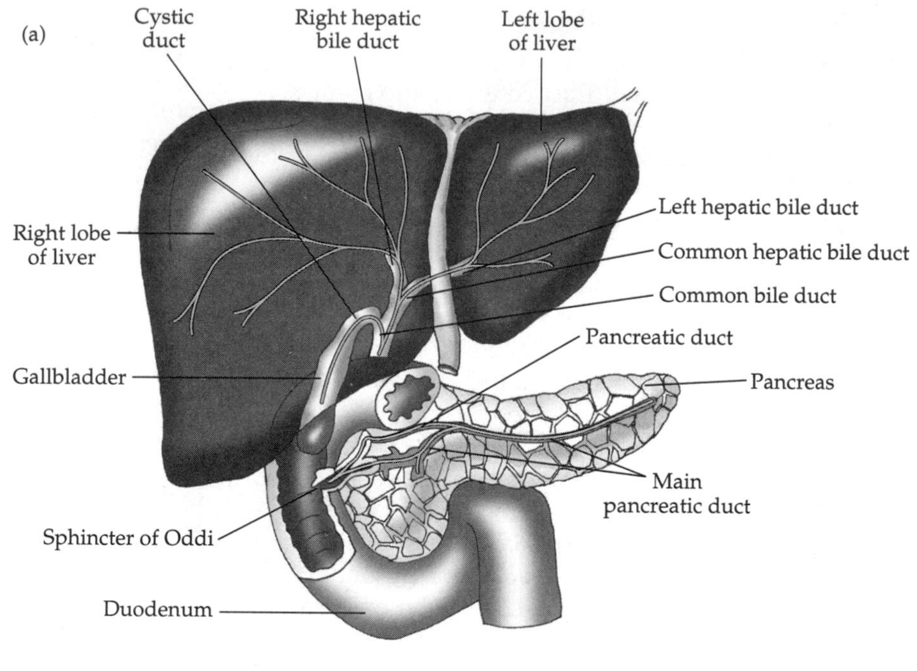

Figure 2.4 (a) The ducts of the gallbladder, liver, and pancreas. (b) Schematic representation of the exocrine and endocrine portions of the pancreas. (Adapted from Stalheim-Smith and Fitch, *Understanding Human Anatomy and Physiology*, St. Paul: West, 1993, p. 808.)

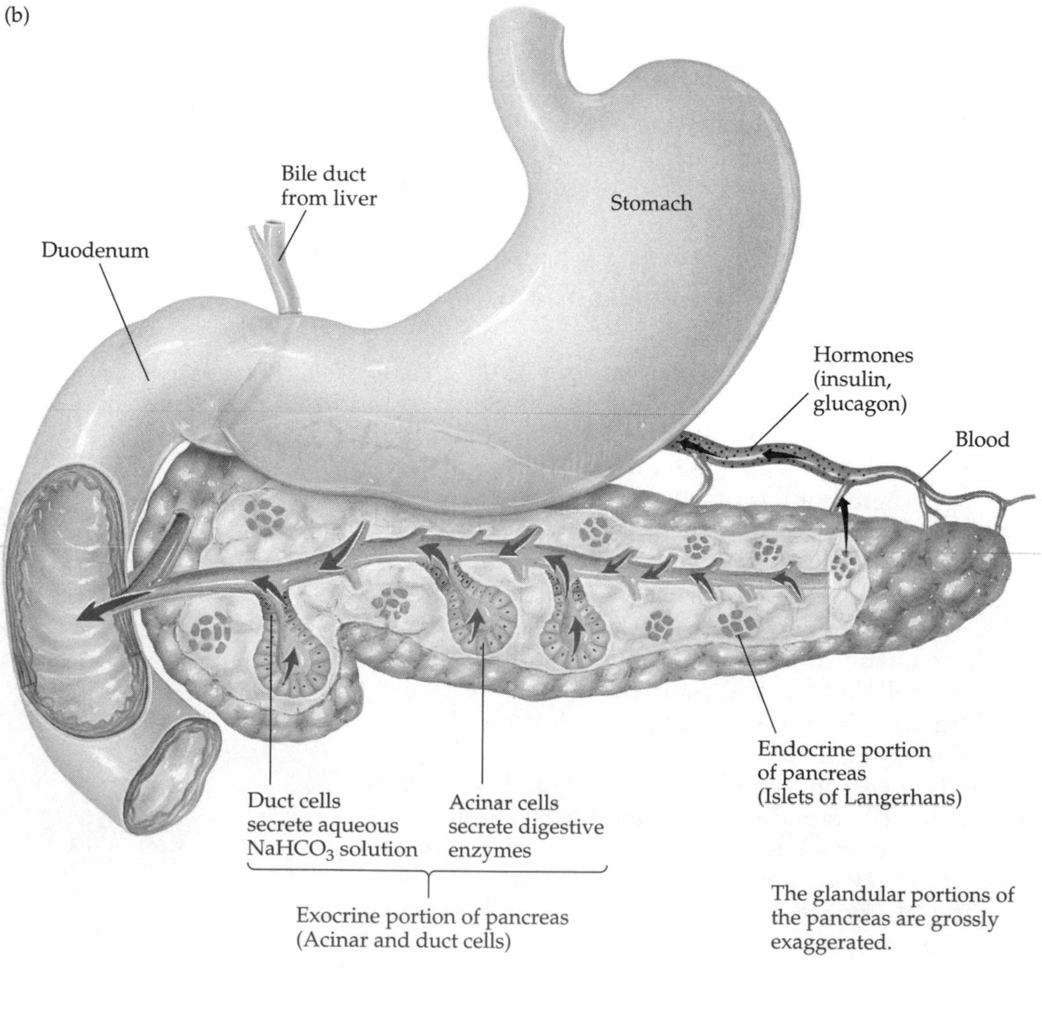

The acinar cells of the pancreas are arranged into circular glands that are attached to small ducts. Enzymes are packaged into secretory structures called granules. Stimulation of pancreatic acinar cells by hormones or the parasympathetic nervous system results in the release of pancreatic digestive enzymes from the granules by **exocytosis.** The digestive enzymes are secreted as part of pancreatic juice. Pancreatic juice contains

- pancreatic digestive enzymes,
- bicarbonate,
- cations such as sodium, potassium, and calcium, and
- the anion chloride in a watery solution.

The pancreatic juice is secreted into small ducts within the pancreas. These small ducts coalesce to form a large main pancreatic duct, which later joins with the common hepatic bile duct to form the bile pancreatic duct. The bile pancreatic duct empties into the duodenum through the sphincter of Oddi (Fig. 2.4a). Blockage of this duct, as may occur with gallstones from the gallbladder, may impair the release of pancreatic juice out of the pancreas and can lead to acute pancreatitis (inflammation of the pancreas), a potentially life-threatening condition.

Although the structure of the small intestine consists of the same layers as identified in Figures 2.2 and 2.5, the epithelial lining or mucosa of the small intestine is structured to maximize surface area and thus maximize its ability to absorb nutrients. The small intestine has a surface area of approximately 300 m^2, an area about equal to a 3-ft-wide sidewalk more than three football fields in length. Contributing to this enormous surface area are

- the large folds of mucosa, called the folds of Kerckring, that protrude into the lumen of the small intestine;
- the fingerlike projections, called villi, that project out into the lumen of the intestine and consist of hundreds of cells (**enterocytes,** also called absorptive epithelial cells) along with blood capillaries and a central lacteal

Figure 2.5 Structure of the small intestine.

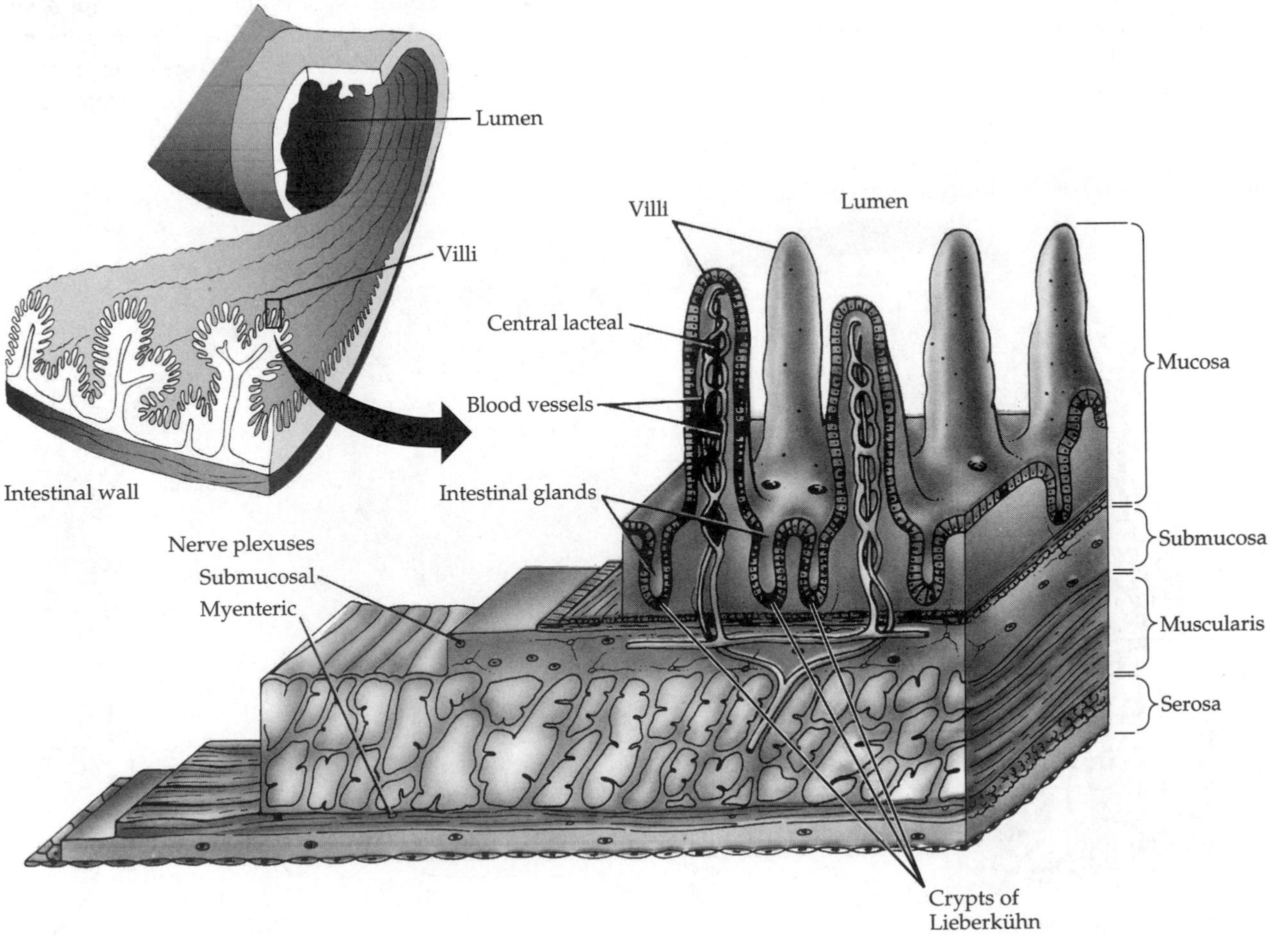

(lymphatic vessel) for transport of nutrients out of the enterocyte (Fig. 2.5);

- the microvilli, hairlike extensions of the plasma membrane of the enterocytes that make up the villi (Fig. 2.6).

The microvilli possess a surface coat, or glycocalyx, as shown in Figure 2.6, and together these comprise the brush border of the enterocytes. Covering the brush border is an unstirred water (fluid) layer. That is, the unstirred water layer lies between the brush border membrane of the intestine and the intestinal lumen. Its presence can have the greatest impact on lipid absorption, and it is discussed further on page 42.

Most of the digestive enzymes produced by the intestinal mucosal cells are found embedded on the brush border, and they function to hydrolyze already partially digested nutrients, mainly carbohydrate and protein. Structurally, the digestive enzymes are **glycoproteins,** compounds consisting of both carbohydrates and protein. The carbohydrate portion or glyco-portion of these glycoprotein enzymes may in part make up the glycocalyx. The glycocalyx, which lines the luminal side of the intestine, is thought to consist of numerous fine filaments that extend almost perpendicular from the microvillus membrane to which it is attached. Digestion of nutrients is usually completed on the brush border but may be completed within the cytoplasm of the enterocytes.

The small intestine also contains small pits called crypts of Lieberkühn (Fig. 2.5) that lie between the villi. Epithelial cells in these crypts continuously undergo mitosis. The new cells gradually migrate upward and out of the crypts toward the tips of the villi. Toward the tip, many former crypt cells function as absorptive enterocytes. Ultimately, the enterocytes will be sloughed off into the intestinal lumen and excreted in the feces. Intestinal cell turnover is rapid, approximately every 3 to 5 days. Cells in the crypts include paneth cells that secrete proteins with unclear functions, goblet cells that secrete mucus, and enterochromaffin (mast) cells with endocrine function. Cells in the crypts of Lieberkühn also secrete fluid and electrolytes into the lumen of the small intestine. This fluid is typically reabsorbed by the villi. The paneth, goblet, and enterochromaffin cells, along with the enterocytes, serve additionally as a protective barrier against pathogens.

Also serving as protection throughout the mucosa and submucosa of the small intestine is mucosa-associated lymphoid tissue, also called gut-associated lymphoid tissue (GALT), if found in the nonmucosal layers of the gastrointestinal tract. GALT is composed of leukocytes (white blood cells). GALT leukocytes are found between intestinal absorptive epithelial cells and make up approximately 15% of the epithelial mucosa. GALT leukocytes include T-lymphocytes, natural killer (NK) cells, and microfold (M) cells, among others, and function in various capacities

Figure 2.6 Structure of the absorptive cell of the small intestine.

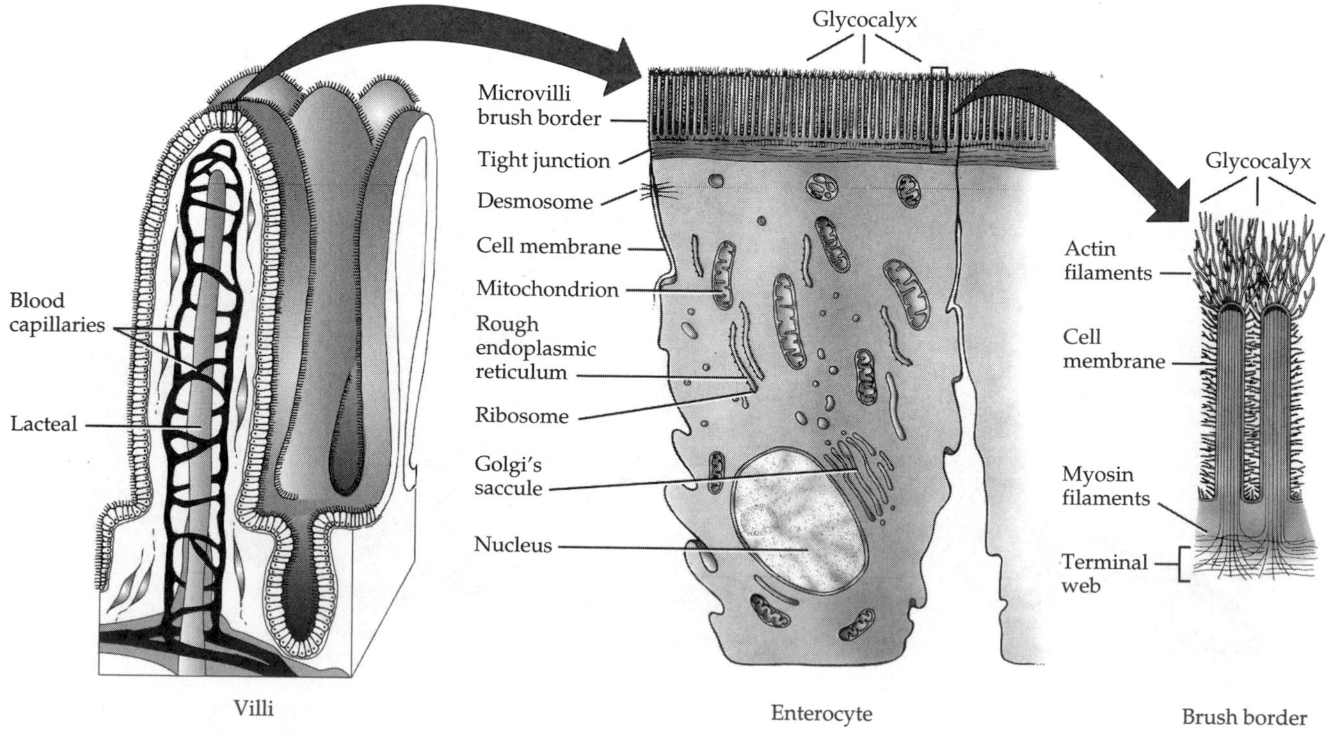

to protect the body against foreign substances. In addition, Peyer's patches, aggregates of lymphoid tissue located in the mucosa and submucosa, contain more T-lymphocytes as well as B-lymphocytes and macrophages to protect the body. The M-cells pass foreign substances to the lymphocytes, which in turn can mount an immune response. Together these leukocytes residing throughout the first two layers of the gastrointestinal tract provide a defense against bacteria or other foreign substances that may have been ingested with consumed food. However, atrophy of the mucosal and submucosal layers of the gastrointestinal tract, which may occur with illness, injury, starvation, or extended periods without food intake, can lead to bacterial translocation. Bacterial translocation is the movement of bacteria and toxins from the gastrointestinal tract into the blood or lymph. The presence of gastrointestinal tract–derived bacteria or its toxins in the blood or lymph can result in sepsis and, potentially, multiple system organ failure.

From the ileum (which is the distal or terminal section of the small intestine), unabsorbed materials empty via the ileocecal valve into the cecum, the right side of the colon (large intestine). From the cecum, materials move sequentially through the ascending, transverse, descending, and sigmoid sections of the colon (Figs. 2.1 and 2.7), which in its entirety is almost 5 ft long. Rather than being a part of the entire wall of the digestive tract as it is in the upper digestive tract, the longitudinal muscle in the colon is gathered into three muscular bands or strips called teniae (also spelled taenia or teneae) coli that extend throughout most of the colon. Contraction of a strip of longitudinal muscle along with contraction of circular muscle causes the uncontracted portions of the colon to bulge outward, creating pouches or haustra (Fig. 2.7). Contractions typically occur in one area of the colon and then move to a different, nearby area. As described by Guyton [1], the fecal material is slowly dug into and rolled over in the colon as one would spade the earth, so that deeper, moister fecal matter is put in contact with the colon's absorptive surface. This process permits dehydration of fecal matter for defecation while increasing fluid and electrolyte absorption.

Figure 2.7 The colon.

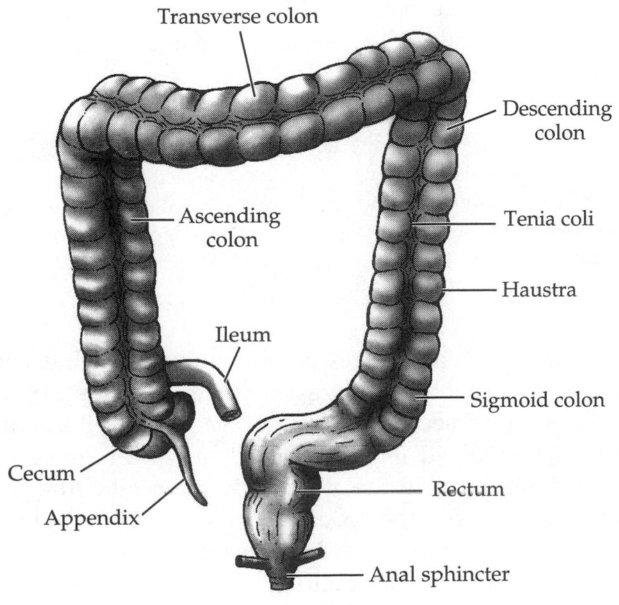

COORDINATION AND REGULATION OF THE DIGESTIVE PROCESS

Regulatory Peptides

Factors influencing digestion and absorption are coordinated, in part, by a group of gastrointestinal tract molecules referred to as regulatory peptides or, more specifically, gastrointestinal hormones and neuropeptides. Together the regulatory peptides affect a variety of digestive functions, including gastrointestinal motility, intestinal absorption, cell growth, and the secretion of digestive enzymes, electrolytes, water, and other hormones.

Some of the regulatory peptides—such as gastrin, cholecystokinin (CCK, also called CCK-pancreozymen and abbreviated CCK-PZ), secretin, gastric inhibitory polypeptide (GIP), and motilin—are considered hormones. Peptides, such as somatostatin, are termed paracrines. When released by endocrine cells, paracrines diffuse through the extracellular space to their target tissues rather than being secreted into the blood for transport. Neurocrines, peptides that originate from nerves of the gut, include vasoactive intestinal peptide (VIP), gastrin-releasing peptide (GRP, also called *bombesin*), neurotensin, and substance P.

The functions of regulatory peptides with respect to the gastrointestinal tract and the digestive process are numerous. Some selected functions follow:

- Gastrin, synthesized primarily by enteroendocrine cells called G-cells in the stomach and proximal small intestine, acts mainly in the stomach. Gastrin release occurs in response to vagal stimulation, ingestion of specific substances or nutrients, gastric distention, hydrochloric acid in contact with gastric mucosa, as well as local and circulating hormones. Gastrin principally stimulates the release of hydrochloric acid, but it also stimulates gastric and intestinal motility and pepsinogen release. Gastrin also stimulates the cellular growth of (that is, has trophic action on) the stomach and both the small and large intestines.

• CCK, secreted into the blood by enteroendocrine cells called I-cells of the proximal small intestine, principally binds to receptors on the pancreas to stimulate the secretion of pancreatic juice and enzymes into the duodenum. It also stimulates the contraction of the gallbladder to facilitate the release of bile into the duodenum. Gastric motility may be slightly inhibited by CCK, whereas intestinal motility is enhanced by CCK.

• Secretin, secreted into the blood by enteroendocrine cells called S-cells found in the mucosa of the proximal small intestine, is secreted in response to the release of acid chyme into the duodenum. Secretin acts primarily on pancreatic acinar cells to stimulate the release of pancreatic juice into the intestine. Secretin is thought to inhibit motility of most of the gastrointestinal tract, especially the stomach and proximal small intestine.

• GIP, produced by enteroendocrine K-cells of the mucosa of the duodenum and jejunum, inhibits gastric secretions and motility. GIP stimulates intestinal secretions and, like the other three hormones, stimulates insulin secretion from the pancreas as well.

Table 2.1 lists additional actions of gastrin, CCK, secretin, and GIP. Other regulatory peptides also affect the digestive process:

• Somatostatin, synthesized by pancreatic and intestinal cells, acts in a paracrine fashion by entering gastric juice. Somatostatin appears to mediate the inhibition of gastrin release as well as the release of GIP, secretin, VIP, and motilin. Gastric acid, gastric motility, pancreatic exocrine secretions, and gallbladder contraction are also inhibited by somatostatin.

• Motilin, a peptide secreted by cells of the duodenum, causes contraction of intestinal smooth muscle and may be involved in regulating different phases of the migrating motility complex (MMC). The MMC is important in maintaining gastrointestinal motility and is described in more detail on page 38 of this chapter.

• VIP is present in neurons within the gut; it is not thought to be present in intestinal endocrine cells. VIP stimulates intestinal secretions, relaxes most gastrointestinal sphincters, inhibits gastric acid secretion, and stimulates pancreatic bicarbonate release into the small intestine.

• Gastrin-releasing peptide (GRP), also called bombesin, released from nerves, stimulates the release of hydrochloric acid, gastrin, and CCK.

• Neurotensin, produced by small intestine mucosa, has no physiological role in digestion at normal circulating concentrations; however, neurotensin may serve to mediate gastric emptying, intestinal motility, and gastric acid secretion after fat ingestion.

• Substance P, another neuropeptide, increases blood flow to the gastrointestinal tract, inhibits acid secretion, increases motility of the small intestine, and binds to pancreatic acinar cells associated with enzyme secretion.

Table 2.1 Actions of Selected Regulatory Peptides

	Hormones			
Action	**Gastrin**	**CCK**	**Secretin**	**GIP**
Acid secretion	S*	S	I*	I*
Gastric emptying	I	I	I*	I
Pancreatic HCO_3^- secretion	S	S*	S*	O
Pancreatic enzyme secretion	S	S*	S	O
Gallbladder contraction	S	S*	S	?
Gastric motility	S	I	I	I
Intestinal motility	S	S	I	?
Insulin release	S	S	S	S*
Mucosal growth	S*	S	I	?
Pancreatic growth	S	S*	S*	?

Abbreviations: S, stimulates; I, inhibits; O, no effect; ?, information unavailable.
*Particularly important function.

Source: Adapted from Johnson LR. Gastrointestinal physiology, 3rd ed. St. Louis: Mosby, 1985, p. 8.

Neural Regulation

The nervous system of the gastrointestinal tract is referred to as the enteric (relating to the intestine) nervous system and lies in the wall of the gastrointestinal tract beginning in the esophagus and extending to the anus. Neural regulation of the gastrointestinal tract involves a combination of neural plexuses (networks) and **reflexes** (involuntary responses to stimuli).

The enteric nervous system can be divided into two neuronal networks, or plexuses: the myenteric plexus (or plexus of Auerbach) and the submucosal plexus (or plexus of Meissner). The location and actions of the two plexuses are given here:

Myenteric Plexus	Submucosal Plexus
Lies in the muscularis externa between longitudinal and circular muscles	Lies in the submucosa
Controls peristaltic activity and/or gastrointestinal motility	Controls mainly gastrointestinal secretions and local blood flow

Gastrointestinal reflexes involving the enteric nervous system are called enterogastric reflexes. They control gastrointestinal secretions and peristalsis as well as other processes involved in digestion. Examples of enterogastric reflexes include the ileogastric reflex and the gastroileal reflex. With the ileogastric reflex, gastric motility is inhibited when the ileum becomes distended. With the gastroileal reflex, ileal motility is stimulated when gastric motility and secretions increase. Other reflexes affect the small and large intestines. For example, the colonoileal reflex from the colon inhibits the emptying of the contents of the ileum into the colon. The intestinointestinal reflex diminishes intestinal motility when a segment of the intestine is overdistended.

THE PROCESS OF DIGESTION: SECRETIONS AND ENZYMES REQUIRED FOR NUTRIENT DIGESTION

Table 2.2 provides a partial list of zymogens/enzymes that participate in the digestion of nutrients in foods. **Zymogens** are often called proenzymes or inactive enzymes because they must be chemically altered to function as an enzyme. We discuss each of these enzymes briefly as we trace nutrient digestion from the oral cavity through the rest of the gastrointestinal tract. The enzymes are discussed again in Chapters 4, 6, and 7, which cover carbohydrates, lipids, and protein, respectively.

The Oral Cavity

On entering the mouth, food is chewed by the actions of the teeth and jaw muscles and is made ready for swallowing by mixing with secretions (saliva) released from the salivary glands. Three pairs of small, bilateral saliva-secreting salivary glands—the parotid, the submandibular, and the sublingual—are located throughout the lining of the oral cavity, along the jaw from the base of the ear to the chin (Fig. 2.8). Secretions (about 1 L/day) from these glands constitute saliva. Specifically, the parotid glands secrete water, electrolytes (sodium, potassium, chloride), and enzymes. The submandibular and sublingual glands secrete water, electrolytes, enzymes, and mucus. Saliva is primarily (99.5%) water, which helps dissolve foods. The principal enzyme of saliva is α amylase (also called ptyalin) (Table 2.2). This enzyme hydrolyzes internal α 1-4 bonds within starch. A second digestive enzyme, lingual lipase, is produced by lingual serous glands on the tongue and in the back of the mouth. This enzyme hydrolyzes dietary triacylglycerols

Table 2.2 Digestive Enzymes and Their Actions

Enzyme or Zymogen/Enzyme	Site of Secretion	Preferred Substrate(s)	Primary Site of Action
Salivary α amylase	Mouth	α 1-4 bonds in starch, dextrins	Mouth
Lingual lipase	Mouth	Triacylglycerol	Stomach, small intestine
Pepsinogen/pepsin	Stomach	Carboxyl end of phe, tyr, trp, met, leu, glu, asp	Stomach
Trypsinogen/trypsin	Pancreas	Carboxyl end of lys, arg	Small intestine
Chymotrypsinogen/chymotrypsin	Pancreas	Carboxyl end of phe, tyr, trp, met, asn, his	Small intestine
Procarboxypeptidase/			
carboxypeptidase A	Pancreas	C-terminal neutral amino acids	Small intestine
carboxypeptidase B	Pancreas	C-terminal basic amino acids	Small intestine
Proelastase/elastase	Pancreas	Fibrous proteins	Small intestine
Collagenase	Pancreas	Collagen	Small intestine
Ribonuclease	Pancreas	Ribonucleic acids	Small intestine
Deoxyribonuclease	Pancreas	Deoxyribonucleic acids	Small intestine
Pancreatic α amylase	Pancreas	α 1-4 bonds, in starch, maltotriose	Small intestine
Pancreatic lipase and colipase	Pancreas	Triacylglycerol	Small intestine
Phospholipase	Pancreas	Lecithin and other phospholipids	Small intestine
Cholesterol esterase	Pancreas	Cholesterol esters	Small intestine
Retinyl ester hydrolase	Pancreas	Retinyl esters	Small intestine
Amino peptidases	Small intestine	N-terminal amino acids	Small intestine
Dipeptidases	Small intestine	Dipeptides	Small intestine
Nucleotidase	Small intestine	Nucleotides	Small intestine
Nucleosidase	Small intestine	Nucleosides	Small intestine
Alkaline phosphatase	Small intestine	Organic phosphates	Small intestine
Monoglyceride lipase	Small intestine	Monoglycerides	Small intestine
Alpha dextrinase or isomaltase	Small intestine	α 1-6 bonds in dextrins, oligosaccharides	Small intestine
Glucoamylase, glucosidase, and sucrase	Small intestine	α 1-4 bonds in maltose, maltotriose	Small intestine
Trehalase	Small intestine	Trehalose	Small intestine
Disaccharidases	Small intestine		Small intestine
Sucrase*		Sucrose	
Maltase		Maltose	
Lactase		Lactose	

*Part of an enzyme complex.

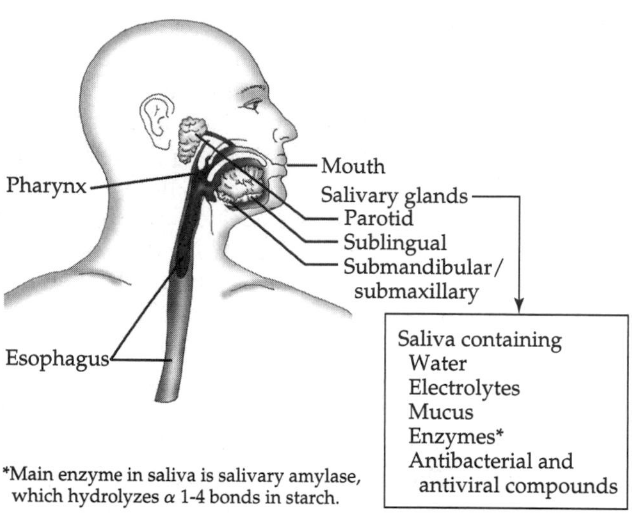

Figure 2.8 Secretions of the oral cavity.

(triglycerides) in the stomach, but its activity is limited due to the coalescing of the fats within the stomach. Activity of the lingual lipase in infants against triglycerides in milk improves digestion of dietary fats. Mucus secretions found in saliva contain glycoproteins, known as **mucins,** that lubricate food and protect the oral mucosa. Antibacterial and antiviral compounds, one example being the antibody IgA (immunoglobulin A), along with trace amounts of organic substances (such as urea) and other solutes (i.e., phosphates, bicarbonate), are also found in saliva. Both the parasympathetic and the sympathetic divisions of the autonomic nervous system affect saliva production and secretion.

The passage of food from the mouth through the pharynx (the oral cavity) into the esophagus constitutes swallowing. Swallowing, which can be divided into several stages—voluntary, pharyngeal, and esophageal—is a reflex response initiated by a voluntary action and regulated by the swallowing center in the medulla of the brain. To swallow food, the esophageal sphincter relaxes, allowing the opening of the esophagus. Food then passes into the esophagus. Simultaneously, the larynx (part of the respiratory tract) moves upward to induce a shift of the epiglottis over the glottis. The closure of the glottis is important in keeping food from entering the trachea, which leads to the lungs. Once food is in the esophagus, the larynx shifts downward to allow the reopening of the glottis.

The Esophagus

When food moves into and down the esophagus, both the striated (voluntary) muscle of the upper portion of the esophagus and the smooth (involuntary) muscle of the distal portion are stimulated by cholinergic (parasympathetic) nerves. The result is peristalsis, a progressive wavelike motion that moves the food (now called a bolus) through the esophagus into the stomach. The process usually takes less than 10 seconds. At the lower (distal) end of the esophagus, just above the juncture with the stomach, lies the lower esophageal sphincter (LES). LES, however, may be a misnomer, because there is no consensus about whether this particular muscle area is sufficiently hypertrophied to constitute a true sphincter. On swallowing, the LES pressure drops. This drop in LES pressure relaxes the sphincter so that food may pass from the esophagus into the stomach.

Multiple mechanisms, including neural and hormonal, regulate LES pressure. The musculature of the LES has a tonic pressure that is normally higher than the intragastric pressure, that is, the pressure within the stomach. This high LES tonic pressure functions to keep the sphincter closed. Closure of the LES sphincter is important because it prevents gastroesophageal reflux, the movement of chyme from the stomach back into the esophagus. The gastric acid in the chyme when present in the esophagus is an irritant to the esophageal mucosa. The individual experiencing reflux feels a burning sensation in the midchest region, a condition referred to as heartburn. Repeated exposure of the esophagus to acid-containing chyme can irritate the esophagus and lead to esophagitis, or inflammation of the esophagus. Foods and/or food-related substances can indirectly affect LES pressure and cause reflux. Smoking, chocolate, high-fat foods, alcohol, and carminatives such as peppermint and spearmint, for example, promote LES relaxation and increase the likelihood of reflux into the esophagus. Gastroesophageal reflux disease, reflux esophagitis, and their treatments are discussed in the perspective at the end of this chapter.

The Stomach

After passage through the LES, food or the bolus enters the stomach. The stomach contains four main regions, shown in Figure 2.9.

- The cardia region lies below the lower esophageal sphincter and receives the swallowed food from the esophagus.
- The fundus lies adjacent to the cardia.
- The large central region of the stomach is called the body. The body of the stomach serves primarily as the reservoir for swallowed food and is the production site for much of the gastric juice.
- The antrum or distal pyloric portion of the stomach extends from the angular notch to the duodenum and functions to grind and mix food with the digestive gastric juices to form semiliquid chyme. The antrum also provides strong peristalsis for gastric emptying through the pyloric sphincter into the duodenum.

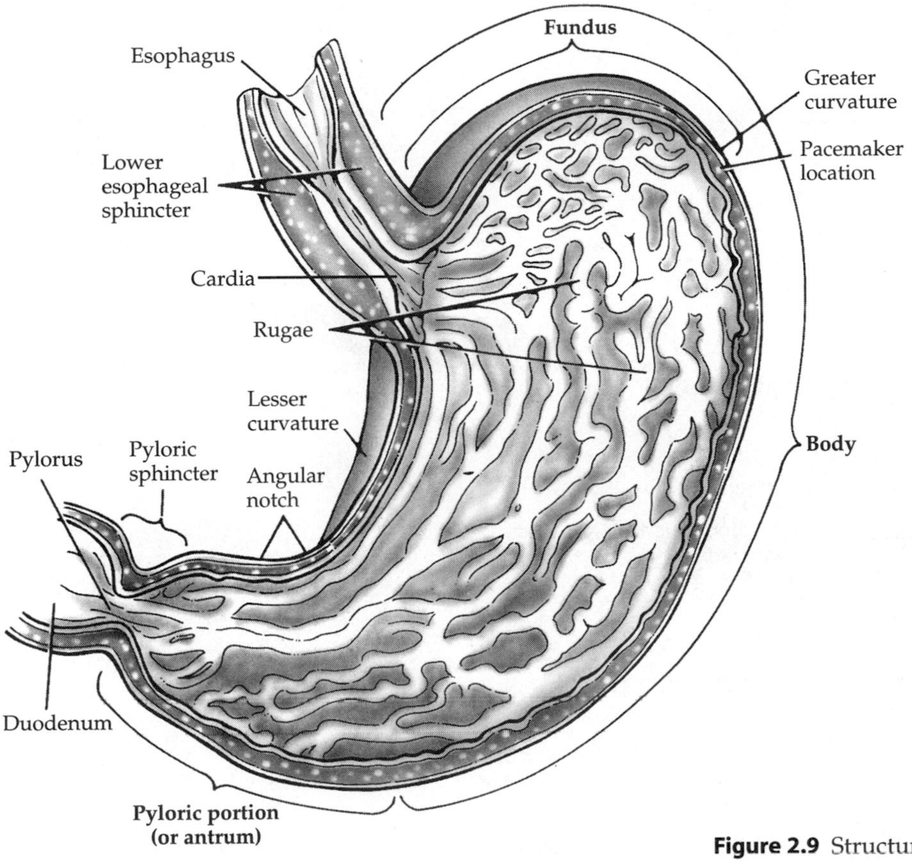

Figure 2.9 Structure of the stomach.

Gastric Juices

Mixing of food with gastric juices begins in the body of the stomach. Gastric juice is produced by three functionally different gastric glands found within the gastric mucosa and submucosa of the stomach. The three gastric glands include

- the cardiac glands, found in a narrow rim at the juncture of the esophagus and the stomach;
- the oxyntic glands, found in the body of the stomach; and
- the pyloric glands, located primarily in the antrum.

Several cell types secreting different substances may be found within a gland. For example, oxyntic glands, depicted in Figure 2.10, contain

- neck (mucus) cells, located close to the surface mucosa, which secrete bicarbonate and mucus;
- parietal (oxyntic) cells, which secrete hydrochloric acid and intrinsic factor;
- chief (peptic or zymogenic) cells, which secrete pepsinogens; and
- enteroendocrine cells, which secrete a variety of hormones.

In contrast to the oxyntic glands, the cardiac glands contain no parietal cells but do possess endocrine and mucus cells. The pyloric glands contain both mucus and parietal cells as well as enteroendocrine cells called G-cells. Gastrin, released from the G-cells into the blood, is carried to its target tissues, including the stomach.

The main constituents of gastric juice produced by the different cells of the gastric glands include water, electrolytes, hydrochloric acid, enzymes, mucus, and intrinsic factor. Some of the main constituents—hydrochloric acid, enzymes, and mucus—of gastric juice are discussed next.

Gastric juice contains an abundance of hydrochloric acid secreted from gastric parietal cells. Parietal cells contain both a potassium chloride transport system and a hydrogen (proton) potassium ATPase exchange system. The potassium chloride system transports both ions into the gastric lumen. The hydrogen potassium ATPase system (H^+, K^+ ATPase), also referred to as a proton pump, allows the exchange of two potassium ions for two hydrogens (protons) for each ATP molecule hydrolyzed. The net effect is the secretion of hydrogen and chloride or hydrochloric acid into the gastric lumen as part of gastric juice. The high concentration of hydrochloric acid in the gastric juice is responsible for its low pH, about 2. The pH

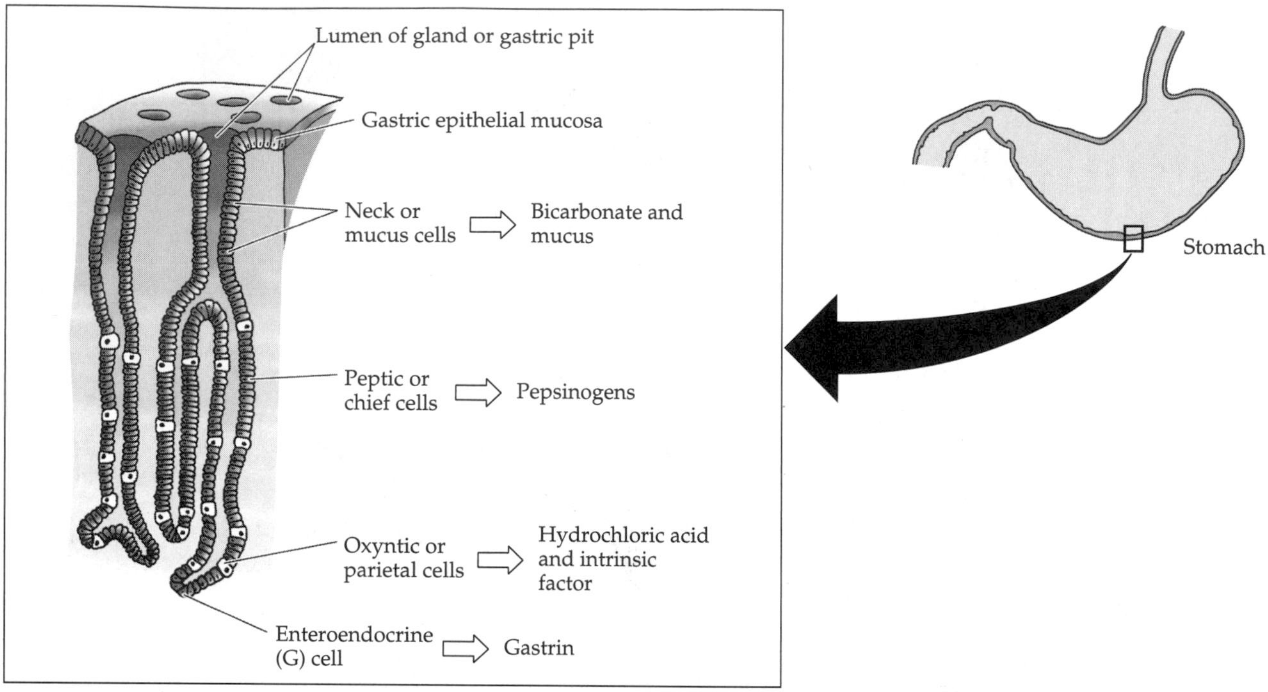

Figure 2.10 An oxyntic gland from the body of the stomach.

value is the negative logarithm of the hydrogen ion concentration. The lower the pH, the more acidic the solution. Figure 2.11 shows the approximate pH values of body fluids and, for comparison, some other compounds and beverages. Notice that the pH of orange juice and typically all fruit juices is higher than that of gastric juice. Thus, the ingestion of such juices cannot lower the gastric pH. Hydrochloric acid has several functions in gastric juice. Some of these functions include

- conversion or activation of the zymogen pepsinogen to form pepsin;
- denaturation of proteins, resulting in the destruction of the tertiary and secondary protein structure and thereby opening interior bonds to the proteolytic effect of pepsin;
- release of various nutrients from organic complexes; and
- acting as bactericide agent, killing many bacteria ingested along with food.

Two enzymes are found in gastric juice. The main enzyme, pepsin, functions as the principal proteolytic enzyme in the stomach and is derived from either of two pepsinogens, I or II. Pepsinogen I is found primarily in the body of the stomach, where most hydrochloric acid is secreted. Pepsinogen II is found in both the body and the antrum of the stomach. The distinction between the two groups of pepsinogens has no known implications for digestion; however, higher concentrations of pepsinogen I correlate positively with acid secretion and have been associated with an increased incidence of peptic ulcers. Pepsinogens are secreted in granules into the gastric lumen from chief cells upon stimulation by acetylcholine and/or acid. Pepsinogens can be converted to pepsin, an active enzyme, in an acid environment (pH $<$ ~5) or in the presence of previously formed pepsin.

$$\text{Pepsinogen} \xrightarrow{\text{Acid or pepsin}} \text{Pepsin}$$

Pepsin functions as a protease, an enzyme that hydrolyzes proteins. Specifically, pepsin is an **endopeptidase,** meaning that it hydrolyzes interior peptide bonds within proteins (Fig. 2.12). More specifically, pepsin appears to have an affinity for peptide bonds adjacent to the carboxyl end of the amino acids methionine and leucine; the dicarboxylic amino acids glutamate and aspartate; and the aromatic amino acids phenylalanine, tyrosine, and tryptophan (Table 2.2). Optimal pepsin activity occurs at about pH 3.5. The second enzyme present in the gastric juice is α amylase that originates from the salivary glands in the mouth. This enzyme, which hydrolyzes starch, retains some activity in the stomach until it is inactivated by the low pH of gastric juice.

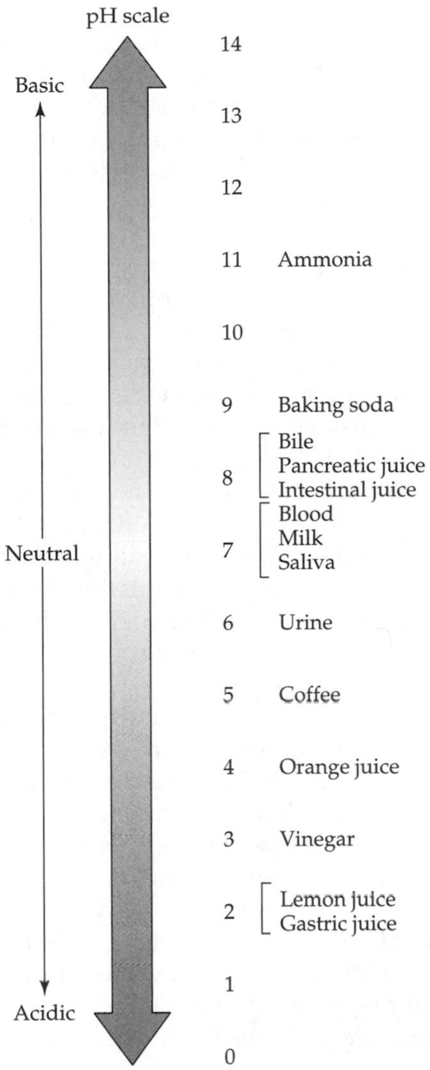

Figure 2.11 Approximate pHs of selected body fluids, compounds, and beverages.

Mucus, secreted by neck or mucus cells, also is found in gastric juice. Secretion of mucus is stimulated by various prostaglandins and by nitric oxide. Mucus, consisting of a network of glycoproteins (mucin), glycolipids, water, and bicarbonate ions (HCO_3^-), serves to lubricate the ingested gastrointestinal contents and to coat and protect the gastric mucosa from mechanical and chemical damage. Mucus forms about a 2-mm-thick layer on top of the gastric mucosa. Tight junctions between gastric cells also help prevent H^+ from penetrating into the gastric mucosa and initiating peptic ulcer formation.

Another constituent of gastric juice is intrinsic factor. Intrinsic factor is secreted by parietal cells and is necessary for the absorption of vitamin B_{12}. Intrinsic factor is discussed in more detail in Chapter 9, "The Water-Soluble Vitamins."

In summary, gastric juice contains several important compounds that aid in the digestive process. However, very little chemical digestion of nutrients occurs in the stomach except for the initiation of protein hydrolysis by the protease pepsin and the limited continuation of starch hydrolysis by salivary α amylase (Fig. 2.12). The only absorption that occurs in the stomach is that of water, alcohol, a few fat-soluble drugs such as aspirin, and a few minerals. The roles of hydrochloric acid and intrinsic factor generated in the stomach are important for iron and vitamin B_{12} status, respectively. With injections of vitamin B_{12}, nourishment and survival are possible without the stomach. Nevertheless, a healthy stomach makes attaining adequate nourishment much easier.

Regulation of Gastric Secretions

Gastric secretion and motility are regulated by multiple mechanisms. As described in a general fashion earlier in this chapter in the section "Coordination and Regulation of the Digestive Process," gastrin, CCK, secretin, and GIP all affect gastric secretion and/or motility to some

Figure 2.12 Digestion in the stomach.

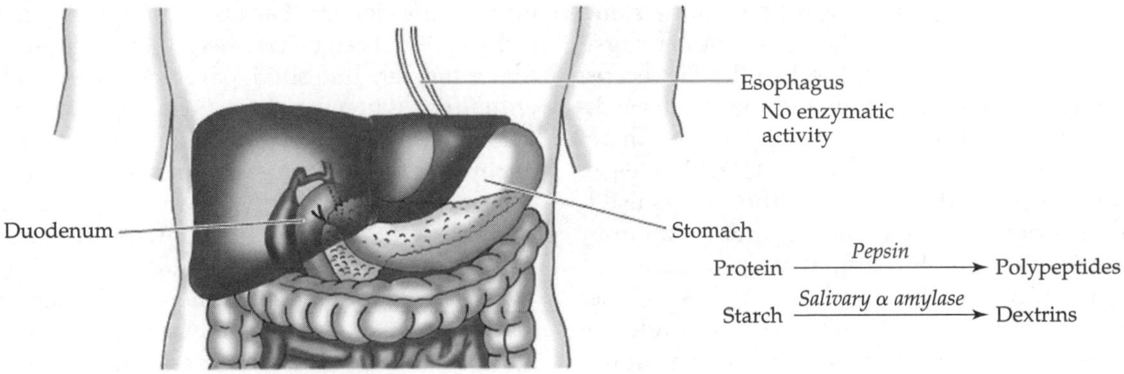

extent. In addition to its inhibition by GIP and secretin, the release of gastric secretions is inhibited by somatostatin, some prostaglandins, and nitric oxide. Gastrin and CCK are main stimulators of gastric acid secretion. Stimulators of gastrin release include gastrin-releasing peptide, epinephrine, coffee, alcohol, calcium, amino acids, and peptides.

Acid release is also stimulated by other means. For example, the vagus nerve releases acetylcholine and stimulates the release of histamine. Both acetylcholine and histamine stimulate acid secretion. Moreover, gastrin also stimulates histamine release. Direct mediators of hydrochloric acid release by the parietal cells include

- gastrin, released by G-cells into the blood, where it acts on parietal cells in the stomach;
- acetylcholine, released, for example, from the vagus nerve to act on parietal cells; and
- histamine, released from gastrointestinal tract mast (enterochromaffin) cells, to bind to H_2 receptors on parietal cells.

Gastrin, acetylcholine, and histamine are potent secretogogues (compounds that stimulate secretion) of hydrochloric acid. Together they prompt the release of substantial amounts of hydrochloric acid from parietal cells.

An understanding of how hydrochloric acid is produced in the body and what stimulates its release is essential to understanding the treatment of peptic ulcers. Peptic ulcers typically result when disruptions occur in the normal defense and repair systems protecting the mucosa of the gastrointestinal tract. The most common cause of peptic ulcers is the bacterium *Helicobacter pylori;* however, chronic use of many substances, including aspirin, alcohol, and nonsteroidal antiinflammatory drugs (NSAID) like ibuprofen, can disrupt the mucosa and deeper layers of the gastrointestinal tract and promote the development of ulcers. Several drugs used to treat peptic ulcers—cimetidine (Tagamet), ranitidine (Zantac), famotidine (Pepcid), and nizatidine (Axid)—act to prevent histamine from binding to H_2 receptors on parietal cells. These drugs, known as H_2 receptor blockers, bind to the H_2 receptors on the parietal cells. When histamine is released, its binding to the H_2 receptor is prevented (the drug blocks histamine's ability to bind), and acid release from the parietal cell is diminished. Other drugs used to treat ulcers—omeprazole (Prilosec) and esomeprazole (Nexium)—work by binding to the proton pump (discussed on p. 35) at the secretory surface of the parietal cell and thus directly inhibit hydrogen release into the gastric juice. Drug therapies are quite effective in the treatment of peptic ulcers; however, foods that act as irritants to the gastric mucosa also need to be avoided during acute peptic ulcer episodes. Further medical nutrition therapy may require increased consumption of nutrients such as protein and iron if the peptic ulcer resulted in bleeding into the gastrointestinal tract.

Gastric Emptying and Motility

When food is swallowed, the proximal portion of the stomach relaxes to accommodate the ingested food. Two processes mediated by the vagus nerve, receptive relaxation and gastric accommodation, influence this relaxation process, considered to be a reflex. Signals for antral contraction, which occur at regular intervals, begin in the proximal stomach at a point along the greater curvature and migrate distally toward the pylorus, the juncture with the small intestine (Fig. 2.9). Response of the antrum to signals by the pacemaker, located between the fundus and body of the stomach, is thought to be affected by a variety of gastrointestinal hormones and neuropeptides.

The pacemaker determines the frequency of the contractions that occur. As the food moves into the antrum, the rate of contractions increases so that in the distal portion of the stomach food is liquefied into chyme. The rate of peristaltic contractions is about 3 per minute in the stomach and increases to about 8 to 12 per minute in the intestine.

The migrating motility complex (MMC), a series of contractions with several phases, moves distally like a wave down the gastrointestinal tract, but mainly in the stomach and intestine. The MMC waves occur approximately every 80 to 120 minutes during interdigestive periods, but their frequency changes during digestive periods. The migrating motility complex functions to sweep out gastrointestinal contents and prevent bacterial overgrowth in the intestine.

Although contractions within the stomach promote physical disintegration of solid foods into liquid form, complete liquefaction is not necessary for the emptying of the stomach contents through the pyloric sphincter into the duodenum. Particles as large as 3 mm in diameter (~1/8 in.) can be emptied from the stomach through the sphincter, but solid particles are usually emptied with fluids when they have been degraded to a diameter of about 2 mm or less. Approximately 1 to 5 mL (~1 tsp) of chyme enters the duodenum about twice per minute. Contraction of the pylorus and proximal duodenum is thought to be coordinated with contraction of the antrum.

Gastric emptying is influenced by several factors. Receptors in the duodenal bulb (the first few centimeters of the proximal duodenum) are sensitive to the volume of chyme and to the osmolarity of the chyme present in the duodenum. Large volumes of chyme, for example, result in increased pressure within the stomach and promote gastric emptying. The presence of hypertonic/hyperosmolar (very concentrated) or hypotonic/hyposmolar (very dilute) chyme in the duodenum results in the activation of osmoreceptors. Activation of the osmoreceptors in turn slows gastric emptying to facilitate the formation of chyme that is isotonic. In addition to volume and osmolarity, the chemical composition of the chyme also affects gastric emptying. Carbohydrate-rich foods and protein-rich foods appear to empty at about the same rate from the stomach; high-fat foods, however, slow gastric emptying into the duodenum. Salts and monosaccharides inhibit gastric emptying, as do many free amino acids such as tryptophan and phenylalanine. Complex carbohydrates, especially soluble fiber, decrease (slow down) the rate of gastric emptying. The presence of acid in the duodenum retards gastric secretions and gastric emptying to allow time for neutralization of the chyme by secretions from accessory organs such as the pancreas and gallbladder. In addition, the presence of acid in the duodenum stimulates the secretion of hormones and regulatory peptides such as CCK and secretin, which promote secretions from accessory organs. With the influence of peptides, neural gastrointestinal reflexes also influence gastric emptying, which following a meal usually takes between 2 and 6 hours.

The Small Intestine

Once in the small intestine, chyme is mixed and moved through the small intestine by various contractions under nervous system influence. Contractions of longitudinal smooth muscles, often referred to as sleeve contractions, function to mix the intestinal contents with the digestive juices. Standing contractions of circular smooth muscles, or segmentation, produces bidirectional flow of the intestinal contents, occurs many times per minute, and serves to mix and churn the chyme with digestive secretions in the small intestine.

Peristaltic waves, or progressive contractions, also accomplished primarily through action of the circular muscles, move the chyme distally along the intestinal mucosa toward the ileocecal valve. Chyme moving from the stomach into the duodenum initially has a pH of about 2 because of its gastric acid content. The duodenum is protected against this gastric acidity by pancreatic secretions with buffering capacity from bicarbonate released into the duodenum and by secretions from the Brunner's glands. The Brunner's glands are located in the mucosa and submucosa of the first few centimeters of the duodenum (duodenal bulb). The mucus-containing secretions are viscous and alkaline, with a pH of approximately 8.2 to 9.3. The mucus itself is rich in glycoproteins and helps protect the epithelial mucosa from damage. Disruptions or inadequate release of these alkaline-rich secretions and/or excessive gastric acid secretion into the duodenum can precipitate the development of duodenal ulcers. Duodenal ulcers typically form distal to the pyloric sphincter in the first few centimeters of the duodenal bulb. As with gastric peptic ulcers, medications to suppress acid production are helpful in the treatment of duodenal ulcers.

Other secretions by intestinal cells include those from glands within the crypts of Lieberkühn. These glands secrete large volumes of intestinal juices, which facilitate digestion of nutrients throughout the small intestine. Distal to the duodenal bulb is a small projection called the duodenal papillae or papillae of Vater, where the bile pancreatic duct carrying secretions from the pancreas and gallbladder empties. These secretions are discussed next.

The Interrelationship Between the Small Intestine and Pancreas in the Digestive Process

The pancreas produces secretions containing fluid, electrolytes (mostly sodium, potassium, and chloride), bicarbonate, and enzymes that are released into the duodenum. The enzymes are responsible for the digestion of approximately half (50%) of all ingested carbohydrates, half (50%) of all proteins, and almost all (90%) of ingested fat. Bicarbonate in pancreatic juice released into the duodenum is important for neutralizing the acid chyme passing into the duodenum from the stomach and for maximizing enzyme activity within the duodenum.

Hormones such as secretin and CCK play important roles in the digestive process occurring in the small intestine. Secretin release is triggered by duodenal acidification with gastric hydrochloric acid. Secretin's major action is to increase the pH of the small intestine by stimulating secretion of water and bicarbonate (pancreatic juice) by the pancreas. This hormone further promotes alkalinization of intestinal contents by inhibiting gastric acid secretion and gastric emptying. CCK further stimulates the secretion of pancreatic juices and enzymes into the duodenum and the contraction of the gallbladder for bile release into the duodenum. CCK is also thought to slightly inhibit gastric motility but to stimulate intestinal motility.

Enzymes produced by the pancreas and necessary for nutrient digestion are listed in Table 2.2, presented earlier. Pancreatic enzymes responsible for the digestion of protein, carbohydrate, and lipid are discussed briefly in the text that follows and in detail in Chapters 4, 6, and 7. **Proteases**—enzymes that digest proteins—found in pancreatic juice and secreted into the duodenum include trypsinogen, chymotrypsinogen, procarboxypeptidases, proelastase, and collagenase.

- Trypsinogen, a zymogen, is converted to its active form, trypsin, by the enzyme enteropeptidase (formerly called enterokinase) and possibly by free trypsin. Enteropeptidase is stimulated by CCK. Trypsin is an endopeptidase specific for peptide bonds at the carboxyl end of basic amino acids (lysine and arginine).
- Chymotrypsinogen is activated to chymotrypsin by trypsin as well as by enteropeptidase. Chymotrypsin, also an endopeptidase, hydrolyzes interior peptide bonds adjacent to the carboxyl end of aromatic amino acids as well as methionine, asparagine, and histidine.
- Procarboxypeptidases are converted to active carboxypeptidases by trypsin. These carboxypeptidases are both **exopeptidases,** enzymes that hydrolyze amino acids off the peptide's terminal end. Carboxypeptidase A cleaves carboxyterminal neutral (including aromatic) amino acids, whereas carboxypeptidase B cleaves carboxyterminal basic amino acids.
- Elastase hydrolyzes fibrous proteins, and collagenase hydrolyzes collagen.

In addition to these zymogens, the pancreas produces trypsin inhibitor, a protein that prevents the activation of proteolytic enzymes within the pancreas.

As a group, proteases hydrolyze peptide bonds, either internally or from the ends, and the net result of their collective actions is the production of polypeptides shorter in length than the original polypeptide, oligopeptides (typically 4–10 amino acids in length), tripeptides, dipeptides, and free amino acids. The latter three may be absorbed into the enterocyte. Oligopeptides and some tripeptides may be further hydrolyzed by brush border aminopeptidases prior to absorption.

Pancreatic α amylase secreted by the pancreas into the duodenum is a principal enzyme necessary for starch digestion. Like the α amylase secreted by salivary glands, pancreatic α amylase hydrolyzes α 1-4 bonds within starch to yield oligosaccharides, dextrins, maltotriose, and maltose. The oligosaccharides and dextrins produced from amylase activity may possess α 1-6 branches, which require further hydrolysis by α dextrinase or isomaltase. The maltotrioses and maltoses will need further hydrolysis by intestinal brush border enzymes prior to absorption.

Enzymes necessary for lipid digestion are also produced by the pancreas. Pancreatic lipase, the major fat-digesting enzyme, hydrolyzes triglycerides, specifically hydrolyzing fatty acids esterified at positions (carbons) 1 and 3 on the glycerol molecule to yield 2-monoacylglycerol and two free fatty acids. With sufficient time, pancreatic lipase may also hydrolyze the fatty acid at the second carbon of the glycerol to yield three free fatty acids and glycerol. In addition to pancreatic lipase, colipase is necessary for some fat digestion. Colipase, secreted in pancreatic juice as a zymogen, is activated by trypsin in the small intestine. Colipase functions by binding to triglycerides and pancreatic lipase, thereby displacing bile. Displacement of bile enables pancreatic lipase to better hydrolyze the triglycerides.

Phospholipid and cholesterol digestion occurs in the small intestine. In the presence of bile, phospholipase A_1 and A_2 hydrolyze fatty acids from phospholipids. Cholesterol esterase hydrolyzes fatty acids from cholesterol esters as well as from triglycerides; however, bile is needed for cholesterol esterase activity. The role of bile in fat digestion is discussed in the next section.

The Interrelationships Among the Small Intestine, Liver, and Gallbladder in the Digestive Process: Bile Synthesis, Storage, Function, Recirculation, and Excretion

Bile Synthesis. **Bile** is a greenish, yellow fluid composed mainly of bile acids (and/or salts) but also cholesterol, phospholipids, and bile pigments (bilirubin and biliverdin) dissolved in an alkaline solution. The bile acids are synthesized in the hepatocytes from cholesterol, which in a series of reactions is oxidized to chenodeoxycholic acid and cholic acid, the two principal or primary bile acids. Chenodeoxycholate and cholate, once formed, conjugate primarily (~75%) with the amino acid glycine to form the conjugated bile acids glycochenodeoxycholic acid (glycochenodeoxycholate) and glycocholic acid (glycocholate), respectively.

Bile Acid		Amino Acid		Conjugated Bile Acid
Cholic acid	+	glycine	⟶	Glycocholic acid
Chenodeoxycholic acid	+	glycine	⟶	Glycochenodeoxycholic acid

Alternately and to a lesser (25%) extent, chenodeoxycholate and cholate conjugate with the amino acid taurine to form two additional primary conjugated bile acids.

Bile Acid		Amino Acid		Conjugated Bile Acid
Cholic acid	+	taurine	⟶	Taurocholic acid
Chenodeoxycholic acid	+	taurine	⟶	Taurochenodeoxycholic acid

Conjugation occurs between the carboxyl group of the bile acid and the amino group of the amino acid as shown in Figure 2.13. Conjugation of the bile acids with

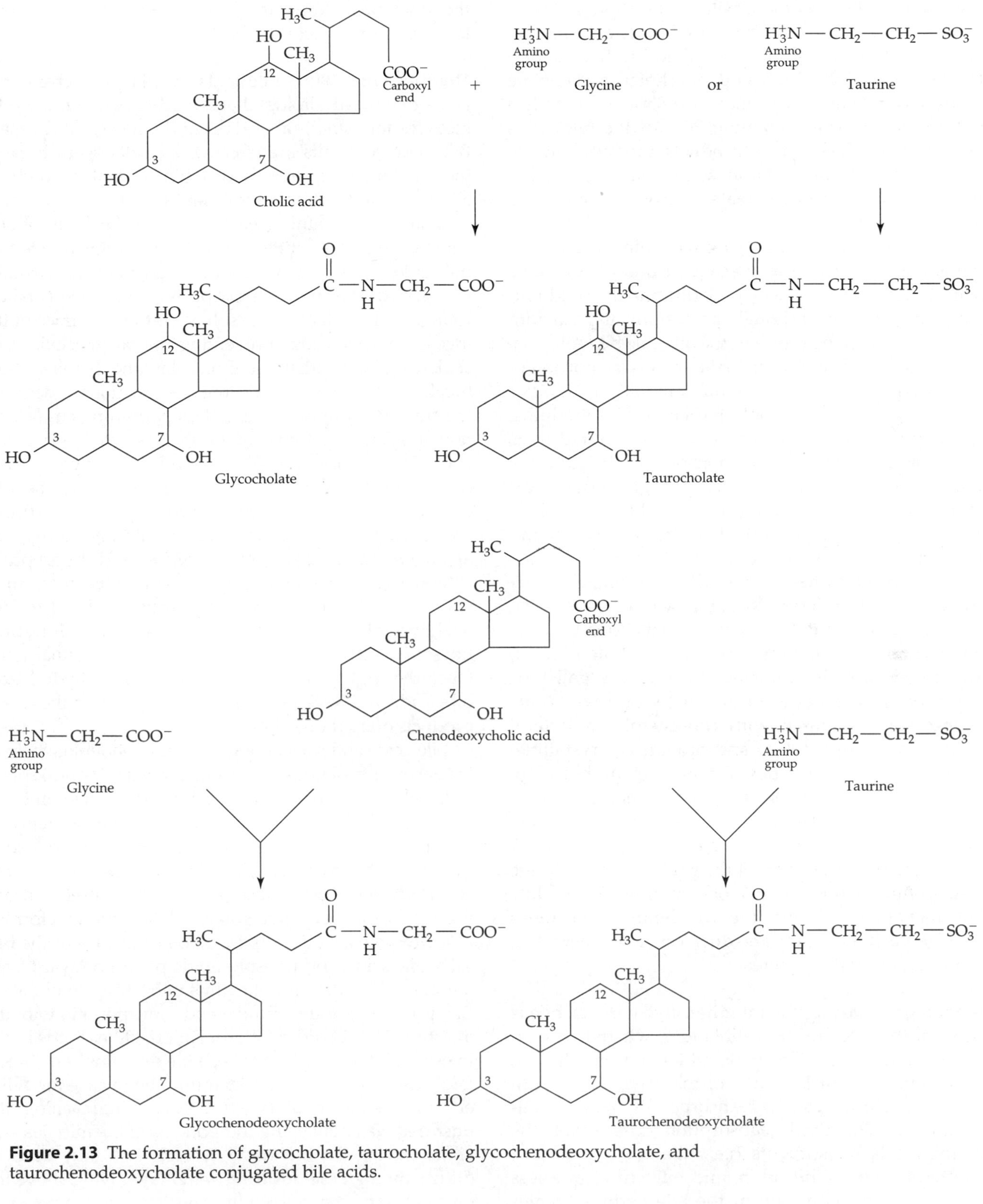

Figure 2.13 The formation of glycocholate, taurocholate, glycochenodeoxycholate, and taurochenodeoxycholate conjugated bile acids.

these amino acids results in better ionization and thus in improved ability to form micelles. The formation and role of micelles are described in the section "The Function of Bile." Chenodeoxycholate and cholate are primary bile acids and make up 80% of the body's total bile acids. The remaining 20% of the bile acids is comprised of secondary products produced in the large intestine from bacterial action on chenodeoxycholic acid to form lithocholate and on cholic acid to form deoxycholate.

In addition to being conjugated to amino acids, most conjugated bile acids are present in bile as bile salts owing to bile's pH (~7.6–8.6). Sodium is the predominant biliary cation, although potassium and calcium bile salts may also be found in the alkaline bile solution.

While bile acids and salts make up a large portion of bile, other substances are also found in bile. These other substances include both cholesterol and phospholipids, especially lecithin, and make up what is referred to as the bile acid–dependent fraction of bile. In addition, water, electrolytes, bicarbonate, and glucuronic acid conjugated bile pigments (mainly bilirubin and/or biliverdin—waste end products of hemoglobin degradation excreted in bile and giving bile its color) are secreted into bile by hepatocytes. This alkaline-rich fraction of the bile is referred to as bile acid–independent. It is important that the bile components remain in the proper ratio to prevent gallstone (cholelithiasis) formation, although other factors influence gallstone production. Gallstones are thought to form when bile becomes supersaturated with cholesterol. Cholesterol precipitates out of solution and provides a crystalline-like structure for the deposition of calcium, bilirubin, phospholipids, and other compounds that ultimately form a "stone." Gallstones may reside silently in the gallbladder; or they may irritate the organ, causing cholecystitis (inflammation of the gallbladder), or lodge in the common bile duct, blocking the flow of bile (choledocholithiasis) into the duodenum. Gallstones also may block the pancreatic duct, causing pancreatitis (inflammation of the pancreas).

Bile Storage. During the interdigestive periods, bile is sent from the liver to the gallbladder, where it is concentrated and stored. The gallbladder concentrates the bile such that as much as 90% of the water, along with some of the electrolytes, is reabsorbed by the gallbladder mucosa. The fluid reabsorption thus leaves the remaining bile constituents (i.e., bile acids and salts, cholesterol, lecithin, bilirubin, and biliverdin) in a less dilute form. Concentration of the bile permits greater storage of bile produced by the liver between periods of food ingestion. Contraction of the gallbladder is stimulated by CCK released in response to chyme entering the duodenum. Bile is secreted into the duodenum through the sphincter of Oddi.

The Function of Bile. Bile acids and bile salts act as detergents to emulsify lipids, that is, to break down large fat globules into small (about 1-mm-diameter) fat droplets. Bile acids and salts are effective as a detergent because they contain both polar (hydrophilic or water "soluble") and nonpolar (hydrophobic or fat "soluble") areas, that is, they are amphipathic (see Fig. 2.14). The hydrophobic (steroid ring) areas of the bile salts attract the ingested fat molecules, which arrive in the small intestine virtually undigested. This hydrophobic portion of the bile salts surrounds and "melts" or "dissolves" into the surface of the ingested fat molecule, preventing the fat molecule from coalescing with other fat molecules and helping them break apart. In other words, the bile functions to decrease the surface tension of the fat, thus permitting emulsification (dispersion of the fat or increase in the exposed surface area of the lipids). Surrounding the hydrophobic center are the polar hydrophilic areas of the bile (the hydroxyl and carboxyl groups and the amino acid) that are directed outward into the watery intestinal juices. This arrangement (hydrophobic interior and hydrophilic exterior) allows the fat to stay in solution. Further, emulsification of fat enables digestion (hydrolysis) of the triacylglycerol molecules by pancreatic and intestinal lipases, which are found in the watery intestinal juice. Once the triglyceride molecules have been hydrolyzed, bile acids and salts help in the absorption of these end products of lipid digestion.

Bile acids and salts, along with phospholipids, help in the absorption of lipids by forming small (<10 nm) spherical, cylindrical, or disklike complexes called micelles (shown in Fig. 2.14). Micelles can contain as many as 40 bile salt molecules. As with emulsification, to form a micelle the hydrophobic steroid portion of bile salts and acids, which is mostly fat soluble, positions itself and surrounds the monoacylglycerols and fatty acids that formed following the action of lipases. Polar portions of the bile salts, bile acids, and phospholipids project outward from the lipid core of the micelle, thus permitting solubility in the watery digestive fluids and transportation to the intestinal brush border for absorption. Other lipids in the intestinal lumen, such as fat-soluble vitamins and cholesterol, also may be incorporated into the micelle for delivery to the intestinal brush border. On reaching the unstirred water layer, the components of the micelles separate, leaving the monoacylglycerols and fatty acids to diffuse through the unstirred water layer lying above the glycocalyx of the microvilli. This transport across the unstirred water layer slows fat absorption into the enterocytes. Figure 2.15 summarizes the digestion and absorption of triacylglycerol.

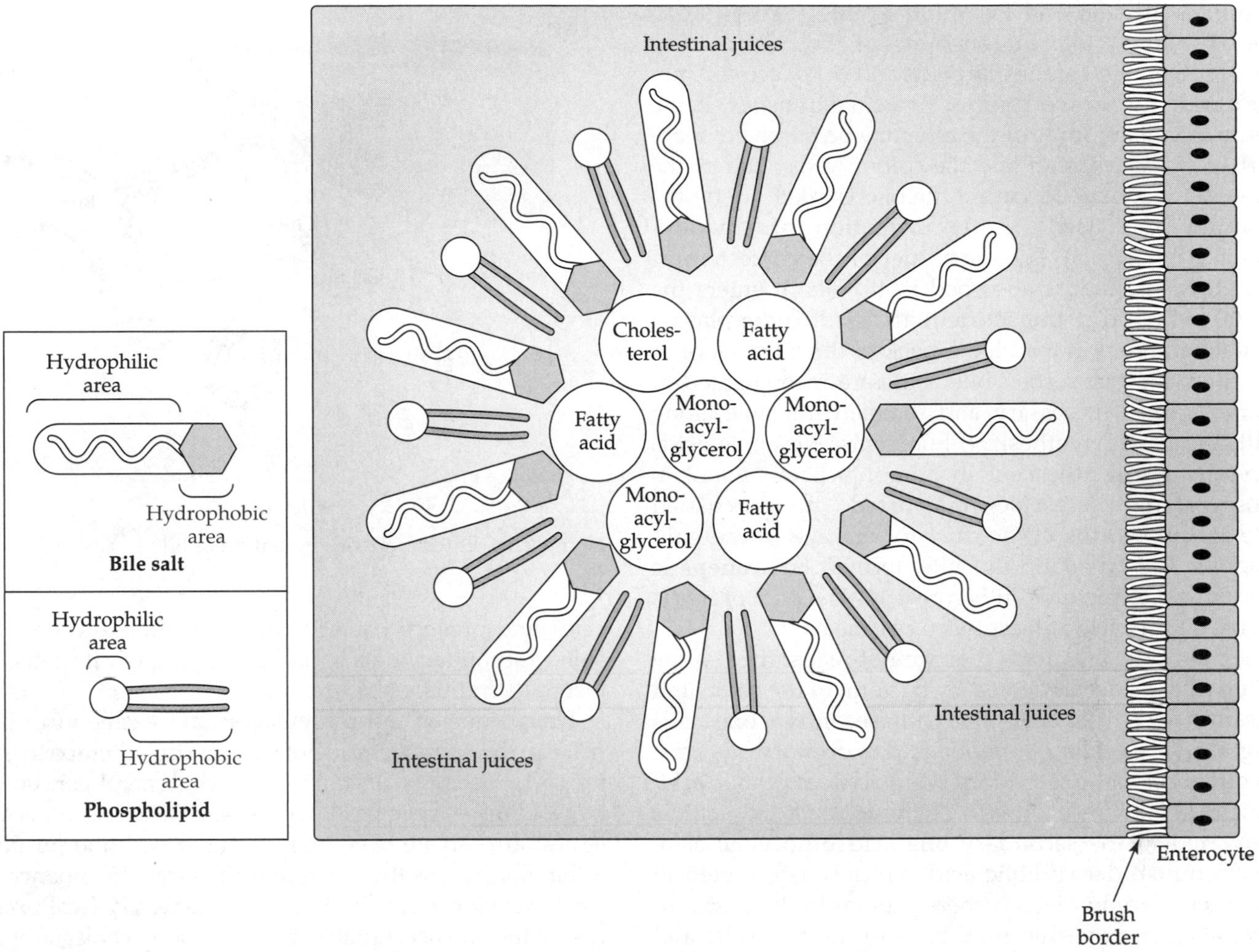

Figure 2.14 A micelle.

Figure 2.15 Digestion and absorption of dietary fat (triacylglycerols).

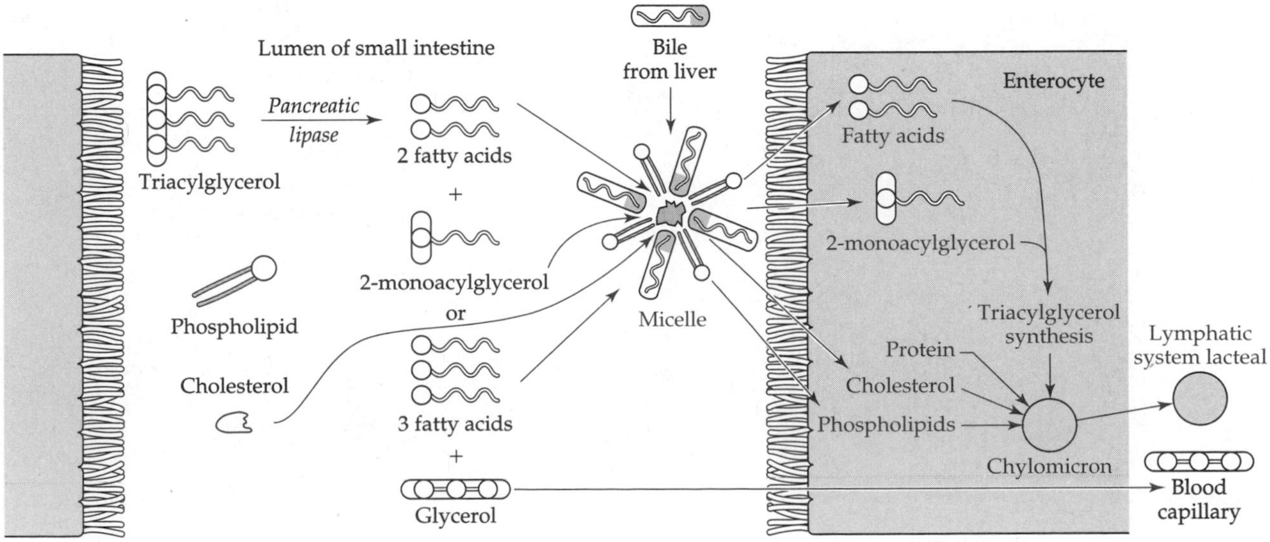

The Recirculation and Excretion of Bile. The human body contains a total bile acid pool of about 2.5 to 5.0 g. Greater than 90% of the bile acids and salts secreted into the duodenum are reabsorbed by active transport in the ileum. Small amounts of the bile may be passively reabsorbed in the jejunum and the colon. About half of the cholesterol contained within the bile is taken up by the jejunum and used in the formation of chylomicrons (see Chap. 6). The remainder of the cholesterol is excreted. Bile that is absorbed in the ileum enters the portal vein and is transported, attached to the plasma protein albumin in the blood, back to the liver. Once in the liver, the reabsorbed bile acids are reconjugated to amino acids if necessary and secreted into bile along with the newly synthesized bile acids. New bile acids typically are synthesized in amounts about equal to those lost in the feces. New bile mixed with recirculated bile is sent via the cystic duct for storage in the gallbladder. The circulation of bile, termed **enterohepatic circulation,** is pictured in Figure 2.16. The pool of bile is thought to recycle at least twice per meal.

Some of the bile acids that are not reabsorbed in the ileum may be deconjugated by bacteria in the colon and possibly the terminal ileum to form secondary bile acids (Fig. 2.17). For example, cholic acid, a primary bile acid, is converted to the secondary bile acid deoxycholic acid, which can be reabsorbed. Chenodeoxycholic acid is converted to the secondary bile acid lithocholic acid, which unlike deoxycholic acid typically is excreted in the feces. Certain dietary fibers present in the gastrointestinal tract, however, may bind to the bile salts and

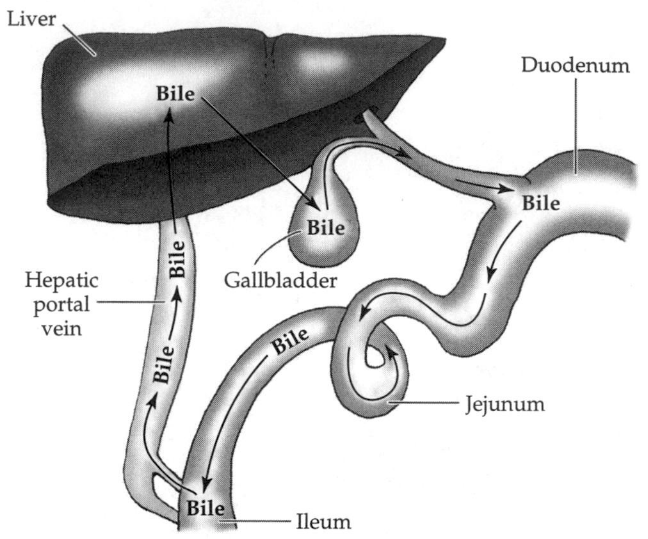

Figure 2.16 Enterohepatic circulation of bile.

acids and prevent bacterial deconjugation and conversion to secondary bile acids. About 0.5 g of bile salts are lost daily in the feces.

Knowledge of the recirculation and excretion of bile helps in the understanding of various drug therapies used for some people with high blood cholesterol concentrations. Drugs—specifically, resins such as cholestyramine (Questran)—have been manufactured with the purpose of binding bile in the gastrointestinal tract to enhance its fecal excretion from the body. The increased fecal excretion of the bile necessitates the use of body cholesterol for

Figure 2.17 The synthesis of secondary bile acids by intestinal bacteria.

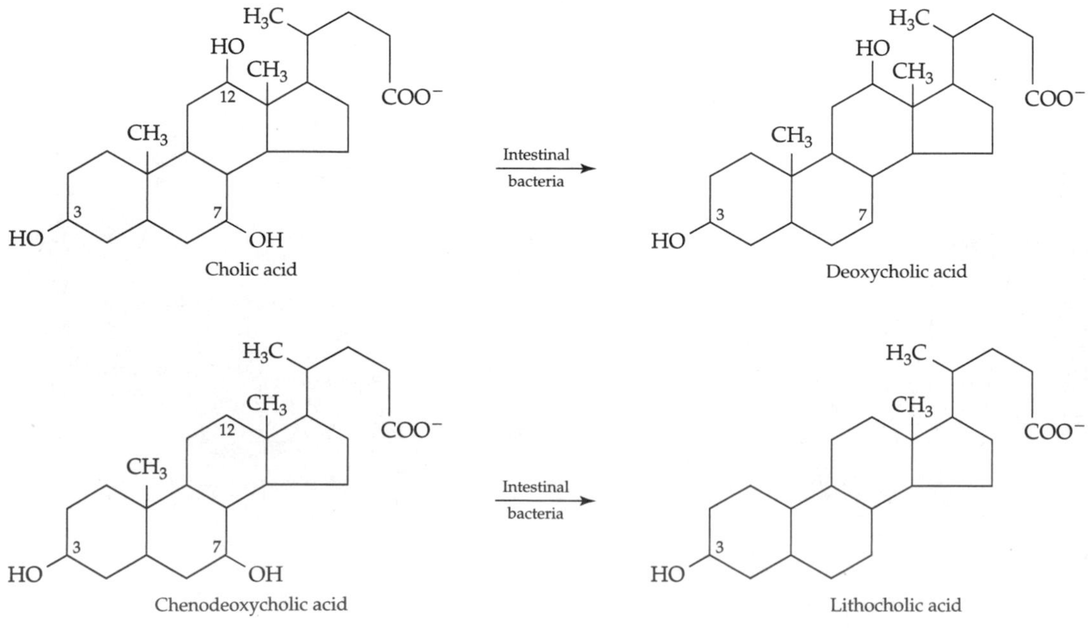

the synthesis of new bile acids. The goal of the use of such drugs is the lowering of blood cholesterol concentrations and a reduced risk of cardiovascular disease.

The Role of the Intestinal Brush Border in the Digestive Process

Several enzymes necessary for digestion, especially carbohydrate and protein, are found on the brush border of the small intestine (Table 2.2). Figure 2.18 shows some enzymes present in the small intestine that are responsible for carbohydrate digestion. Some of these enzymes, including isomaltase, act on α 1-6 bonds. Isomaltase, found on the brush border, functions as part of a complex with sucrase known as the sucrase isomaltase system and hydrolyzes α 1-6 bonds in oligosaccharides and dextrins. To hydrolyze oligosaccharides and dextrins, enzymes capable of breaking α 1-4 bonds are necessary. Glucoamylase, glucosidase, and maltase hydrolyze α 1-4 bonds in oligosaccharides, maltotriose, and maltose. Maltose and maltotriose are generated from the action of pancreatic amylase. Sucrase (invertase) is also active against maltose and maltotriose, as well as hydrolyzing sucrose to yield glucose and fructose. Each of the disaccharidases hydrolyzes disaccharides in two monosaccharides. Maltase hydrolyzes maltose into two glucose molecules. Lactase hydrolyzes lactose into glucose and galactose. Sucrase hydrolyzes sucrose to yield glucose and fructose. Further and more detailed information on carbohydrate digestion is provided in Chapter 4.

The brush border also contains enzymes for protein digestion (Fig. 2.19). These protein-digesting enzymes include

- several aminopeptidases (with different specificities) that hydrolyze N-terminal amino acids from oligopeptides, tripeptides, and dipeptides;
- tripeptidases that hydrolyze tripeptides into free amino acids and a dipeptide; and
- dipeptidases that hydrolyze dipeptides into two free amino acids.

Further information on protein digestion can be found in Chapter 7.

The Interrelationship Between the Digestive and Absorptive Processes in the Small Intestine

Most nutrients must be digested—that is, broken down into smaller pieces—prior to absorption. Digestion of nutrients occurs both in the lumen of the gastrointestinal tract and on the brush border. Although the absorption

Figure 2.18 Summary of luminal digestion of starch and membrane digestion of disaccharides and oligosaccharides. Also indicated are the mechanisms for absorption of digestive products.

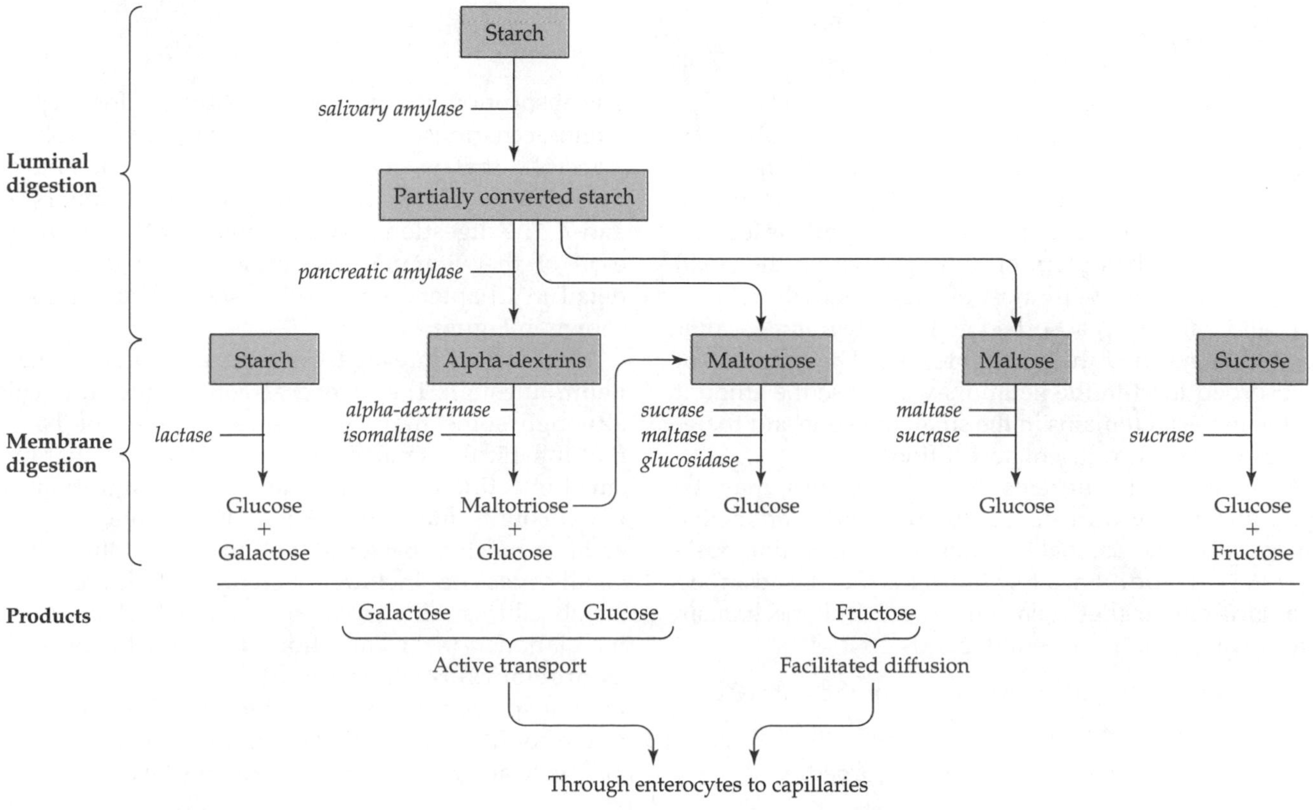

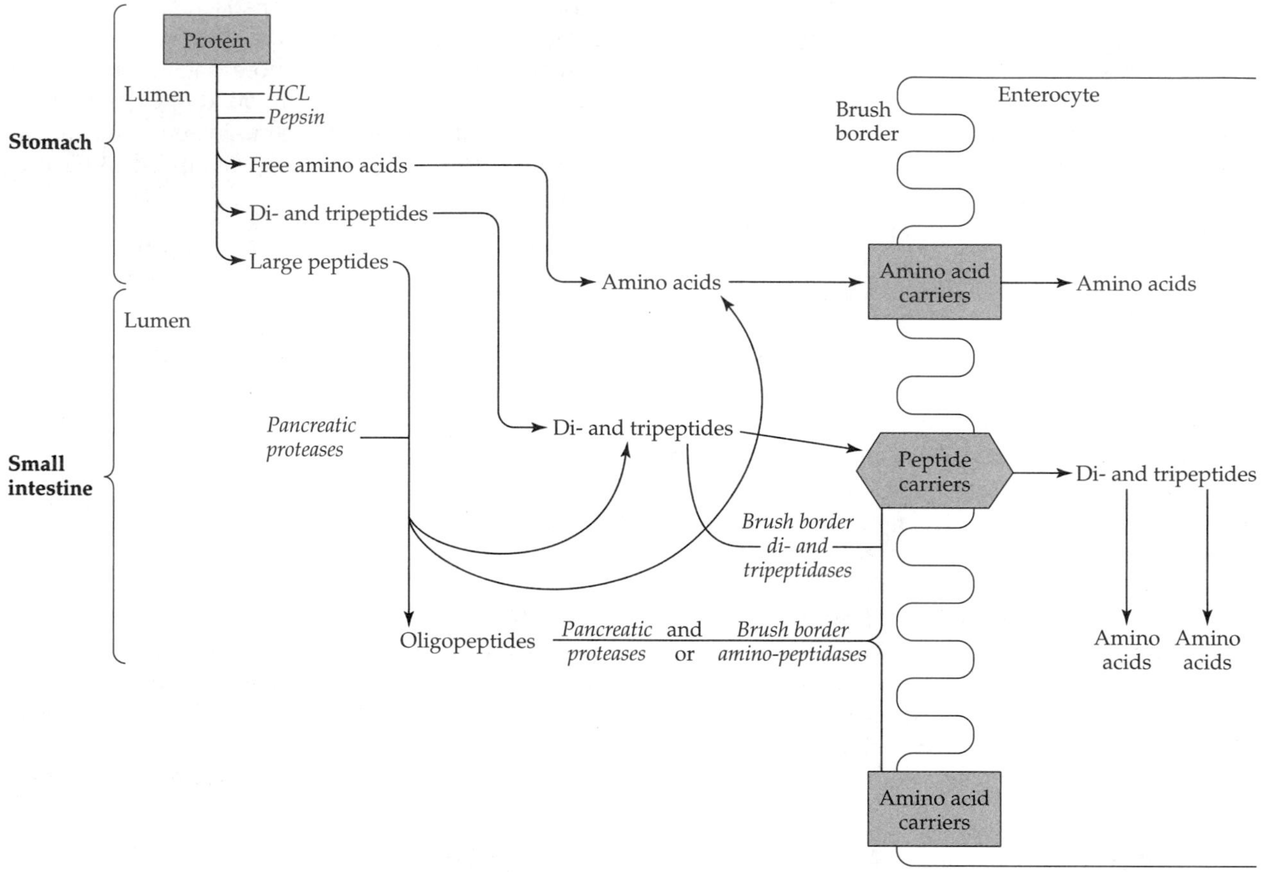

Figure 2.19 Summary of dietary protein digestion and mechanisms for absorption of digestive products.

of some nutrients may occur in the stomach, the absorption of most nutrients begins in the duodenum and continues throughout the jejunum and ileum, as shown in Figure 2.20. Generally, most absorption occurs in the proximal (upper) portion of the small intestine. Digestion and absorption of nutrients within the small intestine are rapid, with most of the carbohydrate, protein, and fat being absorbed within 30 minutes after chyme has reached the small intestine. The presence of unabsorbed food in the ileum may increase the amount of time material remains in the small intestine and therefore may increase nutrient absorption.

Absorption of nutrients into enterocytes may be accomplished by diffusion, facilitated diffusion, active transport, or, occasionally, pinocytosis or **endocytosis** (Fig. 2.21). In addition, a few nutrients may be absorbed by a paracellular (between-cells) route. The mechanism of absorption for a nutrient depends on

- the solubility (fat versus water) of the nutrient,
- the concentration or electrical gradient, and
- the size of the molecule to be absorbed.

The absorption and transport of amino acids, peptides, monosaccharides, fatty acids, monoacylglycerols, and glycerol—that is, the end products of macronutrient digestion—are considered in depth in Chapters 4, 6, and 7. The digestion and mechanisms of absorption for each of the vitamins and minerals are discussed in detail in Chapters 9 to 13; the sites of absorption are shown in Figure 2.20.

Unabsorbed intestinal contents are passed from the ileum through the ileocecal valve into the colon, although some may serve as substrates for bacteria that inhabit the small intestine. Bacterial counts in the small intestine range up to about 10^3/g intestinal contents; counts may be larger than this near the ileocecal sphincter. Bacteria that may be found in the small intestine include bacteroides, enterobacteria, lactobacilli, streptococci, and staphylococci. Recommendations for the ingestion of certain foods (known as **probiotics**), such as yogurt, with live cultures containing specific strains of bacteria to effect an increase in the counts of specific microflora of the gastrointestinal tract are gaining interest in the health field. The

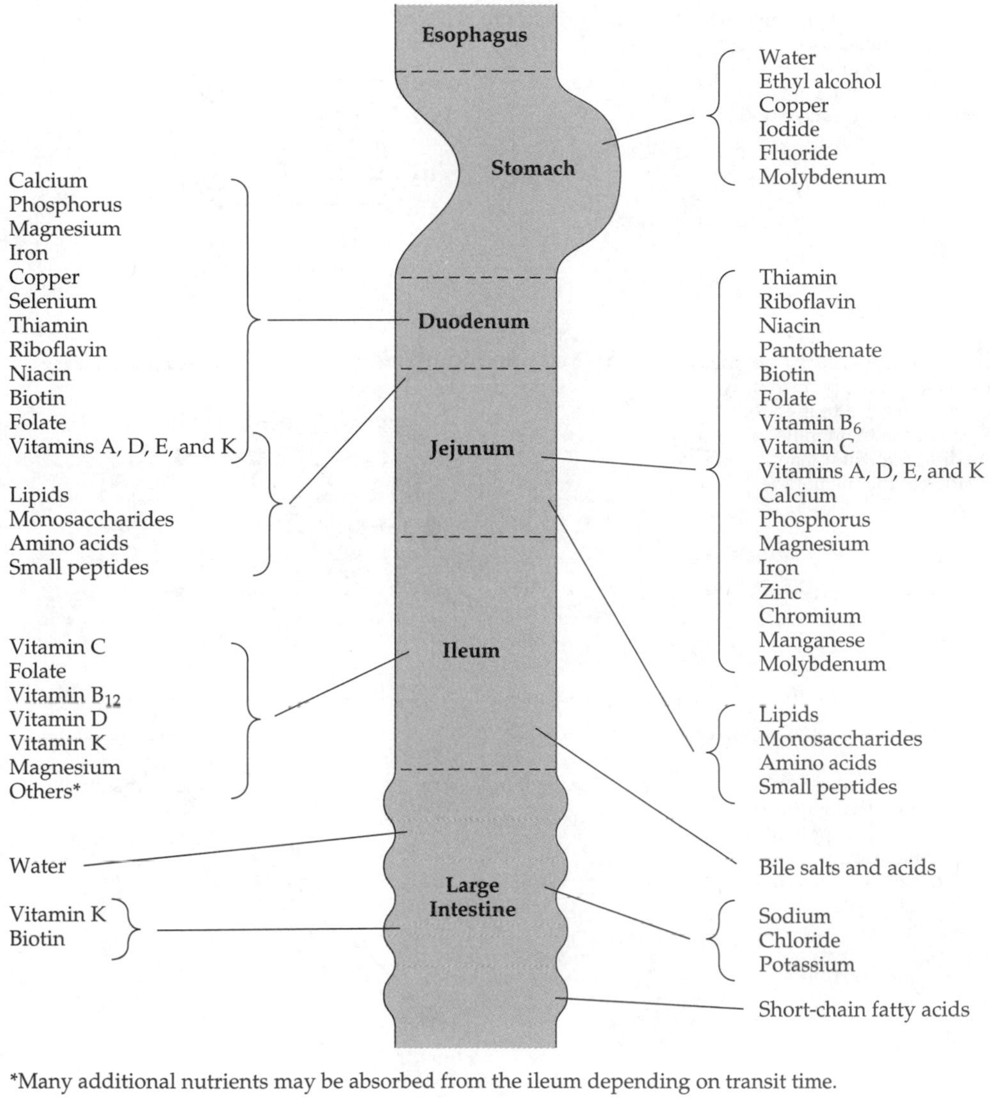

Figure 2.20 Sites of nutrient absorption in the gastrointestinal tract.

intent of probiotics is for the bacteria to survive the passage through the upper digestive tract and then establish themselves in (colonize) the lower gastrointestinal tract, primarily the colon. Also under study is the use of prebiotics, food ingredients that are not digested or absorbed but can stimulate the growth and/or activity of one or more selected species of bacteria in the colon to improve the health of the host. Short-chain, nondigestible oligosaccharide (oligofructose or inulin, for example) ingestion appears to effectively alter selected microbial populations, especially bifido bacteria, in the intestine. The ability to feed prebiotics that selectively promote the growth of certain bacteria, which simultaneously would antagonize the proliferation and growth of other pathogenic strains of bacteria, represents an exciting area of new medical nutrition therapies.

The Colon or Large Intestine

Intestinal material leaving the ileum empties via the ileocecal valve or sphincter into the cecum, the right side of the colon, or large intestine (Fig. 2.7 depicts the anatomy of the human large intestine). On initially entering the colon, the intestinal material is still quite fluid. Contraction of the musculature of the large intestine is coordinated so as to mix the intestinal contents gently and to keep material in the proximal (ascending) colon a sufficient length of time to allow nutrient absorption to occur. The proximal colonic epithelia absorb sodium, chloride, and water more effectively than does the small intestinal mucosa. For example, about 90% to 95% of the water and sodium entering the colon each day is absorbed. Colonic absorption of sodium is influenced by a number of factors, including hormones. Antidiuretic hormone

Diffusion. Some substances, such as water and small lipid molecules, cross membranes freely. The concentration of substances that can diffuse across cell membranes tends to equalize on the two sides of the membrane, so that the substance moves from the higher concentration to the lower; that is, it moves down a concentration gradient.

Facilitated diffusion. Other compounds cannot cross cell membranes without a specific carrier. The carrier may affect the permeability of the membrane in such a way that the substance is admitted, or it may shuttle the compound from one side of the membrane to the other. Facilitated diffusion, like simple diffusion, allows an equalization of the substance on both sides of the membrane. The figure illustrates the shuttle process:

1. Carrier loads particle on outside of cell.
2. Carrier releases particle on inside of cell.
3. Reversal of (1) and (2).

Active transport. Substances that need to be concentrated on one side of the cell membrane or the other require active transport, which involves energy expenditure. The energy is supplied by ATP, and Na^+ is usually involved in the active transport mechanism. The figure illustrates the unidirectional movement of a substance requiring active transport:

1. Carrier loads particle on outside of cell.
2. Carrier releases particle on inside of cell.
3. Carrier returns to outside to pick up another particle.

Pinocytosis. Some large molecules are moved into the cell via engulfment by the cell membrane. The figure illustrates the process:

1. Substance contacts cell membrane.
2. Membrane wraps around or engulfs the substance.
3. The sac formed separates from the membrane and moves into the cell.

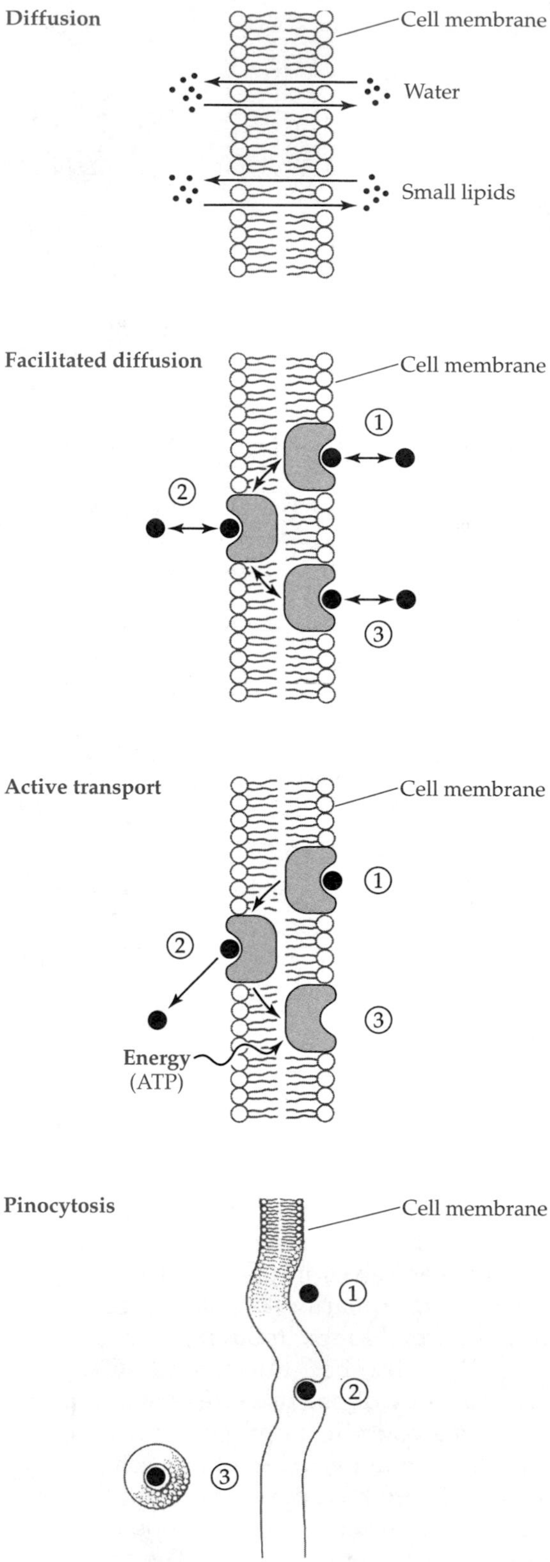

Figure 2.21 Primary mechanisms for nutrient absorption.

(ADH), for example, decreases sodium absorption, while glucocorticoids and mineralocorticoids increase sodium absorption in the colon.

Secretions into the lumen of the colon are few, but some nutrient exchange occurs. Goblet cells in the crypts of Lieberkühn secrete mucus. Mucus protects the colonic mucosa and acts as a lubricant for fecal matter. Potassium is secreted possibly via an active secretory pathway into the colon. Bicarbonate is also secreted in exchange for chloride absorption. Bicarbonate provides an alkaline environment that helps neutralize acids produced by colonic anaerobic bacteria. Sodium and hydrogen ion exchanges also occur, permitting electrolyte absorption. Both gram-negative and gram-positive bacteria strains, representing over 400 species of at least 40 genera, have been isolated from human feces. Intestinal bacterial counts of up to 10^{12}/g gastrointestinal tract contents in the large intestine are reported. Most bacteria found in the ileum and large intestine are anaerobes; the most common include bacteroides, clostridia, lactobacteria, and coliforms. Other examples of bacterial flora that inhabit the large intestine are bifidobacteria, methanogens, eubacteria, and streptococci.

Bacteria gain nutrients for their own growth through unabsorbed food residues in the intestines. Bacteria use primarily dietary carbohydrate, and to a lesser extent amino acids and protein, as substrates necessary for their growth. For example, starch that has not undergone hydrolysis by pancreatic amylase may be used by gram-negative bacteroides or by gram-positive bifidobacteria or eubacteria. Glycoproteins (mainly mucins) found in mucus secretions of the gastrointestinal tract may be broken down and used by bacteria such as bacteroides, bifidobacteria, and clostridia. In addition, sugar alcohols such as sorbitol and xylitol, disaccharides such as lactose, undigested oligosaccharides such as raffinose and stacchyose, and fibers such as some hemicelluloses, pectins, and gums may be degraded by selected bacteria found in the large intestine. Digestive enzymes themselves may even serve as substrate for bacteria such as bacteroides and clostridia. The breakdown of carbohydrate and protein by bacteria is an anaerobic process referred to as **fermentation.**

As described above, bacteria degrade mostly carbohydrate but also some amino acids and protein as substrates for the production of substances, such as energy and carbon atoms, necessary for bacterial growth and maintenance. Acids are one of the principal end products of bacterial carbohydrate fermentation in the large intestine. Specifically, lactate and various **short-chain fatty acids**—acetate, butyrate, and propionate—are generated from bacterial action. These short-chain fatty acids, formerly referred to as volatile fatty acids, serve many purposes. They are thought to stimulate gastrointestinal cell proliferation. The presence of the acids lowers the luminal pH in the colon to effect changes in nutrient absorption and in the growth of certain species of bacteria. In addition, these acids provide substrates for body cell use. Butyrate, for example, may be absorbed via a Na^+/H^+ and/or a K^+/H^+ exchange system in the colon, where it is a preferred energy source for colonic epithelial cells. Butyrate also may regulate gene expression and cell growth. Propionate and lactate are absorbed in the colon and taken up for use by liver cells. Acetate is absorbed and used by muscle and brain cells. Absorption of these acids appears to be concentration-dependent. Other products generated by colonic bacteria include gases such as methane (CH_4), hydrogen (H_2), hydrogen sulfide (H_2S), and/or carbon dioxide (CO_2). Bacterial degradation of branched-chain amino acids generates branched-chain fatty acids such as isobutyrate and isovalerate. Deamination of aromatic amino acids (see Chap. 7) yields phenolic compounds. Amines such as histamine result from the decarboxylation of amino acids such as histidine. Ammonia generated by bacterial deamination of amino acids as well as by bacterial urease action on urea (secreted into the gastrointestinal tract from the blood) can be reabsorbed by the colon and recirculated to the liver, where it can be reused to synthesize urea or amino acids. About 25%, or about 8 g, of the body's urea may be handled in this fashion, and the process must be controlled in people with liver disease to prevent hepatic encephalopathy and coma. Uric acid and creatinine also may be released into the digestive tract and metabolized by colonic bacteria.

As intestinal matter passes through the sections of the colon, contractions by longitudinal and circular muscles promote absorption of water and electrolytes. Fluids from the moist fecal matter are absorbed into the mucosal cells of the colon as the fecal matter moves through the ascending, transverse, and descending sections of the colon. The end result, which usually takes about 12 to 70 hours, is a progressive dehydration of the unabsorbed materials. Typically, the approximately 1 L of chyme that enters the large intestine each day is reduced to less than about 200 g of defecated material containing bacteria, sloughed gastrointestinal cells, inorganic matter, water, small amounts of unabsorbed nutrients/food residue, and constituents of digestive juices.

summary

An examination of the various mechanisms in the gastrointestinal tract that allow food to be ingested, digested, and absorbed and its residue to then be excreted reveals the complexity of the digestion and absorption processes. Normal digestion and absorption of nutrients depend not only on a healthy digestive tract but also on integration of the digestive system with the nervous, endocrine, and circulatory systems.

The many factors influencing digestion and absorption—including the dispersion and mixing of ingested food, the quantity and composition of gastrointestinal secretions, enterocyte integrity, the expanse of intestinal absorptive area, and the transit time of intestinal contents—must be coordinated so that nourishment of the body can occur while homeostasis of body fluids is maintained. Much of the coordination required is provided by regulatory peptides, some of which are provided by the nervous system as well as by the endocrine cells of the gastrointestinal tract.

Although the basic structure of the alimentary canal, which consists of the mucosa, submucosa, muscularis externa, and serosa, remains the same throughout, structural modifications allow for more specific functions by various segments of the gastrointestinal tract. Gastric glands that underlie the gastric mucosa secrete fluids and compounds necessary for digestive functions of the stomach. Also, particularly noteworthy is the presence of the folds of Kerckring, the villi, and the microvilli, all of which serve to dramatically increase the surface area exposed to the contents of the intestinal lumen. This enlarged surface area helps maximize absorption, not only of ingested nutrients but also of endogenous secretions released into the gastrointestinal tract.

Study of the digestive system makes abundantly clear the fact that adequate nourishment of an individual, and therefore his or her health, depends in large measure on a normally functioning gastrointestinal tract. Particularly crucial to nourishment and health is a normally functioning small intestine, because that is where the greatest amount of digestion and absorption occurs. Later chapters expand on the digestion and absorption of the various individual nutrients.

Reference Cited

1. Guyton AC. Textbook of Medical Physiology, 8th ed. Philadelphia: Saunders, 1991.

Web Site

www.nlm.nih.gov/research/visible/visible_human.html

An Overview of Selected Digestive System Disorders with Implications for Nourishing the Body

In Chapter 2, digestion is defined as a process by which food is broken down mechanically and chemically in the gastrointestinal (GI) tract. Digestion ultimately provides nutrients ready for absorption into the body through the cells of the GI tract, principally the cells of the small intestine (enterocytes). Secretions required for the digestion of nutrients are produced by multiple organs of the GI tract. These secretions include principally enzymes but also hydrochloric acid for gastric digestion and bicarbonate and bile for digestion in the intestine. Malfunction of one or more of the organs due to disease can diminish the production and/or release of secretions synthesized and released by these organs into the GI tract. Without secretions or with less than normal amounts of secretions, the digestion of nutrients may be impaired, resulting in nutrient malabsorption.

Many conditions or diseases alter the function of organs of the GI tract and thus affect digestion. For example, some GI tract diseases may cause decreased synthesis and release of secretions needed for nutrient digestion. Other conditions or diseases affecting the GI tract—for example, malfunction of sphincters—can alter motility or clearing of the GI contents through the organs of the GI tract. Clearing problems may cause back fluxes (refluxes) of secretions from, for example, the stomach into the esophagus (remember, normally the contents of the GI tract move from the esophagus to the stomach and not vice versa). Conditions in which the GI mucosa is inflamed or damaged, as well as conditions that increase transit time or speed up the movement of GI contents (food and nutrients) through the GI tract, typically result in nutrient malabsorption due to diminished time for digestion and absorption of nutrients.

An understanding of the physiology of the GI tract and its accessory organs, and of the diseases affecting the GI tract, is essential to understanding how to modify an individual's diet from the standard dietary recommendations for healthy populations of the United States. This perspective addresses, in a general fashion, three disorders affecting the digestive tract and what implications these conditions have with respect to nourishing the body.

Disorder 1: Gastroesophageal Reflux Disease

Gastroesophageal reflux disease (GERD) is a disorder marked by a reflux or backward flow of gastric contents (acidic chyme) from the stomach to the esophagus.

After a person chews and swallows food, the food enters the esophagus and then passes through the lower esophageal sphincter (LES) into the stomach. Normally, the LES displays a relatively high pressure that prevents the reflux of stomach contents into the esophagus. However, changes or decreases in the LES pressure, sometimes called LES incompetence, can ultimately result in GERD. Increases in abdominal pressure, such as may occur with overeating, bending, lifting, lying down, or vomiting or coughing, also can increase reflux and cause GERD.

The recurring reflux of gastric contents, including hydrochloric acid, into the esophagus from the stomach can damage and inflame the esophageal mucosa and result in reflux esophagitis (inflammation of the esophagus due to the refluxed gastric contents). The severity of the esophagitis depends in part on the volume and acidity of the gastric contents that are refluxed and on the length of time the gastric contents are in contact with the esophageal mucosa. The more acidic the contents and the longer the contents are in contact with the mucosa, the more damage will result. Weak peristalsis and delays in gastric emptying are likely to prolong contact time and increase damage. The resistance of the esophageal mucosa also affects the severity of the damage. Repeated bouts of GERD resulting in reflux esophagitis cause, to varying degrees, esophageal edema (swelling); esophageal tissue damage, including erosion and ulceration; blood vessel (usually capillary) damage; spasms; and fibrotic tissue formation, which can cause a narrowing (stricture) within the esophagus.

The individual experiencing GERD and/or reflux esophagitis typically complains of heartburn, that is, a burning sensation in the midchest region. The symptoms usually occur within an hour of eating and worsen if the person lies down soon after eating.

To address nutrition implications of this condition, we first need to reexamine some of the foods, nutrients, or substances in foods that influence LES pressure, that may promote increased acid production, and that may irritate an inflamed esophagus. Several substances decrease LES pressure, including high-fat foods, chocolate, nicotine, alcohol, and carminatives [1–5]. Carminatives refer to volatile oil extracts of plants, most often oils of spearmint and peppermint. Other substances increase gastric secretions, especially acid production. Alcohol, calcium, decaffeinated and caffeinated coffee, and tea (specifically, methylxanthines) stimulate gastric secretions, including hydrochloric acid [6–10]. Citrus products and other acidic foods or beverages, as well as some spices, are known to directly irritate an inflamed esophagus. Ingestion of these substances or foods is likely to aggravate irritated esophageal mucosa.

Based on this knowledge, some of the recommendations for the patient with GERD and/or reflux esophagitis are aimed at

- avoiding substances that can further lower LES pressure, which is already low due to the condition; and, to a lesser extent,
- avoiding substances that may promote the secretion of acid, which would be present in higher concentrations than normal if refluxed, and
- avoiding foods or substances that may irritate an inflamed esophagus.

To implement these recommendations, individuals with GERD or reflux esophagitis must be told which foods or substances to avoid, such as high-fat foods or meals, chocolate, coffee, tea, alcohol, carminatives such as peppermint and spearmint, citrus products, acidic foods, and spices such as red and black pepper, nutmeg, cloves, and chili powder.

In addition to avoiding substances that lower LES pressure, that promote the secretion of acid, and that can irritate an inflamed esophagus, recommendations can also include

- increasing the intake of foods or nutrients that increase LES pressure.

Protein is a nutrient that increases LES pressure [10]. Consequently, a higher-than-normal protein intake is encouraged; however, excessive protein intakes, especially from foods high in calcium such as dairy products, are not recommended. The reason for avoiding excessively high intakes of dairy foods relates to the fact that the amino acids and peptides (generated from digestion of the protein in the dairy products) and calcium in dairy products are known to stimulate gastrin release [11]. Although gastrin increases LES pressure, it is also a potent stimulator of hydrochloric acid secretion.

In addition to noting the previously stated nutrition recommendations, it is important to remember that reflux is more likely to occur with increased gastric volume (i.e., eating large meals), increased gastric pressure (e.g., from obesity), and placement of gastric contents near the sphincter (i.e., bending, lying down, or assuming a recumbent position). Thus, recommendations for individuals with GERD or reflux esophagitis should include

- ingestion of smaller meals (versus consumption of larger meals);
- ingestion of fluids between meals instead of with a meal to help minimize large increases in gastric volume;
- weight loss, if an individual is overweight or obese;
- avoidance of tight-fitting clothes; and
- avoidance of lying down as well as of lifting and bending for at least 2 hours after eating.

Disorder 2: Inflammatory Bowel Diseases

Inflammatory bowel diseases (IBDs) include ulcerative colitis and Crohn's disease (also called regional enteritis) and are characterized by acute, relapsing, or chronic inflammation of various segments of the GI tract, especially the intestines. Although the causes of IBDs are unclear, nutrient malabsorption is a significant problem, for several reasons. First, because of the disease-associated inflammation of the mucosa, brush border disaccharidase and peptidase activities are diminished and thus nutrient digestion is impaired. Second, nutrient transit time is typically decreased/shortened—that is, GI tract contents move through the GI tract more quickly than usual and thus leave little time for absorption. Third, malabsorption occurs due to direct damage to the absorptive mucosa cells. Exacerbating the poor nutrient absorption is poor food intake, which is especially common during acute attacks.

Manifestations of IBDs include excessive diarrhea and/or steatorrhea (high amounts of fat in the feces), which may occur up to 20 times per day. Diarrhea is associated with increased losses of fluid and electrolytes (especially potassium) from the body. Fluid and electrolyte imbalance or even dehydration can result. Blood is often present in the feces, especially with severe inflammation or ulceration of deeper areas of the GI mucosa. Loss of blood impairs the body's protein and mineral (especially iron) status. If IBD has affected the ileum (as is common with Crohn's disease), the absorption of vitamin B_{12} may be impaired (absorption of this vitamin occurs in the ileum), reabsorption of bile salts from the ileum may be diminished, and fat malabsorption may occur. Although pancreatic lipase is available to hydrolyze dietary triglycerides, the lack of sufficient bile or diminished bile function due to bacterial alteration of bile can decrease micelle formation and thus decrease absorption of fatty acids and fat-soluble vitamins into the enterocyte. Unabsorbed fatty acids bind to calcium and magnesium in the lumen of the intestine; the resulting insoluble complex, sometimes called a soap, is excreted in the feces.

Dietary recommendations for people with IBD are aimed at replacing nutrient losses, correcting nutrient imbalances, and improving nutrition status. Some of these dietary recommendations include

- increased iron intake above the RDA, due to increased iron losses with the bloody diarrhea and decreased absorption;
- a low-fat diet, due to impaired fat absorption;
- increased intakes of calcium and magnesium, due to diminished absorption secondary to soap formation and overall malabsorption with diarrhea;
- a high-protein diet to improve protein status diminished by protein loss from the blood into the feces with bloody diarrhea and malabsorption of amino acids;
- fat-soluble vitamin supplements, possibly given in a water-miscible form to improve absorption;
- increased fluids and electrolytes for rehydration and restoration of electrolyte balance, respectively; and
- increased nutrient intake to meet energy and nutrient needs.

Easily digestible carbohydrate-rich foods that are low in fiber, high-protein low-fat foods with minimal residue, and lactose-free foods will need to provide the bulk of the individual's energy needs if oral intake is deemed appropriate. Medium-chain triacylglycerol (MCT) oil, which is absorbed directly into portal blood and does not need bile for absorption, may be added in small amounts to different foods throughout the day to increase energy intake.

Disorder 3: Chronic Pancreatitis

Pancreatitis, or inflammation of the pancreas, provides an excellent example of the nutritional ramifications of a condition affecting an accessory organ of the GI tract. Remember that the exocrine portion of the pancreas produces several enzymes needed for the digestion of all nutrients. *Chronic* refers to an ongoing or long-lasting situation.

Chronic pancreatitis can result from long-time excessive use of alcohol, gallstones, liver disease, viral infections, and use of certain medications, among other factors. With time, sections of pancreatic tissue become dysfunctional. Acinar cells, for example, can ultimately fail to produce sufficient digestive enzymes. Chronic pancreatitis causes severe pain, especially with eating, as well as nausea, vomiting, and diarrhea. Chronic pancreatitis causes maldigestion, with resulting malabsorption of several nutrients. Diminished secretion of pancreatic lipase into the duodenum results in maldigestion of fat and thus malabsorption of fat and fat-soluble vitamins. Fat is malabsorbed because not enough pancreatic lipase is available to hydrolyze the fatty acids from the triglycerides. This hydrolysis is necessary in order for fatty acids and monoacylglycerols to form micelles, the form in which the fatty acids are carried to the enterocyte for absorption. Thus, with pancreatitis, the insufficiency of enzymes available for fat hydrolysis necessitates the consumption of a low-fat diet.

In addition to insufficient pancreatic lipase secretion, bicarbonate secretion into the duodenum is also diminished with pancreatitis. Bicarbonate, in part, functions to increase the pH of the small intestine. Intestinal enzymes function best at an alkaline pH, which is provided by the release of bicarbonate into the intestine. Oral supplements of pancreatic enzymes may be needed to replace the diminished output of these enzymes by the malfunctioning, inflamed pancreas. Medications such as antacids, H_2-receptor blockers, or proton pump inhibitors may also need to be taken. The medications are taken to diminish acid production and thus increase intestinal pH. In effect, they replace the bicarbonate and thus help maintain an appropriate pH for enzyme function. Administration of exogenous insulin also may be needed to replace the insulin no longer produced by damaged pancreatic endocrine cells.

These three conditions have been presented to help you understand how diseases affecting the GI tract — malfunction of a sphincter (GERD and reflux esophagitis), destruction of enterocyte function (IBD), and chronic malfunction of a GI tract accessory organ that provides secretions needed for nutrient digestion (pancreatitis) — affect the body's ability to digest and absorb nutrients. Furthermore, these three conditions illustrate how nutrient intakes need to deviate from recommended levels — in some cases to lower levels and in other cases to higher levels, depending on the condition. Such dietary modifications are typical of many conditions affecting not only the gastrointestinal tract but also other organ systems.

References Cited

1. Babka JC, Castell DO. On the genesis of heartburn: the effects of specific foods on the lower esophageal sphincter. Am J Dig Dis 1973;18:391–97.
2. Wright LE, Castell DO. The adverse effect of chocolate on lower esophageal sphincter pressure. Digest Dis 1975; 20:703–7.
3. Sigmund CJ, McNally EF. The action of a carminative on the lower esophageal sphincter. Gastroenterology 1969; 56:13–18.
4. Dennish GW, Castell DO. Inhibitory effect of smoking on the lower esophageal sphincter. N Engl J Med 1971; 284:1136–37.
5. Hogan WJ, Andrade SRV, Winship DH. Ethanol-induced acute esophageal motor dysfunction. J Appl Physiol 1972;32:755–60.
6. Lenz HJ, Rerrari-Taylor J, Isenberg JI. Wine and five percent alcohol are potent stimulants of gastric acid secretion in humans. Gastroenterology 1983;85:1082–87.
7. Cohen S, Booth GH. Gastric acid secretion and lower esophageal sphincter pressure in response to coffee and caffeine. N Engl J Med 1975;293:897–99.
8. Feldman EJ, Isenberg JI, Grossman MI. Gastric acid and gastrin response to decaffeinated coffee and a peptone meal. JAMA 1981;246:248–50.
9. Thomas FB, Steinbaugh JT, Fromkes JJ, Mekhjian HS, Caldwell JH. Inhibitory effect of coffee on lower esophageal sphincter pressure. Gastroenterology 1980; 79:1262–66.
10. Harris JB, Nigon K, Alonso D. Adenosine-3', 5'-monophosphate: intracellular mediator for methylxanthine stimulation of gastric secretion. Gastroenterology 1969;57:377–84.
11. Levant JA, Walsh JH, Isenberg JI. Stimulation of gastric secretion and gastrin release by single oral doses of calcium carbonate in man. N Engl J Med 1973; 289:555–58.

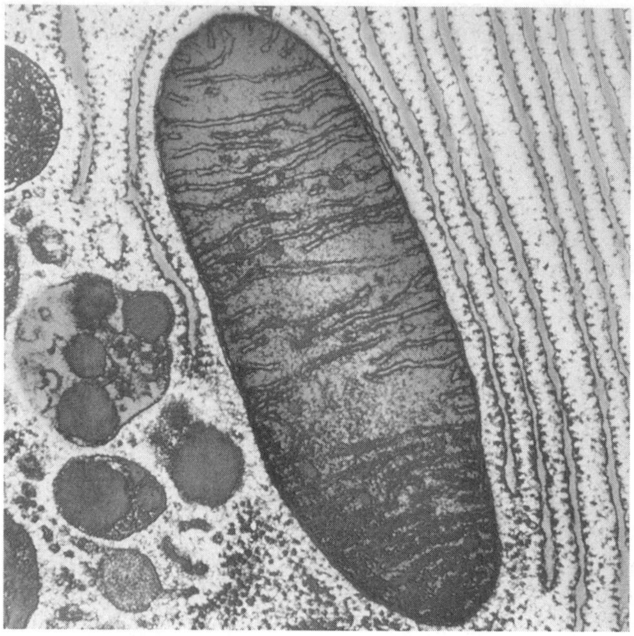

A mitochondrion

chapter 3 Energy Transformation

MOST OF THE PROCESSES THAT SUSTAIN LIFE involve energy. Some processes use energy, while others release it. The term *energy* conjures an image of physical "vim and vigor," the fast runner or the weight lifter straining to lift hundreds of pounds. This notion of energy is accurate insofar as the contraction of muscle fibers associated with mechanical work is an energy-demanding process, requiring adenosine triphosphate (ATP), the major storage form of molecular energy. Beyond the ATP required for physical exertion, however, the living body has other, equally important, requirements for energy, including

- the biosynthetic (anabolic) systems by which substances can be formed from simpler precursors,
- active transport systems by which compounds or ions can be moved across membranes against a concentration gradient (p. 16), and
- the transfer of genetic information.

This chapter addresses the key role of energy transformation and heat production in the use of nutrients and the sustaining of life.

ENERGY RELEASE AND CONSUMPTION IN CHEMICAL REACTIONS

Energy used by the body is ultimately derived from the energy contained in the **macronutrients**—carbohydrate, fat, and protein (and alcohol). If this energy is released, it may simply be expressed as heat, as would occur in the combustion of flammable substances, or be preserved in the form of other chemical energy. The burning of a mole of glucose outside the body liberates heat along with CO_2 and H_2O as products of combustion, as shown:

$$C_6H_{12}O_6 + 6O_2 \longrightarrow 6CO_2 + 6H_2O + \text{heat}$$

The metabolism of glucose to the same CO_2 and H_2O within the cell is nearly identical to that of simple combustion. The difference is that in metabolic oxidation a significant portion of the released energy is salvaged as chemical energy in the form of new, high-energy bonds. These bonds represent a usable source of energy for driving energy-requiring processes. Such stored energy is generally contained in phosphate anhydride bonds, chiefly those of ATP (Fig. 3.1). The analogy between the combustion and the metabolic oxidation of a typical nutrient (palmitic acid) is illustrated in Figure 3.2. The metabolic oxidation illustrated released 59% of the heat that was produced by the combustion.

Units of Energy

The unit of energy used throughout this text is the calorie, abbreviated cal. In the expression of the higher caloric values encountered in nutrition, the unit

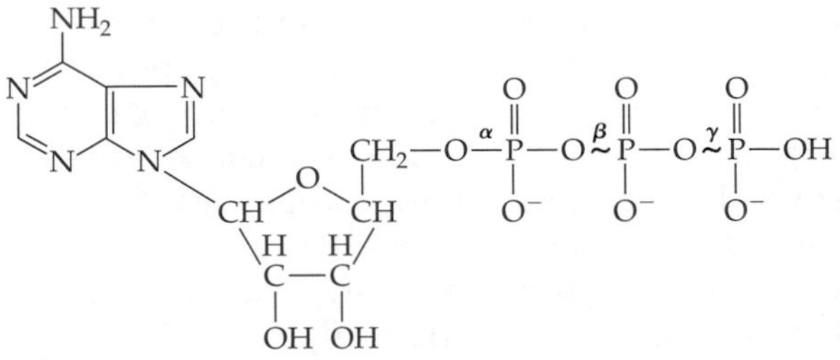

Figure 3.1 Adenosine triphosphate (ATP). The bonds connecting the α- and β-phosphates and the β- and γ-phosphates are anhydride bonds, which release a large amount of energy when hydrolyzed. The bonds are shown as wavy lines, which are customarily used to denote a high-energy source.

kilocalories (kcal) is often used: 1 kcal = 1,000 cal. Students of nutrition should be familiar with another unit of energy called the joule (J). Along with its higher-value counterpart the kilojoule (kJ), the joule has become widely used internationally and is required by many journals. Calories can easily be converted to joules by the factor 4.18:

$$1 \text{ cal} = 4.18 \text{ J, or } 1 \text{ kcal} = 4.18 \text{ kJ}$$

Because nutrition and the calorie have been so closely linked over the years, however, we feel that students of nutrition may be more comfortable with the calorie/kilocalorie unit and digression from this unit may not be appropriate at this time.

FREE ENERGY

The potential energy inherent in the chemical bonds of nutrients is released if the molecules undergo oxidation either through combustion or through oxidation within the cell. This energy is defined as **free energy** (*G*) if, on its release, it is capable of doing work at constant temperature and pressure—a condition that is met within the cell.

Figure 3.2 A comparison of the simple combustion and the metabolic oxidation of the fatty acid palmitate. The energy liberated from combustion assumes the form of heat only, while approximately 40% of the energy released by metabolic oxidation is salvaged as ATP, with the remainder released in the form of heat.

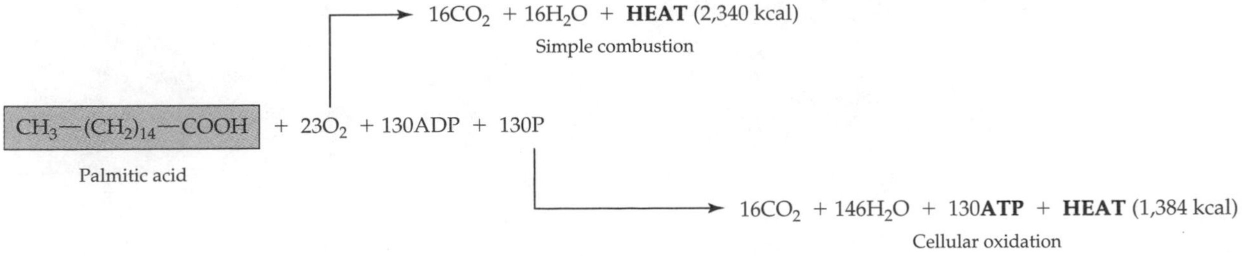

CO_2 and H_2O are the products of the complete oxidation of organic molecules containing only carbon, hydrogen, and oxygen, and they have an inherent free energy. The energy released in the course of oxidation of the organic molecules is in the form of heat or chemical energy. The products have less free energy than do the original reactants. Because energy is neither created nor lost during the reaction, the total energy remains constant. Thus, the difference between the free energy in the products and that in the reactants in a given chemical reaction is a useful parameter for estimating the tendency for that reaction to occur. This difference is symbolized as follows:

$$G_{\text{products}} - G_{\text{reactants}} = \Delta G \text{ of the reaction}$$

where G is free energy and Δ is a symbol signifying change.

Exothermic and Endothermic Reactions

If the G value of the reactants is greater than the G value of the products, as in the case of the oxidation reaction, the reaction is said to be **exothermic,** or energy releasing, and ΔG is negative. In contrast, a positive ΔG indicates that the G value of the products is greater than that of the reactants, indicating that energy must be supplied to the system to convert the reactants into the higher-energy products. Such a reaction is called **endothermic,** or energy requiring.

Exothermic and endothermic reactions are sometimes referred to as downhill and uphill reactions, respectively, terms that help create an image of energy input and release. The free energy levels of reactants and products in a typical exothermic, or downhill, reaction can be likened to a boulder on a hillside that can occupy two positions, A and B, as illustrated in Figure 3.3. As the boulder descends to level B from level A, energy capable of doing work clearly is liberated, and the change in free energy is a negative value. The reverse reaction, moving the boulder uphill to level A from level B, necessitates an input of energy, or an endothermic process, and the change is a positive value. It is important to understand that the quantity of energy released in the downhill reaction is precisely the same as the quantity of energy required for the reverse (uphill) reaction. Only the sign of ΔG changes.

Activation Energy

Although exothermic reactions are favored over endothermic reactions in that they require no external energy input, they do not occur spontaneously. If they did, no energy-producing nutrients or fuels would exist throughout the universe, because they would all have transformed spontaneously to their lower energy level. A certain amount of energy must be introduced into reactant molecules to activate them to what is referred to as their **transition state,** a higher energy level or barrier at which the exothermic conversion to products can indeed take place. The energy that must be imposed on the system to raise the reactants to their transition state is called the **activation energy.** Refer again to the boulder-and-hillside analogy in Figure 3.3. The boulder does not spontaneously descend until the required activation energy can dislodge it from its resting place to the brink of the slope.

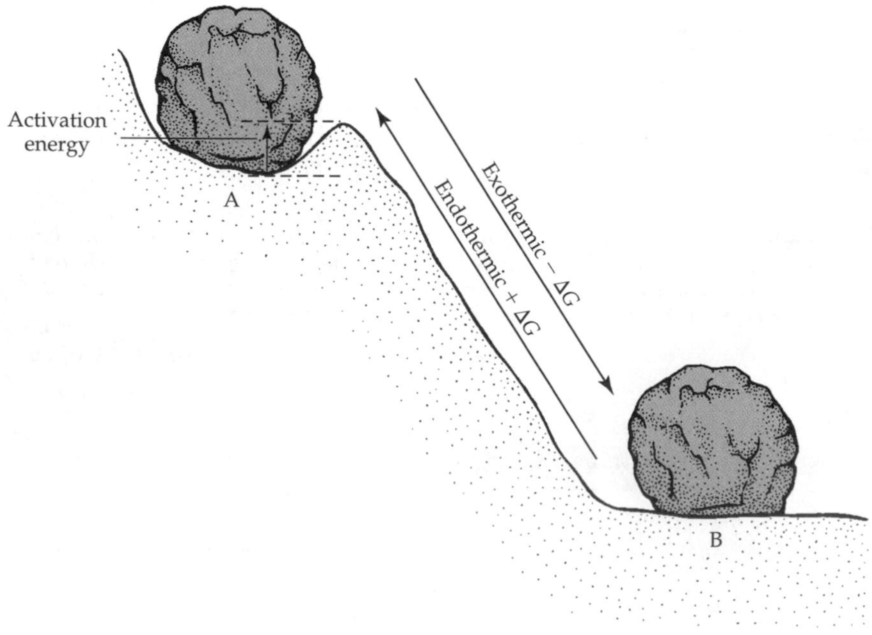

Figure 3.3 The uphill-downhill concept illustrating energy-releasing and energy-demanding processes. Also indicated is the activation energy, which is the amount of energy required to activate the reactant (the boulder, when occupying position A in this case) to its transition state.

Cellular Energy

The cell derives its energy from a series of chemical reactions, each of which exhibits a free energy change. The reactions occur sequentially as nutrients are systematically oxidized ultimately to CO_2 and H_2O. All the reactions are catalyzed by enzymes. Within a given catabolic pathway—for example, the oxidation of glucose to CO_2 and H_2O—some reactions may be energy consuming ($+\Delta G$). However, energy-releasing ($-\Delta G$) reactions are favored, so the net energy transformation for the entire pathway is exothermic.

Reversibility of Chemical Reactions

Most cellular reactions are reversible, meaning that an enzyme (E) that can catalyze the conversion of hypothetical substance A into substance B can also catalyze the reverse reaction, as shown:

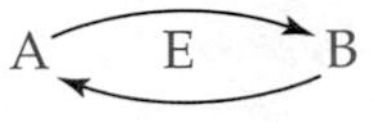

Using the A, B interconversion as an example, we will review the concept of reversibility of a chemical reaction. In the presence of the specific enzyme E, substance A will be converted to substance B. Initially, the reaction is unidirectional because only A is present. However, because the enzyme is also capable of converting substance B to substance A, the reverse reaction becomes significant as the concentration of B increases. From the moment the reaction is initiated, the amount of A will decrease, while the amount of B will increase to the point at which the rate of the two reactions becomes equal. At that point the concentration of A and B will no longer change, and the system is said to be in equilibrium. Whether the A $\longrightarrow$ B reaction or the B $\longrightarrow$ A reaction is energetically favored is indicated by the relative concentrations of A and B at equilibrium.

The equilibrium between reactants and products can be defined in mathematical terms and is called K_{eq}. K_{eq} is simply the ratio of the equilibrium concentration of product B to that of reactant A: $K_{eq} = [B]/[A]$. This ratio reflects the difference in concentrations. From this simple relationship, it can be seen that K_{eq} increases in value when the concentration of A decreases and that of B increases. If K_{eq} has a value greater than 1, substance B is formed from substance A, whereas a value of K_{eq} less than 1 indicates that at equilibrium A will be formed from B. An equilibrium constant equal to 1 indicates that there is no bias for either reaction. The K_{eq} of a reaction can be used to calculate the standard free energy change of the reaction, which is discussed next.

Standard Free Energy Change

In order to compare the energy released or consumed in different reactions, it is convenient to define the free energy at standard conditions. The standard free energy change (ΔG^0) (the superscript zero designates standard conditions) for a chemical reaction is a constant for that particular reaction. It is defined as the difference between the free energy content of the reactants and the free energy content of the products under standard conditions. Standard conditions are defined precisely: a temperature of 25°C (298 K); a pressure of 1.0 atm (atmosphere); and the presence of both the reactants and the products at their standard concentrations, namely, 1.0 mol/L. Under such conditions, ΔG^0 is mathematically related to K_{eq} by the equation

$$\Delta G^0 = -2.3\ RT \log K_{eq}$$

where R is the gas constant (1.987 cal/mol × degrees K) and T is the absolute temperature, 298 K in this case. The factors 2.3, R, and T are constants, and their product is equal to $-2.3(1.987)(298)$, or $-1{,}362$ cal/mol. The equation therefore simplifies to

$$\Delta G^0 = -1{,}362 \log K_{eq}$$

Equilibrium Constant and Standard Free Energy Change

The equilibrium constant of a reaction determines the sign and magnitude of the standard free energy change. For example, referring once again to the A $\longrightarrow$ B reaction, the logarithm of a K_{eq} value greater than 1.0 will be positive, and the sign of ΔG^0 will be negative. We have established that the reaction A $\longrightarrow$ B is energetically favored if ΔG^0 is negative. Conversely, the log of a K_{eq} value less than 1.0 would be negative, and therefore the sign of ΔG^0 would be positive. The $+\Delta G^0$ in this case indicates that the formation of A from B (A $\longleftarrow$ B) is favored in the equilibrium.

Standard pH

Because for most compartments in the body the pH is near neutral, for biochemical reactions a standard pH is also designated. A pH value of 7 is adopted by convention as the standard pH in biochemical reactions. For human nutrition, the free energy change of reactions is designated $\Delta G^{0\prime}$. We will use this notation in our discussion.

Nonstandard Physiological Conditions

Physiologically standard conditions do not often exist. The difference between standard conditions and nonstandard conditions can explain why a reaction having a positive $\Delta G^{0\prime}$ can proceed exothermically ($-\Delta G$) in the cell. For example, consider the reaction catalyzed by the enzyme triosephosphate isomerase (TPI) shown in Figure 3.4. This particular reaction occurs in the glycolytic pathway through which glucose is converted to pyruvate. (The pathway is discussed in detail in

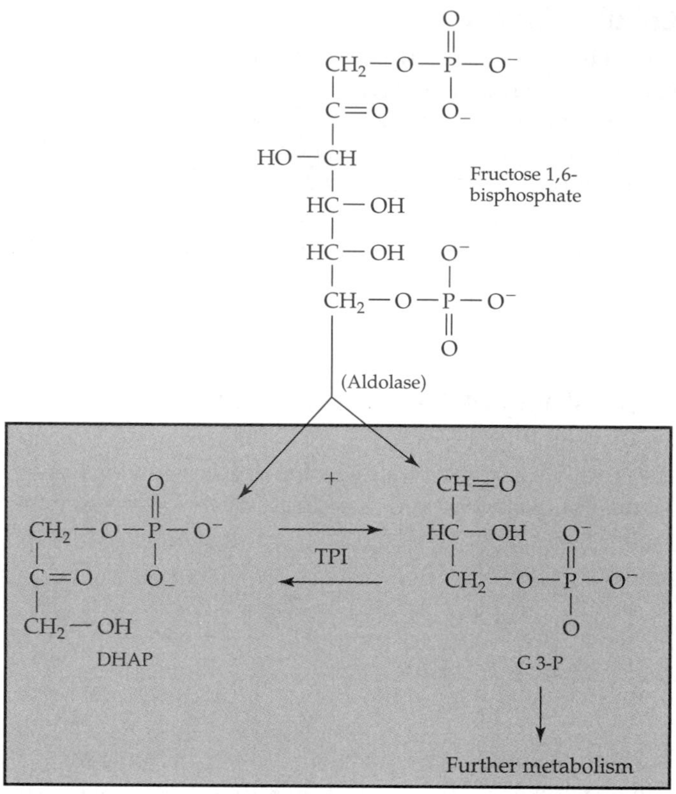

Figure 3.4 A segment of the glycolytic pathway of glucose metabolism, illustrating the interconversion by the enzyme triosephosphate isomerase (TPI) of dihydroxyacetone phosphate (DHAP) and glyceraldehyde 3-phosphate (G 3-P). The two triose phosphates are formed from the splitting of fructose 1,6-bisphosphate by aldolase. Under standard conditions, the TPI equilibrium is shifted toward the formation of DHAP, but in cellular metabolism the further conversion of G 3-P to other metabolites depletes its steady-state concentration and causes the rate of the DHAP $\longrightarrow$ G 3-P reaction to increase.

Chap. 4.) In the glycolytic pathway, the enzyme aldolase produces 1 mol each of dihydroxyacetone phosphate (DHAP) and glyceraldehyde 3-phosphate (G 3-P) from 1 mol of fructose 1,6-bisphosphate. TPI catalyzes an isomerization between the two products of the aldolase reaction. However, of the two products, only the G 3-P is further degraded in the subsequent reactions of glycolysis, resulting in a significantly lower concentration of this metabolite compared with the DHAP.

In this example, two important conditions within the cell deviate from standard conditions: namely, the temperature (~37°C, or 310 K) and the fact that the reactants and products are not both 1.0 mol/L concentrations. To calculate the actual ΔG of the triosephosphate isomerase reaction for the conditions existing in the cell, we use the $\Delta G^{0'}$ of the reaction and the cellular, steady-state concentrations of reactant and product as shown in this equation:

$$\Delta G = \Delta G^{0'} + 2.3 \text{ RT} \log [\text{product}]/[\text{reactant}]$$

The value of $\Delta G^{0'}$ for the reaction DHAP (reactant) $\longrightarrow$ G 3-P (product) is +1,830 cal/mol, indicating that under standard conditions the formation of DHAP is preferred over the formation of G 3-P. For the sake of illustration, however, let us assume that the cellular concentration of DHAP is 50 times that of G 3-P because G 3-P is further metabolized. Substitute these values into the equation:

$$\begin{aligned}\Delta G &= +1{,}830 + 2.3(1.987)(310 \text{ K}) \log 1/50\\ &= +1{,}830 + 1{,}416 \log 0.02\\ &= +1{,}830 + 1{,}416(-1.7)\\ &= +1{,}830 - 2{,}407\\ &= -577 \text{ cal/mol}\end{aligned}$$

The negative ΔG shows that the reaction is indeed proceeding to form G 3-P, as shown, despite the positive $\Delta G^{0'}$ for this reaction.

THE ROLE OF HIGH-ENERGY PHOSPHATE IN ENERGY STORAGE

The preceding section addressed the fundamental principle of free energy changes in chemical reactions and the fact that the cell obtains this free energy through the catabolism of nutrient molecules. It further pointed out that this energy must somehow be used to drive the various energy-requiring processes and anabolic reactions so important in normal cell function. This section explains how ATP can be used as a universal source of

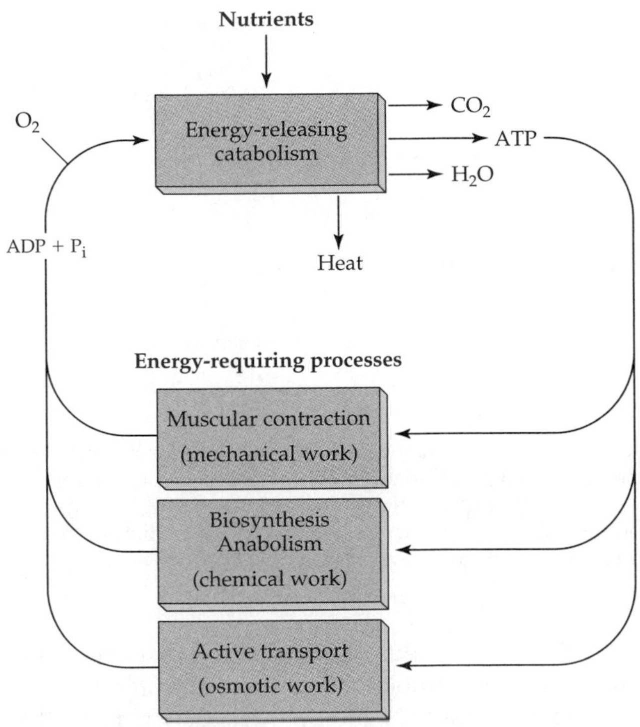

Figure 3.5 An illustration of how ATP is generated from the coupling of ADP and phosphate through the oxidative catabolism of nutrients and how it in turn is used for energy-requiring processes.

energy to drive reactions. The hydrolysis of the phosphate anhydride bonds of ATP can liberate the stored chemical energy when needed. ATP thus can be thought of as an energy reservoir, serving as the major linking intermediate between energy-releasing and energy-demanding chemical reactions in the cell. In nearly all cases, the energy stored in ATP is released by the enzymatic hydrolysis of the anhydride bond connecting the β- and γ-phosphates in the molecule (Fig. 3.1). The products of this hydrolysis are adenosine diphosphate (ADP) and inorganic phosphate (P_i). In certain instances the free phosphate group is transferred to various acceptors, a reaction that activates the acceptors to higher energy levels. The involvement of ATP as a link between the energy-releasing and energy-requiring cellular reactions and processes is summarized in Figure 3.5.

THE HIGH-ENERGY PHOSPHATE BOND

The amount of energy released by phosphate anhydride bonds is large, and several compounds besides ATP possess these bonds. Anhydride bonds are the driving force behind biochemical reactions. Hydrolysis of the anhydride bond connecting the β- and γ-phosphates of ATP is a highly exothermic reaction. The reaction, which releases ADP and P_i, has a $\Delta G^{0\prime}$ of −7,300 cal/mol. The hydrolysis of the anhydride bond connecting the α- and β-phosphates also has a $\Delta G^{0\prime}$ of −7,300 cal/mol. The bond linking the α-phosphate to the adenosine, on the other hand, is a phosphate ester, a bond that characteristically possesses much less free energy than a phosphate anhydride bond. The hydrolysis of adenosine monophosphate (AMP) to yield adenosine and P_i liberates 3,400 cal/mol. This is within the range typical of phosphate ester hydrolysis, which is generally 2,000 to 5,000 cal/mol. As a family, phosphate esters rank below ATP and other nucleoside triphosphates on the release of energy during hydrolysis.

Based on the preceding discussion of phosphate bond energies, it is tempting to think in terms of high-energy and low-energy phosphate bonds, with ATP and other nucleoside triphosphates being high energy and phosphate esters representing low energy. However, the wide range of ester energy, along with the fact that some phosphorylated compounds have even higher energy than ATP, complicates the high energy–low energy concept. Phosphoenolpyruvate and 1,3-diphosphoglycerate, which occur as intermediates in the metabolic pathway of glycolysis, and phosphocreatine, an important source of energy in muscle contraction, are examples of compounds having phosphate bond energies significantly higher than ATP. Their structures are shown in Figure 3.6. Note that "high-energy" bonds are depicted as a wavy line (~, referred to as a tilde), indicating that the free energy of hydrolysis is higher

Figure 3.6 Examples of very high energy phosphate compounds. The phosphate bonds represented by the wavy lines contain more energy than the terminal phosphate bond of ATP, making it energetically possible to transfer these phosphate groups enzymatically to ADP.

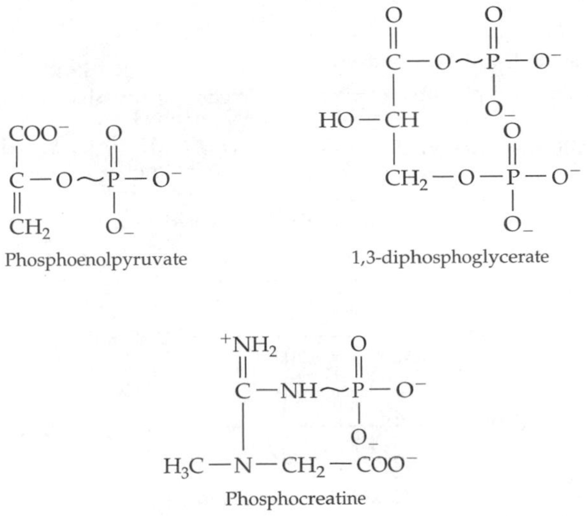

Table 3.1 Free Energy of Hydrolysis of Some Phosphorylated Compounds

Compound	ΔG^0 (cal)
Phosphoenolpyruvate	−14,800
1,3-diphosphoglycerate	−11,800
Phosphocreatine	−10,300
ATP	−7,300
Glucose 1-phosphate	−5,000
Adenosine monophosphate (AMP)	−3,400
Glucose 6-phosphate	−3,300

than it is for the stabler phosphate esters. Table 3.1 lists the standard free energy of hydrolysis of selected phosphate-containing compounds.

COUPLED REACTIONS IN THE TRANSFER OF ENERGY

An understanding of the transformation of chemical energy from macronutrients (food) to storage forms (such as ATP) and the use of the stored energy to synthesize needed compounds for the body is fundamental to the study of human nutrition. These topics are covered in this section as well as throughout this book. It has been pointed out that the $\Delta G^{0'}$ value for the phosphate bond hydrolysis of ATP is intermediate between certain high-energy phosphate compounds and compounds that possess relatively low-energy phosphate esters. ATP's central position on the energy scale lets it serve as an intermediate carrier of phosphate groups. ADP can accept the phosphate groups from high-energy phosphate donor molecules and then, as ATP, transfer them to lower-energy receptor molecules. An example of this is shown in Figure 3.7. By receiving the phosphate groups, the acceptor molecules become activated to a higher energy level, from which they can undergo subsequent reactions.

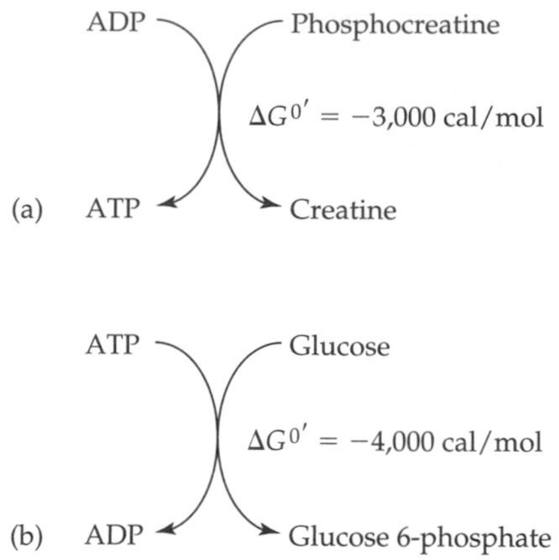

Figure 3.7 (a) Example of high-energy phosphate bond being transferred from high-energy compound phosphocreatine to form ATP. (b) The transfer of the high-energy phosphate bond to a compound that becomes activated, allowing it to enter into the glycolytic pathway.

The end result is the transfer of chemical energy from donor molecules through ATP to receptor molecules.

If a given quantity of energy is released in an exothermic reaction, the same amount of energy must be added to the system for that reaction to be driven in the reverse direction. For example, the hydrolysis of the phosphate ester bond of glucose 6-phosphate liberates 3,300 cal/mol of energy, and the reverse reaction, the addition of the phosphate to glucose to form glucose 6-phosphate, necessitates the input of 3,300 cal/mol. These reactions can be expressed in terms of their standard free energy changes as shown in Figure 3.8. To phosphorylate glucose, the reaction must be coupled with the hydrolysis of ATP, which provides the necessary energy. The additional energy from the reaction is dissipated as heat.

The addition of phosphate to a molecule is called a phosphorylation reaction. It generally is accom-

Figure 3.8 Exothermic reactions.

$$\text{Glucose 6-phosphate} \xrightarrow[\Delta G^{0'} = -3{,}300 \text{ cal/mol}]{} \text{Glucose} + P_i$$

$$\text{Glucose 6-phosphate} \xleftarrow[\Delta G^{0'} = +3{,}300 \text{ cal/mol}]{} \text{Glucose} + P_i$$

Forward reaction favored

(a) The hydrolysis of glucose 6-phosphate to glucose and P_i has a negative $\Delta G^{0'}$ and is favored. The reverse reaction is not energetically favored.

$$\text{ATP} \xrightarrow[\Delta G^{0'} = -7{,}300 \text{ cal/mol}]{} \text{ADP} + P_i$$

$$\text{ATP} \xleftarrow[\Delta G^{0'} = +7{,}300 \text{ cal/mol}]{} \text{ADP} + P_i$$

(b) The hydrolysis of ATP to ADP and P_i has a large negative $\Delta G^{0'}$ and is favored. The reverse reaction occurs with the electron transport chain to provide the energy needed.

$$\text{Glucose} + \text{ATP} \xrightarrow[\Delta G^{0'} = -4{,}000 \text{ cal/mol}]{} \text{Glucose 6-phosphate} + \text{ADP}$$

Coupled reaction favored

(c) The coupled reaction phosphorylating glucose and hydrolysing ATP is energetically favored, with a negative $\Delta G^{0'}$ of 4,000 cal/mol.

plished by the enzymatic transfer of the terminal phosphate group of ATP to the molecule, rather than by the addition of free phosphate as suggested in Figure 3.8a. The reverse reaction is hypothetical, designed only to illustrate the energy requirement for phosphorylation of the glucose molecule. In fact, the enzymatic phosphorylation of glucose by ATP is the first reaction glucose undergoes upon entering the cell (Fig. 3.8c). This reaction promotes glucose to a higher energy level, from which it may be indirectly incorporated into glycogen as stored carbohydrate or systematically oxidized for energy. Phosphorylation therefore can be viewed as occurring in two reaction steps:

1. The hydrolysis of ATP to ADP and phosphate
2. The addition of the phosphate to the substrate (glucose) molecule

A net energy change for the two reactions coupled together is shown in Figure 3.8c. The net $\Delta G^{0\prime}$ for the coupled reaction is −4,000 cal/mol.

It is important to understand the significance of these coupled reactions. They show that even though energy is consumed in the endothermic formation of glucose 6-phosphate from glucose and phosphate, the energy released by the ATP hydrolysis is sufficient to force (or drive) the endothermic reaction that "costs" only 3,300 cal/mol. The coupled reactions result in 4,000 cal/mol left over. The reaction is catalyzed by the enzyme hexokinase or glucokinase, both of which hydrolyze the ATP and transfer the phosphate group to glucose. The enzyme brings the ATP and the glucose into close proximity, reducing the activation energy of the reactants and facilitating the phosphate group transfer. The overall reaction, which results in the activation of glucose at the expense of ATP, is energetically favorable, as evidenced by its high, negative standard free energy change.

FORMATION OF ATP

In the preceding discussion, it was shown that certain molecules can be activated by phosphate group transfer from ATP. The phosphorylation itself is an endothermic reaction but is made possible by the highly exothermic hydrolysis of the terminal phosphate of ATP. For these processes to continue in the body, the ADP produced by the reaction must be reconverted to ATP to maintain the homeostatic concentration of cellular ATP. How is this accomplished, considering the large amount of energy ($\Delta G^{0\prime} = +7{,}300$ cal/mol) required for the reaction?

Obviously, outside sources of considerable energy must be linked to the phosphorylation of ADP. Actually, two such mechanisms function in this respect:

- substrate-level phosphorylation and
- oxidative phosphorylation.

From the standpoint of the amount of ATP produced, oxidative phosphorylation is decidedly the more important of the two mechanisms.

Substrate-Level Phosphorylation

As shown in Table 3.1, phosphorylated molecules have a wide range of free energies of hydrolysis of their phosphate groups. Many of them release less energy than ATP, but some release more. The $\Delta G^{0\prime}$ of hydrolysis of the compounds listed in Table 3.1, called the phosphate group transfer potential, is a measure of the compounds' capacities to donate phosphate groups to other substances. The more negative the transfer potential, the more potent the phosphate donating power. Therefore, a compound that releases more energy on hydrolysis of its phosphate can transfer that phosphate to an acceptor molecule having a relatively more positive transfer potential. For this to occur in actuality, however, there must be a specific enzyme to catalyze the transfer. A phosphate group can be enzymatically transferred from ATP to glucose, a transfer that can be predicted from Table 3.1. It can also be predicted from Table 3.1 that compounds with a more negative phosphate group transfer potential than ATP can transfer phosphate to ADP, forming ATP. This does, in fact, occur in metabolism. The phosphorylation of ADP by phosphocreatine, for example, represents an important mode for ATP formation in muscle, and the reaction exemplifies a **substrate-level phosphorylation** (Fig. 3.7a).

Oxidative Phosphorylation

The major means by which ATP is formed from ADP is through the mechanism of oxidative phosphorylation. This process is discussed in detail here because ATP is the major supplier of energy in metabolism. The required energy is tapped from a pool of energy generated by the flow of electrons from substrate molecules undergoing oxidation. The electrons are then passed through a series of intermediate compounds and ultimately to molecular oxygen, which becomes reduced to H_2O in the process. The compounds participating in this sequential reduction-oxidation constitute the respiratory chain, so named because the electron transfer is linked to the uptake of O_2, which is made available to the tissues by respiration. *Electron transport chain*, a more commonly used alternate term, is used instead throughout this text. The chain functions within the cell mitochondria. These organelles are often referred to as the power plants of the cell based on the large amount of energy liberated by electron transport (p. 6). This energy assumes the form of heat to maintain body temperature and also is used to form ATP from ADP and P_i. Therefore, the term *oxidative phosphorylation* is a descriptive blend of two processes operating simultaneously:

1. The oxidation of a metabolite by O_2 via electron transport
2. The phosphorylation of ADP

The processes of cellular oxidation of nutrients, electron transport, and oxidative phosphorylation perform a unified function and should be thought of together. They are considered next in more detail.

BIOLOGICAL OXIDATION AND THE ELECTRON TRANSPORT CHAIN

Oxidation of the energy nutrients (carbohydrates, protein, lipids, and alcohol) is what releases their inherent chemical energy and makes it available to the body either as heat or as ATP. This section discusses the nature of the oxidative processes that can occur and that are directly involved in energy production.

Cellular oxidation of a compound can occur by several different reactions: the addition of oxygen, the removal of electrons, and the removal of hydrogens. All these reactions are catalyzed by enzymes collectively termed oxidoreductases. Among these, the **dehydrogenases,** which remove hydrogens and electrons from nutrient metabolites, are particularly important in energy transformation. The hydrogens and electrons removed from metabolites by dehydrogenase reactions pass along the components of the electron transport chain and cause the release of large amounts of energy. In reactions in which oxygen is incorporated into a compound or hydrogens are removed by other than dehydrogenases, the electron transport chain is not called into play and no energy is released. Such reactions are catalyzed by a subgroup of oxidoreductase enzymes generally referred to as oxidases; these are not considered further in this section.

The hydrogen ions and electrons removed from a substrate molecule by a dehydrogenase enzyme are transferred to a cosubstrate, such as the vitamin-derived nicotinamide adenine dinucleotide (NAD^+) or flavin adenine dinucleotide (FAD). An example of energy release with oxidation is the oxidation of the fatty acid palmitate shown in Figure 3.2. These reactions occur in the mitochondria. The substrate molecule (M), in its reduced form, will be designated MH_2. As a result of the transfer of hydrogen ions and electrons, the substrate is

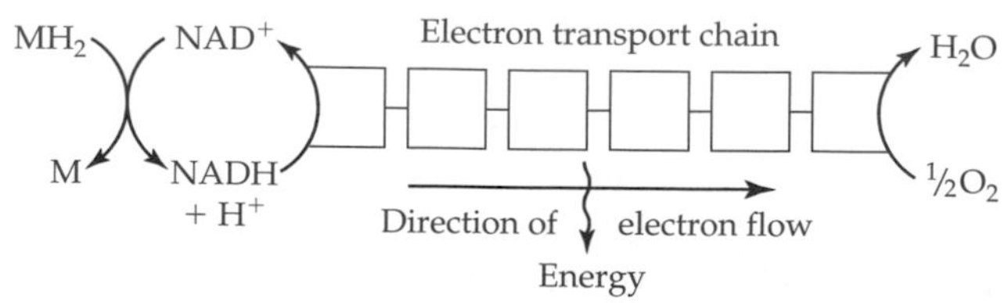

Figure 3.9 The transfer of hydrogen and electrons from MH_2 to NAD^+ and the subsequent oxidation of NADH to H_2O by O_2.

oxidized to M from MH_2, while the oxidized forms of the cosubstrates (either NAD^+ or FAD) become reduced to NADH and $FADH_2$, respectively, upon acceptance of the hydrogens and electrons. The hydrogens and electrons are then enzymatically transferred through the electron transport chain components and eventually to molecular oxygen, which becomes reduced to H_2O. The overall reaction is summarized in Figure 3.9 using the example of NAD^+ as hydrogen acceptor.

Reduction Potentials

The available energy for oxidative phosphorylation is derived from the sequence of individual reduction-oxidation (redox) reactions along the electron transport chain, with each component having a characteristic ability to donate and accept electrons. The released energy is used in part to synthesize ATP from ADP and phosphate. The tendency of a compound to donate and to receive electrons is expressed in terms of its **standard reduction potential,** $E_{0'}$. More negative values of $E_{0'}$ reflect a greater ability of the compound to donate electrons, while increasingly positive values signify an increasing tendency to accept electrons. The reducing capacity of a compound (its tendency to donate H^+ and electrons) can be expressed by the $E_{0'}$ value of its half-reaction, also called the compound's electromotive potential. (In Fig. 3.9, $MH_2 \longrightarrow M$ is a half-reaction; the whole reaction is $MH_2 + NAD^+ \longrightarrow M + NADH_2$.)

Free energy changes accompany the transfer of electrons between electron donor/acceptor pairs of compounds and are related to the measurable electromotive force of the electron flow. It is important to remember that *in electron transfer an electron donor reduces the acceptor and in the process becomes oxidized. Consequently, the acceptor, as it is reduced, oxidizes the donor.* The quantity of energy released is directly proportional to the difference in the standard reduction potentials, $\Delta E_{0'}$, between the partners of the redox pair. The free energy of a redox reaction and the $\Delta E_{0'}$ of the interacting compounds are related by the expression

$$\Delta G^{0'} = -nF\Delta E_{0'}$$

where $\Delta G^{0'}$ is the standard free energy change in calories, n is the number of electrons transferred (in cellular oxidation, assumed to be two), and F is a constant called the faraday (23,062 cal absolute volt equivalent).

An example of a reduction-oxidation reaction that occurs within the electron transport system is the transfer of hydrogen atoms and electrons from NADH through the flavin mononucleotide (FMN)-linked enzyme NADH dehydrogenase to oxidized coenzyme Q (CoQ). The half-reactions and $E_{0'}$ values for each of these reactions follow:

$$NADH + H^+ \longrightarrow NAD^+ + 2H^+ + 2e^-$$
$$E_{0'} = -0.32 \text{ volt}$$
$$CoQH_2 \longrightarrow CoQ + 2H^+ + 2e^-$$
$$E_{0'} = +0.04 \text{ volt}$$

Because the NAD^+ system has a relatively more negative $E_{0'}$ value than the CoQ system, it follows from the preceding discussion that it has a greater reducing potential than the CoQ system, because electrons tend to flow toward the more positive system. The reduction of CoQ by NADH therefore is predictable, and the coupled reaction, linked by the FMN of NADH dehydrogenase, can be written as follows:

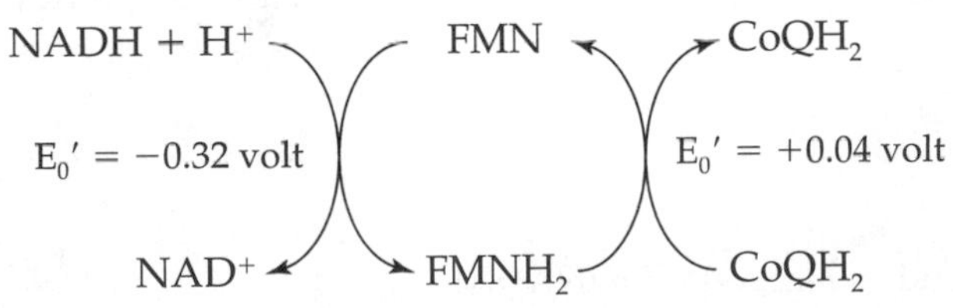

$$\Delta E_{0'} = 0.36 \text{ volt}$$

Inserting this value for ΔE_0 into the energy equation gives

$$\Delta G^{0'} = -2(23{,}062)(0.36) = -16{,}604 \text{ cal/mol}$$

The amount of energy liberated from this single reduction-oxidation reaction within the electron transport chain therefore is more than enough to phosphorylate ADP to ATP, which, it will be recalled, requires approximately 7,300 cal/mol.

Anatomical Site for Oxidative Phosphorylation

To better understand the processes of oxidative phosphorylation, refer back to Figures 1.9 and 1.10, which describe the structure of the mitochondrion. Note that the enzymes of the Krebs cycle, except for one (Chap. 4), and of fatty acid oxidation (Chap. 5) are located in the matrix of the mitochondria. The one enzyme of the Krebs cycle that is an integral part of the inner membrane is succinate dehydrogenase, the importance of which will be discussed later. It is the translocation of H^+ (protons) from within the matrix to the space between the cristae and outer membrane that provides much of the energy that drives oxidative phosphorylation. Note the respiratory stalks on the inner membrane (Fig. 1.9), which also play an important role in the currently accepted mechanism of oxidative phosphorylation.

Dehydrogenase Reactions

The first step in the release of energy from carbohydrates and fat is their oxidation. The reactions involve dehydrogenases to produce NADH and $FMNH_2$. Thus, these reactions will be considered before we look at the electron transport components themselves. Two dehydrogenase reactions occurring in the Krebs cycle are offered as examples of cosubstrate reduction linked to substrate (metabolite) oxidation. The reactions are catalyzed by the enzymes malate dehydrogenase (MDH) and succinate dehydrogenase (SDH) (Fig. 3.10). If dehydrogenation is linked to NAD, hydrogens and electrons flow from the substrate undergoing oxidation through first the NAD^+ system and then the FMN system.

Components of the Oxidative Phosphorylation Chain

After NAD^+ and FMN, the next component in the electron transport chain is an iron sulfur center, which collects only electrons from the FMN system, with the hydrogens being released as protons. The electrons are then passed on to the coenzyme Q (CoQ) system, which also regains two protons, equivalent to the two protons released at the iron sulfur center. Coenzyme Q is also referred to as ubiquinone. Precisely where within their molecular structure these substances accept and release hydrogens and electrons is shown by their reduced and oxidized forms as depicted in Figures 3.11, 3.12, and 3.13.

The components functioning after CoQ, called **cytochromes,** are iron-containing, electron-transferring proteins that act sequentially to carry electrons (only electrons, and not H^+) from CoQ to molecular oxygen. The hydrogens of reduced CoQ are released as protons, and therefore no hydrogen transfer takes place within the cytochrome segment of the chain. The protons collected by CoQ are released into the mitochondrial matrix and ultimately combine with O_2 to form H_2O, as shown later in this chapter. Specifically, the cytochromes are heme proteins in which the iron is bound to porphyrin, forming a heme moiety similar to that found in hemoglobin (Chap. 7). The heme group is a red-brown pigment, and

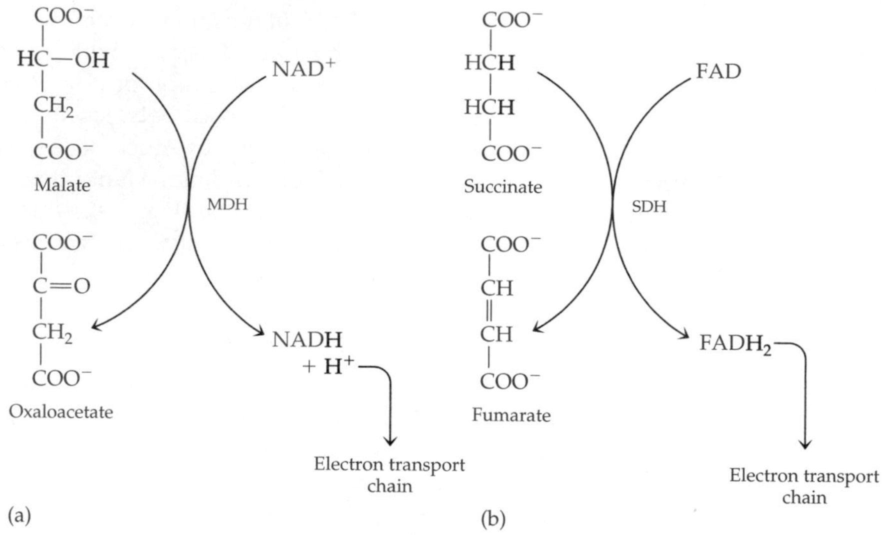

Figure 3.10 Examples of dehydrogenase reactions occurring in the Krebs cycle: malate dehydrogenase (MDH) converting (oxidizing) malate to oxaloacetate (reducing NAD^+) (a), and succinate dehydrogenase (SDH) converting (oxidizing) succinate to fumarate (reducing FAD) (b).

this coloration is imparted to that organelle because of the high concentration of cytochromes in the mitochondrion. Cytochromes designated as cyt a-a3, cyt b, cyt c1, and cyt c function as electron carriers, and although subtle structural differences differentiate them, they share the heme moiety. Among them, the structure of cyt c, shown in Figure 3.14, was the first to be defined. The reduction-oxidation of the cytochromes occurs at the iron atom, which alternates between the ferric (Fe^{+3}) and ferrous (Fe^{+2}) forms as it releases and acquires electrons.

$$Fe^{+2} \longrightarrow Fe^{+3} + e^-$$

Figure 3.11 Nicotinamide adenine dinucleotide (NAD^+) and its reduced form (NADH). The carbon atom (blue shading) is the site of attachment of one of the two hydrogen atoms transferred from a metabolite undergoing dehydrogenation. The hydrogen is actually acquired as a hydride ion (:H^-) that attaches to the nicotinamide ring as shown and neutralizes the positive charge on the ring nitrogen. The remainder of the structure, indicated by the symbol R, is unchanged from that of NAD^+. The second hydrogen transferred from the metabolite is released as a proton. Another dehydrogenase cosubstrate, NADP, differs from NAD^+ only in the attachment of a phosphate group at the position shown by the asterisk.

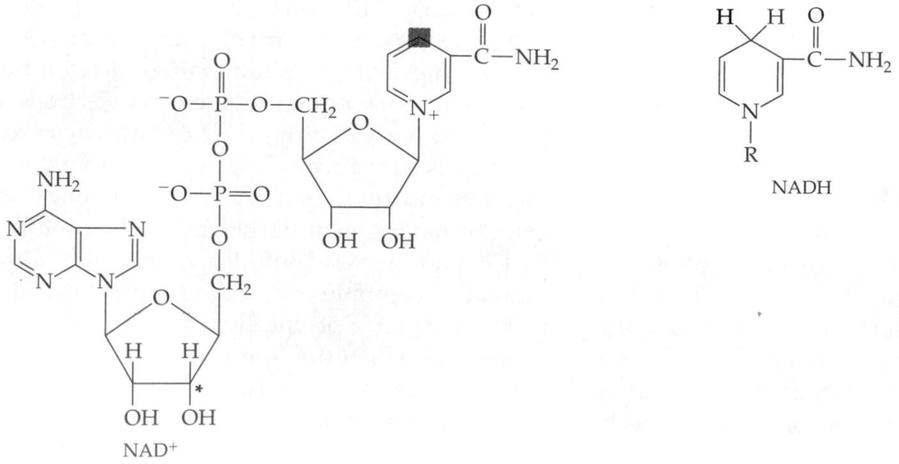

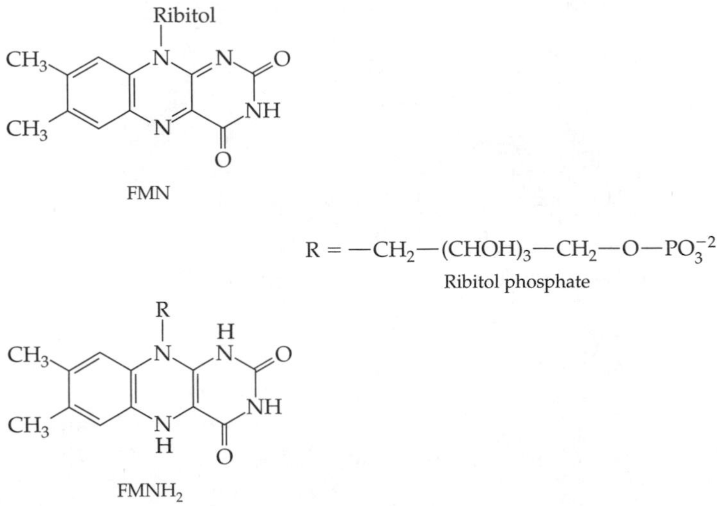

Figure 3.12 Flavin mononucleotide (FMN) and its reduced form ($FMNH_2$). Hydrogens transferred from NADH and H^+ attach to the nitrogen atoms (colored blue in the structures). FMN is the phosphorylated derivative of the vitamin riboflavin (B_2). The cosubstrate FAD differs from FMN in that the ribitol phosphate side chain is linked to adenosine monophosphate (AMP) via a pyrophosphate bond. The site of hydrogen atom attachment to FAD is the same as with FMN.

The iron-sulfur centers, or iron-sulfur proteins, referred to earlier also function as electron carriers in the electron transport chain. The iron in these compounds is not in the form of heme, as it is in the cytochromes, but rather is associated with inorganic sulfur atoms and/or the sulfur atoms in the cysteine amino acid residues of the protein. Two arrangements in which these iron-sulfur centers exist are shown in Figure 3.15.

The components of the electron transport chain are compartmentalized into four different complexes, each of which represents a portion of the chain. Each complex has its own unique composition and catalyzes the transfer of electrons through that portion of the chain. Complexes I and II catalyze electron transfer to CoQ from two different electron donors: NADH (Complex I) and succinate, through $FADH_2$ (Complex II). Complex III carries electrons from CoQ to cytochrome c, and Complex IV completes the sequence by transferring electrons from cytochrome c to O_2. Figure 3.16 shows the sequential order of the electron transport intermediates and their division into the four component complexes. The flow of electrons from NADH to O_2 is "downhill," meaning that each component has a more negative $E_{0'}$ value than its partner on the O_2 side and that energy is released at each step in the sequence. However, the $\Delta E_{0'}$ between the redox pairs varies considerably, and, accordingly, so does the quantity of energy released. The $\Delta G^{0'}$ for each reaction site, calculated from the corresponding $\Delta E_{0'}$ values, is shown in Table 3.2.

At three sites the release of energy is sufficient to effect the phosphorylation of ADP, meaning that for each molecule of NADH reoxidized to NAD^+ by O_2 via the electron transport chain, three ATPs are generated. These sites of oxidative phosphorylation are indicated in Table 3.2 and Figure 3.16. It is important to point out that the number of ATPs produced by oxidative phosphorylation is lower if the dehydrogenase reaction uses the flavin cosubstrate FAD rather than NAD^+. This is because CoQ collects electrons directly from $FADH_2$ through an iron-sulfur center, thereby bypassing the NAD^+-FMN-CoQ phosphorylation site. Therefore, the FAD-requiring succinate dehydrogenase reaction generates only two ATPs rather than three.

Figure 3.13 Oxidized and reduced forms of coenzyme Q, or ubiquinone. The blue groups function in the transfer of hydrogen atoms. The subscript n indicates the number of isoprenoid units in the side chain (most commonly 10).

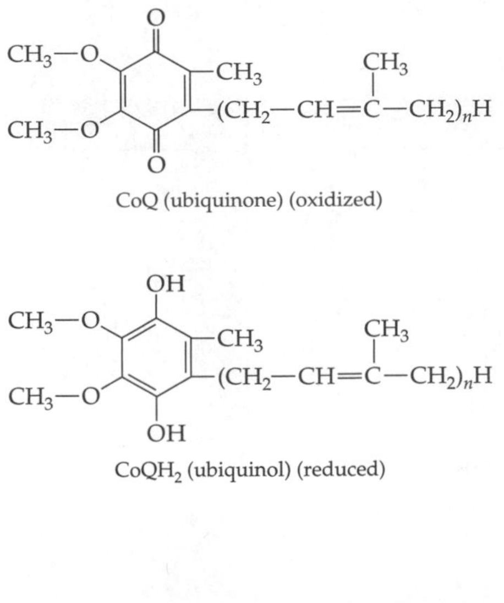

Membrane Location of the Electron Transport Chain

The location of the electron transport chain within the mitochondrion, discussed earlier, is of prime importance

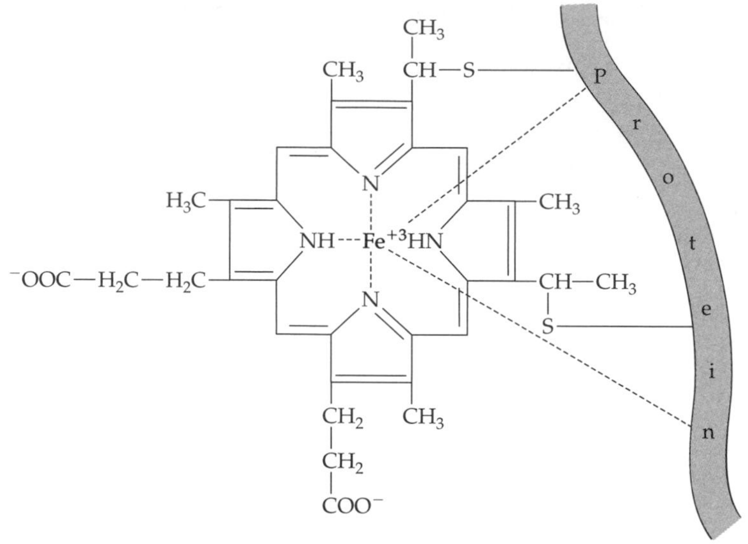

Figure 3.14 Oxidized cytochrome c. In its reduced form, the iron exists as Fe^{+2}.

because it is associated with the predominate theory of the production of ATP. The components of the electron transport chain are positioned within the inner membrane of the mitochondrion and thus are opportunistically situated to facilitate the uptake of electrons from substrates and deliver them to molecular oxygen. Complex I, for example, is oriented so that it can easily interact with the NADH produced by any of the dehydrogenases active in the matrix. The positioning of Complex IV (also called cytochrome oxidase) facilitates its picking up of electrons from Complex III and transferring them to O_2 on the matrix side of the membrane. Cytochrome c, in the intermembrane space, shuttles the electrons from Complex III to Complex IV. The spatial arrangement of the electron transport chain is illustrated schematically in Figure 3.17. Notice that electron flow through Complexes I, III, and IV is accompanied by the translocation of protons from the matrix into the intermembrane space. It is thought that the energy required to phosphorylate ADP to ATP is supplied by this concentration gradient of protons. This theory, known as the **chemiosmotic theory,** will be discussed more in the next section.

The intimate association of energy release with oxidation is exemplified by the oxidation of the fatty acid palmitate shown in Figure 3.2. These reactions occur in the mitochondria. The difference in $E_{0'}$ values between the NAD^+-NADH and the $\frac{1}{2}O_2$-H_2O systems makes it possible to calculate the overall change in free energy across the entire electron transport chain:

$$\Delta E_{0'} = E_{0'}(O_2) - E_{0'}(NAD^+)$$
$$= 0.82 - (-0.32) = 1.14 \text{ volts}$$

Then

$$\Delta G^{0'} = -2(23{,}062)(1.14) = -52{,}581 \text{ cal/mol}$$

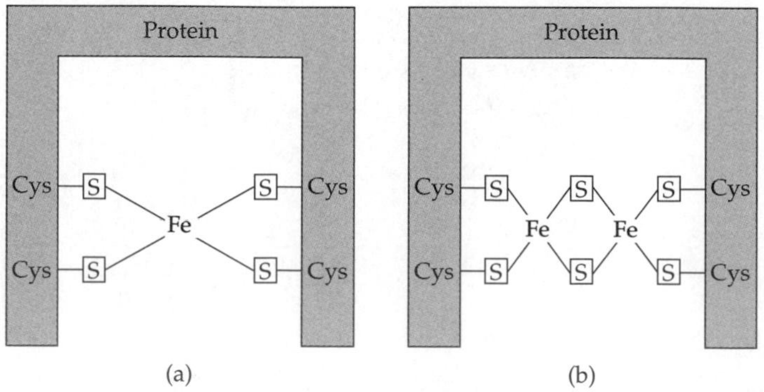

Figure 3.15 A schematic representation of the binding of iron ions in the iron-sulfur centers of the mitochondrial electron transport system. Sulfur atoms can be covalently attached to the protein via cysteine amino acid residues (a), or they can, in addition, be free, as shown in structure (b).

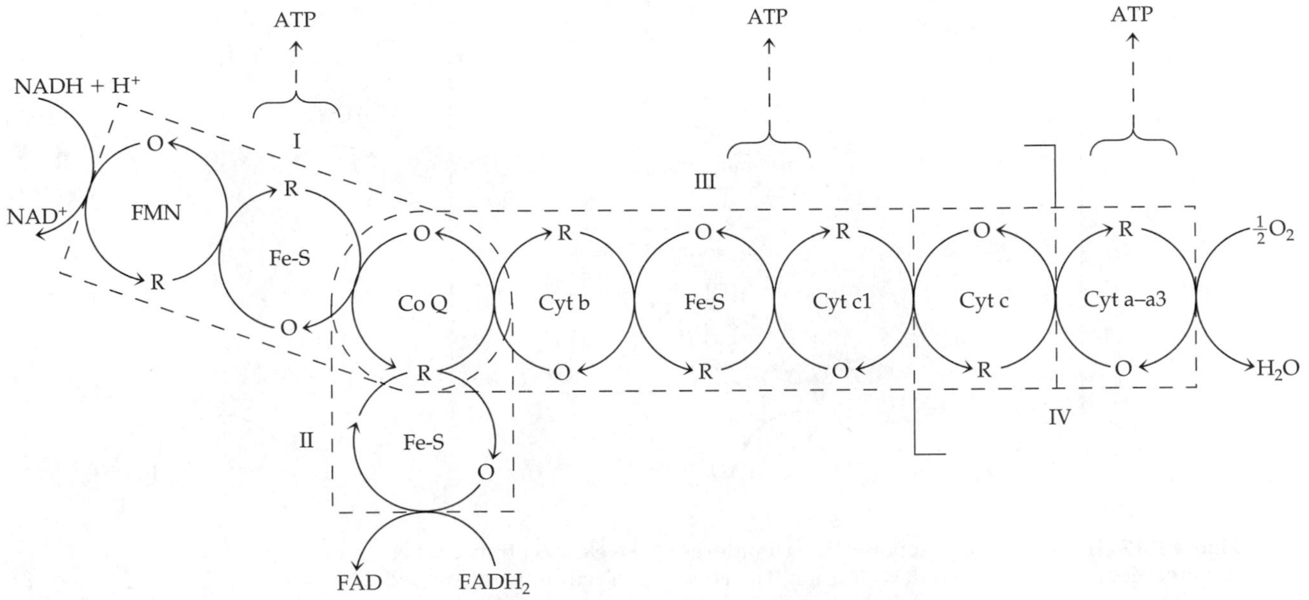

Figure 3.16 The sequential arrangement of the components of the electron transport chain, showing its division into four complexes, I, II, III, and IV. Coenzyme Q (ubiquinone) is shared by Complexes I, II, and III. Cyt c is shared by Complexes III and IV. Reduced cosubstrates, NADH and $FADH_2$, released in the matrix by dehydrogenase enzymes, are ultimately reoxidized by molecular oxygen as the intermediates undergo reversible reduction (R) and oxidation (O). Also indicated are the sites in Complexes I, III, and IV where electron transfers between reduction-oxidation pairs furnish enough energy for the synthesis of ATP from ADP.

Under the standard conditions, 21,900 cal/mol (3 × 7,300) of this total energy is conserved for future use as ATP, while the remaining 30,681 calories, representing close to 60% of the total, is released in the form of heat necessary to help maintain a normal body temperature.

Chemiosmotic Theory

According to the chemiosmotic theory, the precise mechanism by which the energy from electron transport is used to synthesize ATP is thought to be the translocation of the protons. In 1997 Paul Boyer and John Walker shared the Nobel Prize for chemistry for their work on the enzyme ATP synthase, the enzyme that catalyzes the formation of ATP. A review of Paul Boyer's research on ATP synthase is a summation of several decades of work [1]. A brief overview of this theory follows.

Energy released by the downhill (lower to higher $E_{0'}$ values) flow of electrons in Complexes I, III, and IV is used to pump protons, against a concentration gradient, from the matrix into the intermembrane space. This produces a marked disparity in both proton concentration and electrical charge on either side of the membrane. Permeating the membrane are proton channels, through which protons passively diffuse back into the matrix from the intermembrane space (Fig. 3.18). The driving force for the diffusion is the large difference in proton concentration in the two compartments. The channels are constructed from protein aggregates and exist as two distinct sectors designated F_1 and F_0. F_1 is the catalytic sector and resides on the matrix side of the membrane. F_0 is the membrane sector and is involved primarily with proton translocation (Fig. 3.18). Together, these components comprise what is called the F_0F_1 ATPase (or ATP-synthase) aggregate, also referred to as Complex V.

The return flow of protons furnishes the energy necessary for the synthesis of ATP from ADP and P_i. The proton flow is directed by the F_0 sector to the F_1

Table 3.2 Free Energy Changes at Various Sites within the Electron Transport Chain Showing Phosphorylation Sites

Reaction	$\Delta G^{0'}$ (cal/mol)	ADP Phosphorylation
NAD+ ⟶ FMN	−922	
FMN ⟶ CoQ	−15,682	ADP + P ⟶ ATP
CoQ ⟶ cyt b	−1,380	
cyt b ⟶ cyt c1	−7,380	ADP + P ⟶ ATP
cyt c1 ⟶ cyt c	−922	
cyt c ⟶ cyt a	−1,845	
cyt a ⟶ $\frac{1}{2}O_2$	−24,450	ADP + P ⟶ ATP

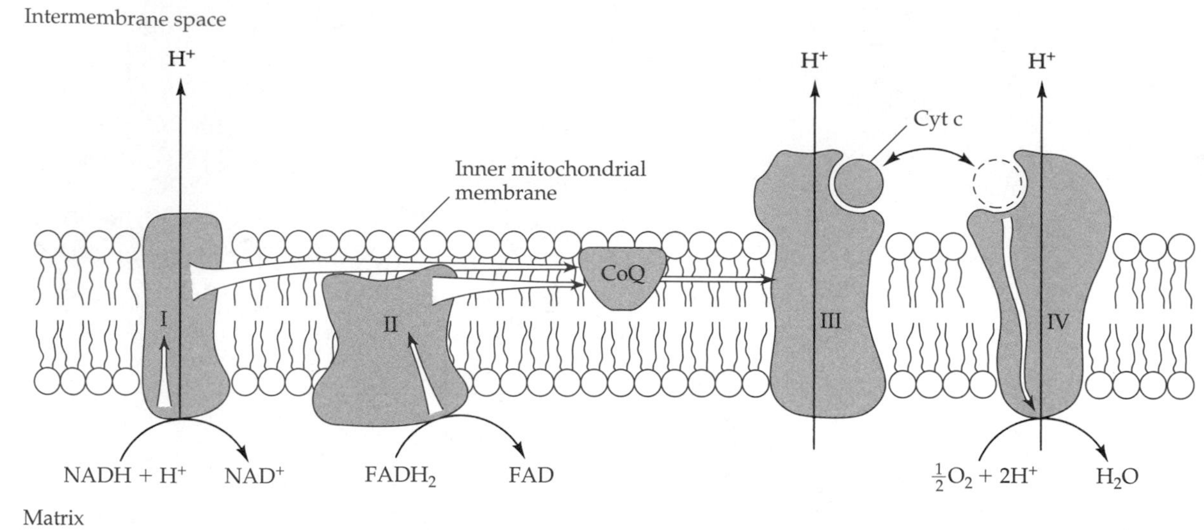

Figure 3.17 The spatial orientation of the complexes of the electron transport chain in the inner membrane of the mitochondrion. The energy of electron flow from reduced cosubstrates (NADH and $FADH_2$) to oxygen, within Complexes I, III, and IV, pumps protons from the matrix to the intermembrane space against a concentration gradient.

headpiece, which has binding sites for ADP and P_i. One oxygen atom of the inorganic phosphate is believed to react with two of the energetic protons, eliminating H_2O from the molecule. The precise mechanism of phosphorylation is complicated and involves the spatial movement of the complex protein. Earlier, it was stated that the energy available from the oxidation of NADH ($+H^+$) is sufficient to produce three ATPs by the phosphorylation of three ADPs. Current research based on the number of protons translocated suggests

Figure 3.18 An illustration of the chemiosmotic theory of oxidative phosphorylation. Energy from electron transport pumps protons into the intermembrane space from the matrix against a concentration gradient. The passive diffusion of protons back into the matrix through the F_0F_1 ATP-synthase aggregate furnishes the energy to synthesize ATP from ADP and inorganic phosphate. For more details, see the text.

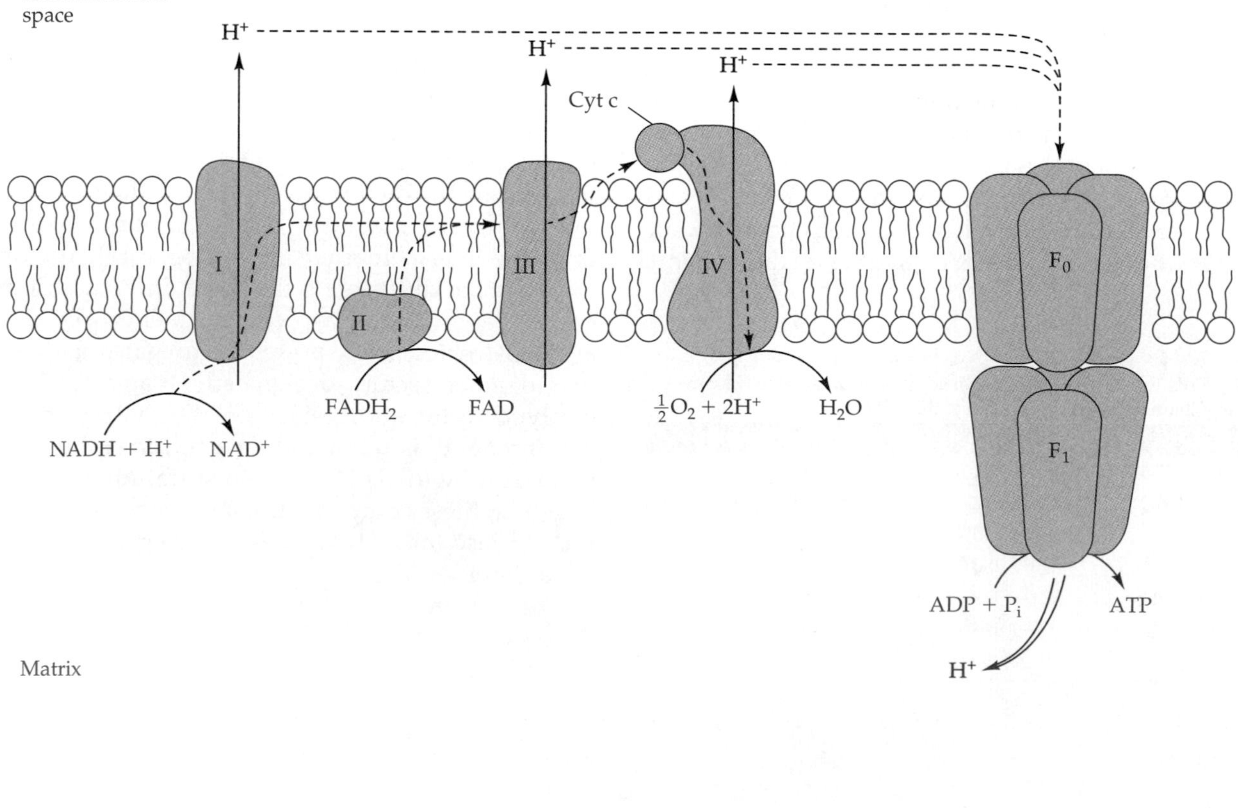

that the theoretical number is 2.5 ATPs produced for each NAD^+. This number accounts for the substrates for ATPase—ADP and P_i—that must be actively transported into the mitochondrion from the cytoplasm, as well as the product, ATP, that must be actively transported out. The estimated number of ATPs formed from NADH oxidation is therefore more realistically 2.5 rather than 3, and from $FADH_2$ the number is 1.5 rather than 2. Throughout this text, however, we will adhere to the convention of ascribing the values 3 and 2 to the number of moles of ATP produced from the oxidation of molar amounts of NADH and $FADH_2$, respectively. A schematic representation of the chemiosmotic theory of oxidative phosphorylation is shown in Figure 3.18. Comprehensive reviews of electron transport, oxidative phosphorylation, and chemiosmotic coupling are available to the interested reader [1–4].

summary

This chapter has dealt with a subject of vital importance in nutrition: the conversion of the energy contained within nutrient molecules into energy usable by the body. The major portion of this energy is needed to maintain normal body temperature, but much of it is also conserved in the form of high-energy phosphate bonds, principally ATP. The ATP can, in turn, activate various substrates by phosphorylation to higher energy levels from which they can undergo metabolism by specific enzymes. The exothermic hydrolysis of the ATP phosphate is sufficient to drive the endothermic phosphorylation, thereby completing the energy transfer from nutrient to metabolite.

ATP can be generated by two distinct mechanisms:

1. The transfer of a phosphate group from a very high energy phosphate donor to ADP, a process called substrate-level phosphorylation
2. Oxidative phosphorylation, by which the energy derived from mitochondrial electron transport is used to unite ADP with inorganic phosphate

Oxidative phosphorylation is the major route for ATP production. Electron flow in the electron transport chain is from reduced cosubstrates to molecular oxygen, which therefore becomes the ultimate oxidizing agent and which becomes reduced to H_2O in the process. The downhill flow of electrons and proton translocation generate sufficient energy to effect oxidative phosphorylation at multiple sites along the chain.

Chapter 4 focuses on carbohydrate metabolism, including the energy-releasing, systematic oxidation of glucose to CO_2 and H_2O. Within this pathway, reactions exemplifying both substrate-level and oxidative phosphorylation are encountered. The reader is encouraged to apply the principles of energy transformation learned in this chapter to the metabolic pathways of the energy nutrients in chapters that follow. More specifically, it should be recalled that electron transport is called into play whenever a mitochondrial dehydrogenation reaction occurs. It is important to understand the link between the controlled oxidation of the energy nutrients and the ultimate uses of the released energy. Reference to this chapter will be made frequently to strengthen this important union of cellular processes.

References Cited

1. Boyer P. The ATP synthase—a splendid molecular machine. Annu Rev Biochem 1997;66:717–49.

2. Trumpower B, Gennis R. Energy transduction by cytochrome complexes in mitochondrial and bacterial respiration: the enzymology of coupling electron transfer reactions to transmembrane proton translocation. Annu Rev Biochem 1994;63:675–702.

3. Tyler D. ATP synthesis in mitochondria. In: The Mitochondrion in Health and Disease. New York: VCH Publishers, Inc., 1992, pp. 353–402.

4. Hatefi Y. The mitochondrial electron transport and oxidative phosphorylation system. Annu Rev Biochem 1985;54:1015–69.

Suggested Readings

Garrett RH, Grisham CM. Electron Transport and Oxidative Phosphorylation in Biochemistry, 2nd ed. Fort Worth: Harcourt College Publishers, 1999, Chap. 21.

Jequier E, Acheson K, Schutz Y. Assessment of energy expenditure and fuel utilization in man. Annu Rev Nutr 1987;7:187–208. The assessment of nutrient energy use is emphasized in this review of energy expenditure.

Web Sites

www.nlm.nih.gov
National Library of Medicine: MEDLINE

www.med.jhu.edu
Johns Hopkins InfoNet

perspective

If Oxidation and Phosphorylation Disconnect: A Waste of Energy!

Revisiting the highlights of Chapter 3, we see that energy transformation in the cell has two major components:

- **oxidation,** which involves removing electrons (and hydrogens) from a substrate molecule and passing them along the components of the electron transport chain to O_2, and
- **phosphorylation,** which involves harnessing the energy released by the electron flow to synthesize ATP from ADP and P_i and applying "leftover" energy (better than 50% of the total energy released) toward the maintenance of normal body temperature.

According to the chemiosmotic theory of ATP synthesis, a substantial disparity of positive electrical charge exists in the matrix and intermembrane space of the mitochondrion. This disparity is the result of proton pumping from the matrix across the inner membrane into the intermembrane space, the energy for which comes from the electron transport (oxidation) component. But the energy used directly to couple ADP with P_i comes from the return, passive coursing of the protons through the F_0F_1 ATPase channels as they move down the concentration gradient back into the matrix compartment.

What if, for any reason, a disruption of the proton gradient in the mitochondrion should arise, so that the difference in proton concentrations between the two compartments is reduced? The consequence would be a reduction in the passive flow of protons through the channels, impeding the synthesis of ATP. In fact, certain chemicals will disrupt the proton gradient. These chemicals are called uncouplers of oxidative phosphorylation because, although they do not interfere with electron flow (oxidation), they hinder ATP synthesis (phosphorylation). In other words, they uncouple oxidation from phosphorylation.

Certain weak organic acids act as chemical uncouplers. The one probably studied most thoroughly and the one first identified as an uncoupler is 2,4-dinitrophenol. It is shown here in its acidic (protonated) form and its basic (dissociated) form:

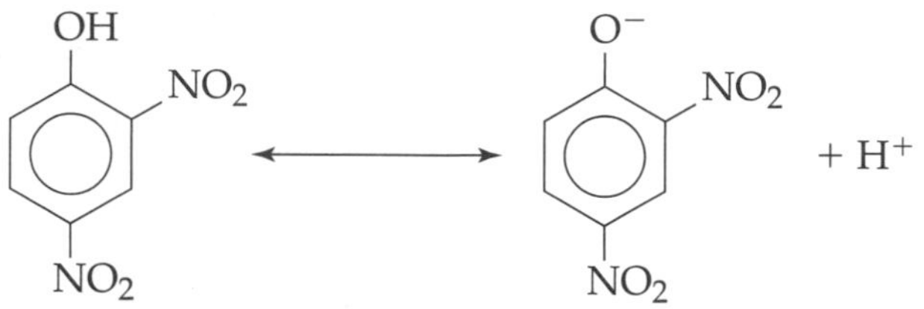

Acid form   Base form

2,4-dinitrophenol is not of particular interest from a nutritional or medicinal standpoint, however, because it is neither a dietary supplement nor a drug. Therefore, the remainder of our discussion focuses on another, more familiar, uncoupler to which any reader of this text can relate, namely, salicylic acid. Salicylic acid is the major metabolite of the wonder drug aspirin (acetylsalicylic acid). As a weak acid, salicylic acid, like 2,4-dinitrophenol, exists in protonated and dissociated forms:

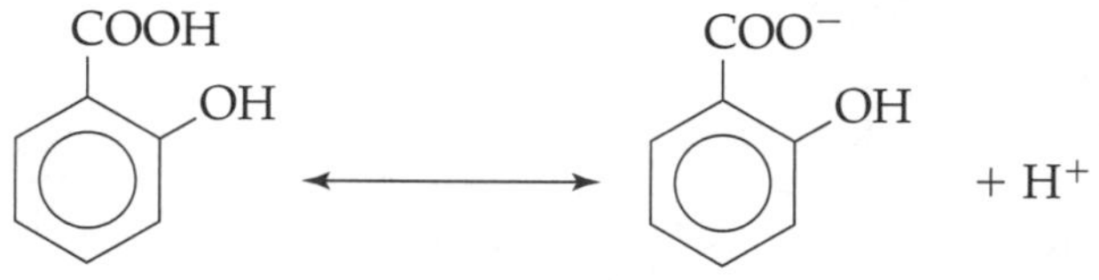

Acid form   Base form

In an environment of low pH (high proton concentration), the basic form of a weak acid acquires a proton and is converted to the acid form. The acid form, in a region of higher pH (low proton concentration), releases its proton and reverts to its basic form. This establishes the premise of how salicylic acid can perturb the delicate proton gradient across the mitochondrial inner membrane. The compound enters the mitochondrion through the outer membrane of the organelle, where it encounters the low pH of the intermembrane space. There it acquires a proton and assumes its acidic, uncharged form. As such, it is quite lipid-soluble and can readily permeate membranes. The protonated salicylic acid passes freely through the inner membrane, carrying with it, of course, the proton it acquired in the intermembrane space. Upon entering the high pH environment of the matrix, the compound releases the proton as it reverts to its basic form. Therefore, the salicylic acid, our example of a chemical uncoupler, acts as a carrier of protons from the intermembrane space across the inner membrane and into the matrix, as illustrated in Figure 1.

The uncoupler's effect of reducing the disparity of proton concentration on either side of the inner membrane reduces the proton flux through the ATPase channels, thereby inhibiting ATP synthesis. It is important to understand, however, that uncouplers do not interfere with electron transport, the source of energy for pumping protons in the first place. Recall from the discussion in Chapter 3 that approximately 40% of the total energy released by electron transport is consumed in the synthesis of ATP, with the remaining 60% manifesting as heat in the maintenance of body temperature. In the wake of the uncoupler effect, which denies ATP synthesis, essentially all oxidation energy manifests as heat. The result is hyperpyrexia (high body temperature)—indeed, a waste of energy and, more important, dangerous physiologically.

It must be emphasized that the hyperpyretic effect of aspirin is incurred only at very high, toxic doses of the drug. However, an interesting dichotomy is associated with aspirin intake. At normal, therapeutic doses, aspirin acts very effectively as an antipyretic, reducing infection-associated fever. On

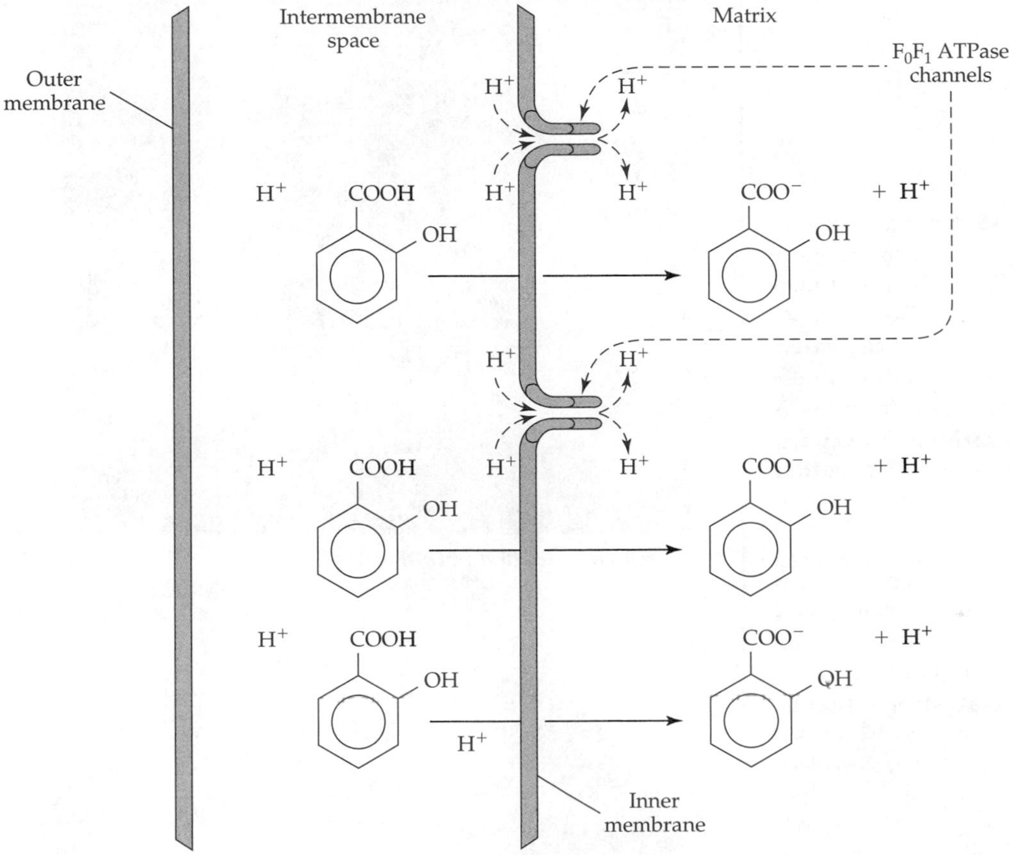

Figure 1 The diffusion of the protonated (acid) form of salicylic acid through the mitochondrial inner membrane and the release of its protons in the matrix. The process reduces the proton concentration gradient across the membrane. This slows the passage of protons through the ATPase channels and interferes with ATP synthesis.

the other hand, as explained in this perspective, toxic levels exhibit the opposite effect. Aspirin overdosing is not common among adults, but it is an all-too-common occurrence with toddlers attracted to its candylike appearance and texture.

Web Site

www.nlm.nih.gov
National Library of Medicine: MEDLINE

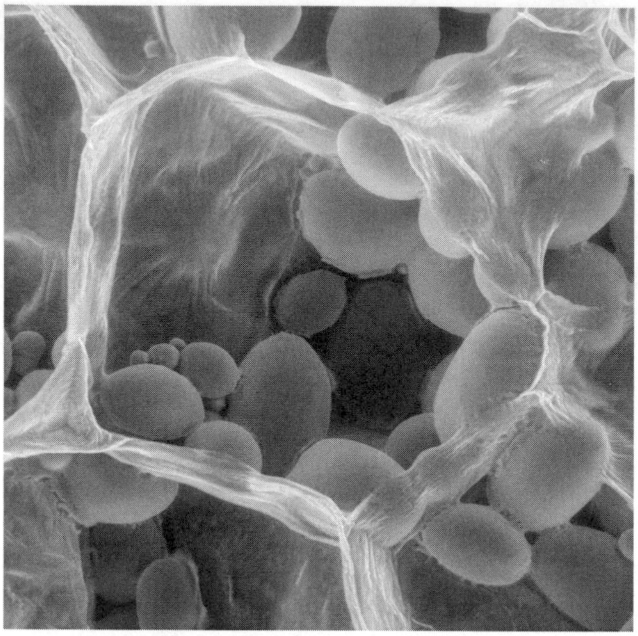

Starch granules in a potato cell

chapter 4 Carbohydrates

THE MAJOR SOURCE OF ENERGY FUEL in the average human diet is carbohydrate, supplying nearly half of the total caloric intake. Roughly half of dietary carbohydrate is in the form of polysaccharides such as starches and dextrins, derived largely from cereal grains and vegetables. The remaining half is supplied as simple sugars, the most important of which include sucrose, lactose, and, to a lesser extent, maltose, glucose, and fructose.

Carbohydrates are polyhydroxy aldehydes or ketones, or substances that produce these compounds when hydrolyzed. They are constructed from the atoms of carbon, oxygen, and hydrogen. These atoms occur in a proportion that approximates that of a "hydrate of carbon," CH_2O, accounting for the term *carbohydrate.* Carbohydrates comprise three major classes: the monosaccharides, the oligosaccharides, and the polysaccharides.

- **Monosaccharides** are structurally the simplest form of carbohydrate in that they cannot be reduced in size to smaller carbohydrate units by hydrolysis. Monosaccharides are called simple sugars and are sometimes referred to as monosaccharide units. The most abundant monosaccharide in nature—and certainly the most important nutritionally—is the 6-carbon sugar glucose.

- **Oligosaccharides** consist of short chains of monosaccharide units joined by covalent bonds. The number of units is designated by the prefixes *di-*, *tri-*, *tetra-*, and so on, followed by the word *saccharide.* Among the oligosaccharides, the disaccharides, with just two monosaccharide units, are the most abundant. Within this group, sucrose, consisting of one glucose and one fructose residue, is nutritionally most significant, furnishing approximately one-third of total dietary carbohydrate in an average diet.
- **Polysaccharides** are long chains of monosaccharide units that may number from several into the hundreds or even thousands. The major polysaccharides of interest in nutrition are glycogen, found in certain animal tissues, and starch and cellulose, both of plant origin. All these polysaccharides consist of only glucose units.

STRUCTURAL FEATURES

Monosaccharides

As monosaccharides occur in nature or arise as intermediate products in digestion, they contain from three to seven carbon atoms and accordingly are termed trioses, tetroses, pentoses, hexoses, and heptoses. In addition to hydroxyl groups, these compounds possess a functional carbonyl group that can be either an aldehyde or a ketone, leading to the additional classification of aldoses, sugars having an aldehyde group, and ketoses, sugars possessing a ketone group. These two classifications together with the number of carbon atoms describe a particular monosaccharide. For example, a five-carbon sugar having a ketone group is a ketopentose, a six-carbon aldehyde-possessing sugar is an aldohexose, and so forth.

Stereoisomerism

A brief discussion of stereoisomerism as it relates to carbohydrates is provided here because most biological systems are stereospecific. (For a more extensive discussion, see Appendix A or a general biochemistry text [1].) Many organic substances, including the carbohydrates, are optically active: if plane-polarized light is passed through a solution of the substances, the plane of light will be rotated to the right (for dextrorotatory substances) or to the left (for levorotatory ones). The direction and extent of the rotation are characteristic of a particular compound and depend on the substance's concentration and temperature and the wavelength of the light. The right or left direction of light rotation is expressed as + (dextrorotatory) or − (levorotatory), and the number of angular degrees indicates the extent of rotation.

Optical activity is attributed to the presence of one or more asymmetrical or chiral carbon atoms in the molecule. **Chiral carbon** atoms have four different atoms or groups covalently attached to them. Because different groups are attached, it is not possible to move any two atoms or groups to other positions and rotate the new structure so it can be superimposed on the original. This moving of groups instead creates a pair of molecules that are mirror images of each other. The molecules are said to be enantiomers, a special class within a broader family of compounds called **stereoisomers.** Stereoisomers are compounds having two or more chiral carbon atoms that have the same four groups attached to those carbon atoms but are not mirror images of each other.

If an asymmetrical substance rotates the plane of polarized light a certain number of degrees to the right, its enantiomer will rotate the light the same number of degrees to the left. Enantiomers exist in D or L orientation, and if a compound is structurally D, its enantiomer will be L. The D and L designation does not predict the direction of rotation of plane-polarized light. Instead, the designation is simply a structural analogy to the reference compound glyceraldehyde, whose D and L forms are by convention drawn as shown in Figure 4.1. The distinction between D and L configurations of enantiomers therefore rests with the direction of the –OH bond on the single chiral carbon of the molecule. Note that in the D configuration it points to the right and in the L configuration to the left. Remember, these forms are not superimposable.

Monosaccharides with more than three carbons will have more than one chiral center. In such cases, the highest-numbered chiral carbon indicates whether the molecule is of the D or the L configuration. (For further explanation, see Appendix A.) Monosaccharides of the D configuration are much more important nutritionally than their L isomers because they exist as such in dietary carbohydrate and are metabolized specifically in that form. The reason for this is that the enzymes involved in carbohydrate digestion and metabolism are stereospecific for D sugars, meaning that they react only with D sugars and are inactive toward L forms.

Figure 4.1 Structural formulas of the D and L configurations of glyceraldehyde.

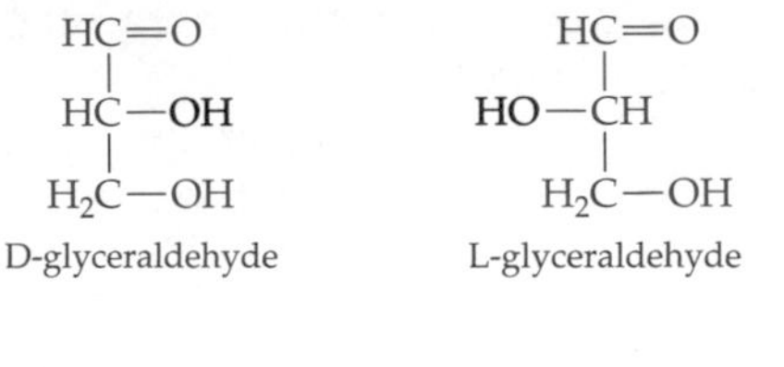

D-glyceraldehyde L-glyceraldehyde

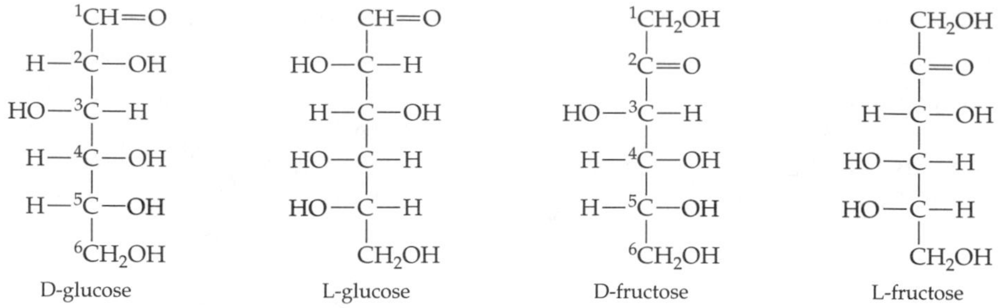

Figure 4.2 Structural (open-chain) models of the D and L forms of the monosaccharides glucose and fructose.

The structures in Figure 4.2 are shown as open-chain models, in which the carbonyl (aldehyde or ketone) functions are free. The monosaccharides generally do not exist in open-chain form, as explained later, but they are shown that way here to clarify the D-L concept and to illustrate the so-called **anomeric carbon,** the carbon atom comprising the carbonyl function. Notice that the anomeric carbon is number 1 in the aldose (glucose) and number 2 in the ketose (fructose).

Ring Structures

In solution, the monosaccharides do not exist in open-chain form, as evidenced by the fact that they do not undergo reactions characteristic of true aldehydes and ketones. Instead, the molecules cyclize, producing forms called hemiacetals if the sugar is an aldose and hemiketals if the sugar is a ketose. The hemiacetal or hemiketal bonds are formed by the reaction of an alcohol group with an aldehyde group or a ketone group, respectively. Therefore, the participating groups within a monosaccharide are the aldehyde or ketone of the anomeric carbon atom and the alcohol group attached to the highest-numbered chiral carbon atom, as illustrated in Table 4.1 using the examples of D-glucose, D-galactose, and D-fructose. The formation of the hemiacetal or hemiketal produces a new chiral center at the anomeric carbon, designated by an asterisk in the structures in Table 4.1, and therefore the bond direction of the newly formed hydroxyl becomes significant. In the cyclized structures shown (known as Fisher projections), the anomeric hydroxyls are arbitrarily positioned to the right, resulting in an alpha (α) configuration. If the anomeric hydroxyl were directed to the left, the structure would be in a beta (β) configuration. Cyclization to the hemiacetal or hemiketal can produce either the α- or the β-isomer. In aqueous solution, however, an equilibrium mixture of the isomers exists, with the concentration of the β form roughly twice that of the α form. In essence, the α-hemiacetal can change to the open structure and again form a ring, with either the α or the β configuration.

Stereoisomerism among the monosaccharides, and also among other nutrients such as amino acids and lipids, has important metabolic implications due to the stereospecificity of certain metabolic enzymes. An interesting example of stereospecificity is the action of the digestive enzyme α-amylase, which hydrolyzes polyglucose molecules such as the starches, in which the glucose units are connected through an α-linkage. Cellulose, also a polymer of glucose but one in which the monomeric glucose residues are connected by β-linkages, is resistant to α-amylase hydrolysis.

Haworth Models

The structures of the cyclized monosaccharides are more conveniently and accurately represented by Haworth models. In such models the carbons and oxygen comprising the five- or six-membered ring are depicted as lying in a horizontal plane, with the hydroxyl groups pointing down or up from the plane. Those groups directed to the right in the open-chain structure point down in the Haworth model, and those directed to the left point up. Table 4.1 shows the structural relationship of simple projection and Haworth formulas for the major naturally occurring hexoses: glucose, galactose, and fructose. Remember that in solution the cyclic monosaccharides open and close to form an equilibrium between the α and the β forms. Regardless of how the cyclic structure is written, the molecule will exist in both forms in solution unless the anomeric carbon has formed a chemical bond and is no longer able to open and close.

Pentoses

Compared to the hexoses (Table 4.1), pentose sugars furnish very little dietary energy due to their low content in the diet. However, they are readily synthesized in the cell from hexose precursors and are incorporated into metabolically important compounds. The aldopentose ribose, for example, is a constituent of key nucleotides such as the adenosine phosphates—adenosine triphosphate (ATP), adenosine diphosphate (ADP), adenosine monophosphate (AMP), cyclic adenosine monophosphate (cAMP), and the nicotinamide adenine dinucleotides (NAD^+, $NADP^+$). Ribose and its deoxygenated form, deoxyribose (Fig. 4.3), are also part of the structures of ribonucleic acid (RNA) and deoxyribonucleic acid (DNA), respectively. Ribitol, a reduction

Table 4.1 Various Structural Representations Among the Hexoses: Glucose, Galactose, and Fructose

Hexose	Fisher Projection	Cyclized Fisher Projection	Haworth	Simplified Haworth
α-D-glucose	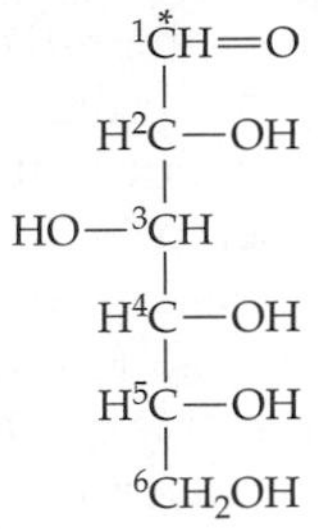	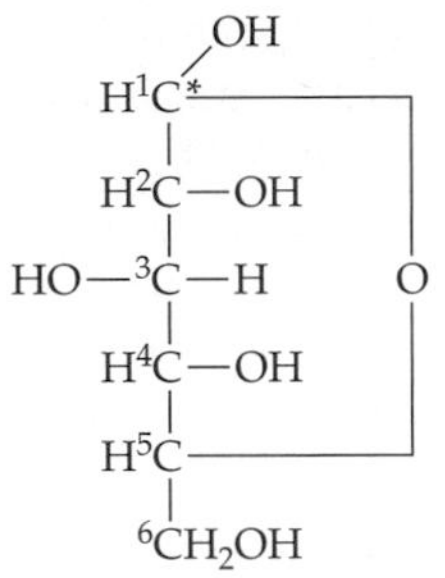	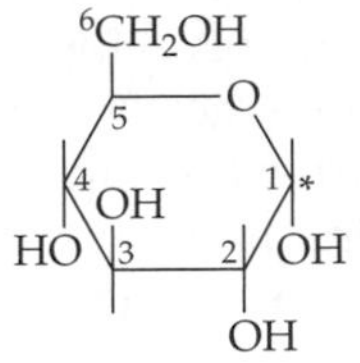	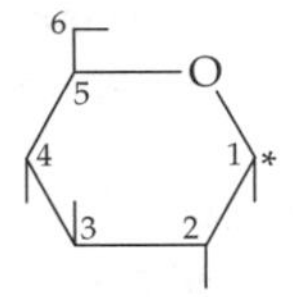
β-D-galactose	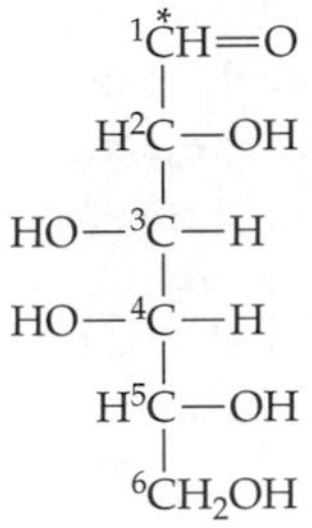	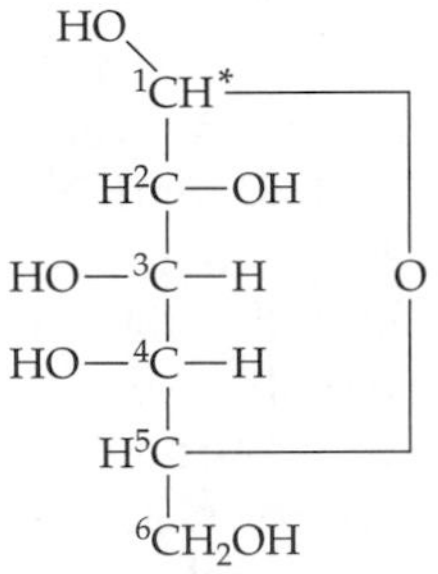	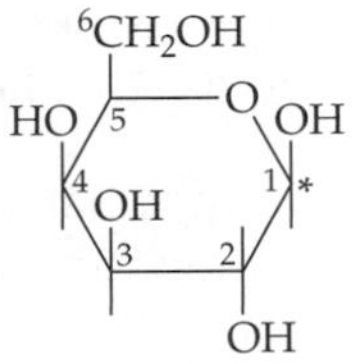	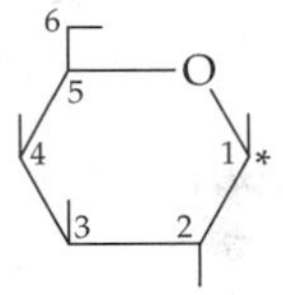
β-D-fructose	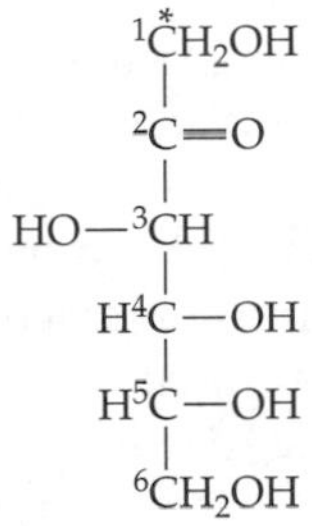	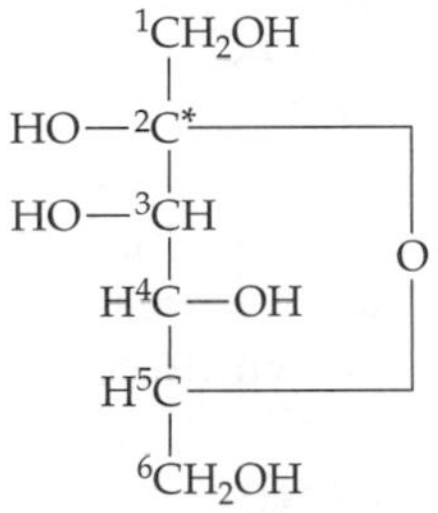	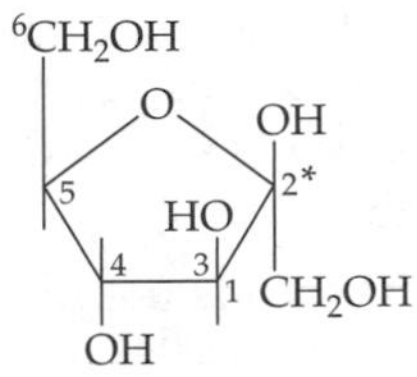	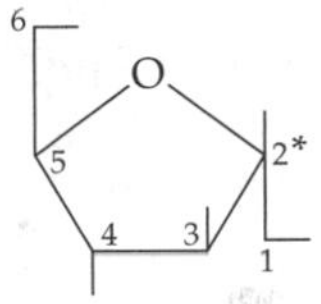

*The anomeric carbon.

product of ribose, is a constituent of the vitamin riboflavin and of the flavin coenzymes, flavin adenine dinucleotide (FAD) and flavin mononucleotide (FMN) (see Fig. 4.3).

Reducing Sugars

Monosaccharides that are cyclized into hemiacetals or hemiketals are sometimes referred to as reducing sugars because they are capable of reducing other substances, such as the copper ion from Cu^{2+} to Cu^{+}. This property is useful in identifying which end of a polysaccharide chain has the monosaccharide unit that can open and close. This role of reducing sugars is discussed in more detail in the section on polysaccharides.

Oligosaccharides

Oligosaccharides are short-chain polymers of monosaccharide units, generally from 2 to about 10 in number, attached to one another through acetal bonds. Acetal bonds, also called glycosidic bonds as they occur in the special case of carbohydrate structures, are formed between a hydroxyl group of one monosaccharide unit

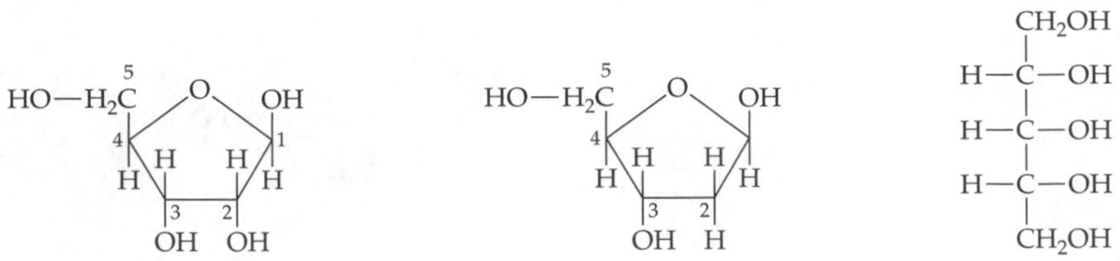

β-D-ribose β-D-2-deoxyribose Ribitol

Figure 4.3 Structural formulas of the pentoses ribose and deoxyribose and of the alcohol ribitol, a reduction product of ribose.

and a hydroxyl group of the next unit in the polymer, with the elimination of one molecule of water. **Disaccharides,** major energy-supplying nutrients, are the most common members of the oligosaccharide family. The glycosidic bonds generally involve the hydroxyl group on the anomeric carbon of one member of the pair of monosaccharides and the hydroxyl group on carbon 4 or 6 of the second member. Furthermore, the glycosidic bond can be α or β in orientation, depending on whether the anomeric hydroxyl group was α or β before the glycosidic bond was formed and on the specificity of the enzymatic reaction catalyzing their formation. Specific glycosidic bonds therefore may be designated α 1-4, β 1-4, α 1-6, and so on. The most common disaccharides are maltose, lactose, and sucrose (see Fig. 4.4).

- *Maltose* is formed primarily from the partial hydrolysis of starch and therefore is found in malt beverages such as beer and malt liquors. It consists of two glucose units linked through an α 1-4 glycosidic bond. The structure on the right in Figure 4.4a is shown in the β form, although it also may exist in the α form.
- *Lactose* is found naturally only in milk and milk products. It is composed of galactose linked by a β 1-4 glycosidic bond to glucose. The glucose can exist in either α or β form (see Fig. 4.4b).
- *Sucrose* (cane sugar, beet sugar) is the most widely distributed of the disaccharides and is the most commonly used natural sweetener. It is composed of glucose and fructose and is structurally unique in that its glycosidic bond involves the anomeric hydroxyl of both residues. The linkage is α with respect to the glucose residue and β with respect to the fructose residue (see Fig. 4.4c). Having no free hemiacetal or hemiketal function, sucrose is not a reducing sugar.

Polysaccharides

The glycosidic bonding of monosaccharide residues may be repeated many times to form high-molecular-weight polymers called polysaccharides. If the structure is composed of a single type of monomeric unit, it is referred to as a homopolysaccharide. If two or more different types of monosaccharides make up its structure, it is called a heteropolysaccharide. Both types exist in nature; however, homopolysaccharides are of far greater importance in nutrition because of their abundance in many natural foods. The polyglucoses starch and glycogen, for example, are the major storage forms of carbohydrate in plant and animal tissues, respectively. Polyglucoses range in molecular weight from a few thousand to 500,000.

The reducing property of a saccharide is useful in describing polysaccharide structure by enabling one end of a linear polysaccharide to be distinguished from the other. In a polyglucose chain, for example, the glucose residue at one end of the chain has a hemiacetal group because its anomeric carbon atom is not involved in acetal bonding to another glucose residue. The residue at the other end of the chain is not in hemiacetal form because it is attached by acetal bonding to the next residue in the chain. A linear polyglucose molecule therefore has a reducing end (the hemiacetal end) and a nonreducing end (at which no hemiacetal exists). This notation is useful in designating at which end of a polysaccharide certain enzymatic reactions occur.

Starch

The most common digestible polysaccharide in plants is starch. It can exist in two forms, amylose and amylopectin, both of which are polymers of D-glucose. The amylose molecule is a linear, unbranched chain in which the glucose residues are attached solely through α 1-4

Figure 4.4 The disaccharides maltose (a), lactose (b), and sucrose (c).

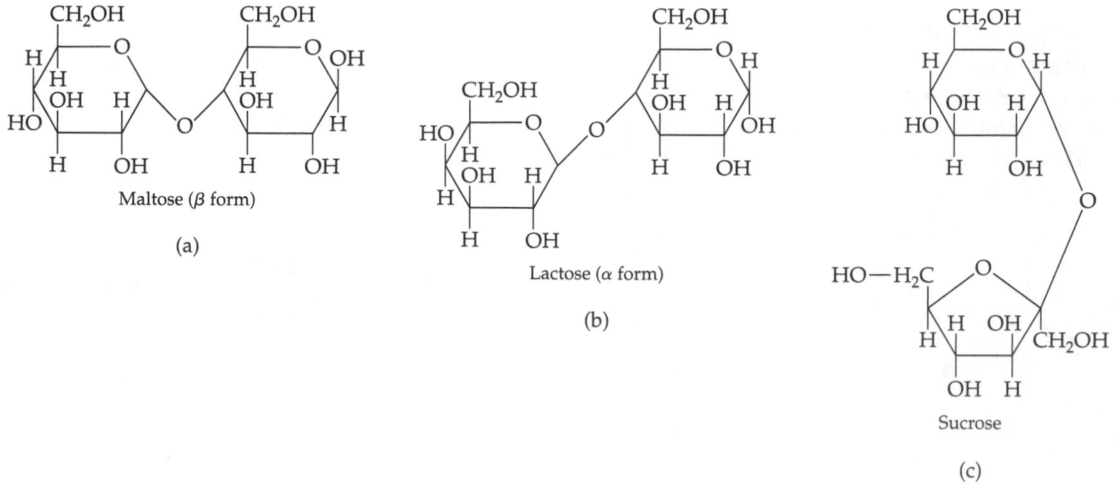

glycosidic bonds. In water, amylose chains adopt a helical conformation. Amylopectin, on the other hand, is a branched-chain polymer, with branch points occurring through α 1-6 bonds, as illustrated in Figure 4.5a. Both forms occur in cereal grains, potatoes, legumes, and other vegetables, with amylose contributing about 15% to 20% and amylopectin 80% to 85% of the total starch content.

Glycogen

The major form of stored carbohydrate in animal tissues is glycogen, which is localized primarily in liver and skeletal muscle. Like amylopectin, it is a highly branched polyglucose molecule. It differs from the starch only in the fact that it is more highly branched (see Fig. 4.5b). The glucose residues within glycogen serve as a readily available source of glucose. When dictated by the body's energy demands, glucose residues are sequentially removed enzymatically from the nonreducing ends of the glycogen chains and enter energy-releasing pathways of metabolism. This process, called **glycogenolysis,** is discussed later in this chapter. The high degree of branching in glycogen and amylopectin offers a distinct metabolic advantage, because it presents a large number of nonreducing ends from which glucose residues can be cleaved.

Figure 4.5 (a) A segment of the amylopectin molecule, illustrating an α 1-6 branch point as well as the α 1-4 linkages along the linear segments. Branch points may occur as frequently as every 25 to 30 residues. (b) Comparison of the gross structures of starch amylopectin and glycogen, showing the difference in the degree of branching. Circles represent glucose residues. Solid circles are those residues located at the nonreducing ends of chains. Only one reducing end is present in each molecule.

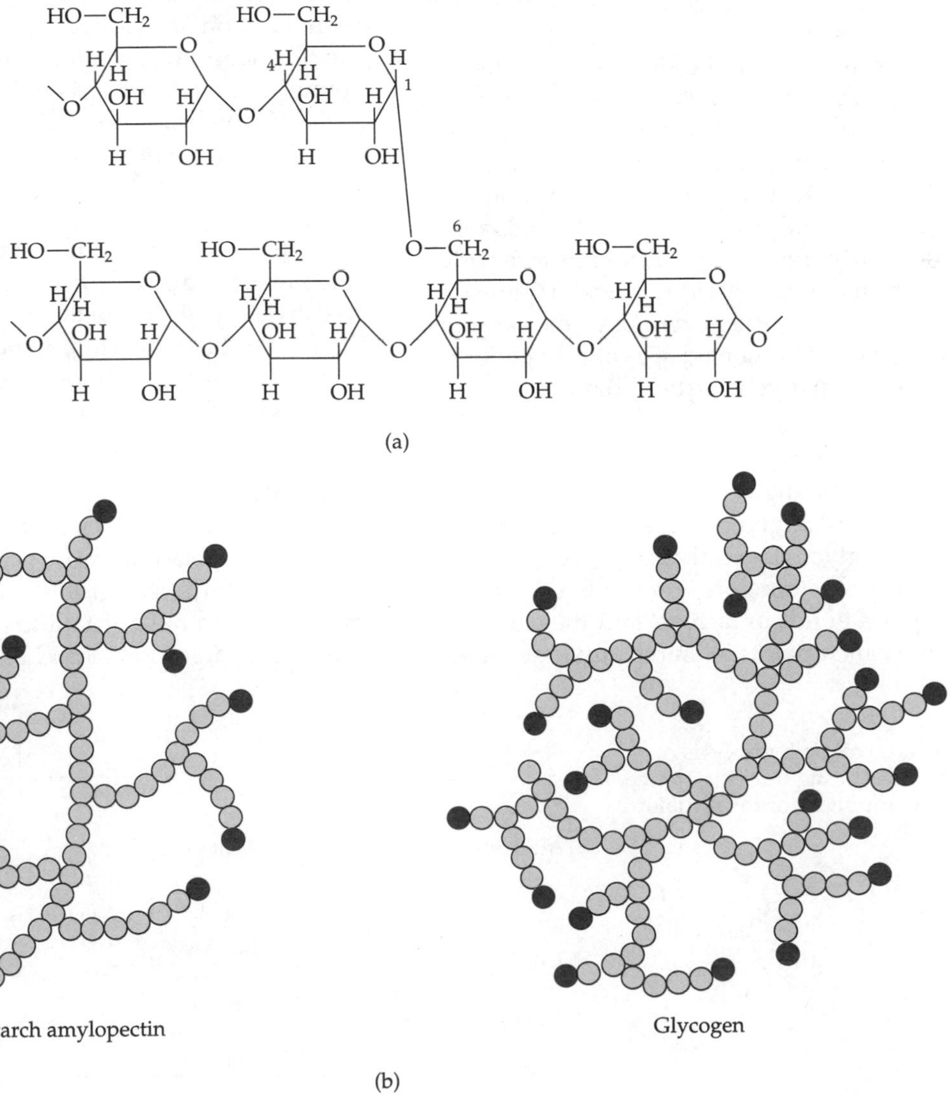

Cellulose

Cellulose is the major component of cell walls in plants. Like the starches, it is a homopolysaccharide of glucose. It differs from the starches in that the glycosidic bonds connecting the residues are β 1-4, rendering the molecule resistant to the digestive enzyme α-amylase, which is stereospecific to favor α 1-4 linkages. Because cellulose is not digestible by mammalian digestive enzymes, it is defined as a dietary fiber and is considered not to provide energy. However, as a source of fiber, cellulose assumes importance as a bulking agent and a potential energy source for some intestinal bacteria that are able to digest it (p. 109). The extent to which the energy is available for absorption in the human is debated. A very limited amount likely is available in the form of short-chain fatty acids.

DIGESTION

The most important dietary carbohydrates nutritionally are polysaccharides and disaccharides, because free monosaccharides are not commonly present in the diet in significant quantities. However, some free glucose and fructose are present in honey, certain fruits, and the carbohydrates added to processed foods. The cellular use of carbohydrates depends on their absorption from the gastrointestinal (GI) tract into the bloodstream, a process normally restricted to monosaccharides. Polysaccharides and disaccharides therefore must be hydrolyzed to their constituent monosaccharide units. The hydrolytic enzymes involved are collectively called **glycosidases** or, alternatively, **carbohydrases.**

Polysaccharides

The key enzyme in the digestion of dietary polysaccharides is α-amylase, a glycosidase that specifically hydrolyzes α 1-4 glycosidic linkages. Resistant to the action of this enzyme, therefore, are the β 1-4 bonds of cellulose, the β 1-4 bonds of lactose, and the α 1-6 linkages that form branch points in starch amylopectin.

Digestion of starches actually begins in the mouth, because α-amylase activity is found in saliva. Given the short period of time that food is in the mouth prior to being swallowed, this phase of digestion produces few monosaccharides. However, the salivary amylase action continues in the stomach until the gastric acid penetrates the food bolus and lowers the pH sufficiently to inactivate the enzyme. By this point, partial hydrolysis of the starches has occurred, with the major products being dextrins, which are short-chain polysaccharides, and maltose. Further digestion of the dextrins is resumed in the small intestine by the α-amylase of pancreatic origin, which is secreted into the duodenal contents. Here the presence of pancreatic bicarbonate elevates the pH to a level favorable for enzymatic function. If the dietary starch form is amylose, which is unbranched, the products of α-amylase hydrolysis are maltose and the trisaccharide maltotriose, which undergoes slower hydrolysis to maltose and glucose. The hydrolytic action of α-amylase on amylopectin, a branched starch, produces glucose and maltose, as it does with amylose. However, the α 1-6 bonds linking the glucose residues at the branch points of the molecule cannot be hydrolyzed by α-amylase. Consequently, disaccharide units called isomaltose, possessing α 1-6 glycosidic bonds, are released.

In summary, the action of α-amylase on dietary starch releases maltose, isomaltose, and glucose as principal hydrolytic products, as illustrated in Figure 4.6. The further breakdown of the disaccharide products to glucose is brought about by specific glycosidases described in the section on disaccharides below.

Resistant Starches

Crystalline starch is insoluble in water and is nondigestible. It is gelatinized by heating (such as in cooking) and in this form is digestible. On cooling, some starch reverts back to the crystalline form and again becomes resistant to digestion. Starches also can be chemically

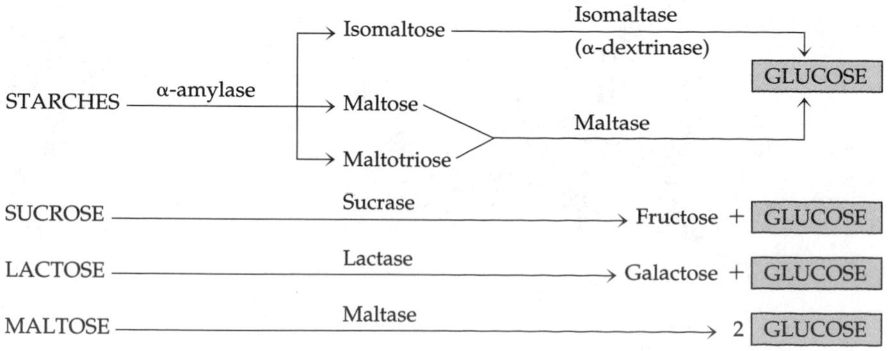

Figure 4.6 The enzymatic hydrolysis of carbohydrates, illustrating the importance of glucose as a component of these major nutrients.

modified to make them more resistant to digestion, for example, modifying the starch by increasing the cross-linking between chains.

Disaccharides

Virtually no digestion of disaccharides or small oligosaccharides occurs in the mouth or stomach. In the human, digestion takes place entirely in the upper small intestine. Unlike α-amylase activity, disaccharidase activity occurs in the microvilli of the intestinal mucosal cells (the brush border) rather than in the intestinal lumen. Among the enzymes located on the mucosal cells are lactase, sucrase, maltase, and isomaltase. Lactase catalyzes the cleavage of lactose to equimolar amounts of galactose and glucose. As was pointed out earlier, lactose is a β 1-4 linkage, and lactase is stereospecific for this beta linkage. Sucrase hydrolyzes sucrose to yield one glucose and one fructose residue. Maltase hydrolyzes maltose to yield two glucose units. Isomaltase (also called α-dextrinase) hydrolyzes the α 1-6 bond of isomaltose, the branch-point disaccharide remaining from the incomplete breakdown of amylopectin; the products are two molecules of glucose.

In summary, nearly all dietary starches and disaccharides ultimately are hydrolyzed completely by specific glycosidases to their constituent monosaccharide units. Monosaccharides, together with small amounts of remaining disaccharides, can then be absorbed by the intestinal mucosal cells. The reactions involved in the digestion of starches and disaccharides are summarized in Figure 4.6.

ABSORPTION, TRANSPORT, AND DISTRIBUTION

The wall of the small intestine is composed of absorptive mucosal cells and mucus-secreting goblet cells that line projections, called villi, that extend into the lumen. On the surface on the lumen side, the absorptive cells have hairlike projections called microvilli (the brush border). A square millimeter of cell surface is believed to have as many as 2×10^5 microvilli projections. The microstructure of the small intestinal wall is illustrated in Figures 2.5 and 2.6. The anatomic advantage of the villi-microvilli structure is that it presents an enormous surface area to the intestinal contents, thereby facilitating absorption. The absorptive capacity of the human intestine has been estimated to amount to about 5,400 g/day for glucose and 4,800 g/day for fructose—a capability that would never be reached in a normal diet.

Absorption of Glucose and Galactose

Glucose and galactose are absorbed into the mucosal cells by active transport, a process that requires energy and the involvement of a specific receptor. The glucose-galactose carrier has been designated sodium-glucose transporter 1 (SGLT1). It is known to be a protein complex dependent on the Na^+/K^+-ATPase pump, which, at the expense of ATP, furnishes energy for the transport of sugar through the mucosal cell. Glucose or galactose cannot attach to the carrier until the carrier has been preloaded with Na^+. Mutation in the SGLT1 gene is associated with glucose-galactose malabsorption.

Glucose appears to leave the mucosal cell at the basolateral surface by three routes. Approximately 15% leaks back across the brush border into the intestinal lumen, about 25% diffuses through the basolateral membrane into the circulation, and the major portion (~60%) is transported from the cell into the circulation via a carrier in the serosal membrane. A small portion of the available glucose may be used by the mucosal cell for its energy needs.

Absorption of Fructose

The absorption mechanism for fructose is not completely resolved. Some evidence suggests active transport, because fructose uptake has been shown to occur against a concentration gradient. Such transport is independent of the active, Na^+-dependent transport of glucose, but the rate of uptake is much slower than that of both glucose and galactose. A large proportion of human subjects studied showed an inability to absorb completely doses of fructose in the range of 20 to 50 g [2]. Fructose, in the absence of glucose, also may be absorbed by facilitated transport involving a specific transporter. In fact, it is likely that GLUT5 (see the section "Glucose Transporters") may be the transporter for fructose [3]. The facilitative transport process can proceed only down a concentration gradient. Because fructose is very efficiently trapped and phosphorylated by the liver, however, there is virtually no circulating fructose in the bloodstream, ensuring its downhill concentration gradient across the intestinal mucosa.

Although fructose absorption takes place more slowly than that of glucose or galactose, which are actively absorbed, it is absorbed faster than sugars such as sorbitol and xylitol, which are absorbed purely by passive diffusion. The extent of the contribution of active transport and facilitative diffusion to fructose absorption has not been established, though both systems are saturable. This accounts for the observations that fructose absorption is limited in nearly 60% of normal adults and that intestinal distress, symptomatic of malabsorption, frequently appears following ingestion of 50 g of pure fructose [4]. This level of intake is commonly found in high-fructose syrups used as sweeteners. Interestingly, coconsumption of glucose with fructose accelerates the absorption of fructose and raises the threshold level of fructose ingestion at which malabsorption symptoms appear [4]. This suggests that the pair of monosaccharides might be absorbed by a so-called disaccharidase-related transport system designed to transport the hydrolytic products of sucrose [2].

Monosaccharide Transport and Cellular Uptake

Following transport across the gut wall, the monosaccharides enter the portal circulation, where they are carried directly to the liver. The liver is the major site of metabolism of galactose and fructose, which are readily taken up by the liver via specific hepatocyte receptors. They enter these cells by facilitated transport and subsequently are metabolized. Both fructose and galactose can be converted to glucose derivatives through pathways that we will discuss later and then stored as liver glycogen, or they may be catabolized for energy according to the liver's energy demand. The blood levels of galactose and fructose are not directly subject to the strict hormonal regulation that is such an important part of glucose homeostasis. However, if their dietary intake is a significantly higher than normal percentage of total carbohydrate intake, they may be regulated indirectly as glucose because of their metabolic conversion to that sugar.

Glucose is nutritionally the most important monosaccharide, because it is the exclusive constituent of the starches and also occurs in each of three major disaccharides (Fig. 4.6). Like fructose and galactose, glucose is extensively metabolized in the liver, but its removal by that organ is not as complete as in the case of fructose and galactose. The remainder of the glucose passes into the systemic blood supply and is then distributed among other tissues, such as muscle, kidney, and adipose tissue. Glucose enters the cells in these organs by facilitated transport. In skeletal muscle and adipose tissue the process is insulin dependent, whereas in the liver it is insulin independent. Because of the nutritional importance of glucose, the facilitated transport process by which it enters the cells of certain organs and tissues warrants a closer look. The following section explores the process in greater detail.

Glucose Transporters

Glucose is effectively used by a wide variety of cell types under normal conditions, and its concentration in the blood must be precisely controlled. The symptoms associated with diabetes mellitus are a graphic example of the consequences of a disturbance in glucose homeostasis. The cellular uptake of glucose requires that it cross the plasma membrane of the cell. This cannot occur by simple diffusion because the highly polar glucose molecule cannot be solubilized in the nonpolar matrix of the lipid bilayer. For glucose to be used by cells, an efficient transport system for moving the molecule into and out of cells is essential. In certain absorptive cells, such as epithelial cells of the small intestine and renal tubule, glucose crosses the plasma membrane (actively) against a concentration gradient, pumped by an Na^+/K^+-ATPase symport system (described in Chap. 1). However, glucose is passively admitted to nearly all cells in the body by a carrier-mediated transport mechanism that does not require energy. The protein carriers involved in this process are called glucose transporters, abbreviated GLUT.

Considered collectively, all transporter proteins share a unique structure. They are integral proteins, penetrating and spanning the lipid bilayer of the plasma membrane. Most transporters, in fact, span the membrane several times. They are oriented such that hydrophilic regions of the protein chain protrude into the extracellular and cytoplasmic media while the hydrophobic regions traverse the membrane, juxtaposed with the membrane's lipid matrix. A model for a glucose transporter, reflecting this spatial arrangement of the molecule, is illustrated in Figure 4.7. In its simplest form, a transporter

- has a specific combining site for the molecule being transported;
- undergoes a conformational change upon binding the molecule, allowing the molecule to be translocated to the other side of the membrane and released; and
- has the ability to reverse the conformational changes without the molecule's being bound to the transporter, so that the process can be repeated.

Six isoforms of glucose transporters have been described: GLUT1, GLUT2, GLUT3, GLUT4, GLUT5, and GLUT7 are designated according to the order of their discovery. GLUT6 possesses structural homology to GLUT3 but is not a functioning transporter. All cells express at least one of these GLUT isoforms on their plasma membranes. The different isoforms have distinct tissue distribution and biochemical properties, and they contribute to the precise disposal of glucose according to varying physiological conditions. Tissue distribution of the glucose transporters is summarized in Table 4.2.

The GLUT1 and GLUT3 isoforms are believed to be responsible for basal, or constitutive, glucose uptake. The number of these transporter molecules on a given area of cell surface is relatively static and does not

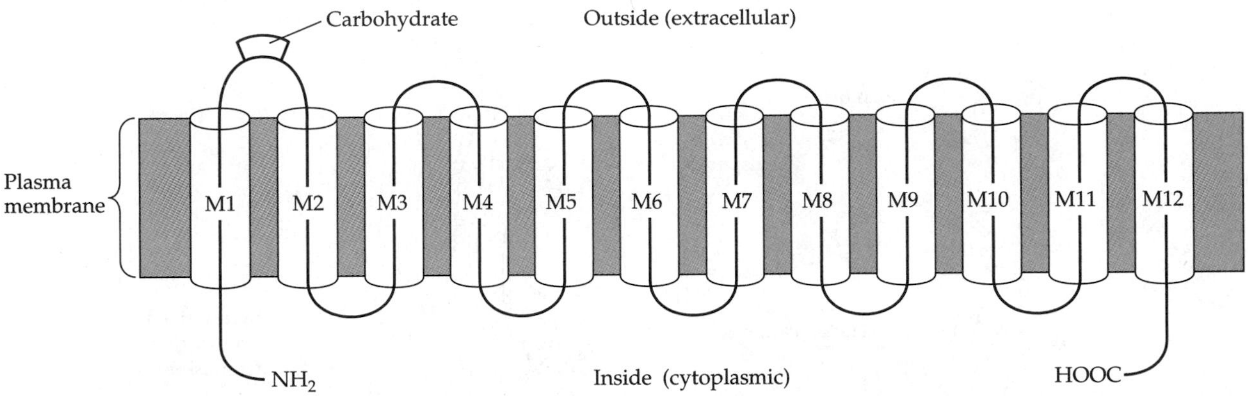

Figure 4.7 A model of a glucose transporter (GLUT1), showing its structural orientation in the plasma membrane. Alpha helical regions of the protein span the membrane 12 times at transmembrane sites designated M1 through M12. Transmembrane segments consist largely of hydrophobic amino acids, whereas the loops on the extracellular and cytoplasmic sides of the membrane are primarily hydrophilic. The transporter is a single polypeptide chain composed of approximately 500 amino acid residues.

increase on insulin stimulation. The same is true for the liver isoform (GLUT2), which is responsible for the bidirectional transport of glucose by the hepatocyte. (GLUT2 may also be involved in the movement of glucose out of absorptive epithelial cells and into the circulation following the active transport of the glucose into the cells by symporters, moving Na^+/K^+ and glucose across the membrane in the same direction.) GLUT4, in contrast, is quite sensitive to insulin, and its concentration on the plasma membrane increases dramatically in response to the hormone. The increase in the membrane transporter population is accompanied by an accelerated increase in the uptake of glucose by the insulin-stimulated cells. The presence of GLUT4 in skeletal muscle and in adipose tissue is what makes these tissues responsive to insulin. Liver, brain, and erythrocytes lack the GLUT4 isoform and therefore are not sensitive to insulin. A feature of non-insulin-dependent diabetes mellitus (NIDDM), described in the Chapter 8 perspective "Diabetes: Metabolism Out of Control," is a resistance to insulin. The disease is believed to arise from abnormalities in the synthesis or activity of GLUT4. An excellent review of the GLUT isoform family is found in Baldwin [5].

Synthesis and storage of the insulin-responsive transporter GLUT4, as for the other transporter isoforms, occur as described in Chapter 1 for all proteins. Following its synthesis from mRNA on the ribosomes of the rough endoplasmic reticulum, the transporter enters the compartments of the Golgi apparatus, where it is ultimately packaged in tubulovesicular structures in the trans-Golgi network. In the basal, unstimulated state of the adipocyte, GLUT4 resides in these structures as well as, to some extent, in small cytoplasmic vesicles [6]. This subcellular distribution of GLUT4 is also found in skeletal muscle cells [7]. On stimulation by insulin, the tubulovesicle-enclosed transporters are translocated to the plasma membrane, where they become expressed on the cell surface. The proposed mechanism is illustrated in Figure 4.8.

The endothelial tissue of which blood vessel walls are constructed is freely permeable to metabolites such as glucose. Some tissues, most notably the brain, possess an additional layer of epithelial tissue between the

Table 4.2 Human Glucose Transporters

Designation	Insulin Regulatable	Major Sites of Expression
GLUT1	No	Erythrocyte (human), blood-brain barrier, placenta, fetal tissues in general
GLUT2	No	Liver, pancreatic β-cell, kidney, small intestine
GLUT3	No	Brain (neurons)
GLUT4	Yes	Brown and white adipocytes, heart and skeletal muscle
GLUT5	No	Small intestine
GLUT7	No	Endoplasmic reticulum of hepatocytes

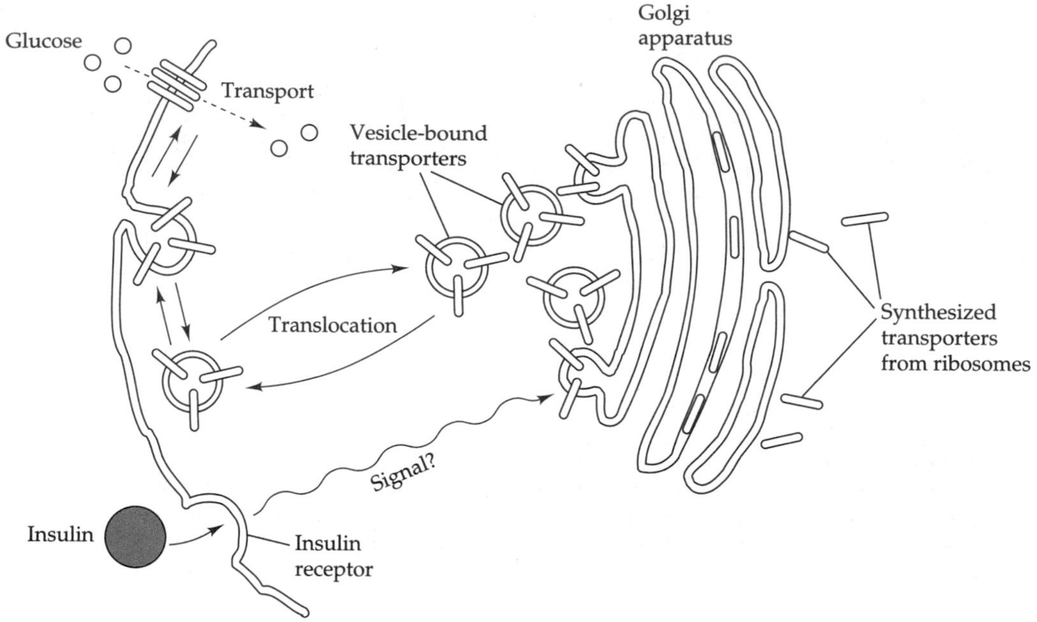

Figure 4.8 Proposed mode of insulin action on glucose transport. The theoretical sequence of events is as follows: (1) The binding of insulin to its specific receptor induces a signal of as yet unknown nature that stimulates the translocation of vesicles containing the glucose transporters to the plasma membrane. (2) The vesicles fuse with the plasma membrane, releasing the transporters and allowing them to position themselves in the membrane. (3) On removal of insulin from its receptor, membrane-bound transporters are retranslocated back to the intracellular pool by an endocytosis-like mechanism.

blood vessel and the cells of the brain. Unlike endothelium, epithelial layers are not readily permeable, and the passage of metabolites through them requires active transport or facilitative diffusion. For this reason, epithelium is referred to as the blood tissue barriers of the body. Among the blood tissue barriers studied—including those of brain, cerebrospinal fluid, retina, testes, and placenta—GLUT1 appears to be the prime isoform for glucose transport [8].

In summary, glucose is transported into cells in the body by the isoforms of glucose transport proteins, and cells of the various organs have specific glucose transporters associated with them. The level of GLUT4, found primarily in skeletal muscle and adipose tissue, is insulin dependent.

Maintenance of Blood Glucose Levels

Maintenance of normal blood glucose concentration is a major function of the liver. Regulation is the net effect of the organ's metabolic processes that remove glucose from the blood either for glycogen synthesis or for energy release and of processes that return glucose to the blood, such as glycogenolysis and **gluconeogenesis.** These pathways, which are examined in detail in the section "Integrated Metabolism in Tissues," are hormonally influenced, primarily by the antagonistic pancreatic hormones insulin and glucagon and the glucocorticoid hormones of the adrenal cortex. The rise in blood glucose following the ingestion of carbohydrate, for example, triggers the release of insulin while reducing the secretion of glucagon. These changes in the two hormone levels increase the uptake of glucose by muscle and adipose tissue, returning blood glucose to homeostatic levels. A fall in blood glucose concentration, conversely, signals a reversal of the pancreatic hormonal secretions—that is, decreased insulin and increased glucagon release. In addition, an increase in the secretion of glucocorticoid hormones, primarily cortisol, occurs in answer to—and to offset—a falling blood glucose level. Glucocorticoids cause increased activity of hepatic gluconeogenesis, a process described in detail in a later section.

Glycemic Response to Carbohydrates

The rate at which glucose is absorbed from the intestinal tract appears to be an important parameter in controlling the homeostasis of blood glucose. This relationship involving dietary carbohydrates is important, because current research suggests a role for elevated blood glucose in the development of chronic diseases and obesity. This topic, discussed in this section, also has direct implications for diabetes mellitus (see the Chap. 8 perspective on diabetes). An alternative way to classify dietary carbohydrates is by their ease of absorption and their impact on the elevation of blood glucose levels. The implications of consuming high-glycemic index foods for chronic disease and obesity have recently been reviewed [9,10]. These reviews suggest that the glycemic index and glycemic load (defined below) offer a way to examine the relative risks of diets designed to prevent coronary heart disease (CHD) and/or obesity.

The effect that carbohydrate-containing foods have on blood glucose concentration, referred to as the glycemic response of the food, varies with the time course of digestion and absorption of the carbohydrates in that food. Some foods cause a rapid rise and fall in blood glucose levels, while others cause a slower and more extended rise and fall. The glycemic index of a food, a classification proposed to provide quantitative comparisons between foods, is defined as the increase in blood glucose level over the baseline level during a 2-hour period for a defined amount of carbohydrate (usually 50 g) compared with the same amount of carbohydrate in a reference food. The reference food is typically either glucose or white bread. In practice, the glycemic index is measured by determining the area under the curve after plotting the blood glucose level following ingestion of the food and comparing that area to the area under the curve for the reference food (Fig. 4.9). For individuals with diabetes mellitus (see the Chap. 8 perspective on diabetes), the area under the curve is much steeper; in other words, the area under the curve is much greater. The reviews suggest that the longer and higher the elevation of blood glucose, the greater the risk of developing chronic diseases and obesity [9,10]. The extent of the risk is better defined by glycemic load, a weighted average of the glycemic indexes of all foods eaten throughout the day. In summary, the risk of chronic disease and obesity appears to be related to the degree of blood glucose elevation and the percentage of time over which glucose levels are elevated.

INTEGRATED METABOLISM IN TISSUES

The metabolic fate of the monosaccharides depends to a great extent on the body's energy needs at the time. The activity of certain metabolic pathways is regulated according to these needs in such a way that some may be stimulated while others may be suppressed. The major regulatory mechanisms are hormonal (involving the action of hormones such as insulin, glucagon, epinephrine, and the corticosteroid hormones) and allosteric enzyme activation or suppression.

Allosteric enzymes provide regulation for some pathways because their activities can be altered by compounds called modulators. A negative modulator of an allosteric enzyme reduces the activity of the enzyme and slows the velocity of the reaction it catalyzes, whereas a positive modulator increases the activity of an allosteric enzyme and thus increases the velocity of the reaction. The effect of a modulator, whether negative or positive, is exerted on its allosteric enzyme as a result of changes in the concentration of the modulator. The mechanisms of regulation of metabolism, including induction, post-translational modification, and translocation, are discussed in detail in the section "Regulation of Metabolism."

The metabolic pathways of carbohydrate use and storage consist of **glycogenesis** (the making of glycogen), glycogenolysis (the breakdown of glycogen), **glycolysis** (the oxidation of glucose), the **hexosemonophosphate shunt** (the production of 5-carbon monosaccharides and NADPH), the **Krebs cycle** (oxidation of pyruvate and

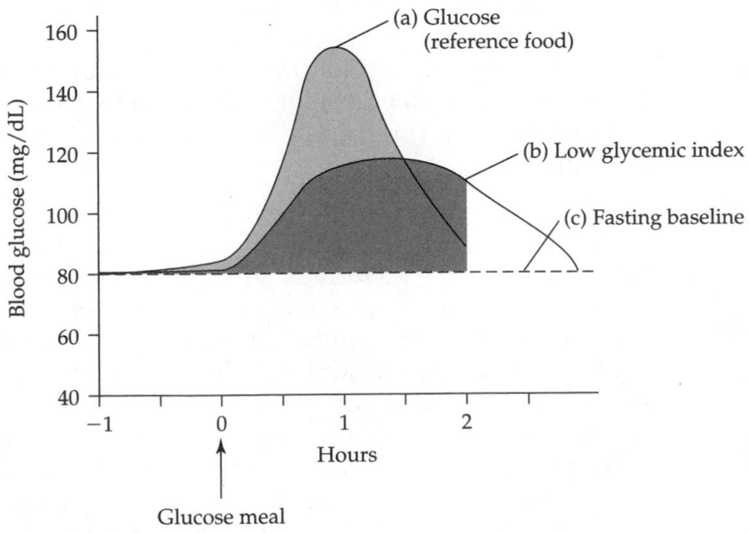

Figure 4.9 (a) The elevation in blood glucose level following 50 g of glucose (glycemic index = 100 by definition). (b) The elevation of blood glucose levels above the baseline (c) following the intake of 50 g of low-glycemic-index food. The glycemic index for this food is determined by dividing the area under the curve for the test food (b) by the area under the curve for the reference food (a) and then multiplying by 100.

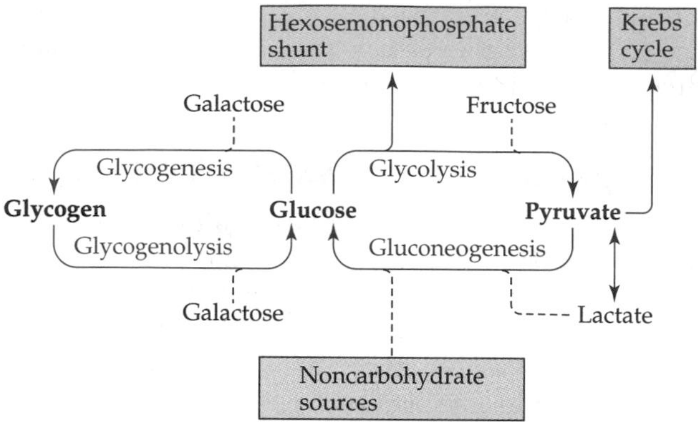

Figure 4.10 An overview of the major pathways of carbohydrate metabolism, emphasizing the fate of glucose but also indicating the sites of entry of galactose and fructose into the pathways.

acetyl CoA), and gluconeogenesis (the making of glucose from noncarbohydrate precursors). An integrated overview of these pathways is given in Figure 4.10. A detailed review of the pathways' intermediary metabolites, sites of regulation, and, most important, functions in the overall scheme of things are considered in the sections that follow. Reactions within these pathways are numbered to allow elaboration on those reactions that are particularly significant from a nutritional standpoint. Because of the central role of glucose in carbohydrate nutrition, its metabolic fate is featured here. The entry of fructose and galactose into the metabolic pathways is introduced later in the discussion.

Glycogenesis

The term *glycogenesis* refers to the pathway by which glucose ultimately is converted into glycogen. This pathway is particularly important in hepatocytes because the liver is a major site of glycogen synthesis and storage. Glycogen accounts for as much as 7% of the wet weight of this organ. The other major sites of glycogen storage are skeletal muscle and, to a lesser extent, adipose tissue. In human skeletal muscle, glycogen generally accounts for a little less than 1% of the wet weight of the tissue. The glycogen stores in muscle can be used as an energy source in that muscle fiber when the body is confronted by an energy demand such as physical exertion. The glycogenic pathway therefore is of vital importance in ensuring a reserve of instant energy. The pathway is illustrated in Figure 4.11a. Following are comments on selected reactions.

1. Upon entering the cell, glucose is first phosphorylated, producing a phosphate ester at the number 6 carbon of the glucose. In muscle cells, the enzyme catalyzing this phosphate transfer from ATP is hexokinase, an allosteric enzyme that is negatively modulated by the product of the reaction, glucose 6-phosphate. Glucose phosphorylation in the liver is catalyzed primarily by glucokinase (sometimes referred to as hexokinase D). Although the reaction product, glucose 6-phosphate, is the same, interesting differences distinguish it from hexokinase. For example, hexokinase is negatively modulated by glucose 6-phosphate, while glucokinase is not. Also, glucokinase has a much higher K_m than hexokinase, meaning that it can convert glucose to its phosphate form at a higher velocity should the cellular concentration of glucose rise significantly (e.g., after a carbohydrate-rich meal). The much lower K_m of hexokinase indicates that it is catalyzing at maximum velocity even at average glucose concentrations. In the presence of high blood glucose, the production of glucose 6-phosphate initiates glycogen synthesis (glycogenesis), which keeps the level of free glucose low and enhances the entry of glucose into the liver cell down a concentration gradient. Therefore, the liver has the capacity to reduce blood glucose concentration when it becomes high. Furthermore, glucokinase is inducible by the hormone insulin, whose levels are increased by elevated blood glucose levels. In diabetes mellitus, type 1 (see the Chap. 8 perspective on diabetes), glucokinase activity is therefore below normal values, because patients have low insulin levels. The low glucokinase activity contributes to the liver cell's inability to rapidly take up and metabolize glucose. The concept of K_m and its significance as it applies to this reaction were discussed in Chapter 1. The hexokinase/glucokinase reaction is energy consuming, because the glucose is activated (phosphorylated) at the expense of ATP.

2. The phosphate is transferred from the 6-carbon of the glucose to the 1-carbon in a reaction catalyzed by the enzyme phosphoglucomutase.

3. Nucleoside triphosphates other than ATP sometimes function as activating substances in intermediary metabolism. In this reaction, energy derived from the hydrolysis of the α-β-phosphate anhydride bond of uridine triphosphate (UTP to UMP) allows the coupling of the resulting uridine monophosphate to the glucose 1-phosphate to form uridine diphosphate glucose (UDP-glucose).

4. Glucose is incorporated into glycogen as UDP-glucose. The reaction is catalyzed by glycogen synthase and requires some preformed glycogen (primer) to which the incoming glucose units can be attached. The nature of the glycogen primer has become understood only in recent years. Previously, the unanswered question was how a new glycogen molecule is initiated if glycogen synthase requires a primer. The answer lies in an intriguing protein called glycogenin. Glycogenin itself acts as the primer to which the first glucose residue is covalently attached, and it also catalyzes (is

(a)

(b)

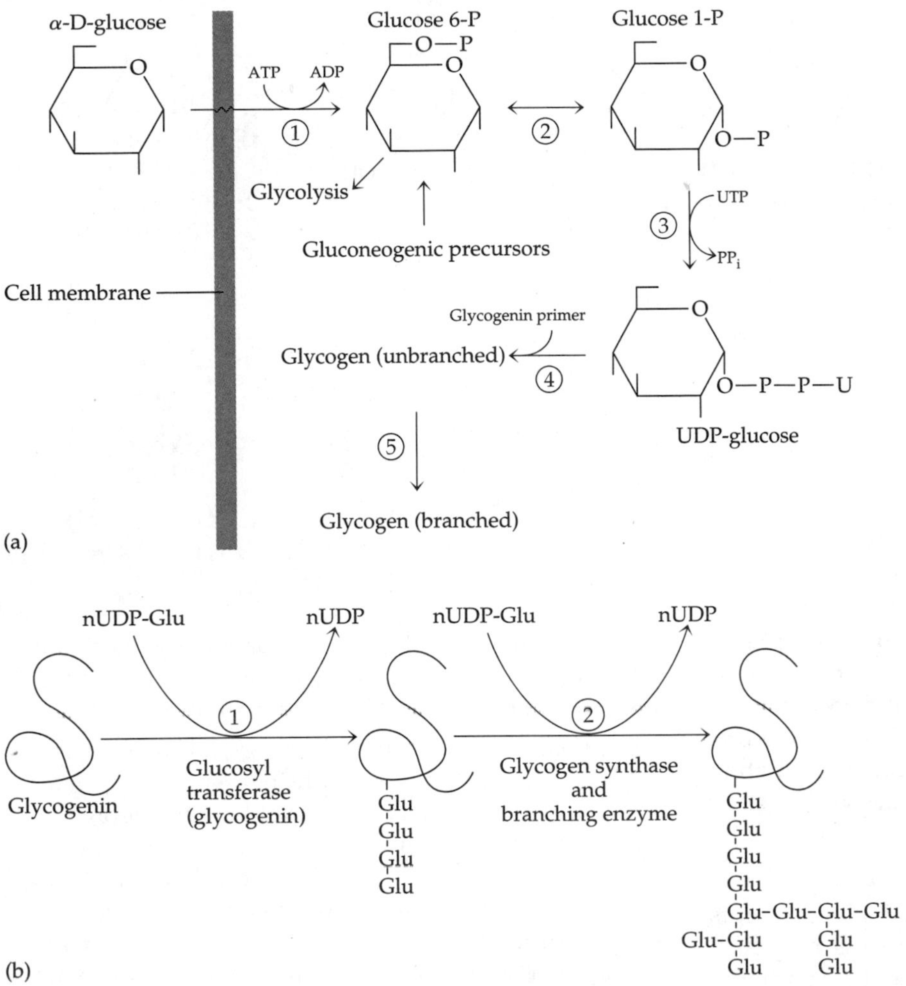

Figure 4.11 (a) Reactions of glycogenesis, by which the formation of glycogen from glucose occurs. Glycogen appears to be formed principally from gluconeogenic precursor substances rather than from glucose directly [11]. (b) The primer function of glycogenin. The glucosyl transferase activity of glycogenin catalyzes the attachment to itself of from two to seven glucose residues transferred from UDP-glucose (reaction 1). Remaining glucose units of the glycogen molecule are incorporated into the molecule by glycogen synthase and linked together by glycogen synthase and the branching enzyme (reaction 2). The letter *n* represents an unspecified number of UDP-glucose molecules.

the enzyme for) the reaction by which the attachment occurs. In addition, glycogenin catalyzes the attachment of additional glucose residues to form chains of up to eight units. At that point, glycogen synthase takes over, extending the glycogen chains further. The role of glycogenin in glycogenesis has been reviewed [12], and a simplified view of the process is shown schematically in Figure 4.11b. Glycogen synthase exists in an active (dephosphorylated) form and a less active (phosphorylated) form. Insulin facilitates glycogen synthesis by stimulating the dephosphorylation of glycogen synthase. The glycogen synthase reaction is the primary target of insulin's stimulatory effect on glycogenesis.

5. Branching within the glycogen molecule is very important, because it increases the molecule's solubility and compactness. Branching also makes available many nonreducing ends of chains from which glucose residues can be cleaved and used for energy, in the process known as glycogenolysis and described in the following section. Glycogen synthase cannot form the α 1-6 bonds of the branch points. This is left to the action of the branching enzyme, which transfers small oligosaccharide segments from the end of the main glycogen chain to carbon number 6 hydroxyl groups throughout the chain. The overall pathway of glycogenesis, like most synthetic pathways, consumes energy, because an ATP (reaction 1) and a UTP (reaction 3) are consumed for each molecule of glucose introduced.

Glycogenolysis

The potential energy of glycogen is contained within the glucose residues that comprise its structure. In accordance with the body's energy demands, the residues can be systematically cleaved one at a time from the ends of the glycogen branches and routed through energy-releasing pathways. The breakdown of glycogen into individual glucose units, in the form of glucose 1-phosphate, is called glycogenolysis. Like its counterpart, glycogenesis, glycogenolysis is regulated by hormones, most importantly glucagon (of pancreatic

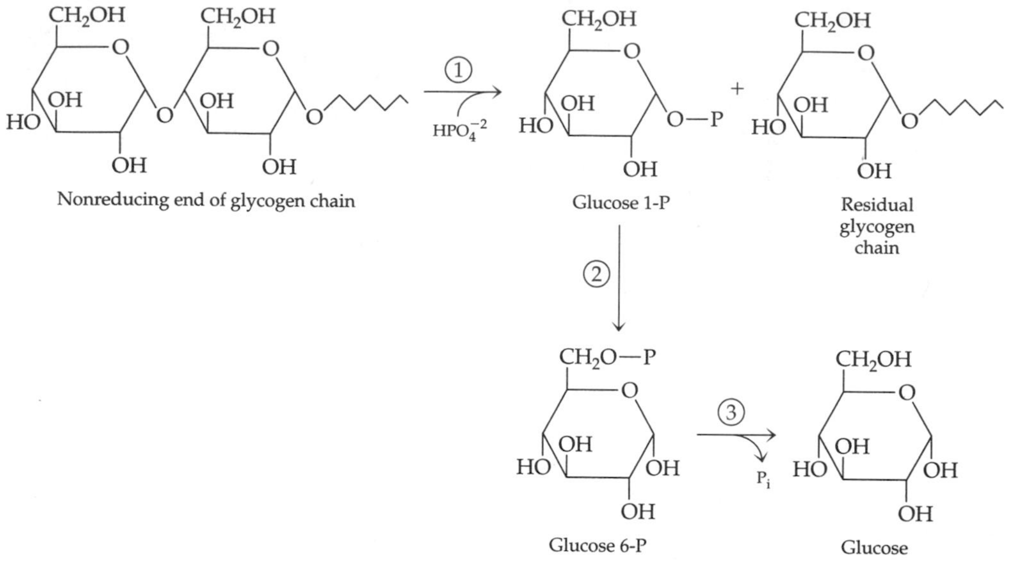

Figure 4.12 The reactions of glycogenolysis, by which glucose residues are sequentially removed from the nonreducing ends of glycogen segments. Reactions 1 and 2 are shared by both liver and muscle cells. In liver cells, glucose 6-phosphate can be converted to free glucose (reaction 3) by glucose 6-phosphatase. Muscle cells lack glucose 6-phosphatase and therefore cannot carry out reaction 3.

origin) and the catecholamine hormone epinephrine (produced in the adrenal medulla). Both of these hormones stimulate glycogenolysis and are directed at the initial reaction, glycogen phosphorylase. Therefore, they function antagonistically to insulin in regulating the balance between free and stored glucose. The steps involved in glycogenolysis are shown in Figure 4.12. Comments on selected reactions follow.

1. The sequential release of individual glucose units from glycogen is a **phosphorolysis** process by which the glycosidic bonds are cleaved by phosphate addition. The products of one such cleavage reaction are glucose 1-phosphate and the remainder of the intact glycogen chain minus the one glucose residue. The reaction is catalyzed by glycogen phosphorylase, an important site of metabolic regulation by both hormonal and allosteric enzyme modulation. Glycogen phosphorylase can exist as either phosphorylase a (a phosphorylated active form) or phosphorylase b (a dephosphorylated, inactive form). The two forms are interconverted by other enzymes, which can either attach phosphate groups to the phosphorylase enzyme or remove phosphate groups from it. The enzyme catalyzing the phosphorylation of phosphorylase b to its active "a" form is called phosphorylase b kinase. The enzyme that removes phosphate groups from the active "a" form of phosphorylase, producing the inactive "b" form, is called phosphorylase a phosphatase. The rate of glycogen breakdown to glucose 1-phosphate therefore depends on the relative activity of these enzymes.

The regulation of phosphorylase activity in the breakdown of liver and muscle glycogen is complex. It can involve covalent regulation, which is the phosphorylation-dephosphorylation regulation just described, and may also involve allosteric regulation by modulators. These and other mechanisms of regulation are broadly reviewed in the section "Regulation of Metabolism."

- *Covalent regulation* is strongly influenced by the hormones epinephrine (which stimulates glycogenolysis in muscle) and glucagon (which stimulates glycogenolysis in liver). Both of these hormones exert their effect by stimulating phosphorylase b kinase, thereby promoting the formation of the more active ("a") form of the enzyme. This hormonal activation of phosphorylase b kinase is mediated through cAMP, the cellular concentration of which is increased by the action of the same hormones, epinephrine and glucagon.
- *Allosteric regulation* of phosphorylase generally involves the positive modulator AMP, which induces a conformational change in the inactive "b" form, resulting in a fully active "b" form. ATP competes with AMP for the allosteric site of the enzyme. High ATP levels prevent the shift to the enzyme's active form and tend to keep it in its inactive form. No covalent (phosphorylation) regulation is involved in allosteric modulations.

The interconversion of phosphorylases a and b, along with the active and inactive forms of phosphorylase b by covalent and allosteric regulation, respectively, is shown in Figure 4.13. For the interested reader, a biochemistry text (for example, [1]) includes a more detailed account of the regulation of the phosphorylase reaction.

Although glycogen phosphorylase cleaves α 1-4 glycosidic bonds, it cannot hydrolyze α 1-6 bonds. The

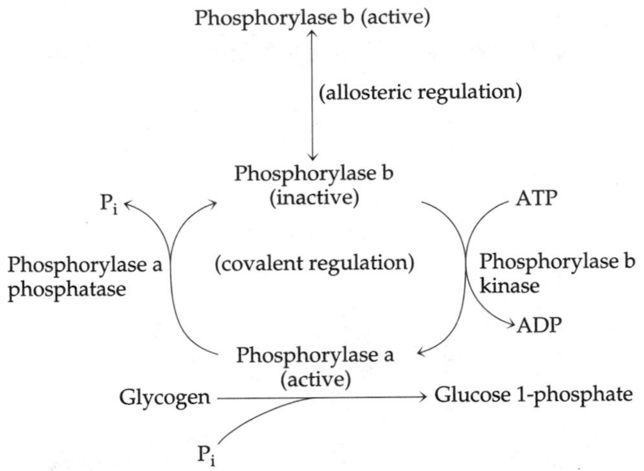

Figure 4.13 An overview of the regulation of glycogen phosphorylase. The enzyme is regulated covalently by phosphorylation to an active "a" form and by dephosphorylation to an inactive "b" form, reactions mediated through cAMP by hormones such as epinephrine and glucagon. It is also regulated allosterically by AMP and ATP, which cause shifts in the equilibrium between inactive and active "b" forms. AMP positively modulates the enzyme by shifting the equilibrium toward its active "b" form. ATP inhibits the effect of AMP, thereby favoring the formation of the inactive "b" form. For more details, see the text under the description for reaction 1 of glycogenolysis.

enzyme acts repetitively along linear portions of the glycogen molecule until it reaches a point four glucose residues from an α 1-6 branch point. Here the degradation process stops, resuming only after an enzyme called the debranching enzyme cleaves the α 1-6 bond at the branch point.

2. At times of heightened glycogenolytic activity, the formation of increased amounts of glucose 1-phosphate shifts the glucose phosphate isomerase reaction toward production of the 6-phosphate isomer (Fig. 4.12).

3. The conversion of glucose 6-phosphate to free glucose requires the action of glucose 6-phosphatase. This enzyme functions in liver and kidney cells but is not expressed in muscle cells or adipocytes. Therefore, free glucose can be formed from liver glycogen and transported via the bloodstream to other tissues for oxidation, but muscle glycogen cannot contribute to the blood glucose level. Thus, the liver, but not muscle, can control the concentration of glucose in the blood. Although muscle and, to some extent, adipose tissue have glycogen stores, these stores can be broken down to glucose only for use within the cells of these tissues.

Glycolysis

Glycolysis is the pathway by which glucose is degraded into two units of pyruvate, a triose. From pyruvate, the metabolic course of the glucose depends largely on the availability of oxygen within the cell, and therefore the course is said to be either aerobic or anaerobic. Under anaerobic conditions—that is, in a situation of oxygen debt—pyruvate is converted to lactate. Under otherwise normal conditions, this would occur mainly in times of strenuous exercise when the demand for oxygen by the working muscles exceeds that which is available. The lactate can also diffuse from the muscle to the bloodstream and be carried to the liver for conversion to glucose. Under anaerobic conditions, glycolysis releases a small amount of usable energy that can help sustain the muscles even in a state of oxygen debt. Providing this energy is the major function of the anaerobic pathway to lactate.

Pyruvate can also follow an aerobic course of reactions. It can be transported into the mitochondria and participate in the Krebs cycle, in which it becomes completely oxidized to CO_2 and H_2O. Complete oxidation is accompanied by the release of relatively large amounts of energy, much of which is salvaged as ATP by the mechanism of oxidative phosphorylation. The glycolytic enzymes function within the cytoplasmic matrix of the cell, while the enzymes catalyzing the Krebs cycle reactions are located within the mitochondrion. Therefore, pyruvate must enter the mitochondrion for complete oxidation. Glycolysis followed by Krebs cycle activity (aerobic catabolism of glucose) demands an ample supply of oxygen, a condition that generally is met in normal, resting mammalian cells. In a normal, aerobic situation, complete oxidation of pyruvate generally occurs, with only a small amount of lactate being formed. The primary importance of glycolysis in energy metabolism, therefore, is in providing the initial sequence of reactions (to pyruvate) necessary for the complete oxidation of glucose via the Krebs cycle, which supplies relatively large quantities of ATP.

In cells that lack mitochondria, such as the erythrocyte, the pathway of glycolysis is the sole provider of ATP by the mechanism of substrate-level phosphorylation of ADP, as discussed in Chapter 3. Nearly all cell types conduct glycolysis, but most of the energy derived from carbohydrates originates in liver, muscle, and adipose, which together constitute a major portion of total body mass. The pathway of glycolysis, under both aerobic and anaerobic conditions, is summarized in Figure 4.14. Also indicated in the figure is the mode of entry of dietary fructose and galactose into the pathway for metabolism. Following are comments on selected reactions.

1. The hexokinase/glucokinase reaction consumes 1 mol ATP/mol glucose. Hexokinase (but not glucokinase) is negatively regulated by the product of the reaction,

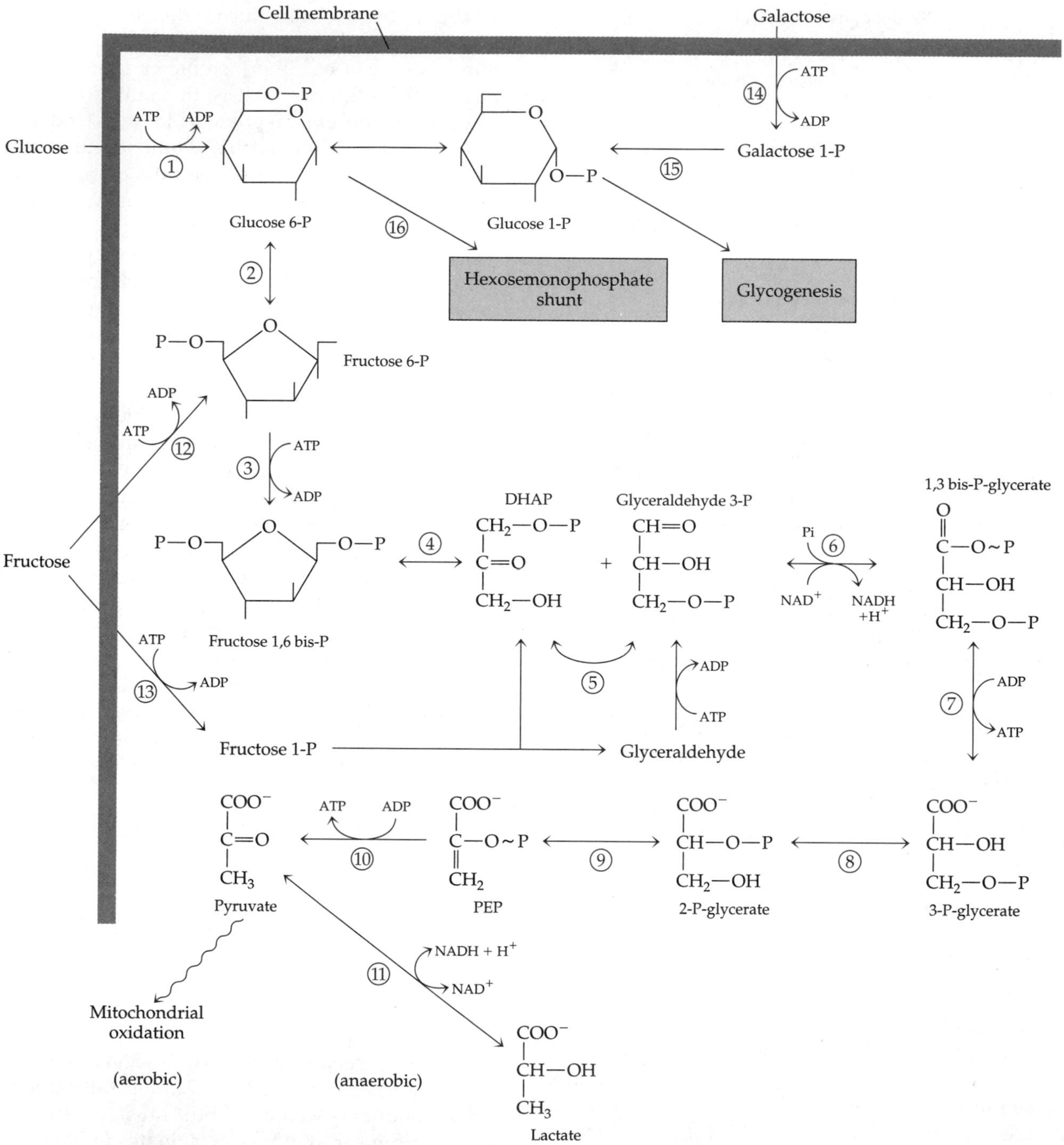

Figure 4.14 Glycolysis, indicating the mode of entry of glucose, fructose, and galactose into the pathway, as well as the alternative entry of glucose 6-phosphate into the hexosemonophosphate shunt. Under conditions of oxygen debt (anaerobic), pyruvate is converted to lactate. If the supply of oxygen is adequate, pyruvate can be oxidized completely in the mitochondrion to carbon dioxide and water.

glucose 6-phosphate. Glucokinase (but not hexokinase) is induced by insulin.

2. Glucose phosphate isomerase (also called hexose phosphate isomerase) catalyzes this interconversion of isomers—glucose 6-P to fructose 6-P.

3. The phosphofructokinase reaction, an important regulatory site, is modulated (by allosteric mechanisms) negatively by ATP and citrate and positively by AMP and ADP. Another ATP is consumed in the reaction. This important reaction is also regulated hormonally by glucagon (by induction), as described later in this chapter.

4. The aldolase reaction results in the splitting of a hexose (fructose) bisphosphate into two triose phosphates, glyceraldehyde 3-phosphate and dihydroxyacetone phosphate (DHAP).

5. The isomers glyceraldehyde 3-phosphate and dihydroxyacetone phosphate are interconverted by the enzyme triosephosphate isomerase. In an isolated system, the equilibrium favors DHAP formation. In the cellular environment, however, it is shifted completely toward the production of glyceraldehyde 3-phosphate, because this metabolite is continuously removed from the equilibrium by the subsequent reaction catalyzed by glyceraldehyde 3-phosphate dehydrogenase.

6. In this reaction, glyceraldehyde 3-phosphate is oxidized to a carboxylic acid, while inorganic phosphate is incorporated as a high-energy anhydride bond. The enzyme is glyceraldehyde 3-phosphate dehydrogenase, which uses NAD^+ as its hydrogen-accepting cosubstrate. Under aerobic conditions, the NADH formed is reoxidized to NAD^+ by O_2 via the electron transport chain in the mitochondria, as explained in the next section. The reason why O_2 is not necessary to sustain this reaction under anaerobic conditions is that the NAD^+ consumed is restored by a subsequent reaction converting pyruvate to lactate (see reaction 11, following).

7. This reaction, catalyzed by phosphoglycerate kinase, exemplifies a substrate-level phosphorylation of ADP. Refer to Chapter 3 for a more detailed review of this mechanism, which forms ATP from ADP by the transfer of a phosphate from a high-energy donor molecule.

8. Phosphoglyceromutase catalyzes the transfer of the phosphate group from the number 3 carbon to the number 2 carbon of the glyceric acid.

9. Dehydration of 2-phosphoglycerate by the enzyme enolase introduces a double bond that imparts high energy to the phosphate bond.

10. The product of reaction 9, phosphoenolpyruvate (PEP), donates its phosphate group to ADP in a reaction catalyzed by pyruvate kinase. This is the second site of substrate-level phosphorylation of ADP in the glycolytic pathway.

11. The lactate dehydrogenase reaction transfers two hydrogens from NADH and H^+ to pyruvate, reducing it to lactate. NAD^+ is formed in the reaction and can replace the NAD^+ consumed in reaction 6 under anaerobic conditions. It must be emphasized that this reaction is most active in situations of oxygen debt, as occurs in prolonged muscular activity. Under normal, aerobic conditions, pyruvate enters the mitochondrion for complete oxidation. A third important option available to pyruvate is its conversion to the amino acid alanine by transamination, a reaction by which pyruvate acquires an amino group from the amino acid glutamate (Chap. 7). This, together with the fact that pyruvate is also the product of the catabolism of various amino acids, makes pyruvate an important link between protein (amino acid) and carbohydrate metabolism.

12 and **13.** These two reactions provide the means by which dietary fructose enters the glycolytic pathway. Fructose is an important factor in the average American diet, as nearly half the carbohydrate consumed is sucrose and high-fructose corn syrup is becoming more popular as a food sweetener. Reaction 12, which functions in extrahepatic tissues, involves the direct phosphorylation by hexokinase to form fructose 6-phosphate. This is a relatively unimportant reaction. It is slow and occurs only in the presence of high levels of fructose. Reaction 13 is the major means by which fructose is converted to glycolysis metabolites. The phosphorylation occurs at the number 1 carbon and is catalyzed by fructokinase, an enzyme found only in liver cells. The fructose 1-phosphate subsequently is split by aldolase (designated aldolase B to distinguish it from the enzyme acting on fructose 1,6-bisphosphate), forming DHAP and glyceraldehyde. The latter can then be phosphorylated by glyceraldehyde kinase (or triokinase) at the expense of a second ATP to produce glyceraldehyde 3-phosphate. This reaction converts fructose to glycolytic intermediates, which can then follow the pathway to pyruvate formation and Krebs cycle oxidation. Alternatively, the three-carbon intermediates can be used in the liver to produce free glucose by a reversal of the first part of the glycolytic pathway through the action of gluconeogenic enzymes. Glucose formation from fructose is particularly important if fructose provides the major source of carbohydrate in the diet.

Because the phosphorylation of fructose is essentially the liver's responsibility, eating large amounts of fructose can deplete hepatocyte ATP and thus reduce the rate of various biosynthetic processes, such as protein synthesis.

14. Like glucose and fructose, galactose is first phosphorylated. The transfer of the phosphate from ATP is catalyzed by galactokinase, and the resulting phosphate ester is at the number 1 carbon of the sugar. The major dietary source of galactose is lactose, from which the galactose is released hydrolytically by lactase.

15. Galactose 1-phosphate can be converted to glucose 1-phosphate through the intermediates uridine diphosphate (UDP)-galactose and uridine diphosphate (UDP)-glucose. The enzyme galactose 1-phosphate uridyl transferase transfers a uridyl phosphate residue from UDP-glucose to the galactose 1-phosphate, yielding glucose 1-phosphate and UDP-galactose. In a reaction catalyzed by epimerase, UDP-galactose can then be converted to UDP-glucose, in which form it can be converted to glucose 1-phosphate by the uridyl transferase reaction already referred to or be incorporated into glycogen by glycogen synthase, as described previously in the section "Glycogenesis." It can also enter the glycolytic pathway as glucose 6-phosphate, made possible by the reaction series UDP-glucose ⟶ glucose 1-phosphate ⟶ glucose 6-phosphate. As glucose 6-phosphate, it can also be hydrolyzed to free glucose in liver cells (but not muscle).

16. This indicates the entry of glucose 6-phosphate into a pathway called the hexosemonophosphate shunt (the pentose phosphate pathway), which we will discuss later.

The Krebs Cycle

The Krebs cycle, also referred to as the tricarboxylic acid cycle or the citric acid cycle, is at the forefront of energy metabolism in the body. It can be thought of as the common and final catabolic pathway, because products of carbohydrate, fat, and amino acids that enter the cycle can be completely oxidized to CO_2 and H_2O, with the accompanying release of energy. Over 90% of the energy released from food is estimated to occur as a result of Krebs cycle oxidation. Not all the substances entering the cycle are totally oxidized, however. Some Krebs cycle intermediates are used in the formation of glucose by the process of gluconeogenesis (discussed later), and some can be converted to certain amino acids by transamination (Chap. 7).

The Krebs cycle is located within the matrix of the mitochondria. The high energy output of the Krebs cycle is attributed to mitochondrial electron transport, with oxidative phosphorylation being the source of ATP formation, as discussed in Chapter 3. The oxidation reactions occurring in the cycle are actually dehydrogenations in which an enzyme catalyzes the removal of two hydrogens to an acceptor cosubstrate such as NAD^+ or FAD. Because both the enzymes of the cycle and the enzymes and electron carriers of electron transport are compartmentalized within the mitochondria, the reduced cosubstrates, NADH and $FADH_2$, are readily reoxidized by O_2 via the electron transport chain, located in the mitochondrial inner membrane.

In addition to its production of the reduced cosubstrates NADH and $FADH_2$, which furnish the energy through their oxidation via electron transport, the Krebs cycle produces most of the carbon dioxide through decarboxylation reactions. In terms of glucose metabolism, recall that two pyruvates are produced from one glucose molecule during cytoplasmic glycolysis. These pyruvates in turn are transported into the mitochondria, where decarboxylation leads to the formation of two acetyl CoA units and two molecules of CO_2. The two carbons represented by the acetyl CoA are incorporated into citric acid and sequentially lost as CO_2 through Krebs cycle decarboxylations. Most of the CO_2 produced is exhaled through the lungs, although some is used in certain synthetic reactions called carboxylations.

The Krebs cycle is shown in Figure 4.15. The acetyl CoA, which couples with oxaloacetate to begin the pathway, is formed from numerous sources, including the breakdown of fatty acids, glucose (through pyruvate), and certain amino acids. We will consider the formation from pyruvate here, because pyruvate links cytoplasmic glycolysis to the Krebs cycle. The reaction shown in Figure 4.16 is referred to as the pyruvate dehydrogenase reaction. The reaction is actually a complex one requiring a multienzyme system and various cofactors, with the enzymes and cofactors contained within an isolatable unit called the pyruvate dehydrogenase complex. The cofactors include coenzyme A (CoA), thiamin pyrophosphate (TPP), Mg^{2+}, NAD^+, FAD, and lipoic acid. Four vitamins therefore are necessary for the activity of the complex: pantothenic acid (a component of CoA), thiamin, niacin, and riboflavin. The role of these vitamins and others as precursors of coenzymes is discussed in Chapter 9. The enzymes in the complex include pyruvate decarboxylase, dihydrolipoyl dehydrogenase, and dihydrolipoyl transacetylase. The net effect of the complex is decarboxylation and dehydrogenation of pyruvate, with NAD^+ serving as the terminal hydrogen acceptor. This reaction therefore yields energy, because the reoxidation of the NADH by electron transport produces 3 mol of ATP by oxidative phosphorylation. Allosterically, the reaction is regulated negatively by acetyl CoA and by NADH, and positively by ADP and Ca^{2+}.

The condensation of acetyl CoA with oxaloacetate initiates the Krebs cycle reactions. Following are comments on the reactions (Fig. 4.15).

1. The formation of citrate from oxaloacetate and acetyl CoA is catalyzed by citrate synthase. The reaction is regulated negatively by ATP.

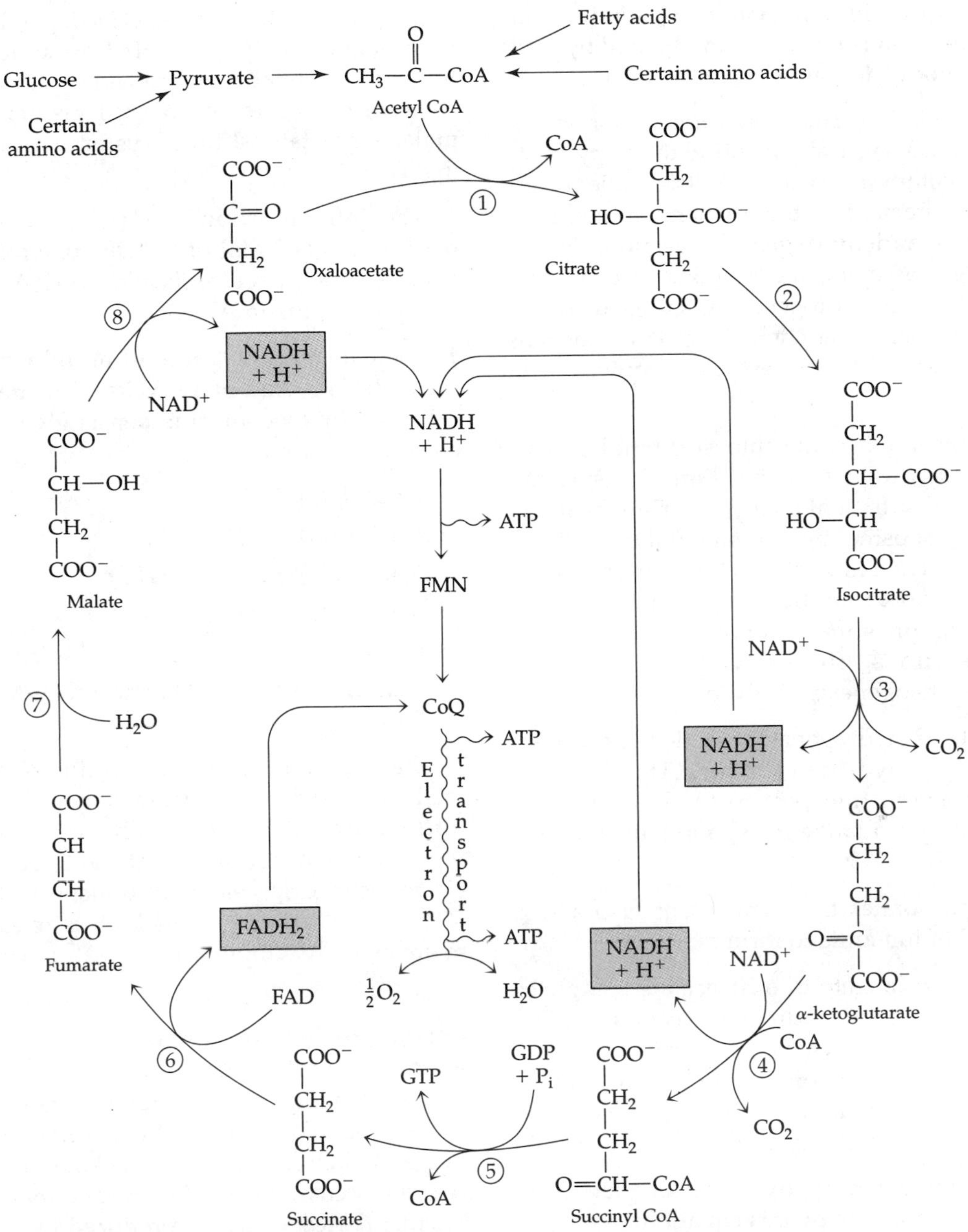

Figure 4.15 The Krebs (citric acid) cycle. This representation of the cycle is designed to emphasize the formation of reduced coenzymes and how their reoxidation by electron transport contributes to the synthesis of ATP.

2. The isomerization of citrate to isocitrate involves *cis* aconitate as an intermediate. The isomerization, catalyzed by aconitase, involves dehydration followed by sterically reversed hydration, resulting in the repositioning of the –OH group onto an adjacent carbon.

3. The isocitrate dehydrogenase reaction, the first of four dehydrogenation reactions within the cycle, supplies energy through the respiratory chain reoxidation of the NADH. Note that the first loss of CO_2 in the cycle occurs at this site. The CO_2 arises from the spontaneous

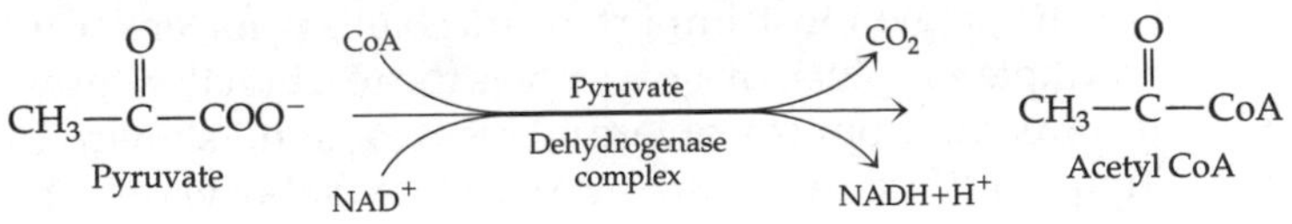

Figure 4.16 The pyruvate dehydrogenase reaction.

decarboxylation of an intermediate compound, oxalosuccinate. The reaction is positively modulated by ADP and negatively modulated by ATP and NADH.

4. The decarboxylation and dehydrogenation of α-ketoglutarate is mechanistically identical to the pyruvate dehydrogenase complex reaction in its multienzyme-multicofactor requirement. In the reaction, referred to as the α-ketoglutarate dehydrogenase reaction, NAD^+ serves as hydrogen acceptor, and a second carbon is lost as CO_2. The pyruvate dehydrogenase, isocitrate dehydrogenase, and α-ketoglutarate dehydrogenase reactions account for the loss of the three-carbon equivalent of pyruvate as CO_2.

5. Energy is conserved in the thioester bond of succinyl CoA. The hydrolysis of that bond by succinyl thiokinase releases sufficient energy to drive the phosphorylation of guanosine diphosphate (GDP) by inorganic phosphate. The resulting GTP is a high-energy phosphate anhydride compound like ATP. As such, GTP can serve as phosphate donor in certain phosphorylation reactions, for example, in reactions involved in gluconeogenesis or glycogenesis.

6. The succinate dehydrogenase reaction uses FAD instead of NAD^+ as hydrogen acceptor. The $FADH_2$ is reoxidized by electron transport to O_2, but only two ATPs are formed by oxidative phosphorylation instead of three.

7. Fumarase incorporates the elements of H_2O across the double bond of fumarate to form malate.

8. The conversion of malate to oxaloacetate completes the cycle. NAD^+ acts as hydrogen acceptor in this dehydrogenation reaction, which is catalyzed by malate dehydrogenase. This reaction is the fourth site of reduced cosubstrate formation and thus results in additional energy release in the cycle.

In summary, the complete oxidation of glucose to CO_2 and H_2O can be shown by this equation:

$$C_6H_{12}O_6 + 6\,O_2 \longrightarrow 6\,CO_2 + 6\,H_2O + \text{energy}$$

Complete oxidation is achieved by the combined reaction sequences of the glycolytic and Krebs cycle pathways. Therefore, under aerobic conditions, the amount of released energy conserved as ATP is as follows:

1. The glycolytic sequence, glucose $\longrightarrow$ two pyruvates, produces two ATPs by substrate-level phosphorylation (2 ATPs).

2. The two NADHs formed in the glycolytic sequence at the glyceraldehyde 3-phosphate dehydrogenase reaction yield either four or six ATPs depending on the shuttle system for moving the NADH-reducing equivalents into the mitochondria for reoxidation. Generally six will be formed, due to the overall greater activity of the malate-aspartate shuttle system, as discussed later (6 ATPs).

3. The intramitochondrial pyruvate dehydrogenase reaction yields 2 mol of NADH, one for each pyruvate oxidized, and therefore six additional ATPs by oxidative phosphorylation (6 ATPs).

4. The oxidation of 1 mol of acetyl CoA in the Krebs cycle yields a total of 12 ATPs. The sites of formation, indicated by reaction number as given in Figure 4.15, follow:

Reaction (3) 3 ATPs
Reaction (4) 3 ATPs
Reaction (5) 1 ATP (as GTP)
Reaction (6) 2 ATPs
Reaction (8) 3 ATPs
Total: 12 ATPs × 2 mol of acetyl CoA per mole of glucose = 24 ATPs

The total number of ATPs produced for the complete oxidation of 1 mol of glucose is therefore 38, equivalent to 262.8 kcal. Recall from Chapter 3 that this figure represents only about 40% of the total energy released by mitochondrial electron transport. The remaining 60%, or approximately 394 kcal, is released as heat to maintain body temperature.

Acetyl CoA Oxidation and Krebs Cycle Intermediates

A steady supply of four-carbon units is needed for the Krebs cycle to oxidize all of the acetyl CoA produced to CO_2 and H_2O. In their absence, ketoacidosis will result. We will discuss this briefly here and more extensively in Chapter 6. Acetyl CoA is produced by fatty acid oxidation and amino acid catabolism as well as from the pyruvate derived from glycolysis (see Chaps. 6 and 7). This clearly leads to an imbalance between the amounts of acetyl CoA and oxaloacetate, which condense one-to-one stoichiometrically in the citrate synthase reaction. To keep the Krebs cycle functioning, oxaloacetate and/or other Krebs cycle intermediates that can form oxaloacetate must be replenished in the cycle. Such a mechanism does exist. Oxaloacetate, fumarate, succinyl CoA, and α-ketoglutarate can all be formed from certain amino acids, but the single most important mechanism for ensuring an ample supply of oxaloacetate is the reaction that forms it directly from pyruvate. This reaction, shown in Figure 4.17, is catalyzed by pyruvate carboxylase. The

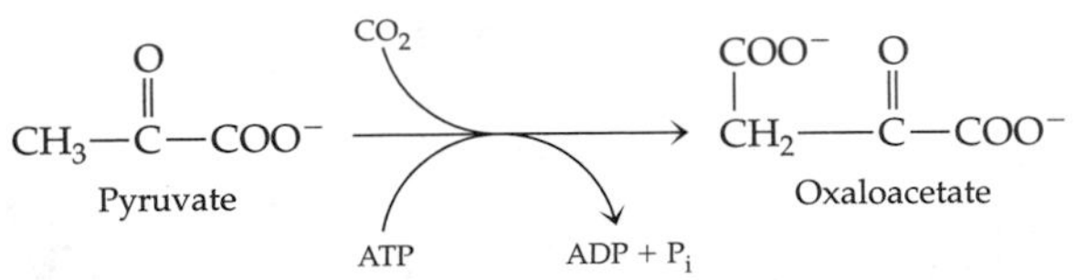

Figure 4.17 The reaction by which oxaloacetate is formed directly from pyruvate, thereby restoring oxaloacetate to the Krebs cycle.

"uphill" incorporation of CO_2 is accomplished at the expense of ATP, and the reaction requires the participation of biotin. The conversion of pyruvate to oxaloacetate is called an anaplerotic (filling-up) process because of its role in restoring oxaloacetate to the cycle. It is interesting that pyruvate carboxylase is regulated positively by acetyl CoA, thereby accelerating oxaloacetate formation in response to increasing levels of acetyl CoA.

NADH in Anaerobic and Aerobic Glycolysis: The Shuttle Systems

Under anaerobic conditions, the NADH produced in the pathway of glycolysis (the glyceraldehyde 3-phosphate dehydrogenase reaction) cannot undergo reoxidation by mitochondrial electron transport because molecular oxygen is the ultimate oxidizing agent in that system. Instead, NADH is used in the lactate dehydrogenase reduction of pyruvate to lactate, thereby becoming reoxidized to NAD^+ without the involvement of oxygen. In this manner, NAD^+ is restored to sustain the glyceraldehyde 3-phosphate dehydrogenase reaction, allowing the production of lactate to continue in the absence of oxygen.

When the system is operating aerobically and the supply of oxygen is ample to allow total oxidation of incoming glucose, lactic acid is not formed. Instead, pyruvate enters the mitochondrion, as does a carrier molecule of hydrogen atoms that were transferred to it from NADH. NADH cannot enter the mitochondrion directly. Rather, reducing equivalents in the form of carriers of hydrogen atoms removed from the NADH in the cytoplast are shuttled across the mitochondrial membrane. Once in the mitochondrial matrix, the carriers are enzymatically dehydrogenated, and NAD^+ becomes reduced to NADH. The latter can then become oxidized by electron transport and consequently can generate about three ATPs per mole of NADH by oxidative phosphorylation. In this manner, six ATPs are formed aerobically per mole of glucose. The result of the shuttle system is therefore equivalent to a transfer of NADH from the cytoplasm into the mitochondrion, although the transfer does not occur directly.

Shuttle substances that transport the hydrogens removed from cytoplasmic NADH into the mitochondrion are malate and glycerol 3-phosphate. Figure 4.18 illustrates how these shuttle systems function in the reoxidation of cytoplasmic NADH. The shuttle systems are specific to certain tissues. The more active malate-aspartate shuttle functions in the liver, kidney, and heart, whereas the glycerol 3-phosphate shuttle functions in the brain and skeletal muscle.

Malate-Aspartate Shuttle System

The most active shuttle compound, malate, is freely permeable to the inner mitochondrial membrane. The malate is oxidized by the enzyme malate dehydrogenase to oxaloacetic acid in the matrix of the mitochondria, using NADH as a cofactor and generating three ATPs per mole. The oxaloacetic acid undergoes transamination by aspartate aminotransferase to form aspartic acid, which is freely permeable to the inner membrane and can move back out into the cytosol. The effect is movement of NADH into the mitochondria even though the inner mitochondrial membrane is impermeable to it.

Glycerol 3-Phosphate Shuttle System

Glycerophosphate produced by glycolysis is oxidized by two glycerophosphate dehydrogenases, one in the cytoplasm and the other on the outer face of the inner mitochondrial membrane. The glycerol 3-phosphate shuttle, in contrast to the malate-aspartate shuttle, leads to only two ATPs per mole of cytosol-produced NADH because the intramitochondrial reoxidation of glycerol 3-phosphate is catalyzed by glycerol phosphate dehydrogenase, which uses FAD instead of NAD^+ as hydrogen acceptor. Therefore, if the glycerol 3-phosphate shuttle is in effect, only four ATPs will be formed aerobically per mole of glucose by oxidative phosphorylation.

Energy Production in Glycolysis

To summarize energy release from glycolysis in terms of ATP produced, substrate-level phosphorylation reactions result in a net of two ATPs. This is all that is produced from anaerobic glycolysis. If the starting point of glycolysis is glycogen rather than free glucose, the hexokinase reaction is bypassed and the energy yield is therefore increased by one ATP for glycolysis of glycogen glucose, under either aerobic or anaerobic conditions.

Under aerobic conditions, in contrast, additional ATPs are formed by oxidative phosphorylation. This is because the cytoplasmic NADH produced is not used in the (anaerobic) lactate dehydrogenase reaction but is reoxidized via the shuttle systems to NAD^+ by electron transport and oxygen. The number of additional ATPs formed depends on which shuttle system is used to move the NADH hydrogens into the mitochondrion. If the malate-aspartate shuttle is in effect, six ATPs are produced, bringing the total to eight. In tissues using

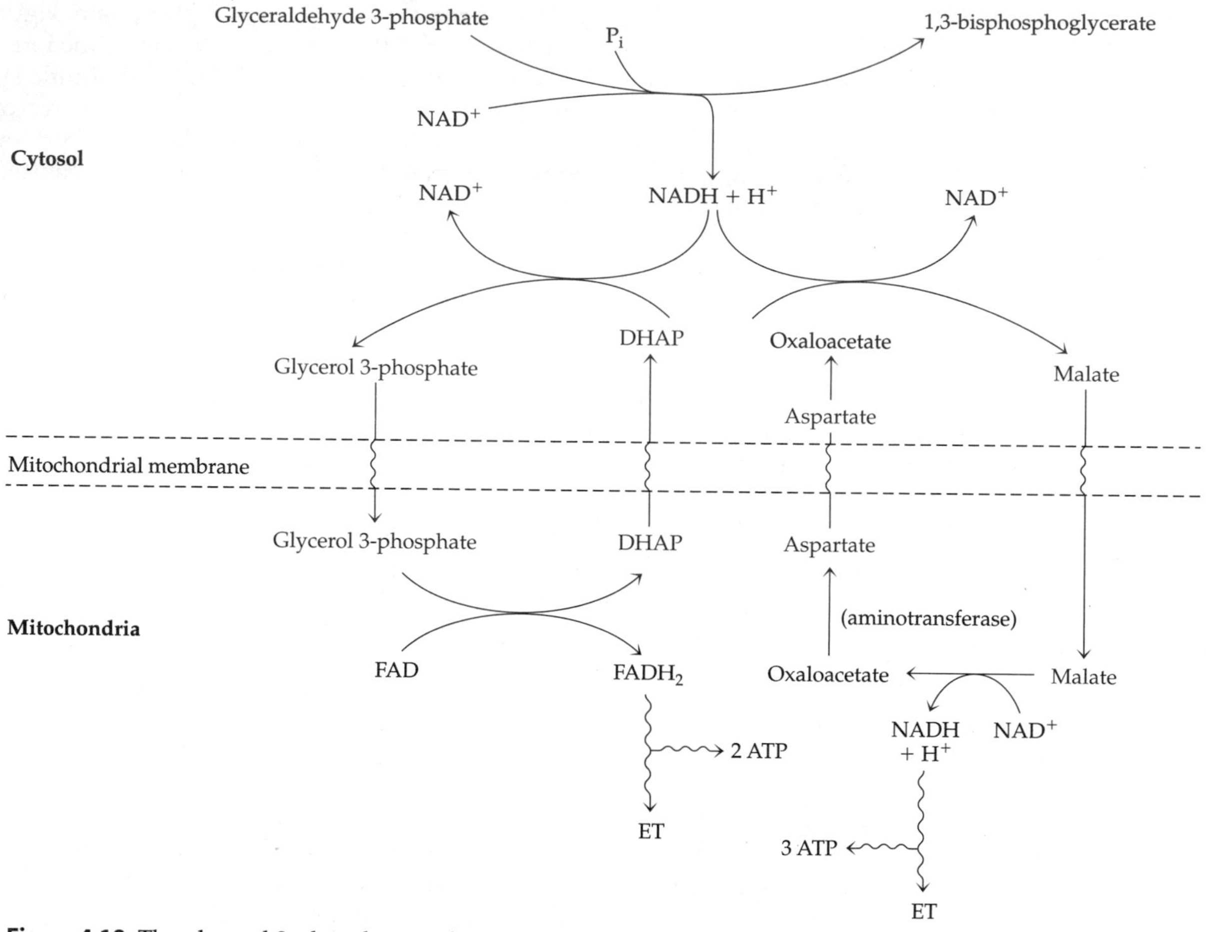

Figure 4.18 The glycerol 3-phosphate and malate-aspartate shuttle systems by which cytosolic NADH can be indirectly reoxidized by mitochondrial electron transport. Reducing equivalents of NADH are reoxidized by either FAD- or NAD^+-requiring enzymes, leading to the production of either two or three ATPs, respectively, per mole of cosubstrate. Abbreviations: DHAP, dihydroxyacetone phosphate; ET, electron transport.

the glycerol 3-phosphate shuttle, just four ATPs are formed by oxidative phosphorylation, for a glycolytic total of six.

The Hexosemonophosphate Shunt (Pentose Phosphate Pathway)

The purpose of a metabolic shunt is to generate important intermediates not produced in other pathways. Two very important products of the hexosemonophosphate shunt are

- pentose phosphates, necessary for the synthesis of the nucleic acids found in DNA and RNA and for other nucleotides (Fig. 4.3); and
- the reduced cosubstrate NADPH, used for important metabolic functions, including the biosynthesis of fatty acids (Chap. 6), the maintenance of reducing substrates in red blood cells necessary to ensure the functional integrity of the cells, and drug metabolism.

The hexosemonophosphate shunt begins with two consecutive dehydrogenase reactions catalyzed by glucose 6-phosphate dehydrogenase (G-6-PD) and 6-phosphogluconate dehydrogenase (6-PGD). Both reactions require $NADP^+$ as cosubstrate, accounting for the formation of NADPH as a reduction product. Pentose phosphate formation is achieved by the decarboxylation of 6-phosphogluconate to form the pentose phosphate ribulose 5-phosphate, which in turn is isomerized to its aldose isomer, ribose 5-phosphate. Pentose phosphates can subsequently be "recycled" back to hexose phosphates through the transketolase and transaldolase reactions illustrated in Figure 4.19. This recycling of pentose phosphates therefore does not result in pentose utilization, but it does assure generous production of NADPH as the cycle repeats.

The cells of some tissues have a high demand for NADPH, particularly those that are active in the synthesis of fatty acids, such as the mammary gland,

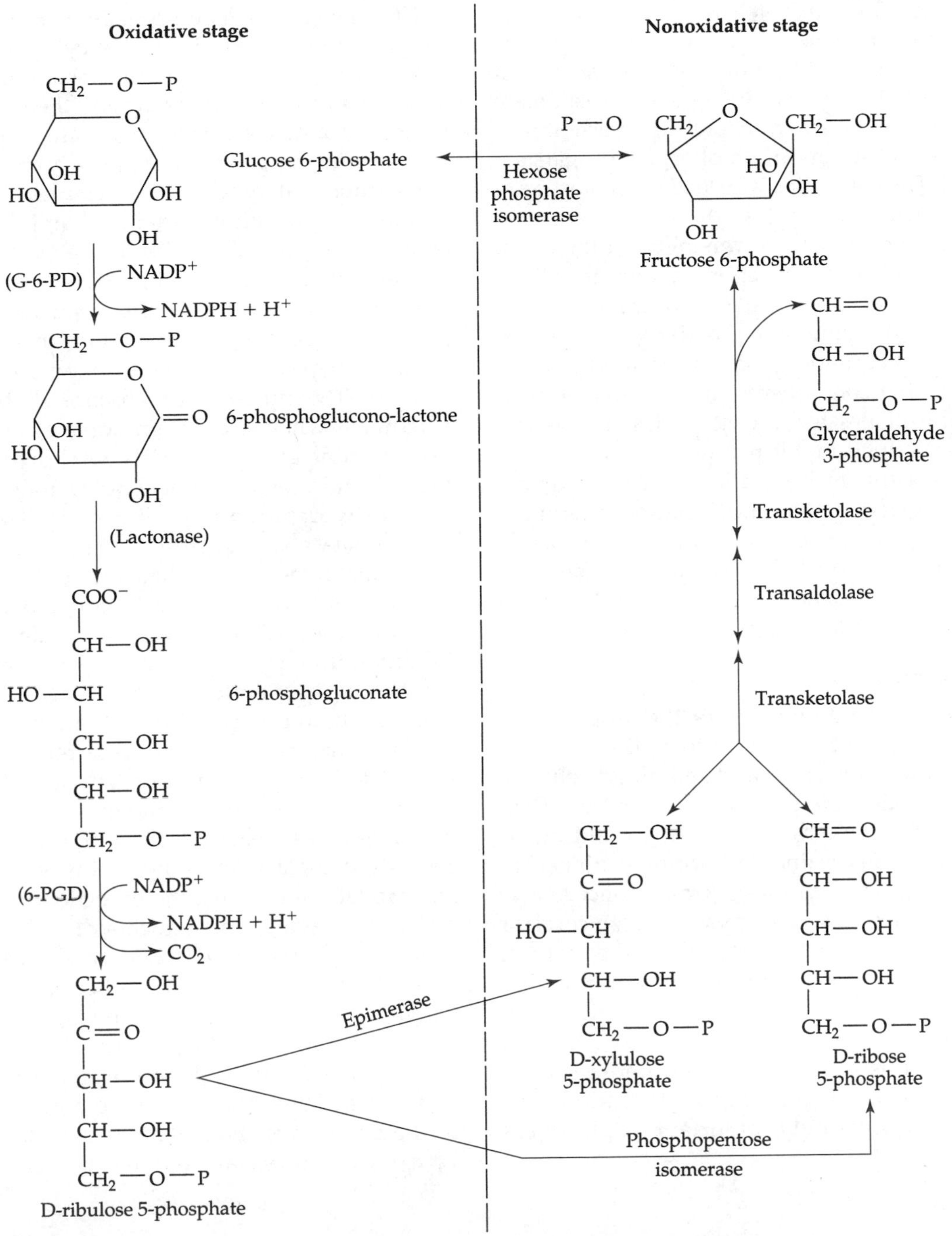

Figure 4.19 The hexosemonophosphate shunt, showing the oxidative stage (left side of diagram) and the nonoxidative stage (right side of diagram). The reversibility of the transketolase and transaldolase reactions makes it possible to form pentose phosphates directly from hexose phosphates (the nonoxidative pathway) while bypassing the dehydrogenation reactions of the oxidative pathway. For an explanation of how the shunt and its stages relate to cell specialization, see the text. Abbreviations: G-6-PD, glucose 6-phosphate dehydrogenase; 6-PGD, 6-phosphogluconate dehydrogenase.

adipose tissue, the adrenal cortex, and the liver. These tissues predictably engage the entire pathway, recycling pentose phosphates back to glucose 6-phosphate to repeat the cycle and assure an ample supply of NADPH. The pathway reactions that include the dehydrogenase reactions and therefore the formation of NADPH from $NADP^+$ are referred to as the oxidative reactions of the pathway. This segment of the pathway is illustrated on the left in Figure 4.19. The re-formation of glucose 6-phosphate from the pentose phosphates, through reactions catalyzed by transketolase, transaldolase, and hexose phosphate isomerase, are referred to as the nonoxidative reactions of the pathway and are shown on the right in Figure 4.19. Transketolase and transaldolase enzymes catalyze complex reactions in which three-, four-, five-, six-, and seven-carbon phosphate sugars are interconverted. These reactions are detailed in most comprehensive biochemistry texts [1].

It should be noted that the reversibility of the transketolase and transaldolase reactions allows the direct conversion of hexose phosphates into pentose phosphates while bypassing the oxidative reactions. Therefore, cells that undergo a more rapid rate of replication and that consequently have a greater need for pentose phosphates for nucleic acid synthesis can produce these products in this manner.

The shunt is active in liver, adipose tissue, adrenal cortex, thyroid gland, testis, and lactating mammary gland. Its activity is low in skeletal muscle because of the limited demand for NADPH (fatty acid synthesis) in this tissue and also because of muscle's reliance on glucose and fatty acids for energy metabolism.

Gluconeogenesis

D-glucose is an essential nutrient for the proper function of most cells. The brain and other tissues of the central nervous system (CNS) and red blood cells are particularly dependent on glucose as a nutrient. When dietary intake of carbohydrate is reduced and blood glucose concentration declines, a hormonal triggering of accelerated glucose synthesis from noncarbohydrate sources occurs. Lactate, pyruvate, glycerol (a catabolic product of triacylglycerols), and certain amino acids represent the important noncarbohydrate sources. The process of producing glucose from such compounds is termed gluconeogenesis. The liver is the major site of this activity, although under certain circumstances, such as prolonged starvation, the kidneys become increasingly important in gluconeogenesis.

Gluconeogenesis is essentially a reversal of the glycolytic pathway. Most of the cytoplasmic enzymes involved in the conversion of glucose to pyruvate catalyze their reactions reversibly and therefore provide the means for also converting pyruvate to glucose. Three reactions in the glycolytic sequence are *not* reversible: the reactions catalyzed by the enzymes glucokinase and hexokinase, phosphofructokinase, and pyruvate kinase (sites 1, 3, and 10 in Fig. 4.14). These reactions all involve ATP and are unidirectional by virtue of the high, negative free energy change of the reactions. Therefore, the process of gluconeogenesis requires that these reactions be either bypassed or circumvented by other enzyme systems. The presence or absence of these enzymes determines whether a certain organ or tissue is capable of conducting gluconeogenesis. As shown in Figure 4.20, the glucokinase and phosphofructokinase reactions can be bypassed by specific phosphatases (glucose 6-phosphatase and fructose 1,6-bisphosphatase, respectively) that remove phosphate groups by hydrolysis.

The bypass of the pyruvate kinase reaction involves the formation of oxaloacetate as an intermediate. Mitochondrial pyruvate can be converted to oxaloacetate by pyruvate carboxylase, a reaction that was discussed earlier as an anaplerotic process. Oxaloacetate, in turn, can be decarboxylated and phosphorylated to phosphoenolpyruvate (PEP) by PEP carboxykinase, thereby completing the bypass of the pyruvate kinase reaction. The PEP carboxykinase reaction is a cytoplasmic reaction, however, and therefore oxaloacetate must leave the mitochondrion to be acted on by the enzyme. The mitochondrial membrane, however, is impermeable to oxaloacetate, which therefore must first be converted to either malate (by malate dehydrogenase) or aspartate (by transamination with glutamate; see Chap. 7), both of which freely traverse the mitochondrial membrane. This mechanism is similar to the malate-aspartate shuttle previously discussed. In the cytoplasm, the malate or aspartate can be converted to oxaloacetate by malate dehydrogenase or

Figure 4.20 Glucokinase and phosphofructokinase reactions.

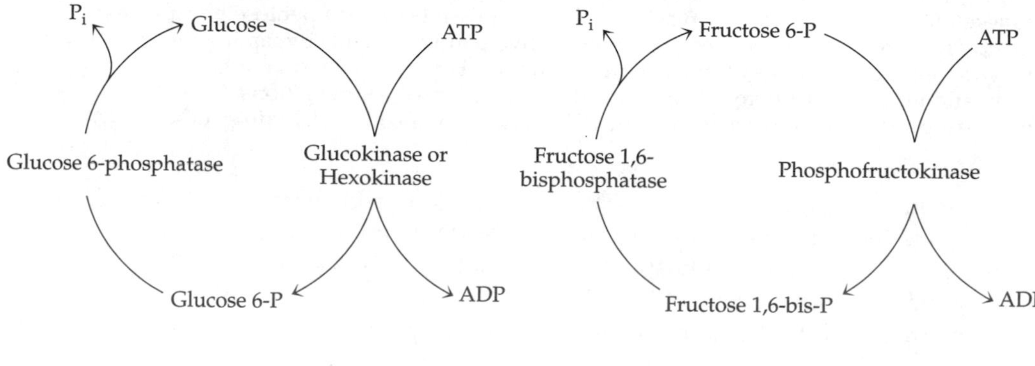

aspartate aminotransferase (glutamate oxaloacetate transaminase), respectively.

The reactions of the pyruvate kinase bypass also allow the carbon skeletons of various amino acids to enter the gluconeogenic pathway, leading to a net synthesis of glucose. Such amino acids accordingly are called glucogenic. Glucogenic amino acids can be catabolized to pyruvate or to various Krebs cycle intermediates or be anaerobically converted to glucose by leaving the mitochondrion in the form of malate or aspartate, as described. Reactions showing the entry of noncarbohydrate substances into the gluconeogenic system are shown in Figure 4.21, along with the bypass of the pyruvate kinase reaction.

Lactate Utilization

Effective gluconeogenesis accounts for the liver's ability to control the high levels of blood lactate that may accompany strenuous physical exertion. Muscle and adipose tissue, for example, lack the ability to form free glucose from noncarbohydrate precursors because they lack glucose 6-phosphatase. Thus, muscle and adipose lactate cannot serve as a precursor for free glucose within these tissues or contribute to the maintenance of

Figure 4.21 The reactions of gluconeogenesis, showing the bypass of the unidirectional pyruvate kinase reaction and the entry into the pathway of noncarbohydrate substances such as glycerol, lactate, and amino acids. Abbreviations: G6P, glucose 6-phosphate; F6P, fructose 6-phosphate; FBP, fructose 1,6-bisphosphate; DHAP, dihydroxyacetone phosphate; G3P, glyceraldehyde 3-phosphate; BPG, 1,3-bisphosphoglycerate; 3PG, 3-phosphoglycerate; 2PG, 2-phosphoglycerate; PEP, phosphoenolpyruvate.

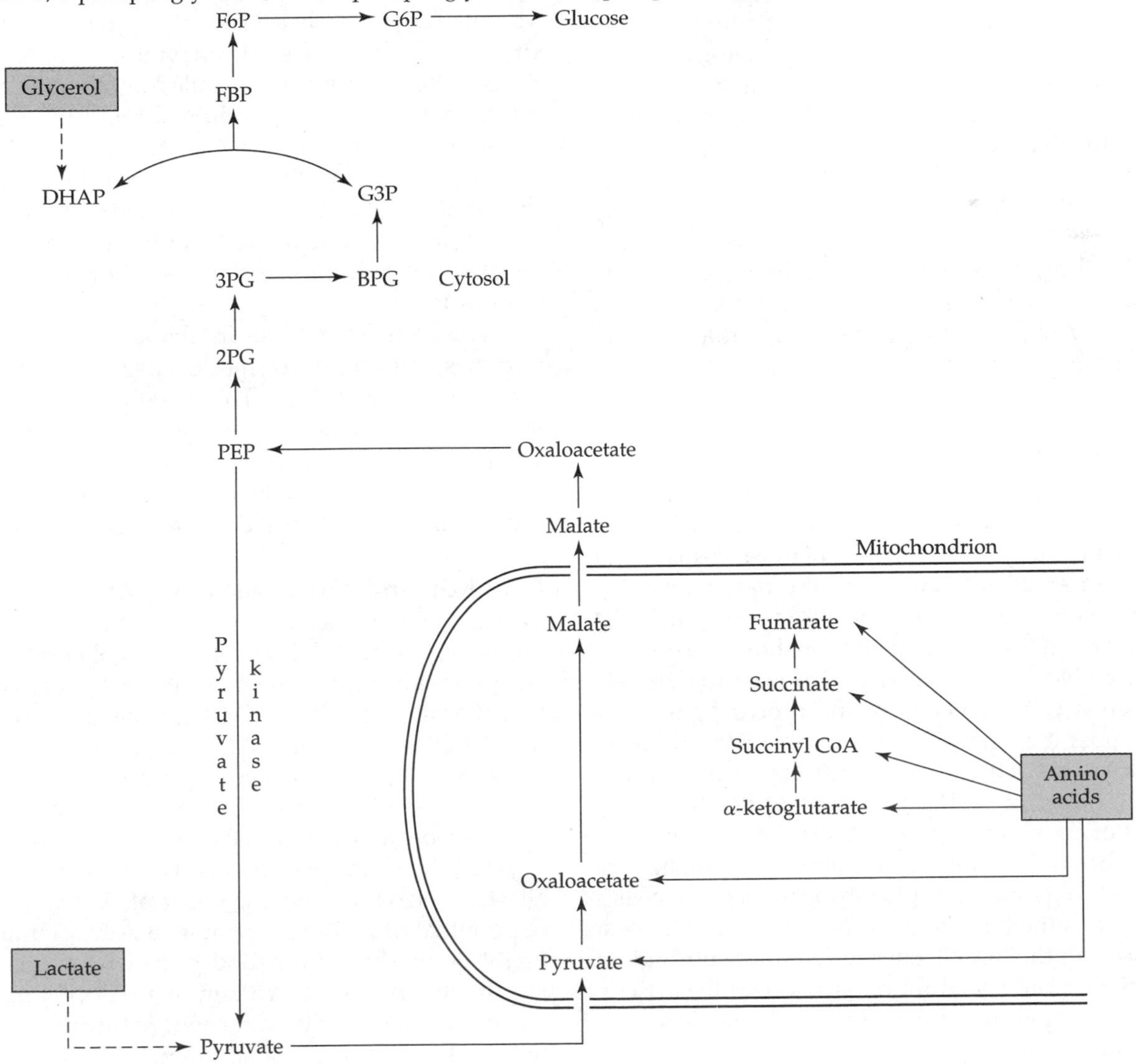

blood glucose levels. Also, muscle cells convert lactate to glycogen only very slowly, especially in the presence of glucose (as when glucose enters muscle or adipose cells from the blood). How, then, is the high level of muscle lactate that can be encountered in situations of oxygen debt dealt with? Recovery is accomplished by the gluconeogenic capability of the liver. The lactate leaves the muscle cells and is transported via the general circulation to the liver, where it can be converted to glucose. The glucose can then be returned to the muscle cells to reestablish homeostatic concentrations there. This circulatory transport of muscle-derived lactate to the liver and the return of glucose to the muscle is referred to as the Cori cycle.

Efficient Glycogenesis

During the past decade, evidence has emerged from in vitro studies that glucose has limited use by the liver as the sole substrate at physiological concentrations and is, in fact, a poor precursor of liver glycogen. However, glucose use is greatly enhanced if additional gluconeogenic substances such as fructose, glycerol, or lactate are available along with the glucose. The term *glucose paradox* [12] refers to the limited incorporation of glucose into glycogen in the absence of other gluconeogenic substances in vivo. It is now believed that glucose ingested during a meal takes a somewhat roundabout path to glycogen. First it is taken up by red blood cells in the bloodstream and converted to lactate by glycolysis. Then the lactate is taken up by the liver and converted to glucose 6-phosphate by gluconeogenesis (and ultimately to glycogen).

REGULATION OF METABOLISM

The purpose of regulation is both to maintain homeostasis and to alter the reactions of metabolism in such a way as to meet the nutritional and biochemical demands of the body. An excellent example is the reciprocal regulation of the glycolysis and Krebs cycle (catabolic) pathways and the gluconeogenic (anabolic) pathways. Because the glycolytic conversion of glucose to pyruvate liberates energy, the reversal of the process, gluconeogenesis, must be energy consuming. The pyruvate kinase bypass in itself is energetically expensive, considering that 1 mol of ATP and 1 mol of GTP must be expended in converting intramitochondrial pyruvate to extramitochondrial PEP. It follows that among the factors that regulate the glycolysis : gluconeogenesis activity ratio is the body's need for energy. Our discussion focuses on the body's energy requirements and on how regulation can speed up or slow down the activity of the metabolic pathways contributing to release or consumption of energy.

In a broad sense, regulation is achieved by four mechanisms:

- negative or positive modulation of allosteric enzymes by effector compounds,
- hormonal activation by covalent modification or induction of specific enzymes,
- directional shifts in reversible reactions by changes in reactant or product concentrations, and
- translocation of enzymes within the cell (covered in Chap. 1).

Allosteric Enzyme Modulation

Allosteric enzymes can be stimulated or suppressed by certain compounds, usually formed within the pathway in which the enzymes function. An allosteric, or regulatory, enzyme is said to be positively or negatively modulated by a substance (modulator) according to whether the effect is stimulation or suppression, respectively. Modulators generally act by altering the conformational structure of their allosteric enzymes, causing a shift in the equilibrium between so-called tight and relaxed conformations of the enzyme (these terms refer to the three-dimensional structure of the enzyme). Assume the enzyme is functionally more active in its relaxed form than in its tight form. A positive modulator then causes a shift toward the relaxed configuration, whereas a negative modulator shifts the equilibrium toward the tight form.

As discussed previously in Chapter 1 (in the section on enzymes), allosteric enzymes catalyze unidirectional, or nonreversible, reactions. This is because modulators of those enzymes must either stimulate or suppress a reaction in one direction only. The stimulation or suppression of an enzyme that catalyzes both the forward and the reverse direction of a reaction would have little value.

AMP, ADP, and ATP as Allosteric Modulators

Cellular energy has a profound influence on energy-producing cycles. An important regulatory system in energy metabolism is the ratio of the cellular concentration of ADP (or AMP) to ATP. The usual breakdown product of ATP is ADP, but as ADP increases in concentration some of it becomes enzymatically converted to AMP. Therefore, ADP and/or AMP accumulation can signify an excessive breakdown of ATP and a depletion of ATP.

AMP, ADP, and ATP all act as modulators of certain allosteric enzymes, but the effect of AMP or ADP will oppose that of ATP. For example, if ATP accumulates, as might occur during a period of muscular relaxation, it negatively modulates certain regulatory enzymes in energy-releasing (ATP-producing) pathways. This acts to reduce the production of additional ATP. An increase in

AMP (or ADP) concentration conversely signifies a depletion of ATP and the need to produce more of this energy source. In such a case, AMP or ADP can positively modulate allosteric enzymes functioning in energy-releasing pathways as their concentration increases. Two examples of positive modulation by AMP are

- its ability to bring about a shift from the inactive form of phosphorylase b to an active form of phosphorylase b (see Fig. 4.13) in glycogenolysis and
- its stimulation, by a similar mechanism, of the enzyme phosphofructokinase, which catalyzes a reaction in the glycolytic pathway.

It can be reasoned that increased levels of AMP are accompanied by an enhanced activity of either of these reactions that encourages glucose catabolism. The resulting shift in metabolic direction, as signaled by the AMP buildup, causes the release of energy as glucose is metabolized and helps restore depleted ATP stores.

In addition to being positively modulated by AMP, phosphofructokinase is modulated positively by ADP and negatively by ATP. As the store of ATP increases and further energy release is not called for, ATP can thus signal the slowing of the glycolytic pathway at that reaction. Phosphofructokinase is an extremely important rate-controlling allosteric enzyme and is modulated by a variety of substances. Its regulatory function has already been described in Chapter 1.

Other regulatory enzymes in carbohydrate metabolism are modulated by ATP, ADP, or AMP. Pyruvate dehydrogenase complex, citrate synthase, and isocitrate dehydrogenase are all negatively modulated by ATP. Pyruvate dehydrogenase complex is positively modulated by AMP, and citrate synthase and isocitrate dehydrogenase are positively modulated by ADP.

Regulatory Effect of NADH : NAD^+ Ratio

The ratio of NADH to NAD^+ also has an important regulatory effect. Certain allosteric enzymes are responsive to an increased level of NADH or NAD^+. These coenzymes regulate their own formation through negative modulation. Because NADH is a product of the oxidative catabolism of carbohydrate, its accumulation would signal for a decrease in catabolic pathway activity. Conversely, higher proportions of NAD^+ signify that a system is in an elevated state of oxidation readiness and would send a modulating signal to accelerate catabolism. Stated differently, the level of NADH in the fasting state is markedly lower than in the fed state because the rate of its reoxidation by electron transport would exceed its formation from substrate oxidation. Fasting, therefore, logically encourages glycolysis and Krebs cycle oxidation of carbohydrates. Dehydrogenase reactions, which involve the interconversion of the reduced and oxidized forms of the cosubstrate, are reversible. If metabolic conditions lead to the accumulation of either NADH or NAD^+, the equilibrium is shifted so as to consume more of the predominant form. Pyruvate dehydrogenase complex is positively modulated by NAD^+, while pyruvate kinase, citrate synthase, and α-ketoglutarate dehydrogenase are negatively modulated by NADH.

Hormonal Regulation

Hormones can regulate specific enzymes either by covalent regulation or by enzyme induction. Covalent regulation refers to the binding of a group by a covalent bond. An example of this type of regulation is the phosphorylation and dephosphorylation of the enzymes, which converts them to active or inactive forms. In some instances, phosphorylation activates and dephosphorylation inactivates the enzyme. In other cases, the reverse may be true. Examples may be found in the covalent regulation of glycogen synthase and glycogen phosphorylase, enzymes discussed in the sections on glycogenesis and glycogenolysis, respectively. Phosphorylation inactivates glycogen synthase, whereas dephosphorylation activates it. In contrast, phosphorylation activates glycogen phosphorylase, and dephosphorylation inactivates it.

Another important example of covalent regulation by a hormone is the control by glucagon of the relative rates of liver glycolysis and gluconeogenesis. The control is directed at the opposing reactions of the phosphofructokinase (PFK) and fructose bisphosphatase (FBPase) site and is mediated through a compound called fructose 2,6-bisphosphate. Unlike fructose 1,6-bisphosphate, fructose 2,6-bisphosphate is not a normal glycolysis intermediate but instead serves solely as a regulator of pathway activity. *Fructose 2,6-bisphosphate stimulates PFK activity and suppresses FBPase activity, thereby stimulating glycolysis and reducing gluconeogenesis.* Cellular concentration of fructose 2,6-bisphosphate is set by the relative rates of its formation and breakdown. The compound is formed by phosphorylation of fructose 6-phosphate by phosphofructokinase 2 (PFK-2) and is broken down by fructose bisphosphatase 2 (FBPase-2). The designation 2 distinguishes these enzymes from PFK and FBPase, which catalyze the formation and breakdown, respectively, of fructose 1,6-bisphosphate. PFK-2 and FBPase-2 activities are expressed by a single (bifunctional) enzyme, and the relative activity of each is controlled by glucagon. Glucagon stimulates the phosphorylation of the bifunctional enzyme, resulting in sharply increased FBPase-2 activity and suppression of PFK-2 activity. *Glucagon therefore stimulates hepatic gluconeogenesis and suppresses glycolysis by reducing the concentration of fructose 2,6-bisphosphate, a positive modulator of the glycolytic enzyme PFK.* The end result is that in response to falling blood glucose levels, the release of glucagon encourages hepatic gluconeogenesis and thus restoration of blood glucose levels.

Covalent regulation is usually mediated through cAMP, which acts as a second messenger in the hormones' action on the cell. Recall that insulin strongly affects the glycogen synthase reaction positively and that epinephrine and glucagon positively regulate glycogen phosphorylase in muscle and the liver, respectively. Each of these hormonal effects is mediated through covalent regulation.

The control of enzyme activity by hormone induction represents another mechanism of regulation. Enzymes functioning in the glycolytic and gluconeogenic pathways can be divided into three groups:

Group 1: *Glycolytic enzymes*
- Glucokinase
- Phosphofructokinase
- Pyruvate kinase

Group 2: *Bifunctional enzymes*
- Phosphoglucoisomerase
- Aldolase
- Triosephosphate isomerase
- Glyceraldehyde 3-phosphate dehydrogenase
- Phosphoglycerate kinase
- Phosphoglyceromutase
- Enolase
- Lactate dehydrogenase

Group 3: *Gluconeogenic enzymes*
- Glucose 6-phosphatase
- Fructose bisphosphatase
- PEP carboxykinase
- Pyruvate carboxylase

As discussed in Chapter 1, enzyme (protein) synthesis is either constitutive (at a constant rate) or adaptive (in response to a stimulus, i.e., inductive). Groups 1 and 3 are inducible enzymes, meaning that their concentrations can rise and fall in response to molecular signals such as a sustained change in the concentration of a certain metabolite. Such a change might arise through a prolonged shift in the dietary intake of certain nutrients. Induction results in the stimulated transcription of new messenger RNA programmed to produce the hormone. Glucocorticoid hormones are known to stimulate gluconeogenesis by inducing the formation of the key gluconeogenic enzymes, and insulin may stimulate glycolysis by inducing an increased synthesis of key glycolytic enzymes. Enzymes in group 2 are not inducible and are produced at a steady rate under the control of constitutive, or basal, gene systems. Noninducible enzymes are required all the time at a relatively constant level of activity, and their genes are expressed at a more or less constant level in virtually all cells. Genes for enzymes that are not inducible are sometimes called housekeeping genes.

The interrelationship among pathways of carbohydrate metabolism is exemplified by the regulation of blood glucose concentration. The interconversion of the pathways, the topic of discussion for Chapter 8, is best understood after metabolism of lipids and amino acids has been discussed (Chaps. 6 and 7). Largely through the opposing effects of insulin and glucagon, fasting serum glucose level normally is maintained within the approximate range of 60 to 90 mg/dL. Whenever blood glucose levels are excessive or sustained at high levels due to an insufficiency of insulin, other insulin-independent pathways of carbohydrate metabolism for lowering blood glucose become increasingly active. Such insulin-independent pathways are indicated in Figure 4.22. The overactivity of these pathways is believed to be partly responsible for the clinical manifestations of diabetes mellitus, type 1 (see the Chap. 8 perspective on diabetes).

Directional Shifts in Reversible Reactions

Most enzymes catalyze reactions reversibly, and the preferred direction a reversible reaction is undergoing at a particular moment is largely dependent on the relative concentration of each reactant and product. A buildup in concentration of one of the reactants will drive or force the reaction toward formation of the other. For example, consider the hypothetical pathway intermediates A and B, which are interconverted reversibly.

Reaction 1 ⟵ A ⟵ B ⟵
→

Reaction 2 ⟶ A ⟶ B ⟶
←

Reaction 1 may represent the reaction in a metabolic steady state in which the formation of A from B is preferred over the formation of B from A. It shows a net formation of A from B, as indicated by the size of the directional arrows. Reaction 2 shows that the steady state shifts toward the formation of B from A if some metabolic event or demand causes the concentration of A to rise above its homeostatic levels.

This concept is exemplified by the phosphoglucomutase reaction, which interconverts glucose 6-phosphate and glucose 1-phosphate and which functions in the pathways of glycogenesis and glycogenolysis (see Figs. 4.11 and 4.12). At times of heightened glycogenolytic activity (rapid breakdown of glycogen), glucose 1-phosphate concentration rises sharply, driving the reaction toward the formation of glucose 6-phosphate. With the body at rest,

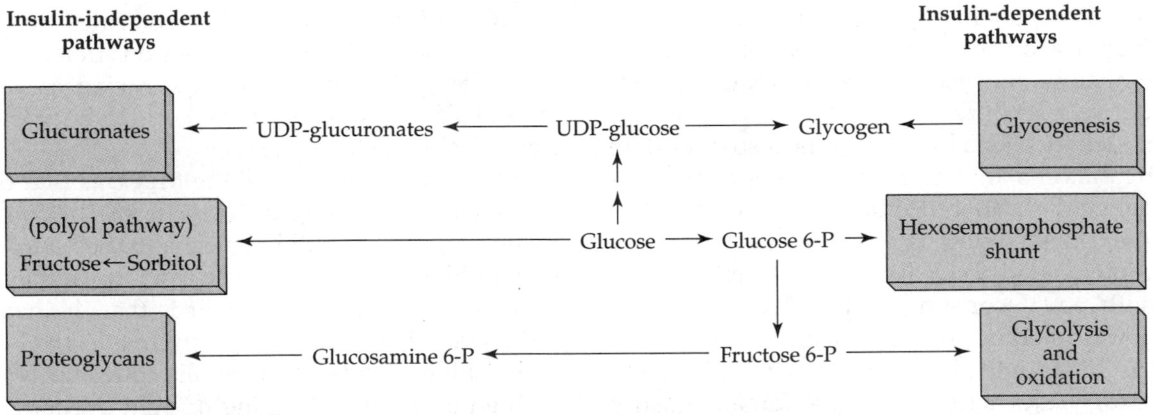

Figure 4.22 Insulin-independent and insulin-dependent pathways of glucose metabolism.

glycogenesis and gluconeogenesis are accelerated, increasing the concentration of glucose 6-phosphate. This in turn shifts the phosphoglucomutase reaction toward the formation of glucose 1-phosphate and ultimately glycogen.

ETHYL ALCOHOL: METABOLISM AND BIOCHEMICAL IMPACT

Ethyl alcohol is not a carbohydrate. Empirically, however, ethanol's structure (CH_3–CH_2–OH) most closely resembles a carbohydrate, and we have chosen to review it in this chapter for several reasons. First, it is a common dietary component, being consumed in the form of alcoholic beverages such as beer, wines, and distilled spirits. Second, the pathways that oxidize ethyl alcohol also oxidize (or detoxify) other exogenous substances in the body. Although ethanol is not a "natural" nutrient, it does have caloric value (its calories are "empty," that is, devoid of beneficial nutrients). Each gram of ethanol yields 7 kcal, and ethanol may account for up to 10% of the total energy intake of moderate consumers and up to 50% for alcoholics. Because of its widespread consumption and relatively high caloric potency, it commands attention in a nutrition textbook.

Ethanol is readily absorbed throughout the entire gastrointestinal tract. It is transported unaltered in the bloodstream and then oxidatively degraded in tissues, primarily the liver, first to acetaldehyde and then to acetate. In tissues peripheral to the liver, as well as in the liver itself, the acetate subsequently is converted to acetyl CoA and oxidized via the Krebs cycle. At least three enzyme systems are capable of ethanol oxidation:

- alcohol dehydrogenase (ADH),
- the microsomal ethanol oxidizing system (MEOS; also known as the cytochrome P-450 system), and
- catalase, in the presence of hydrogen peroxide.

Of these, the catalase-H_2O_2 system is the least active, probably accounting for <2% of in vivo ethanol oxidation. Therefore, we will not discuss it further. Nearly all ingested ethanol is oxidized by hepatic (and, to some extent, gastric) alcohol dehydrogenase and hepatic microsomal cytochrome P-450 systems.

The Alcohol Dehydrogenase (ADH) Pathway

ADH is a soluble enzyme functioning in the cytoplasm of liver cells. It is an ordinary NAD^+-requiring dehydrogenase and is known to be able to oxidize ethanol to acetaldehyde. The NADH formed by the reaction can be oxidized by mitochondrial electron transport by way of the NADH shuttle systems, thereby giving rise to ATP formation by oxidative phosphorylation. The K_m of alcohol dehydrogenase for ethanol is approximately 1 mM, or about 5 mg/dL. (K_m is reviewed in Chapter 1, in the section dealing with enzymes.) This means that at that cellular concentration of ethanol, ADH is functioning at half its maximum velocity. At concentrations three or four times the K_m, the enzyme is saturated with the ethanol substrate and is catalyzing at its maximum rate. Concentrations of ethanol in the cell more than four times the K_m level cannot be oxidized by ADH.

Because ethanol is an exogenous dietary ingredient, there is no "normal" concentration of ethanol in the cells or the bloodstream. The so-called toxic level of blood ethanol, however, is considered to be in the range of 50 to 100 mg/dL and is defined by its pharmacological actions. The high lipid solubility of ethanol allows it to enter cells passively with ease. If its cellular concentration were to reach a level even one-third or one-fourth that in blood, ADH would be saturated by the substrate and would be functioning at its maximum velocity. The excess, or "spillover," ethanol then must be metabolized by alternate systems, the most important of which is the microsomal ethanol oxidizing system (MEOS), described next. Another factor forcing a shift to the microsomal metabolizing system is a depletion of NAD^+, brought about by the high level of activity of ADH. The microsomal system does not require NAD^+ for its oxidative reactions.

Alcohol dehydrogenase activity is also found in gastric mucosal cells. Interestingly, there appears to be a significant gender difference in the level of its activity in these cells. Young (premenopausal) females develop higher blood alcohol levels than male counterparts with equal consumption and consequently display a lower tolerance for alcohol and are at greater risk of toxic effects in the liver. The lower level of alcohol dehydrogenase activity in the female gastric mucosa is believed to account for this observation [13,14].

The Microsomal Ethanol Oxidizing System (MEOS)

Despite its name, the microsomal ethanol oxidizing system (MEOS) is able to oxidize a wide variety of compounds in addition to ethanol, including fatty acids, aromatic hydrocarbons, steroids, and barbiturate drugs. The oxidation occurs through a system of electron transport, similar to the mitochondrial electron transport system described in detail in Chapter 3. Because the MEOS is microsomal and is associated with the smooth endoplasmic reticulum, it is sometimes referred to as the microsomal electron transport system. Another distinction of the system is its requirement for a special cytochrome called cytochrome P-450, which acts as an intermediate electron carrier. Cytochrome P-450 is not a singular compound but rather exists as a family of structurally related cytochromes, the members of which share the property of absorbing light having a wavelength of 450 nm.

Ethanol oxidation by the MEOS is linked to the simultaneous oxidation of NADPH by molecular oxygen. Because two substrates therefore are oxidized concurrently, the enzymes involved in the oxidations are commonly called mixed-function oxidases. One oxygen atom of the oxygen molecule is used to oxidize NADPH to $NADP^+$, and the second oxidizes the ethanol substrate to acetaldehyde. Both oxygen atoms are reduced to H_2O, and therefore two H_2O molecules are formed in the reactions. Microsomal electron transport of the MEOS is shown in Figure 4.23. Acting as carriers of electrons from NADPH to oxygen are FAD, FMN, and a cytochrome P-450 system.

An important feature of the MEOS is that certain of its enzymes, including the cytochrome P-450 units, are inducible by ethanol. This means that ethanol, particularly at higher concentrations, can induce the synthesis of these substances. The result is that the hepatocytes can metabolize ethanol much more effectively, thereby establishing a state of metabolic tolerance. Compared with a normal (nondrinking or light-drinking) subject, an individual in a state of metabolic tolerance to ethanol can ingest larger quantities of the substance before showing the effects of intoxication. When enzyme induction occurs, however, it can also accelerate the metabolism of other substances metabolized by the microsomal system. In other words, tolerance to ethanol induced by heavy drinking can render a person tolerant to other substances in addition to ethanol.

Alcoholism: Biochemical and Metabolic Alterations

Excessive consumption of ethanol can lead to alcoholism, defined by the National Council on Alcoholism as consumption that is capable of producing pathological changes. Alcoholism is a serious socioeconomic and health problem, exemplified by the fact that in the United States alcohol-related liver disease has been reported as the sixth leading cause of death [15]. The well-known consequences of alcoholism—fatty liver, hepatic disease (cirrhosis), lactic acidosis, and metabolic tolerance—can be explained by the manner in which ethanol is metabolized. Basically, the consequences of excessive alcohol intake are explainable by metabolic effects of (1) acetaldehyde toxicity, (2) elevated NADH : NAD^+ ratio, (3) metabolic competition, and (4) induced metabolic tolerance.

A comprehensive review of the association of nutritional and biochemical alterations with alcoholism is available [16].

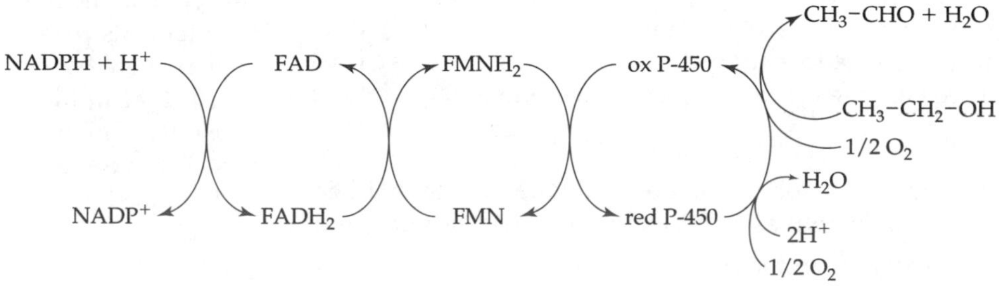

Figure 4.23 The microsomal ethanol oxidizing system (MEOS). Both ethanol and NADPH are oxidized by molecular oxygen in this electron transfer scheme. Because two substrates are oxidized, enzymes involved in the oxidation are referred to as mixed-function oxidases.

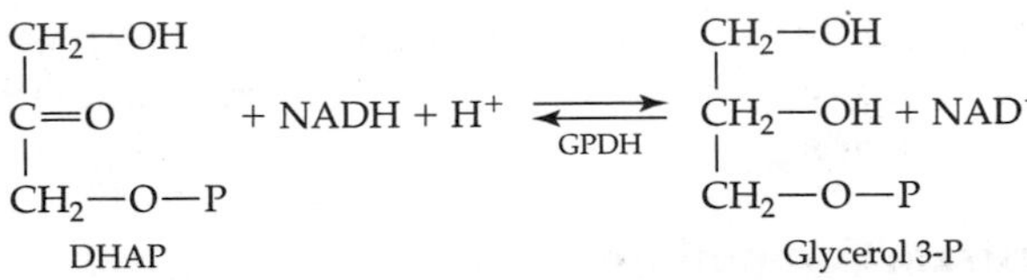

Figure 4.24 The reaction of dihydroxyacetone (DHAP) to glycerol 3-P, producing NAD^+ from NADH.

Acetaldehyde Toxicity

Both the ADH and the MEOS routes of ethanol oxidation produce acetaldehyde, which is believed to exert direct adverse effects on metabolic systems. For example, acetaldehyde is able to attach covalently to proteins, forming protein adducts. Should the adduct involve an enzyme, the activity of that enzyme could be impaired. Acetaldehyde has also been shown to impede the formation of microtubules in liver cells and to cause the development of perivenular fibrosis, either of which is believed to initiate the events leading to cirrhosis. These and other possible adverse effects of acetaldehyde are reviewed by Lieber [17].

It was once thought that alcoholic cirrhosis was caused by malnutrition, as the drinker satisfied his or her caloric needs with the "empty" calories of alcohol at the expense of a nutritionally balanced diet. In view of the effect of high levels of acetaldehyde on hepatocyte structure and function, however, it is now known that chronic overindulgence can cause cirrhosis in the absence of nutritional deficiency and even when the alcohol is coingested with an enriched diet.

High NADH : NAD^+ Ratio

The oxidation of ethanol increases the concentration of NADH at the expense of NAD^+, therefore elevating the NADH : NAD^+ ratio. This is because both ADH and acetaldehyde dehydrogenase use NAD^+ as cosubstrate. NADH is an important regulator of certain dehydrogenase reactions. The rise in concentration of NADH represents an overproduction of reducing equivalents, which in turn acts as a signal for a metabolic shift toward reduction—namely, hydrogenation. Such a shift can account for fatty liver (through the anabolic activity producing fatty acids) and lactic acidemia (high blood-lactate levels), which often accompany alcoholism, by increasing the reduction of pyruvate to lactic acid. For example, lactic acidemia can be attributed in part to the direct effect of NADH in shifting the lactate dehydrogenase (LDH) reaction toward the formation of lactate. The reaction, which follows, is driven to the right by the high concentration of NADH:

$$\text{Pyruvate} + \text{NADH} + \text{H}^+ \xrightarrow[\text{LDH}]{\longrightarrow} \text{Lactate} + \text{NAD}^+$$

Lipids accumulate in most tissues in which ethanol is metabolized, resulting in fatty liver, fatty myocardium, fatty renal tubules, and so on. The mechanism appears to involve both increased lipid synthesis and decreased lipid removal and can be explained in part by the increased NADH : NAD^+ ratio. As NADH accumulates, it slows dehydrogenase reactions of the Krebs cycle, such as the isocitrate dehydrogenase and α-ketoglutarate dehydrogenase reactions, thereby slowing the overall activity of the cycle. This results in an accumulation of citrate, which positively regulates acetyl CoA carboxylase. Acetyl CoA carboxylase converts acetyl CoA into malonyl CoA by the attachment of a carboxyl group. It is the key regulatory enzyme for the synthesis of fatty acids from acetyl CoA (Chap. 6). The high NADH : NAD^+ ratio therefore directs metabolism away from Krebs cycle oxidation and toward fatty acid synthesis.

Also contributing to the lipogenic effect of alcoholism is the effect of NADH on the glycerophosphate dehydrogenase (GPDH) reaction. The reaction, shown in Figure 4.24, favors the reduction of dihydroxyacetone phosphate (DHAP) to glycerol 3-phosphate if NADH concentration is high. Glycerol 3-phosphate provides the glycerol component in the synthesis of triacylglycerols. Therefore, a high NADH : NAD^+ ratio stimulates the synthesis of both the fatty acids and the glycerol components of triacylglycerols, contributing to the cellular fat accumulation that develops in alcoholism.

The glutamate dehydrogenase (GluDH) reaction (Fig. 4.25) also is affected by a rise in NADH concentration, resulting in impaired gluconeogenesis. The GluDH reaction is extremely important in gluconeogenesis because of the role it plays in the conversion of amino acids to their carbon skeletons by transamination and in the release of their amino groups as NH_3. A shift in the reaction toward glutamate due to elevated NADH

Figure 4.25 The reversible reaction of glutamate and NAD^+ forming α-ketoglutarate, NADH, and ammonia, catalyzed by glutamate dehydrogenase (GluDH).

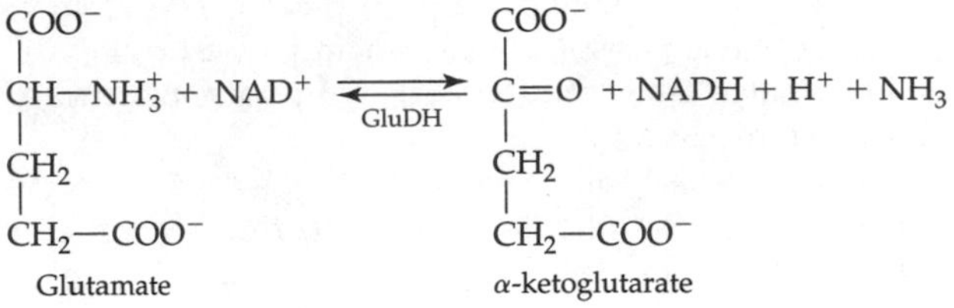

depletes the availability of α-ketoglutarate, which is the major acceptor of amino groups in the transamination of amino acids.

Substrate Competition

A well-established nutritional problem associated with excessive alcohol metabolism is a deficiency of vitamin A. Two aspects of ethanol interference with normal metabolism probably can account for this problem. One is the effect of ethanol on retinol dehydrogenase, the cytoplasmic enzyme that converts retinol to retinal. Retinal is required for the synthesis of photopigments used in vision. Retinol dehydrogenase is thought to be identical to ADH, and therefore ethanol competitively inhibits the hepatic conversion of retinol to retinal. In addition to this substrate competition effect, ethanol may interfere with retinol metabolism through induced metabolic tolerance.

Induced Metabolic Tolerance

As explained earlier, ethanol can induce enzymes of the MEOS, causing an increased rate of metabolism of substrates oxidized by this system. Retinol, like ethanol, spills over into the MEOS when ADH is saturated and NAD^+ stores are low because of heavy ingestion of ethanol. Ethanol induction of retinol-metabolizing enzymes then can occur. The specific component of the MEOS known to be induced by heavy consumption of ethanol has been designated cytochrome P-450IIE1. Although induction accelerates the hepatic oxidation of retinol, the oxidation product is not retinal but other polar, inert products of oxidation. The hepatic depletion of retinol can therefore be attributed to its accelerated metabolism, which is secondary to ethanol induction of a metabolizing enzyme. In effect, the alcoholic subject becomes tolerant to vitamin A, necessitating a higher dietary intake of the vitamin to maintain normal hepatocyte concentrations.

Alcohol in Moderation: The Brighter Side

Alcohol is a nutritional "Jekyll and Hyde," and which face it flaunts is clearly a function of the extent to which it is consumed. We focused earlier on the effects of alcohol at high intake levels and the negative impact of alcoholism on metabolism and nutrition. Many studies, however, have suggested that alcohol consumed in moderation may have beneficial effects, particularly in its ability to improve plasma lipid profiles and reduce the risk of cardiovascular disease.

Ethanol is known to elevate the level of high-density lipoprotein (HDL) in serum and to lower the amount of serum lipoprotein a [18,19]. Both effects favor a decrease in cardiovascular disease risk. This is because HDL protects against the deposition of arterial fatty plaque (atherogenesis), whereas high levels of lipoprotein a appear to promote it. The effect of these and other lipoproteins on atherogenesis will be discussed in Chapter 6. Other mechanisms for the apparent protective action of alcohol against atherogenesis have been suggested. A well-recognized component of the atherogenic process is the proliferation of smooth muscle cells underlying the endothelium of arterial walls. Studies have shown that alcohol may suppress the proliferation of smooth muscle cells, thereby slowing the atherogenic process [20].

summary

The major sources of dietary carbohydrate are the starches and the disaccharides. In the course of digestion, these are hydrolyzed by specific glycosidases to their component monosaccharides, which are absorbed into the circulation from the intestine. The monosaccharides then are transported to the cells of various tissues, passing through the cells' outer membrane by facilitative transport via transporters. Glucose is transported into the cells of many different tissues by the GLUT family of transporters. In the cells, monosaccharides first are phosphorylated at the expense of ATP and then can follow any of several integrated pathways of metabolism. Glucose is phosphorylated in most cells by hexokinase, but in the liver it is phosphorylated by glucokinase. Fructose is phosphorylated mainly by fructokinase in the liver. Galactose is phosphorylated by galactokinase, also a liver enzyme.

Cellular glucose can be converted to glycogen, primarily in liver and skeletal muscle, or it can be routed through the energy-releasing pathways of glycolysis and the Krebs cycle in these and other tissues for ATP production. Glycolytic reactions convert glucose (or glucose residues from glycogen) to pyruvate. From pyruvate, either an aerobic course (complete oxidation in the Krebs cycle) or an anaerobic course (to lactate) can be followed. Nearly all the energy formed by the oxidation of carbohydrates to CO_2 and H_2O is released in the Krebs cycle, as reduced coenzymes are oxidized via mitochondrial electron transport. On complete oxidation, approximately 40% of this energy is retained in the high-energy phosphate bonds of ATP. The remaining energy supplies heat to the body.

Noncarbohydrate substances derived from the other major nutrients, fats and proteins, can be converted to glucose or glycogen by the pathways of gluconeogenesis. The reverse is not true in that the basic carbon skeleton of fatty acids cannot be converted to a net synthesis of glucose. Basically, the reactions are the reversible reactions of glycolysis, shifted toward glucose synthesis in accordance with reduced energy demand by the body. Three kinase reactions occurring in glycolysis are not reversible, however, requiring the involvement of different enzymes and pathways to circumvent those reactions in the process of gluconeogenesis. Muscle glycogen provides a source of glucose for energy only for muscle fiber, because muscle lacks the enzyme glucose 6-phosphatase, which forms free glucose from glucose 6-phosphate. Glucose 6-phosphatase is active in liver, however, which means that the liver can release free glucose from its glycogen stores into the circulation for use by other tissues. The Cori cycle describes the liver's uptake and gluconeogenic conversion of muscle-produced lactate to glucose.

A metabolic pathway is regulated according to the body's need for energy or for maintaining homeostatic cellular concentrations of certain metabolites. Regulation is exerted mainly through hormones, through substrate concentrations (which can affect the velocity of enzyme reactions), and through allosteric enzymes that can be modulated negatively or positively by certain pathway products.

Ethanol is catabolized ultimately to acetyl CoA, furnishing calories through Krebs cycle oxidation. The nutritional complexities of alcohol abuse were discussed.

In Chapters 6 and 7, we will see that fatty acids and the carbon skeleton of various amino acids also are ultimately oxidized through the Krebs cycle. The amino acids that do become Krebs cycle intermediates, however, may not be completely oxidized to CO_2 and H_2O but instead may leave the cycle to be converted to glucose or glycogen (by gluconeogenesis) should dietary intake of carbohydrate be low. The glycerol portion of triacylglycerols enters the glycolytic pathway at the level of dihydroxyacetone phosphate, from which point it can be oxidized for energy or used to synthesize glucose or glycogen. The fatty acids of triacylglycerols enter the Krebs cycle as acetyl CoA, which is oxidized to CO_2 and H_2O but cannot contribute carbon for the net synthesis of glucose. This topic is considered further in Chapter 6.

These examples of the entrance of noncarbohydrate substances into the pathways discussed in this chapter are cited here to remind the reader that these pathways are not singularly committed to carbohydrate metabolism. Rather, they must be thought of as common ground for the interconversion and oxidation of fats and proteins as well as carbohydrate. It is essential to maintain this broad perspective when we move on to Chapters 6 and 7, which examine the metabolism of lipids and proteins, respectively.

References Cited

1. Garrett RH, Grisham CM. Biochemistry, 2nd ed. Fort Worth: Harcourt College Publishers, 1999.

2. Riby J, Fujisawa T, Kretchmer N. Fructose absorption. Am J Clin Nutr 1993;58(suppl 5):748S–53S.

3. Burant C, Takeda J, Brot-Laroche E, Bell G, Davidson N. Fructose transporter in human spermatozoa and small intestine is GLUT5. J Biol Chem 1992;267:14523–26.

4. Truswell AS, Seach JM, Thorburn AW. Incomplete absorption of pure fructose in healthy subjects and the facilitating effect of glucose. Am J Clin Nutr 1988;48:1424–30.

5. Baldwin SA. Mammalian passive glucose transporters: members of a ubiquitous family of active and passive transport proteins. Biochim et Biophysica Acta 1993;1154:17–49.

6. Bloc J, Gibbs EM, Lienhard GE, Slot JW, Geuze HJ. Insulin-induced translocation of glucose transporters from post-Golgi compartments to the plasma membrane of 3T3-L1 adipocytes. J Cell Biol 1988;106:69–76.

7. Freidman JE, Dudek RW, Whitehead DS, et al. Immunolocalization of glucose transporter GLUT4 within human skeletal muscle. Diabetes 1991;40:150–54.

8. Takata K, Hirano H, Kasahara M. Transport of glucose across the blood-tissue barriers. Int Rev Cyt 1997;172:1–53.

9. Ludwig, DS. The glycemic index: physiological mechanism relating to obesity, diabetes and cardiovascular disease. JAMA 2002; 287:2414–24.

10. Augustin LS, Francesch IS, Jenkins DJA, Kendall CWC, Lavecchia C. Glycemic index in chronic disease: a review. Euro J Clin Nutr 2002;56:1049–71.

11. Katz J, McGarry JD. The glucose paradox: is glucose a substrate for liver metabolism? J Clin Invest 1984;74:1901–9.

12. Smythe C, Cohen P. The discovery of glycogenin and the priming mechanism for glycogen biosynthesis. Eur J Biochem 1991;200: 625–31.

13. Frezza M, di Padova C, Pozzato G, Terpin M, Baraona E, Lieber C. High blood alcohol levels in women. The role of decreased alcohol dehydrogenase activity and first pass metabolism. N Engl J Med 1990;322:95–99.

14. Thomasson R. Gender differences in alcohol metabolism: physiological responses to ethanol. Recent Dev Alcohol 1995; 12:163–79.

15. US Bureau of the Census: Statistical Abstract of the United States, 1975. Washington, DC: US Government Printing Office, 1975.

16. Mendenhall C, Weesner R. Alcoholism. In: Kaplan LA, Pesce AJ, eds. Clinical Chemistry: Theory, Analysis, Correlation, 3rd ed. St. Louis: Mosby, 1996, pp. 682–95.

17. Lieber CS. Biochemical and molecular basis of alcohol-induced injury to liver and other tissues. N Engl J Med 1988;319: 1639–50.

18. Valimaki M, Laitinen K, Ylikahri R, et al. The effect of moderate alcohol intake on serum apolipoprotein A-I-containing lipoproteins and lipoprotein-(a). Metabolism 1991;40:1168–72.

19. Jackson R, Scragg R, Beaglehole R. Alcohol consumption and risk of coronary heart disease. BMJ 1991;303:211–16.

20. Locher R, Suter P, Vetter W. Ethanol suppresses smooth muscle cell proliferation in the post-prandial state: a new antiatherosclerotic mechanism of ethanol? Am J Clin Nutr 1998;67: 338–41.

Suggested Readings

McGarry JD, Kuwajima M, Newgard CB, Foster DW. From dietary glucose to liver glycogen: the full circle round. Ann Rev Nutr 1987;7:51–73.

The glucose paradox is emphasized, from the standpoint of its emergence, as are the attempts to resolve it.

Pilkis SJ, El-Maghrabi MR, Claus TH. Hormonal regulation of hepatic gluconeogenesis and glycolysis. Ann Rev Biochem 1988;57:755–83.

This is a brief, clearly presented summary of the effect of certain hormones on the important regulatory enzymes in these major pathways of carbohydrate metabolism.

Web Sites

www.medscape.com
Medscape

www.cdc.gov
Centers for Disease Control and Prevention

www.ama-assn.org
American Medical Association

www.wadsworth.com/nutrition
Wadsworth Publishing Company

Hypoglycemia: Fact or Fall Guy?

Maintenance of normal blood glucose concentration (normoglycemia) is essential to good health. The consequences of abnormally high levels (**hyperglycemia**), such as occur in diabetes, are well established. Concentrations that are significantly below the normal range (**hypoglycemia**) introduce a well-recognized syndrome as well. This perspective deals with the latter situation.

Glucose is our most important carbohydrate nutrient. Its concentration in the blood is established by a balance between processes that infuse glucose into the blood and those that remove it from the blood for use by the cells. The primary sources of blood glucose are

- exogenous (dietary sugars and starches),
- hepatic glycogenolysis, and
- hepatic gluconeogenesis.

The primary glucose-requiring tissues are the brain, erythrocytes, and muscle.

Preprandial (before-meals) serum glucose levels generally range from 70 to 105 mg/dL in patients who have no disorder of glucose metabolism (1 dL = 100 mL). If whole blood is the specimen, the range is somewhat lower, approximately 60 to 90 mg/dL. Should levels drop below this range, glucoreceptors in the hypothalamus stimulate the secretion of counterregulatory hormones to try to return the glucose to homeostatic levels. Such hormones include

- glucagon, which increases hepatic glycogenolysis and gluconeogenesis;
- epinephrine, which inhibits glucose use by muscle and increases muscle glycogenolysis; and
- cortisol and growth hormone, although these have a delayed release and do not contribute significantly to acute recovery.

The major hormone acting antagonistically to those listed is insulin, which has the opposing effect of increasing cellular uptake of glucose, thereby reducing its serum concentration.

If, in spite of counterregulatory hormone response, subnormal concentrations of glucose persist, a state of clinical hypoglycemia can possibly result. This, in turn, can give rise to any number of associated symptoms. Symptoms may be attributable to the low glucose level or to the hormonal response to the low glucose level and are broadly categorized as adrenergic or neuroglucopenic.

Adrenergic symptoms arise as a result of increased activity of the autonomic nervous system, coincident with accelerated release of epinephrine. Adrenergic symptoms include weakness, sweating/warmth, tachycardia (rapid heart rate), palpitation, and tremor.

Neuroglucopenic symptoms are usually associated with a more severe hypoglycemic state. They include headache, hypothermia, visual disturbances, mental dullness, and seizures. During insulin-induced hypoglycemia, adrenergic symptoms may manifest at serum glucose concentrations of about 60 mg/dL, and neuroglucopenic symptoms at approximately 45 to 50 mg/dL.

Many of the symptoms listed here are nonspecific and somewhat vague, and they may arise as a result of any number of unrelated disorders. For this reason, hypoglycemia is among the most overdiagnosed ailments. Before it can be diagnosed as bona fide clinical hypoglycemia, a condition must comply with the following contingencies:

1. A low serum glucose level
2. Presence of adrenergic or neuroglucopenic symptoms
3. Relief of symptoms upon ingestion of carbohydrate and a return of glucose levels toward normal

Patients commonly may have serum glucose concentrations as low as 50 mg/dL and yet be asymptomatic (without symptoms), while others may be normoglycemic but have any number of the symptoms congruent with hypoglycemia. In neither case is true clinical hypoglycemia verifiable.

Two types of hypoglycemia exist:

- *Fasting hypoglycemia* is usually caused by drugs, such as exogenous insulin, used in the treatment of type 1 diabetes, or the sulfonylureas, which stimulate the secretion of insulin. It can also be caused by insulinomas (β cell tumors) or excessive intake of alcohol.
- *Fed (reactive) hypoglycemia* has two possible causes in patients who have not undergone certain gastrointestinal surgical procedures: impaired glucose tolerance (IGT) and the more common idiopathic postprandial syndrome.

Some patients with IGT or early stages of diabetes experience **postprandial** (after-meals) hypoglycemia due to an initially delayed insulin response to food, followed by excessive insulin release that drives glucose levels down to hypoglycemic concentrations. This condition can be diagnosed by the oral glucose tolerance test (OGTT), in which serum glucose levels are observed following an oral load of glucose over an extended period of time (often as long as 5 hours).

Much attention has been paid to the putative idiopathic (of unknown origin) postprandial form of hypoglycemia. It has been difficult to document that adrenergic symptoms occur simultaneously with the analytical finding of hypoglycemia. As discussed earlier, adrenergic symptoms frequently do not correlate with low glucose levels. Furthermore, feeding may not relieve the symptoms or elevate serum glucose. This is the form of hypoglycemia that has been overdiagnosed as such. The actual cause is more complex, and other factors may be players in the game.

Diet therapy is the cornerstone of treatment for all forms of reactive (fed) hypoglycemia. Patients should avoid simple or refined carbohydrates and may also benefit from frequent, small feedings of snacks containing a mixture of carbohydrate, protein, and fat.

Suggested Reading

Andreoli T, Bennett J, Carpenter C, and Plum F. Hypoglycemia. In: Cecil Essentials of Medicine, 5th ed. Philadelphia: W. B. Saunders, 2001, Chap. 69.

Web Site

www.betterhealth.com
Better Health

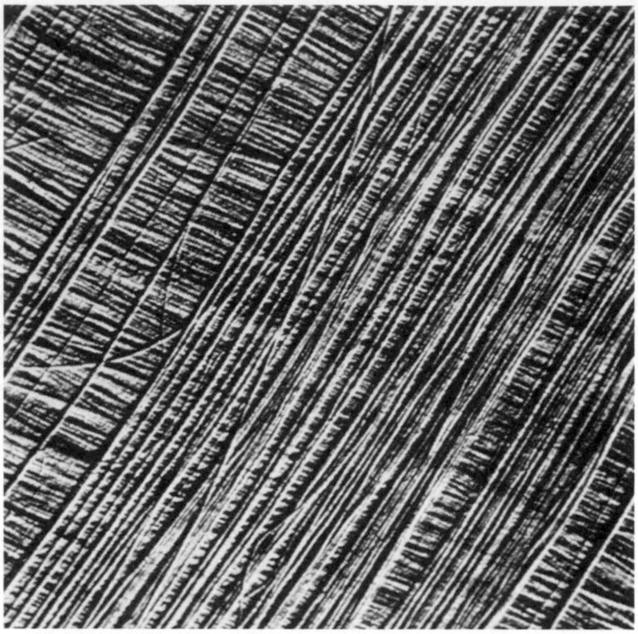

Cellulose fibers in a plant cell wall

chapter 5 Fiber

DIETARY FIBER WAS RECOGNIZED AGAIN as an important food component in about the mid-1970s. Yet the concept of fiber, originally referred to as crude fiber or indigestible material, and its extraction from animal feed and forages were introduced in Germany during the 1850s. The crude fiber extraction method was used, even for human food, into the 1990s, despite the existence of better methodology and the inconsistent relationship between crude fiber and dietary fiber. Today, soluble and insoluble fibers may be extracted or, in some cases, manufactured in laboratories and added as an ingredient to create foods containing what we now call functional fiber.

Results from extensive research devoted to dietary fiber during the last 25 or so years have implicated dietary fiber as an important component in various aspects of gastrointestinal tract function and in the prevention and/or management of a variety of disease states. The varying effects of fiber observed by researchers are related to the fact that dietary fiber consists of different components, each with its own distinctive characteristics. Examining these many components plus their various distinctive characteristics emphasizes the fact that dietary fiber cannot be considered a single entity. This chapter addresses the definitions of dietary fiber and functional fiber; the relationship between plants and fiber; and the chemistry, intraplant functions, and properties of fiber. It also provides recommendations for fiber intake.

DEFINITIONS OF DIETARY FIBER AND FUNCTIONAL FIBER

With the publication of the 2002 Dietary Reference Intakes for Energy, Carbohydrate, Fiber, Fat, Protein and Amino Acids by the National Academy of Sciences Food and Nutrition Board, uniform definitions for dietary fiber and functional fiber were established. **Dietary fiber** refers to nondigestible (by human digestive enzymes) carbohydrates and lignin that are intact and intrinsic in plants [1]. **Functional fiber** consists of nondigestible carbohydrates that have been isolated, extracted, or manufactured and have been shown to have beneficial physiological effects in humans [1]. Table 5.1 lists dietary and functional fibers. Each fiber listed in Table 5.1 is discussed in this chapter in the section "Chemistry and Characteristics of Dietary and Functional Fibers."

FIBER AND PLANTS

The plant cell wall contains >95% of dietary fibers, including cellulose, hemicellulose, lignin, and pectins as well as some nonstarch polysaccharides. The plant cell wall consists of both a primary and a secondary wall. The primary wall is a thin envelope surrounding the contents of the growing cell. The secondary wall develops as the cell matures. The secondary wall of a mature plant contains many strands of cellulose arranged in an orderly fashion within a matrix of noncellulosic polysaccharides. The primary wall also contains cellulose, but in smaller amounts and less well organized. The hemicellulose content of plants varies but can make up 20% to 30% of the cell walls. Starch, the energy storage product of the cell, is found within the cell walls.

Table 5.1 Dietary and Functional Fibers

Dietary Fibers	Functional Fibers
Cellulose	Cellulose
Hemicellulose	Pectin
Pectin	Lignin*
Lignin	Gums
Gums	β-glucans
β-glucans	Fructans*
Fructans	Chitin and chitosan*
Resistant starches	Polydextrose and polyols*
	Psyllium
	Resistant dextrins*
	Resistant starches

*Data showing positive physiological effects in humans are needed.

Lignin deposits form in specialized cells whose function is to provide structural support to the plant. As the plant matures, lignin spreads through the intracellular spaces, penetrating the pectins. Pectins function as intercellular cement and are located between and around the cell walls. Lignin continues dispersing through intracellular spaces, but it also permeates the primary wall and then spreads into the developing secondary wall. As plant development continues further, suberin is deposited in the cell wall just below the epidermis and skin. Suberin is made up of a variety of substances, including phenolic compounds as well as long-chain alcohols and polymeric esters of fatty acids. Cutin, also made of polymeric esters of fatty acids, is a water-impermeable substance that is secreted onto the plant surface. Both suberin and cutin are enzyme- and acid-resistant. In addition to suberin and cutin, waxes (consisting of complex hydrophobic, hydrocarbon compounds) are found in many plants and function to coat the external surfaces.

The consumption of plant foods provides fiber in the diet. The plant species, the part of the plant (leaf, root, stem), and the plant's maturity all influence the composition (cellulose, hemicellulose, pectin, lignin, etc.) of the fiber that is consumed. For example, consumption of cereal bran (which consists of the outer layers of cereal grains) such as wheat bran provides primarily hemicellulose along with lignin. Consumption of fruits and vegetables provides almost equal quantities (~30%) of cellulose and pectin. In contrast, cereals are quite low in cellulose. We will review each of the dietary fibers, including their characteristics and functions, as well as foods rich in the particular fiber. Identifying the chemical characteristics and various intraplant functions and properties of these plant cell wall substances (and/or substances in contact with the wall) promotes conceptualization of how fiber components may affect physiological and metabolic functions in humans.

CHEMISTRY AND CHARACTERISTICS OF DIETARY AND FUNCTIONAL FIBERS

Cellulose

Cellulose is considered a dietary fiber as well as a functional fiber when added to foods. Chemical analysis shows cellulose (Fig. 5.1a) to be a long, linear **polymer** (a high-molecular-weight substance made up of a chain of repeating units) of β 1-4 linked glucose units (alternately stated, a D-glucopyranosyl homopolymer in β 1-4 glycosidic linkages). Cellulose is a main component of plant cell walls. Hydrogen bonding between sugar residues in adjacent parallel running cellulose chains imparts a microfibril three-dimensional structure to cellulose. Being a large,

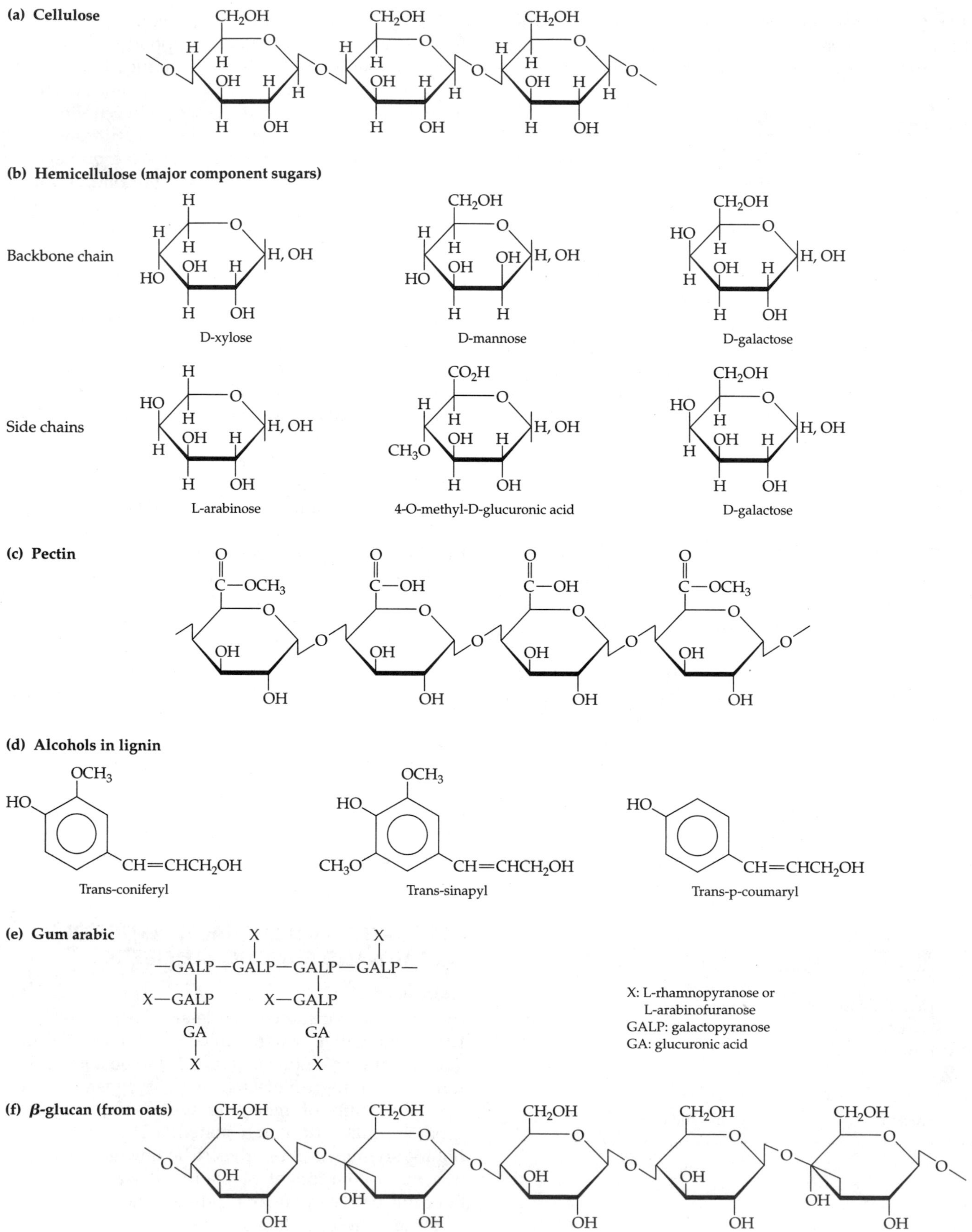

Figure 5.1 Chemical structures of dietary fibers and some functional fibers.

linear, neutrally charged molecule, cellulose is water-insoluble, although it can be modified chemically (e.g., carboxymethylcellulose, methylcellulose, and hydroxypropylmethylcellulose) to be more water-soluble for use as a food additive. Degradation of cellulose by colonic bacteria varies, but generally it is poorly fermented. Some examples of foods high in cellulose relative to other fibers include bran, legumes, nuts, peas, root vegetables, vegetables of the cabbage family, the outer covering of seeds, and apples. Purified, powdered cellulose (usually isolated from wood) and modified celluloses are often added to foods, for example, as a thickening or texturing agent or to prevent caking or syneresis (leakage of liquid). Some examples of foods to which cellulose or a modified form of cellulose is added include breads, cake mixes, sauces and sandwich spreads, dips, frozen meat products (e.g., chicken nuggets), and fruit juice mixes.

Hemicellulose

Hemicellulose, a dietary fiber and a component of plant cell walls, consists of a heterogeneous group of polysaccharide substances that vary both between different plants and within a plant depending on location. Hemicelluloses contain a number of sugars in their backbone and side chains. The sugars, which form a basis for hemicellulose classification, include xylose, mannose, and galactose in the hemicellulose backbone and arabinose, glucuronic acid, and galactose in the hemicellulose side chains. The number of sugars in the side chains varies such that some hemicelluloses are relatively linear while others are highly branched. Some of the sugars found in hemicelluloses are shown in Figure 5.1b. One example of a hemicellulose structure is β 1-4 linked D-xylopyranose units with branches of 4-O-methyl D-glucopyranose uronic acids linked by α 1-2 bonds or with branches of L-arabinofuranosyl units linked by α 1-3 bonds. The sugars in the side chains confer important characteristics on the hemicellulose. For example, hemicelluloses that contain acids in their side chains are slightly charged and water-soluble. Other hemicelluloses are water-insoluble. Fermentability of the hemicelluloses by intestinal **microflora,** bacteria adapted to living in that specific environment, is also influenced by the sugars and their positions. For example, hexose and uronic acid components of hemicellulose are more accessible to bacterial enzymes than are the other hemicellulose sugars. Foods that are relatively high in hemicellulose include bran and whole grains as well as nuts, legumes, and some vegetables and fruits.

Pectins

Pectins are a family of compounds that in turn make up a larger family of pectic substances including pectins, pectic acids, and pectinic acids. Pectin is both a dietary fiber and a functional fiber. Pectinic acids represent polygalacturonic acids that either are partly esterified with methanol or have no or negligible amounts of methyl esters. Pectins typically represent a complex group of polysaccharides referred to as galacturonoglycans, which also vary in methyl ester content. Galacturonic acid is a primary constituent of pectin and makes up its backbone structure. The backbone is usually an unbranched chain of α 1,4-linked D-galacturonic acid units (polygalactopyranosyluronic acids), as shown in Figure 5.1c. Many of the carboxyl groups of the uronic acid moieties exist as methyl esters. Other carbohydrates may be linked to the galacturonic acid chain. These additional sugars, sometimes found attached as side chains, include rhamnose, arabinose, xylose, fucose, and galactose; galactose may be present in a methylated form. Pectins form part of the primary cell wall of plants and part of the middle lamella. They are water-soluble and gel-forming and have high ion-binding potential. Because they are stable at low pH values, pectins perform well in acidic foods. In the body, pectins are almost completely metabolized by colonic bacteria and are not a good fecal bulking agent. Rich sources of pectins include apples, strawberries, and citrus fruits. Legumes, nuts, and some vegetables also provide pectins. Commercially, pectins are usually extracted from citrus peel or apples and added to many products. Pectin is added to jellies and jams to promote gelling. It is also added to fruit roll-ups, fruit juices, and icings or frostings, among other products. Pectin is added to some enteral nutrition formulas administered to tubefed hospital patients to provide a source of fiber in their diets.

Lignin

Lignin is a three-dimensional (highly branched) polymer composed of phenol units with strong intramolecular bonding. The primary phenols composing lignin include trans-coniferyl, trans-sinapyl, and trans-p-coumaryl, shown in Figure 5.1d. Lignin forms the structural components of plants and is thought to attach to other noncellulose polysaccharides such as heteroxylans found in plant cell walls. Lignin is insoluble in water, has hydrophobic binding capacity, and is not digested (is poorly fermented) by colonic bacterial microflora. Lignin is both a dietary fiber and a functional fiber. Mature root vegetables such as carrots, wheat, and fruits with edible seeds (e.g., strawberries) are high in lignin.

Gums

Gums, also referred to as *hydrocolloids,* represent a group of substances. Gums are secreted at the site of plant injury by specialized secretory cells and can be exuded from plants (i.e., forced out of plant tissues). Gums that function as tree **exudates** include gum arabic, gum karaya, and gum ghatti; gum tragacanth is a shrub exudate. Gums are composed of a variety of sugars and sugar derivatives. Occurring prominently in the gums are galactose and glucuronic acid, as well as uronic acids, arabinose, rhamnose, and mannose, among others. Within the large intestine, gums are highly fermented by colonic bacteria. Of the tree exudates, gum arabic is most commonly used as a food additive to promote gelling, thickening, and stabilizing. Gum arabic, shown in Figure 5.1e, contains a main galactose backbone joined by β 1-3 linkages and β 1-6 linkages along with side chains of galactose, arabinose, rhamnose, glucuronic acid, and/or methylglucuronic acid joined by β 1-6 linkages. The nonreducing ends terminate with a rhamnopyrosyl unit. The popularity of gum arabic is due to its physical properties, which include high water solubility, pH stability, and gelling characteristics. It is found in candies such as caramels, gumdrops, and toffees, as well as in other assorted products.

The water-soluble gums guar gum and locust bean gum (also called carob gum) are made from the ground endosperm of guar seeds and locust bean seeds, respectively. These gums consist mostly of galactomannans, the main component of the endosperm. Galactomannans contain a mannose backbone in 1-4 linkages and in a 2:1 or 4:1 ratio with galactose present in the side chains. Guar galactomannans have more branches than locust bean galactomannans. Both guar gum and locust bean gum are added as a thickening agent and water-binding agent (among other roles) to products such as bakery goods, sauces, dairy products, ice creams, dips, and salad dressings. Gums are also found naturally in foods such as oatmeal, barley, and legumes. Some gums (xanthan gum and gellan gum) can be synthesized by microorganisms. Gums are considered to be both dietary and functional fibers.

β-glucans

β-glucans are homopolymers of glucopyranose units (Fig. 5.1f). This water-soluble dietary fiber is found in relatively high amounts in cereal brans, especially oats and barley. Oat β-glucan consists of a chain of β-D-glucopyranosyl units joined mostly in 1-4 linkages but also some 1-3 linkages. β-glucans, extracted from cereals, are used commercially as a functional fiber due to their effectiveness in reducing serum cholesterol and postprandial blood glucose concentrations. β-glucans are highly fermentable in the colon.

Fructans — Inulin, Oligofructose, and Fructooligosaccharides

Fructans, including inulin, oligofructose, and fructooligosaccharides, are chemically composed primarily of fructose units in chains of varying length. Inulin consists of a fructose chain, containing from 2 to 60 units, with β 2-1 linkages and a glucose molecule linked to the C-2 position of the terminal fructofuranose unit to create a nonreducing unit at the end of the molecule. While human digestive enzymes are not able to hydrolyze the β 2-1 linkage, bifidobacteria have β-fructosidase, which can hydrolyze the β 2-1 linkage. Oligofructose is formed from the partial hydrolysis of inulin and typically contains between 2 and 8 fructose units; it may or may not contain an end glucose molecule. Fructooligosaccharides (FOS) are similar to oligofructose except that polymerization ranges from 2 to 4. Ingestion of fructooligosaccharides has been shown to promote the growth of bifidobacteria (act as a prebiotic). Whether the increased presence of such bacteria is beneficial requires additional studies [2–4]. Fructans are found naturally in plants and are considered dietary fibers, but at present they are not reported in most food composition databases. The most common food sources of inulin include chicory, onions, and Jerusalem artichokes. Inulin and oligofructose also may be synthesized from sucrose. The fibers can be extracted and purified from plant sources for commercial use. Inulin is used to replace fat in fillings, dressings, and frozen dessert, to name a few examples. Oligofructose is added, for example, to cereals, yogurt, dairy products, and frozen desserts. With sufficient data showing positive physiological effects, fructans added to foods could be considered a functional fiber.

Resistant Starch

Resistant starch is starch that is unable to be enzymatically digested. Starch found in plant cell walls that is inaccessible to amylase activity is one type of resistant starch, designated RS_1. Gelatinization of starch can increase its accessibility to enzymes; such starch is designated RS_2. Resistant starch also may be formed during food processing. The cooking and cooling of starchy foods or the extrusion of starchy foods, for example, generates retrograde starch referred to as RS_3. Chemical modifications of starch, such as the formation of starch esters, or cross-bonded starches also result in resistant starch (referred to as RS_4). Neither RS_3 nor RS_4 is digested by human digestive enzymes, but both may be partially fermented by colonic bacteria. RS_1 and RS_2 are considered dietary fibers, while RS_3 and RS_4 are considered functional fibers [1].

Chitin and Chitosan

Chitin is an amino-polysaccharide containing β 1-4 linked glucose units. It is similar in structure to cellulose, but an N-acetyl amino group substitutes for the hydroxyl group at the C-2 of the D-glucopyranose residue. Chitin is insoluble in water. Chitosan is a deacetylated form of chitin. Chitin can replace cellulose in the cell walls of some lower plants. It is also a component of the exoskeleton of insects and is found in the shells of crustaceans such as crabs and lobsters. Chitin and chitosan are sold as supplements. Chitosan in some studies has been shown to effectively reduce serum cholesterol concentrations [5,6]. With additional data showing physiological benefits in humans, chitosan and chitin may be considered functional fibers [1].

Polydextrose and Polyols

Polydextrose is a polysaccharide consisting of glucose and sorbitol units that have been polymerized at high temperatures and under a partial vacuum. Polydextrose, available commercially, is added to foods as a bulking agent or as a sugar substitute. The polysaccharide is neither digested nor absorbed by the human gastrointestinal tract; however, it can be partially fermented by colonic bacteria and contributes to fecal bulk. Polyols such as polyglycitol and malitol are found in syrups. With sufficient data on physiological benefits, some polyols and polydextrose may be classified as functional fibers [1].

Psyllium

Psyllium is obtained from the husk of psyllium seeds (also called plantago or fleas seed). Products containing psyllium have high water-binding properties and thus provide viscosity in solutions. Psyllium is considered a functional fiber. It is added, for example, to health products such as Metamucil for its laxative properties [1]. Foods containing psyllium and bearing a health claim are required to state on the label that the food should be eaten with at least a full glass of liquid and that choking may result if the product is not ingested with enough liquid [7]. In addition, the label should state that the food should not be eaten if a person has difficulty swallowing [7].

Resistant Dextrins

Resistant dextrins, also called *resistant maltodextrins,* are generated by treating cornstarch with heat and acid and then enzymes (amylase). The resistant dextrins consist of glucose polymers containing α 1-4 and α 1-6 glucosidic bonds and α 1-2 and α 1-3 bonds. With sufficient data showing beneficial physiological effects, resistant dextrins may be considered functional fibers [1].

SELECTED PROPERTIES AND PHYSIOLOGICAL AND METABOLIC EFFECTS OF FIBER

The physiological and metabolic effects of fiber vary based on the type of ingested fiber. Significant characteristics of dietary fiber that affect its physiological and metabolic roles include its solubility in water, its hydration or water-holding capacity and viscosity, its adsorptive attraction or ability to bind organic and inorganic molecules, and its degradability or fermentability by intestinal bacteria. We will review each of these characteristics and their effects on various physiological and metabolic processes. Figure 5.2 diagrams their relationships. However, as you study these characteristics and their effects on the body, it is important to remember that we eat foods with a mixture of dietary fiber, not foods with just cellulose, hemicellulose, pectins, gums, and so forth. Thus, the effects on the various body processes are not as straightforward as presented in this chapter and vary considerably based on the foods ingested.

Figure 5.2 Gastrointestinal response to soluble and insoluble fibers.

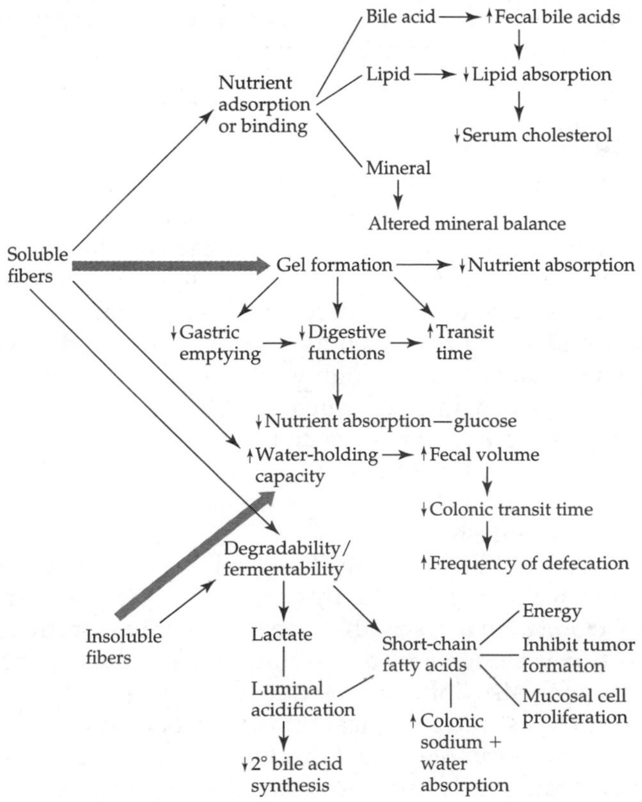

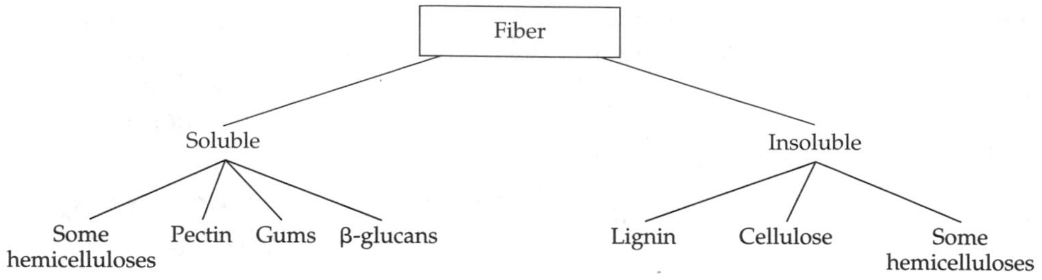

Figure 5.3 Soluble and insoluble fibers.

Solubility in Water

Fiber is often classified as water soluble or water insoluble (Fig. 5.3). Fibers that dissolve in hot water are soluble, and those that will not dissolve in hot water are insoluble. In general, water-soluble fibers include some hemicelluloses, pectin, gums, and β-glucans. Cellulose, lignin, and some hemicelluloses are examples of dietary fibers classified as insoluble. Generally, vegetables and wheat, along with most grain products, contain more insoluble fibers than soluble fibers.

Solubility in water also may be used as a basis for broadly dividing the characteristics of fibers. For example, soluble fibers generally delay gastric emptying, increase transit time (through slower movement) through the intestine, and decrease nutrient (e.g., glucose) absorption. In contrast, insoluble fibers decrease (speed up) intestinal transit time and increase fecal bulk. These actions (discussed in the following section) of the soluble and insoluble fibers in turn induce other physiological and metabolic effects.

Water-Holding/Hydration Capacity and Viscosity

Water-holding or hydration capacity of foods refers to the ability of fiber in food to bind water; think of fiber as a dry sponge moving through the digestive tract hydrating or soaking up water and digestive juices as it moves through the digestive tract. Many of the water-soluble fibers such as pectins, gums, and some hemicelluloses have a high water-holding capacity in comparison with fibers such as cellulose and lignin, which have a lower water-holding capacity. In addition, some water-soluble fibers such as pectins, psyllium, and gums form viscous (thick) solutions within the gastrointestinal tract.

Water-holding capacity, however, is not just dependent on the fiber's solubility in water. The pH of the gastrointestinal tract, the size of the fiber particles, and/or the degree of processing of the foods providing fiber also influence water-holding capacity and in turn its physiological effects. Coarsely ground bran, for example, has a higher hydration capacity than bran that is finely ground. Consequently, coarse bran with large particles holds water, increases fecal volume, and speeds up the rate of fecal passage through the colon. Maintaining the integrity of cells in grains and legumes rather than subjecting them to traditional milling processes also appears to affect the water-holding capacity of fibers.

The gastrointestinal effects from the ingestion of fibers that can hold water and create viscous solutions within the gastrointestinal tract include

- delayed (slowed) emptying of food from the stomach;
- reduced mixing of gastrointestinal contents with digestive enzymes;
- reduced enzyme function;
- decreased nutrient diffusion rate (and thus delayed nutrient absorption), resulting in attenuation of the blood glucose response; and
- altered small intestine transit time.

We will discuss each of these effects.

Delayed (Slowed) Gastric Emptying

When fibers form viscous gels or hydrate within the stomach, the release of the chyme from the stomach (gastric emptying) into the duodenum (proximal small intestine) is delayed (slowed). Thus, nutrients remain in the stomach longer with these fibers than they would in the absence of the ingested fiber. This effect creates a feeling of postprandial (after-eating) satiety (fullness) as well as slows down the digestion process, because carbohydrates and lipids that remain in the stomach undergo no digestion in the stomach and must move into the small intestine for further digestion to occur.

Reduced Mixing of Gastrointestinal Contents with Digestive Enzymes

The presence of viscous gels or hydrated fiber in the gastrointestinal tract provides a physical barrier that can impair the ability of the nutrients in the food to interact with the digestive enzymes. This interaction is critical for digestion to occur.

Reduced Enzyme Function

Viscous gel-forming fibers have been shown to interfere with the enzymatic hydrolysis of nutrients within the gastrointestinal tract. For example, gums may inhibit intestinal peptidases that are necessary for the digestion of peptides to amino acids [8,9]. The activity of pancreatic lipase also has been diminished because of ingestion of viscous gel-forming fibers and has thus resulted in inhibition of lipid digestion [8]. It is unclear whether fiber directly decreases the activity of these digestive enzymes or acts by reducing the rate of enzyme penetration into the food.

Decreased Nutrient Diffusion Rate — Attenuation of the Blood Glucose Response

Remember that for nutrients to be absorbed they must move from the lumen of the small intestine through a glycoprotein- (mucin-)rich water layer lying on top of the enterocytes. The fiber-associated decreased diffusion rate of nutrients through this layer is probably due to an increased thickness of the unstirred water layer. In other words, the unstirred water layer becomes more resistant to nutrient movement, and without this movement nutrients cannot be absorbed into the enterocyte.

Another mechanism may also be responsible for decreased nutrient diffusion. Gums appear to slow glucose absorption by decreasing the convective movement of glucose within the intestinal lumen. Convective currents induced by peristaltic movements are responsible for bringing nutrients from the lumen to the epithelial surface for absorption. Decreasing the convective solute movement also may help explain the decreased absorption of amino acids and fatty acids caused by viscous fiber [8]. Ingestion of viscous fibers such as gums, pectin, β-glucans, psyllium, and to a variable extent fructooligosaccharides and polydextrose has been shown to slow transit, delay glucose absorption, lower blood glucose concentrations, and affect hormonal (especially insulin) response to the absorbed nutrient [10–20]. Such effects are beneficial to individuals with diabetes mellitus and reduce postprandial blood glucose concentrations and insulin needs/response.

A decreased nutrient diffusion rate may in turn result in nutrients "missing" their normal site of maximal absorption. For example, if a nutrient is normally absorbed in the proximal intestine but because of gel formation is "trapped" as part of the gel, then absorption cannot occur at this site. Should the nutrient be released from the gel, the release is most likely going to occur at a site distal to where the nutrient would normally have been absorbed. The extent to which nutrients are absorbed throughout the digestive tract varies with the individual nutrient.

Altered Small Intestine Transit Time

In general, soluble fibers typically delay (slow down or increase) small intestine transit time versus insoluble fibers, which decrease (speed up or shorten) transit time within the small intestine. As with decreased diffusion rates, the changes in transit time, especially if it is shortened, may result in decreased nutrient absorption due to insufficient time for the nutrients to be in contact with enterocytes.

Adsorption or Binding Ability

Some fiber components, especially lignin, gums, pectins, and some hemicelluloses but also some Maillard products, have the ability to bind (adsorb) substances such as enzymes and nutrients in the gastrointestinal tract. Maillard products result from food processing and consist of enzyme-resistant linkages between the amino group ($-NH_2$) of amino acids, especially the amino acid lysine, and the carboxyl groups (–COO–) of reducing sugars. Maillard products are formed during heat treatment, particularly in the baking and frying of foods, and typically cannot be digested by human digestive enzymes. The ability of some Maillard products and fibers to adsorb substances depends in part on gastrointestinal pH as well as particle size, food processing, and fermentability [21]. The physiological effects of the ingestion of fibers with adsorption properties within the gastrointestinal tract may include

- diminished absorption of lipids,
- increased fecal bile acid excretion,
- lowered serum cholesterol concentrations (hypocholesterolemic properties), and
- altered mineral balance.

The mechanisms by which these effects occur vary considerably and will be reviewed next.

Diminished Absorption of Lipids

Soluble fibers (e.g., pectin, gums, and β-glucans) but also the insoluble fiber lignin may affect lipid absorption by adsorbing fatty acids, cholesterol, and/or bile acids within the digestive tract. Fatty acids and cholesterol that are bound to fiber cannot form micelles and cannot be absorbed in this bound form; only free fatty acids, monoacylglycerols, and cholesterol can be incorporated into micelles. Remember that micelles are needed for these end products of fat digestion to be transported through the unstirred water layers and into the enterocyte. Thus, fiber-bound lipids typically are not absorbed in the small intestine and pass into the large intestine where they will be excreted in the feces or degraded by intestinal bacteria.

Increased Fecal Bile Acid Excretion

Adsorption of bile acids to fibers prevents the use of the bile acids for micelle formation. And, like fiber-bound fatty acids, bile acids bound to fiber cannot be reabsorbed and recirculated (enterohepatic recirculation). Fiber-bound bile acids are typically sent into the large intestine for either fecal excretion or degradation by colonic microflora.

Lowered Serum Cholesterol Concentrations (Hypocholesterolemic Properties)

The ability of fibers to lower serum cholesterol concentrations is based on a series of events. First, with the increased excretion of bile acids and cholesterol in the feces, less bile undergoes enterohepatic recirculation. A decrease in the bile acids returned to the liver and decreased cholesterol absorption lead to a decreased cholesterol content of liver cells. Decreased hepatic cholesterol promotes removal of LDL cholesterol from the blood. The decrease in returned bile acids to the liver also necessitates the use of cholesterol for synthesis of new bile acids. The net effect is a lower serum cholesterol. A second proposed mechanism for the hypocholesterolemic (lower blood cholesterol) effect of fiber is the shift of bile acid pools away from cholic acid and toward chenodeoxycholic acid. Chenodeoxycholic acid appears to inhibit 3-hydroxy 3-methylglutaryl (HMG) CoA reductase, a regulatory enzyme necessary for cholesterol biosynthesis [9]. Decreased HMG CoA reductase activity results in reduced hepatic cholesterol synthesis and theoretically lower blood cholesterol concentrations. A third mechanism, shown in animal studies, suggests that production of propionate or other short-chain fatty acids from bacterial degradation of fiber (discussed in the next section) lowers serum cholesterol concentrations through inhibitory effects on fatty acid synthesis. However, propionate fed to humans has had varying effects on serum cholesterol concentrations.

Studies have demonstrated that ingestion of psyllium, some gums (especially guar gum), β-glucan and oat products, resistant dextrins, and pectin can result in lower serum cholesterol concentrations to varying degrees [16,22–36]. Variable effects on blood lipid concentrations also have been shown with ingestion of inulin and fructooligosaccharides [11,14,20]. From a food perspective, ingestion of fruits and vegetables, soy products, and oat products such as oatmeal and oat bran has been shown to decrease serum cholesterol concentrations to variable degrees. Corn, wheat, rice bran, and cellulose, however, are less effective [19,35,36]. The cholesterol-lowering effects observed in studies of humans fed chitosan supplements are equivocal [5,6].

Altered Mineral Balance

Some fibers—especially those with uronic acid, such as hemicellulose, pectins, and gums—can form cationic bridges with minerals within the gastrointestinal tract. Lignin, which has both carboxyl and hydroxyl groups, is also thought to play a role in mineral adsorption. The overall effect (positive or negative) that fiber has on mineral balance depends to some extent on its degree of fermentability or its accessibility to bacterial enzymes in the colon. Microbial proliferation from slowly fermentable fibers may result in increased binding of minerals within the new microbial cells and in the loss of minerals from the body, assuming colonic mineral absorption. In contrast, the more rapidly fermentable fibers (such as pectins) appear to have a favorable effect on mineral balance. Calcium, zinc, and iron bound to these fiber components are released as fermentation occurs and may possibly be absorbed in the colon [9].

Degradability/Fermentability

Chapter 2 discussed the microflora of the gastrointestinal tract. Recall that both the small and large intestines contain numerous microflora, although most are found in the large intestine. Many of these microflora are capable of degrading (fermenting) fiber, especially pectins and gums. In addition to these fibers, some cellulose and some hemicelluloses are also fermentable, but their fermentation is much slower than that of the other fibers. This section discusses first fermentable fibers and their effects on the body. A discussion of the effects of fibers that are not fermentable then follows.

Fermentable Fibers

The principal metabolites of fermentable fibers (including any starch that has passed into the cecum and been degraded by bacteria) are lactate and short-chain fatty acids (SCFAs), formerly called volatile fatty acids (VFAs) because of their volatility in acidic aqueous solutions. Many different fibers, such as pectin, gums, psyllium, some hemicelluloses, polydextrose, and resistant starch, are degraded to short-chain fatty acids. The short-chain fatty acids include primarily acetic, butyric, and propionic acids. In addition to these acids, other products of fiber fermentation are hydrogen, carbon dioxide, and methane gases that are excreted as flatus or expired by the lungs. Different fibers are fermented to different short-chain fatty acids in different amounts by different bacteria. For example, ingestion of pectin resulted in higher propionate concentrations in the colon of rats versus wheat bran, which resulted in higher butyrate concentrations [37]. Bacteria that act on pectin include, for example,

- bacteroides that generate acetate, propionate, and succinate;
- eubacteria that yield acetate, butyrate, and lactate; and
- bifidobacteria that produce acetate and lactate.

Some general effects of short-chain fatty acids generated from fiber fermentation by intestinal microbes include

- increased water and sodium absorption in the colon,
- mucosal cell proliferation,
- provision of energy, and
- acidification of luminal environment.

We will briefly review each of these general effects.

Increased Water and Sodium Absorption in the Colon. Short-chain fatty acids produced by fermentation are rapidly absorbed, and their absorption in turn stimulates water and sodium absorption in the colon.

Mucosal Cell Proliferation. Substrates generated from the degradation of dietary fiber in the colon stimulate the proliferation of mucosal cells in the gastrointestinal tract.

Provision of Energy. Short-chain fatty acids provide body cells with substrate for energy production. Butyric acid provides an energy source for colonic epithelial cells. Those fatty acids not used by the colonic cells, primarily the propionic and acetic acids, are carried by the portal vein to the liver, where the propionate and some of the acetate are taken up and metabolized. Most of the acetate, however, passes to the peripheral tissues, where it is metabolized by skeletal and cardiac muscle. Remember from the section on lowered serum cholesterol that it is the propionic acid generated from fiber fermentation that in rats inhibited hepatic cholesterol biosynthesis.

Fermentation of carbohydrates by colonic anaerobic bacteria makes available to the body some of the energy contained in undigested food reaching the cecum. The exact amount of energy realized depends mostly on the amount and type of dietary fiber that is ingested. It is estimated that in developed countries as much as 10% to 15% of ingested carbohydrate may be fermented in the colon; in the third-world (developing) countries, this percentage may be considerably higher [38].

Acidification of Luminal Environment. The generation of short-chain fatty acids in the colon from bacterial fermentation of carbohydrate results in a decrease in the pH of the colon's luminal environment. With the more acidic pH, free bile acids become less soluble. Furthermore, the activity of 7 α dehydroxylase diminishes (optimal pH ~6–6.5) and thus decreases the rate of conversion of primary bile acids to secondary bile acids. With the lower pH, calcium also becomes more available (soluble) to bind bile and fatty acids [39]. These latter two changes may be protective against colon cancer.

Nonfermentable Fibers

Fiber components that are nonfermentable, principally cellulose and lignin, or that are more slowly fermentable, such as some hemicelluloses, are particularly valuable in promoting the proliferation of microbes in the colon. Microbial proliferation may be important both for detoxification and as a means of increasing fecal volume (bulk).

Detoxification. The detoxification role is based on the theory that the synthesis of increased microbial cells (i.e., microbial proliferation) could result in the increased microbial scavenging and sequestering of substances or toxins, which eventually are excreted. Alternately, certain colonic bacteria appear to inhibit proliferation of tumor cells and/or delay tumor formation. In addition, bacteria such as *L. acidophilus* reduced the activity of enzymes that catalyze the conversion of procarcinogens to carcinogens [40].

Increased Fecal Volume (Bulk). In addition to its detoxifying role, microbial proliferation may promote increased fecal volume or bulk. Fecal bulk consists of unfermented fiber, salts, and water as well as bacterial mass. In general, fecal bulk increases with increased bacterial proliferation. This occurs not only because of the mass of the bacteria but also because bacteria are about 80% water. Thus, with increased fecal bacteria present, there is an increase in mass and in the water-holding capacity of the feces.

In general, fecal bulk increases as fiber fermentability decreases. The rapidly fermentable fibers, such as pectins, gums, and β-glucans, appear to have little or no effect on fecal bulk. Wheat bran is one of the most effective fiber laxatives because it can absorb three times its weight of water, thereby producing a bulky stool. Gastrointestinal responses to wheat bran include

- increased fecal bulk,
- greater frequency of defecation,
- reduced intestinal transit time, and
- decreased intraluminal pressure.

Rice bran has been found to be even more effective than wheat bran in eliciting an increased fecal bulk and a reduced intestinal transit time; both rice and wheat bran are helpful in treating constipation [41]. Other fibers that have been shown to increase fecal bulk and decrease stool transit time to improve laxation include cellulose, psyllium, inulin, and oligosaccharides [42–46].

ROLES OF FIBER IN DISEASE PREVENTION AND MANAGEMENT

The importance to health of an adequate fiber intake is demonstrated by some of the physiological effects exerted by the various dietary fibers. Particularly noteworthy are the hypoglycemic and hypolipidemic effects of soluble fibers. Slowing the absorption rate of carbohydrate can help the individual with diabetes mellitus in regulating blood glucose concentrations. Serum cholesterol concentrations in excess of 200 mg/dL are considered a risk factor for heart disease. Thus, ingestion of soluble fibers that can lower serum cholesterol to acceptable concentrations is beneficial against heart disease. Adequate intake of fiber, especially insoluble, nonfermentable fiber, also has been implicated in the treatment of several gastrointestinal disorders, including diverticular disease, gallstones, irritable bowel syndrome, and constipation. Evidence for the effectiveness of fiber in the control of other diseases appears equivocal; however, populations with higher fiber intakes have a lower incidence of gastrointestinal disorders, heart disease, and breast and colon cancers [47–65]. A generous fiber intake also appears to benefit some people in their efforts at weight control. The bulk provided by fiber may have some satiety value. High-fiber foods may reduce the hunger associated with caloric restriction while simultaneously delaying gastric emptying and somewhat reducing nutrient utilization [64–66]. The effectiveness of a high-fiber diet as a treatment for obesity remains unclear.

While different fibers exhibit different characteristics, in some cases it is ingestion of foods, and not just fiber, that has been shown to influence disease risk. Ingestion of whole-grain cereals, not just cereal fiber, for example, has been shown to negatively correlate with risk of death from heart disease [51]. Similarly, the postprandial insulin response, which in turn influences plasma glucose concentrations, has been shown to be influenced by the form of food and botanical structure rather than by the amount of fiber or type of grain product [67].

The U.S. Food and Drug Administration has approved several health claims related to fiber. The claims typically focus on fruits, vegetables, and grain products. For example, for one claim the food requirements include fruits, vegetables, or grain products that are low in fat and a good source of dietary fiber without fortification. An example of such a claim is "Low fat diets rich in fiber-containing grain products, fruits and vegetables may reduce the risk of some types of cancer, a disease associated with many factors" [7]. Another sample claim for fruits, vegetables, and grain products that are low in fat (saturated and total) and cholesterol and contain at least 0.6 g soluble fiber per reference amount without fortification is "Diets low in saturated fat and cholesterol and rich in fruits and vegetables and grain products that contain some types of dietary fiber, particularly soluble fiber, may reduce the risk of heart disease, a disease associated with many factors" [7]. Another model claim—"Low fat diets rich in fruits and vegetables (foods that are low in fat and may contain dietary fiber, vitamin A, or vitamin C) may reduce the risk of some types of cancer, a disease associated with many factors"—has also been approved for fruits and vegetables that are a good source of vitamin A or C or dietary fiber [7]. A fourth claim is associated with β-glucan from oat bran (containing at least 5.5% β-glucan soluble fiber), rolled oats or oatmeal (containing at least 4% β-glucan soluble fiber), whole oat flour (providing at least 4% β-glucan soluble fiber), or psyllium husk with a purity of no less than 95%. An example related to this claim is "Soluble fiber from foods such as [name of soluble fiber source and food product], as part of a diet low in saturated fat and cholesterol, may reduce the risk of heart disease. A serving of [name of food product] supplies [amount] grams of the [necessary daily dietary intake for the benefit] soluble fiber from [name of soluble fiber source] necessary per day to have this effect" [7].

Mechanisms by which dietary fibers prevent disease are multiple and varied [1,39,53–59,63,68,69]. Some of the many mechanisms of action by which fiber has been proposed to prevent colon cancer are highlighted here.

- High bile acid concentrations are associated with a high risk of colon cancer. Thus, fibers that adsorb bile acids to promote fecal excretion have a protective effect by decreasing free concentration and the availability of bile acids for conversion to secondary bile acids, which are thought to promote colon carcinogenesis.
- Fibers that increase fecal bulk decrease the intraluminal concentrations of procarcinogens and carcinogens and thereby reduce the likelihood of interactions with colonic mucosal cells.
- Provision of a fermentable substrate to colonic bacteria alters species and numbers of bacteria and/or their metabolism, which may inhibit proliferation or development of tumor cells or conversion of procarcinogens to carcinogens.

- A shortened fecal transit time decreases the time during which toxins can be synthesized and in which they are in contact with the colon.
- Fiber fermentation to short-chain fatty acids decreases the interluminal pH, thereby decreasing synthesis of secondary bile acids, which have been shown to promote the generation of tumors.
- Degradation of fiber by fermentation may release fiber-bound calcium. The increased calcium in the colon may help eliminate the mitogenic advantage that cancer cells have over normal cells in a low-calcium environment.
- Butyric acid appears to slow the proliferation and differentiation of colon cancer cells.
- Insoluble fibers, such as lignin, that resist degradation bind carcinogens, thereby minimizing the chances of interactions with colonic mucosal cells.

Not all studies show anticarcinogenic effects with fiber. In some studies, soluble fibers enhance the development of colorectal cancers. Proposed mechanisms for such action include these: (1) soluble fibers reduce the ability of insoluble fibers to adsorb hydrophobic carcinogens and thus more carcinogens may enter the colon maintained in solution than adsorbed onto insoluble fibers; (2) on degradation of soluble fibers, carcinogens are released and deposited on the colonic mucosal surface; (3) soluble fibers may cross the intestinal epithelium and transport with them carcinogens maintained in solution; (4) soluble fibers may reduce absorption of bile salts and thereby increase the chance for conversion to secondary bile acids [39,59].

There is little agreement among the numerous studies designed to determine the effect of fiber in the development of colon cancer. Most of the evidence for the positive role of fiber in colon cancer prevention has come from epidemiological observations. Unfortunately, in these epidemiological studies variation in many dietary factors other than fiber intake has been noted. The dietary factors most often identified as being involved in variations in the incidence of colorectal cancer among different population groups are too many total calories, high fat, too much protein, low fiber, low intake of vitamin D and calcium, and low intake of antioxidants [53]. Meta-analyses, however, of both epidemiological and case-controlled studies that investigated dietary fiber and colon cancer found that fiber-rich diets were associated with a protective effect against colon cancer in the majority of studies [63,69]. Furthermore, risk of colorectal cancer in the United States is thought to be reducible by up to 31% with a 13-g daily increase in dietary fiber intake [63].

RECOMMENDED FIBER INTAKE

Recommendations for increasing the amount of fiber in the U.S. diet have come from several governmental and private organizations, each with a concern for improving the health of the U.S. public [70–74]. In 2002, the National Academy of Sciences Food and Nutrition Board established Dietary Reference Intakes, specifically adequate intakes (AI), for fiber. Adequate intakes of total fiber, representing the sum of dietary fiber and functional fiber, were established based on amounts of fiber shown to protect against heart disease [1]. For men aged 19 to 50 years, 38 g total fiber is recommended, and for men ≥51 years of age, 31 g total fiber is recommended. For women aged 19 to 50 years, 25 g total fiber is recommended, and for women ≥51 years, 21 g total fiber is recommended. Recommendations for total fiber intake for children aged 1 to 3 and 4 to 8 years are 19 g and 25 g, respectively. For girls 9 to 18 years old, total fiber intake recommendations are 26 g; for boys 9 to 13 and 14 to 18 years of age, recommendations are 31 g and 38 g, respectively. No Tolerable Upper Intake Level for dietary fiber or functional fiber has been established [1].

Dietary changes encouraged in order to accomplish an increased fiber intake are consistent with the Food Guide Pyramid [75]. Individuals should consume

- fiber-rich legumes, which may serve as the primary source of protein in a meal;
- at least 5 servings of fruits and vegetables per day; and
- at least 2 to 3 servings per day of whole grains as part of the 6 to 11 servings recommended by the Food Guide Pyramid [75].

Notice that recommendations that fiber intake be increased are interpreted in terms of dietary change rather than addition to the diet of fiber supplements, which more than likely are devoid of other nutrients. As a person incorporates high-fiber foods, the percentage of complex carbohydrates increases in relation to the amount of fat and protein in the diet, making an increase in fiber almost inevitable. It remains important, however, to eat a variety of cereals, legumes, fruits, and vegetables so that variety in dietary fibers is maximized.

Although many tables now provide the soluble and insoluble fiber composition of foods (thus allowing calculation of total dietary fiber intake) a quick method for calculating typical dietary fiber intakes is available that allows for assessment in a clinical setting from a food history, 24-hour diet recall, or food record [76]. Because fiber-rich foods consist primarily of fruits, vegetables, grains, legumes, nuts, and seeds, the number of servings from each of these groups can be multiplied by the mean total fiber content of each food group [76]. For example, numbers of servings (size determined from the U.S. Department of Agriculture data or food label) of fruits (not including juices) and vegetables are each multiplied by 1.5 g. The 1.5 g represents the average amount of dietary fiber per serving of fruit and per serving of vegetable. Numbers of servings of refined grains are multiplied by 1.0 g, and numbers of servings of whole grains are multiplied by 2.5 g. The totals from each of the four categories are summed and added to food-specific fiber values for legumes, nuts, seeds, and concentrated fiber sources; food-specific fiber values are obtained from databases [76]. The values calculated using this quick method were within 10% of the results obtained by looking up each individual food's fiber content [76].

summary

Definitions have now been established for dietary and functional fibers. Dietary fibers are nondigestible carbohydrates and lignin that are intact and intrinsic in plants. Examples of dietary fibers include cellulose, hemicellulose, lignin, pectin, gums, β-glucans, fructans, and resistant starches. Functional fibers are nondigestible carbohydrates that have been isolated, extracted, or manufactured and have been shown to have beneficial physiological effects in humans. Note that functional fibers, unlike dietary fibers, do not have to be intact or intrinsic only to plants. Functional fibers shown to have beneficial effects are cellulose, pectins, gums, β-glucans, psyllium, and resistant starches. Other fibers, including lignin, fructans, chitin and chitosan, polydextrose and polyols, and resistant dextrins, require additional studies.

The physiological effects of fiber in the gastrointestinal tract are as varied as the number of fiber components and are determined to a large extent by the types and amounts present. Some of the many characteristics of dietary and functional fibers shown to be beneficial include water-holding/hydration capacity and viscosity, adsorption or binding ability, and degradation/fermentability. To obtain fiber via the diet, food sources of fiber need to be varied and complementary. Assurance of a good intake of fiber requires consumption of a variety of high-fiber foods including whole-grain cereals and breads, legumes, fruits, and vegetables.

References Cited

1. Food and Nutrition Board. Dietary Reference Intakes for Energy, Carbohydrate, Fiber, Fat, Protein and Amino Acids. Washington DC: National Academy of Sciences, 2002.

2. Tuohy K, Kolida S, Lustenberger A, Gibson G. The prebiotic effects of biscuits containing partially hydrolyzed guar gum and fructo-oligosaccharides—a human volunteer study. Br J Nutr 2001;86: 341–48.

3. Bouhnik Y, Vahedi K, Achour L, Attar A, Salfati J, Pochart P, Marteau P, Flourie B, Bornet F, Rambaud J-C. Short-chain fructo-oligosaccharides administration dose-dependently increases fecal bifidobacteria in healthy humans. J Nutr 1999;129:113–16.

4. Gibson G, Beatty E, Wang X, Cummings J. Selective stimulation of bifidobacteria in the human colon by oligofructose and inulin. Gastroenterology 1995;108:975–82.

5. Guerciolini R, Radu-Radulescu L, Boldrin M, Dallas J, Moore R. Comparative evaluation of fecal fat excretion induced by orlistat and chitosan. Obes Res 2001;9:364–67.

6. Wuolijoki E, Hirvela T, Ylitalo P. Decrease in serum LDL cholesterol with microcrystalline chitosan. Methods Find Exp Clin Pharmacol 1999; 21:357–61.

7. www.cfsan.fda.gov

8. Ink SL, Hurt HD. Nutritional implications of gums. Food Tech 1987;41:77–82.

9. Jenkins D, Jenkins A, Wolever T, Rao A, Thompson L. Fiber and starchy foods: gut function and implications in disease. Am J Gastroenterol 1986;81:920–30.

10. Jie Z, Bang-yao L, Ming-jie X, Hai-wei L, Zu-kang Z, Ting-song W, Craig S. Studies on the effects of polydextrose intake on physiologic functions in Chinese people. Am J Clin Nutr 2000;72:1503–9.

11. Brighenti F, Casiraghi M, Canzi E, Ferrari A. Effect of consumption of a ready-to-eat breakfast cereal containing inulin on the intestinal milieu and blood lipids in healthy male volunteers. Eur J Clin Nutr 1999;53:726–33.

12. Groop P-H, Aro A, Stenman S, Groop L. Long-term effects of guar gum in subjects with non-insulin dependent diabetes mellitus. Am J Clin Nutr 1993;58:513–18.

13. Hallfrisch J, Scholfield D, Behall K. Diets containing soluble oat extracts improve glucose and insulin responses of moderately hypercholesterolemic men and women. Am J Clin Nutr 1995;61:379–84.

14. Jackson K, Taylor G, Clohessy A, Williams C. The effect of the daily intake of inulin on fasting lipid, insulin and glucose concentrations in middle-aged men and women. Br J Nutr 1999;82:23–30.

15. Landin K, Holm G, Tengborn L, Smith U. Guar gum improves insulin sensitivity, blood lipids, blood pressure, and fibrinolysis in healthy men. Am J Clin Nutr 1992;56:1061–65.

16. Anderson J, Algood L, Turner J, Oeltgen P, Daggy B. Effects of psyllium on glucose and serum lipid responses in men with type 2 diabetes and hypercholesterolemia. Am J Clin Nutr 1999;70:466–73.

17. Wolever T, Jenkins D. Effect of dietary fiber and foods on carbohydrate metabolism. In: Spiller G, ed. CRC Handbook of Dietary Fiber in Human Nutrition. Boca Raton, FL: CRC Press, 1993, pp. 111–62.

18. Luo J, Rizkalla S, Alamowitch C, Boussairi A, Blayo A, Barry J-L, Laffitte A, Guyon F, Bornet F, Slama G. Chronic consumption of

short-chain fructooligosaccharides by healthy subjects decreased basal hepatic glucose production but had no effect on insulin-stimulated glucose metabolism. Am J Clin Nutr 1996;63:939–45.

19. Niemi M, Keinanen-Kiukaanniemi S, Salmela P. Long-term effects of guar gum and microcrystalline cellulose on glycaemic control and serum lipids in type 2 diabetes. Eur J Clin Pharmacol 1988;34:427–29.

20. VanDokkum W, Wezendonk B, Srikumar TS, van den Heuvel EGHM. Effect of nondigestible oligosaccharides on large-bowel functions, blood lipid concentrations and glucose absorption in young healthy male subjects. Eur J Clin Nutr 1999;53:1–7.

21. Eastwood M, Passmore R. A new look at dietary fiber. Nutr Today 1984;19:6–11.

22. Ripsin C, Keenan J, Jacobs D, Elmer P, Welch R, VanHorn L, Liu K, Turnbull W, Thye F, Kestin M, Hegsted M, Davidson DM, Davison MH, Dugan LD, Demark-Wahnefried W, Beling S. Oat products and lipid lowering: A meta-analysis. JAMA 1992;267:3317–25.

23. Brown L, Rosner B, Willett W, Sacks F. Cholesterol-lowering effects of dietary fiber: a meta-analysis. Am J Clin Nutr 1999;69:30–42.

24. Davidson M, Dugan L, Burns J, Bova J, Story K, Drennan K. The hypocholesterolemic effects of β-glucan in oatmeal and oat bran: a dose controlled study. JAMA 1991;265:1833–39.

25. Davidson M, Maki K, Kong J, Dugan L, Torri S, Hall H, Drennan K, Anderson S, Fulgoni V, Saldanha L, Olson B. Long-term effects of consuming foods containing psyllium seed husk on serum lipids in subjects with hypercholesterolemia. Am J Clin Nutr 1998;67:367–76.

26. Anderson J, Tietyen-Clark J. Dietary fiber: hyperlipidemia, hypertension, and coronary heart disease. Am J Gastroenterol 1986; 81:907–19.

27. Penagini R, Velio P, Vigorelli R, Bozzani A, Castagnone D, Ranzi T, Bianchi PA. The effect of dietary guar on serum cholesterol, intestinal transit, and fecal output in man. Am J Gastroenterol 1986;81:123–25.

28. Anderson J, Davidson M, Blonde L, Brown W, Howard J, Ginsberg H, Allgood L, Weingand K. Long-term cholesterol-lowering effects of psyllium as an adjunct to diet therapy in the treatment of hypercholesterolemia. Am J Clin Nutr 2000;71:1433–38.

29. Aro A, Uusitupa M, Voutilainen E, Korhonen T. Effects of guar gum in male subjects with hypercholesterolemia. Am J Clin Nutr 1984; 39:911–16.

30. Blake D, Hamblett C, Frost P, Judd P, Ellis P. Wheat bread supplemented with depolymerized guar gum reduces the plasma cholesterol concentration in hypercholesterolemic human subjects. Am J Clin Nutr 1997;65:107–13.

31. Braaten J, Wood P, Scott F, Wolynetz M, Lowe M, Bradley-White P, Collins M. Oat beta-glucan reduces blood cholesterol concentration in hypercholesterolemic subjects. Eur J Clin Nutr 1994;48:465–74.

32. Cerda J, Robbins F, Burgin C, Baumgartner T, Rice R. The effects of grapefruit pectin on patients at risk for coronary heart disease without altering diet or lifestyle. Clin Cardiol 1988;11:589–94.

33. MacMahon M, Carless J. Ispaghula husk in the treatment of hypercholesterolemia: a double-blind controlled study. J Cardiovasc Risk 1998;5:167–72.

34. Beer M, Arrigoni E, Amado R. Effects of oat gum on blood cholesterol levels in healthy young men. Eur J Clin Nutr 1995;49:517–22.

35. Anderson J, Jones A, Riddell-Mason S. Ten different dietary fibers have significantly different effects on serum and liver lipids of cholesterol-fed rats. J Nutr 1994;124:78–83.

36. Hillman L, Peters S, Fisher C, Pomare E. The effects of the fiber components pectin, cellulose and lignin on serum cholesterol levels. Am J Clin Nutr 1985;42:207–13.

37. Lupton J, Kurtz P. Relationship of colonic luminal short chain fatty acids and pH to *in vivo* cell proliferation in rats. J Nutr 1993;123: 1522–30.

38. McNeil N. The contribution of the large intestine to energy supplies in man. Am J Clin Nutr 1984;39:338–42.

39. Harris P, Ferguson L. Dietary fibre: its composition and role in protection against colorectal cancer. Mut Res 1993;290:97–110.

40. Gorbach SL. Lactic acid bacteria and human health. Ann Med 1990;22:37–41.

41. Tomlin T, Read N. Comparison of effects on colonic function caused by feeding rice bran and wheat bran. Eur J Clin Nutr 1988; 42:857–61.

42. Ashraf W, Park F, Lof J, Quigley E. Effects of psyllium therapy on stool characteristics, colon transit time and anorectal function in chronic idiopathic constipation. Aliment Pharmacol Ther 1995;9: 639–47.

43. Gibson G, Willems A, Reading S, Collins MD. Fermentation of non-digestible oligosaccharides by human colonic bacteria. Proc Nutr Soc 1996;55:899–912.

44. Kleessen B, Sykura B, Zunft H, Blaut M. Effects of inulin and lactose on fecal microflora, microbial activity, and bowel habits in elderly constipated persons. Am J Clin Nutr 1997;65:1397–1402.

45. McRorie J, Daggy B, Morel J, Diersing P, Miner P, Robinson M. Psyllium is superior to docusate sodium for treatment of chronic constipation. Aliment Pharmacol Ther 1998;12:491–97.

46. Cummings JH. The effect of dietary fiber on fecal weight and composition. In: Spiller GA, ed. CRC Handbook of Dietary Fiber in Human Nutrition, 2nd ed. Boca Raton, FL: CRC Press, 1993, pp. 263–349.

47. Pietinen P, Malila N, Virtanen M, Hartman TJ, Tangrea JA, Albanes D, Viramo J. Diet and risk of colorectal cancer in a cohort of Finnish men. Cancer Causes Control 1999;10:387–96.

48. Rimm E, Ascherio A, Giovannucci E, Spiegelman D, Stampfer M, Willett W. Vegetable, fruit, and cereal fiber intake and risk of coronary heart disease among men. JAMA 1996;275:447–51.

49. Wolk A, Manson J, Stampfer M, Colditz G, Hu F, Speizer F, Hennekens C, Willett W. Long-term intake of dietary fiber and decreased risk of coronary heart disease among women. JAMA 1999; 281:1998–2004.

50. Todd S, Woodward M, Tunstall-Pedoe H, Bolton-Smith C. Dietary antioxidant vitamins and fiber in the etiology of cardiovascular disease and all-causes mortality: results from the Scottish Heart Health Study. Am J Epidemiol 1999;150:1073–80.

51. Jacobs DR, Meyer KA, Kushi LH, Folsom AR. Whole-grain intake may reduce the risk of ischemic heart disease death in postmenopausal women: The Iowa Women's Health Study. Am J Clin Nutr 1998;68:248–57.

52. Olesen M, Gudmand-Hoyer E. Efficacy, safety, and tolerability of fructooligosaccharides in the treatment of irritable bowel syndrome. Am J Clin Nutr 2000;72:1570–75.

53. Jenkins D, Jenkins A, Rao A, et al. Cancer risk: possible role of high carbohydrate, high fiber diets. Am J Gastroenterol 1986;81: 931–35.

54. Ausman L. Fiber and colon cancer: does the current evidence justify a preventive policy? Nutr Rev 1993; 51:57–63.

55. Klurfeld D. Dietary fiber-mediated mechanisms in carcinogenesis. Cancer Res (suppl) 1992;52:2055s–59s.

56. Hill M. Bile acids and colorectal cancer. Eur J Canc Prevent 1991; 1:69–72.

57. Van Munster I, Nagengast F. The influence of dietary fiber on bile acid metabolism. Eur J Cancer Prevent 1991;1:35–44.

58. Potter J. Colon cancer—do the nutritional epidemiology, the gut physiology and the molecular biology tell the same story? J Nutr 1993; 123:418–23.

59. Harris P, Roberton A, Watson M, Triggs C, Ferguson L. The effects of soluble fiber polysaccharides on the adsorption of a hydrophobic carcinogen to an insoluble dietary fiber. Nutr Cancer 1993;19:43–54.

60. Aldoori W, Giovannucci E, Rockett H, Sampson L, Rimm E, Willett W. A prospective study of dietary fiber types and symptomatic diverticular disease in men. J Nutr 1998;128:714–19.

61. Brodribb A. Treatment of symptomatic diverticular disease with a high-fibre diet. Lancet 1977;1:664–66.

62. Cummings J. Nutritional management of diseases of the gut. In: Garrow JS, James WPT, Ralph A, eds. Human Nutrition and Dietetics, 10th ed. Edinburgh: Churchill Livingston, 2000, pp. 547–73.

63. Howe G, Benito E, Castelleto R, Cornee J, Esteve J, Gallagher R, Iscovich J, Dengao J, Kaaks R, Kune G, et al. Dietary intake of fiber and decreased risk of cancers of the colon and rectum: evidence from the combined analysis of 13 case-controlled studies. J Natl Cancer Inst 1992;84:1887–96.

64. Anderson J, Bryant C. Dietary fiber: diabetes and obesity. Am J Gastroenterol 1986;81:898–906.

65. Kritchevsky D. Dietary fiber. Ann Rev Nutr 1988;8:301–28.

66. Rigaud D, Paycha F, Meulemans A, Merrouche M, Mognon M. Effect of psyllium on gastric emptying, hunger feeling and food intake in normal volunteers: a double blind study. Eur J Clin Nutr 1998;52:239–45.

67. Juntunen K, Niskanen L, Liukkonen K, Poutanen K, Holst J, Mykkunen H. Postprandial glucose, insulin, and incretin responses to grain products in healthy subjects. Am J Clin Nutr 2002;75:254–62.

68. Lupton JR. Butyrate and colonic cytokinetics: differences between *in vitro* and *in vivo* studies. Eur J Cancer Prev 1995;4:373–78.

69. Trock B, Lanza E, Greenwald P. Dietary fiber, vegetables, and colon cancer: critical review and meta-analyses of the epidemiologic evidence. J Natl Cancer Inst 1990;82:650–61.

70. Ad Hoc Expert Panel on Dietary Fiber, Federation of American Societies for Experimental Biology. Physiologic and Health Consequences of Dietary Fiber. Rockville, MD: FASEB, 1987.

71. Butrum RR, Clifford CK, Lanza E. NCI dietary guidelines: rationale. Am J Clin Nutr 1988;48:888–95.

72. Diabetes Care and Education Practice Group, the American Diabetes Association. Nutritional recommendations and principles for individuals with diabetes mellitus. J Am Diet Assoc 1994;4:504–6.

73. American Dietetic Association. Position of the American Dietetic Association: health implications of dietary fiber. J Am Diet Assoc 1997;97:1157–59.

74. Beebe CA, Pastors JG, Powers MA, Wylie-Rosett J. Nutrition management for individuals with non-insulin dependent diabetes mellitus in the 1990s: a review by the Diabetes Care and Education Dietetic Practice Group. J Am Diet Assoc 1991;91:196–202,205–7.

75. U.S. Department of Agriculture. The Food Guide Pyramid. Washington, DC: Home and Garden Bulletin Number 252, 1992.

76. Marlett JA, Cheung TF. Database and quick methods of assessing typical dietary fiber intakes using 228 commonly consumed foods. J Am Diet Assoc 1997;97:1139–48, 1151.

perspective

Phytochemicals and Herbal Supplements in Health and Disease

Over the past decade, the market for herbal supplements has exploded, with more than 500 herbs marketed in the United States and sales in excess of \$3 billion/year [1]. The public's enthusiasm stems from a number of benefits purported to be derived from the use of various herbs (plants or particular parts of a plant such as the leaf, stem, root, bark, seed, flower, etc.). The top seven selling herbs in America include ginkgo biloba, St. John's wort, ginseng, garlic, echinacea, saw palmetto, and kava [2]. Benefits derived from the use of these herbs range from effects on the brain to improve memory or treat depression to the treatment of the common cold. This perspective will review some of the active ingredients—that is, the phytochemicals—in herbs (as well as in many other plant foods) and provide an overview of some of the more common herbal supplements used to maintain health and/or treat disease.

Phytochemicals

Phytochemicals consist of a large group of nonnutrient compounds that are biologically active in the body. As implied by the name, phytochemicals are found in plants, including fruits, vegetables, legumes, grains, herbs, tea, and spices. Of the tens of thousands of phytochemicals, polyphenolic phytochemicals make up the largest group. The polyphenols, which include more than 8,000 compounds, can be divided into a variety of classes depending on the classification system. One of the largest of these classes is the flavonoids, which includes several subclasses listed in Table 1. Table 1 also provides examples of foods rich in flavonoids. Among the flavonoids, the flavanols are more widely distributed. In contrast, the isoflavones are found mostly in soybeans and its products.

Other phytochemicals, listed in Table 2 with some of their food sources, include carotenoids (see also Chapter 10), terpenes, organosulphides, phenolic acids, phytosterols, glucosinolates, and isothiocyanates, among others.

While Tables 1 and 2 list examples of foods containing some of the phytochemicals, it is important to note that most plant foods contain multiple phytochemicals. Tomatoes, for example, may contain as many as 10,000 different phytochemicals. Moreover, many of the phytochemicals are found in foods in a variety of forms, such as various glycoside conjugates. Upon ingestion of the foods, the glycosides are metabolized to varying degrees to produce aglycones (unconjugated forms). The differences in the metabolism of these phytochemicals in the body complicate the interpretation of research studies and recommendations. Moreover, in addition to differences in the metabolism of phytochemicals, phytochemical composition is affected by environmental conditions, plant genetics, degree of ripeness, and processing and storage of the plant foods.

Phytochemicals are thought to play several important roles in the body. Flavonoids, for example, are found in cell membranes between the aqueous and lipid bilayers, where they exhibit antioxidant functions in the body. Specifically, flavonoids can scavenge free radicals such as hydroxyl, peroxyl, alkyl peroxyl, and superoxide and can terminate chain reactions (see the Chapter 10 perspective for a discussion of free radicals and termination). It is first the ability of the flavonoid to donate a hydrogen atom from its phenolic hydroxyl group to the free radical (similar to vitamin E) and second the ability of the phenolic ring to stabilize the unpaired electron that makes flavonoids good antioxidants. Polyphenols other than flavonoids, as well as other classes of phytochemicals, also exhibit antioxidant activity, including lignans, carotenoids, and resveratrol, found in grapes and peanuts.

Table 1 Flavonoid Phytochemicals and Their Sources [3–6]

Flavonoid Subclass	Phytochemicals	Sources
Flavonols	Quercetin, kaempferol, myricetin	Onions, tea, olive, kale, leaf lettuce, cranberry, tomato, apple, turnip green, endive, ginkgo biloba, St. John's wort
Flavanones	Tangeritin, naringenin, hesperitin, hesperedin	Citrus fruits
Flavanols	Catechins, epicatechins	Green tea, pear, wine, apple
Isoflavones	Genistein, daidzein, equol	Legumes, especially soy beans, nuts, milk, cheese, flour, tofu, miso, soy sauce
Flavones	Apigenin, luteolin	Celery, olives, ginkgo biloba

Table 2 Phytochemicals and Their Sources [3–6]

Phytochemical Class	Phytochemicals	Sources
Carotenoids	β-carotene, α-carotene, lutein, lycopene	Tomato, pumpkin, squash, carrot, watermelon, papaya, guava
Terpenes	Limonene, carvone	Citrus fruits, cherries, ginkgo biloba
Organosulphides	Diallyl sulphide, allyl methyl sulphide, S-allylcysteine	Garlic, onions, leeks, cruciferous vegetables: broccoli, cabbage, Brussels sprouts, mustard, watercress
Phenolic acids	Hydroxycinnamic acids: caffeic, ferulic, chlorogenic, neochlorogenic, curcumin Hydroxybenzoic acids: ellagic, gallic	Blueberry, cherry, pear, apple, orange, grapefruit, white potato, coffee bean, St. John's wort, echinacea Raspberry, strawberry, grape juice
Lignans	Secoisolariciresinol, mataresinol	Berries, flaxseed/oils, nuts, rye bran
Saponins	Panaxadiol, panaxatriol	Alfalfa sprouts, potato, tomato, ginseng
Phytosterols	β-sitosterol, campesterol, stigmasterol	Vegetable oils (soy, rapeseed, corn, sunflower)
Glucosinolates	Glucobrassicin, gluconapin, sinigrin, glucoiberin	Cruciferous vegetables: broccoli, cabbage, Brussels sprouts, mustard, watercress
Isothiocyanates	Allylisothiocyanates, indoles, sulforaphane	Cruciferous vegetables (see above)

In addition to antioxidant roles, some lignans and flavonoids—such as the isoflavones, flavones, and flavanols—exhibit antiestrogenic effects. Phytoestrogens such as the isoflavones are structurally similar to estrogen in that the phenol ring can bind to estrogen receptors on cells. Soy products, rich in isoflavones, have been marketed for use by women during perimenopause to help alleviate some of the side effects of diminished natural estrogen in the body. In addition, the isoflavone genestein, along with lignans and some flavonoids, has been shown to inhibit tumor formation and proliferation. Thus, teas, especially black and green teas that are especially rich in flavonoids, are enjoying increased popularity. Glucosinolates and isothiocyanates, along with terpenes and some phenolic acids such as hydroxycinnamic acid, also appear to have some protective effects against cancer (tumor formation), while phytosterols and isoflavones exhibit cholesterol-lowering effects that may be protective against heart disease. In fact, soy products rich in isoflavones and margarines with added phytosterols are being marketed for use in the diets of individuals with hypercholesterolemia.

Herbs are rich sources of many phytochemicals. They have been used for decades, and sometimes centuries, in Asia and other parts of the world to prevent and/or treat a variety of health problems. The purported benefits of five commonly used herbs—ginkgo biloba, St. John's wort, ginseng, garlic, and echinacea—will be discussed here.

Ginkgo Biloba

Ginkgo biloba, from the *Ginkgoaceae* family, is a tall, long-living (as long as 1,000 years), deciduous tree with gray-colored bark. The tree is native to China and was introduced into North America in the 18th century. The fan-shaped leaves of ginkgo biloba are cultivated, formulated, and concentrated into an extract containing the active compounds. Pharmacologically active flavonoids found in the leaves include, for example, tannins and their glycosides. Some flavonoid glycosides and glucosides are quercetin and kaempferol 3-rhamnosides and 3-rutinosides. Terpenes, which are also active, consist of ginkgolides A, B, C, J, and M and bilobalides. Active ingredients in ginkgo biloba have been shown to induce peripheral vasodilation, reduce red blood cell aggregation and platelet activating factor, alter neurotransmitter receptors and levels, and exhibit antioxidant actions.

Ginkgo biloba is purported to improve arterial and venous blood flow, especially cerebral and peripheral vascular circulation, and to improve neurosensory function. Thus, the herb is often recommended for conditions in which poor circulation is a factor, such as intermittent claudication (pain, cramping, and fatigue in the leg muscles, which is usually a symptom of peripheral arterial occlusive disease), memory impairment, dementia, vertigo (dizziness), and tinnitus (ringing in the ears). Conclusions of meta-analyses and extensive reviews of studies examining the efficacy of gingko biloba are varied. For example, some, but not all, controlled clinical studies suggest that ginkgo extracts are more effective than a placebo in the treatment of some cognitive disorders, some cerebral disorders, intermittent claudication, and vertigo; however, further clinical trials are needed. Generally, the uses of ginkgo biloba for cerebral insufficiency/memory impairment in the elderly and for the treatment of intermittent claudication are promising, but the data are not considered to be fully convincing.

Typical daily dosages of standardized gingko biloba extracts used in most clinical studies totaled about 120 mg (although higher dosages have been used). The ginkgo biloba dosages generally are divided and administered three times daily. Ginkgo biloba extracts typically are standardized to contain 22% to 27% flavonoids and 5% to 7% terpene lactones, of which 2.8% to 3.4% are ginkgolides and 2.6% to 3.6% are bilobalides. Benefits may not be observed for at least 6 weeks. Side effects that may be associated with the use of ginkgo biloba include headache, dizziness, palpitations, and mild gastrointestinal distress (nausea and abdominal pain). Contact with the whole plant may be associated with an allergic skin reaction. Interactions have been reported between ginkgo biloba and aspirin, warfarin (anticoagulant), and Vioxx (rofexocib, antiarthritic).

St. John's Wort

St. John's wort (*Hypericum perforatum*) is a perennial herb that produces golden yellow flowers. The flowers are typically harvested, dried, and extracted using alcohol and water. Major ingredients include naphthodianthrones (such as hypericin and pseudohypericin), phloroglucinols (such as hyperforin and adhyperforin), various flavonoids/flavonols (such as hyperoside, quercitrin, rutin, and kaempferol, among others), proanthocyanidins, xanthones, and phenolic acids (including caffeic acid, chlorogenic acid, and ferulic acid). Hypericin and hyperforin are thought to be the main active ingredients. Extracts of St. John's wort (*wort* is an Old English word for "plant") are usually standardized to provide 0.3% hypericin.

St. John's wort has been shown to inhibit neurotransmitter metabolism (especially of norepinephrine, dopamine, and serotonin), modulate neurotransmitter receptor concentrations and sensitivity, and alter neurotransmitter reuptake in the central nervous system. Oral consumption of St. John's extracts is recommended in the treatment of depression and anxiety. Oily hypericum preparations also are used topically to relieve inflammation and promote healing of, for example, first-degree burns, hemorrhoids, or minor wounds. Numerous studies and meta-analyses of studies have shown that use of St. John's wort is more effective than a placebo and similarly as effective as many antidepressant therapies in the treatment of mild to moderate depressive disorders. Moreover, the herb is often safer with respect to the side effects typically associated with the use of some antidepressant drug regimens.

Daily dosages of up to about 1,000 mg standardized extract (administered in divided doses) are commonly recommended, with therapeutic regimens of 2–3 weeks needed before effects are expected. The herb is sold in tablets and capsules and in tea and tincture forms. Adverse effects associated with the use of St. John's wort may include headache, fatigue, gastrointestinal distress (nausea, abdominal pain), dizziness, confusion, restlessness, and photosensitivity. The photosensitivity occurs with high dosages or prolonged use and is manifested as dermatitis and mucous membrane inflammation with sunlight exposure. Interactions have been reported between St. John's wort and anticoagulants, oral contraceptive (birth control) agents, theophylline (used for asthma), cyclosporin (used to diminish risk of transplant rejection), digoxin (heart contractility drug), and indinavir (antiviral drug).

Ginseng

Ginsengs are derived from several different species of the genus *Panax*. It is from the genus *Panax* that Asian (*P. ginseng* C. A. Meyer) and American (*P. quinquefolium*) ginsengs are derived. However, these species should not be confused with Siberian or Russian ginsengs or with Brazilian and Indian ginsengs, which are derived from a different plant. Ginsengs are perennial shade plants native to Korea and China. Ginseng has been used as an herbal remedy in Asia for centuries. All parts of the plant contain pharmacologically active components; however, the root is the most often used portion of the herb. The active components of ginseng (roots) are a group of triterpenoid saponin glycosides collectively called ginsenosides. Two saponins in ginseng are panaxadiol and panaxatriol (panaxans).

Ginseng is purported to reduce fatigue and improve stamina and well-being and thus to serve as an energy enhancer, or adaptogen. In other words, ginseng is said to increase the body's ability to resist or cope with stress and to help the body build vitality. In addition, it has been suggested that ginseng is anticarcinogenic. While a few studies have demonstrated that ginseng modulates some central nervous system activities to enhance performance, improve mood, diminish fatigue, and improve reaction time, among other effects, results of numerous other studies and meta-analyses assessing the effects of ginseng on the body do not support the claims. In other words, the efficacy of ginseng has not been clearly established for any indication.

Recommended dosages of ginseng (as tablets) range from about 100 to 300 mg/day to be taken in divided doses. Tinctures and fluid extracts also are available. Ginseng extracts usually contain 4% to 7% ginsenosides. Ginseng root also is available and is used in dosages of 0.6 to 2 g. For those using ginseng, daily use for a short duration is suggested. Problems with product quality are common; despite label reports, products often contain negligible to no ginseng. Side effects most often observed from the use of ginseng include headache, diarrhea, insomnia, and nervousness. Negative interactions have been reported between ginseng and warfarin (anticoagulant), the monoamine oxidase inhibitor phenelzine, and alcohol. In addition, germanium, an ingredient in some ginseng preparations, has been reported to induce resistance to diuretics.

Garlic

Garlic (*Allium sativum*) is part of the *Liliaceae* family, belonging specifically to the genus *Allium*. Garlic is similar to onions (also members of the *Liliaceae* family), chives, and leeks; all contain derivatives of the sulfur-containing amino acid cysteine, mainly S-allyl-L-cysteine sulfoxide, also known as *alliin*. Alliin may be converted to allicin (diallyldisulfide-S-oxide) in the presence of alliinase, which is exposed when garlic cells are destroyed by cutting or chewing, for example. Allicin degrades to diallyl disulfide, the main component in the odor of garlic, and to ajoene.

These active components of garlic (classified as organosulphides) have been shown in various studies to be antilipidemic, antithrombotic, antihypertensive, anticarcinogenic, antiglycemic, antioxidant, and immune-enhancing. However, meta-analyses of controlled clinical trials suggest promising but not conclusive benefits of garlic only as a modest blood lipid–lowering agent (total and LDL cholesterol and triglycerides) and as an antithrombotic agent.

Garlic is available naturally (in bulbs) or in more concentrated form as tablets or capsules. Typical daily dosages of garlic used in the studies ranged from about 600 to 900 mg of powdered garlic per day, equivalent to about 1.8 to 2.7 g or one-half to one clove of fresh garlic. Commercial garlic preparations, however, may not contain all of garlic's active compounds. Garlic cloves, for example, contain about 0.8% alliin; however, not all the alliin is usually retained in the making of garlic powder. Losses of allicin to varying degrees also occur. Side effects most commonly associated with garlic consumption include unpleasant body and breath odor, heartburn, flatulence, and other gastrointestinal-tract problems. Individuals on aspirin or anticoagulant therapies typically should avoid ingestion of large amounts of garlic.

Echinacea

Echinacea is derived from a native North American plant species characterized by spiny cone flowering heads, similar in appearance to the daisy. Three types of echinacea, *Echinacea angustifolia*, *E. pallida*, and *E. purpurea*, are available commercially. Several parts of the plant, including the roots, flowers (tops), or leaves either alone or in combination, are used in the preparation of dietary echinacea supplements. Liquid alcohol–based extracts of the roots (*E. angustifolia*) or the expressed juice of the aerial portion (*E. purpurea*) are commonly sold forms of the herb.

Several active ingredients are found in echinacea. Some of these are thought to include high-molecular-weight polysaccharides (such as heteroxylans, arabinogalactans, and rhamnogalactans), glycoproteins, flavonoids, alkamides (such as isoburylamide), alkenes, alkynes (such as polyacetylenes), and phenolic acids (caffeic and ferulic acid derivatives such as cichoric acid, echinacosides, and cynarin). One or more of these active ingredients are thought to stimulate components of the immune system. Examples of enhancement of the immune system include increased production of cytokines by macrophages, activation of T-cells, and increased phagocytic activity, among others. Because of these actions, the herb typically is recommended for the treatment of colds, upper-respiratory infections, or flulike symptoms. Its topical application also is recommended as an aid in the healing of superficial wounds as well as for psoriasis and eczema. Meta-analyses and reviews of studies examining the effectiveness of echinacea in the treatment of colds and upper-respiratory infections suggest promising but inconclusive results.

Daily doses of the herb usually consist of 500 to 1,000 mg of ground herb or root in tablets or capsules or brewed as a tea, or 0.5 to 4 mL of liquid extracts or tinctures (depending on strength). Dosages are generally divided and ingested two to three times daily. A consecutive maximum limit of echinacea use of 6 to 8 weeks has been suggested, with use for 10 to 14 days thought to be sufficient, as the effectiveness of echinacea is thought to diminish over time. Major side effects from the use of echinacea have not been reported; however, allergic reactions may occur. Echinacea use by individuals with systemic or immune system dysfunction disorders is contraindicated.

Regulation of Herbal Supplements

The Dietary Supplement Health and Education Act of 1994 allows herbs and phytomedicinals to be sold as dietary supplements as long as health or therapeutic claims do not appear on the product label [7]. The act defines dietary supplements to include vitamins, minerals, herbal or botanical products, amino acids, metabolites, extracts, and other substances alone or in combination that are added to the diet [7]. Because herbal supplements need not comply with other laws, the consumer and retailer have no assurance that the herb in the supplement corresponds with the label description. Thus, the reputation of the producer becomes extremely important. Herbs may be contaminated or adulterated in the manufacturing process. Incorrect parts of the herb, such as the stem versus the root, or an incorrect stage of ripeness may be used in production of the supplement [8,9]. In other words, quality assurance of herbs and phytomedicinals is generally lacking in the United States [8–10]. The act itself or reviews of the Dietary Supplement Health and Education Act of 1994 are available for additional or more specific information [8,11,12].

References Cited

1. Glaser V. Billion-dollar market blossoms as botanicals take root. Nat Biotechnol 1999;17:17–18.
2. Ernst E. The risk-benefit profile of commonly used herbal therapies: gingko, St. John's wort, ginseng, echinacea, saw palmetto, and kava. Ann Intern Med 2002;136:42–53.
3. Rowland I. Optimal nutrition: fibre and phytochemicals. Proc Nutr Soc 1999;58:415–19.
4. King A, Young G. Characteristics and occurrence of phenolic phytochemicals. J Am Diet Assoc 1999;99:213–18.
5. www.nal.usda.gov/fnic/foodcomp/Data/isoflav/isoflav.html
6. www.nal.usda.gov/fnic/foodcomp/Data/car98/car98.html
7. Dietary Supplement Health and Education Act, 103-417, 3.(a). 1994 bill/resolution.
8. Drew A, Myers S. Safety issues in herbal medicine: implications for the health professions. Med J Australia 1997;166:538–41.
9. Gilroy C, Steiner J, Byer T, Shapiro H, Georgian W. Echinacea and truth in labeling. Arch Intern Med 2003;163:699–704.
10. Tyler V. Herbal remedies. J Pharm The 1995;11:214–20.
11. Dietary supplements: recent chronology and legislation. Nutr Rev 1995;53:31–36.
12. www.cfsan.fda.gov/~dms/supplmnt.html

Recommended Books

American Herbal Products Association. Botanical Safety Handbook. CRC Press LLC, 1997.

Blumenthal M (ed.). The Complete German Commission E Monographs: Therapeutic Guide to Herbal Medicines. Austin, TX: American Botanical Council Publisher, 1998.

Gruenwald J, Brendler T, Jaenicke C, eds. PDR for Herbal Medicines, 2nd ed. Medical Montvale, NJ: Economic Co. Publisher, 2000.

Newall C, Anderson L, Phillipson J. Herbal Medicines: A Guide for Health-Care Professionals. London, UK: The Pharmaceutical Press, 1996.

Upton R. The American Herbal Pharmacopoeia. Santa Cruz: AHP, 2002.

General Reviews with Information on Phytochemicals and Herbs

Assemi M. Herbs affecting the central nervous system: gingko, kava, St. John's wort, and valerian. Clin Obstet Gynec 2002;44:824–35.

Barrett B, Kiefer D, Rabago D. Assessing the risks and benefits of herbal medicine: an overview of scientific evidence. Altern Ther Hlth Med 1999;5:40–49.

Bartels C, Miller S. Herbal and related remedies. Nutr Clin Pract 1998;13:5–19.

Bisset N. Herbal Drugs and Phytopharmaceuticals. Boca Raton, FL: CRC Press, 1994.

Bradlow H, Telang N, Sepkovic D, Osborne M. Phytochemicals as modulators of cancer risk. Adv Exp Med Biol 1999;472:207–21.

Briskin DP. Medicinal plants and phytomedicines. Plant Physiol 2000;124:507–14.

Dennehy C. Botanicals in cardiovascular health. Clin Obstet Gynec 2001;44:814–23.

DeSmet PAGM. Herbal remedies. New Engl J Med 2002;347:2046–56.

Hasler C, Blumberg J. Phytochemicals. J Nutr 1999;129:756S–57S.

Rhodes M. Physiologically active compounds in plant foods: an overview. Proc Nutr Soc 1996;55:371–84.

Rivlin RC. Nutrition and cancer prevention: new insights into the role of phytochemicals. Adv Exp Med Biol 2001;492:255–62.

Ross J, Kasum C. Dietary flavonoids: bioavailability, metabolic effects, and safety. Ann Rev Nutr 2002:22:19–34.

Setchell K. Phytoestrogens: the biochemistry, physiology, and implications for human health of soy isoflavones. Am J Clin Nutr 1998:68(suppl):1333S-46S.

Setchell K, Cassidy A. Dietary isoflavones: biological effects and relevance to human health. J Nutr 1999;129:758S–67S.

Visioli F, Borsani L, Galli C. Diet and prevention of coronary heart disease: the potential role of phytochemicals. Cardio Res 2000;47:419–25.

Yeum K, Russell R. Carotenoid bioavailability and bioconversion. Ann Rev Nut 2002:22:483–504.

Web Sites with Information on Phytochemicals and Herbs

www.herbs.org
www.herbalgram.org
www.ars-grin.gov/duke/
www.nccam.nih.gov
www.ibismedical.com
www.naturaldatabase.com
www.nal.usda.gov/fnic/foodcomp/Data/isoflav/isoflav.html
www.nal.usda.gov/fnic/foodcomp/Data/car98/car98.html
www.usp.org
www.cfsan.fda.gov/~dms/supplement.html

Ginkgo Biloba

Haguenauer J, Cantenot F, Koshas H, Pierart H. Treatment of equilibrium disorders with ginkgo biloba. Presse Medicale 1986;15:1569–72.

Kleijnen J, Knipschild P. Ginkgo biloba. Lancet 1992;340:1136–39.

Kleijnen J, Knipschild P. Ginkgo biloba for cerebral insufficiency. Br J Clin Pharmacol 1992;34:352–58.

LeBars P, Kastelan J. Efficacy and safety of ginkgo biloba extract. Pub Hlth Nutr 2000;3:495–99.

Mahady G. Ginkgo biloba for the prevention and treatment of cardiovascular disease. J Cardiovasc Nurs 2002;16:21–32.

McKenna D, Jones K, Hughes K. Efficacy, safety, and use of ginkgo biloba in clinical and preclinical applications. Altern Ther Hlth Med 2001;7:70–90.

Salvador R. Ginkgo. Can Pharm J 1995;128:39–41,52.

Taillandier J, Ammar A, Rabourdin J, Ribeyre J, Pichon J, Niddam S, Pierart H. Treatment of cerebral aging disorders with ginkgo biloba. Presse Medicale 1986;15:1583–87.

St. John's Wort

Anonymous. Final report on the safety assessment of hypericum perforatum extract and hypericum perforatum oil. Int J Toxicol 2001;20(suppl 2):31–39.

Barnes J, Anderson LA, Phillipson JD. St. John's wort: a review of its chemistry, pharmacology, and clinical properties. J Pharm Pharmacol 2001;53:583–600.

Bilia AR, Gallori S, Vincieri FF. St. John's wort and depression efficacy, safety, and tolerability—an update. Life Sci 2002;70:3077–96.

Greeson JM, Sanford B, Monti DA. St. John's wort (*Hypericum perforatum*): a review of the current pharmacological, toxicological, and clinical literature. Psychopharmacology 2001;153:402–14.

Linde K, Mulrow CD. St. John's wort for depression. Cochrane Database of Systematic Reviews 2000;2:CD000448.

McIntyre M. A review of the benefits, adverse effects, drug interactions, and safety of St. John's wort. J Alt Comp Med 2000;6:115–24.

Upton R, Graff A, Williamson E, et al. American Herbal Pharmacopoeia and therapeutic compendium: St John's wort, *Hypericum perforatum.* HerbalGram 1997;40:S1–32.

Ginseng

Bahrke M, Morgan W. Evaluation of the ergogenic properties of ginseng. Sports Med 1994;18:229–48.

Becker B, Greene J, Evanson J, Chidsey G, Stone W. Ginseng-induced diuretic resistance. JAMA 1996;276:606–7.

Coon JT, Ernst E. *Panax* ginseng. Drug Safety 2002;25:323–44.

Cui J, Garle M, Eneroth P, Bjorkhem I. What do commercial ginseng preparations contain? Lancet 1994;344:134.

Janetzky K, Morreale A. Probable interaction between warfarin and ginseng. Am J Health Syst Pharm 1997;54:692–93.

McRae S. Elevated serum digoxin levels in a patient taking digoxin and Siberian ginseng. Can Med Assoc 1996;155:293–95.

Shibata S. Chemistry and cancer preventing activities of ginseng saponins and some related triterpenoid compounds. J Korean Med Sci 2001;16(suppl):S28–37.

Siegel R. Ginseng abuse syndrome: problems with the panacea. JAMA 1979;241:1614–15.

Sorensen H, Sonne J. A double-masked study of the effects of ginseng on cognitive functions. Curr Ther Res 1996;57:959–68.

Yun TK. Experimental and epidemiological evidence of the cancer-preventive effects of *Panax ginseng* C. A. Meyer. Nutr Rev 1996;54:S71–81.

Garlic

Ackermann RT, Mulrow CD, Ramirez G, Gardner CD, Morbidoni L, Lawrence VA. Garlic shows promise for improving some cardiovascular risk factors. Arch Intern Med 2001;161:813–24.

Block E. The chemistry of garlic and onions. Sci Am 1985;252:114–19.

Jepson RG, Kleijnen J, Leng GC. Garlic for peripheral arterial occlusive disease. Cochrane Database Syst Rev 2000; 2:CD000095.

Journal of Nutrition 2001;131(3S):951S–1119S.

Kerckhoffs DA, Brounds F, Hornstra G, Mensink RP. Effects of the human serum lipoprotein profile of beta-glucan, soy protein and isoflavones, plant sterols and stanols, garlic and tocotrienols. J Nutr 2002;132: 2494–2505.

Kik C, Kahane R, Gebhardt R. Garlic and health. Nutr Metab Cardiovasc Dis 2001;11:57–65.

Spigelski D, Jones PJ. Efficacy of garlic supplementation in lowering serum cholesterol levels. Nutr Rev 2001; 59:236–41.

Stevinson C, Pittler M, Ernst E. Garlic for treating hypercholesterolemia: a meta-analysis of randomized clinical trials. Ann Intern Med 2000;133:420–29.

Echinacea

Giles JT, Palat CT, Chien SH, Chang ZG, Kennedy DT. Evaluation of echinacea for treatment of the common cold. Pharmacotherapy 2000;20:690–97.

Gilroy C, Steiner J, Byer T, Shapiro H, Georgian W. Echinacea and truth in labeling. Arch Intern Med 2003; 163:699–704.

Hobbs C. Echinacea: a literature review. Herbal Gram 1994;30:33–47.

Melchart D, Linde K, Fischer P, Kaesmayr J. Echinacea for preventing and treating the common cold. Cochrane Database of Systematic Reviews 2000;2: CD000530.

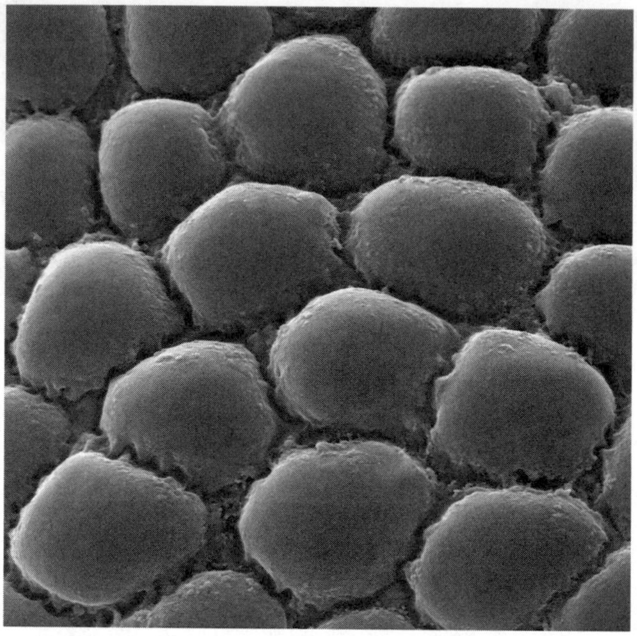

© Dr. Dennis Kunkel/Visuals Unlimited

Fat cells in connective tissue

chapter 6 Lipids

THE PROPERTY THAT SETS LIPIDS APART from other major nutrients is their solubility in organic solvents such as ether, chloroform, and acetone. If lipids are defined according to this property, which is generally the case, the scope of their function becomes quite broad. It encompasses not only dietary sources of energy and the lipid constituents of cell and organelle membranes but also the fat-soluble vitamins, corticosteroid hormones, and certain mediators of electron transport such as coenzyme Q.

Among the many compounds classified as lipids, only a small number are important as dietary energy sources or as functional or structural constituents within the cell. The following classification is limited to those lipids germane to this section of the text, which deals with energy-releasing nutrients. Fat-soluble vitamins are discussed in Chapter 10.

1. Simple lipids
   a. Fatty acids
   b. Triacylglycerols, diacylglycerols, and monoacylglycerols

c. Waxes (esters of fatty acids with higher alcohols)
   (1) Sterol esters (cholesterol–fatty acid esters)
   (2) Nonsterol esters (vitamin A esters, and so on)

2. Compound lipids
   a. Phospholipids
      (1) Phosphatidic acids (i.e., lecithin, cephalins)
      (2) Plasmalogens
      (3) Sphingomyelins
   b. Glycolipids (carbohydrate containing)
   c. Lipoproteins (lipids in association with proteins)

3. Derived lipids: derivatives such as sterols and straight-chain alcohols obtained by hydrolysis of those lipids in groups 1 and 2 that still possess general properties of lipids

In the discussion of the structure and physiological function of lipids that follows, lipids have been grouped arbitrarily according to fatty acids, triacylglycerols (triglycerides), sterols and steroids, phospholipids, and glycolipids. This grouping is more functional than structural.

STRUCTURE AND BIOLOGICAL IMPORTANCE

Fatty Acids

As a class, the fatty acids are the simplest of the lipids. They are composed of a straight hydrocarbon chain terminating with a carboxylic acid group. Therefore, they create within the molecules a polar, hydrophilic end and a nonpolar, hydrophobic end that is insoluble in water (Fig. 6.1). Fatty acids are components of the more complex lipids, discussed in later sections. They are of vital importance as an energy nutrient, furnishing most of the calories from dietary fat.

The length of the carbon chains of fatty acids found in foods and body tissues varies from 4 to about 24 carbon atoms. The fatty acids may be saturated (SFA), monounsaturated (MUFA, possessing one carbon-carbon double bond), or polyunsaturated (PUFA, having two or more carbon-carbon double bonds). PUFAs of nutritional interest may have as many as six double bonds. Where a carbon-carbon double bond exists, there is an opportunity for either a *cis* or a *trans* geometric isomerism that significantly affects the molecular configuration of the molecule. The *cis* isomerism form results in a folding back and kinking of the molecule into a U-like orientation, whereas the *trans* form has the effect of extending the molecule into a linear shape similar to that of saturated fatty acids. The structures in Figure 6.1 illustrate saturation and unsaturation in an 18-carbon fatty acid and show how *cis* or *trans* isomerization affects the molecular configuration.

The more carbon-carbon double bonds occurring within a chain, the more pronounced is the bending effect. The amount of bending plays an important role in the structure and function of cell membranes. Most naturally occurring unsaturated fatty acids are of the *cis* configuration, although the *trans* form does exist in some natural fats and oils. Most fatty acids are derived from partially hydrogenated fats and oils. Partial hydrogenation, a process commonly used in making margarine, is designed to solidify vegetable oils. Double bonds of *cis* orientation, not reduced by hydrogen in the process, undergo an electronic rearrangement to the *trans* form, which is energetically stabler. The availability of *trans* fatty acids in the typical U.S. diet has been estimated to be approximately 8.1 g/person/day, the major source of which is margarines and spreads [1].

Concerns have been raised about the possible adverse nutritional effects of dietary *trans* fatty acids, particularly their reputed role in the etiology of cardiovascular disease. This topic is discussed in the section "Lipids, Lipoproteins, and Cardiovascular Disease Risk" in this chapter.

Fatty Acid Nomenclature

Two systems have been developed to provide a shorthand way to understand the chemical structure of a fatty acid. Both systems are used regularly and will be used interchangeably in the text for different purposes.

The delta (Δ) system is a notation system that has been established to denote the chain length of the fatty acids and the number and position of any double bonds that may be present. For example, the notation 18:2 $\Delta^{9,12}$ describes linoleic acid. The first number, 18 in this case, represents the number of carbon atoms; the number following the colon refers to the number of double bonds present; and the superscript numbers following the delta symbol designate the carbon atoms at which the double bonds begin. In this system, the numbering starts from the carboxyl end of the fatty acid.

A second commonly used system of notation locates the position of double bonds on carbon atoms counted from the methyl, or omega (ω), end of the carbon chain. For instance, the notation for linoleic acid would be 18:2 ω-6. Substitution of the omega symbol with the letter *n* has been popularized. Using this designation, the notation for linoleic acid would be expressed as 18:2 n-6. In this system, the total number of carbon atoms in the chain is given by the first number, the number of double bonds is given by the number following the colon, and the location (carbon atom number) of the first double bond is given by the number following ω- or n-. This system of notation takes into account the fact that double bonds in a fatty acid are always separated by three carbons. Thus, if you know the location of the first double bond, you can determine the remaining double bonds.

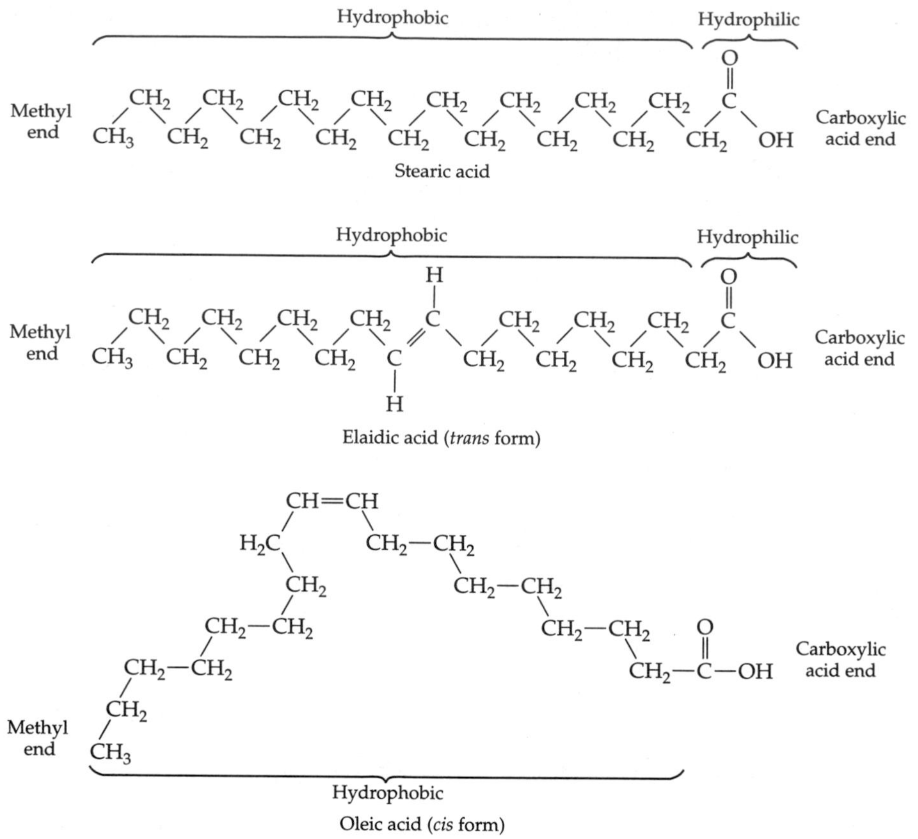

Figure 6.1 Structures of selected fatty acids.

$$-CH{=}CH-CH_2-CH{=}CH-$$

The location of multiple double bonds is unambiguous given their total number and the location of the one closest to either the methyl end or the carboxylic acid end, depending on the nomenclature system used.

A comparison of the two systems is shown in Figure 6.2. The designation of linoleic acid by each of the two systems is 18:2 $\Delta^{9,12}$ or 18:2 ω-6 (n-6). The fatty acid α-linolenic acid, which contains three double bonds, is identified as 18:3 $\Delta^{9,12,15}$ or 18:3 ω-3 (n-3).

Table 6.1 lists some naturally occurring fatty acids and their dietary sources. For unsaturated fatty acids, the table shows both the Δ system and the ω system. The list includes only those fatty acids having chain lengths of 14 or more carbon atoms, because these are most important both nutritionally and functionally. For example, palmitic acid (16:0), stearic acid (18:0), oleic acid (18:1), and linoleic acid (18:2) together account for >90% of the fatty acids in the average U.S. diet. However, it should be understood that shorter-chain fatty acids do occur in nature. Butyric acid (4:0) and lauric acid (12:0) occur in large amounts in milk fat and coconut oil, respectively.

Most fatty acids have an even number of carbon atoms. The reason for this will be evident in the discussion of fatty acid synthesis. Odd-numbered-carbon fatty acids occur naturally to some extent in some sources. For example, certain fish, such as menhaden, mullet, and tuna, as well as the bacterium *Euglena gracilis*, contain fairly high concentrations of odd-numbered-carbon fatty acids.

Essential Fatty Acids

If fat is entirely excluded from the diet of humans, a condition develops that is characterized by retarded growth, dermatitis, kidney lesions, and early death. Studies have shown that the feeding of certain unsatu-

Figure 6.2 The structure of linoleic acid, showing the two systems for nomenclature. The delta (Δ) system counts from the carboxylic acid end of the carbon chain, and the omega (ω) system counts from the methyl end.

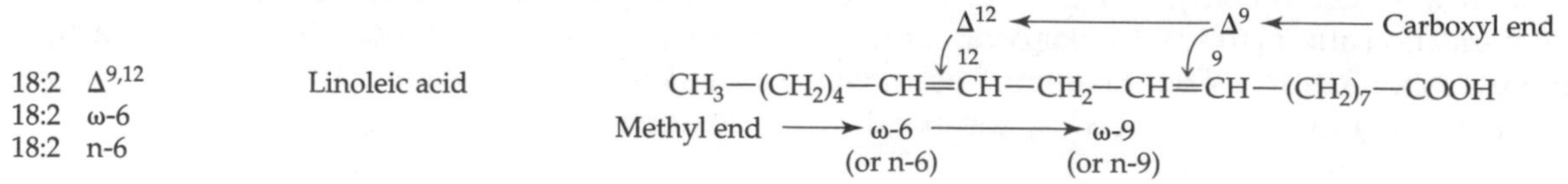

Table 6.1 Some Naturally Occurring Fatty Acids

Notation	Common Name	Formula	Source
Saturated Fatty Acids			
14:0	Myristic acid	$CH_3–(CH_2)_{12}–COOH$	Coconut and palm nut oils, most animal and plant fats
16:0	Palmitic acid	$CH_3–(CH_2)_{14}–COOH$	Animal and plant fats
18:0	Stearic acid	$CH_3–(CH_2)_{16}–COOH$	Animal fats, some plant fats
20:0	Arachidic acid	$CH_3–(CH_2)_{18}–COOH$	Peanut oil
24:0	Lignoceric acid	$CH_3–(CH_2)_{22}–COOH$	Most natural fats, peanut oil in small amounts
Unsaturated Fatty Acids			
16:1 Δ^9 (n-7)	Palmitoleic acid	$CH_3–(CH_2)_5–CH=CH–(CH_2)_7–COOH$	Marine animal oils, small amount in plant and animal fats
18:1 Δ^9 (n-9)	Oleic acid	$CH_3–(CH_2)_7–CH=CH–(CH_2)_7–COOH$	Plant and animal fats
18:2 $\Delta^{9,12}$ (n-6)	Linoleic acid	$CH_3–(CH_2)_4–\overset{6*}{C}H=\overset{12\dagger}{C}H–CH_2–CH=\overset{9\dagger}{C}H–(CH_2)_7–COOH$	Corn, safflower, soybean, cottonseed, sunflower seed, and peanut oil
18:3 $\Delta^{9,12,15}$ (n-3)	α-linolenic acid	$CH_3–(CH_2–CH=CH)_3–(CH_2)_7–COOH$	Linseed, soybean, and other seed oils
20:4 $\Delta^{5,8,11,14}$ (n-6)	Arachidonic acid	$CH_3–(CH_2)_3–(CH_2–CH=CH)_4–(CH_2)_3–COOH$	Small amounts in animal fats
20:5 $\Delta^{5,8,11,14,17}$ (n-3)	Eicosapentaenoic acid	$CH_3–(CH_2–CH=CH)_5–(CH_2)_3–COOH$	Marine algae, fish oils
22:6 $\Delta^{4,7,10,13,16,19}$ (n-3)	Docosahexaenoic acid	$CH_3–(CH_2–CH=CH)_6–(CH_2)_2–COOH$	Animal fats as phospholipid component, fish oils

*Number of first carbon double bond from methyl end (*n* system). †Number of carbon double bond from carboxylic acid end (Δ system).

rated fatty acids such as linoleic, α-linolenic, and arachidonic acids is effective in curing the conditions related to the lack of these fatty acids. Some unsaturated fatty acids thus cannot be synthesized in animal cells but must be acquired in the diet from plant foods. The two essential fatty acids are linoleic acid (18:2 n-6) and α-linolenic acid (18:3 n-3). From linoleic acid, γ-linolenic (18:3 n-6) and arachidonic acids (20:4 n-6) can be formed in the body. An intermediate fatty acid in the pathway is eicosatrienoic acid. The pathway is

linoleic acid (18:2 n-6)

↓

γ-linolenic acid (18:3 n-6)

↓

eicosatrienoic acid (20:3 n-6)

↓

arachidonic acid (20:4 n-6)

The essentiality of linoleic and α-linolenic acids is due to the fact that humans lack enzymes called Δ^{12} and Δ^{15} desaturases, which incorporate double bonds at these positions. These enzymes are found only in plants. Humans are incapable of forming double bonds beyond the Δ^9 carbon in the chain. If a $\Delta^{9,12}$ fatty acid is obtained from the diet, however, additional double bonds can be incorporated at Δ^6 (desaturation). Fatty acid chains can also be elongated by the enzymatic addition of two carbon atoms at the carboxylic acid end of the chain. These reactions are discussed further in the section on fatty acid synthesis and are illustrated later in Figure 6.31.

n-3 Fatty Acids

Nutritional interest in the n-3 fatty acids has escalated enormously in recent years because of their reported hypolipidemic and antithrombotic effects. An n-3 fatty acid of particular interest is eicosapentaenoic acid (20:5 n-3) because it is a precursor of the physiologically important eicosanoids, discussed later in this chapter. Fish oils are particularly rich in these unique fatty acids and therefore are the dietary supplement of choice in research designed to study their effects. Food sources and tissue distribution of a few commonly occurring n-3 polyunsaturated fatty acids are given in Table 6.2.

Table 6.2 Dietary Sources and Tissue Distribution of the Major n-3 Polyunsaturated Fatty Acids

Fatty Acid Series	Major Members of Series	Tissue Distribution in Mammals	Dietary Sources
n-3	α-linolenic acid 18:3 n-3	Minor component of tissues	Some vegetable oils (soy, canola, linseed, rapeseed) and leafy vegetables
	Eicosapentaenoic acid 20:5 n-3	Minor component of tissues	Fish and shellfish
	Docosahexaenoic acid 22:6 n-3	Major component of membrane phospholipids in retinal photoreceptors, cerebral gray matter, testes, and sperm	Fish and shellfish

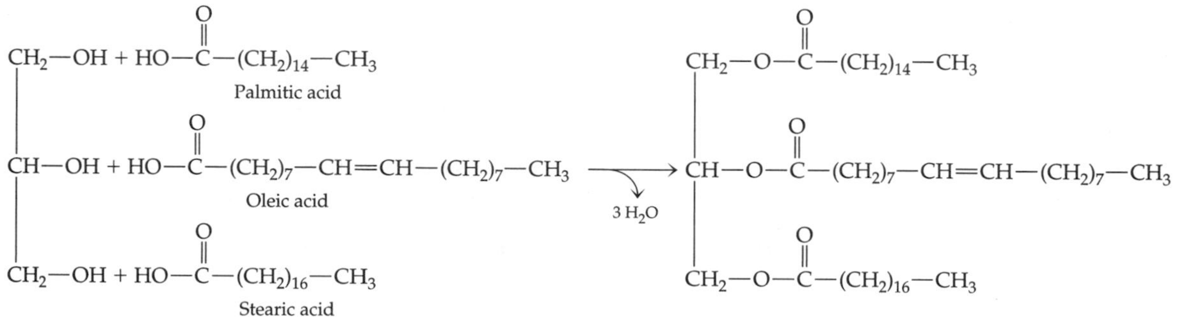

Figure 6.3 Linkage of palmitic, oleic, and stearic acid, forming a triacylglycerol.

Triacylglycerols (Triglycerides)

Most stored body fat is in the form of triacylglycerols, which represent a highly concentrated form of energy. They account for nearly 95% of dietary fat. Structurally, they are composed of a trihydroxy alcohol, glycerol, to which are attached three fatty acids by ester bonds. The fatty acids may be all the same (a simple triacylglycerol) or different (a mixed triacylglycerol). The linking of the fatty acids palmitic, oleic, and stearic to glycerol, with the liberation of three water molecules, is shown in Figure 6.3.

Acylglycerols composed of glycerol esterified to a single fatty acid (a monoacylglycerol) or to two fatty acids (a diacylglycerol) are shown in Figure 6.4. The fatty acids can be on any of the three carbons of glycerol. The mono- and diacylglycerols occur in negligible amounts in tissues. However, they are important intermediates in some metabolic reactions and may be components of other lipid classes. They also may occur in processed foods, to which they can be added as emulsifying agents.

Figure 6.4 Chemical structure of a monoacylglycerol (left) and a diacylglycerol (right).

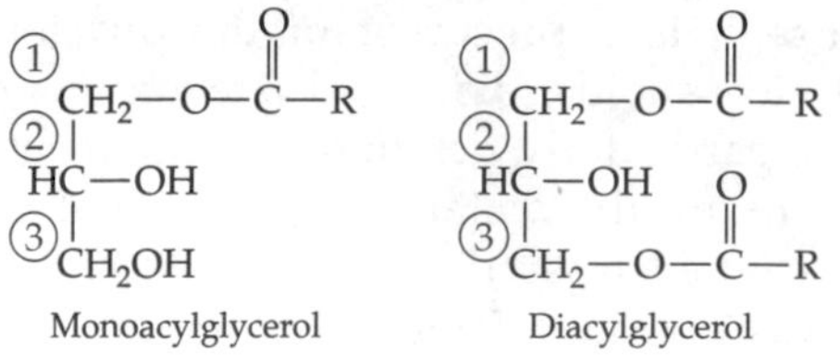

The specific glycerol hydroxyl group to which a certain fatty acid is attached is indicated by a numbering system for the three glycerol carbons. This system is complicated somewhat by the fact that the central carbon of the glycerol is asymmetrical when different fatty acids are esterified at the two end carbon atoms and therefore may exist in either the D or the L form (Appendix). Unfortunately, this means that the same monoacylglycerol may be written in two ways (see Fig. 6.5a). To resolve this ambiguity, a system of nomenclature called stereospecific numbering (*sn*) has been adopted whereby the

Figure 6.5 Monoacylglycerol structure and stereospecific numbering.

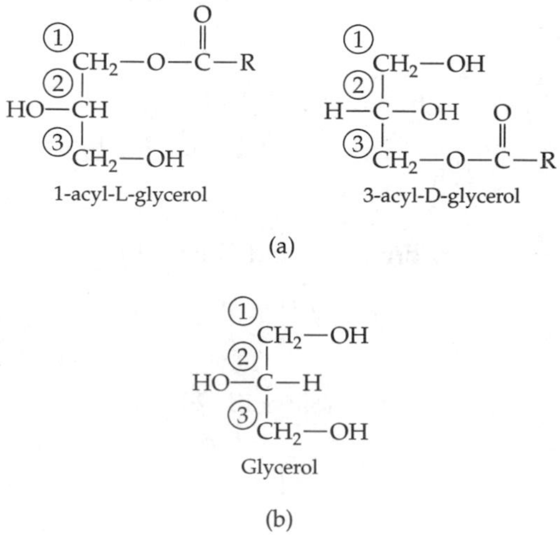

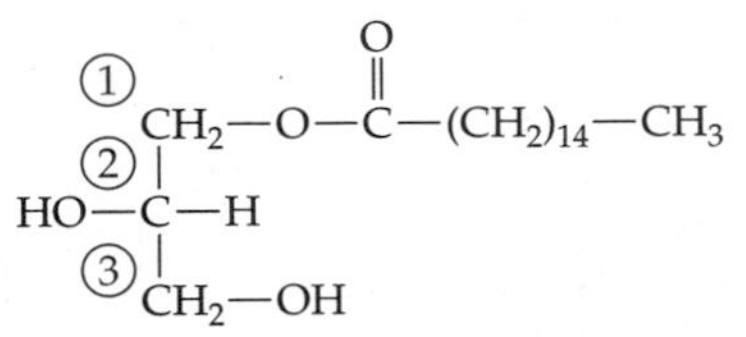

Figure 6.6 Structural formula of the monoacylglycerol 1-monopalmitoyl glycerol.

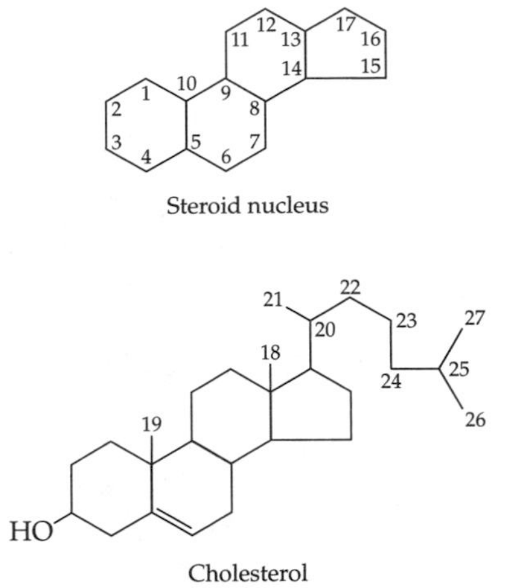

Figure 6.7 Structure of cholesterol, with numbering system for carbons in the steroid nucleus.

glycerol is always written as in Figure 6.5b, with the C-2 hydroxyl group oriented to the left (L) and the carbons numbered 1 through 3 beginning at the top. Accordingly, 1-monopalmitoyl glycerol (Fig. 6.6) can be drawn in either of the ways shown in Figure 6.5a. Using this system, the naming of the triacylglycerol shown in Figure 6.3 is 1-palmitoyl-2-oleoyl-3-stearoyl-L-glycerol.

Triacylglycerols exist as fats (solid) or oils (liquid) at room temperature depending on the nature of the component fatty acids. Triacylglycerols containing a high proportion of relatively short chain fatty acids or unsaturated fatty acids tend to be liquid (oils) at room temperature. Saturated fatty acids of longer chain length have a higher melting point and exist as solids at room temperatures. When used for energy, fatty acids are released in free (nonesterified) form as free fatty acids (FFA) from the triacylglycerols in adipose tissue cells by the activity of lipases, and the FFA are then transported by albumin to various tissues for oxidation.

Sterols and Steroids

This class of lipid is characterized by a four-ring core structure called the cyclopentanoperhydrophenanthrene, or steroid, nucleus. **Sterols** are monohydroxy alcohols of steroidal structure, with cholesterol being the most common example. Cholesterol is present only in animal tissues. It can exist in free form, or the hydroxyl group can be esterified with a fatty acid. Many sterols other than cholesterol are found in plant tissues. The structure of cholesterol is shown in Figure 6.7, along with the numbering system for the carbons in the steroid nucleus.

Meats, egg yolk, and dairy products, the common dietary sources of cholesterol, contain fairly large amounts. In the body, this sterol is an essential component of cell membranes, particularly the membranes of nerve tissue. Despite the bad press that cholesterol has garnered over the years because of its implication in cardiovascular disease, it serves as the precursor for many other important steroids in the body, including the bile acids; steroid sex hormones such as estrogens, androgens, and progesterone; the adrenocortical hormones; and the vitamin D of animal tissues (cholecalciferol). These steroids differ from one another in the arrangement of double bonds in the ring system, the presence of carbonyl or hydroxyl groups, and the nature of the side chain at C-17. All these structural modifications are mediated by enzymes that function as dehydrogenases, isomerases, hydroxylases, or desmolases. Desmolases remove or shorten the length of side chains on the steroid nucleus. The derivation of the various types of steroids from cholesterol is diagramed in Figure 6.8. Although many physiologically active corticosteroid hormones, sex hormones, and bile acids exist, only representative compounds are shown. The biological importance and metabolic reactions of these compounds will be discussed later in this chapter.

Sterols, together with phospholipids (considered next), comprise only about 5% of dietary lipid.

Phospholipids

As the name implies, lipids belonging to the **phospholipids** contain phosphate. They also possess one or more fatty acid residues. Phospholipids are categorized into one of two groups called glycerophosphatides and sphingophosphatides, depending on whether their core structure is glycerol or the amino alcohol sphingosine (Fig. 6.9), respectively.

Glycerophosphatides

The building block of a glycerophosphatide is phosphatidic acid, formed by the esterification of two fatty acids at C-1 and C-2 of glycerol and the esterification of the C-3 hydroxyl with phosphoric acid. In most cases, glycerophosphatides have a saturated fatty acid on position 1 and an unsaturated fatty acid on position 2. The structure in Figure 6.10 typifies a phosphatidate, a term that does not define a specific structure because different fatty acids may be involved. The conventional numbering of the glycerol carbon atoms is the same as that for triacylglycerols. From top to bottom, the numbering is *sn*-1, *sn*-2, and *sn*-3, provided the glycerol is written in the

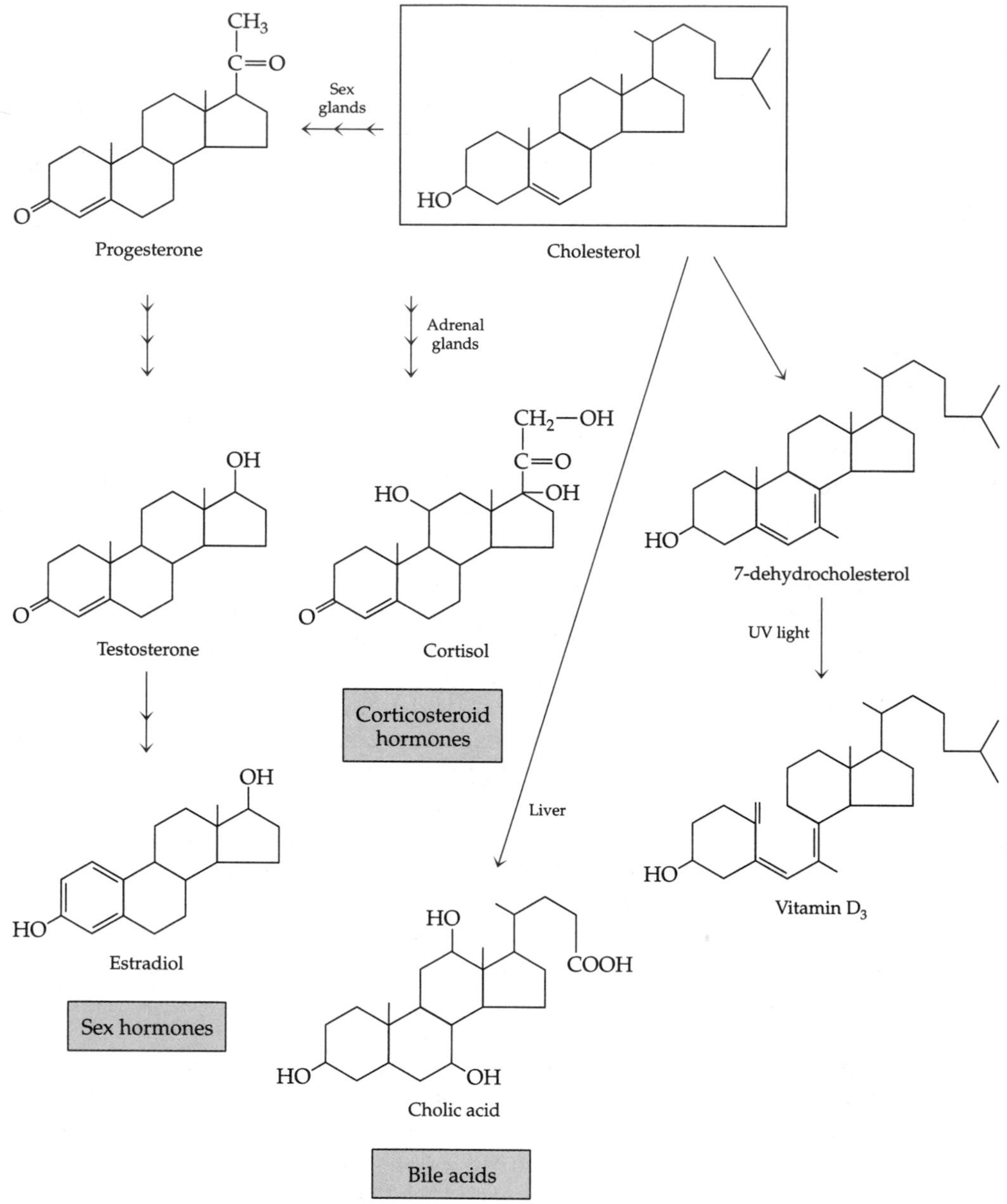

Figure 6.8 The formation of physiologically important steroids from cholesterol. Only representative compounds from each category of steroid are shown.

Figure 6.9 Structure of the amino alcohol sphingosine.

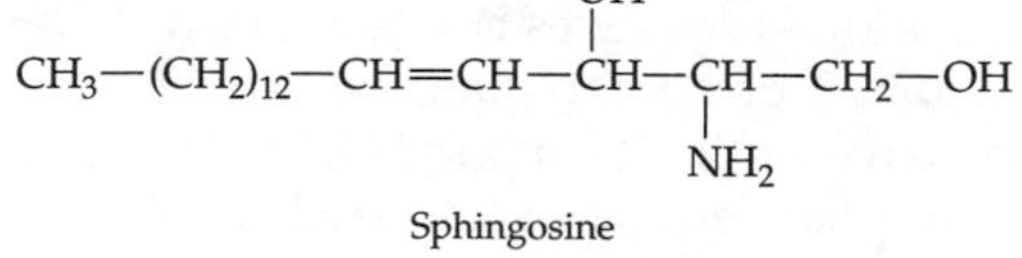

Figure 6.10 Typical structure of a phosphatidate (in L configuration).

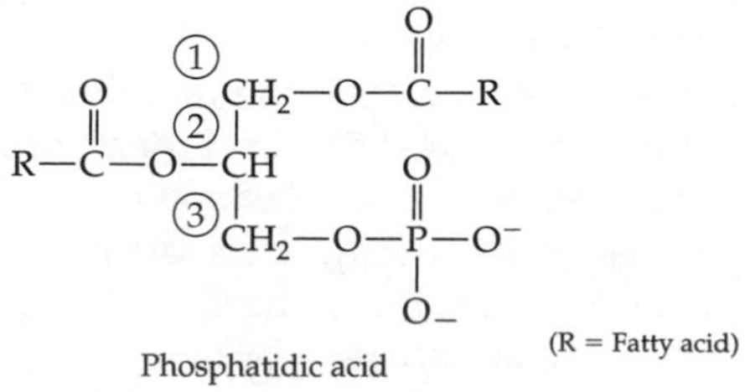

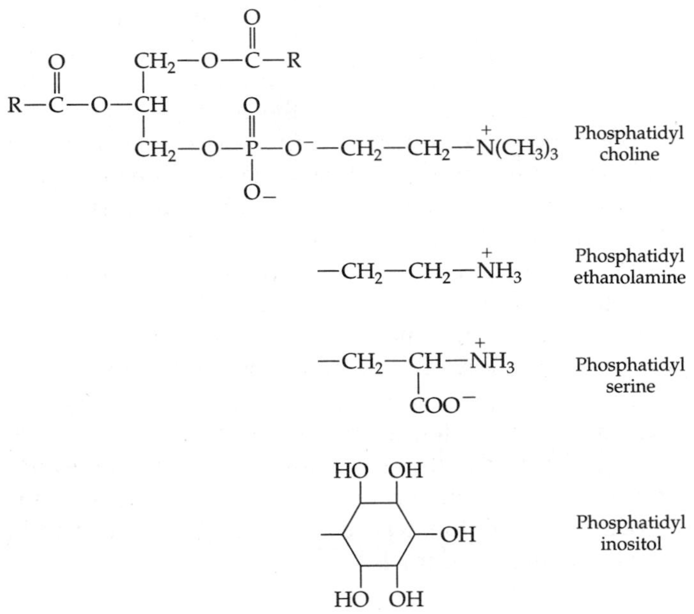

Figure 6.11 Structure of phosphatidylcholine (lecithin), along with alcohols that form other phospholipids.

L configuration so that the C-2 fatty acid constituent is directed to the left, as shown. Phosphatidic acids form a number of derivatives with compounds such as choline, ethanolamine, serine, and inositol, each of which possesses an alcohol group through which a second esterification to the phosphate takes place (Fig. 6.11). The compounds are named as the phosphatidyl derivatives of the alcohols, as indicated in the figure. The structure shown is phosphatidylcholine, which probably is better known by its common name, lecithin. The other phospholipids are formed by replacing the choline, as shown.

Phospholipids are more polar than the triacylglycerols and sterols and therefore tend to attract water molecules. Because of this hydrophilic property, phospholipids are commonly expressed on the surface of blood-borne lipid particles, such as chylomicrons, thereby stabilizing the particles in the aqueous medium. Furthermore, as a constituent of cell and organelle membranes, phospholipids serve as a conduit for the passage of water-soluble and fat-soluble materials across the membrane.

Biological Roles of Phospholipids

Phospholipids play several important roles in the body. Glycerophosphatides, for example, are very important components of cell membranes. In addition to lending structural support to the membrane, they serve as a source of physiologically active compounds. We will see later how arachidonate can be released on demand from membrane-bound phosphatidylcholine and phosphatidylinositol when it is needed for synthesis of **eicosanoids** (20-carbon fatty acids).

Another phospholipid, phosphatidylinositol, also participates in cell functions. For example, it plays a specific role in the anchoring of membrane proteins when the proteins are covalently attached to lipids. This has been demonstrated by the release of certain membrane proteins when cells are treated with a phosphatidylinositol-specific phospholipase C, which hydrolyzes the ester bond connecting the glycerol to the phosphate. Phosphatidylinositols anchor a wide variety of surface antigens and other surface enzymes in eukaryotic cells. In addition, certain hydrolytic products of phosphatidylinositol are active in intracellular signaling and act as second messengers in hormone stimulation. Phosphatidylinositol in the plasma membrane can be doubly phosphorylated by ATP, forming phosphatidylinositol-4,5-bisphosphate. Stimulation of the cell by certain hormones activates a specific phospholipase C, which produces inositol-1,4,5-trisphosphate and diacylglycerol from phosphatidylinositol-4,5-bisphosphate. Both of these products function as second messengers in cell signaling. Inositol-1,4,5-trisphosphate causes the release of Ca^{2+} held within membrane-bounded compartments of the cell, triggering the activation of a variety of Ca^{2+}-dependent enzymes and hormonal responses [2]. Diacylglycerol binds to and activates an enzyme, protein kinase C, that transfers phosphate groups to several cytoplasmic proteins, thereby altering their enzymatic activities [3]. This dual signal hypothesis of phosphatidylinositol hydrolysis is represented in Figure 6.12.

Sphingolipids

The 18-carbon amino alcohol sphingosine forms the backbone of the **sphingolipids.** Sphingosine (Fig. 6.9) typically combines with a long-chain fatty acid through

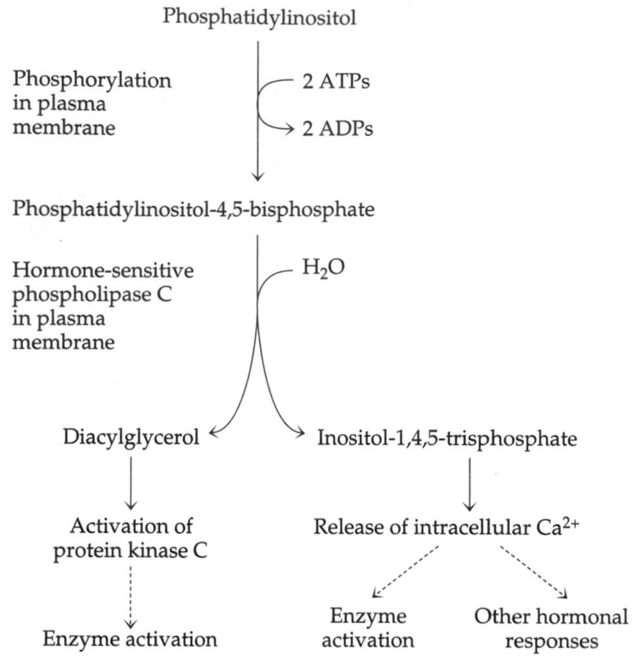

Figure 6.12 Phosphatidylinositol-4,5-bisphosphate, formed in the plasma membrane by phosphorylation of phosphatidylinositol, is hydrolyzed by a specific phospholipase C in response to hormonal signals. Both products of hydrolysis act as intracellular messengers.

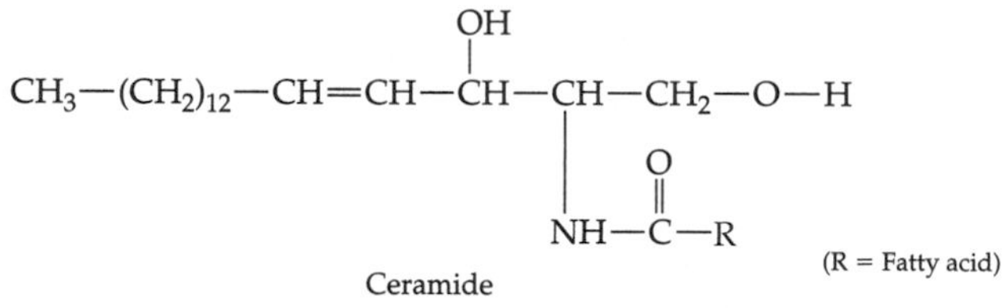

Figure 6.13 Structure of the sphingolipid ceramide.

an amide linkage to form ceramide (Fig. 6.13). Lipids formed from sphingosine (Fig. 6.9) are categorized into three subclasses: sphingomyelins, cerebrosides, and gangliosides. Of these, only the sphingomyelins are sphingophosphatides. The other two subclasses of sphingolipids contain no phosphate but instead possess a carbohydrate moiety. They are referred to as glycolipids and are discussed in the next section.

Sphingomyelins occur in plasma membranes of animal cells and are found in particularly large amounts in the myelin sheath of nerve tissues. The sphingomyelins contain ceramide (a fatty acid residue attached in an amide linkage to the amino group of the sphingosine), which in turn is esterified to phosphorylcholine (see Fig. 6.14). Sphingomyelins can combine with either phosphorylcholine or phosphorylethanolamine. Sphingomyelins are important in the nervous system (e.g., in the myelin sheath) in higher animals.

Glycolipids

Glycolipids can be subclassified into cerebrosides and gangliosides. They are so named because they have a carbohydrate component within their structure. Like the phospholipids, their physiological role is principally structural, contributing little as an energy source. They occur in the medullary sheaths of nerves and in brain tissue, particularly the white matter. As in the case of sphingomyelin, the sphingosine moiety provides the backbone for glycolipid structure. It is attached to a fatty acid by an amide bond, forming ceramide, as discussed previously. The glycolipids do not contain phosphate.

A cerebroside is characterized by the linking of ceramide to a monosaccharide unit such as glucose or galactose, producing either a glucocerebroside or a galactocerebroside (Fig. 6.15).

Gangliosides resemble cerebrosides except that the single monosaccharide unit of the cerebroside is replaced by an oligosaccharide containing various monosaccharide derivatives such as N-acetyl neuraminic acid and N-acetyl galactosamine. Gangliosides are known to be involved in certain recognition events occurring at the cell surface. For example, they provide the carbohydrate determinants of the human blood groups A, B, and O.

Figure 6.14 The structure of sphingomyelin.

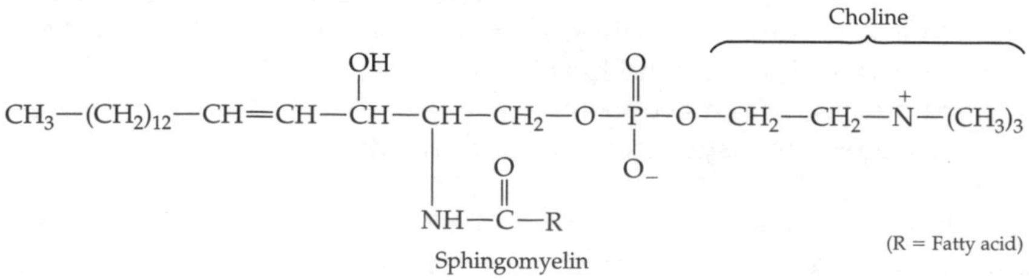

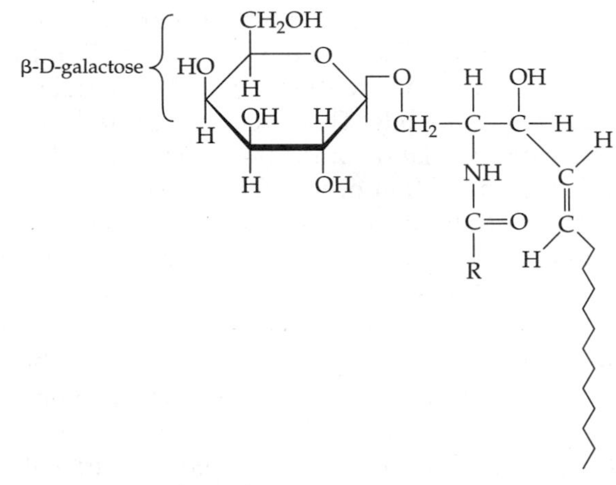

Figure 6.15 A cerebroside.

DIGESTION

Because fats are hydrophobic, their digestion poses a special problem in that their digestive enzymes, like all proteins, are hydrophilic and normally function in an aqueous environment. However, the surface area of dietary lipid, targeted for digestion, is greatly enhanced by a very efficient emulsification process mediated mainly by the bile salts. Consequently, the accessibility of the fat to digestive enzymes is greatly increased by bile salt action.

Triacylglycerols, phospholipids (primarily phosphatidylcholine), and sterols (mainly cholesterol) provide the lipid component of the typical Western diet. Of these, triacylglycerols, customarily called fats, are by far the major contributor, with a consumption rate of about 150 g daily on average. Compare this to the intake of cholesterol, which is typically 300 to 600 mg depending on the quantity of fatty animal products in the diet. Digestive enzymes involved in the breakdown of dietary lipids in the gastrointestinal tract are esterases that cleave the ester bonds within triacylglycerols (lipase), phospholipids (phospholipases), and cholesteryl esters (cholesterol esterase).

Triacylglycerol Digestion

Most dietary triacylglycerol digestion is completed in the lumen of the small intestine, although the process actually begins in the stomach. Digestive activity at these two sites is attributed to two different forms of lipases: (1) lingual lipase, secreted by serous glands lying beneath the tongue, and (2) pancreatic lipase. Basal secretion of lingual lipase apparently occurs continuously but can be stimulated by neural (sympathetic agonists), dietary (high fat), and mechanical (sucking and swallowing) factors. Lingual lipase accounts for the limited digestion of fat in the stomach, made possible by the enzyme's particularly high stability at the low pH of the gastric juices. It can readily penetrate milk fat globules without substrate stabilization by bile salts, a feature that makes it particularly important for fat digestion in the suckling infant, whose pancreatic function may not be fully developed. Lingual lipases act preferentially on triacylglycerols containing medium- and short-chain fatty acids. It preferentially hydrolyzes fatty acids at the *sn*-3 position, releasing fatty acid and 1,2-diacylglycerol as products. This specificity again is advantageous for the suckling infant because in milk triacylglycerols short- and medium-chain fatty acids are usually esterified at the *sn*-3 position. Short- and medium-chain fatty acids are metabolized more directly than are long-chain fatty acids.

For dietary fat in the stomach to be hydrolyzed by lingual lipase, some degree of emulsification must occur to expose a sufficient surface area of the substrate. Muscle contractions of the stomach and the squirting of the fat through a partially opened pyloric sphincter produce shear forces sufficient for emulsification. Also, potential emulsifiers in the acid milieu of the stomach include complex polysaccharides, phospholipids, and peptic digests of dietary proteins. The presence of undigested lipid in the stomach delays the rate of emptying of the stomach contents, presumably by way of the hormone enterogastrone (GIP and secretin; Chap. 2), which inhibits gastric motility. Fats therefore have a "high satiety value."

Significant hydrolysis and absorption, especially of the long-chain fatty acids, require less acidity, appropriate lipases, more effective emulsifying agents (bile salts), and specialized absorptive cells. These conditions are provided in the lumen of the upper small intestine. The partially hydrolyzed lipid emulsion leaves the stomach and enters the duodenum as fine lipid droplets. Effective emulsification takes place because as mechanical shearing continues, it is complemented by bile that is released from the gallbladder as a result of stimulation by the hormone cholecystokinin (CCK). Refer to page 42 for a discussion of the role of bile in digestion and the synthesis of bile from cholesterol (see also Figs. 2.13–2.17). Bicarbonate is simultaneously released from the pancreas, elevating the pH to a level suitable for pancreatic lipase activity. In combination with triacylglycerol breakdown products, bile salts are excellent emulsifying agents. Their emulsifying effectiveness is due to their **amphipathic** properties, that is, their possessing both hydrophilic and hydrophobic "ends." Such molecules tend to arrange themselves on the surface of small fat particles with their hydrophobic ends turned inward and their hydrophilic regions turned outward toward the water phase. This chemical action, together with the help of peristaltic agitation, converts the fat into small droplets with a greatly increased surface area. The particles then can be readily acted on by pancreatic lipase.

The Role of Colipase

Pancreatic lipase activation is complex, requiring the participation of the protein colipase, calcium ions, and bile salts. Colipase is formed by the hydrolytic activation by trypsin of procolipase, also of pancreatic origin. It contains approximately 100 amino acid residues and possesses distinctly hydrophobic regions that are believed to act as lipid-binding sites. Colipase has been shown to associate strongly with pancreatic lipase and therefore may act as an anchor, or linking point, for attachment of the enzyme to the bile salt–stabilized micelles (described later).

The action of pancreatic lipase on ingested triacylglycerols results in a complex mixture of diacylglycerols, monoacylglycerols, and free fatty acids. Its specificity is primarily toward *sn*-1-linked fatty acids and secondarily to *sn*-3 bonds. Therefore, the main path of this digestion progresses from triacylglycerols to 2,3-diacylglycerols to 2-monoacylglycerols. Only a small percentage of the triacylglycerols is hydrolyzed totally to free glycerol. The complete hydrolysis of triacylglycerols that does occur probably follows the isomerization of the 2-monoacylglycerol to 1-monoacylglycerol, which is then hydrolyzed.

Cholesterol and Phospholipid Digestion

Cholesterol esters and phospholipids are hydrolyzed by a specific process described here. Esterified cholesterol undergoes hydrolysis to free cholesterol and a fatty acid in a reaction catalyzed by the enzyme cholesterol esterase. The C-2 fatty acid of lecithin is hydrolytically removed by a specific esterase, phospholipase A_2 producing lysolecithin and yet another free fatty acid. The products of the partial digestion of lipids, primarily 2-monoacylglycerols, lysolecithin, cholesterol, and fatty acids, combine with bile salts to form negatively charged polymolecular aggregates called micelles. These have a much smaller diameter (~5 nm) than the unhydrolyzed precursor particles, allowing them access to the intramicrovillus spaces (50–100 nm) of the intestinal membrane (Fig. 2.15).

ABSORPTION

Stabilized by the polar bile salts, the micellar particles are sufficiently water-soluble to penetrate what is called the unstirred water layer bathing the absorptive cells of the small intestine. The absorptive cells are called intestinal mucosal cells, or enterocytes. Micelles interact at the brush border of these cells, whereupon the lipid contents of the micelles (which include FFA, 2-monoacylglycerols, cholesterol, cholesterol esters, and lysolecithin) diffuse out of the micelles and into the enterocytes, moving down a concentration gradient. Although this process occurs in the distal duodenum and the jejunum, the bile salts are not absorbed at this point but instead are absorbed in the ileal segment of the small intestine. There they are returned to the liver via the portal vein to be resecreted in the bile. This circuit is referred to as the enterohepatic circulation of the bile salts (Chap. 2).

After the absorption of free fatty acids, 2-monoacylglycerols, cholesterol, and lysophosphatidylcholine into the enterocytes, intracellular re-formation of triacylglycerols, phosphatidylcholine, and cholesteryl esters takes place. The process, however, is a function of the chain length of the fatty acids involved. Fatty acids having more than 10 to 12 carbon atoms are first activated by being coupled to coenzyme A by the enzyme acyl CoA synthetase. They are then reesterified into triacylglycerols, phosphatidylcholine, and cholesteryl esters as mentioned earlier. Short-chain fatty acids, those containing fewer than 10 to 12 carbon atoms, in contrast, pass from the cell directly into the portal blood, which takes them directly to the liver. In the blood, short-chain fatty acids attach to albumin for transport to other tissues for processing. The different fates of the long- and short-chain fatty acids are due to the specificity of the acyl CoA synthetase enzyme for long-chain fatty acids only. Key features of intestinal absorption of lipid digestion products are depicted in Figure 6.16.

It should be pointed out that triacylglycerols can also be synthesized from α-glycerophosphate in the enterocytes. This metabolite can be formed either from the phosphorylation of free glycerol or from reduction of dihydroxyacetone phosphate, an intermediate in the pathway of glycolysis (see Fig. 4.14). Triacylglycerol synthesis by this route is also shown in Figure 6.16.

Lipids resynthesized in the enterocytes, together with fat-soluble vitamins, are collected in the cell's endoplasmic reticulum as large fat particles. While still in the endoplasmic reticulum, the particles receive a layer of protein on their surface. This tends to stabilize the particles in the aqueous environment of the circulation, which they eventually enter. The particles are pinched off as lipid vesicles that then fuse with the Golgi apparatus. There carbohydrate is attached to the protein coat, and the completed particles, called chylomicrons, are transported to the cell membrane and exocytosed into the lymphatic circulation. Chylomicrons therefore belong to a family of compounds called **lipoproteins,** which get their name from the fact that lipid and protein comprise their composition. Recall the discussion of lipid digestion in Chapter 2 and Figure 2.14, which describes micelle formation, and Figure 2.15, which describes transport of fatty acids, glycerol, triacylglycerols, and lipoprotein in the intestinal enterocytes. Lipoproteins play an important role in the transport of lipids, and serum lipoprotein patterns have been implicated as risk factors in chronic cardiovascular disease.

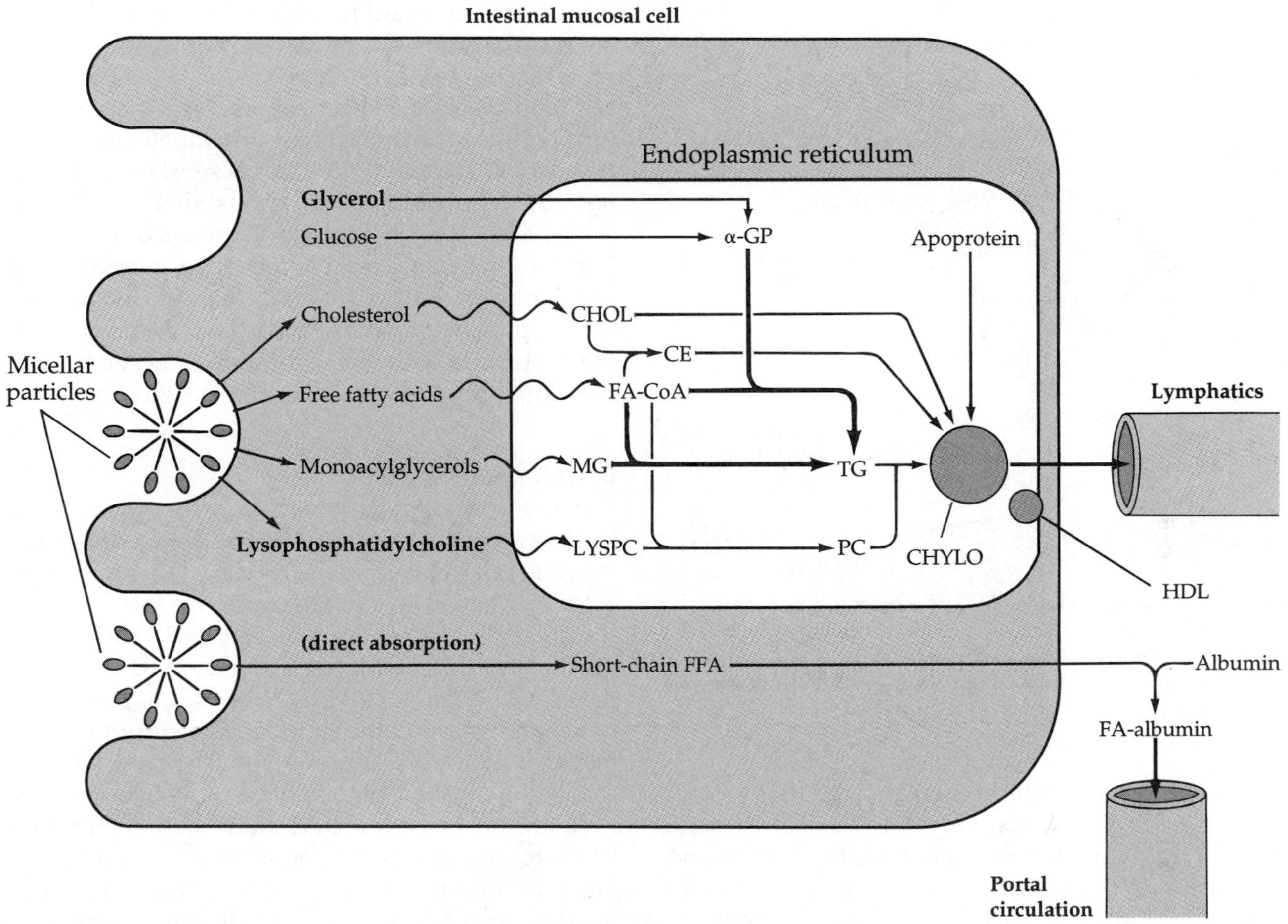

Figure 6.16 The uptake of micellar lipid particles by the intestinal mucosal cell, and the reassembly of the lipid components within the endoplasmic reticulum (shown as white area) of the cell. The reassembly of the lipids produces principally chylomicrons, although small amounts of HDL can be formed in this manner. Following their combination with apoproteins, the lipoprotein particles are released into the lymphatic circulation and ultimately the portal blood. Short-chain free fatty acids enter the portal circulation directly, as shown. Abbreviations: CHOL, cholesterol; CE, cholesteryl ester; FA-CoA, CoA-activated fatty acids; MG, monoacylglycerol; LYSPC, lysophosphatidylcholine; α-GP, α-glycerophosphate; CHYLO, chylomicrons; TG, triacylglycerol; PC, phosphatidylcholine.

The protein portion only of any lipoprotein is called the **apolipoprotein.** Apolipoproteins play a very important role in the structural and functional relationship among the lipoproteins (discussed in the next section).

TRANSPORT AND STORAGE

Lipoproteins

Chylomicrons are the primary form of lipoprotein formed from exogenous (dietary) lipids. Lipoproteins other than chylomicrons transport endogenous lipids, which are circulating lipids that do not arise directly from intestinal absorption but instead are processed through other tissues, such as the liver. Several types of lipoproteins exist, differing in their chemical composition, physical properties, and metabolic function. The role shared by all the lipoproteins, however, is the transport of lipids from tissue to tissue to supply the lipid needs of different cells. The arrangement of the lipid and protein components of a typical lipoprotein particle is represented in Figure 6.17. It can be seen from the figure that the more hydrophobic lipids are located in the core of the particle, while the relatively more polar proteins and phospholipids are situated on the surface to enhance aqueous stability.

Lipoproteins differ according to the ratio of lipid to protein within the particle as well as in having different proportions of lipid types: triacylglycerols, cholesterol and cholesteryl esters, and phospholipids. Such compositional differences influence the density of the particle, which has become the physical characteristic used to differentiate and classify the various lipoproteins. In the

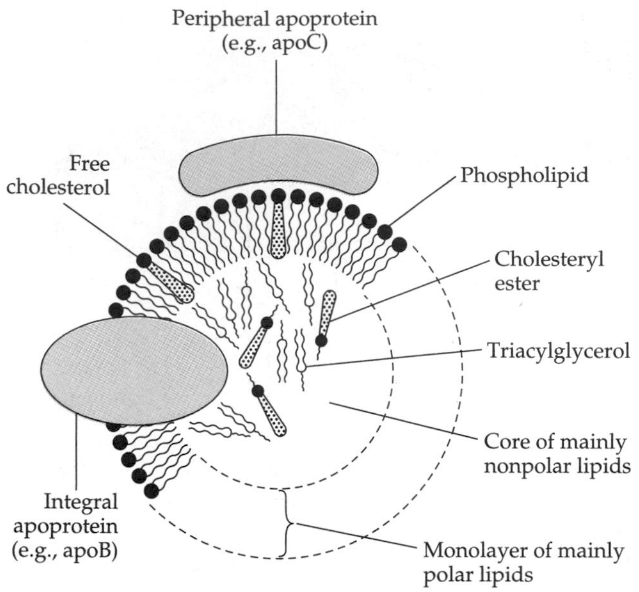

Figure 6.17 Generalized structure of a plasma lipoprotein. Note the similarities with the structure of the plasma membrane. A small amount of cholesteryl ester and triacylglycerol is found in the surface layer and a little free cholesterol in the core.

order of lowest to highest density, the lipoprotein fractions are chylomicrons, very low density lipoproteins (VLDLs), low-density lipoproteins (LDLs), and high-density lipoproteins (HDLs). There is also an intermediate-density particle (IDL), having a density between that of VLDL and LDL. The IDL particles are very short lived in the bloodstream, however, and have little nutritional or physiological importance. Table 6.3 summarizes several physical and chemical characteristics of the lipoproteins.

Apolipoproteins

Apolipoproteins, the protein components of lipoproteins, tend to stabilize the lipoproteins as they circulate in the aqueous environment of the blood, but they also have other important functions. They confer specificity on the lipoprotein complexes, allowing them to be recognized by specific receptors on cell surfaces. They also stimulate certain enzymatic reactions, which in turn regulate the lipoproteins' metabolic functions.

A series of letters (A to E), with subclasses of each, are now used to identify the various apolipoproteins. For convenience, they are usually abbreviated "apo" and followed by the identifying letter—that is, apoA-1, apoB-100, apoC-2, and so on. A partial listing of the apolipoproteins, together with their molecular weight, the lipoprotein with which they are associated, and their postulated physiological function, is found in Table 6.4.

Distribution of Lipids

The re-formed lipid derived from exogenous sources leaves the enterocytes (intestinal mucosal cells) largely in the form of chylomicrons, which then undergo intravascular conversion to chylomicron remnants (structurally similar to VLDL). To some extent, HDL can be synthesized within the enterocytes and released directly into the mesenteric lymph. The lipoproteins first appear in the lymphatic vessels of the abdominal region and then enter the bloodstream at a slow rate so as to prevent large-scale changes in the lipid content of peripheral blood. Entry of chylomicrons into the blood from the lymph continues for up to 14 hours after consumption of a meal rich in fat. The peak level of lipid in blood plasma usually occurs 30 minutes to 3 hours after a meal and returns to near normal within 5 to 6 hours. This can vary, however, depending on the stomach emptying time, which in turn is dependent on the size and composition of the meal.

Chylomicrons and VLDL, which is formed endogenously in the liver, are transported by the blood throughout all tissues in the body while undergoing intravascular hydrolysis at certain tissue sites. This hydrolysis occurs through the action of the enzyme lipoprotein lipase, which is associated with the endothelial cell surface of the small blood vessels and capillaries within adipose and

Table 6.3 Chemical and Physical Properties of Plasma Lipoproteins in Humans

Property	Chylomicrons	VLDL	IDL	LDL	HDL
Density (g/mL)	<1.006	<1.006	1.006–1.019	1.019–1.063	1.063–1.21
Diameter (nm)	80–500	40–80	24.5	20	7.5–12
Lipids (% by wt.)	98	92	85	79	50
Cholesterol	9	22	35	47	19
Triglyceride	82	52	20	9	3
Phospholipid	7	18	20	23	28
Apoproteins (%)	2	8	15	21	50
Major	A-1, A-2 B-48 C-1,2,3 E	B-100 C-1,2,3 E	B-100 C-1,2,3 E	B-100	A-1, A-2 C-1,2,3 E

Table 6.4 Apolipoproteins of Human Plasma Lipoproteins

Apolipoprotein	Lipoprotein	Molecular Mass (Da)	Additional Remarks
apoA-1	HDL, chylomicrons	28,000	Activator of lecithin: cholesterol acyltransferase (LCAT). Ligand for HDL receptor.
apoA-2	HDL, chylomicrons	17,000	Structure is two identical monomers joined by a disulfide bridge. Inhibitor of LCAT?
apoA-4	Secreted with chylomicrons but transfers to HDL	46,000	Associated with the formation of triacylglycerol-rich lipoproteins. Function unknown.
apoB-100	LDL, VLDL, IDL	550,000	Synthesized in liver. Ligand for LDL receptor.
apoB-48	Chylomicrons, chylomicron remnants	260,000	Synthesized in intestine.
apoC-1	VLDL, HDL, chylomicrons	7,600	Possible activator of LCAT.
apoC-2	VLDL, HDL, chylomicrons	8,916	Activator of extrahepatic lipoprotein lipase.
apoC-3	VLDL, HDL, chylomicrons	8,750	Several polymorphic forms depending on content of sialic acids.
apoD	Subfraction of HDL	20,000	Function unknown.
apoE	VLDL, HDL, chylomicrons, chylomicron remnants	34,000	Present in excess in the β-VLDL of patients with type III hyperlipoproteinemia. The sole apoprotein found in HDL_c of diet-induced hypercholesterolemic animals. Ligand for chylomicron remnant receptor in liver and LDL receptor.

muscle tissue. Its extracellular action on the circulating particles releases free fatty acids and diacylglycerols, which are quickly absorbed by the tissue cells.

Storage of Triglycerides

The large, triacylglycerol-laden chylomicrons account for the turbidity (milky appearance) of postprandial plasma. Because lipoprotein lipase is the enzyme that solubilizes these particles by its lipolytic action, it is sometimes referred to as "clearing factor." The part of the chylomicron that is left following this lipolytic action is called a **chylomicron remnant**—a smaller particle relatively less rich in triacylglycerol but richer in cholesterol. These remnants are removed from the bloodstream by liver cell endocytosis following interaction of the remnant particles with specific receptors for apolipoprotein E or B/E on the cells [4]. Nascent VLDL of liver origin also undergoes triacylglycerol stripping by lipoprotein lipase at extracellular sites, resulting in the formation of a transient IDL particle and, finally, a cholesterol-rich LDL. The apolipoprotein apoC-2 is an activator of lipoprotein lipase and a component of both chylomicrons and VLDL, as indicated in Table 6.4. This accounts for the susceptibility of these particles to lipoprotein lipase action and is an example of the regulatory function of an apolipoprotein. Figure 6.18 summarizes the formation of the lipoproteins and their interconversions, along with their lipid-protein composition.

Within the muscle cells, the free fatty acids and those derived from the hydrolysis of the absorbed diacylglycerols are primarily oxidized for energy, with only limited use for the resynthesis and storage of triacylglycerols. Aerobically trained muscle, however, does contain triacylglycerol deposits. In adipose tissue, in contrast, the absorbed fatty acids are largely used for the synthesis of triacylglycerols, in keeping with that tissue's storage role. In this manner, chylomicrons and VLDL are cleared from the plasma in a matter of minutes and a few hours, respectively, from the time they enter the bloodstream.

Role of the Liver and Adipose Tissue in Lipid Metabolism

Liver

The liver plays a very important role in the body's use of lipids and lipoproteins. Hepatic synthesis of the bile salts, indispensable for digesting and absorbing dietary lipids, is one of its functions. In addition, the liver is the key player in lipid transport, because it is the site of synthesis of lipoproteins formed from endogenous lipids and apoproteins. The liver is capable of de novo synthesis of lipids from nonlipid precursors such as glucose and amino acids. It can also take up and catabolize exogenous lipids delivered to it in the form of chylomicron remnants, repackaging their lipids into HDL and VLDL forms. Lipid metabolism in the liver is summarized in Figure 6.19. Also shown in Figure 6.19 is a glimpse of the reactions by which glucose and amino acids can be converted into lipid. They are included as a reminder to the reader that pathways of lipid, carbohydrate, and protein metabolism are integrated and cannot stand alone. These interrelationships will be discussed further in Chapter 8.

In the postprandial state, glucose, amino acid, and short-chain fatty acid concentrations rise in portal blood.

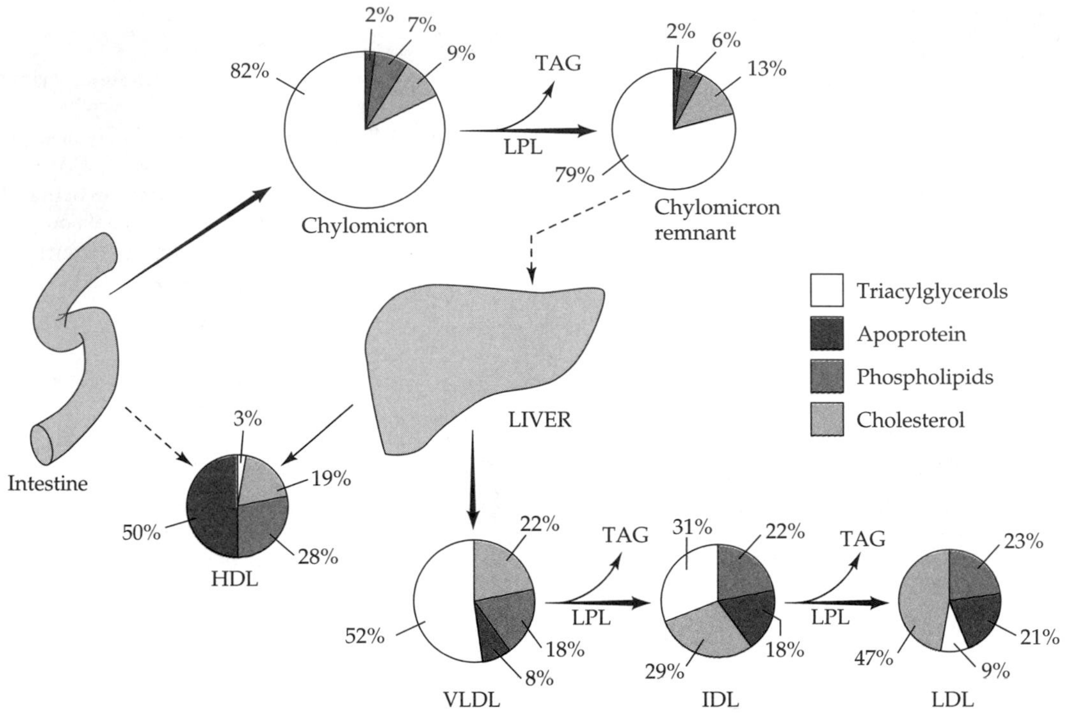

Figure 6.18 Conversion pathways of lipoproteins formed from exogenous sources (intestinal absorption) and from endogenous formation (synthesis in liver). Although small amounts of HDL are synthesized within the enterocytes of the small intestine, its major site of synthesis is the liver. Relative particle size of the lipoproteins is shown along with their approximate composition. Abbreviations: TAG, triacylglycerols; LPL, lipoprotein lipase.

In the hepatocyte, glucose is phosphorylated for use, and glycogen subsequently is synthesized until the hepatic stores are repleted. If portal hyperglycemia persists (more glucose comes from the digestive system), glucose is converted to fatty acids via acetyl CoA and also to triose phosphates (such as glycerol 3-phosphate), from which the glycerol portion of triglycerides is derived. Amino acids can also serve as precursors for lipid synthesis because they can be metabolically converted to acetyl CoA and pyruvate. The synthesis of fatty acids, triacylglycerols, and glycerophosphatides is described in detail later in this chapter.

In addition to the newly synthesized lipid derived from nonfatty precursors, there is also the exogenous lipid delivered to the liver in the form of chylomicron remnants as well as short-chain fatty acids. The mechanism for the hepatic uptake and hydrolysis of chylomicron remnants is not entirely clear, although these particles are believed to first interact, via the apolipoprotein E on their surface, with specific receptors for apoE in the vascular endothelial cells of the liver. The lipid portion of the chylomicron remnant is hydrolyzed in the hepatocyte to free fatty acids, monoacylglycerols and diacylglycerols, glycerol, and cholesterol, but resynthesis of these compounds promptly occurs in a manner analogous to the events in the intestinal mucosal cell. An alternate fate of the lipid entering the hepatocyte is for the fatty acids to be used for energy.

Exogenous free fatty acids of short-chain length delivered directly to the hepatic tissue can be used for energy or, following chain elongation, for resynthesis of other lipid fractions. Chylomicron remnant cholesterol and cholesteryl esters may be

- converted to bile salts and secreted in the bile,
- secreted into the bile as neutral sterol (such as cholesterol or cholesterol ester), or
- incorporated into VLDL or HDL and released into the plasma.

Newly synthesized triacylglycerol is combined with phospholipid, cholesterol, and proteins to form VLDL and HDL, which are released into the circulation. The HDL, small and triacylglycerol poor relative to the VLDL, possesses phospholipids and cholesterol as its major lipid constituents. Because triacylglycerols can be formed from glucose, hepatic triacylglycerol production is accelerated when the diet is rich in carbohydrate. This results in VLDL overproduction and may account for the occasional transient hypertriacylglycerolemia in

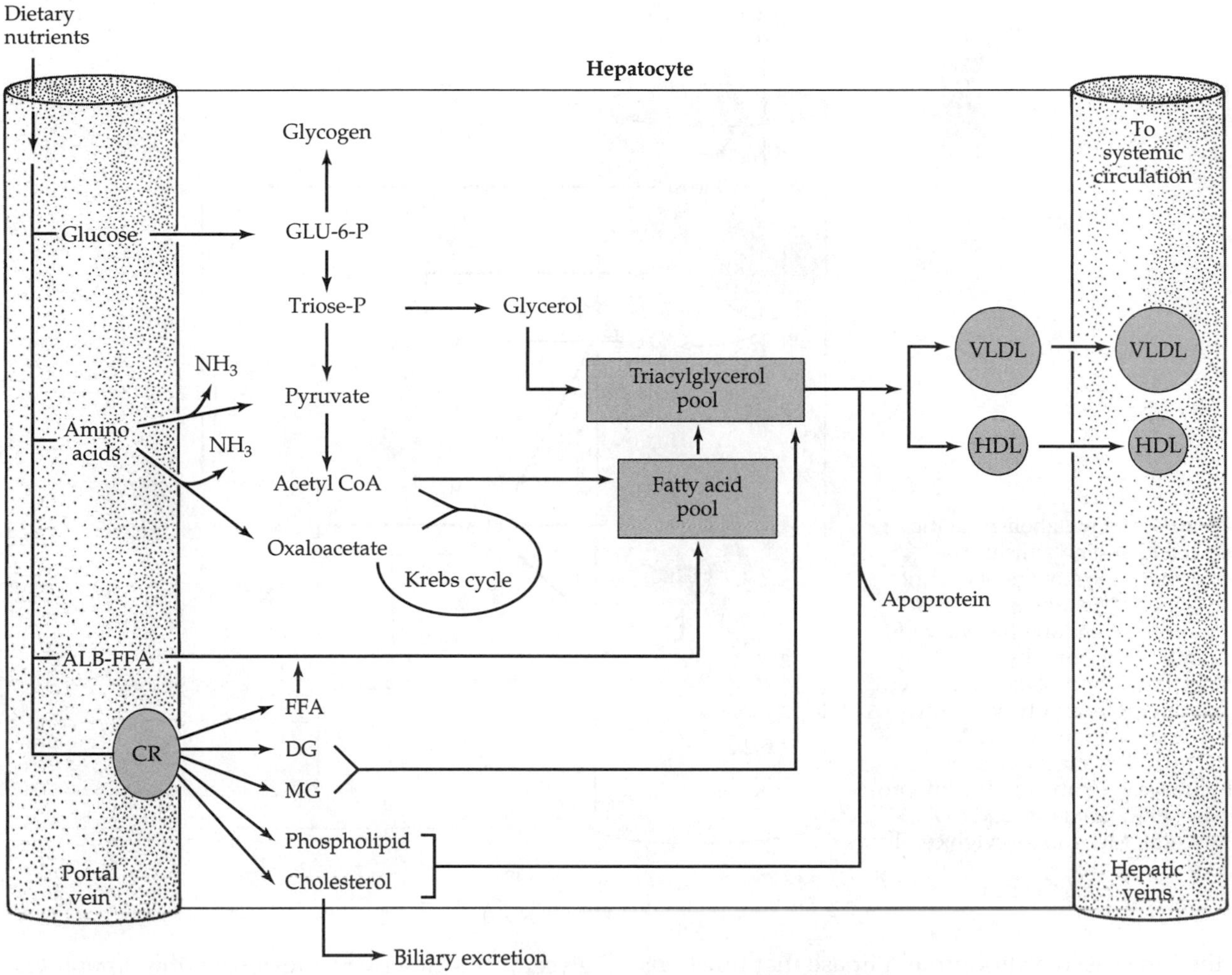

Figure 6.19 Lipid metabolism in the liver following a meal, showing its relationship to carbohydrate and amino acid metabolism. Abbreviations: ALB-FFA, albumin-bound free fatty acids; CR, chylomicron remnants; DG, diacylglycerols; MG, monoacylglycerols.

normal people when they consume diets rich in simple sugars.

Adipose Tissue

Adipose tissue shares with the liver an extremely important role in fat metabolism. Unlike the liver, it is not involved in the uptake of chylomicron remnants or the synthesis of endogenous lipoproteins. Instead, adipocytes are the major storage site for triacylglycerol, which is in a continuous state of turnover in the cells: lipolysis (hydrolysis), countered by reesterification. These two processes are not simply forward and reverse directions of the same reactions but are different pathways involving different enzymes and substrates. Each of the processes is regulated separately by nutritional, metabolic, and hormonal factors, the net effect of which determines the level of circulating fatty acids and the extent of adiposity. A single large globule of fat constitutes over 85% by volume of the adipose cell.

In the fed state, metabolic pathways in adipocytes favor triacylglycerol synthesis. As in the liver, adipocyte triacylglycerol can be synthesized from glucose, a process strongly influenced by insulin. Insulin accelerates the entry of glucose into the adipose cells (the liver does not respond to this action of the hormone) and also increases the availability and uptake of fatty acids by stimulating lipoprotein lipase. Cellular glucose, via its glycolytic breakdown, provides a source of glycerophosphate for reesterification with the fatty acids to form triacylglycerols. Absorbed monoacylglycerols and diacylglycerols also furnish the glycerol building block for this resynthesis. Insulin exerts its lipogenic action further by inhibiting intracellular lipase, which hydrolyzes stored triacylglycerols. Intracellular lipase is insulin sensitive, distinguishing it

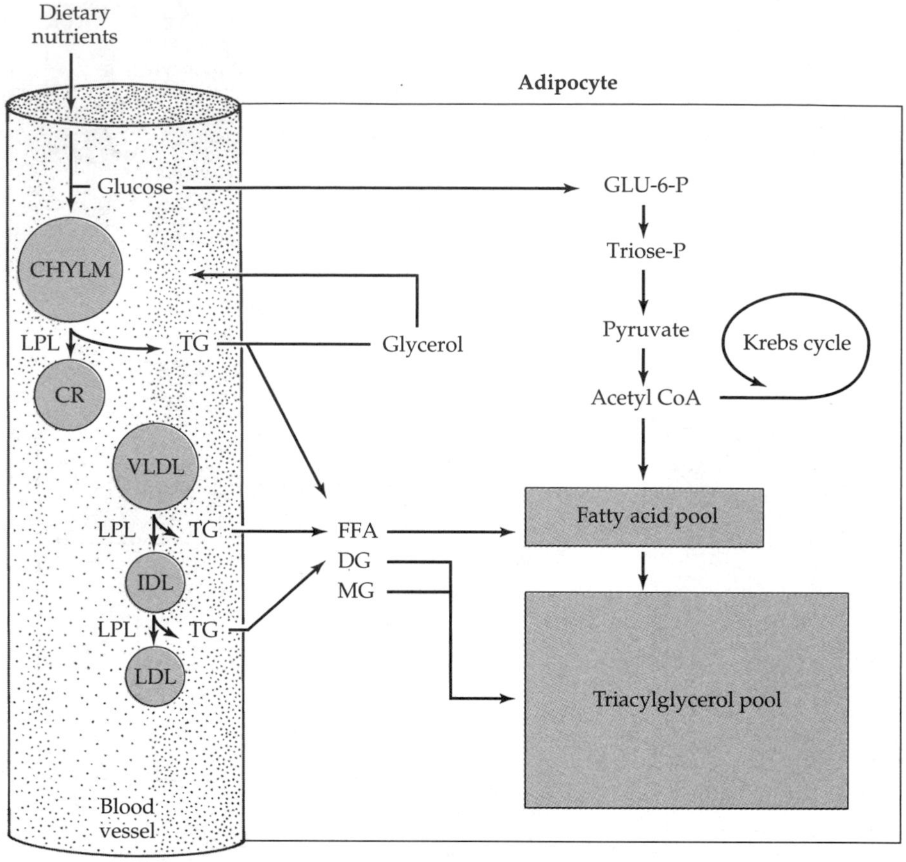

Figure 6.20 Lipid metabolism in the adipose cell following a meal. The pathways favor the storage of energy as triacylglycerol. Insulin stimulates lipogenesis by promoting the entry of glucose into the cell and by inhibiting the lipase, which hydrolyzes the stored triacylglycerol to free fatty acids and glycerol. Abbreviations: CHYLM, chylomicrons; TG, triacylglycerol; CR, chylomicron remnant; LPL, lipoprotein lipase; FFA, free fatty acids; DG, diacylglycerol; MG, monoacylglycerol.

from the intravascular lipoprotein lipase that functions extracellularly. Postprandial fat metabolism is summarized in Figure 6.20.

Metabolism of Triacylglycerol during Fasting

To this point, the discussion has dealt with the role of the liver and adipose tissue in the fed state. In the fasting state, shifts in the metabolic scheme occur in these tissues. For example, as blood glucose levels diminish, insulin concentration falls, accelerating lipolytic activity in adipose tissue. The lipolytic activity produces free fatty acids and glycerol. Free fatty acids derived from adipose tissue circulate in the plasma in association with albumin and are taken up by the liver or muscle cells and oxidized for energy by way of acetyl CoA formation. In the liver, some of the acetyl CoA is diverted to the production of the ketone bodies, which can serve as important energy sources for muscle tissue and the brain during fasting and starvation. The liver continues the synthesis of VLDL and HDL and releases them into circulation, though these processes are diminished in a fasting situation. Glucose derived from liver glycogen and free fatty acids transported to the liver from adipose tissue become the major precursors for the synthesis of endogenous VLDL triacylglycerol. As described previously, this lipoprotein then undergoes catabolism to IDL, transiently, and to LDL by lipoprotein lipase. Most of the plasma HDL is endogenous and is composed mostly of phospholipid and cholesterol, along with apoproteins (chiefly of the A series).

Metabolism of Lipoproteins

Chylomicrons and chylomicron remnants normally are not present in the blood serum during the fasting state. The fasting serum concentration of VLDL is relatively quite low compared with its concentration in postprandial serum because of VLDL's rapid conversion to IDL and LDL. Therefore, the major lipoproteins in fasting serum are LDL (derived from VLDL), HDL (synthesized mainly in the liver), and a very small amount of VLDL. As discussed earlier and summarized in Table 6.4, the apolipoproteins may regulate metabolic reactions within the lipoprotein particles and determine to a great extent how the particles interact with each other and with receptors on specific cells.

Low-Density Lipoprotein (LDL)

The LDL fraction is the major carrier of cholesterol, binding about 60% of the total serum cholesterol. Its function is to transport the cholesterol to tissues, where it may be used for membrane construction or for conversion into other metabolites such as the steroid hormones. LDL interacts with LDL receptors on cells via its apoB, specifically apoB-100, an event that culminates in the removal of the lipoprotein from the circulation. LDL receptors are located on liver cells as well as on cells of tissues peripheral to the liver, but the liver does not effectively remove the LDL from circulation. The distribution of LDL among tissues may depend on its rate of transcapillary transport as well as on the activity of the LDL receptors on cell surfaces. Once bound to the receptor, the receptor and the LDL particle, complete with its lipid cargo, are internalized together by the cell. The particle's component parts are then degraded by lysosomal enzymes in the cell. The LDL receptor is examined in greater detail in the next section. Its discovery in the late 1970s and early 1980s was a significant biochemical event.

The LDL Receptor: Structure and Genetic Aberrations

The discovery of the LDL receptor is credited to Michael S. Brown, M.D., and Joseph L. Goldstein, M.D., who received the 1985 Nobel Prize in Physiology or Medicine. The discovery stemmed from their seeking the molecular basis for the clinical manifestation of hypercholesterolemia, and their research revealed the following facts about LDL and its connection to cholesterol metabolism.

LDL binds to normal fibroblasts (and other cells, particularly the hepatocytes and cells of the adrenal gland and ovarian corpus luteum) with high affinity and specificity. In mutant cells, however, the binding is very inefficient. Although deficient binding of LDL is characteristic of all mutant cells, much variation in binding ability exists among different patients with familial homozygous hypercholesterolemia.

Membrane-bound LDL is internalized by endocytosis made possible by receptors that cluster in coated pits. Figure 6.21 depicts the fate of the LDL particle following its binding to the membrane receptor. The receptor, having released its LDL, returns to the surface of the cell, making a round-trip into and out of the cell every 10 minutes during its 20-hour life span [5]. The dissociated LDL moves into the lysosome, where its protein and cholesteryl ester components are hydrolyzed by lysosomal enzymes into amino acids, FFAs, and free cholesterol. The resulting free cholesterol exerts the following regulatory functions:

- It modulates the activity of two microsomal enzymes, 3-hydroxy-3-methylglutaryl CoA reductase (HMG CoA reductase) and acyl CoA: cholesteryl acyl transferase (ACAT).

Figure 6.21 (a) Sequential steps in endocytosis of LDL leading to synthesis of cholesteryl ester. (b) Effect of cholesteryl ester on HMG CoA reductase, ACAT, and the concentration of LDL receptors in the cell. (Brown M, Goldstein J. Receptor mediated endocytosis: insights from the lipoprotein receptor system. © The Noble Foundation 1986.)

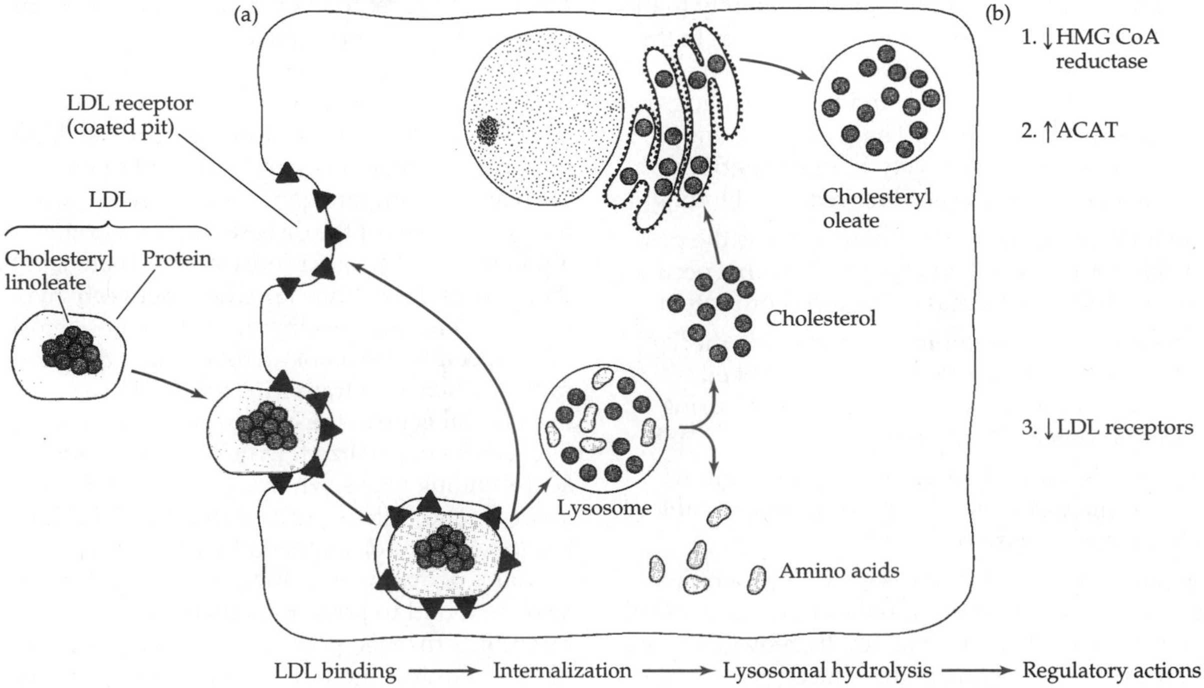

- By lowering the concentration of receptor mRNA, it suppresses synthesis of LDL receptors so as to prevent further entry of LDL into the cell.

Activity of the HMG CoA reductase, the rate-limiting enzyme in cholesterol synthesis, is suppressed through decreased transcription of the reductase gene and the concomitant increased degradation of the enzyme. In contrast, ACAT is activated, promoting formation of cholesteryl esters that can be stored as droplets in the cytoplasm of the cell.

Mutant cells unable to bind and/or internalize LDL efficiently and thus deprived of the cholesterol needed for membrane synthesis must obtain the needed cholesterol via de novo synthesis. In these cells, HMG CoA reductase is activated while ACAT is depressed.

LDL receptors interact with apoB-100, the protein carried on the surface of the LDL. The interaction between the receptors and the apoB-100 is the key to the cell's internalization of the LDL. The number of receptors synthesized by cells varies according to cholesterol requirements.

The LDL receptor has been found to be a transmembrane glycoprotein that, in the course of its synthetic process, undergoes several carbohydrate-processing reactions. The carbohydrate moiety is important for proper functioning of the receptor, and its location on the molecule has been mapped. Five domains of the LDL receptor have been identified.

- Domain 1, which is furthest from the membrane and contains the NH_2 terminal of the receptor protein, is rich in cysteine residues. These residues allow the formation of many disulfide bonds that give stability to the molecule. Many of the other amino acid residues in this cysteine-rich domain have negatively charged side chains. This first domain, then, could be the binding site for apoB-100, with its positively charged lysine and arginine residues. These positively charged residues of apoB-100 are known to be crucial for receptor binding.
- Domain 2, made up of 350 amino acids, is the possible location for the N-linked glycosylation that occurs during the maturation process of the receptor protein.
- Domain 3 is located immediately outside the plasma membrane and is the site of the O-linked glycosylation. This glycosylation, too, occurs during the maturation process of the receptor.
- Domain 4 is made up of 22 hydrophobic amino acids that, because of their affinity for lipids, are able to span the plasma membrane.
- Domain 5, the final domain, is the COOH terminal end of the protein and projects into the cytoplast. This tail enables the receptors to move laterally, thereby mediating the clustering of the receptors in the coated pits.

Along with the delineation of the structure of the normal LDL receptor, knowledge of the structural defects existing in mutants has developed. Although a gene on chromosome 19 encodes the protein of the LDL receptor, the mutations of the gene are not always the same. How the normal functioning of the receptor is affected depends on what particular domain(s) of the receptor have undergone mutation. The term *familial hypercholesterolemia* has been used for a variety of conditions that result in greatly elevated serum cholesterol levels and are due to genetic metabolic defects. These defects can be either homozygous or heterozygous. The defects commonly involve the dysfunction or absence of LDL receptors. Of the 110 familial hypercholesterolemia homozygotes studied, 10 different abnormal forms of the LDL receptors have been identified. These can be divided into four classes:

- class 1, in which no receptors are synthesized;
- class 2, in which precursors of the receptors are synthesized but then are not processed properly and fail to move into the Golgi apparatus;
- class 3, in which the precursors for the LDL receptors are synthesized and processed but the processing is faulty, preventing the receptors from binding LDL normally; and
- class 4, mutations that allow production of receptors that reach the surface of the cell and bind LDL but are unable to cluster in the coated pits.

Maturation of the LDL receptor precursor proteins, like that of other proteins synthesized on the endoplasmic reticulum of the cell, occurs in the cell's Golgi apparatus. There the LDL receptors are targeted for their final destination (Chap. 1). Incomplete or improper processing can prevent the receptor from reaching its proper destination on the plasma membrane.

Relatively few people (1 in 1 million) are homozygous for familial hypercholesterolemia, but many people (1 in 500) carry one mutant gene for the disease. Knowledge of the mechanisms of the disease can be of tremendous benefit in treating the latter individuals. There is little doubt that a causal relationship exists between hypercholesterolemia and the development of atherosclerosis.

Reducing serum cholesterol through drug therapy can cause an increased transcription for LDL receptors by the one normal gene in the heterozygotes, and serum cholesterol can be normalized. Drug therapy includes both bile acid–binding resins, which increase fecal removal of cholesterol, and HMG CoA reductase inhibitors, which reduce cholesterol synthesis in the liver.

Many people who exhibit no clear-cut genetic defect also are found to possess an inadequate number of LDL receptors. In this population group, nutrition could be the environmental factor leading to decreased production of LDL receptors. A diet high in saturated fats and cholesterol appears to be one of the culprits.

The concentration of many cell receptors can be regulated. For example, the number of receptors present in target cells can be decreased if the concentration of an agonist circulating in the blood remains high for an extended period of time. This is referred to as down-regulation.

To summarize the role of the LDL fraction in normal lipid metabolism, it can be thought of as a depositor of cholesterol and other lipids in peripheral cells possessing the LDL receptor. Cells targeted by LDL include the cells of the vascular endothelium. It therefore follows that a high concentration and activity of LDL have implications in the etiology of cardiovascular disease.

High-Density Lipoprotein (HDL)

Opposing LDL's cholesterol-depositing role is the HDL fraction of serum lipoproteins. An important function of HDL is to remove unesterified cholesterol from cells and other lipoproteins where it may have accumulated and return the cholesterol to the liver for excretion in the bile. Two key properties of HDL are necessary for this process to occur.

The first key property is HDL's ability to bind to receptors on both hepatic and extrahepatic cells. Receptors may be specific for HDL, but they also include the LDL receptor to which HDL can bind via its apoE component. In other words, the LDL receptor recognizes both apoE and apoB-100 and consequently is referred to as the apoB,E receptor. The implication is that HDL can compete with LDL at its receptor site.

The second key property of HDL is mediated through its apoA-1 component, which stimulates the activity of the enzyme lecithin : cholesterol acyltransferase (LCAT). This enzyme forms cholesteryl esters from free cholesterol by catalyzing the transfer of fatty acids from the C-2 position of phosphatidylcholine to free cholesterol. The free cholesterol (recipient) substrate is derived from the plasma membrane of cells or surfaces of other lipoproteins. Cholesteryl esters resulting from this reaction can then exchange readily among plasma lipoproteins, mediated by a transfer protein called cholesteryl ester transfer protein (CETP). LCAT, by taking up free cholesterol and producing its ester form, thus promotes the net transfer of cholesterol out of nonhepatic cells and other lipoproteins. Cholesteryl esters can then be transported directly to the liver in association with HDL or indirectly by LDL, following CETP transfer from HDL to LDL. Recall that either lipoprotein can bind to LDL (apoB,E) receptors.

Following their deposition in the liver cells, the esters are hydrolyzed by cholesteryl esterase, and the free cholesterol is excreted in the bile as bile salt (Fig. 6.8). This is the major route of cholesterol excretion from the body.

The net effect of these properties of HDL is the retrieval of cholesterol from peripheral cells and other lipoproteins and its return, as cholesteryl ester, to the liver. The process is referred to as reverse cholesterol transport. Its benefit to the cardiovascular system is that by reducing the amount of deposited cholesterol in the vascular endothelium, it also reduces the risk of fatty plaque formation and atherosclerosis. This delivery of cholesteryl esters to the liver presumably explains the correlation of high HDL levels with reduced risk of cardiovascular disease, a topic reviewed in the next section.

LIPIDS, LIPOPROTEINS, AND CARDIOVASCULAR DISEASE RISK

Atherosclerosis is a degenerative disease of vascular endothelium. The principal players in the atherogenic process are cells of the immune system and lipid material, primarily cholesterol and cholesteryl esters. An early response to arterial endothelial cell injury is an increased adherence of monocytes and T lymphocytes to the area of the injury. **Cytokines,** protein products of the monocytes and lymphocytes, mediate the atherogenic process by their chemotactic attraction of phagocytic cells to the area.

Additional exposure to a high level of circulating LDL and the deposition and oxidative modification of cholesteryl esters further promote the inflammatory process. The process is marked by the uptake of LDL by phagocytic cells that become engorged with lipid, called foam cells. Phagocytic uptake is accelerated if the apoB component of the LDL is modified by oxidation. Lipid material in the form of foam cells may then infiltrate the endothelium. As lipid accumulates, the lumen of the blood vessel involved is progressively occluded. The deposited lipid, known to be derived from blood-borne lipids, is called fatty plaque. The pathophysiology of atherosclerosis has been reviewed [6] and is the subject of this chapter's first perspective.

Ever since it was discovered that plaque composition is chiefly lipid, an enormous research effort has been undertaken to investigate the possible link between dietary lipid and the development of atherosclerosis. The existence of such a link has come to be known as the lipid hypothesis, which maintains that dietary lipid intake can alter blood lipid levels, which in turn initiate or exacerbate atherogenesis. Following is a brief account of the alleged involvement of certain dietary lipids and fatty acids and of genetically acquired apolipoproteins in atherogenesis.

Cholesterol

At center stage in the lipid hypothesis controversy is cholesterol. The effects of dietary interventions designed to improve serum lipid profiles are generally measured by the extent to which the interventions raise or lower serum cholesterol. There is some justification for this reasoning in that cholesterol is a major component of atherogenic fatty plaque and many studies have linked cardiovascular disease risk to chronically elevated serum cholesterol levels. Receiving the greatest attention, however, is not so much the change in total cholesterol concentration but how the cholesterol is distributed between its two major transport lipoproteins, LDL and HDL. Because it is commonly and conveniently quantified in clinical laboratories, cholesterol assays can be used to establish LDL:HDL ratios by measuring the amount of cholesterol in each of the two fractions. Assayed cholesterol associated with the LDL fraction is designated LDLC by laboratory analysts, and cholesterol transported in the HDL fraction is designated HDLC.

Because in the interest of wellness it is desirable to maintain relatively low serum levels of LDL and relatively high levels of HDL (a low LDL : HDL ratio), the concept of "good" and "bad" cholesterol emerged. The "good" form is that associated with HDL, and the "bad" form is transported as LDL. It is important to understand, however, that the cholesterol per se is not "good" or "bad"; rather, it serves as a proxy for the relative concentrations of LDL and HDL, ratios of which can indeed be good or bad. LDL : HDL ratios are, in fact, determined more reliably by measurements other than cholesterol content. For example, immunological methods for quantifying apoB (the major LDL apoprotein) and apoA (the primary HDL apoprotein) are now widely used. Ratios of apoA to apoB then serve as an indicator of cardiovascular disease risk, with risk increasing as the ratio decreases.

Among the reasons for cholesterol's "bad press" as it is considered in connection with cardiovascular disease is the fact that cholesterol and especially cholesteryl esters are major components of fatty plaque. Contrary to widespread belief, changing the amount of cholesterol in the diet has only a minor influence on blood cholesterol concentration in most people. This is because compensatory mechanisms are engaged, such as HDL activity in scavenging excess cholesterol and the down-regulation of cholesterol synthesis by dietary cholesterol (discussed in the section "Synthesis of Cholesterol"). It is well known, however, that certain individuals respond strongly, and others weakly, to dietary cholesterol (hyper- and hyporesponders). This phenomenon, which may have a genetic basis, is further complicated by the observation that significant within-person variability exists independent of diet, a fact that clearly confounds the results of intersubject studies.

Several mechanisms may be considered when trying to account for differences in individual responses to dietary cholesterol, including

- differences in absorption or biosynthesis,
- differences in the formation of LDL and its receptor-mediated clearance, and
- differences in its rates of removal and excretion.

These considerations have been extensively reviewed [7].

Saturated and Unsaturated Fatty Acids

Research dealing with the influence of various kinds of fatty acids on cardiovascular disease risk has focused on the effect that each kind has on serum cholesterol levels. The literature dealing with the effect of dietary fats containing primarily saturated fatty acids (SFAs), monounsaturated fatty acids (MUFAs), polyunsaturated fatty acids (PUFAs), or *trans* fatty acids is as extensive as that related to the consuming of cholesterol itself. Early research results generally led to the conclusion that SFAs are hypercholesterolemic and PUFAs are hypocholesterolemic. Furthermore, it was assumed that MUFAs were neutral in this regard, neither increasing nor lowering serum cholesterol.

Current research focuses not so much on total cholesterol effects but rather on how LDLC : HDLC ratios are shifted by the test lipids. For example, studies have shown diets rich in MUFA to be as effective as PUFA-rich diets in lowering LDL cholesterol and triacylglycerols without significant change in HDL [8,9]. There has also been interest in how the position of the double bonds in PUFA (n-3 vs. n-6 species), as well as their *cis/trans* isomerism, relates to lipoprotein ratio effects. The effect of *trans* fats is discussed in the next section.

The understanding of the role of dietary intake of lipids in cardiovascular disease risk has changed over time [10,11]. Consumption of the following lipids shows a *positive* correlation with the risk of cardiovascular disease (CVD), primarily due to a hypercholesterolemic effect or to unfavorable shifts in LDLC : HDLC ratios:

- total fat,
- saturated fatty acids,
- cholesterol, and
- *trans* fat.

Consumption of the following lipids shows a *negative* correlation with CVD risk, primarily due to a hypocholesterolemic effect or to favorable shifts in LDL : HDL ratios:

- Monounsaturated fatty acids (provided adjustments are made for coconsumed cholesterol and saturated fatty acids).
- Polyunsaturated fatty acids (if adjusted for cholesterol and saturated fatty acids). Both n-3 and n-6 types are effective. The linoleic acid (18:2 n-6) content in adipose tissue was found to be inversely associated with CVD risk. The greater the content of 18:2 n-6, the lower the risk for CVD.
- n-3 fatty acids. The n-3 PUFAs exert antiatherogenic properties by various mechanisms, including the following:
  - Interference with platelet aggregation, due in part to inhibition of thromboxane (TXA_2) production. This is thought to be caused by displacement of the TXA_2 precursor, arachidonic acid, from platelet phospholipid stores by the fatty acids. Eicosapentaenoic acid (EPA; 20:5 n-3), docosahexaenoic acid (DHA; 20:6 n-3), and α-linolenic acid (18:3 n-3) exerted similar antiaggregatory effects [11].
  - Reduction in the release of proinflammatory cytokines from cells involved in fatty plaque formation (see this chapter's perspective "The Role of Lipids and Lipoprotein in Atherogenesis").
  - Sharp reduction (25%–30%) in serum triacylglycerol concentration. α-linoleate was less effective than EPA or DHA, and plant n-3 fatty acids were generally less effective than marine n-3 fatty acids in their capacity to reduce triacylglycerols [12,13].

The potential risk of CVD is actually more complicated than what is implied by listing positive and negative correlates. It involves a combination of dietary factors along with exercise and other life-style determinants and genetics. For instance, there is heterogeneity in the cholesterolemic response to individual fatty acids even within a fatty acid class. This is particularly true among the long-chain saturated fatty acids. Strong evidence indicates that lauric (12:0), myristic (14:0), and palmitic (16:0) acids are all hypercholesterolemic, specifically raising LDLC, with myristic acid (14:0) being the most potent in this respect. On the other hand, stearic acid (18:0), neutral in its effect, in fact is reputed to lower total cholesterol and LDLC relative to carbohydrate. Therefore, stearic acid should not be grouped with shorter-chain SFAs with respect to LDLC effects. Oleic acid (18:1) and linoleic acid (18:2 n-6) are hypocholesterolemic compared to 12:0 and 16:0 fatty acids. Linoleate (18:2 n-6) is the more potent of the two, independently lowering total and LDL cholesterol [14].

Despite years of investigation, the mechanism by which hypercholesterolemic fatty acids exert their effects has not been conclusively defined. However, they have been alleged to operate in one or more of the following ways:

- by suppressing the excretion of bile acids, thereby lowering lipid absorption;
- by enhancing the synthesis of cholesterol and LDL, either by reducing the degree of control exerted on the regulatory enzyme HMG CoA reductase or by affecting apoB synthesis;
- by retarding LCAT activity or receptor-mediated uptake of LDL; or
- by acting as regulators of gene expression.

Trans Fatty Acids

Double-bonded carbon atoms can exist in either a *cis* or a *trans* orientation, as described on page 129. Most natural fats and oils contain only *cis* double bonds. The much smaller number of naturally occurring *trans* fats are found mostly in the fats of ruminants, for example, in milk fat, which contains 4% to 8% *trans* fatty acids. Much larger amounts are found in certain margarines and margarine-based products, shortenings, and frying fats as a product of the partial hydrogenation of PUFA. The process of hydrogenation imparts to the product a higher degree of hardness (remaining solid at room temperature) and plasticity (spreadability), which is more desirable to both the consumer and the food manufacturer. In the process, however, as hydrogen atoms are catalytically added across double bonds, electronic shifts take place that cause remaining, unhydrogenated *cis* double bonds to revert to a *trans* configuration that is energetically stabler.

The most abundant *trans* fatty acids in the diet are elaidic acid (Fig. 6.1) and its isomers, which are of an 18:1 structure. It has been reported that diets rich in these fatty acids are as hypercholesterolemic as saturated fatty acids [15]. In fact, serum lipid profiles following feeding of a diet high in *trans* fatty acids may be even more unfavorable than saturated fatty acids because not only are total cholesterol and LDL cholesterol levels elevated, but HDL cholesterol level is lowered. The study cited was criticized for using *trans* elaidic acids obtained by a process not typical of the hydrogenation of margarines and shortenings and also for including uncharacteristically large dietary amounts of the *trans* fatty acids in the study diet. However, reports from subsequent studies confirm that *trans* fat consumption elevates serum LDLC while decreasing HDLC and also raises total cholesterol : HDLC ratios [16]. Another confirmatory investigation, conducted on a large group of healthy women over an 8-year period, matched *trans* fat intake with the incidence of nonfatal myocardial infarction or death from coronary heart disease [17]. Although the study indicated a positive correlation between *trans* fat intake and coronary heart disease, it was not free of criticism due to the fact that the data were obtained by consumer questionnaires rather than by a randomized control study, in which intake could be precisely monitored by researchers [18]. Furthermore, there was a high degree of variability of *trans* fatty acids in the foods consumed by the subjects, and a clear-cut dose-response relationship could not be demonstrated [19].

Some reports exonerate *trans* fat in regard to its alleged hypercholesterolemic properties. In a randomized crossover study involving hypercholesterolemic subjects, the replacement of butter with margarine in a low-fat diet actually lowered LDLC and apolipoprotein B by 10%, while HDLC and apolipoprotein A levels were unaffected [20].

Current guidelines issued by the Institute of Medicine of the National Academy recommend keeping the intake of *trans* fatty acids as low as is reasonable. Reducing *trans* fatty acid intake to zero is impossible, because *trans* fats occur naturally. Labeling requirements for *trans* fatty acids will make the consumer more aware of foods that contain them. The adverse findings on *trans* fats represent an about-face from the long-standing nutrition dogma that unsaturated fats are invariably preferred over saturated fats.

Lipoprotein a

In the 1960s, a genetic variant of LDL was discovered in human serum. The particle differs from normal LDL in that it is attached to a unique marker protein of high molecular weight (513,000 D). The marker protein is currently referred to as apolipoprotein a, or apo(a), and the complete lipoprotein particle is called lipoprotein a, or Lp(a).

At the time of the discovery of Lp(a), it was evident that not all people had the lipoprotein in their serum. Also, in many of those who did, its concentration was very low compared with other lipoproteins. Consequently, it was dismissed as having little importance. However, interest in Lp(a) was renewed during the following two decades, when numerous studies suggested a positive correlation between Lp(a) concentration and atherosclerotic disease.

Structurally, Lp(a) is assembled from LDL and the apo(a) protein. The LDL component of the complex possesses apoB-100 as its only protein component. Linkage of the LDL portion of the particle to apo(a) is through a disulfide bond connecting the two proteins apo(a) and apoB-100. A strong structural homology (similar amino acid sequence) has recently been discovered between apo(a) and plasminogen. Plasminogen is the inactive precursor of the enzyme plasmin, which dissolves blood clots by its hydrolytic action on fibrin. This discovery has stimulated extensive research into the genetics, metabolism, function, and clinical significance of Lp(a).

The physiological function of Lp(a) is not yet defined with certainty, although it is tempting to speculate that its role may be linked to the two functional systems from which the particle was derived: a lipid transport system and the blood-clotting system. It has been proposed that Lp(a) may bind to fibrin clots via its plasminogen-like apo(a) and therefore may deliver cholesterol to regions of recent injury and wound healing.

Reviews of Lp(a) cite numerous epidemiological studies [21] that show a positive correlation between Lp(a) concentration and premature myocardial infarction, a blocking of blood vessels in the heart due to clot formation. This finding has led to the conclusion that Lp(a) may represent an independent genetic risk for atherosclerotic disease. Unfortunately, blood levels of the lipoprotein do not respond to dietary intervention and respond only very weakly to lipid-lowering drugs. One of the many open questions is whether Lp(a) is linked to atherogenesis over an extended period of time because of its lipoprotein properties or instead plays a role in the sudden development of a clot due to the binding of its plasminogen-like apo(a) component to fibrin. Perhaps both mechanisms apply.

Apolipoprotein E

Recall that the term *apolipoprotein* refers to the protein moiety of a lipoprotein. Studies have shown that one apolipoprotein, apolipoprotein E (apoE), may have a role in the etiology of atherogenesis. As shown in Table 6.4, apoE is a structural component of VLDL, HDL, chylomicrons, and chylomicron remnants. The most important physiological function of apoE is that it is the component recognized by the LDL receptor-related protein (also referred to as the postulated apoE receptor) and the LDL receptor (Fig. 6.21). By way of interaction with these receptors, apoE mediates the uptake of apoE-possessing lipoproteins into the liver.

ApoE exists in three isoforms: E2, E3, and E4. They are genetically encoded by three alleles, E2, E3, and E4, respectively. A single individual inherits one allele from each parent and therefore will become one of the following six possible phenotypes: E2,2; E3,2; E3,3; E3,4; E4,2; E4,4. The effects of apoE polymorphism on plasma lipids and a predisposition to cardiovascular disease have been well studied [22]. There is evidence that E4 phenotypes have an increased risk of developing cardiovascular disease, apparently due to elevation of the LDL serum level. The apoE phenotype alone is associated with a stepwise increase in LDLC (cholesterol that is contained within the LDL fraction). LDLC increased in the order of phenotypes E3,2 < E3,3 < E4,3. This relationship is independent of the ratio of polyunsaturated to saturated fats consumed [23].

Based on the link between the E4 allele and a predisposition to cardiovascular disease, the allele is considered to be a predictor of latent atherogenesis. A longitudinal study of elderly men conducted over a 5-year period revealed a doubling of the frequency of the E4 allele among those who died of coronary heart disease during the study period [24].

INTEGRATED METABOLISM IN TISSUES

Catabolism of Triacylglycerols and Fatty Acids

The complete hydrolysis of triacylglycerols yields glycerol and three fatty acids. In the body, this occurs largely through the activity of lipoprotein lipase of vascular endothelium and through an intracellular lipase that is active in the liver and particularly active in adipose tissue. The glycerol portion can be used for energy by the liver and by other tissues having activity of the enzyme glycerokinase, through which glycerol is converted to glycerol phosphate. Glycerol phosphate can enter the glycolytic pathway at the level of dihydroxyacetone phosphate, from which point either energy oxidation or gluconeogenesis can occur (review Fig. 4.14).

Fatty acids are a very rich source of energy, and on an equal-weight basis they surpass carbohydrates in this property. This is because fatty acids exist in a more reduced state than that of carbohydrate and therefore undergo a greater extent of oxidation en route to CO_2 and H_2O. Many tissues are capable of oxidizing fatty acids by way of a mechanism called β-oxidation, described below. On entry into the cell of the metabolizing tissue, the fatty acid is first activated by coenzyme A, an energy-requiring reaction catalyzed by cytoplasmic fatty acyl CoA synthetase (see Fig. 6.22). The reaction actually consumes the equivalent of two ATPs, because the pyrophosphate must also be hydrolyzed to ensure irreversibility of the reaction.

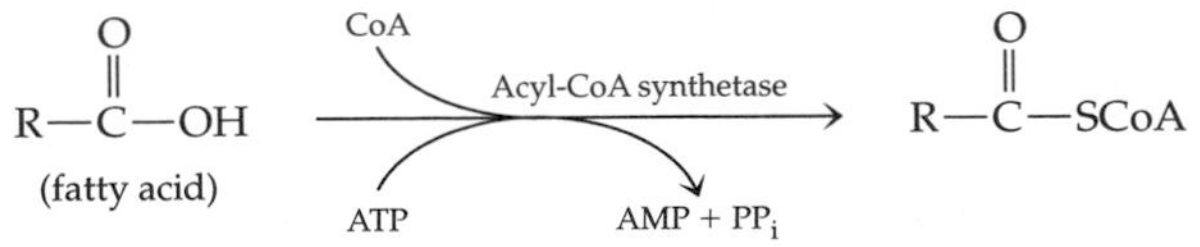

Figure 6.22 Activation of fatty acid by coenzyme A.

Mitochondrial Transfer of Acyl CoA

The oxidation of fatty acids occurs within the mitochondrion. Long-chain fatty acids and their CoA derivatives are incapable of crossing the inner mitochondrial membrane (but can cross the permeable outer membrane), necessitating a membrane transport system. The carrier molecule for this system is carnitine (Chap. 9), which can be synthesized in humans from lysine and methionine and is found in high concentration in muscle. The activated fatty acid is joined covalently to carnitine at the cytoplasmic side of the mitochondrial membrane by the transferase enzyme carnitine acyltransferase I (CAT I). A second transferase, acyltransferase II (CAT II), located on the inner face of the inner membrane, releases the fatty acyl CoA and carnitine into the matrix (see Fig. 6.23).

β-Oxidation of Fatty Acids

The oxidation of the activated fatty acid in the mitochondrion occurs via a cyclic degradative pathway by which two-carbon units in the form of acetyl CoA are cleaved one by one from the carboxyl end. The reactions of β-oxidation are summarized in Figure 6.24 and discussed in the following list.

1. The formation of a double bond between the α- and β-carbons, catalyzed by acyl CoA dehydrogenase. There are four such dehydrogenases, each specific to a range

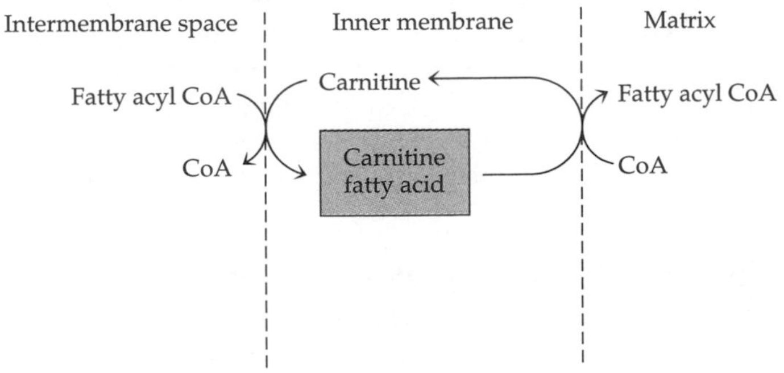

Figure 6.23 Membrane transport system for transporting fatty acyl CoA across the inner mitochondrial membrane.

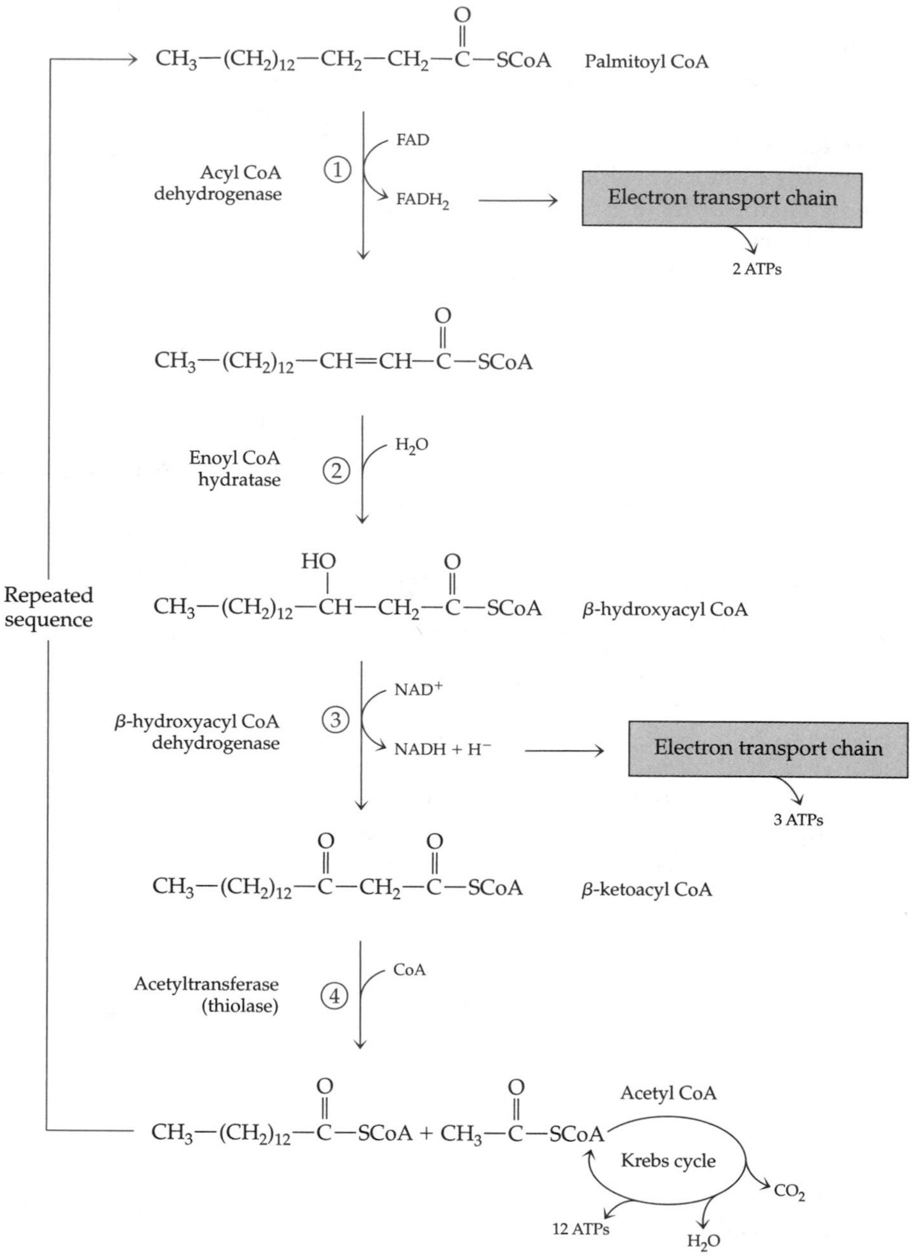

Figure 6.24 The mitochondrial β-oxidation of an activated fatty acid using palmitate as an example. The yield of ATPs from the oxidation of each acetyl group is indicated. The name of the enzyme catalyzing each reaction is written to the left of each reaction arrow.

of chain lengths. The $FADH_2$ yields its two hydrogens to CoQ and therefore feeds two electrons into the electron transport system (ETS), which, it will be recalled, is also compartmentalized in the mitochondrion. The ETS oxidation of $FADH_2$ yields two ATPs.

2. The unsaturated acyl CoA accepts a molecule of water, a reaction catalyzed by enoyl CoA hydratase, sometimes called crotonase.

3. The β-hydroxy group is oxidized to the ketone by the NAD^+-requiring enzyme β-hydroxyacyl CoA dehydrogenase. The ETS oxidation of the NADH leads to the formation of three ATPs.

4. The β-ketoacyl CoA is cleaved by acyltransferase (also called thiolase), resulting in the insertion of CoA and cleavage at the β-carbon. The products of this reaction are acetyl CoA and a saturated CoA-activated fatty acid having two fewer carbons than the original fatty acid. This reaction completes one cycle of the degradative pathway. The entire sequence of reactions is repeated, with two carbons being removed with each cycle.

Energy Considerations in Fatty Acid Oxidation

The activation of a fatty acid requires two high-energy bonds per mole of fatty acid oxidized. Each cleavage of a saturated carbon-carbon bond yields five ATPs, two by oxidation of $FADH_2$ and three by oxidation of NADH via oxidative phosphorylation. The acetyl CoAs produced are oxidized to CO_2 and water in the Krebs cycle, and for each acetyl CoA oxidized, 12 ATPs (or their equivalent) are produced (Chap. 4). Using the example of palmitate (16 carbons), we can summarize the yield of ATP as follows:

7 carbon-carbon cleavages	$7 \times 5 = 35$
8 acetyl CoAs oxidized	$8 \times 12 = 96$
Total ATPs produced	131
2 ATPs for activation	−2
Net ATPs	129

Nearly one-half of dietary and body fatty acids, however, are unsaturated and therefore must provide a considerable portion of lipid-derived energy. They are catabolized by β-oxidation in the mitochondrion in nearly identical fashion as their saturated counterparts, except that one fatty acyl CoA dehydrogenase reaction is not required for each double bond present. This is because the double bond introduced into the saturated fatty acid by the reaction occurs naturally in unsaturated fatty acids. However, the specificity of the enoyl CoA hydratase reaction requires that the double bond be between the second and third carbon in order for the hydration to take place, and the "natural" double bond may not occupy the Δ^2 position. For example, after three cycles of β-carbon oxidation, the position of the double bond in what was originally a Δ^9 monounsaturated fatty acid will occupy a Δ^3 position. Figure 6.25 shows 18:1 Δ^9 undergoing three cycles of β-oxidation. At the end of the third cycle, the fatty acid is a Δ^3 fatty acid. The presence of a specific enoyl CoA transisomerase then shifts the double bond from Δ^3 to Δ^2, allowing the hydrase and subsequent reactions to proceed. The oxidation of an unsaturated fatty acid results in somewhat less energy production than oxidation of a saturated fatty acid of the same chain length, because for each double bond present one $FADH_2$-producing fatty acyl CoA dehydrogenase reaction is bypassed, resulting in two fewer ATPs.

Although most fatty acids metabolized are composed of an even number of carbon atoms, small amounts of fatty acids having an odd number of carbon atoms are also used for energy. β-oxidation occurs as described, with the liberation of acetyl CoA until a residual propionyl CoA remains. The subsequent oxidation of propionyl CoA requires reactions that use the vitamins biotin and B_{12} in a coenzymatic role (see Fig. 6.26). Because the succinyl CoA formed in the course of these reactions can be converted into glucose, the odd-numbered carbon fatty acids are uniquely glucogenic among all the fatty acids.

Formation of the Ketone Bodies

In addition to its direct oxidation via the Krebs cycle, acetyl CoA may follow other catabolic routes in the liver, one of which is the pathway by which the so-called **ketone bodies** (acetoacetate, β-hydroxybutyrate, and acetone) are formed. Acetoacetate and β-hydroxybutyrate are not oxidized further in the liver but instead are transported by the blood to peripheral tissues, where they can be converted back to acetyl CoA and oxidized via the Krebs cycle. The steps in ketone body formation occur as shown in Figure 6.27. The reversibility of the β-hydroxybutyrate dehydrogenase reaction, together with enzymes present in extrahepatic tissues that convert acetoacetate to acetyl CoA (shown by broken arrows in Fig. 6.27), reveals how the ketone bodies can serve as a source of fuel in these tissues.

Ketone body formation is actually an "overflow" pathway for acetyl CoA use, providing another way for the liver to distribute fuel to peripheral cells. Normally, the concentration of the ketone bodies in the blood is very low, but it may reach very high levels in situations of accelerated fatty acid oxidation combined with low carbohydrate intake or impaired carbohydrate use.

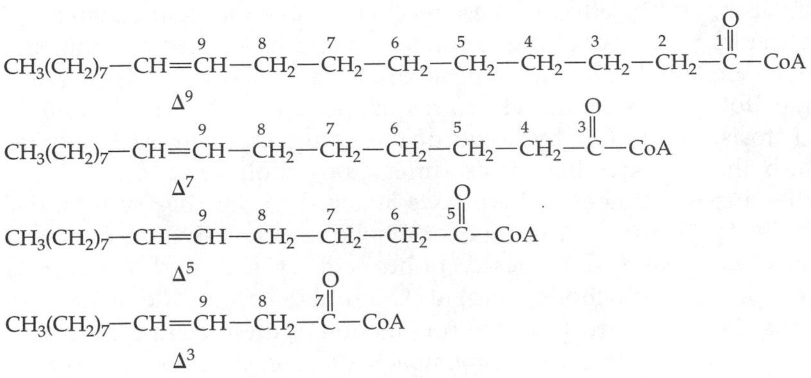

Figure 6.25 Sequential β-oxidation of oleic acid, showing the location of the double bond using the Δ nomenclature system. Numbers above the carbons represent the original carbon numbers of oleic acid.

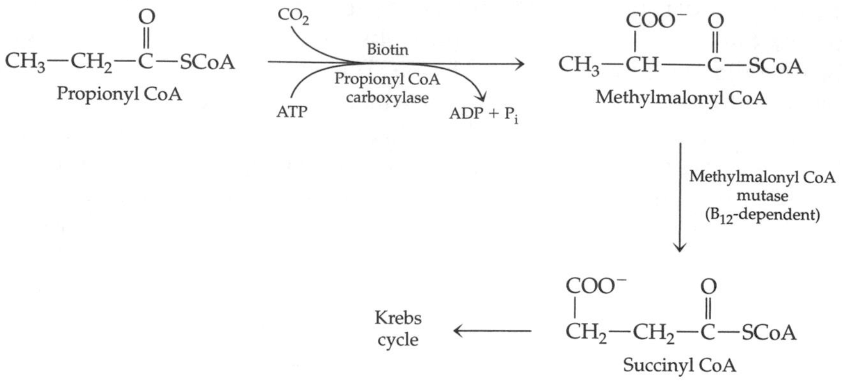

Figure 6.26 Oxidation of propionyl CoA.

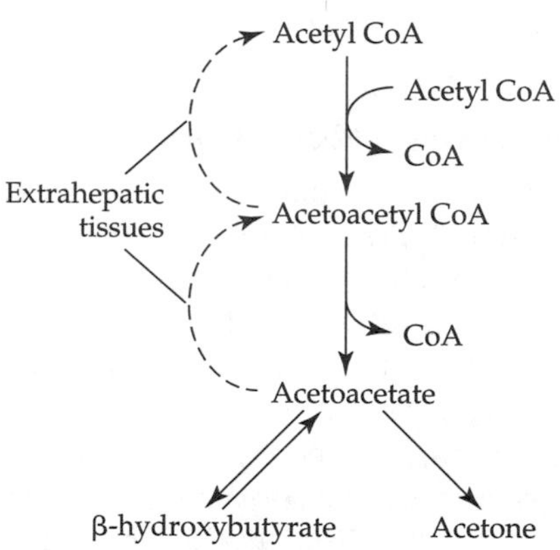

Figure 6.27 Steps in ketone body formation.

Such a situation would occur in diabetes mellitus, starvation, or simply a very low carbohydrate diet. Recall that it was pointed out in Chapter 4 that for the Krebs cycle to function there must be an adequate supply of four-carbon units. These are formed mainly from pyruvate (formed during glycolysis). Without the oxidation of glucose, there is an inadequate supply of carbohydrate and thus a reduced pool of oxaloacetate, with which the acetyl CoA would normally combine for oxidation in the Krebs cycle. As carbohydrate use is diminished, oxidation of fatty acids accelerates to provide energy through the production of Krebs cycle substrates (acetyl CoA). This shift to fat catabolism, coupled with reduced oxaloacetate availability, results in an accumulation of acetyl CoA. As would be expected, a sharp increase in ketone body formation follows, resulting in the condition known as ketosis. Ketosis can be dangerous in that it can disturb the body's acid-base balance (two of the ketone bodies are, in fact, organic acids). However, the liver's ability to deliver ketone bodies to peripheral tissues such as the brain and muscle is an important mechanism for providing fuel in periods of starvation. In short, it is the lesser of two evils.

Catabolism of Cholesterol

Unlike the triacylglycerols and fatty acids, cholesterol is not an energy-producing nutrient. Its four-ring core structure remains intact in the course of its catabolism and is eliminated as such through the biliary system, as described in detail in Chapter 2. Cholesterol, primarily in the form of its ester, is delivered to the liver chiefly in the form of chylomicron remnants, as well as in the form of LDL and HDL. The cholesterol that is destined for excretion either is hydrolyzed by esterases to the free form, which is secreted directly into the bile canaliculi, or is first converted into bile acids prior to entering the bile. It is estimated that neutral sterol, most of which is cholesterol, represents about 55% and bile acids (salts) 45% of total sterol excreted.

The key metabolic changes in the cholesterol-to-bile acid transformation are

- reduction in the length of the hydrocarbon side chain at C-17,
- addition of a carboxylic acid group on the shortened chain, and
- addition of hydroxyl groups to the ring system of the molecule.

The effect of these reactions is to enhance the water solubility of the sterol, facilitating its excretion in the bile. Cholic acid, whose structure is shown in Figure 6.8, has hydroxyl groups at C-7 and C-12 in addition to the C-3 hydroxyl of the native cholesterol. The other major bile acids differ from cholic acid only in the number of hydroxyls attached to the ring system. For example, chenodeoxycholic acid has hydroxyls at C-3 and C-7, deoxycholic acid at C-3 and C-12, and lithocholic acid at C-3 only. Other bile acids are formed from the conjugation of these compounds with glycine or taurine, which attaches through the carboxyl group of the steroid. These reactions are shown in Figure 2.13.

It has already been pointed out that the enterohepatic circulation can return absorbed bile salts to the liver. Bile salts returning to the liver from the intestine repress the formation of an enzyme catalyzing the rate-limiting step in the conversion of cholesterol into bile acids. If the bile salts are prevented from returning to the liver, the activity of this enzyme increases, stimulating the conversion of cholesterol to bile acids and leading to their excretion. The removal of bile salts is exploited therapeutically in the treatment of hypercholesterolemia by the use of unabsorbable, cationic resins that bind bile salts in the intestinal lumen and prevent their return to the liver.

Synthesis of Fatty Acids

Aside from linoleic acid and α-linolenic acid, which are essential and must be acquired from the diet, the body is capable of synthesizing fatty acids from simple precursors. The basic process involves the sequential assembly of a "starter" molecule of acetyl CoA with units of malonyl CoA, the CoA derivative of malonic acid. Ultimately, however, all the carbons of a fatty acid are contributed by acetyl CoA, because malonyl CoA is formed from acetyl CoA and CO_2. This reaction occurs in the cytoplasm. It is catalyzed by acetyl CoA carboxylase, a complex enzyme containing biotin as its prosthetic group. The role of biotin in **carboxylation reactions** (such as this one), which involve the incorporation of a carboxyl group into a compound, is discussed in Chapter 9. ATP furnishes the driving force to attach the new carboxyl group to acetyl CoA (see Fig. 6.28).

Nearly all the acetyl CoA formed in metabolism occurs in the mitochondria. It is formed there from pyruvate oxidation, from the oxidation of fatty acids, and from the degradation of the carbon skeletons of some amino acids (Chap. 7). The synthesis of fatty acids is localized in the cytoplast, but acetyl CoA as such is not able to pass through the mitochondrial membrane. The major mechanism for the transfer of acetyl CoA to the cytoplast is by way of its passage across the mitochondrial membrane in the form of citrate. In the cytoplast, citrate lyase converts the citrate to oxaloacetate and acetyl CoA. This reaction, shown here, is essentially the reversal of the citrate

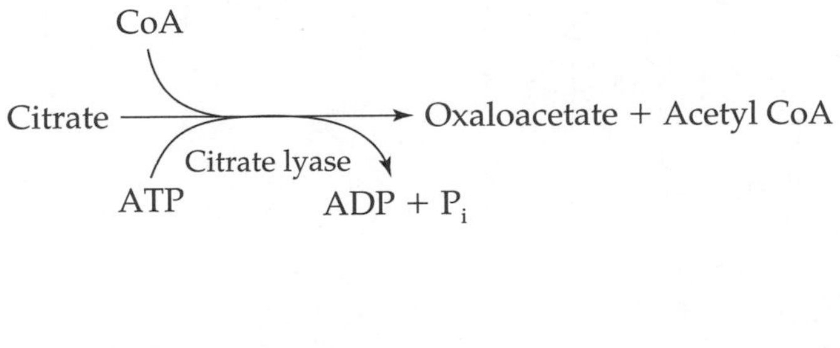

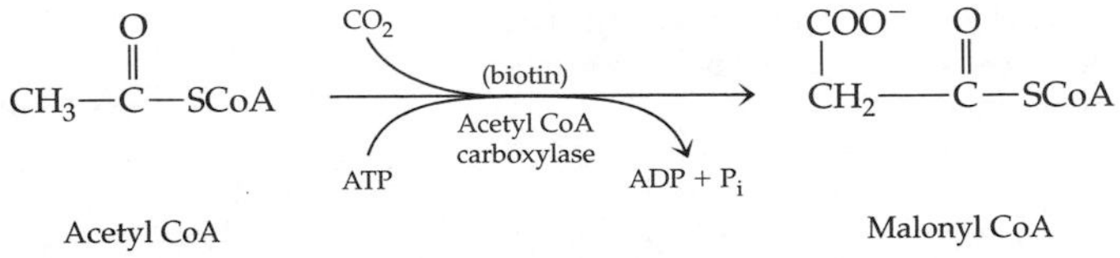

Figure 6.28 Formation of malonyl CoA from acetyl CoA and CO_2 (carboxylation reaction).

synthetase reaction of the Krebs cycle, except that it requires expenditure of ATP.

The enzymes involved in fatty acid synthesis are arranged in a complex called the fatty acid synthase system. Key components of this complex are the acyl carrier protein (ACP) and the condensing enzyme (CE), both of which possess free –SH groups to which the acetyl CoA and malonyl CoA building blocks attach. ACP is structurally similar to CoA (Fig. 9.21). Both possess a 4′-phosphopantetheine component (pantothenic acid coupled through β-alanine to thioethanolamine) and phosphate. The thioethanolamine contributes the free –SH group to the complex. The free –SH of the condensing enzyme is contributed by the amino acid cysteine.

Before the actual steps in the elongation of the fatty acid chain can begin, the two sulfhydryl groups must be "loaded" correctly with malonyl and acetyl groups. Acetyl CoA is transferred to ACP, with the loss of CoA, to form acetyl ACP. The acetyl group is then transferred again to the –SH of the condensing enzyme, leaving available the ACP–SH, to which malonyl CoA attaches, again with the loss of CoA. This loading of the complex can be represented as in Figure 6.29.

The extension of the fatty acid chain then proceeds through the following sequential steps, which also are shown schematically in Figure 6.30. The enzymes catalyzing these reactions are also part of the fatty acid synthase complex along with ACP and CE.

1. In the condensation reaction, the carbonyl carbon of the acetyl group is coupled to C-2 of malonyl ACP with the elimination of the malonyl carboxyl group as CO_2. The reaction is catalyzed by β-ketoacyl-ACP synthase.

2. The β-ketone is reduced, with NADPH serving as hydrogen donor. The reduction is catalyzed by β-ketoacyl-ACP reductase.

3. The alcohol is dehydrated, yielding a double bond. The reaction is catalyzed by β-hydroxyacyl-ACP dehydratase.

4. The double bond is reduced to butyryl-ACP, again with NADPH acting as reducing agent. Enoyl-ACP reductase catalyzes the reaction.

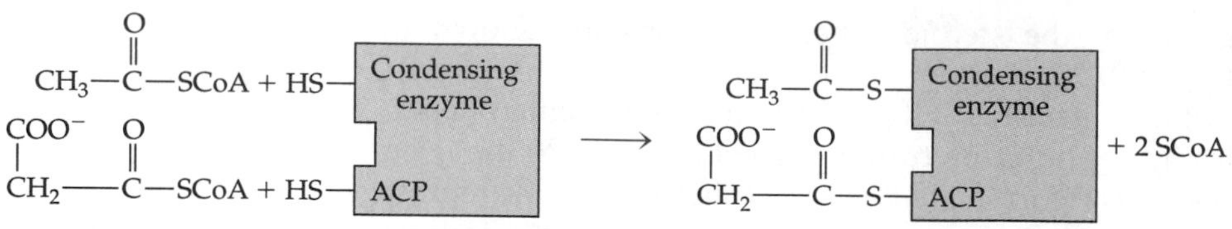

Figure 6.29 "Loading" of sulfhydryl groups into the fatty acid synthase system.

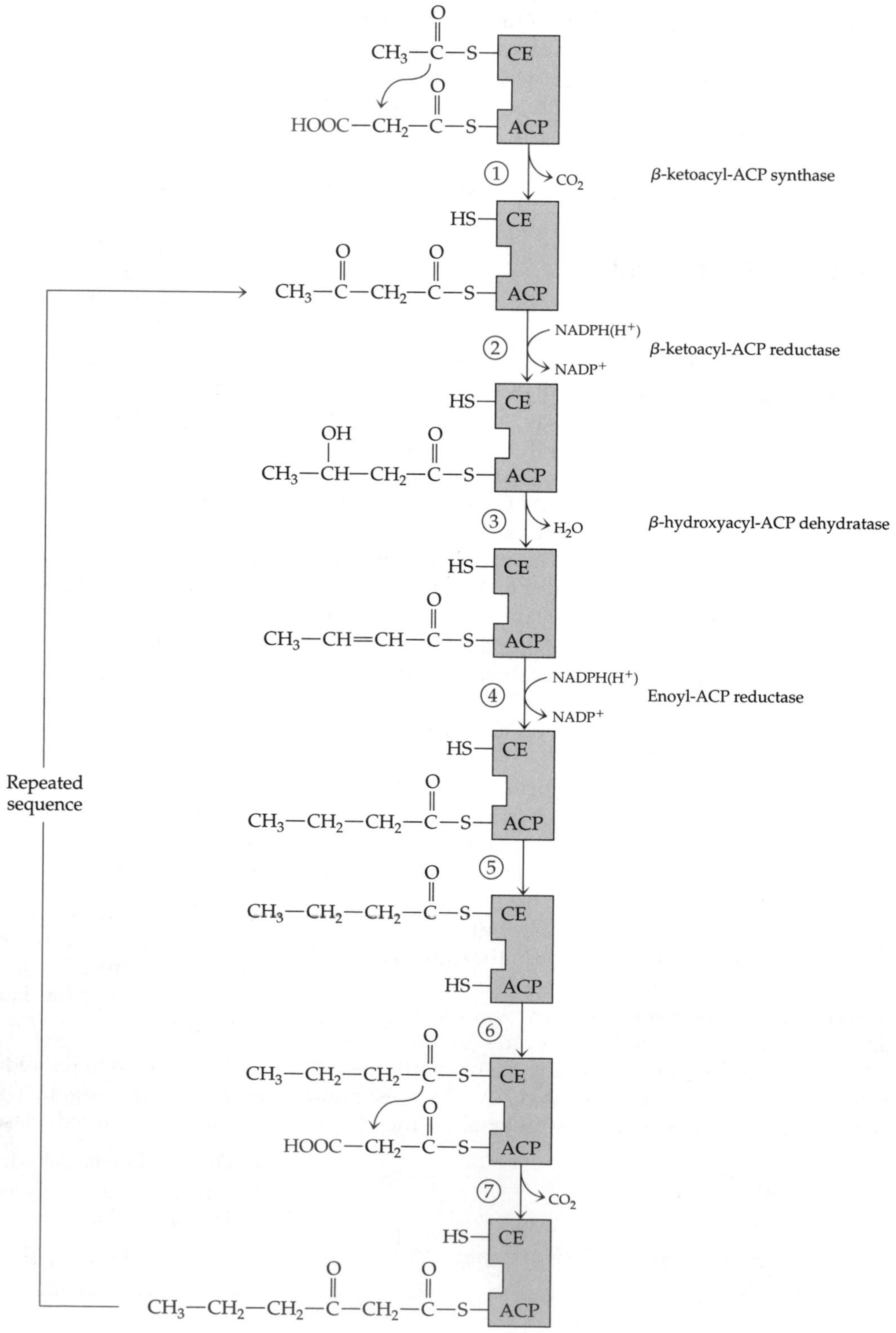

Figure 6.30 The steps in the synthesis of fatty acid. CE (condensing enzyme) and ACP (acyl carrier protein) are members of a complex of enzymes referred to as the fatty acid synthase system.

5. The butyryl group is transferred to the CE, exposing the ACP sulfhydryl site to a second molecule of malonyl CoA.

6. Malonyl ACP forms for a second time.

7. A second condensation reaction takes place, with coupling of the butyryl group on the CE to C-2 of the malonyl ACP. The six-carbon chain is then reduced and transferred to CE in a repetition of steps 2 through 5. A third molecule of malonyl CoA attaches at ACP–SH, and so forth. The completed fatty acid chain is hydrolyzed from the ACP without transfer to the CE.

The normal product of the fatty acid synthase system is palmitate, 16:0. It can in turn be lengthened by fatty acid elongation systems to stearic acid, 18:0, and even longer saturated fatty acids. Elongation occurs by the addition of two-carbon units at the carboxylic acid end of the chain. Furthermore, by **desaturation** reactions, palmitate and stearate can be converted to their corresponding Δ^9 monounsaturated fatty acids, palmitoleic acid (16:1) and oleic acid (18:1), respectively. Fatty acid desaturation reactions are catalyzed by enzymes referred to as mixed-function oxidases, so called because two different substrates are oxidized: the fatty acid (by removal of hydrogen atoms to form the new double bond) and NADPH. Oxygen is the terminal hydrogen and electron acceptor to form H_2O.

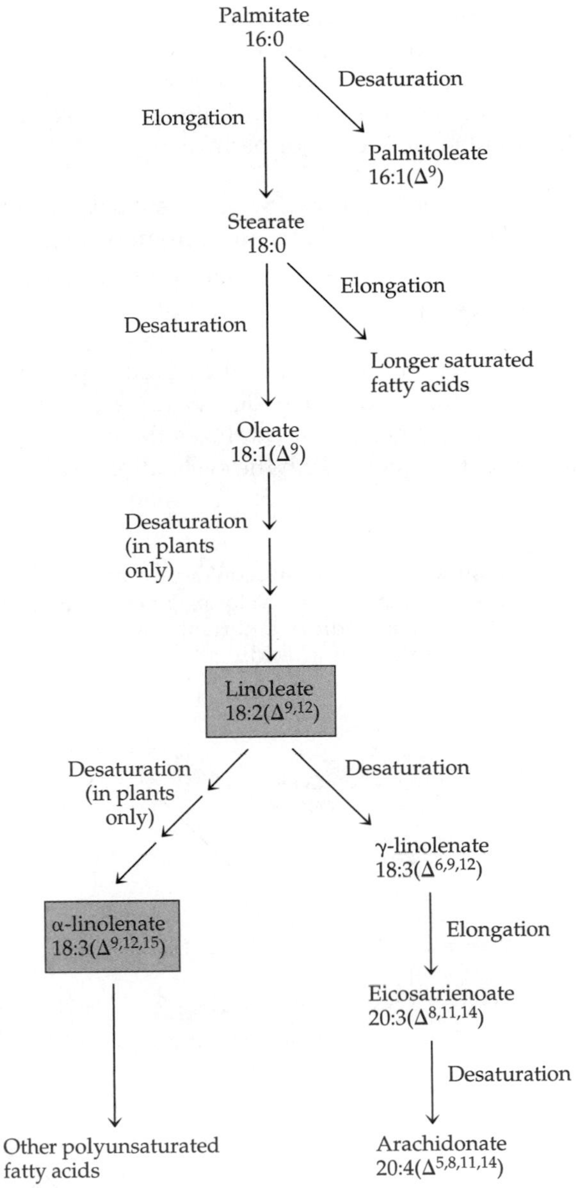

Figure 6.31 Routes of synthesis of other fatty acids from palmitate as precursor. Elongation and desaturation reactions allow palmitate to be converted into longer and more highly unsaturated fatty acids. Mammals cannot convert oleate into linoleate or α-linolenate (shaded in figure). These fatty acids are therefore essential and must be acquired in the diet.

Essential Fatty Acids

As pointed out previously human cells cannot introduce additional double bonds beyond the Δ^9 site because they lack enzymes called Δ^{12} and Δ^{15} desaturases. That is why linoleic acid (18:2 $\Delta^{9,12}$) and α-linolenic acid (18:3 $\Delta^{9,12,15}$) are essential fatty acids. They can be acquired from plant sources because plant cells do have the desaturase enzymes. Once linoleic acid is acquired, longer, more highly unsaturated fatty acids can be formed from it by a combination of elongation and desaturation reactions. Figure 6.31 illustrates the elongation and desaturation of palmitate and linoleate. These elongation reactions produce fatty acids that are metabolized to biologically active compounds that play a significant physiological role, described next.

Eicosanoids: Fatty Acid Derivatives of Physiological Significance

The essentiality of linoleic acid and α-linolenic acid is due to the fact that they act as precursors for some longer, more highly unsaturated fatty acids, which in turn are necessary

- for the formation of cell membranes and
- as precursors of compounds called eicosanoids.

Eicosanoids are fatty acids composed of 20 carbon atoms. They include the physiologically potent families of substances called **prostaglandins, thromboxanes,** and **leukotrienes,** all of which are formed from precursor fatty acids by the incorporation of oxygen atoms into the fatty acid chains. Reactions of this sort are often referred to as **oxygenation reactions,** and the enzymes catalyzing the reactions are named oxygenases.

The most important fatty acid serving as a precursor for eicosanoid synthesis is arachidonate. Its oxygenation follows either of two major pathways:

- the "cyclic" pathway, which results in the formation of prostaglandins and thromboxanes, and
- the "linear" pathway, which produces leukotrienes.

The featured enzyme in the cyclic pathway is prostaglandin endoperoxide synthase, sometimes called cyclo-oxygenase. It catalyzes the oxygenation of arachidonate together with the cyclization of an internal segment of the arachidonate chain, the hallmark structural feature of the prostaglandins and thromboxanes. The enzyme that converts arachidonate to the leukotrienes in the linear pathway is lipoxygenase, and the pathway is often referred to as the lipoxygenase pathway. Figure 6.32 is an overview of the reactions of the cyclic and linear pathways of arachidonic acid.

Prostaglandins (PG) are 20-carbon fatty acids having a 5-carbon ring in common but displaying modest structural differences among themselves. As shown in Figure 6.32, they are designated PGD, PGE, PGF, PGI, PGG, and PGH; subscripts indicate the number of double bonds, with the "2" series being the most important. These compounds, along with the thromboxanes, exhibit a wide range of physiological actions, including the lowering of

Figure 6.32 The formation of prostaglandins, thromboxanes, and leukotrienes from arachidonic acid via cyclo-oxygenase and lipoxygenase pathways. Abbreviations: PG, prostaglandin; TX, thromboxane; 5-HPETE, 5-hydroperoxy-6, 8, 11, 14-eicosatetraenoic acid.

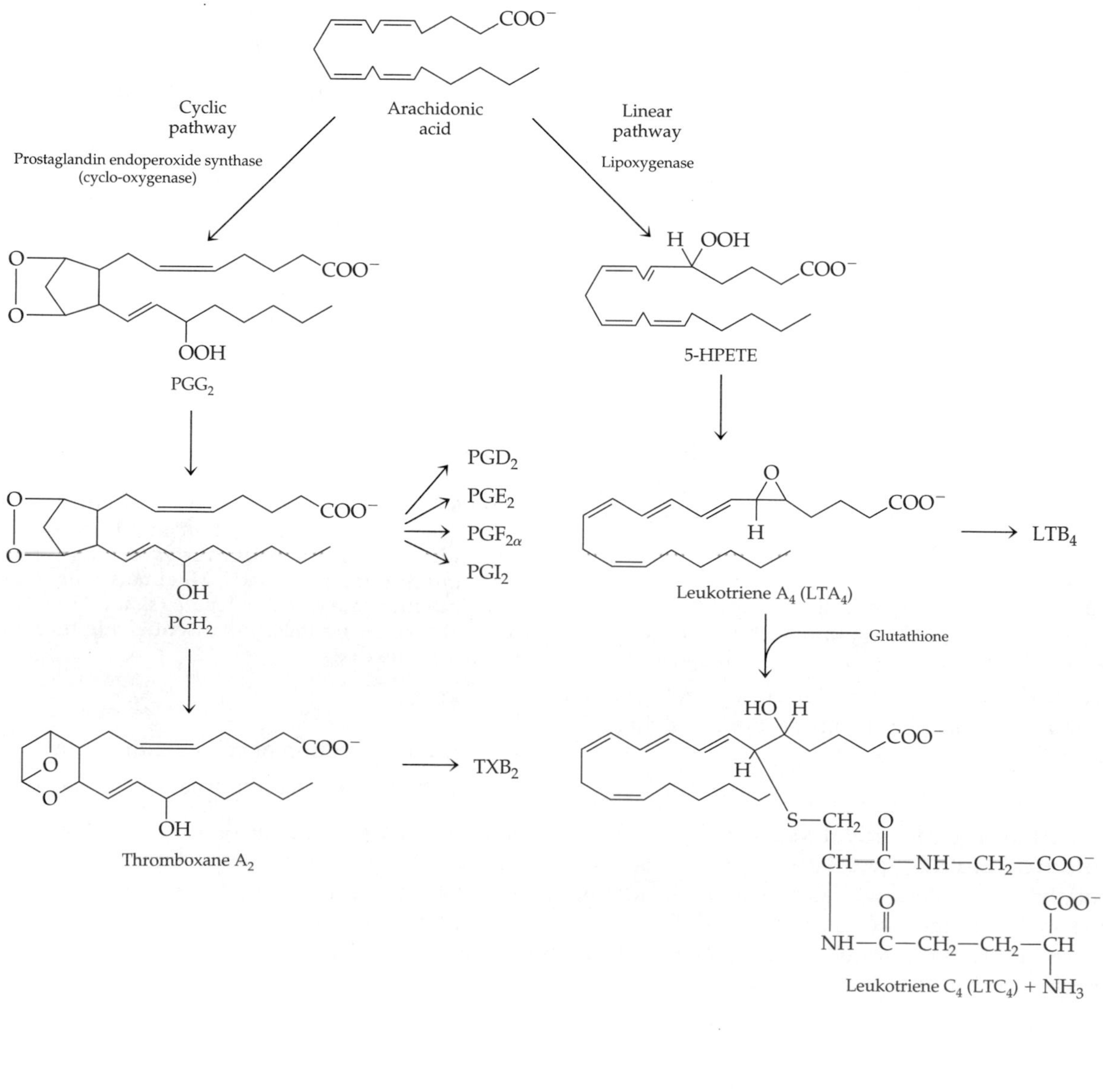

blood pressure, diuresis, blood platelet aggregation, effects on the immune and nervous systems as well as gastric secretions, and the stimulation of smooth muscle contraction, to name several. They are described as being "hormonelike" in function. However, hormones originate from a specific gland and their actions are the same for all their target cells, while prostaglandins are widely distributed in animal tissues but affect only the cells in which they are synthesized. They do appear to alter the actions of hormones, often through their modulation of cAMP levels and the intracellular flow of calcium ions.

Certain combinations of prostaglandins and thromboxanes may exhibit antagonistic effects. For example, prostacyclin (PGI_2) is a potent stimulator of adenylate cyclase and thereby acts as a platelet "antiaggregating" factor, because platelet aggregation is inhibited by cAMP. Opposing this action is thromboxane A_2, which inhibits adenylate cyclase and consequently serves as a "proaggregating" force. Another example of opposing actions of the prostaglandins is the vasodilation of blood vessels by PGE_2 and their vasoconstriction by PGF_2.

Certain prostaglandins produce a rise in body temperature (fever) and can cause inflammation and therefore pain. The anti-inflammatory and antipyretic (fever-reducing) activity of aspirin, acetaminophen, and indomethacin is due to their inhibitory effect on prostaglandin endoperoxide synthase (cyclo-oxygenase), which results in reduced prostaglandin and thromboxane synthesis. The 5-lipoxygenase pathway of leukotriene (LTC_4) formation from arachidonate is shown in Figure 6.32. Although not shown in the pathway, LTC_4 is further metabolized to other leukotrienes in the following order:

$$LTC_4 \longrightarrow LTD_4 \longrightarrow LTE_4 \longrightarrow LTF_4$$

The structures of LTA_4 and LTC_4 are shown because they exemplify a leukotriene and a peptidoleukotriene, respectively. Note that LTC_4 is formed from LTA_4 by incorporation of the tripeptide glutathione (γ-glutamylcysteinyl-glycine). LTD_4, LTE_4, and LTF_4 are peptidoleukotrienes produced from LTC_4 by peptidase hydrolysis of bonds within the glutathione moiety. Like the prostaglandins, these substances share structural characteristics but are classified within the A, B, C, D, and E series according to their structural differences. As for prostaglandins, the subscript number represents the number of double bonds in the compound.

Leukotrienes have potent biological actions. Briefly, they contract respiratory, vascular, and intestinal smooth muscles. The effects on the respiratory system include constriction of bronchi and increased mucus secretion. These actions, which are known to be expressed through binding to specific receptors, have implicated the leukotrienes as mediators in asthma, immediate hypersensitivities, inflammatory reactions, and myocardial infarction. In fact, one of the major chemical mediators of anaphylactic shock—the so-called slow-reacting substance of anaphylactic shock, or SRS-A—has been found to be a mixture of the peptidoleukotrienes LTC_4, LTD_4, and LTE_4. Anaphylactic shock is a life-threatening response to chemical substances, primarily histamine, that are released as a result of a severe allergic reaction.

A necessity for eicosanoid formation is the availability of an appropriate amount of free (unesterified) arachidonate. Cellular concentration of the free fatty acid is not adequate and therefore must be released from membrane glycerophosphatides by a specific hydrolytic enzyme called phospholipase A_2. Structural features of glycerophosphatides were reviewed in the section on phospholipids. The most important glycerophosphatides acting as sources of arachidonate in cells are phosphatidylcholine and phosphatidylinositol. When present in these structures, arachidonate normally occupies the *sn*-2 position. Recall that the *sn*-2 position of phospholipids normally is occupied by a polyunsaturated fatty acid.

The release of arachidonate from membrane glycerophosphatides, for eicosanoid synthesis, is influenced by stimuli. These stimuli are of two main types, physiological (specific) and pathological (nonspecific). Physiological stimulation, a natural occurrence, is brought about by stimulatory compounds such as epinephrine, angiotensin II, and antigen-antibody complexes. Pathological stimuli, which result in a more generalized release of all fatty acids from the *sn*-2 position, include mechanical damage, ischemia, and membrane-active venoms. Table 6.5 lists the precursors, sites of synthesis, and physiological effects of a few major eicosanoid groups.

In addition to the prostaglandins made from arachidonic acid, an n-6 fatty acid, there is another series made from eicosapentaenoic acid, an n-3 fatty acid. A few of the major compounds in this series are shown in Table 6.5. The physiological action of these two series of hormonelike substances is too extensive to be covered here. In general, the two series have opposing actions.

Impact of Diet on Fatty Acid Synthesis

The rate of fatty acid synthesis can be influenced by diet. Diets high in simple carbohydrates and low in fats induce a set of lipogenic enzymes in the liver. This induction is exerted through the process of transcription, leading to elevated levels of the mRNA for the enzymes. The transcriptional response is triggered by an increase in glucose metabolism, and the triggering substance, though not positively identified, is thought to be glucose 6-phosphate [25]. Other studies have confirmed that a very low fat/high sugar diet causes an increase in fatty

Table 6.5 Physiological Characteristics of Eicosanoids

Eicosanoid Family	Precursor: Arachidonate (20:4 n-6)	Precursor: Eicosapentaenoate (20:5 n-3)	Site of Synthesis	Mode of Action
Prostacyclins	PGI_2	PGI_3	Vascular endothelium	Vasodilator, platelet antiaggregator
Thromboxanes	TXA_2	TXA_3	Platelet	Vasoconstrictor, platelet aggregator
Leukotrienes	LTB_4	LTB_4	Leukocytes	Chemotaxis

Source: Anderson PA, Sprecher HW. Omega-3 fatty acids in nutrition and health. *Dietetic Currents* 14 (no. 2), 1987. Reprinted with permission of Ross Laboratories, Columbus, OH 43216.

acid synthesis and in palmitate-rich, linoleate-poor VLDL triacylglycerols. Furthermore, the effect may be reduced if starch is substituted for the sugar, possibly owing to the slower absorption of starch glucose and a lower postprandial insulin response [26].

Synthesis of Triacylglycerols (Triglycerides)

The biosyntheses of triacylglycerols and glycerophosphatides share common precursors and can be considered together in this section. The precursors are CoA-activated fatty acids and glycerol 3-phosphate, the latter being produced either from the reduction of dihydroxyacetone phosphate or from the phosphorylation of glycerol. These and subsequent reactions of the pathways are shown in Figure 6.33. The figure depicts two pathways for lecithin synthesis from diacylglycerol. The de novo pathway of lecithin synthesis is the major route. However, the importance of the salvage pathway increases when there is a deficiency of the essential amino acid methionine.

Synthesis of Cholesterol

Nearly all the tissues in the body are capable of synthesizing cholesterol from acetyl CoA. The liver accounts for about 20% of endogenous cholesterol. Among the extrahepatic tissues, which are responsible for the remaining 80% of synthesized cholesterol, the intestine is probably the most active. The cholesterol production rate, which includes both absorbed cholesterol and endogenously synthesized cholesterol, approximates 1 g/day. Compare this with the recommended dietary intake of about 300 mg/day. The average cholesterol intake is considered to be about 600 mg/day, only about half of which is absorbed. Endogenous synthesis therefore accounts for more than two-thirds of the daily total.

At least 26 steps are known to be involved in the formation of cholesterol from acetyl CoA. The individual steps are not provided here, but the synthesis of cholesterol can be thought of as occurring in three stages:

1. A cytoplasmic sequence by which 3-hydroxy-3-methylglutaryl CoA (HMG CoA) is formed from 3 mol of acetyl CoA
2. The conversion of HMG CoA to squalene, including the important rate-limiting step of cholesterol synthesis in which HMG CoA is reduced to mevalonic acid by HMG CoA reductase
3. The formation of cholesterol from squalene

Figure 6.33 A schematic summary of the synthesis of triacylglycerols and lecithin showing that precursors are shared. In lecithin formation, three moles of activated methionine (S-adenosylmethionine) introduce three methyl groups in the de novo pathway, and choline is introduced as CDP (cytidine diphosphate) choline in the so-called salvage pathway.

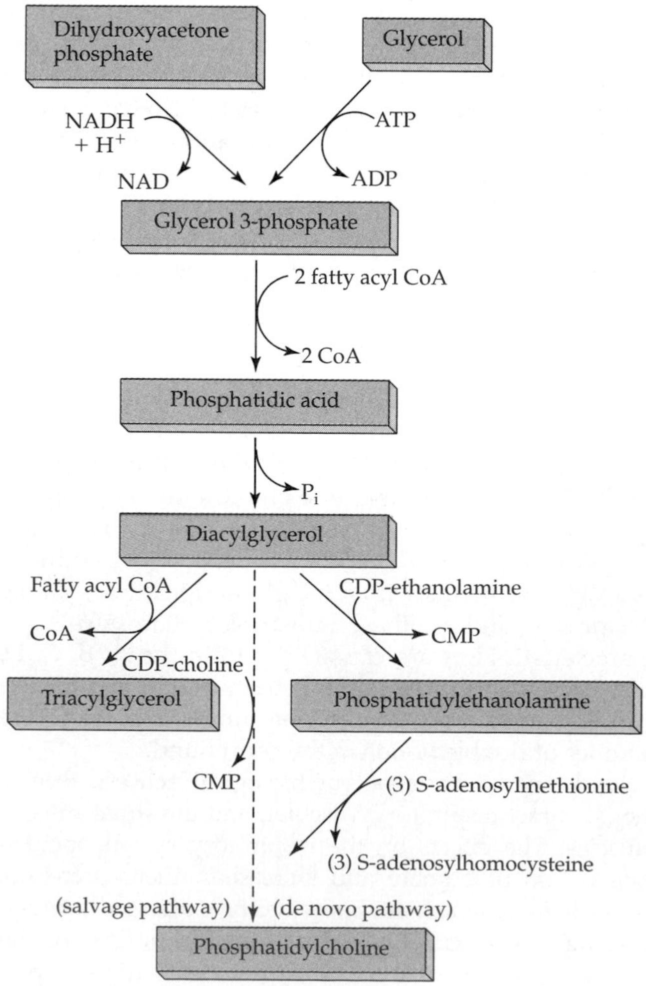

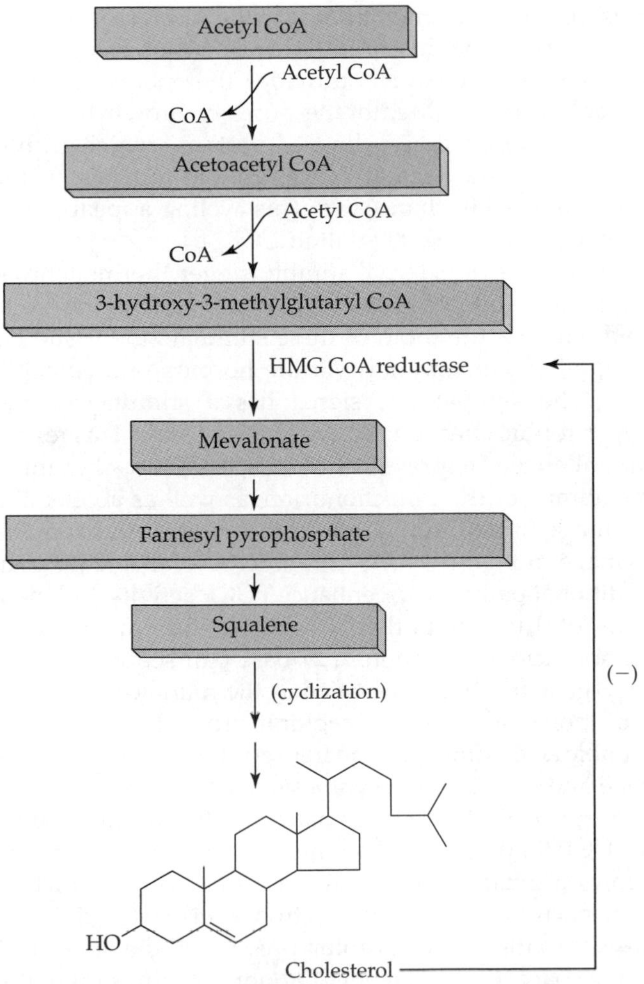

Figure 6.34 An overview of the pathway of cholesterol biosynthesis in the hepatocyte indicating the negative regulatory effect of cholesterol on the HMG CoA reductase reaction.

As total body cholesterol increases, the rate of synthesis tends to decrease. This is known to be due to a negative feedback regulation of the HMG CoA reductase reaction. This suppression of cholesterol synthesis by dietary cholesterol seems to be unique to the liver and is not much evident in other tissues. The effect of feedback control of biosynthesis depends to a great extent on the amount of cholesterol absorbed. The suppression is not sufficient to prevent an increase in the total body pool of cholesterol when dietary intake is high. A brief scheme of hepatic cholesterolgenesis and its regulation is shown in Figure 6.34.

REGULATION OF LIPID METABOLISM

The regulation of fatty acid oxidation is closely linked to carbohydrate status. Fatty acids formed in the cytoplast of liver cells can either be converted into triacylglycerols and phospholipids or be transported via carnitine into the mitochondrion for oxidation. Carnitine acyl transferase I, which catalyzes the transfer of fatty acyl groups to carnitine (see Fig. 6.23), is specifically inhibited by malonyl CoA. Recall that malonyl CoA is the first intermediate in the synthesis of fatty acids. Therefore, it is logical that an increase in its concentration would promote fatty acid synthesis while inhibiting fatty acid oxidation. Malonyl CoA concentration increases whenever a person is well supplied with carbohydrate, because excess glucose that cannot be oxidized or stored as glycogen is converted to triacylglycerols for storage, increasing the demands for malonyl CoA. Therefore, glucose-rich cells do not actively oxidize fatty acids for energy. Instead, a switch to lipogenesis is stimulated, accomplished in part by inhibition of the entry of fatty acids into the mitochondrion.

Blood glucose levels can affect lipolysis and fatty acid oxidation by other mechanisms as well. Hyperglycemia triggers the release of insulin, which promotes glucose transport into the adipose cell and therefore lipogenesis. The hormone also exerts a pronounced antilipolytic effect. Hypoglycemia results in a reduced intracellular supply of glucose, thereby suppressing lipogenesis. Furthermore, the low level of insulin accompanying the hypoglycemic state would favor lipolysis, with a flow of free fatty acids into the bloodstream. Low glucose levels also stimulate the rate of fatty acid oxidation in the manner described in the section dealing with the ketone bodies. In this case, accelerated oxidation of fatty acids follows the reduction in Krebs cycle activity, which in turn results from inadequate oxaloacetate availability.

The key enzyme for the mobilization of fat is hormone-sensitive triacylglycerol lipase, found in adipose tissue cells. Lipolysis is stimulated by hormones such as epinephrine and norepinephrine, adrenocorticotropic hormone (ACTH), thyroid-stimulating hormone (TSH), glucagon, growth hormone, and thyroxine. Insulin, as mentioned earlier, antagonizes the effects of these hormones by inhibiting the lipase activity.

A very important allosteric enzyme involved in the regulation of fatty acid biosynthesis is acetyl CoA carboxylase, which forms malonyl CoA from acetyl CoA (Fig 6.28). The enzyme, which functions in the cytoplast, is positively stimulated by citrate. In the absence of this modulator, the enzyme is barely active. Citrate is continuously produced in the mitochondrion as a Krebs cycle intermediate, but its concentration in the cytoplast is normally low. However, should mitochondrial citrate concentration increase, the compound can escape to the cytoplast. There it acts as a positive allosteric signal to acetyl CoA carboxylase, thereby increasing the rate of formation of malonyl CoA, which results in lipogenesis. Also, recall that citrate is the precursor for cytoplasmic acetyl CoA. Therefore, the result of citrate accumulation is that excess acetyl CoA is diverted to fatty acid synthesis and away from Krebs cycle activity.

Acetyl CoA carboxylase can be modulated negatively by palmitoyl CoA, which is the product of fatty acid synthesis. This situation would most likely arise when fatty acid concentrations increase as a result of insufficient glycerophosphate, with which fatty acids must combine to form triacylglycerols. Deficient glycerophosphate levels would likely be due to inadequate carbohydrate availability. In such a situation, regulation would logically favor fatty acid oxidation rather than synthesis.

A great deal of interest in serum cholesterol levels has been generated because of the alleged correlation of the compound to the predisposition to cardiovascular disease. The regulation of cholesterol homeostasis is associated with its effect on LDL receptor concentration and on the activity of regulatory enzymes such as acyl CoA:cholesterol acyltransferase (ACAT) and hydroxymethylglutaryl CoA (HMG CoA) reductase. Cholesterol's feedback suppression of HMG CoA reductase has been discussed and is shown in Figure 6.34. The combination of increasing ACAT activity (the conversion of free cholesterol to cholesteryl esters) and decreasing the amount of LDL receptors reduces the accumulation of cholesterol in vascular endothelial and smooth muscle cells. Figure 6.21 illustrates these mechanisms of control.

BROWN FAT THERMOGENESIS

Brown adipose tissue obtains its name from its high degree of vascularity and the abundant mitochondria present in the adipocytes. Recall that the mitochondria are pigmented, owing to the cytochromes and perhaps other oxidative pigments associated with electron transport. Not only are there larger numbers of mitochondria in brown fat cells compared with white fat cells, but the mitochondria also are structurally different so as to promote **thermogenesis** (heat production) at the expense of producing ATP.

Brown fat mitochondria have special H^+ pores in their inner membrane, formed by an integral protein called thermogenin, or the uncoupling protein (UCP). UCP is a translocator of protons, allowing the external H^+ pumped out by electron transport to flow back into the mitochondria rather than through the F_0F_1 ATP-synthase site of phosphorylation. Remember that it is the H^+ gradient that brings about the conformational changes that result in the phosphorylation of ADP to produce ATP. Figure 6.35 illustrates how the proposed mechanism of brown fat thermogenesis relates to the chemiosmotic theory of oxidative phosphorylation. Protons within the mitochondrial matrix are pumped outside the inner membrane by the electron transport energy. Then the downhill flow of protons through the F_0F_1 aggregate channels provides the energy for ADP phosphorylation. Membrane pores of brown fat mitochondria allow the cycling of protons, which results in lowering the proton concentration and heat being generated rather than ATPs. This cycling appears to be regulated by the 32,000-dalton UCP.

Two types of external stimuli trigger thermogenesis: (1) the ingestion of food and (2) prolonged exposure to cold temperature. Both of these stimulate the tissue via sympathetic innervation via the hormone norepinephrine. The sympathetic signal has a stimulatory and hypertrophic effect on brown adipose tissue. This results in enhanced expression of the UCP in the inner membrane of the mitochondrion, as well as accelerated synthesis of lipoprotein lipase and glucose transporters to make more fatty acids and glucose available [27]. An additional pathway for enhanced UCP activity, independent of the sympathetic nervous system, involves retinoic acid stimulation. A 27-base-pair sequence in the UCP gene has been identified as the retinoic acid receptor. Upon binding to its receptor in brown fat adipocytes, retinoic acid stimulates the transcriptional activity of the gene and therefore the synthesis of UCP [28].

Figure 6.35 includes the pathways for the stimulation of UCP expression. The higher UCP concentration allows a greater proton flux into the matrix, which in turn encourages greater electron transport activity in answer to the reduced proton pressure in the intermembrane space. Enhancement of lipoprotein lipase and glucose transporters provides fuel (fatty acids and glucose, respectively) to meet the higher metabolic demand. The end result of this stimulation is that the phosphorylation of ADP by electron transport in the mitochondria of the brown fat cells becomes "uncoupled," which leads to less ATP formation but considerably more heat production. As ATP production diminishes, the dynamics of the catabolic breakdown and the anabolic biosynthesis of stored nutrients will shift to catabolism in an effort to replenish the ATP.

Theoretically, then, weight reduction should accompany a higher activity of brown fat, and, indeed, a possible link between obesity and deficient brown fat cell function has been researched. For example, evidence indicates that thermogenesis is defective in instances of obesity. However, direct evidence that the defect resides in brown adipose tissue is tenuous. Studies using thermographic skin measurements have shown defective thermogenesis in the brown fat depots of obese subjects who had received catecholamine hormone, but such measurements are imprecise because of the insulation provided by the thick, subcutaneous adipose tissue of obese people. In fact, some researchers are of the

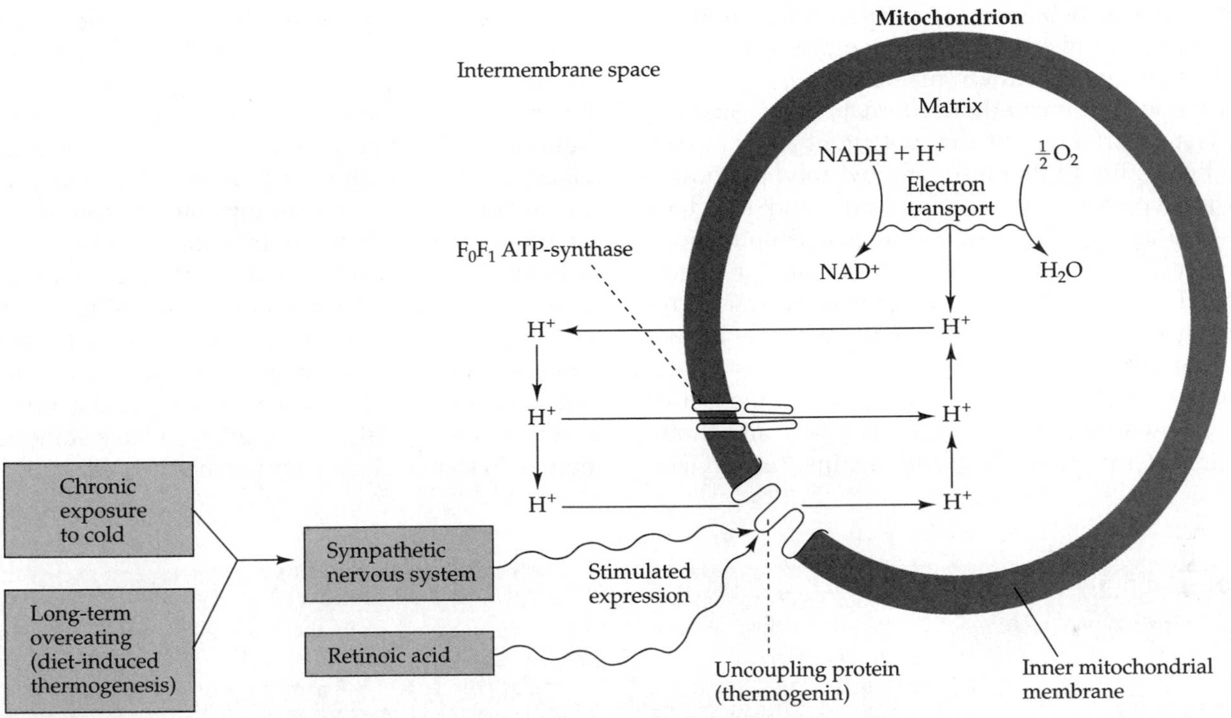

Figure 6.35 The stimulatory effect of some mediators on brown adipocyte thermogenesis. Retinoic acid has recently been shown to act independently of the sympathetic nervous system. Enhanced activity of the uncoupling protein, which translocates protons from the intermembrane space of the mitochondrion to the matrix, shifts the energy released from the proton flow toward thermogenesis and away from ATP synthesis.

opinion that a simple, single test to assess appropriate brown fat function in obese subjects is lacking. Despite this shortcoming, the demonstration of the catecholamine stimulation of brown fat thermogenesis deserves further investigation. It raises the tempting possibility that brown adipose tissue may relate to human obesity both in a causal way and as a focus for diet therapy.

THERAPEUTIC INHIBITION OF FAT ABSORPTION: OLESTRA AND ORLISTAT

Because of the association between dietary fat and obesity—and even cardiovascular disease—reduction in fat intake is a logical nutritional recourse. This has been difficult to achieve, however, because fat enhances palatability, which is a major driving force in food selection. The synthetic compound olestra was developed as a fat replacement to impart palatability to a food without the consequences of high-calorie fat. Orlistat has a different mode of action, interfering with the absorption of natural dietary fat.

Olestra is a mixture of hexa-, hepta-, and octaesters of sucrose with long-chain fatty acids. It imparts a taste essentially indistinguishable from fat, yet it is not hydrolyzable by the pancreatic lipases and therefore has no caloric value. Technically, it can replace fat in a wide variety of foods and can be used to reduce fat-derived calories in cooked, baked, or fried foods. Because undigested food entering the bowel can cause intestinal irritability, olestra was viewed unfavorably as a probable contributor to such discomfort. In fact, some early reports linked olestra with colonic irritability, with accompanying gas and diarrhea. While this issue remains under debate, most well-designed studies have exonerated olestra in this regard. In one such investigation, substitution of up to 30 g of olestra in a meal of 45 g fat had no effect on gastric, small intestinal, or colonic transit time [29]. This finding has been corroborated by numerous other studies. Furthermore, there have been positive findings as to the overall safety of olestra, not only from the standpoint of its harmlessness to the gastrointestinal tract but also regarding areas such as metabolism and absorption, mutagenicity, carcinogenicity, and nutrition [30].

Still under study, however, is whether reduction in fat energy intake may positively influence appetite such that an energy-compensatory mechanism stimulates an enhanced intake of carbohydrate. Pronounced compensatory biobehavioral responses may accompany severe reductions in energy from fat, making adherence to the low-fat diet difficult to maintain [31].

Orlistat is a semisynthetic derivative of lipstatin, which is a naturally occurring, potent inhibitor of pancreatic lipase. Recall that although hydrolytic products of triacylglycerols—monoacylglycerols and free fatty acids—are absorbed across the intestinal epithelium, intact triacylglycerols are not. The rationale for orlistat use, therefore, is that by restricting the hydrolysis of triacylglycerols, the compound will sharply reduce absorption of fat.

Orlistat acts by binding covalently to the serine residue of the active site of pancreatic lipase and shows little or no inhibitory activity against α-amylase, trypsin, chymotrypsin, or the phospholipases. Dose-response curves show that a plateau of inhibition of dietary fat absorption occurs at high levels of the drug (>400 mg/day), corresponding to approximately 35% inhibition. At therapeutic doses (300–400 mg/day) taken in conjunction with a well-balanced, mildly hypocaloric diet, orlistat inhibits fat absorption as much as approximately 30%, contributing to a caloric deficit of about 200 calories. Preliminary tests have shown that orlistat may indeed represent a promising alternative approach to the management of obesity. It does not cause significant gastrointestinal disturbances and does not appear to affect gastric emptying and acidity, gallbladder motility, bile composition, biliary stone formation, or systemic electrolyte balance [32,33].

summary

The hydrophobic character of lipids makes them unique among the major nutrients, requiring special handling in the body's aqueous milieu. Ingested fat must be finely dispersed in the intestinal lumen in order to present a sufficiently large surface area for enzymatic digestion to occur. In the bloodstream, reassembled lipid must be associated with proteins to ensure its solubility in that environment while undergoing transport.

The major sites for the formation of lipoproteins are the intestine, which produces them from exogenously derived lipids, and the liver, which forms lipoproteins from endogenous lipids. Central to the processes of fat transport and storage is adipose tissue, which accumulates fat as triacylglycerol when the intake of energy-producing nutrients is greater than the body's caloric needs. When the energy demand so dictates, fatty acids are released from storage and transported to other tissues for oxidation. The mobilization follows the adipocyte's response to specific hormonal signals that stimulate the activity of the intracellular lipase.

Fatty acids are a rich source of energy. Their mitochondrial oxidation furnishes large amounts of acetyl CoA for Krebs cycle catabolism, and in situations of low carbohydrate intake or use, as occurs in starvation or diabetes, the rate of fatty acid oxidation increases significantly with concomitant acetyl CoA accumulation. This causes a rise in the level of the ketone bodies—organic acids that can be deleterious through their disturbance of acid-base balance but that also are beneficial as sources of fuel to tissues such as muscle and brain in periods of starvation.

Although the lipids are thought of first and foremost as energy sources, some can be identified with intriguing hormonelike functions ranging from blood pressure alteration and platelet aggregation to enhancement of immunological surveillance. These potent bioactive substances are the prostaglandins, thromboxanes, and leukotrienes, all of which are derived from the fatty acids, arachidonate, and certain other long-chain PUFAs.

Dietary lipid has been implicated in atherogenesis, the process leading to development of the degenerative cardiovascular disease called atherosclerosis. A major consideration in the prevention and control of this disease has been the concentration of cholesterol in the blood serum and the relative hypocholesterolemic or hypercholesterolemic effect of certain diets. Saturated fatty acids having medium-length chains, along with unsaturated *trans* fatty acids, are alleged to be hypercholesterolemic, while mono- and polyunsaturated *cis* fats tend to lower serum cholesterol.

Fats can be synthesized by cytoplasmic enzyme systems when energy production by carbohydrate is adequate. The synthesis begins with simple precursors such as acetyl CoA and can be triggered by hormonal signals or by elevated levels of citrate, which acts as a regulatory substance. Blood glucose concentration also acts as a sensitive regulator of lipogenesis, which is stimulated when a hyperglycemic state exists.

Protein metabolism will be surveyed in Chapter 7. There it will be seen that amino acids, like carbohydrates and lipids, can furnish energy through their oxidation or can be metabolically converted into other substances of biochemical importance. Once again, it should be emphasized that the metabolic pathways of the energy nutrients are linked through common metabolites. Gluconeogenesis, discussed in Chapter 4, illustrates this integration through the formation of carbohydrate from the glycerol moiety of lipids and certain amino acids. Chapter 7 will demonstrate how protein can be converted into fat through common intermediates. The expression "A rose is a rose is a rose" applies quite appropriately to intermediary metabolites. For example, if acetyl CoA is the substrate for an enzyme, the enzyme will convert it with no regard as to whether it originated through carbohydrate, lipid, or protein metabolism.

References Cited

1. Hunter JE, Applewhite TH. Reassessment of transfatty acid availability in the U.S. diet. Am J Clin Nutr 1991;54:363–69.

2. Berridge M. Inositol triphosphate and calcium signalling. Nature 1993;361:315–25.

3. Berridge MJ. Inositol triphosphate and diacylglycerol: two intersecting second messengers. Ann Rev Biochem 1987;56:159–93.

4. Borensztajn J, Getz GS, Kotlar TJ. Uptake of chylomicron remnants by the liver: further evidence for the modulating role of phospholipids. J Lipid Res 1988;29:1087–96.

5. Brown MS, Goldstein JL. A receptor-mediated pathway for cholesterol homeostasis. Science 1986;232:34–47.

6. Ross R. The pathogenesis of atherosclerosis: a prospective for the 90s. Nature 1993;362:801–9.

7. Beynen AC, Katan MB, Van Zutphen LFM. Hypo- and hyperresponders: individual differences in the response of serum cholesterol concentration to changes in diet. Adv in Lipid Res 1987;22:115–71.

8. Mensink RP, Katan MB. Effect of a diet enriched with monounsaturated or polyunsaturated fatty acids on levels of low-density and high-density lipoprotein cholesterol in healthy women and men. N Engl J Med 1989;321:436–41.

9. Berry EM, Eisenberg S, Haratz D, et al. Effects of diets rich in monounsaturated fatty acids on plasma lipoproteins—the Jerusalem Nutrition Study: high MUFAs vs. high PUFAs. Am J Clin Nutr 1991; 53:899–907.

10. Caggiula A, Mustad V. Effects of dietary fat and fatty acids on coronary artery disease risk and total and lipoprotein cholesterol concentrations: epidemiologic studies. Am J Clin Nutr 1997;65(suppl): 1597S–610S.

11. Freese R, Mutanen M. α-linolenic acid and marine long chain n-3 fatty acids differ only slightly in their effects on hemostatic factors in healthy subjects. Am J Clin Nutr 1997;66:591–98.

12. Harris W. n-3 fatty acids and serum lipoproteins: human studies. Am J Clin Nutr 1997;65(suppl):1645S–54S.

13. Connor WE. Importance of n-3 fatty acids in health and disease. Am J Clin Nutr 2000;71:171S–75S.

14. Kris-Etherton P, Yu Shaomei. Individual fatty acid effects on plasma lipids and lipoproteins: human studies. Am J Clin Nutr 1997;65(suppl):1628S–44S.

15. Mensink RP, Katan MB. Effect of dietary *trans* fatty acids on high density and low density lipoprotein cholesterol levels in healthy subjects. N Engl J Med 1990;323:439–45.

16. Ascherio A, Willett W. Health effects of *trans* fatty acids. Am J Clin Nutr 1997;66(suppl):1006S–10S.

17. Willett W, Stampfer M, Manson J, Colditz G, et al. Intake of *trans* fatty acids and risk of coronary heart disease among women. Lancet 1993;341:581–85.

18. Shapiro S. Do *trans* fatty acids increase the risk of coronary artery disease? A critique of the epidemiologic evidence. Am J Clin Nutr 1997;66(suppl):1011–17.

19. Kris-Etherton P, Dietschy J. Design criteria for studies examining individual fatty acid effects on cardiovascular disease risk factors: human and animal studies. Am J Clin Nutr 1997;65(suppl): 1590S–96S.

20. Chisholm A, Mann J, Sutherland W, Duncan A, et al. Effect on lipoprotein profile of replacing butter with margarine in a low fat diet: randomized crossover study with hypercholesterolaemic subjects. BMJ 1996;312:931–34.

21. Harris E. Lipoprotein (a): a predictor of atherosclerotic disease. Nutr Rev 1997;55:61–64.

22. Lehtinen S, Lehtimki T, Sisto T, Salenius J, et al. Apolipoprotein E polymorphism, serum lipids, myocardial infarction and severity of angiographically verified coronary artery disease in men and women. Atherosclerosis 1995;114:83–91.

23. Cobb M, Teitlebaum H, Risch N, Jekel J, Ostfeld A. Influence of dietary fat, apolipoprotein E phenotype, and sex on plasma lipoprotein levels. Circulation 1992;86:849–57.

24. Stengard J, Zerba K, Pekkanen J, Ehnholm C, et al. Apolipoprotein E polymorphism predicts death from coronary heart disease in a longitudinal study of elderly Finnish men. Circulation 1995;91:265–69.

25. Towle H, Kaytor E, Shih H. Regulation of the expression of lipogenic enzyme genes by carbohydrate. Annu Rev Nutr 1997; 17:405–33.

26. Hudgins L, Seidman C, Diakun J, Hirsch J. Human fatty acid synthesis is reduced after the substitution of dietary starch for sugar. Am J Clin Nutr 1998;67:631–39.

27. Himms-Hagan J. Brown adipose thermogenesis: interdisciplinary studies. FASEB J 1990;4:2890–98.

28. Alvarez R, DeAndres J, Yubero P, et al. A novel regulatory pathway of brown fat thermogenesis: retinoic acid is a transcriptional activator of the mitochondrial uncoupling protein. J Biol Chem 1995;270:5666–73.

29. Aggarwal AM, Camilleri M, Phillips SF, Schlagheck TG, et al. Olestra, a nondigestible, nonadsorbable fat. Effects on gastrointestinal and colonic transit. Dig Dis Sci 1993;38:1009–14.

30. Bergholz CM. Safety evaluation of olestra, a nonabsorbed, fatlike fat replacement. Crit Rev Food Sci Nutr 1992;32:141–46.

31. Cotton J, Weststrate J, Blundell J. Replacement of dietary fat with sucrose polyester: effects on energy intake and appetite control in non-obese males. Am J Clin Nutr 1996;63:891–96.

32. Guerciolini R. Mode of action of orlistat. Int J Obes Relat Metab Disord 1997;21(suppl3):S12–S23.

33. Sjostrom L, Rissaned A, Anderson T. Randomized placebo-controlled trial of orlistat for weight loss and prevention of weight regain in obese patients. Lancet 1998;352:167–72.

Suggested Readings

Brown MS, Goldstein JL. A receptor-mediated pathway for cholesterol homeostasis. Science 1986;232:34–47. This is an excellent step-by-step review of the research resulting in the delineation of the LDL receptor, its mechanisms of cholesterol homeostasis, and the therapeutic implications of these mechanisms.

Budowski P. Omega-3 fatty acids in health and disease. In: Bourne GH, ed. World Review of Nutrition and Dietetics, 1988;57:214–74. The structural aspects, sources, and antithrombotic actions of the omega-3 fatty acids are thoroughly reviewed, along with the eicosanoids and their multiplicity of physiological functions.

Web Sites

www.nal.usda.gov/fnic
U.S. Government Food and Nutrition Information Center

www.amhrt.org
American Heart Association

www.eatright.org
American Dietetic Association

The Role of Lipids and Lipoproteins in Atherogenesis

Atherogenesis is a degenerative systemic process involving arteries. If unchecked, the process becomes symptomatic, as vascular damage and impeded blood flow develop. The resulting disease state is called atherosclerosis. Although the disease is generally associated with old age, lesions begin to develop many years before symptoms become evident.

The innermost layer of the arterial wall, that which is in direct contact with the flowing blood, is called the intima. The intima consists of a layer of endothelial cells that act as a barrier to blood-borne cells and other substances. Underlying the intima is the media, consisting of layers of smooth muscle cells that make up the muscular component of the arterial wall. The atherogenic process is believed to begin in the endothelium, with subsequent or concurrent involvement of the medial smooth muscle cells.

The mechanism of atherogenesis is complex and not yet fully understood. However, two major components appear to be implicated:

- cells of the immune system, primarily monocytes and macrophages that are phagocytic cells, and T lymphocytes; and
- lipids and lipoproteins, most importantly LDL, oxidized or otherwise modified.

These components function together in the disease process.

It has been known for some time that a high level of circulating cholesterol is a major risk factor for cardiovascular disease. More recently, however, convincing experimental evidence has implicated LDL more specifically as the prime contributor to the process. LDL is the major transporter of cholesterol in the serum. The concentration of circulating LDL is controlled by two factors:

- Its rate of formation from VLDL (see this chapter). Normally, about one-third of VLDL is converted to LDL, and two-thirds is removed by the liver via apoE receptors.
- Its fractional clearance rate. LDL is removed by LDL receptors primarily (75%) in the liver but also in other tissues. A small amount is removed by cellular endocytosis, the so-called scavenger process.

Initiation of the atherogenic process may begin in response to some form of endothelial cell injury. This could result from mechanical stress such as hypertension or a high level of oxidized LDL, known to be toxic to endothelial cells. An increased adherence of monocytes and T lymphocytes to the affected area follows, along with infiltration of platelets. Activation of these cells is believed to occur as a result of concurrent penetration of the endothelium by LDL. The following events, also illustrated in Figure 1, then occur, although not necessarily in the order listed:

- Growth factors released from platelets stimulate the proliferation of smooth muscle cells in the arterial media. The smooth muscle cells accumulate lipid presented to them as LDL, transforming them into lipid-laden foam cells.
- Monocytes (or macrophages) also take up LDL particles, becoming foam cells. This uptake of LDL at the arterial wall is the scavenger pathway of LDL removal. It works independently of the LDL receptor.
- Macrophages, stimulated by the uptake of LDL, release additional growth factors and chemotactic factors (cytokines) that attract more macrophages to the site, creating more foam cells.
- Most of the lipid in foam cells is cholesterol and cholesteryl esters. As the foam cells proliferate, their lipid contents accumulate in the form of fatty streaks. These ultimately enlarge, occluding, to a matter of degree, the arterial lumen, which can become narrowed to the extent that blood flow is compromised.

Figure 1 Proposed events in the process of atherogenesis. Native LDL ([N]LDL) penetrates the arterial intima, becoming oxidized ([O]LDL) or otherwise modified to a form readily phagocytosed by macrophages that become lipid-engorged foam cells. Oxidized LDL is also cytotoxic to endothelial cells, creating an endothelial injury (EI) that attracts platelets. Platelets release platelet-derived growth factor (PDGF) that stimulates the proliferation of smooth muscle cells, which also can take up oxidized LDL by endocytosis and become foam cells. Macrophages, activated by the phagocytosis of oxidized LDL, release macrophage (or monocyte) chemotaxins (MC), which attract additional macrophages to the site, thereby perpetuating the process. Eventually, the proliferation of foam cells and smooth muscle cells impacts on the arterial lumen, narrowing it to the point that blood flow is compromised.

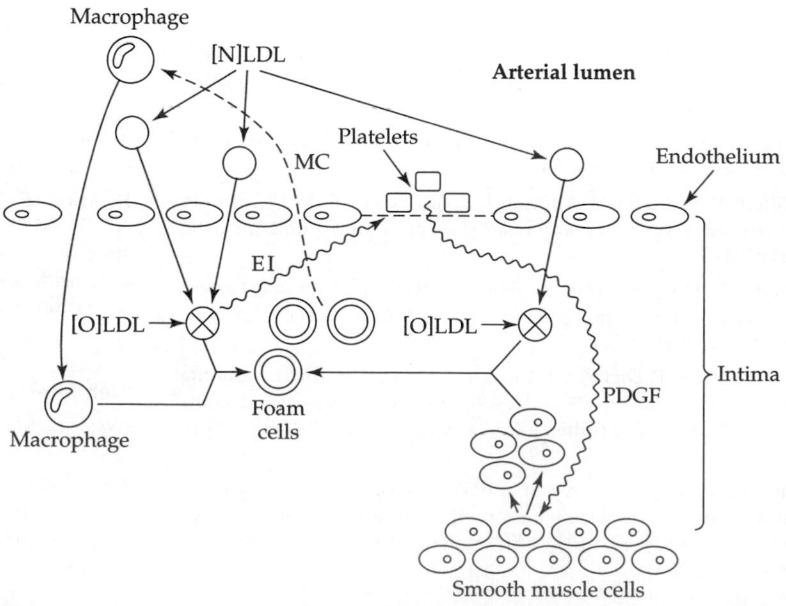

LDL modified by oxidation is a stronger contributor to atherogenesis than is native LDL. Uptake of oxidized LDL by macrophages is much more rapid than uptake of native LDL. In fact, cultured macrophages do not take up native LDL in vitro. Also, oxidized LDL has a considerably stronger proliferative effect on smooth muscle cells, and it is more toxic to endothelial cells [1]. It has been proposed that oxidized LDL may play a central role in atherogenesis in at least three additional ways [2]:

- It acts as a chemoattractant for the blood-borne monocytes to enter the subendothelial space.
- It causes the transformation of monocytes into macrophages.
- It causes the trapping of macrophages in the endothelial spaces by inhibiting their motility.

The oxidizing power in the cells involved has not been identified, but metal ions such as Cu^{2+} and Fe^{3+}, superoxide radicals, and heme-containing compounds have been suggested. Oxidation results in peroxidation of double bonds in the lipid moiety of the LDL particle. Cholesterol and cholesteryl esters can be converted into 7-keto derivatives, and unsaturated fatty acids are oxidatively fragmented into shorter-chain aldehydes. The toxicity of 7-ketocholesterol is believed to induce apoptosis in smooth muscle cells, a process associated with the release of oxidizing species that can contribute further to lipid peroxidation [3]. It has been suggested that the shorter-chain aldehydes resulting from peroxidation of unsaturated fatty acids may attach covalently to the apoprotein B-100 component of the particle through lysine side chains. In its chemically modified form, but not in its unaltered form, the protein is recognized by receptors on scavenger cells such as macrophages. Therefore, uptake of LDL, and consequently foam cell production, is accelerated [2].

A recent overview of atherosclerosis published in a lay journal provides an understandable and well-illustrated look at current understanding of the development of atherosclerosis [4]. Evidence for the participation of oxidized LDL in the atherogenic process is certainly convincing. Although the benefit of supplementation with antioxidants such as vitamin E to slow the process, and therefore reduce the risk of cardiovascular disease, has yet to be determined, the rationale for doing so is sound. The role of dietary intervention in reducing oxidized LDL and its atherogenic effects has been reviewed [5].

References Cited

1. Aug N, Pieraggi MT, Thiers JC, Ngre-Salvayre A, et al. Proliferative and cytotoxic effects of mildly oxidized low-density lipoproteins on vascular smooth-muscle cells. Biochem J 1995;309:1015–20.

2. Steinberg D, Parthasarathy S, Carew T, Kjoo J, Witztum J. Beyond cholesterol: modifications of low density lipoprotein that increase its atherogenicity. N Engl J Med 1989;320:915–24.

3. Nishio E, Arimura S, Watanabe Y. Oxidized LDL induces apoptosis in cultured smooth muscle cells: a possible role for 7-ketocholesterol. Biochem Biophys Res Commun 1996;223:413–18.

4. Libby P. Atherosclerosis: the new view. Sci Amer 2002;286:47–55.

5. Reaven P, Witztum J. Oxidized low density lipoproteins in atherogenesis: role of dietary intervention. Annu Rev Nutr 1996;16:51–71.

Web Sites

www.cspinet.org
Center for Science in the Public Interest

www.amhrt.org
American Heart Association

Nutrigenomics: The Foundation for Individualized Nutrition, by Ruth M. DeBusk, Ph.D., R.D.

What Is Nutrigenomics?

Nutrigenomics, also called "nutritional genetics" and "genomic nutrition," is an emerging discipline. Nutrigenomics is concerned with the role of genes in diet-related disease, the impact of genetic variability on an individual's risk of developing such a disease, and the ability of bioactive components in the diet to influence physiological function through their effects on genetic outcomes. (Refer to Table 1 for a listing of key terms related to nutrigenomics.)

At one end of the spectrum, nutrigenomics focuses on understanding (1) the mechanisms by which genes play a role in diet-related disease, (2) the complex biochemical pathways that result from decoding the information within the genes, (3) the intricate nutritional sensor system that communicates environmental signals to cells and the genes they contain, and (4) the ability of bioactive components in the diet to influence these various processes. At the other end of the spectrum, nutrigenomics encompasses the process of developing foods that contain these bioactive components that in turn influence the physiological outcomes encoded in an individual's genes. Nutrigenomics is causing diet to be viewed in a new context. Food components influence, both positively and negatively, the risk of developing diet-related diseases and also serve as signals that are detected by cellular sensor systems and thereby influence gene and protein expression and, ultimately, metabolite production.

In all cases, tools commonly employed in genetic research are being used to study the mechanisms by which diet affects genetic outcomes and to develop functional foods containing bioactive components that can minimize the risk of diet-related disease. By helping us understand how dietary choices influence the health of individuals and providing us with a means to exert control over

Table 1 Glossary of Nutritional Genetics Terminology

Food-related Terminology	Bioactive food components	Dietary components, both nutritive and nonnutritive, that can influence genetic outcomes through their effects on gene or protein expression or metabolite production and usage
	Functional foods	Foods that confer health benefits beyond their traditional nutrient content
Research Disciplines	Metabolomics	The study of the influence of the genome on an organism's metabolite profile
	Nutrigenomics	The application of genetic research to nutritional science to study a variety of aspects of diet-related disease, from mechanisms by which dietary components influence genetic outcomes to the development of functional foods containing specific dietary components that reduce the risk of particular diet-related disease
	Pharmacogenomics	The study of how genetic variations influence how individuals respond to drugs
	Proteomics	The study of the protein products of gene expression (also called "expression profiling"), with the goal of identifying the proteins and understanding their role in the functioning of an organism
	Transcriptomics	The study of the relative amounts of RNA expressed in cells or tissues
Research Methodology	DNA microarray technology	A laboratory technique that allows monitoring of an entire genome on a single chip
	In vitro expression systems	A laboratory tool for studying gene expression isolated from the complexity of the whole organism
	Knockout mouse	A mouse in which a single gene is inactivated or "knocked out" in a manner that leaves all other genes unaffected
	Transgenic organism	A plant or animal into which foreign genes have been inserted; the transgenic mouse is a frequently used model system for studying the role of a human gene in the overall functioning of the mouse
Genetics and Cell Biology Terminology	Dietary sensor/sensing system	The mechanism by which cells and organisms measure the nutritional sufficiency of the environment in which they find themselves; information is typically conveyed through the process of signal transduction
	Dietary signatures	The effect of one or more dietary components on the pattern of gene expression, protein expression, and metabolite production in different tissues
	Genotype	The genetic makeup of an organism, in contrast to its phenotype
	Polymorphism	A common variation of a gene's normal sequence that occurs in greater than 1% of a population
	Phenotype	The physical and functional characteristics of the organism that result from the expression of the genes in that organism
	Single nucleotide polymorphisms (SNPs)	The most common form of polymorphism, in which a single nucleotide in the genetic material is altered and the specific alteration occurs in greater than 1% of a population
	Transcriptome	The sum total of all the RNA species expressed by the genome of an organism
	Signal transduction	The transmission, through a series of biochemical reactions, of a signal at the surface of a cell to its interior; often involves the sensing of a triggering event at the cell surface that leads to changes in gene expression in the nucleus of the cell

these influences, nutrigenomics holds the promise of enabling individuals to personalize their diets in order to promote maximal life expectancy and the highest possible quality of life.

Impact of Nutrigenomics

Nutrigenomics is expected to have a significant impact on nutrition research, nutrition therapy, the food industry, and nutrition policy. Nutrigenomics research is proceeding on two levels: the molecular level and the systems biology level. Molecular studies focus on mechanisms involving gene-diet interactions. Systems biology approaches, in contrast, are whole organism oriented and are concerned with the response of the organism to bioactive food components.

At the molecular level, nutrigenomics research addresses how bioactive components in the diet affect metabolism, a field of study called metabolomics. The potential exists for using nutrition therapy to compensate for faulty genes and their resultant metabolic defects, which in turn result in physiological dysfunction. Also at the molecular level, nutrigenomics is concerned with determining the dietary signatures of various tissues in response to specific food components. Nutrigenomics research also incorporates proteomics, particularly the impact of genetic variation on the function of proteins associated with diet-related diseases.

At the systems biology level, nutrigenomics addresses the role of bioactive dietary components in the sensing systems that monitor the nutritional sufficiency of the environment in which an organism finds itself. This type of research also focuses on identifying the genes that influence the risk of developing diet-related diseases and on determining how dietary manipulation can reduce risk.

The outcome of the shift in nutrition research to a nutrigenomics focus is expected to have a significant impact on the clinical practice of nutrition. To date, nutrition therapy has been focused at the population level, developing recommendations that fit the general population. In the future, nutrition therapy will be focused at the individual level, with nutrigenomics providing insight into the genetic makeup of the individual and the appropriate nutritional therapy. The diet will supply the necessary bioactive components to effect the therapeutic intervention. Nutrition therapy will increase its emphasis on preventing disease in addition to managing disease. It will enable individuals to minimize genetic susceptibilities and optimize wellness. Through an understanding of how nutrition influences metabolic pathways, signal transduction, and gene expression, methods can be developed that will detect early pathological changes. Timely nutritional intervention strategies will improve outcomes, for both disease management and disease prevention.

The impact on the food industry is expected to be similarly dramatic. Specific dietary components will be identified as health-promoting metabolites, signal transducers, and influencers of gene and protein expression and will be linked to specific subpopulations with particular genetic susceptibilities for disease. The food industry is expected to respond by developing functional foods that have specific molecular targets, such as increasing the expression of a beneficial gene or filling a metabolic gap that results from a defective gene.

Health policy in general, and nutrition policy in particular, will evolve as the understanding of the role of genes in health progresses. With the shift to nutrigenomics as the cornerstone of personalized nutrition, blanket dietary generalizations and one-size-fits-all recommendations will give way to dietary recommendations tailored to the individual's genetic makeup. Genomic research is identifying the genes that predispose different populations to health disparities. Nutrigenomics will determine how genes, diet, and disease interact to bring about these disparities and offer options for minimizing them. Rather than being stratified by race, people will instead be sorted into genetic subpopulations. Individuals within a genetic subpopulation will be more alike than different in terms of their responses to food.

Major Issues in Nutrigenomics

Understanding the relationships among genes, dietary components, and health holds the potential for preventing diet-related diseases. This is arguably the most important goal of nutrigenomics and certainly its greatest potential. Considerable basic research is needed before this potential can be realized, however. Research is focused primarily on gene/diet-related disease associations and their underlying mechanisms and on the role of food components in dietary sensor systems. Among the specific research goals for the focus on gene/diet-related disease associations is identification of

- the genotypes that increase risk of diet-related disease and quantification of their impact,
- the genes associated with each diet-related disease and their products,
- the mechanisms by which these genes influence the development of diet-related disease and confer susceptibility on individuals,
- the levels of nutrients appropriate to specific alterations in the genetic material and the consequences for the proteins they encode (e.g., alterations in K_m), and
- the bioactive food components that influence the development of each of these diseases.

With respect to the focus on dietary sensor systems, specific research goals include

- identification of the bioactive food components that serve as dietary signals;
- elucidation of the mechanisms by which these signals influence gene and protein expression and metabolite production (e.g., as transcription cofactors);
- the quantification of the impact of these signals on gene and protein expression and metabolite production in different cells, tissues, and organs (i.e., characterization of these "dietary signatures"); and
- the development of biomarkers that identify early diet-related metabolic dysfunction.

Once these fundamentals are in place, nutrigenomics can provide the basis for therapeutic interventions that target specific steps in the sequence of events leading to homeostasis within an organism. Coupling knowledge of an individual's genotype and its inherited disease susceptibilities with the detection of early-stage pathological changes provides an opportunity for effective dietary intervention strategies designed to restore homeostasis and prevent diet-related disease.

Genetic Tools Used in Nutrigenomics

The Human Genome Project has provided the impetus for the development of a number of tools for genetic research. The tools employed in nutrigenomics are similar to the tools used in pharmacogenomics. In addition to standard chemical and biochemical techniques, key technologies include recombinant DNA technology, polymerase chain reaction (PCR), sequencing, single nucleotide polymorphism (SNP) analysis, gene expression profiling using DNA microarrays, in vitro systems, model systems, and transgenic organisms. Whereas pharmacogenomics uses these tools to examine an individual's response to a drug, nutrigenomics is concerned with the individual's response to his or her nutritional environment.

The basic tools of recombinant DNA technology, such as cloning, PCR, and DNA sequencing, are used to create new combinations of DNA molecules and to identify each nucleotide building block of the DNA. These tools have been central to the success of the Human Genome Project in identifying the nature and order of the approximately 3 billion nucleotides in the human genome. In an equally important application, a DNA sequence containing a human gene can be excised, reproduced many times using PCR until a suitable amount of the gene is available, and then inserted into another organism. That organism may be a microorganism capable of serving as a factory for producing large quantities of a valuable molecule or a mammalian organism such as the laboratory mouse. An alternative is an in vitro system such as a tissue culture in which gene function and the regulation of gene expression can be studied. Each type of system has its utility. For example, in vitro systems are useful for studying the effect of bioactive dietary components on gene expression. An intact organism, such as the mouse model system, more closely simulates the human and is helpful in determining a gene's function.

One classical approach to studying the role of a gene in a metabolic process is to alter the gene and observe the effect. The mouse model system is particularly well suited to this approach. A human gene replaces the mouse version of that same gene at each of the two locations in the mouse genome. To determine the role of the gene in the phenotype of the mouse, both copies of the human gene are inactivated to create a "knockout mouse" and the effect on the phenotype of the mouse is observed.

Single nucleotide polymorphisms (SNPs) are useful as genetic markers and, as such, are helpful in predicting disease susceptibility and metabolic capability. Single changes in the nucleotide structure of DNA lead to variant forms, many of which are thought to predispose individuals to disease or alter their ability to metabolize particular substances, such as drugs, food, or environmental toxins. The vast majority of DNA is the same between individuals. The differences, which are the basis for phenotypic variation, are believed to be due to SNPs. These gene variants are quite stable from one generation to the next, so their transmission through multiple generations can be traced. When a change is shared by greater than 1% of the population, it becomes a common variant that's useful for diagnostic purposes. An SNP map of the human genome is being constructed, with over a million SNPs already identified.

DNA microarray technology allows an entire genome to be captured onto a single "chip," a glass plate the size of a microscope slide. The development of this technology has allowed researchers to move beyond one-gene-at-a-time experimentation to assessment of multiple genes at once. Important practical applications include the ability to identify the genes expressed in a particular tissue or at specific times during development or in response to an environmental signal. Microarrays have been useful in distinguishing different types of cancer that, on the surface, appear to be the same but are genetically distinct and respond to different therapies.

Nutrigenomics and Nutrition Therapy

As nutrigenomics research identifies the key players in diet-related disease and the details of their roles and interactions with one another, the expectation is that the approach to developing nutritional interventions will change significantly. Among the more significant contributions is increased effectiveness of interventions for the chronic diseases, such as coronary heart disease, hypertension, stroke, type 2 diabetes, cancer, inflammatory disorders, obesity, and osteoporosis. These diseases result from the interaction of multiple genes and multiple environmental factors. In most cases, neither the genes nor the environmental factors have yet been identified, making it particularly challenging to determine effective interventions.

As an example, the response of individuals with coronary heart disease to nutrition therapy is notoriously heterogeneous. In some the atherogenic profile responds positively to dietary fat manipulation, whereas in others there is no effect. In still others, the profile actually worsens in response to a diet low in saturated fat and cholesterol. At the other end of the spectrum are individuals for whom the fat content of the diet appears to be irrelevant to heart health. In an era of population-based dietary recommendations, these types of heterogeneous responses have been baffling and more than a little frustrating to practitioners. The response is variable at the population level but not at the individual level. Each individual has a reproducible response to diet, based on his or her genetic makeup.

Several genes have already been identified as contributing to the heterogeneity in responses to dietary fat manipulation. In an extensive examination of the literature relating serum lipid response to dietary intervention, Masson et al. found that variation in the genes that code for lipoproteins A-I, A-IV, B, and E leads to a variable dietary response to lipids. In particular, the presence of the A allele (variant) of apoA-I-75 caused a greater response in LDL levels compared to the G (normal) allele. In the apoA-IV gene, polymorphisms resulting in the substitution of histidine for glutamine at position 360 or of serine for threonine at position 347 had altered responses to the dietary fat manipulation. At least three variants of the apoB gene have been found to affect response to dietary fat: the R-allele of the apoB EcoRI polymorphism, the I-allele of the apoB signal peptide I/D polymorphism, and the XbaI X-allele. However, no consistent pattern has yet emerged. The impact of genetic variation in the apoE gene suggests that individuals with the E4 allele have the greatest response in total, LDL, and HDL cholesterol and those with the normal (E2) allele have the least response.

Nutrigenomics research will continue to identify the genes involved in coronary heart disease and the response of each genetic variant to dietary manipulation. This knowledge, coupled with knowledge of an individual's genetic makeup, will position the nutrition practitioner to develop interventions targeted to the specific needs of the individual. Such targeted therapy is expected to improve clinical outcomes for those in which coronary heart disease has already manifested. The even greater promise of nutrigenomics is the early identification of individuals at risk for developing heart disease and the ability to offer these individuals interventions that will prevent disease manifestation.

Nutrigenomics and Food Development

The identification of components in food that are capable of triggering signal transduction, changing gene expression, supplying needed metabolites, or otherwise modifying disease sets the stage for the development of functional foods containing bioactive components. Such foods can be used to minimize the impact of disease or, ultimately, to help prevent disease. Functional foods have no official definition in the United States but are generally considered to be those foods that have health benefits beyond the traditional nutrients they contain. Functional foods are eagerly anticipated for different stages of life, such as childhood development and menopause, and for the management and prevention of coronary heart disease, hypertension, stroke, diabetes, cancer, gastrointestinal disorders, obesity, and osteoporosis. Besides offering health benefits, the demand by consumers for functional foods or their isolated bioactive components can help growers diversify their crop offerings and also help create niche markets for high-value products.

A number of bioactive components have already been identified, but they're believed to be just a small proportion of the large number of bioactive components present in food. Examples include conjugated linolenic acid, docosapentaenoic acid, eicosapentaenoic acid, curcumin, genistein, ginger, lutein, lycopene, psyllium, stanols and sterols, sulforaphane, theanine, and various classes of compounds, such as catechins, flavonoids, fructooligosaccharides, gallic acids, isoflavones, lignans, saponins, terpenes, thiols, tocopherols, and tocotrienols. Research is under way to identify the health-promoting components and to develop products and crops that incorporate these components.

Preparation for Careers in Nutrigenomics

Common to all the applications of nutrigenomics is a solid foundation in biology, chemistry, genetics, nutrition, medicine, and food science. Critical thinking skills and an understanding of research study design and analysis are essential regardless of the particular specialty area of nutrigenomics a person might enter. Opportunities for nutrition professionals versed in genomics are expanding and promise to be an integral part of future nutrition practice in all its manifestations.

Resources

Ames BN, Elson-Schwab I, Silver EA. High-dose vitamin therapy stimulates variant enzymes with decreased coenzyme binding affinity (increased K_m): relevance to genetic disease and polymorphisms. Am J Clin Nutr 2002;75:616–58.

Clarke SD, Thuillier P, Baillie RA, Sha X. Peroxisome proliferator–activated receptors: a family of lipid-activated transcription factors. Am J Clin Nutr 1999;70:566–71.

DeBusk RM. Genetics: The Nutrition Connection. Chicago, IL: American Dietetic Association, 2002.

Elliott R, Ong TJ. Nutritional genomics. BMJ 2002;324: 1438–42.

Fogg-Johnson N, Kaput J. Nutrigenomics: an emerging scientific discipline. Food Technol 2003;57:60–67.

Guengerich FP. Functional genomics and proteomics applied to the study of nutritional metabolism. Nutr Rev 2001;59:259–63.

Kim YS, Milner JA. Nutritional genomics and proteomics in cancer prevention. J Nutr 2003;133(suppl).

King HC, Sinha AA. Gene expression profile analysis by DNA microarrays. JAMA 2001;286:2280–88.

Masson LF, McNeil G, Avenell A. Genetic variation and the lipid response to dietary intervention: a systematic review. Am J Clin Nutr 2003;77:1098–1111.

Müller M, Kersten S. Nutrigenomics: goals and strategies. Nat Rev Genet 2003;4:315–22.

Nabel EG. Cardiovascular disease. N Engl J Med 2003; 349:60–72.

NCMHD Center of Excellence for Nutritional Genomics, University of California at Davis. www.nutrigenomics-UCDavis.edu; accessed Nov. 13, 2003.

Simopoulos AP. Genetic variation and dietary response: utrigenetics/nutrigenomics. Asia Pacific J Clin Nutr 2002; 1:S117–S128.

Wargovich MJ, Cunningham JE. Diet, individual responsiveness and cancer prevention. J Nutr 2003;133: 2400S–2403S.

Wei LN. Retinoid receptors and their coregulators. Ann Rev Pharmacol Toxicol 2003;43:47–74.

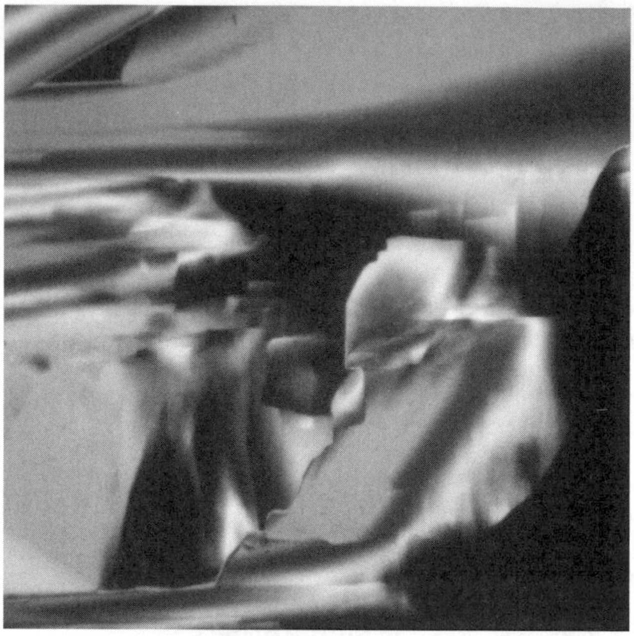

Polarized light micrograph of crystalline arginine

chapter 7 Protein

THE IMPORTANCE OF PROTEIN IN NUTRITION and health cannot be overemphasized. It is quite appropriate that the Greek word chosen as a name for this nutrient is *proteos*, meaning "primary" or "taking first place." Proteins are found throughout the body, with over 40% of body protein found in skeletal muscle, over 25% found in body organs, and the remaining found mostly in the skin and blood. Proteins are essential nutritionally because of their constituent amino acids, which the body must have in order to synthesize its own variety of proteins and nitrogen-containing molecules that make life possible. Each body protein is unique in the characteristics and pattern of sequencing of the amino acids that comprise its structure.

In a review of protein, an appropriate focus is the functional roles of various body proteins. Also needed is an examination of the digestion of protein and the subsequent absorption and metabolism of amino acids. Protein needs as they are affected by tissue protein synthesis and catabolism are addressed. Lastly, recommended intakes of protein and protein quality are reviewed.

FUNCTIONAL CATEGORIES

The molecular architecture and activity of living cells are largely dependent on proteins, which make up over half of the solid content of cells and which show great variability in size, shape, and physical properties. Their physiological roles also are quite variable, and because of this variability a categorization of proteins according to their functions can be helpful in the study of human metabolism. This type of categorization demonstrates the body's dependence on properly functioning proteins and provides a basis for understanding the significance of protein structure.

Enzymes

Enzymes are protein molecules (generally designated by the suffix *-ase*) that act as catalysts to change the rate of reactions occurring in the body. Enzymes are found both intracellularly and extracellularly, such as in the blood. Enzymes are frequently classified according to the type of reactions that they catalyze. For example:

- hydrolases cleave compounds;
- isomerases transfer atoms within a molecule;
- ligases (synthases) join compounds;
- oxidoreductases transfer electrons;
- transferases move functional groups.

Enzymes are necessary for sustaining life. They are constructed so that they combine selectively with other molecules (called substrates) in the cell. The active site on the enzyme (a small region usually in a crevice of the enzyme) is where the enzyme and substrate bind and the product is generated. Some enzymes, however, require a cofactor or coenzyme for carrying out the reaction. Minerals such as zinc, iron, and copper function as cofactors for some enzymes. B vitamins serve as coenzymes for many enzymes. Most human physiological processes require enzymes for promotion of chemical changes that could not otherwise occur. Some examples of physiological processes dependent on enzyme function include digestion, tissue energy production, blood coagulation, and excitability and contractibility of neuromuscular tissue. Additional information on enzymes (catalytic proteins) is found in Chapter 1.

Hormones

Hormones are chemical messengers that are synthesized and secreted by endocrine tissue (glands) and transported in the blood to target tissue(s) or organ(s), where they bind to protein receptors. Hormones generally regulate metabolic processes, for example, through promotion of the synthesis of enzymes or effects on enzyme activity.

Whereas some hormones are derived from cholesterol and classified as steroid hormones, others are derived from one or more amino acids. The amino acid tyrosine, for example, is used along with the mineral iodine for the synthesis of the thyroid hormones. Tyrosine is also used for the synthesis of the catecholamines, including dopamine, norepinephrine, and epinephrine. The hormone melatonin is derived in the brain from the amino acid tryptophan. Other hormones are made up of one or more polypeptide chains. Insulin, for example, consists of two polypeptide chains linked by a disulfide bridge. Glucagon, parathyroid hormone, and calcitonin each consist of a single polypeptide chain. There are many other peptide hormones, such as adrenocorticotropic hormone (ACTH), somatotropin (growth hormone), and vasopressin (also known as antidiuretic hormone, ADH), that have important roles in human metabolism and nutrition. These hormones are discussed throughout this chapter and the book.

Structural Proteins

Proteins with structural roles include

- the contractile proteins and
- the fibrous proteins.

The two main contractile proteins include actin and myosin, both found in muscles. Fibrous proteins include collagen, elastin, and keratin and are found in bone, teeth, skin, tendons, cartilage, blood vessels, hair, and nails. Collagen is a group of well-studied proteins. Each type of collagen is made of three polypeptide chains that are cross-linked for strength. The amino acid composition of the chains is high in the amino acids glycine and proline. In addition, collagen contains two amino acids—hydroxylysine and hydroxyproline—that are not found in other proteins. Collagen polypeptides are also attached to carbohydrate chains and thus are considered to be glycoproteins. Other structural proteins, such as elastin, are associated with proteoglycans. Both glycoproteins and proteoglycans are conjugated proteins and are discussed further in the section "Other Roles."

Immunoproteins

Immunoproteins may also be referred to as immunoglobulins (Ig) or antibodies (Ab). Immunoproteins, of which there are five major classes (IgG, IgA, IgM, IgE, and IgD), are Y-shaped proteins made of four polypeptide chains. The immunoglobulins are produced by plasma cells derived from B-lymphocytes, a type of white blood cell. Immunoglobulins function by binding to antigens and inactivating them. Antigens typically consist of foreign substances such as bacteria or viruses that have entered the body. By complexing with antigens, immunoglobulin-antigen complexes can be recognized and destroyed through reactions with either complement proteins or cytokines. The complement proteins (approximately 20) are produced primarily in the liver and circulate in the blood and extracellular fluid. Cytokines are produced by white blood cells such as T-helper (CD_4) cells and macrophages. In addition, white blood cells such as macrophages and neutrophils also destroy foreign antigens through the process of phagocytosis.

Transport Proteins

Transport proteins are a diverse group of proteins that combine with other substances in the blood or within cells to provide a mode of transport for those substances. Transport proteins in cell membranes, for example, carry and thus regulate the flow of nutrients into and out of cells. Some transport proteins that are found in blood and are of particular importance are

- albumin, which transports a variety of nutrients such as calcium, zinc, and vitamin B_6;
- transthyretin (formerly called prealbumin), which complexes with another protein, retinol-binding protein, for the transport of retinol (vitamin A);
- hemeproteins, iron-containing proteins that bind and/or transport oxygen;
- transferrin, an iron transport protein; and
- ceruloplasmin, a copper transport protein.

Albumin and transthyretin are discussed further in this chapter under the heading "Plasma Proteins" in the section "Amino Acid Metabolism." Hemeproteins such as hemoglobin and myoglobin, as well as the transport proteins transferrin and ceruloplasmin, are discussed in more detail in Chapter 12, "Microminerals," under the topics of iron and copper. Additional information on transport proteins is also found in Chapter 1.

Other Roles

Proteins, because of their constituent amino acids, can serve as a buffer in the body. A **buffer** is a compound that ameliorates a change in pH that would otherwise occur in response to the addition of alkali or acid to a solution. The pH of the blood and other body tissues must be maintained within an appropriate range. Blood pH ranges from about 7.35 to 7.45, whereas cellular pH levels are often more acidic. For example, the pH of red blood cells is about 7.2, and that of muscle cells is about 6.9. The H^+ concentration within cells is buffered by both the phosphate system and the amino acids in proteins. The protein hemoglobin, for example, functions as a buffer in red blood cells. In the plasma and extracellular fluid, proteins and the bicarbonate system serve as buffers. Amino acids act as acids or bases in aqueous solutions such as those in the body by releasing and accepting hydrogen ions, thereby contributing to the buffering capacity of proteins in the body. The buffering ability of proteins can be illustrated by the reaction H^+ + protein $\leftrightarrow$ Hprotein.

Conjugated proteins also play important and diverse roles in the body. Conjugated proteins are proteins that are conjugated (joined) to nonprotein components. Examples of some conjugated proteins include glycoproteins, proteoglycans, lipoproteins, flavoproteins, and metalloproteins.

- **Glycoproteins** consist of a protein covalently bound to a carbohydrate component. The carbohydrate in glycoproteins generally includes short chains of glucose, galactose, mannose, fucose, N-acetylglucosamine, N-acetylgalactosamine, and acetylneuraminic (sialic) acid, present at the terminal end of the oligosaccharide chain. The carbohydrate portion of the glycoprotein can make up as much as 85% of the weight of the glycoprotein. The carbohydrate component is bound typically through an N-glycosidic linkage with asparagine's amide group in its side chain or through an O-glycosidic linkage with the hydroxy group in serine's or threonine's side chain. Glycoproteins are found in body secretions such as mucus, connective tissue such as collagen and elastin, and bone matrix. In fact, the continuous secretion of mucus glycoproteins from the lungs and small intestine represents a constant drain on an individual's amino acid supplies, especially threonine. Many plasma proteins such as transthyretin and hormones such as thyrotropin are glycoproteins.
- **Proteoglycans** are macromolecules with proteins covalently conjugated via O-glycosidic or N-glycosylamine linkages to glycosaminoglycans (formerly called mucopolysaccharides). Glycosaminoglycans consist of long chains of repeating disaccharides and comprise up to 95% of the weight of the proteoglycan. Proteoglycans make up, in part, the extracellular matrix (ground substance) that surrounds many mammalian tissues or cells such as skin, bone, and cartilage. Examples of proteoglycans include hyaluronic acid, chondroitin sulfate, keratan sulfate, dermatan sulfate, and heparan sulfate.
- Lipoproteins consist of a hydrophobic core of lipids, including cholesterol and triglycerides, surrounded by phospholipids and a protein "coat." The proteins in the lipoproteins are actually a group of about 10 different apoproteins that enable transport of the lipid in the blood and help direct the lipoproteins to target cells for use by body tissues. There are four

main types of lipoproteins: chylomicrons, very low density, low-density, and high-density lipoproteins (discussed in detail in Chap. 6).

- Flavoproteins generally refer to protein enzymes bound to flavin mononucleotide (FMN) or flavin adenine nucleotide (FAD). Flavoproteins are discussed in more detail in Chapter 9 under the vitamin riboflavin, page 284.
- Metalloproteins, as their name implies, are proteins to which minerals are complexed. Some metalloproteins have enzymatic activity, and some serve as a transport or storage protein for the metal. Metalloproteins are discussed under each of the trace minerals (microminerals) presented throughout Chapter 12.

PROTEIN STRUCTURE AND ORGANIZATION

The functional role of protein is determined by its basic structure and organization. The primary, secondary, and tertiary structures of proteins illustrate their three key levels of organization. Some proteins have an additional fourth level of organization, the quaternary structure.

Primary Structure

The primary structure of a protein is the sequencing and strong covalent bonding of amino acids that occur as the polypeptide chain is synthesized on the ribosomes. The primary structure of a protein is shown in Figure 7.1. The various amino acids making up the polypeptide are labeled in sequence and represent the primary structure. The side chain of one amino acid differs from that of another amino acid, thus making each amino acid different. Polypeptide backbones do not differ between polypeptide chains. The side chains of the amino acids of the polypeptide chain or chains making up the total protein molecule account for the differences among proteins. Moreover, the side chains affect the coiling and folding of a protein on itself to (in effect) help determine the final form (structure) of the protein molecule.

Secondary Structure

The secondary structure of a protein is achieved through weaker bonding, such as hydrogen bonding, than the bonding that characterizes the primary structure. Weak repeating linkages between nearby amino acids account for this second level of protein organization.

One type of secondary structure of proteins is the α-helix, a cylindrical-like shape formed by a coiling of the polypeptide chain on itself, with interactions (H bonds between the hydrogen atom attached to the amide nitrogen and the carbonyl oxygen atom) occurring at every fourth peptide linkage (Fig. 7.2a). The side chains of the amino acids in the α-helix structure extend outward. Varying degrees of the α-helix appear in widely divergent proteins, depending on their function. In those regions where it occurs, the α-helix provides some rigidity to that portion of the molecule.

Another type of secondary protein structure is the β-conformation, or β-pleated sheet. In this structure, the polypeptide chain is fully stretched out, with the side chains positioned either up or down. The stretched polypeptide can fold back on itself with its segments packed together, as shown in Figure 7.2b. Both this structure and the α-helix are quite stable and provide strength and rigidity to proteins. These two secondary structures, α-helix and β-pleated sheet, are particularly abundant in proteins with structural roles, such as collagen, elastin, and keratin. Collagen, for example, is a triple helix composed of three long polypeptide α-chains. Each of the long polypeptide chains is "twisted" and covalently cross-linked within and between the triple helix units. The structure resembles a tough, rodlike structure.

The random coil is the third type of secondary structure (Fig. 7.2c). Little stability exists in this structure because of the presence of certain amino acids whose side chains interfere with one another.

Tertiary Structure

The third level of organization in proteins is the tertiary structure. Many proteins, including enzymes, transport proteins, and immunoproteins, exist in a tertiary

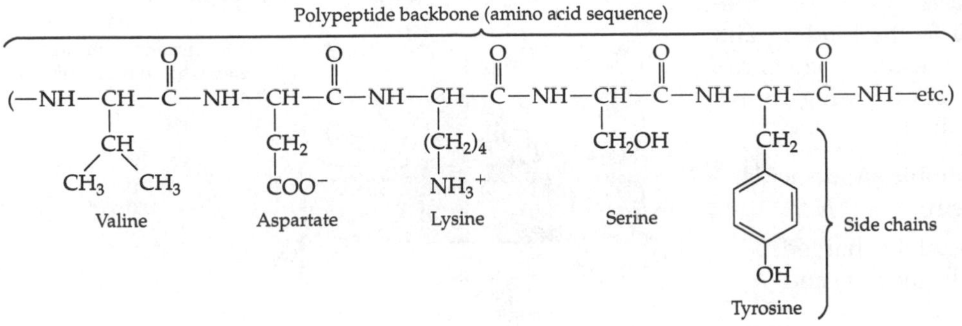

Figure 7.1 The primary structure of a protein.

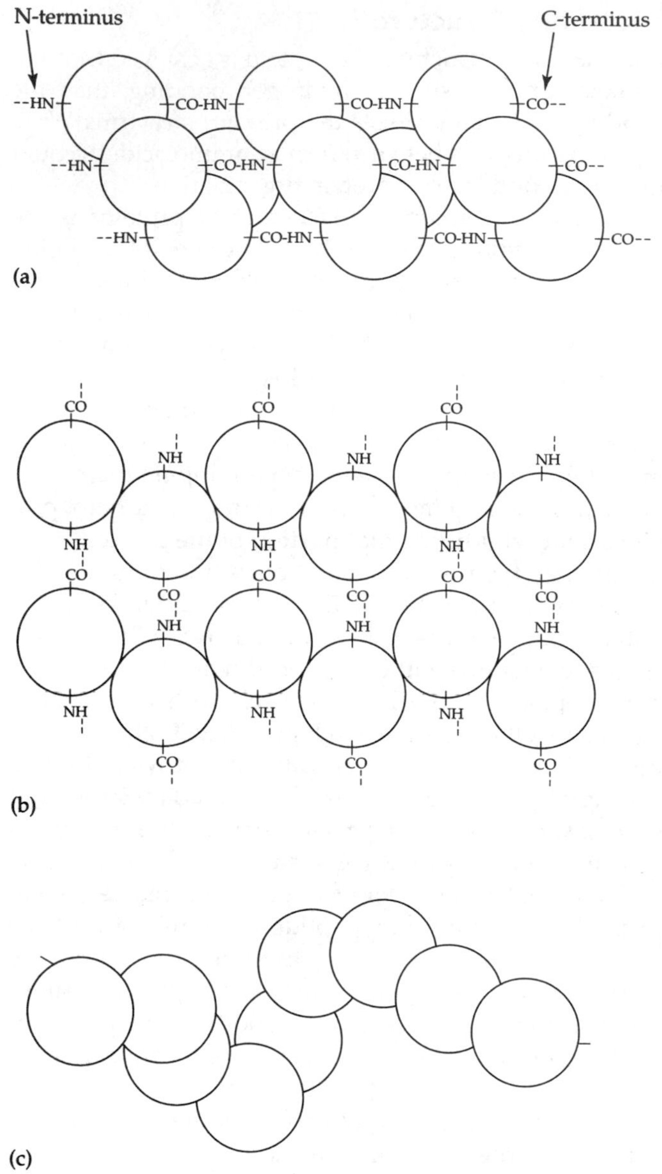

Figure 7.2 The secondary structure of proteins: (a) the α-helix, (b) the β-pleated sheet, and (c) the random coil.

structure in the body. This structure results from interactions among amino acid residues or side chains that are located at considerable linear distances from each other along the peptide chain. These interactions produce a globular-like structure due to the binding and looping of the protein molecule, the result of which can be seen in Figure 7.3. Interactions contributing to this third level of organization include the

- clustering together of hydrophobic amino acids toward the center of the protein;
- electrostatic attraction of oppositely charged amino acid residues, such as lysine ($^+1$) and glutamate ($^-1$); and

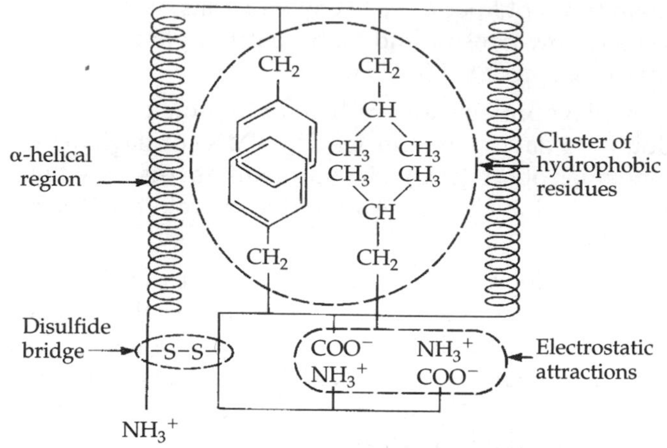

Figure 7.3 Tertiary structure of proteins.

- strong covalent bonding between cysteine residues where the —SH groups are oxidized to form disulfide bridges (—S—S—).

Other, weaker attractions among amino acid residues may also occur along the chain. Together, these interactions among the amino acid residues determine the protein's overall shape and, therefore, the particular function of the protein in the cell.

Quaternary Structure

The final level of protein organization, quaternary structure, involves anywhere from two to several polypeptide chains. Proteins with a quaternary structure most commonly are composed of either two or four polypeptide chains, and the aggregate formed is called an **oligomer.** The polypeptides making up the oligomer, commonly termed subunits, are held together by hydrogen bonds and electrostatic salt bridges or attractions. Oligomeric proteins are particularly important in intracellular regulation because the subunits can assume different spatial orientations relative to each other and in so doing change the properties of the oligomer. Hemoglobin (Fig. 7.4), an oligomer with four subunits, illustrates this point. Each subunit of hemoglobin

Figure 7.4 Quaternary structure of a protein.

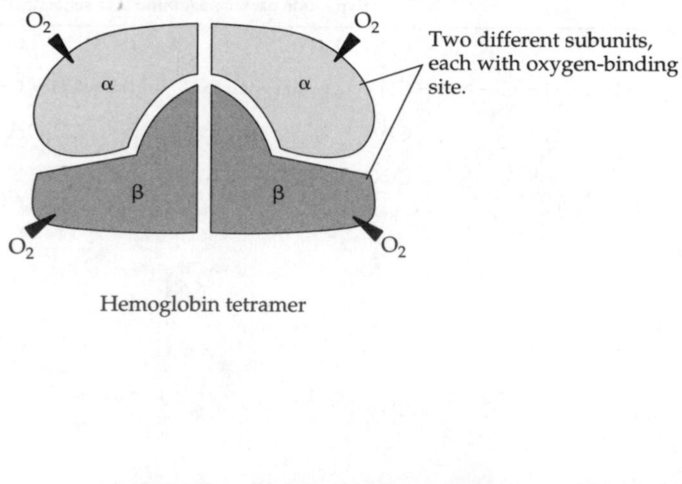

can bind 1 molecule of oxygen. Rather than acting independently, however, the subunits cooperate by conformational changes so as to enhance the affinity of hemoglobin for oxygen in the lungs and to increase its ability to unload oxygen in the peripheral tissues.

Other very important oligomers, such as regulatory enzymes, similarly undergo conformational changes on interaction with substrate molecules. In so doing, they enhance the formation of enzyme-substrate complexes whenever the concentration of substrate presented to the cell begins to increase or inhibit the formation of complexes when the substrate concentration falls to a low level.

AMINO ACID CLASSIFICATION

Amino acids may be classified in a variety of ways, including by structure, net charge, polarity, and essentiality. We will address each of these four classifications.

Structure

Structurally, all amino acids have a central carbon (C), at least one amino group ($-NH_2$), at least one carboxy (acid) group ($-COOH$), and a side chain (R group) that makes each amino acid unique. The generic amino acid may be represented as follows:

$$H_2N{-}\underset{\displaystyle R}{\underset{|}{CH}}{-}COOH$$

The distinctive characteristics of the side chains of the amino acids making up a polypeptide bestow on a protein its structure and consequently its functional role in the body. These same distinctive characteristics determine whether certain amino acids can be synthesized in the body or must be ingested. Furthermore, these characteristics program the various amino acids for their specific metabolic pathways in the body. The differences among the side chains of the amino acids commonly found in body proteins are shown in the structural classification of amino acids in Table 7.1. The division of amino acids based on structural similarities is one approach used for classification of amino acids. The division of amino acids based on the presence or absence of net charge is another classification system used for amino acids.

Net Electrical Charge

The amino acids listed in Table 7.1 and discussed here are shown based on their structures as they would exist in an aqueous solution at the physiological pH, approximately 6 to 8, of the human body. Amino acids in aqueous solution are ionized. The term **zwitterion** or dipolar ion is applied to amino acids with no carboxy or amino groups in their side chain to generate an additional charge to the molecule. Zwitterions have no net electrical charge because their side chains are not charged and the one positive and one negative charge from the amino and carboxy group, respectively, in their base structure cancel each other out. Amino acids with no net charge do not migrate substantially if placed in an electric field.

$$H_3N^+{-}\underset{\displaystyle R}{\underset{|}{CH}}{-}COO^-$$

Amino acids with neutral side chains (listed below) have no net electrical charge.

Neutral Amino Acids			
Alanine	Glycine	Methionine	Threonine
Asparagine	Hydroxylproline	Phenylalanine	Tryptophan
Cysteine	Isoleucine	Proline	Tyrosine
Glutamine	Leucine	Serine	Valine

Two groups of amino acids (listed below) exhibit a net charge. Because of the presence of additional carboxyl groups in the side chains, the dicarboxylic amino acids aspartic acid and glutamic acid exhibit a net negative charge. Amino acids or proteins with a high content of dicarboxylic amino acids exhibit a negative charge and will migrate toward the anode if placed in an electric field. In contrast, because of the presence of additional amino groups in their side chains, the basic amino acids, also called dibasic, (lysine, arginine, histidine, hydroxylysine) exhibit a net positive charge.

Negatively Charged Amino Acids	Positively Charged Amino Acids
Aspartic acid	Arginine
Glutamic acid	Histidine
	Hydroxylysine
	Lysine

Polarity

The tendency of an amino acid to interact with water at physiological pH—that is, its polarity—represents another means of classifying amino acids. Polarity is dependent on the side chain/R group of the amino acid. Amino acids are classified as polar or nonpolar, although they can have varying levels of polarity. Both the dicarboxylic (aspartic acid and glutamic acid) and basic (lysine, arginine, histidine, hydroxylysine) amino acids are polar; that is, they interact with water. The neutral amino acids interact with water to different

Table 7.1 Structural Classification of Amino Acids

1. *With aliphatic side chains*

Glycine (Gly)

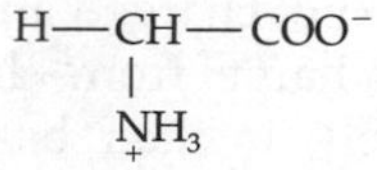

Alanine (Ala)

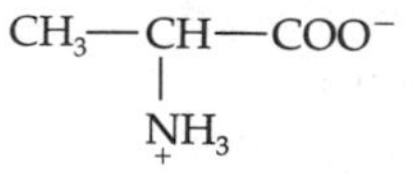

Valine (Val)

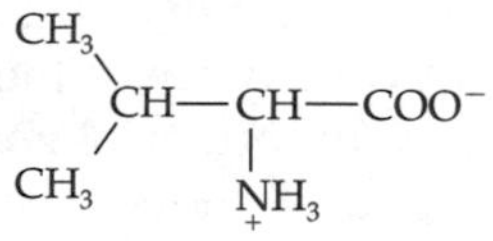

Leucine (Leu)

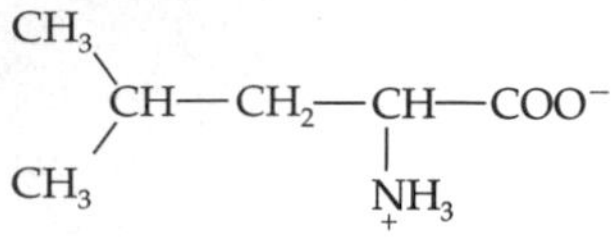

Isoleucine (Ile)

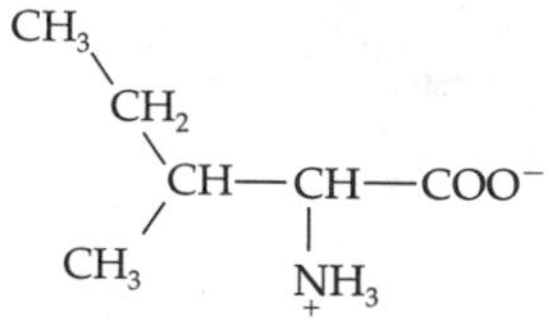

2. *With side chains containing hydroxylic (OH) groups**

Serine (Ser)

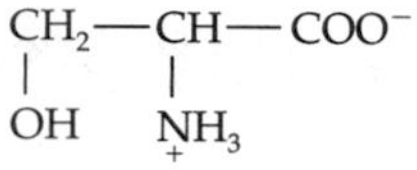

Threonine (Thr)

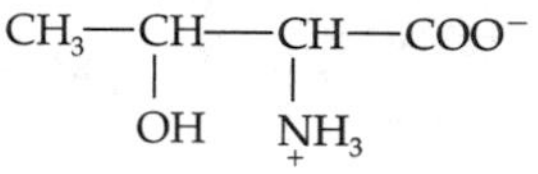

3. *With side chains containing sulfur atoms*

Cysteine (Cys)

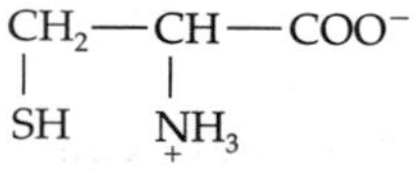

Methionine (Met)

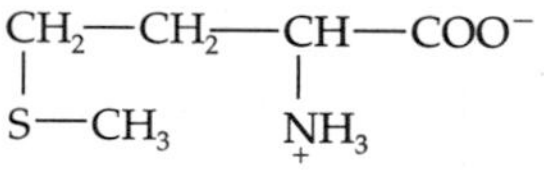

4. *With side chains containing acidic groups or their amides*

Aspartic acid (Asp)

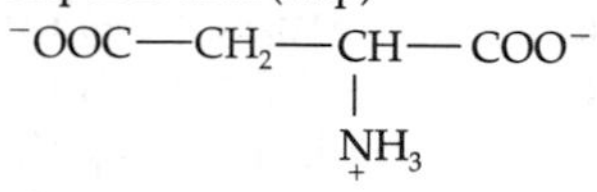

Glutamic acid (Glu)

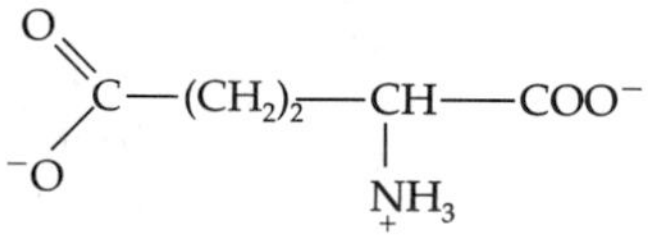

Asparagine (Asn)

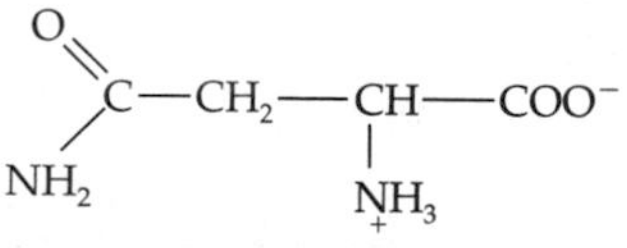

Glutamine (Gln)

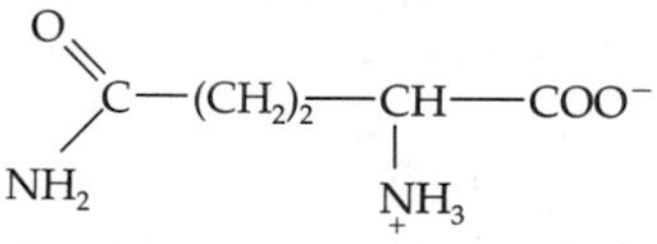

5. *With side chains containing basic groups*

Arginine (Arg)

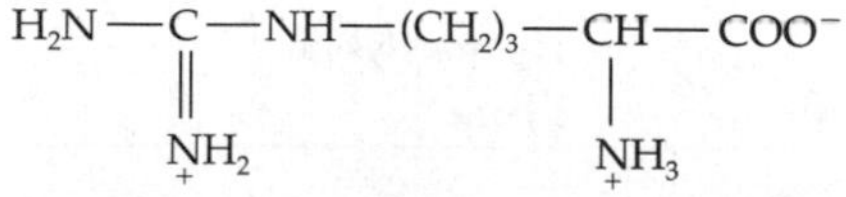

Lysine (Lys)

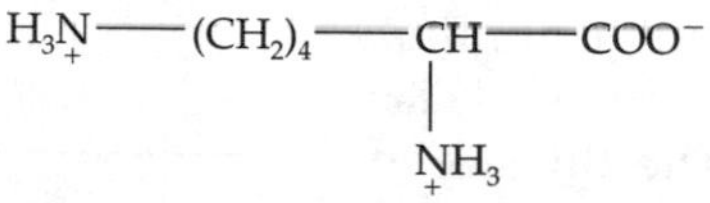

Histidine (His)

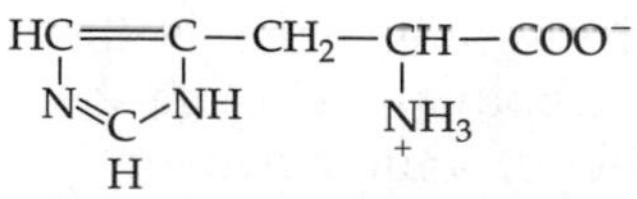

6. *With side chains containing aromatic ring*

Phenylalanine (Phe)

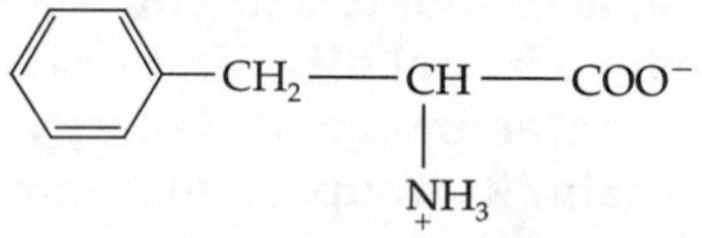

Tyrosine (Tyr)

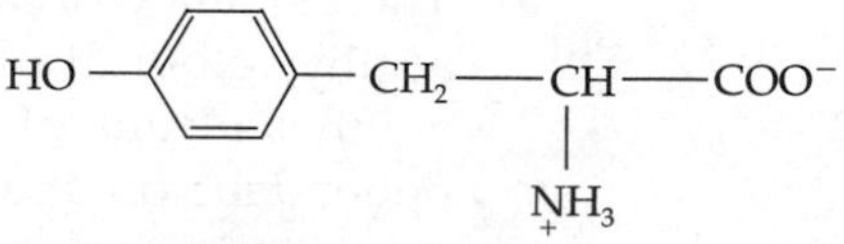

Tryptophan (Trp)

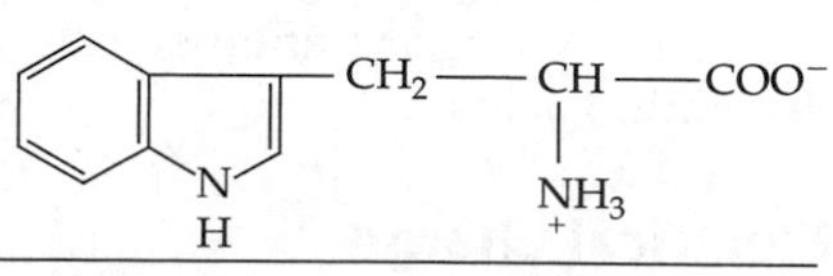

* Although tyrosine contains a hydroxyl group, it is classified as an amino acid containing an aromatic ring (see Group 6).

Table 7.1 *(Continued)*

7. *Imino acids*
Proline (Pro)

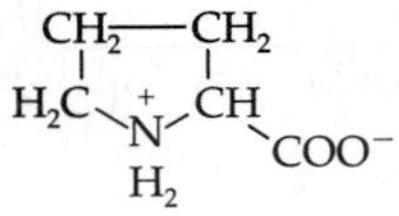

8. *Amino acids formed posttranslationally*
Cystine (Cys-S-S-Cys)

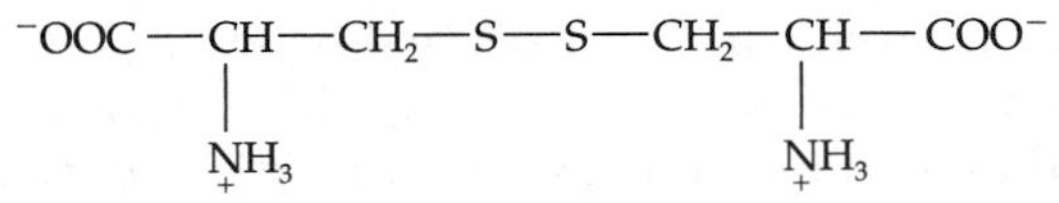

Hydroxylysine (Hyl)

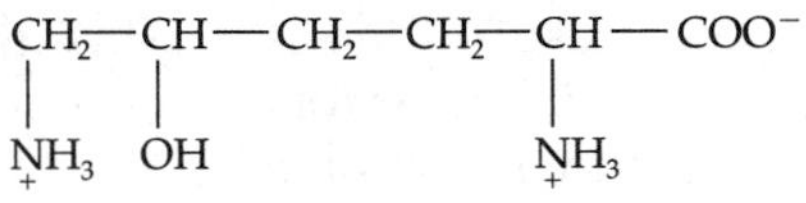

Hydroxyproline (Hyp)

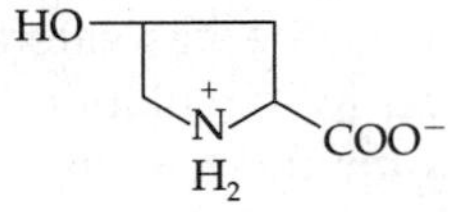

3-methylhistidine (3-meHis)

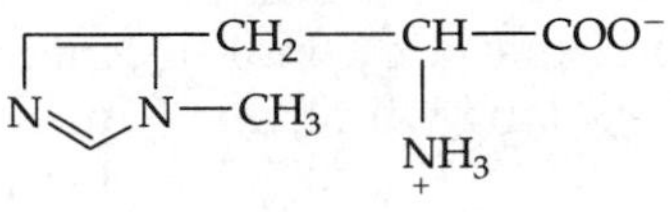

degrees and can be divided into polar, nonpolar, and relatively nonpolar categories, as listed below.

Polar Neutral Amino Acids	Nonpolar Neutral Amino Acids	Relatively Nonpolar Amino Acids
Asparagine	Alanine	Phenylalanine
Cysteine	Glycine	Tryptophan
Glutamine	Isoleucine	Tyrosine
Methionine	Leucine	
Serine	Proline	
Threonine	Valine	

The polar neutral amino acids contain functional groups in their side chains, such as the hydroxyl group for serine and threonine, the sulfur atom for cysteine and methionine, and the amide group for asparagine and glutamine, that can interact through hydrogen bonds with water; thus, we categorize them as polar. In contrast, the nonpolar amino acids listed in the second column above contain side chains that do not interact with water. Thus, these amino acids typically do not interact with water and are categorized as nonpolar or hydrophobic (water fearing). The aromatic amino acids are relatively nonpolar. Tyrosine for example, because of its hydroxyl group on the phenyl ring, can to a limited extent form hydrogen bonds with water—hence the term "relatively nonpolar."

Essentiality

While amino acids can be classified based on structure or properties such as net charge or polarity, in 1957 Rose [1] categorized the amino acids found in proteins as nutritionally essential (indispensable) or nutritionally nonessential (dispensable). At that time only eight amino acids—leucine, isoleucine, valine, lysine, tryptophan, threonine, methionine, and phenylalanine—were found to be essential for adult humans. Histidine was later added as an essential amino acid. We now know that if we give an α-keto or hydroxy acid of leucine, isoleucine, valine, tryptophan, methionine, or phenylalanine (as may be done with individuals with renal failure), the α-keto or hydroxy acid form of these amino acids can be transaminated to form the respective amino acid. Three amino acids—lysine, threonine, and histidine—cannot undergo transamination to any appreciable extent. Thus, lysine, threonine, and histidine are totally indispensable.

Identifying amino acids strictly as dispensable or indispensable, however, is an inflexible classification that allows no gradations, even in decidedly different and/or changing physiological circumstances. Newer categories added to the essential/indispensable and nonessential/dispensable categories include conditionally or acquired indispensable amino acids. A dispensable amino acid may become indispensable should an organ fail to function properly, as in the case of infants born prematurely or in the case of disease-associated organ malfunction. For example, neonates born prematurely often have immature organ function and are unable to synthesize many nonessential amino acids such as cysteine and proline. Immature liver function or liver malfunction due to cirrhosis, for example, impairs phenylalanine and methionine metabolism, which occurs primarily in the liver. Consequently, the amino acids tyrosine and cysteine normally synthesized from phenylalanine and methionine catabolism, respectively, become indispensable until normal organ function is established. Inborn errors of amino acid metabolism resulting from genetic disorders in which key enzymes in amino acid metabolism lack sufficient enzymatic activity illustrate another situation in which dispensable amino acids become indispensable. Individuals with classical phenylketonuria (PKU) exhibit little to no phenylalanine hydroxylase activity. This enzyme converts phenylalanine to tyrosine. Without hydroxylase activity, tyrosine is not synthesized in the body and must be provided completely by diet; thus, it is indispensable for this condition (PKU). In other inborn errors of metabolism, amino acids such as cysteine become indispensable. Thus, amino acids that normally are dispensable may become indispensable under certain physiological conditions. Amino acids that are conditionally indispensable are listed below, along with their usual amino acid precursors.

Conditionally Indispensable Amino Acids and Their Precursors

Amino Acid	Precursor(s)
Tyrosine	Phenylalanine
Cysteine	Methionine, serine
Proline	Glutamate
Arginine	Glutamine or glutamate, aspartate
Glutamine	Glutamate, ammonia

SOURCES OF PROTEIN

Ingested or exogenous proteins serve as sources of the essential amino acids and are the primary source of the additional nitrogen needed for the synthesis of the nonessential amino acids and nitrogen-containing compounds. Dietary or exogenous sources of protein include

- animal products such as meat, poultry, fish, and dairy products, with the exception of butter, sour cream, and cream cheese; and
- plant products such as grains, grain products, legumes, and vegetables.

A discussion of protein quality is found at the end of this chapter, page 218.

Endogenous proteins presented to the digestive tract represent another source of amino acids and nitrogen, and they mix with exogenous nitrogen sources [2]. Endogenous proteins include

- desquamated mucosal cells, which generate about 50 g of protein per day; and
- digestive enzymes and glycoproteins, which generate about 17 g of protein per day.

The digestive enzymes and glycoproteins are derived from digestive secretions of the salivary glands, stomach, intestine, biliary tract, and pancreas. Most of these endogenous proteins, which may total about 70 g or more per day, are digested and provide amino acids available for absorption. Digestion of protein and absorption of amino acids are crucial for optimal protein nutriture.

DIGESTION AND ABSORPTION

This section of the chapter focuses first on the digestion of protein in the digestive tract. Next, the mechanisms by which the end products of protein digestion are transported across the brush border membrane of the intestinal cell (absorption) are reviewed. From within the intestinal cell, amino acids must cross the basolateral membrane to gain access to the blood for circulation to tissues. Thus, the transport systems for the ferrying of amino acids across the basolateral membrane and other extraintestinal tissue membranes are presented. Lastly, because not all amino acids entering the intestinal cells get into the blood, the use of amino acids by the intestinal cells themselves is discussed.

Protein Digestion

Although macronutrient digestion was covered in Chapter 2, this chapter outlines digestion with respect solely to protein within the gastrointestinal tract organs.

Mouth and Esophagus

No appreciable digestion of protein occurs in the mouth or esophagus.

Stomach

The digestion of exogenous protein begins in the stomach, with the action of hydrochloric acid (HCl) in gastric juice. Hydrochloric acid release from gastric parietal (also called oxyntic) cells is stimulated by a variety of compounds, including the hormone gastrin, the neuropeptide gastrin-releasing peptide (GRP), the neurotransmitter acetylcholine, and the amine histamine. Hydrochloric acid denatures (disrupts) the quaternary, tertiary, and secondary structures of protein and begins the activation of pepsinogen to pepsin, which is secreted by gastric chief cells. Denaturants such as hydrochloric acid break apart hydrogen and electrostatic bonds to "unfold or uncoil" the protein; peptide bonds, however, are not affected by the hydrochloric acid. Pepsin, once formed, is catalytic against pepsinogen as well as other proteins.

$$\text{Pepsinogen} \xrightarrow{\text{HCl}} \text{Pepsin}$$

Pepsin functions as an endopeptidase at a pH $<\sim 3.5$ to hydrolyze peptide bonds in proteins or polypeptides.

Pepsin attacks peptide bonds adjacent to the carboxyl end of a relatively wide variety of amino acids (i.e., pepsin has low specificity), including leucine; methionine; aromatic amino acids consisting of phenylalanine, tyrosine, and tryptophan; and the dicarboxylic amino acids glutamate and aspartate. The end products of gastric protein digestion with pepsin include primarily large polypeptides along with some oligopeptides and free amino acids. These end products in an acid chyme are emptied through the pyloric sphincter into the duodenum (the proximal or upper part of the small intestine) for further digestion.

Small Intestine

The end products in the acid chyme that are delivered into the duodenum further serve to stimulate the release of regulatory hormones/peptides such as secretin and cholecystokinin (CCK) from the mucosal endocrine cells. Secretin and CCK are carried by the blood to the pancreas, where the acinar cells are stimulated to secrete alkaline pancreatic juice containing bicarbonate, electrolytes, water, and digestive proenzymes/zymogens. In addition to pancreatic juice, the Brunner's glands of the small intestine release mucus-rich secretions.

Digestive proenzymes/zymogens secreted by the pancreas, and further responsible for protein and polypeptide digestion, include

- trypsinogen,
- chymotrypsinogen,
- procarboxypeptidases A and B,
- proelastase, and
- collagenase.

Within the small intestine, these inactive zymogens must be chemically altered to be converted into their respective active enzymes capable of substrate hydrolysis. The following reactions occur in the small intestine to activate the zymogens:

$$\text{Trypsinogen} \xrightarrow{\text{Enteropeptidase}} \text{Trypsin}$$

Enteropeptidase (an endopeptidase formerly known as enterokinase) is secreted from the intestinal brush border in response to CCK and secretin. Once trypsin is formed, it can act on more trypsinogen as well as on chymotrypsinogen to yield active proteolytic enzymes.

$$\text{Trypsinogen} \xrightarrow{\text{Trypsin}} \text{Trypsin}$$

$$\text{Chymotrypsinogen} \xrightarrow{\text{Trypsin}} \text{Chymotrypsin}$$

Trypsin and chymotrypsin are both endopeptidases. Trypsin is specific for peptide bonds adjacent to basic amino acids (lysine and arginine). Excess free trypsin generated from trypsinogen also acts by negative feedback to inhibit pancreatic cell trypsinogen synthesis, thereby regulating pancreatic zymogen secretion [2]. Chymotrypsin is specific for peptide bonds adjacent to aromatic amino acids (phenylalanine, tyrosine, and tryptophan), as well as for methionine, asparagine, and histidine.

Both elastase, an endopeptidase derived from proelastase, and collagenase hydrolyze polypeptides into smaller fragments such as oligopeptides and tripeptides. Procarboxypeptidases are converted to carboxypeptidases by trypsin and serve as exopeptidases.

$$\text{Procarboxypeptidases} \xrightarrow{\text{Trypsin}} \text{Carboxypeptidases}$$

These exopeptidases attack peptide bonds at the C-terminal end of polypeptides to release free amino acids. Carboxypeptidases are zinc-dependent enzymes, specifically requiring zinc at the active site. Carboxypeptidase A hydrolyzes peptides with C-terminal aromatic neutral or aliphatic neutral amino acids. Carboxypeptidase B cleaves basic amino acids from the C-terminal end, generating free basic amino acids as end products.

Several peptidases are produced by the brush border of the small intestine, including the ileum, enabling peptide digestion and amino acid absorption to occur in the distal small intestine. Some of these peptidases include

- aminopeptidases, which vary in specificity and cleave amino acids from the N-terminal end of oligopeptides;
- dipeptidylaminopeptidases, some of which are magnesium-dependent and hydrolyze N-terminal amino acids from dipeptides; and
- tripeptidases, which are specific for selected amino acids and hydrolyze tripeptides to yield a dipeptide and a free amino acid.

Some tripeptides, such as trileucine, undergo brush border hydrolysis, whereas other tripeptides, such as triglycine or proline-containing peptides, are absorbed intact and hydrolyzed within the intestinal cell. Amino acids (an end product of protein digestion) have also been shown to inhibit the activity of brush border peptidases (end product inhibition). Table 7.2 outlines the process of protein digestion, which yields two main end products: peptides, principally dipeptides and tripeptides, and free

Table 7.2 Some Enzymes Responsible for the Digestion of Protein

Zymogen	Enzyme or Activator	Enzyme	Site of Activity	Substrate (peptide bonds adjacent to)
Pepsinogen	HCl or pepsin ⟶	Pepsin	Stomach	Most amino acids, including aromatic, dicarboxylic, leu, met
Trypsinogen	Enteropeptidase ⟶ or Trypsin	Trypsin	Intestine	Basic amino acids
Chymotrypsinogen	Trypsin ⟶	Chymotrypsin	Intestine	Aromatic amino acids, met, asn, his
Procarboxypeptidases	Trypsin ⟶	Carboxypeptidase	Intestine	
		A		C-terminal neutral amino acids
		B		C-terminal basic amino acids
		Aminopeptidases	Intestine	N-terminal amino acids

amino acids. To be utilized by the body, these end products must now be absorbed across the brush border of the intestinal epithelial mucosal cells (also called enterocytes).

Intestinal Brush Border Membrane Amino Acid and Peptide Absorption

Absorption represents the passage of a substance (such as an amino acid or peptide) from the lumen of the gastrointestinal tract, most often the intestine, across the brush border membrane of the intestinal cell and into the cell. This section addresses the mechanisms by which amino acids and peptides are absorbed into intestinal cells.

Amino Acid Transport

Amino acid absorption, shown in generic fashion without the roles of sodium and pump systems in Figure 7.5, occurs along the entire small intestine, but sites of maximal absorption of peptides and their component amino acids differ. In general, most amino acids are absorbed in the proximal (upper) small intestine.

Figure 7.5 Amino acid absorption: a generic diagram without showing the roles of sodium and pump systems.

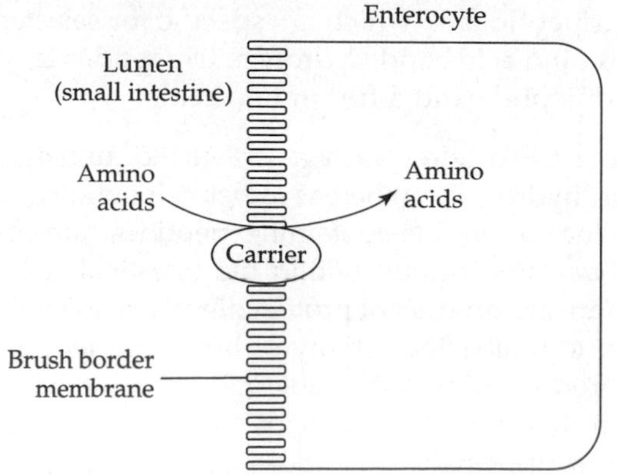

Multiple energy-dependent (requiring ATP hydrolysis) transport systems with overlapping specificity for amino acids have been demonstrated in the intestinal brush border [3]. Both sodium-dependent and sodium-independent transport systems exist. Figure 7.6 represents a schematic of sodium-dependent amino acid transport, which can be broken down into five stages [4]:

1. Sodium binds to the carrier.
2. This binding of sodium appears to increase the affinity of the carrier for the amino acid, which then binds to the carrier.
3. Next, a sodium–amino acid–cotransporter complex forms.
4. A conformational change in the complex results in the delivery of the sodium and amino acid into the cytoplasm of the enterocyte.
5. Lastly, sodium is pumped out of the cell by Na1/K1 -ATPase.

However, for the transport of some amino acids, steps 1 and 2 may be reversed; that is, the binding of the amino acid may precede the binding of the sodium.

Carrier systems are thought to be present in enterocytes for the basic amino acids lysine and arginine plus cystine and ornithine, the dicarboxylic amino acids aspartate and glutamate, as well as the neutral amino acids. In fact, several neutral transport systems are thought to exist in the brush border of the intestine.

Transport systems for amino acids are designated using a lettering system with a further distinction that uppercase letters be used for sodium dependence and lowercase letters for sodium independence [5]; however, not all systems (e.g., the L, which is sodium-independent) follow this rule. Most amino acids are thought to be transported across the brush border by sodium-dependent

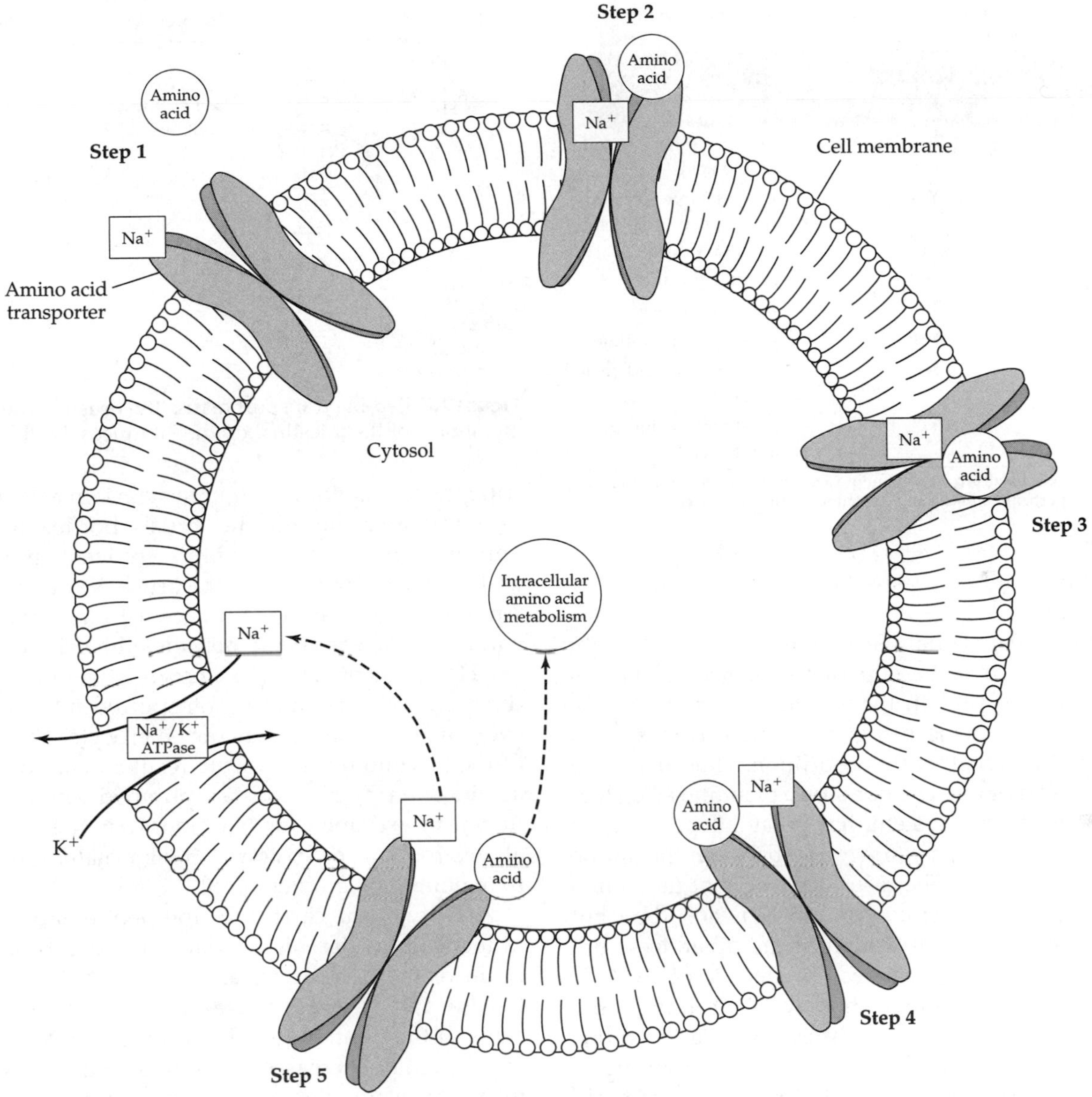

Figure 7.6 Conceptual schematic of a membrane-bound sodium(Na^+)-dependent amino acid carrier (transporter).

transporters, which include the B, IMINO, X^-_{AG} and $B^{o,+}$ system transporters. Table 7.3 lists some of the sodium-dependent and -independent transport systems responsible for carrying amino acids across the brush border into the intestinal cell and some examples of amino acids that are carried by each of these transport systems. Not all systems, however, have been identified in humans.

Competition between amino acids for transport by a common carrier has been documented. In addition, regulation (both induced de novo synthesis of specific amino acid carriers and decreased carrier synthesis) of transport carriers has been shown and helps to ensure adequate capacity [3].

The affinity (K_m) of a carrier for an amino acid is influenced both by the hydrocarbon mass of the amino acid's side chain and by the net electrical charge of the amino acid. As the hydrocarbon mass of the side chain increases, affinity increases [6]. Thus, the branched-chain amino acids typically are absorbed faster than smaller amino acids. Neutral amino acids also tend to be absorbed at higher rates than dibasic (basic) or dicarboxylic (acidic) amino acids. Essential amino acids are absorbed faster than nonessential amino acids, with methionine, leucine, isoleucine, and valine being the most rapidly absorbed [6]. The most slowly absorbed amino acids are the two dicarboxylic (acidic) amino

Table 7.3 Some Systems Transporting Amino Acids across the Intestinal Cell Brush Border Membrane

Amino Acid Transport Systems	Sodium Required	Examples of Substrates Carried
L	No	Leucine, other neutral amino acids
B	Yes	Phenylalanine, tyrosine, tryptophan, isoleucine, leucine, valine
IMINO	Yes	Proline, glycine
y^{+}*	No	Basic amino acids
X^{-}_{AG}	Yes	Aspartate, glutamate
$B^{o,+}$	Yes	Most neutral and basic amino acids
$b^{o,+}$	No	Most neutral and basic amino acids

*In the presence of sodium, neutral amino acids can competitively inhibit the y^{+} system and participate in exchange reactions with the basic substrates [3].

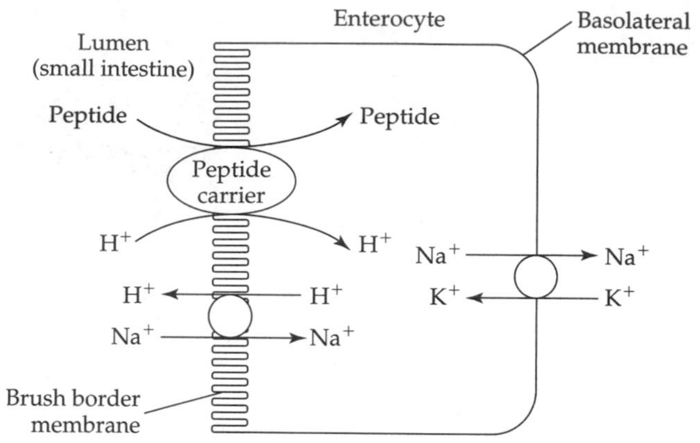

Figure 7.7 Peptide transport across the brush border membrane of the intestinal epithelial mucosal cell.

acids, glutamate and aspartate, both of which are nonessential [6].

Ingesting free, crystalline L-amino acids is thought by many athletes to be superior to ingesting natural foods containing protein for muscle protein synthesis. However, amino acids using the same carrier system compete with each other for absorption. Thus, ingesting one amino acid or a particular group of amino acids that use the same carrier system may create, depending on the amount ingested, a competition between the amino acids for absorption. The result may be that the amino acid present in highest concentration is absorbed but also may impair the absorption of the other, less concentrated amino acids carried by that same system. Thus, amino acid supplements may result in impaired or imbalanced amino acid absorption. Furthermore, absorption of peptides (which are obtained from digestion of natural protein-containing foods) is more rapid than absorption of an equivalent mixture of free amino acids. Also, nitrogen assimilation following ingestion of protein-containing foods is superior to that following ingestion of free amino acids. In other words, free amino acids have no absorptive advantage. Moreover, the supplements are usually expensive, typically taste terrible, and may cause gastrointestinal distress.

Peptide Transport

Peptide (primarily dipeptide and tripeptide) transport across the brush border membrane of the enterocyte occurs by transport systems different from those that transport amino acids. The number of transport systems for peptides has not been determined, but peptides appear to be absorbed more rapidly than free amino acids. Sodium has been shown to be required for one of the carrier systems that transports both dipeptides and tripeptides, but not for other systems. In addition, peptide transport across the brush border membrane appears to be associated with the movement of protons and thus depolarization of the brush border membrane. An area of low pH lying adjacent to the brush border surface of the enterocyte provides the driving force for the H^{+} gradient. Thus, as shown in Figure 7.7, as the dipeptide or tripeptide is transported into the enterocyte, an H^{+} ion also enters the enterocyte. The transport of the H^{+} into the enterocyte results in an intracellular acidification. The H^{+} ions are pumped back out into the lumen in exchange for Na^{+} ions. An Na^{+}/K^{+}-ATPase allows for Na^{+} extrusion at the basolateral membrane to maintain the gradient [7,8].

Affinity of the carrier for the peptide appears to be influenced by stereoisomerism, the length of the side chain of the N-terminal amino acid, substitutions on the N- and C-terminals, and the number of amino acids in the peptide [9,10]. For example, as the length of the peptide increases above three amino acids, affinity for transport decreases. In addition, peptides, like amino acids, compete with one another for transporters.

Peptide transport is thought to represent the primary system for amino acid absorption. Sixty-seven percent of amino acids are absorbed in the form of small peptides, with the remaining 33% absorbed as free amino acids [11]. Peptides, once within the enterocytes, are hydrolyzed by cytoplasmic peptidases to generate free intracellular amino acids.

Intestinal Basolateral Membrane Transport of Amino Acids

The transport of the amino acids across the basolateral membrane of the enterocyte (Fig. 7.8) into the interstitial fluid appears to be the same as the transport of amino acids across the membrane of nonepithelial cells. Diffusion and sodium-independent transport

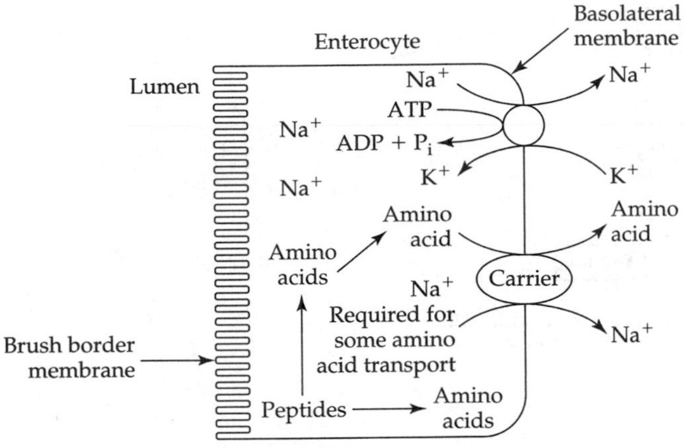

Figure 7.8 Amino acid transport across the basolateral membrane of the intestinal mucosal cell.

Table 7.4. Some Systems Transporting Amino Acids across the Intestinal Cell Basolateral Membrane

Amino Acid Transport System	Sodium Required	Examples of Substrates Carried
L	No	Leucine, other neutral amino acids
y^+	No	Basic amino acids
$b^{o,+}$	No	Neutral and basic amino acids
X^-_{AG}	Yes	Aspartate and glutamate
A	Yes	Alanine, other short-chain, polar, neutral amino acids
ASC	Yes	Alanine, cysteine, serine, other three- and four-carbon amino acids
asc	No	Same substrates as ASC

are thought to be the primary modes of amino acid transport across the basolateral membrane of the enterocyte. Sodium-dependent pathways are quantitatively important when the amino acid concentrations in the gut lumen are low. Active transport of amino acids into the enterocytes is necessary to provide the enterocyte with amino acids to meet its own needs. Some of the basolateral transport systems include those listed in Table 7.4.

Intestinal Cell Amino Acid Use

Although the preceding sections have covered amino acid absorption across the brush border and basolateral membranes, it must be remembered that not all amino acids are transported out of the intestinal cell and into circulation. Many of the amino acids absorbed following protein digestion are used along the villus for protein synthesis. Within the intestinal cell, amino acids may be used for energy or for synthesis of compounds such as

- apoproteins necessary for lipoprotein formation,
- new digestive enzymes,
- hormones, or
- nitrogen-containing compounds.

In addition, amino acids may be partially metabolized either to other amino acids or to other compounds that may be released into portal blood.

Glutamine, for example, is utilized in several ways by the intestinal cell (Fig. 7.9). It is used extensively by intestinal cells as a primary source of energy and has been shown to have trophic (growth) effects, such as stimulating cell proliferation, on the gastrointestinal mucosa cells [12,13]. In addition, glutamine has been shown to enhance the synthesis of heat shock proteins. These roles of glutamine in the gastrointestinal tract have prompted several companies to enrich enteral nutrition products with glutamine. Glutamine is also being added to parenteral (intravenous) nutritional mixtures and used for hospitalized patients. When glutamine is fed through tube feedings, over 50% of glutamine is extracted by the splanchnic (visceral) bed. In addition to dietary glutamine, much of the body's glutamine is produced by the lungs and skeletal muscles and then released and taken up mostly by the intestinal cells. Glutamine not used for energy production within the intestine also may be partially catabolized to generate ammonia and glutamate [14]. Ammonia enters the portal blood for uptake by the liver or may be used within the intestinal cell for carbamoyl phosphate synthesis. Glutamate may undergo transamination in which its amino group is removed and α-ketoglutarate, an intermediate in the Krebs cycle, remains. The amino group is transferred to the compound pyruvate (which is present in the intestinal cell from glucose metabolism) to form the amino acid alanine, as shown below.

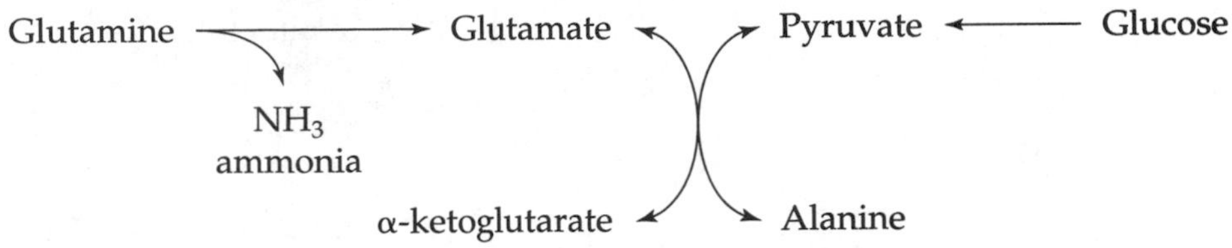

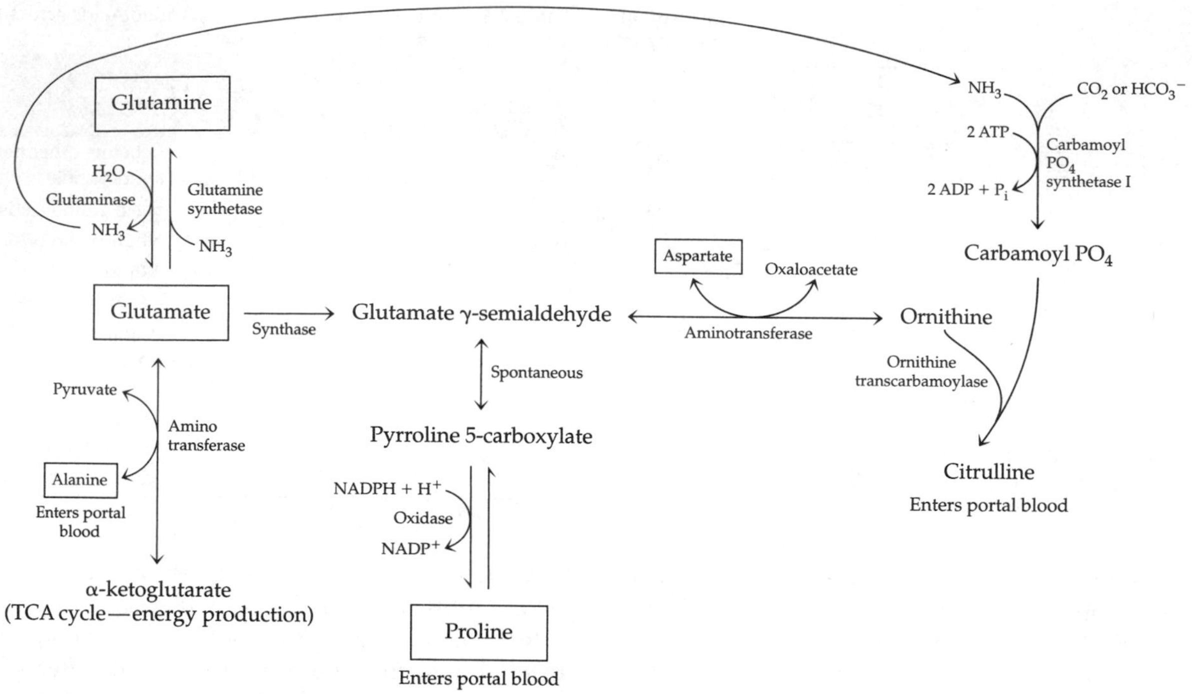

Figure 7.9 A partial overview of amino acid metabolism in the intestinal cell.

Once formed, alanine leaves the intestinal cell, enters portal blood, and subsequently is taken up along with ammonia by periportal hepatocytes. The periportal hepatocytes funnel the ammonia into urea synthesis.

Glutamate (in the intestinal cell) not used for alanine synthesis can be used in the intestinal cell to synthesize proline, as shown in Figure 7.9 and in these reactions:

Glutamate ⟶ Glutamate γ-semialdehyde
⟶ Pyrroline 5-carboxylate ⟶ Proline

Proline is then released into portal blood for delivery to the liver. Glutamate not used for proline synthesis may be used to synthesize ornithine, which in turn may be released into portal blood or can be used to make citrulline (Fig. 7.9).

Glutathione (a tripeptide) can be made in the enterocyte from glutamate and two other amino acids, glycine and cysteine (Fig. 7.10) [15]. Glutathione functions with the selenium-dependent enzyme glutathione peroxidase to destroy lipid peroxides (LOOH) and hydrogen peroxides (H_2O_2). Glutathione also can reduce reactive oxygen species (e.g., $O_2\cdot$ and $OH\cdot$) in the intestinal cell. Unless these reactive species are destroyed, they can damage cellular DNA, proteins, and polyunsaturated fatty acids in intestinal cell membranes to cause membrane peroxidation and cell necrosis (death). Glutathione is discussed in more detail later in the chapter on page 189 and in Chapter 12 under selenium. In addition, the perspective at the end of Chapter 10 provides a discussion of glutathione and other cell antioxidant systems.

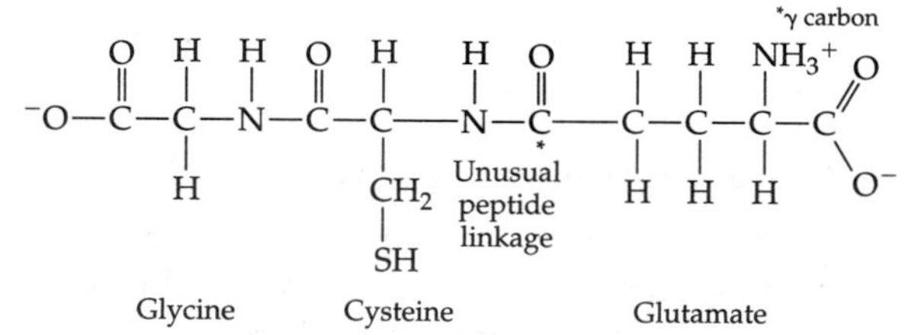

Figure 7.10 The structure of reduced glutathione (GSH).

In addition to metabolism of glutamine and glutamate, metabolism of aspartate from the diet generally occurs within intestinal cells. Aspartate most often undergoes transamination with α-ketoglutarate or pyruvate to generate oxaloacetate and either glutamate or alanine, respectively.

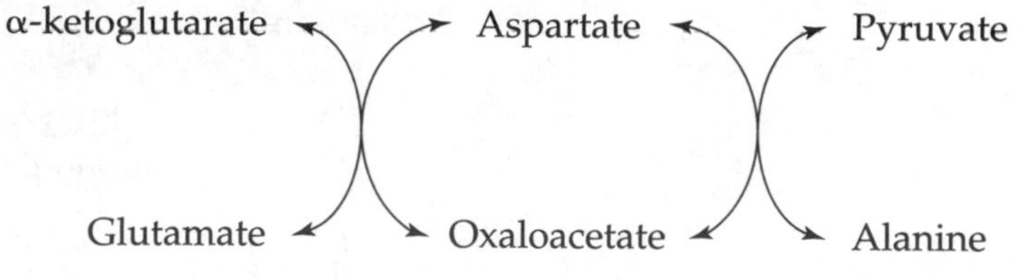

Along with amino acid catabolism and synthesis, two enzymes (carbamoyl phosphate synthetase I and ornithine transcarbamoylase) and possibly all five enzymes of the urea cycle are present in intestinal cells [16]. Carbamoyl phosphate synthetase I catalyzes the synthesis of carbamoyl phosphate from NH_3 (ammonia), bicarbonate (HCO_3^-), and ATP in mucosal epithelial cells, as shown in Figure 7.9 and here:

$$NH_3 + HCO^{2}_{3} + ATP \longrightarrow \text{Carbamoyl phosphate}$$

Ornithine transcarbamoylase synthesizes citrulline from ornithine and carbamoyl phosphate as follows:

$$\text{Carbamoyl phosphate} + \text{Ornithine} \longrightarrow \text{Citrulline}$$

Citrulline, once made, is released into blood and then typically taken up by the kidney, which has a high capacity for arginine synthesis.

Amino Acid Absorption into Extraintestinal Tissues

Amino acids not used by the intestinal cell are transported across the basolateral membrane of the enterocyte into interstitial fluid, where they enter the capillaries of the villi and eventually the portal vein for transport to the liver. Most peptides that have been absorbed intact into the intestinal cell undergo hydrolysis by proteases present within the cytoplasm of the enterocyte. Thus, primarily free amino acids are found in portal circulation. Occasionally, however, small oligopeptides can be found in splanchnic circulation and are thought to have entered circulation by paracellular or intercellular routes—that is, by passing through tight junctions of mucosal cells or by transcellular endocytosis [17]. The ability to administer peptides that can be used by body tissues directly into the blood (parenteral nutrition) is of nutritional significance in many clinical conditions in which amino acids (e.g., tyrosine, cysteine, and glutamine) need to be provided but cannot easily be given in an oral/enteral capacity because they are insoluble or unstable in their free form. The ability to provide these insoluble or unstable amino acids in peptide form that can be utilized by tissue would allow nutrient provision in situations in which traditional free amino acid parenteral mixtures are ineffective.

Hydrolysis of peptides is thought to occur by peptidases or proteases in the plasma, at the cell membrane (especially the liver, kidney, and muscle), or intracellularly in the cytosol or various organelles following transport as an intact peptide [9,17,18]. Peptide transport in renal tubular cells, for example, has been demonstrated and is influenced by molecular structure and the **lipophilicity** (hydrophobicity) of the amino acids at both the N- and the C-terminal of the peptide [19,20]. Peptides with either basic or acidic amino acids at either the N- or C-terminal have lower affinity for transport than peptides with neutrally charged side chains at these positions.

Amino acid transport into liver cells (hepatocytes) occurs by some carrier systems similar to those within the intestinal basolateral membrane. Additional systems, however, also transport amino acids into the liver. The sodium-dependent N system transports glutamine and histidine into hepatocytes [3]. Hormones and cytokines, such as interleukin-1 and tumor necrosis factor alpha, have been shown to influence amino acid transport. System A in hepatocytes, for example, is induced by glucagon [3] and provides amino acid substrates for gluconeogenesis. System Gly is sodium-dependent and specific for glycine; two sodium ions are transported for each glycine. Extrahepatic tissues such as the kidneys are also thought to transport amino acids by systems similar to those described for the intestinal basolateral membrane. However, an additional system, the γ-glutamyl cycle, is thought to be important in transporting amino acids through membranes of renal tubular cells, erythrocytes, and perhaps neurons.

In the γ-glutamyl cycle, glutathione acts as a carrier of selected neutral amino acids into cells. Glutathione, found in most cells of the body, is a tripeptide consisting of glycine, cysteine, and glutamate. As shown in Figure 7.10, an unusual peptide linkage occurs in glutathione between the γ-carboxyl group of glutamate and the α-amino group of cysteine. In the γ-glutamyl cycle (Fig. 7.11), glutathione in its reduced form reacts with γ-glutamyl transpeptidase located in cell membranes to form a γ-glutamyl enzyme complex. The glutamate part of the glutathione molecule remains with the enzyme complex, while cysteinylglycine is released into the cell cytoplasm and eventually cleaved into its constituent amino acids by a cytosolic peptidase. The γ-glutamyl enzyme complex functions by binding to a neutral amino acid at the cell surface and carrying it via a γ-carboxyl peptide linkage into the cell. Within the cell, γ-glutamyl cyclotransferase can cleave the peptide bond between the neutral amino acid and the γ-carbon of glutamate. Glutathione is resynthesized within the cell from cysteine, glutamate, and glycine in a series of energy-dependent reactions. The neutral amino acid that has just been released within the cell may function in the synthesis of new proteins or nitrogen-containing molecules or may be catabolized.

AMINO ACID METABOLISM

The liver is the primary site for the uptake of most (about 50%–65%) amino acids following ingestion of a meal. The liver is thought to monitor the absorbed amino acids and

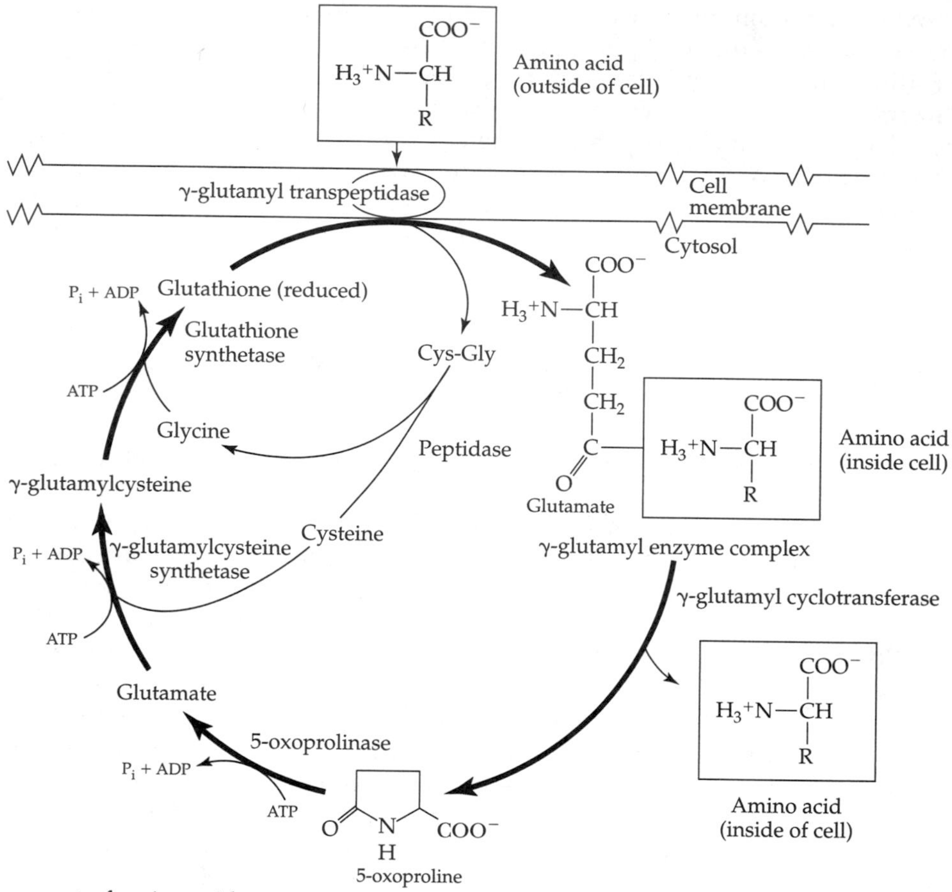

Figure 7.11 The γ-glutamyl cycle for transport of amino acids.

to adjust the rate of their metabolism (including catabolism, or breakdown of amino acids, and anabolism, or use of amino acids for synthesis) according to the needs of the body. Typically, of the amino acids entering the liver after a meal, about 20% are used for the synthesis of proteins and nitrogen-containing compounds; of this 20% of amino acids used for synthesis, most of what is synthesized will remain in the liver and the rest will be released into the plasma. Each of these areas—the synthesis of proteins, nitrogen-containing nonprotein compounds, and purine and pyrimidine bases; the catabolism of amino acids; and the metabolism of amino acids—will be addressed in this section.

Synthesis of Plasma Proteins, Nitrogen-Containing Nonprotein Compounds, and Purine and Pyrimidine Bases

The liver cells, like other body cells, use the amino acids they receive from portal blood and general circulation to synthesize protein [21]. Many of the proteins, such as enzymes, that are made in the liver will remain in the liver; other proteins, however, are released into the plasma. The concentration of total protein in human plasma typically ranges up to about 7.5 g/dL. The proteins found in plasma consist of primarily glycoproteins but also include simple proteins and lipoproteins. These plasma proteins perform a variety of functions.

Plasma Proteins

Several of the proteins in the plasma are used to assess an individual's protein status, specifically visceral (internal organ) protein status. Albumin, the most abundant of the plasma proteins, is synthesized by the liver and released into the blood. Albumin functions in the plasma to maintain oncotic pressure as well as to transport nutrients such as vitamin B_6; minerals including zinc, calcium, and small amounts of copper; nutrients such as fatty acids; and the amino acid tryptophan. Some drugs and hormones are also transported by albumin. Because of albumin's relatively long half-life (~14–18 days), it is not as good or as sensitive an indicator of visceral protein status as some of the other plasma proteins. The half-life is the time it takes for 50% of the amount of a protein such as albumin (or nonprotein compound) to be degraded.

Other proteins synthesized by the liver and released into plasma include transthyretin (formerly called prealbumin), retinol-binding protein (complexed together and involved with retinol, or vitamin A, and thyroid hormone transport), blood-clotting proteins, and globulins. There are several classes of globulins:

- α1-globulins include various glycoproteins and high-density lipoproteins (HDLs).
- α2-globulins include various glycoproteins, haptoglobin for free hemoglobin transport, ceruloplasmin for copper transport and oxidase activity, prothrombin for blood coagulation, and very low density lipoproteins (VLDLs).
- β-globulins include transferrin for iron and other mineral transport and low-density lipoproteins (LDLs).
- γ-globulins include immunoglobulins or antibodies.

Transthyretin and retinol-binding protein, like albumin, are used as indicators of visceral protein status. Because transthyretin and retinol-binding protein have relatively shorter half-lives (~2 days and 12 hours, respectively) than albumin, they are more sensitive indicators of changes in visceral protein status than is albumin.

Another group of proteins synthesized in the liver and released in large quantities into the blood as part of the systemic inflammatory response syndrome to infection (sepsis), injury, and/or inflammation is referred to as acute phase proteins or acute phase reactant proteins. Some examples of these acute phase proteins are C-reactive protein, fibronectin, orosomucoid (also called α1 acid glycoprotein), α1 antitrypsin, haptoglobin, α2 macroglobulin, ceruloplasmin, metallothionein, and serum amyloid A. Collectively, these proteins perform a variety of functions aimed at protecting the body, including stimulation of the immune system, promotion of wound healing, and chelation and removal of free iron from circulation to prevent its use by bacteria for growth. The perspective at the end of this chapter provides a more detailed discussion of some of the functions of these acute phase proteins.

The body also generates another group of proteins, referred to as stress or (heat) shock proteins (abbreviated *hsp*). These proteins are synthesized in response to stress, including heat stress and oxidative stress. Exercise or other physical activity in warm environments, among other conditions, promotes the synthesis of these proteins. While the proteins are categorized by molecular weight (e.g., hsp 60, hsp 70, hsp 90, etc.), their functions remain unclear. Hypothesized roles include repair of denatured or injured proteins.

Nitrogen-Containing Nonprotein Compounds

Nitrogen-containing nonprotein compounds or molecules, of which there are several, are also synthesized in the liver (and often in other sites) from amino acids and perform a number of functions in the body. Some of these compounds (listed below) and their functions are described in this section.

Sources of Nitrogen for Some Nitrogen-Containing Nonprotein Compounds

Nitrogen-Containing Nonprotein Compound	Constituent Amino Acids
Glutathione	Cysteine, glycine, glutamate
Carnitine	Lysine, methionine
Creatine	Arginine, glycine, methionine
Carnosine	Histidine, β-alanine
Choline	Serine

Not included in this list are a number of biogenic amines, neurotransmitters/hormones, and neuropeptides that are synthesized from amino acids in many glands, tissues, and organs throughout the body. A discussion of these compounds is found in this chapter in the section "Brain and Accessory Tissues," page 214. Some of the compounds also are mentioned in sections that discuss the metabolism of amino acids.

Glutathione. Glutathione is a tripeptide synthesized from three amino acids: glycine, cysteine, and glutamate. Glutathione (Fig. 7.10) is referred to as a thiol because it contains a sulfhydryl (-SH) group in its reduced form (GSH). It is found in most cells of the body and has several functions. Glutathione transports amino acids as part of the γ-glutamyl cycle (Fig. 7.11). It participates in the synthesis of leukotriene (LT) C4, which mediates the body's response to inflammation. With the enzyme glutathione peroxidase, glutathione protects cells by reacting with hydrogen peroxides (H_2O_2) and lipid hydroperoxides (LOOHs) before they can cause damage to cells. Glutathione also acts as a scavenger of free radicals ($O_2\cdot$ and $OH\cdot$) to protect cells and cell membranes. Glutathione synthesis is sensitive to protein intake and pathological conditions. Hepatic GSH and mucosal and systemic GSH concentrations decline with poor protein intake as well as during inflammation and disease; this decline negatively impacts the body, necessitating strategies to enhance or at least maintain GSH concentrations [22]. Glutathione is discussed in further detail in a discussion of selenium and glutathione peroxidase in Chapter 12, as well as in the perspective at the end of Chapter 10.

Carnitine. Carnitine, another nitrogen-containing compound (Fig. 7.12), is made in the liver from lysine, which has been methylated using methyl groups from SAM (S-adenosyl methionine), made from the amino acid methionine. Following lysine methylation, trimethyllysine undergoes hydroxylation at the 3 position to form 3-OH trimethyllysine. This latter

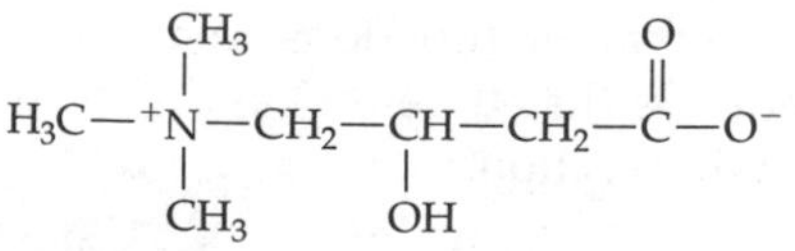

Figure 7.12 Carnitine.

compound is further metabolized to generate γ-butyrobetaine and subsequently carnitine. Iron and vitamins B_6, C, and niacin participate in the synthesis of carnitine, which is shown in Figure 9.5. In addition to its synthesis in the liver and kidney, carnitine is found in foods such as beef and pork. In these foods, carnitine may be free or bound (as acylcarnitine) to long- or short-chain fatty acid esters. Carnitine from food is absorbed in the proximal small intestine by sodium-dependent active transport and possibly also by passive diffusion. Approximately 54% to 87% of carnitine intake is absorbed. Muscle represents the primary carnitine pool, although no carnitine is made there. Intramuscular concentrations of carnitine are generally 50 times greater than usual plasma concentrations. Carnitine homeostasis is maintained principally by the kidney, with >90% of filtered carnitine and acylcarnitine being reabsorbed.

Carnitine, found in most body tissues, is needed for the transport of fatty acids, especially long-chain fatty acids, across the inner mitochondrial membrane for oxidation. The inner mitochondrial membrane is impermeable to long-chain (≥10) fatty acyl CoAs. This role of carnitine is discussed in more detail on page 151. Carnitine also forms acylcarnitines from short-chain acyl CoAs. These acylcarnitines may serve to buffer the free coenzyme (Co) A pool.

Carnitine deficiency, though quite rare, results in impaired energy metabolism [23]. Advertisements marketing carnitine supplements to help burn fat or supply energy are making false claims. Furthermore, although use of carnitine supplements has been shown to increase plasma and muscle carnitine, studies have not uniformly shown improved physical performance [24–28].

Creatine. Creatine (Fig. 7.13), a key component of the energy compound creatine phosphate, also called phosphocreatine, can be obtained from foods (primarily meat and fish) or synthesized in the body. The first step in the synthesis of creatine occurs in the kidney, where arginine and glycine react to form guanidoacetate. In this reaction, the guanidinium group of arginine is transferred to glycine; the remainder of the arginine molecule is released as ornithine. The next step in the synthesis of creatine is the methylation of guanidoacetate. This step occurs in the liver using SAM (S-adenosyl methionine) as a methyl donor (see also Fig. 7.27).

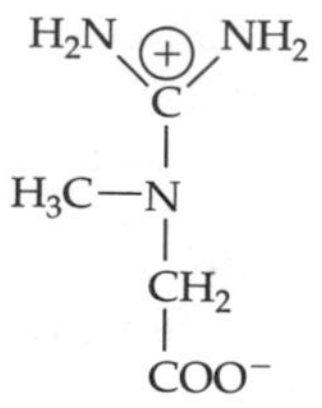

Figure 7.13 Creatine.

Once synthesized, creatine is released into the blood for transport to tissues. About 95% of body creatine is in muscle, with the remaining 5% in organs such as the kidneys and brain. In tissues, creatine is found both in free form as creatine and in its phosphorylated form. The phosphorylation of creatine to form phosphocreatine is shown here:

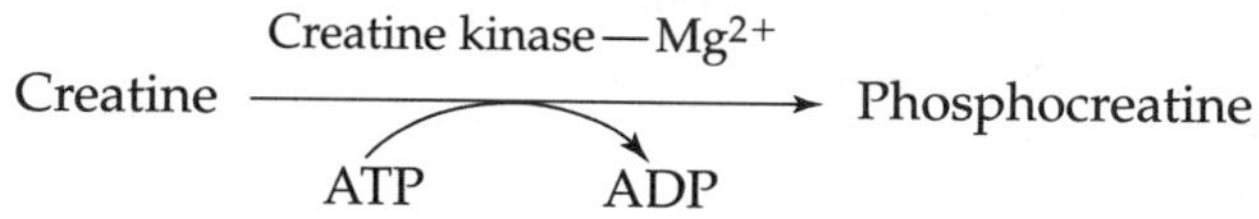

Phosphocreatine functions as a "storehouse for high-energy phosphate." In fact, over half of the creatine in muscle at rest is in the form of phosphocreatine.

Phosphocreatine replenishes ATP in a muscle that is rapidly contracting. Remember, muscle contraction requires energy. This energy is obtained with the hydrolysis of ATP. However, ATP in muscle can suffice for only a fraction of a second. Phosphocreatine, stored in the muscle and possessing a higher phosphate group transfer potential than ATP, can transfer a phosphoryl group to ADP, thereby forming ATP or assisting in ATP regeneration, providing energy for muscular activity. Creatine kinase catalyzes the phosphate transfer in active muscle as shown here:

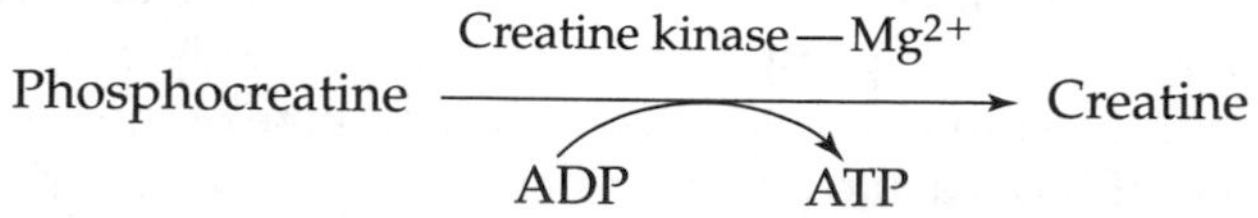

The availability and use of phosphocreatine by muscle are thought to delay the breakdown of muscle glycogen stores, which upon further catabolism also can be used by muscle for energy. See the section "Skeletal Muscle" in this chapter (p. 208) for additional information on phosphocreatine.

Phosphocreatine and creatine do not remain in the muscle for extended periods of time. Both compounds spontaneously cyclize in a nonreversible, nonenzymatic reaction to form creatinine, which is excreted by the kidneys into the urine. Urinary creatinine excretion is often used as an indicator of somatic muscle mass, as discussed in the section "Nitrogen-Containing

Compounds as Indicators of Muscle Mass and Muscle Catabolism," page 212.

Creatine supplements have been shown to increase (~20%–50%) muscle total creatine concentrations and the amount of short-duration maximal exercise that can be performed [29–32]. Typical dosages were 5 g creatine monohydrate taken four times per day for a total of 20 g/day; supplements generally were consumed for 5 or 6 days. Ingestion of a carbohydrate solution with creatine supplements resulted in greater muscle creatine accumulation than did ingestion of creatine alone [33]. Some short-term positive effects of creatine included reduced decline in peak muscle torque production during repeat bouts of high-intensity isokinetic contractions, higher peak isokinetic torque production sustained during repeat bouts of maximal voluntary contraction, and increased whole-body exercise performance during two initial bouts of maximal isokinetic cycling lasting 30 seconds [30,32,34]. Other studies, for example among endurance athletes and highly trained swimmers, however, have reported no effects on performance [31,35,36]. Furthermore, side effects associated with long-term use of creatine are unknown.

Carnosine. Carnosine (β-alanyl histidine; Fig. 7.14) is made in the body from histidine and β-alanine via an energy-dependent reaction catalyzed by carnosine synthetase. In the body, carnosine is found mainly in skeletal muscle, cardiac muscle, and the brain, as well as in the kidneys and stomach. Related compounds include a methylated form of carnosine known as anserine (β-alanyl methylhistidine) and homocarnosine (γ-aminobutyryl histidine), among others. Carnosine also is available in foods, primarily meats, and can be absorbed intact from the intestine via peptide transporters. While not all the functions of carnosine have been identified, some studies show carnosine to exhibit antioxidant activity, both scavenging hydroxyl and superoxide radicals and quenching singlet oxygen [37,38]. In addition, carnosine appears to suppress lipid peroxidation and react with protein carbonyl. In muscle, carnosine regulates intracellular calcium and contractility [37–39].

Choline. Choline (Fig. 7.15) is made in the body from methylation of serine using S-adenosyl methionine (SAM). Choline is also found in foods, in small amounts in free form and more commonly as part of the phospholipid lecithin (phosphatidyl choline). Foods rich in lecithin include eggs, liver and other organ meats, muscle meats, wheat germ, and legumes such as soybeans and peanuts. Lecithin is also added to many foods as an emulsifier.

In the body, choline functions as a methyl donor and as part of the neurotransmitter acetylcholine, the phospholipid phosphatidyl choline (commonly called lecithin), and spingomyelin. To be converted to acetylcholine, free choline crosses the blood-brain barrier and enters cerebral cells from the plasma via a specific choline transport system. Within the presynaptic terminal of the neuron, acetylcholine is formed by the action of choline acetyltransferase as follows:

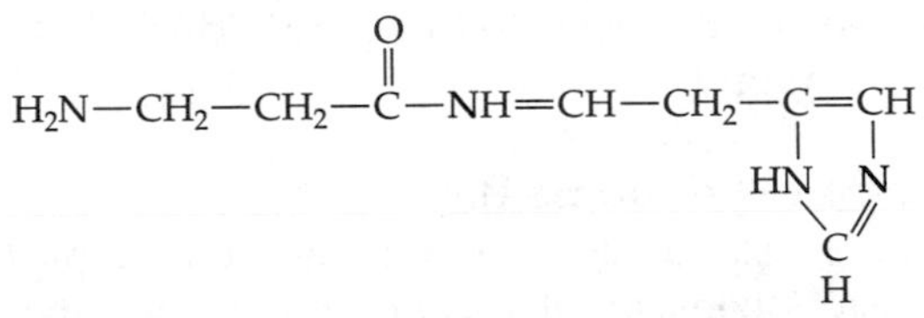

Figure 7.14 Carnosine.

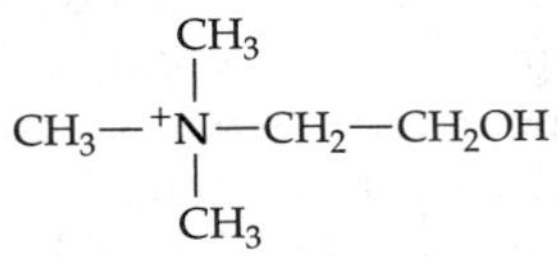

Figure 7.15 Choline.

$$\text{Choline} + \text{acetyl CoA} \longrightarrow \text{Acetylcholine} + \text{CoA}$$

Concentrations of choline in cholinergic neurons typically are below the K_m of choline acetyltransferase; thus, the enzyme normally is not saturated. Acetyl CoA is thought to arise from glucose metabolism by neural glycolysis and the action of the pyruvate dehydrogenase complex. Choline also can be recycled—that is, phospholipases can liberate choline from lecithin and spingomyelin as needed, and acetylcholinesterase can hydrolyze acetylcholine following synaptic transmission.

Choline is oxidized in the liver and kidneys. In the liver, choline oxidation generates betaine, which functions as a methyl donor to regenerate methionine from homocysteine (see p. 203). Further metabolism of betaine generates dimethyl glycine, which may be catabolized to glycine, methylene tetrahydrofolate, carbon dioxide, and ammonium ion (see p. 205).

Experimental diets devoid of choline can result in decreases in plasma choline and phosphatidylcholine concentrations as well as alterations in some liver enzymes. Animals devoid of dietary choline develop a fatty liver accompanied by some hepatic necrosis. The Food and Nutrition Board has suggested that an adequate intake consists of 425 mg and 550 mg choline for adult females and males, respectively [40]. Such intakes are easily obtained through dietary consumption of animal products and foods containing fats. A tolerable upper intake level of 3.5 g choline daily also has been set [40]. The **tolerable upper intake level** represents the highest level of daily intake that is likely to pose no risks of adverse health effects to most individuals in the general population [40].

Purine and Pyrimidine Bases

Another group of compounds derived in part from amino acids consists of purine and pyrimidine bases. A brief review of purine and pyrimidine synthesis and degradation follows.

The synthesis of the nitrogen-containing bases of nucleotides occurs for the most part de novo in the liver. Synthesis of the pyrimidines uracil, cytosine, and thymine is initiated by the formation of carbamoyl phosphate from glutamine, CO_2, and ATP. The enzyme carbamoyl phosphate synthetase II catalyzes this reaction in the cytoplasm and is distinct from carbamoyl phosphate synthetase I, which is needed in the initial step of urea synthesis and is found in the mitochondria. Carbamoyl phosphate reacts with the amino acid aspartate to form N-carbamoylaspartate. Aspartate transcarbamoylase catalyzes the reaction, which is the committed step in pyrimidine biosynthesis. Synthesis of the pyrimidine bases is illustrated in Figure 7.16. Once uridine monophosphate (UMP) is formed, it may react with other nucleoside di- and triphosphates. The formation of thymidine monophosphate (TMP) from deoxyuridine monophosphate (dUMP) should particularly be noted. ATP can phosphorylate TMP to form TTP. In the synthesis of DNA, dTTP (deoxythymidine triphosphate) replaces UTP, uridine triphosphate.

The purine bases adenine and guanine are synthesized de novo as nucleoside monophosphates by sequential addition of carbons and nitrogens to ribose-P that has originated from the hexose monophosphate shunt. As shown in Figure 7.17a, ribose 5-P reacts with ATP to form phosphoribosyl pyrophosphate (PPRP). Glutamine then donates a nitrogen to form 5-phosphoribosylamine (PRPP). This step represents the committed step in purine nucleotide synthesis. Next in a series of reactions, nitrogen and carbon atoms from glycine are added, formylation occurs by tetrahydrofolate (THF, a form of the B vitamin folate), another nitrogen atom is donated by the amide group of glutamine, and ring closure occurs. Another set of reactions occurs involving the addition of carbons from CO_2 and from 10-formyl THF (from folate) and a nitrogen from aspartate. Thus, the purine ring as shown in Figure 7.17b is derived from amino acids, including glutamine, glycine, and aspartate, as well as from folate and CO_2.

The formation of individual purine bases and nucleotides is shown in Figure 7.17c. Inosine monophosphate (IMP) is used to synthesize adenosine monophosphate (AMP) and guanosine monophosphate (GMP).

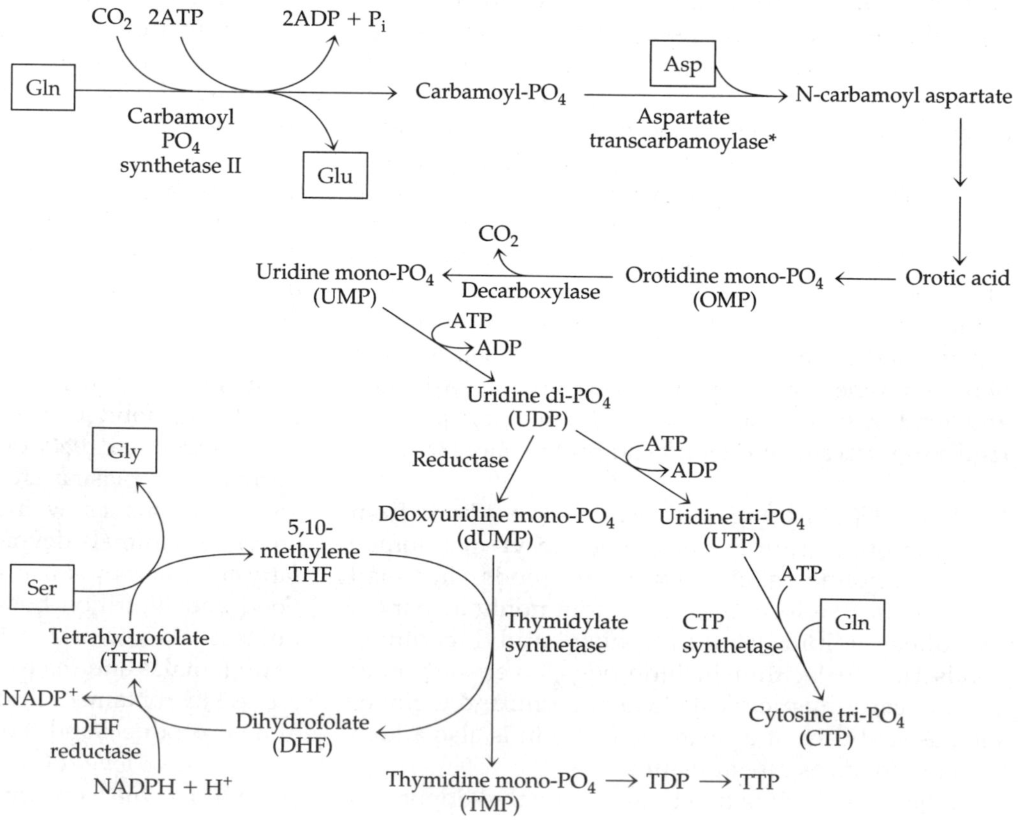

Figure 7.16 Pyrimidine synthesis.

*Aspartate transcarbamolyase catalyzes the commited step in pyrimidine biosynthesis.

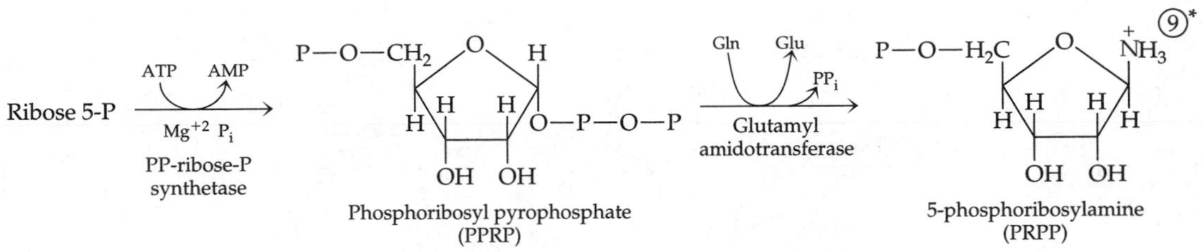

(a) Initiation of biosynthesis by reaction between PPRP and glutamine (Gln).

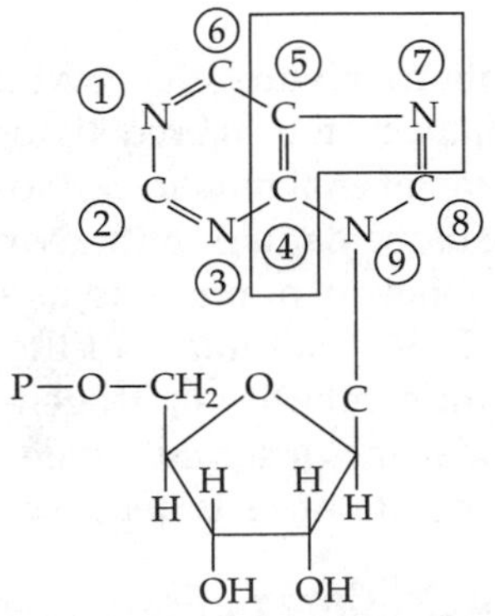

*Nitrogen (9) is donated by amide group from *glutamine*. Donors of other atoms in order of introduction:

a. *Glycine:* N (7) and C (4) and (5) introduced as single unit.

b. *Formate:* C (8) donated via 10-formyl THF (tetrahydrofolic acid)

c. *Glutamine* amide group: N (3)

d. *Respiratory CO_2* as "active CO_2": C (6)

e. *Aspartic acid:* N (1)

f. *Formate:* C (2) via 10-formyl THF

(b) Sources of carbon and nitrogen atoms in purine ring.

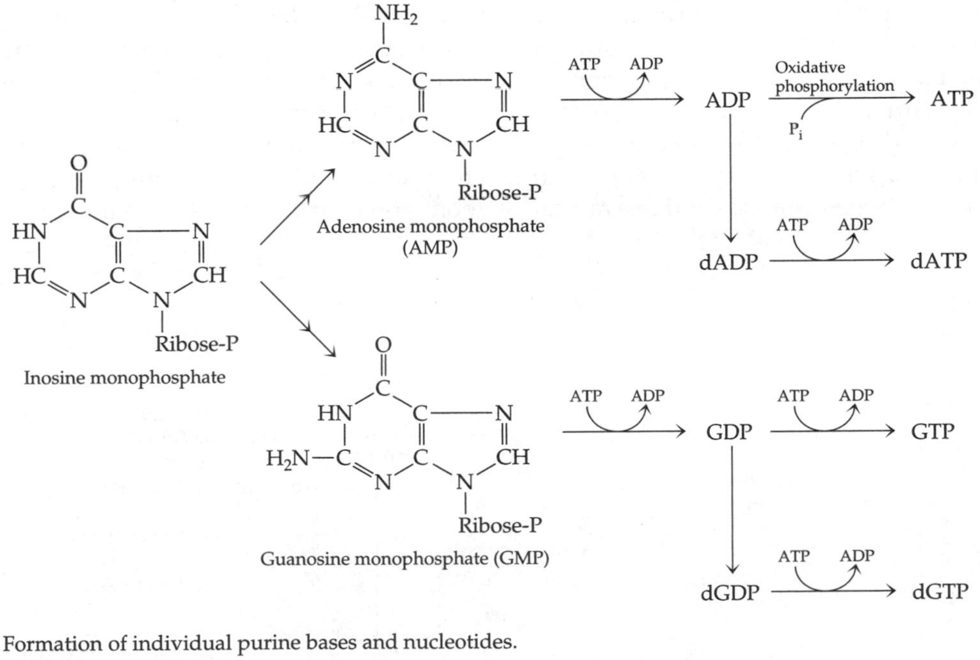

(c) Formation of individual purine bases and nucleotides.

Figure 7.17 Synthesis of purines and sources of carbon and nitrogen atoms.

AMP and GMP are phosphorylated to ADP and GDP, respectively, by ATP. The deoxyribotides are formed at the diphosphate level by converting ribose to deoxyribose, thereby producing dADP and dGDP. ADP can be phosphorylated to ATP via oxidative phosphorylation; the remaining nucleotides are phosphorylated to their triphosphate form by ATP. Purine nucleotides can also be synthesized by the salvage pathways, whereby purine bases react with PRPP to form the mononucleotides.

Degradation of pyrimidines involves the sequential hydrolysis of the nucleoside triphosphates to mononucleotides, nucleosides, and, finally, free bases. This process can be accomplished in most cells by lysosomal enzymes. During catabolism of pyrimidines, the

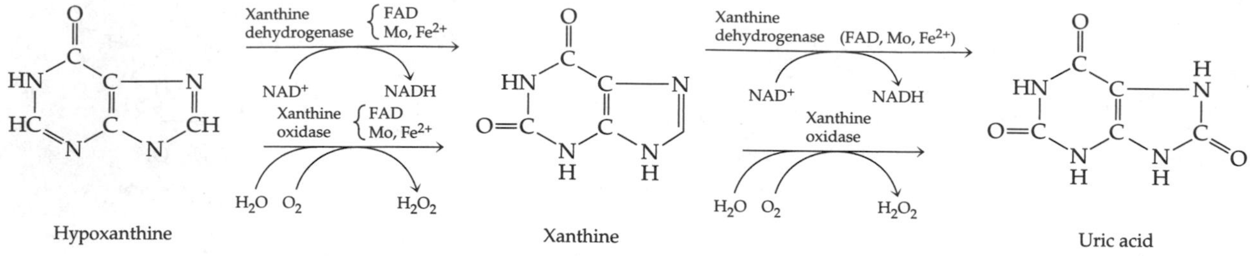

Figure 7.18 Purine catabolism yields uric acid.

ring is opened with the production of CO_2 and ammonia from the carbamoyl portion of the molecule. The ammonia can be converted to urea and excreted. Malonyl CoA and methylmalonyl CoA, produced from the remainder of the ring, follow their normal metabolic pathways, thus requiring no special excretion route.

Purines are progressively oxidized primarily in the liver, yielding hypoxanthine, xanthine, and uric acid. Xanthine dehydrogenase or oxidase, molybdenum- and iron-dependent enzymes, catalyze these two reactions, shown in Figure 7.18. Uric acid normally is excreted in the urine; however, up to 200 mg of uric acid may be excreted daily into the digestive tract. Under pathological conditions such as gout or renal failure, the uric acid may accumulate in the blood and be deposited in and around joints. Furthermore, under conditions of oxygen deprivation (as with a myocardial infarction or an intestinal ischemia), xanthine dehydrogenase may be converted to xanthine oxidase. Reperfusion of the tissue with oxygen can result in increased hydrogen peroxide and free radical concentrations. Hydrogen peroxide and free radicals may further damage the injured tissues. Research involving introduction of enzymes and antioxidant nutrients to help minimize tissue damage with reoxygenation is ongoing.

An overview of amino acid use for anabolism is given in Figure 7.19. A summary of the use of selected amino acids for the synthesis of nitrogen-containing nonprotein compounds and selected biogenic amines, hormones and neuromodulators is depicted in Figure 7.20.

Amino Acid Catabolism Overview

Liver cells have a high capacity for the uptake and catabolism of all amino acids. In fact, after a meal, the liver takes up about 50% to 65% of amino acids from portal blood. The liver is the main site for the catabolism of indispensable amino acids, with the exception of the branched-chain amino acids. The rate of hepatic catabolism for the amino acids, however, differs. Branched-chain amino acids, for example, are catabolized much more slowly in the liver than in muscle. Furthermore, not

Figure 7.19 Use of amino acids for anabolism.

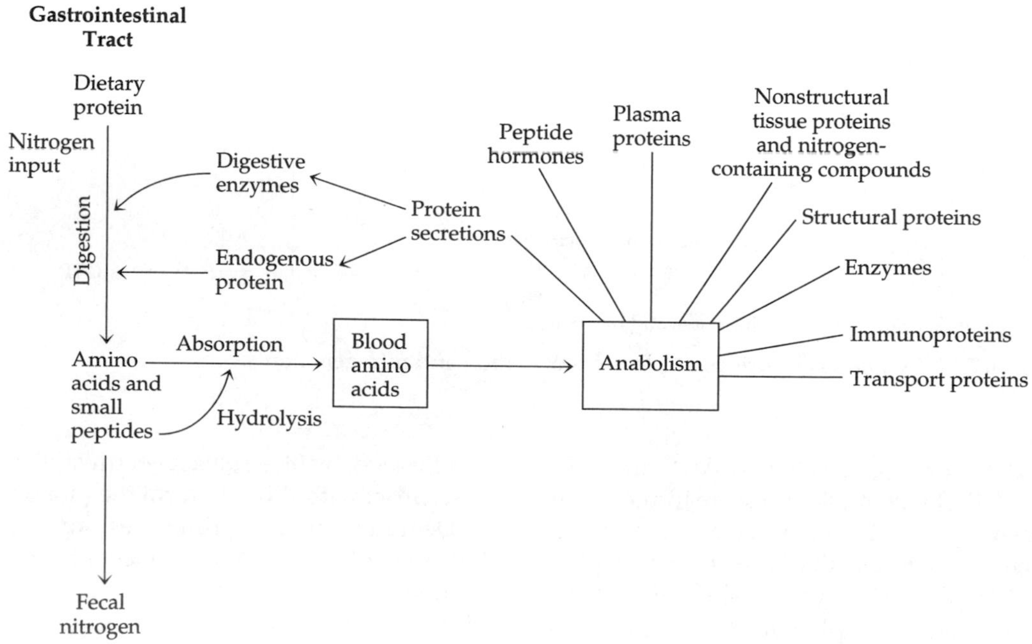

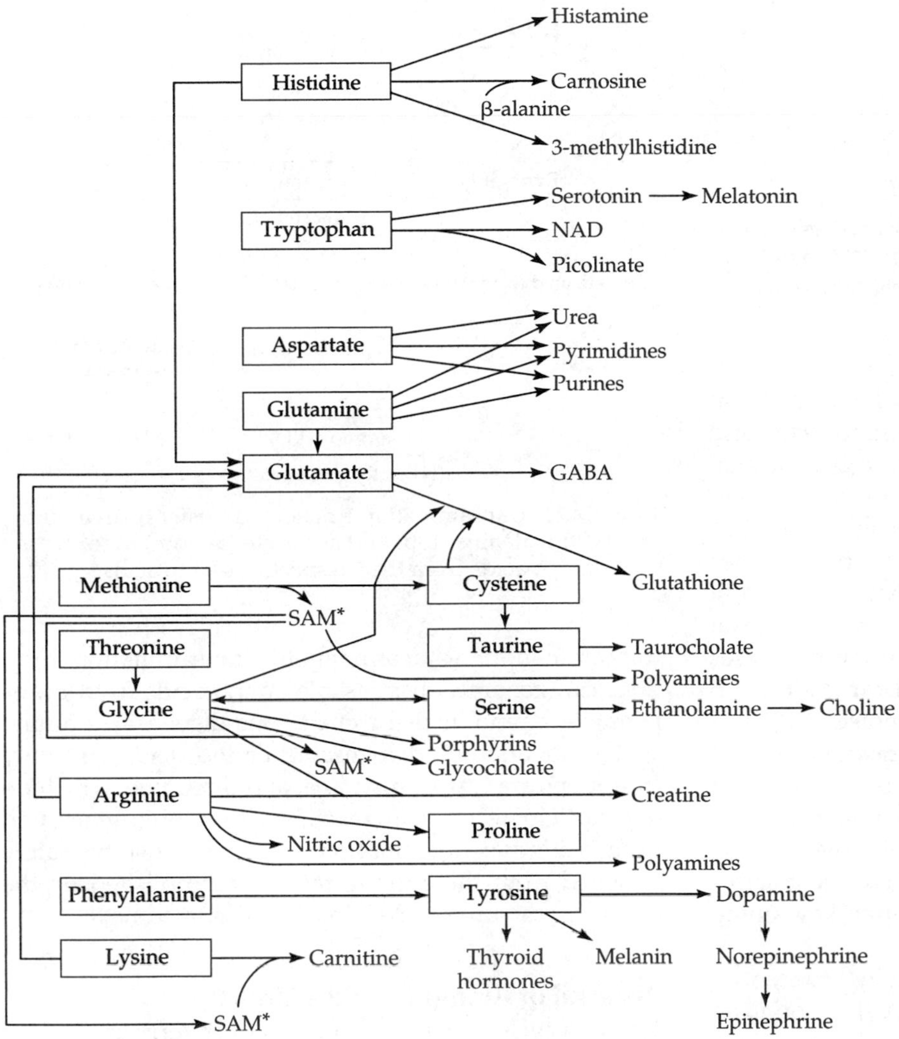

Figure 7.20 A summary of the use of selected amino acids for the synthesis of nitrogen-containing compounds and selected biogenic amines, hormones and neuromodulators.

*SAM = s-adenasyl methionine.

all amino acids are catabolized in the same regions of the liver. Periportal hepatocytes, for example, catabolize most amino acids—with the exception of glutamate and aspartate—that are metabolized by perivenous hepatocytes. The liver derives up to 50% of its energy (ATP) from amino acid oxidation; the energy generated in turn may be used for gluconeogenesis or urea synthesis, among other needs, depending on the body's state of nutriture. This section on amino acid catabolism first focuses on the reactions that occur as amino acids are broken down in liver cells, including first the transamination and deamination of amino acids and then the urea cycle. It next discusses the uses of the carbon skeleton of amino acids.

Transamination and Deamination of the Amino Acids

Usually, the first step in the metabolism of amino acids not used for the synthesis of proteins or nitrogen-containing compounds is the removal of the amino group from the amino acid. Amino acids can undergo deamination and/or transamination to remove amino groups. Deamination reactions involve only the removal of an amino group, with no direct transfer to another compound. Some amino acids that are more commonly deaminated include glutamate, histidine, serine, glycine, and threonine; however, many of these same amino acids also can be transaminated. The enzymes carrying out the deamination reactions are generally lyases, dehydratases, or dehydrogenases. Figure 7.21 shows the deamination of the amino acid threonine by threonine dehydratase to form α-ketobutyrate (another α-keto acid) and ammonium. Ammonia is readily used by periportal hepatocytes for urea synthesis. The synthesis of urea in the liver is addressed in the next subsection, "Disposal of Ammonia—the Urea Cycle."

Transamination reactions involve the transfer of an amino group from one amino acid to an amino acid carbon skeleton or α-keto acid (an amino acid without an

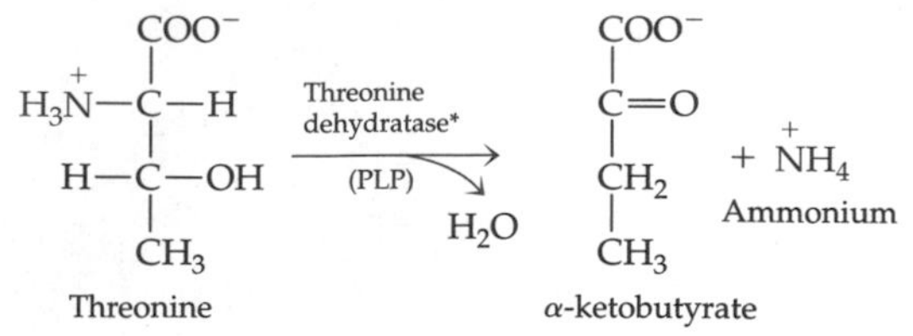

*The enzyme is called *dehydratase* rather than *deaminase* because the reaction proceeds by loss of elements of water.

Figure 7.21 The deamination of the amino acid threonine.

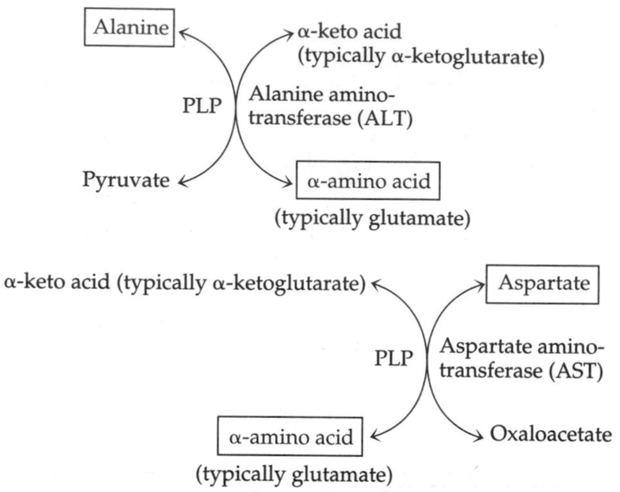

Figure 7.22 Transamination reactions. Transfer of an amino group from alanine (top) and aspartate (bottom) to form other amino acids from their respective α-keto acids.

amino group). The carbon skeleton/α-keto acid that gains the amino group becomes an amino acid, and the amino acid that loses its amino group becomes an α-keto acid. These reactions are important for the synthesis of many of the body's dispensable amino acids.

Transamination reactions are catalyzed by enzymes called aminotransferases. These enzymes typically require vitamin B_6 in its coenzyme form, pyridoxal phosphate (PLP). Some examples of aminotransferases include tyrosine aminotransferase, branched-chain aminotransferases, alanine aminotransferase (ALT; formerly called glutamate pyruvate transaminase and abbreviated GPT), and aspartate aminotransferase (AST; formerly called glutamate oxaloacetate transaminase and abbreviated GOT). These latter two aminotransferases (ALT and AST) are among the most active of the aminotransferases and involve three key amino acids: alanine, glutamate, and aspartate.

Aminotransferases are found in varying concentrations in different tissues. For example, AST is found in higher concentrations in the heart than in the liver, muscle, and other tissues. In contrast, ALT is found in higher concentrations in the liver than in the heart but is also found in moderate amounts in the kidney and small amounts in other tissues. Normal serum concentrations of these enzymes are low; however, with trauma or disease to an organ, serum enzyme concentrations rise and serve as an indicator of both which organ has been damaged and the severity of the organ damage.

Reactions catalyzed by ALT and AST are shown in Figure 7.22. ALT transfers amino groups from alanine to an α-keto acid (e.g., α-ketoglutarate), forming pyruvate and another amino acid (e.g., glutamate), respectively. AST transfers amino groups from aspartate also to an α-keto acid (e.g., α-ketoglutarate), yielding oxaloacetate and another amino acid (e.g., glutamate), respectively. These reactions are reversible. Because glutamate and α-ketoglutarate readily transfer and/or accept amino groups, these compounds play central roles in amino acid metabolism.

In summary, the first step in the utilization of amino acids, for functions other than the synthesis of proteins or nitrogen-containing compounds, requires either transamination or deamination. Transamination reactions can generate dispensable amino acids from indispensable amino acids or create one dispensable amino acid from another dispensable amino acid. The only exceptions are lysine, histidine, and threonine, which do not participate in such reactions. Ammonia generated from oxidative deamination reactions must be safely removed from the system; this is accomplished by the actions of the urea cycle, which is discussed next.

Disposal of Ammonia—the Urea Cycle

The urea cycle, which functions in the liver, is important for the removal of ammonia from the body. Too much ammonia in the body is toxic and can lead to brain malfunction and coma. Some of the sources of ammonia in the body include

- ammonia formed in the body from chemical reactions such as deamination,
- ammonia ingested and absorbed from the foods we eat, and
- ammonia generated in the gastrointestinal tract from bacterial lysis of urea and amino acids and subsequently absorbed through the enterocyte.

The liver has two systems in place to deal with ammonia. First and foremost, periportal hepatocytes are active in ureagenesis. Ammonia from the diet or from intestinal bacterial synthesis enters portal blood and first comes in contact with hepatocytes, specifically, periportal hepatocytes capable of urea synthesis. These same periportal cells are responsible for almost all amino acid catabolism, so ammonia generated during amino acid degradative reactions can be immediately taken up for urea synthesis. However, should the periportal cells fail to use all the ammonia, a second group of hepatocytes, the perivenous hepatocytes, are capable of utilizing the ammonia for glutamine synthesis. The perivenous cells thus provide a "backup" system for ammonia that escaped involvement in urea production [41].

Figure 7.23 reviews key compounds of the urea cycle and shows its relationship with amino acids and the Krebs cycle. The reactions of the urea cycle are broken down in the following list:

- Ammonia (NH_3) combines with CO_2 or HCO_3^- to form carbamoyl phosphate in a reaction catalyzed by mitochondrial carbamoyl phosphate synthetase I (CPSI) and using 2 mol of ATP and Mg^{2+}. N-acetylglutamate (NAG), made in the liver and intestine, is required as an allosteric activator to allow ATP binding.
- Carbamoyl phosphate reacts with ornithine in the mitochondria, using the enzyme ornithine transcarbamoylase (OTC) to form citrulline. Citrulline in turn inhibits OTC activity.
- Aspartate reacts with citrulline once it has been transported into the cytosol. This step, catalyzed by argininosuccinate synthetase, is the rate-limiting step of the cycle. ATP (two high-energy bonds) and Mg^{2+} are required for the reaction, and argininosuccinate is formed. Argininosuccinate, arginine, and AMP + PP_i inhibit the enzyme.
- Argininosuccinate is cleaved by argininosuccinase in the cytosol to form fumarate and arginine. Both fumarate and arginine inhibit argininosuccinase activity. Argininosuccinase is found in a variety of tissues throughout the body, especially the liver and kidneys. High concentrations of arginine increase the synthesis of N-acetylglutamate (NAG), which is needed for the synthesis of carbamoyl phosphate in the mitochondria.
- Urea is formed and ornithine is re-formed from the cleavage of arginine by arginase I, a manganese-requiring hepatic enzyme. Arginase activity is inhibited by both ornithine and lysine and may become rate limiting under conditions that limit manganese availability or that alter its affinity for manganese [16,42].

Overall, the urea cycle uses four high-energy bonds. Oxidations in the Krebs cycle coupled with

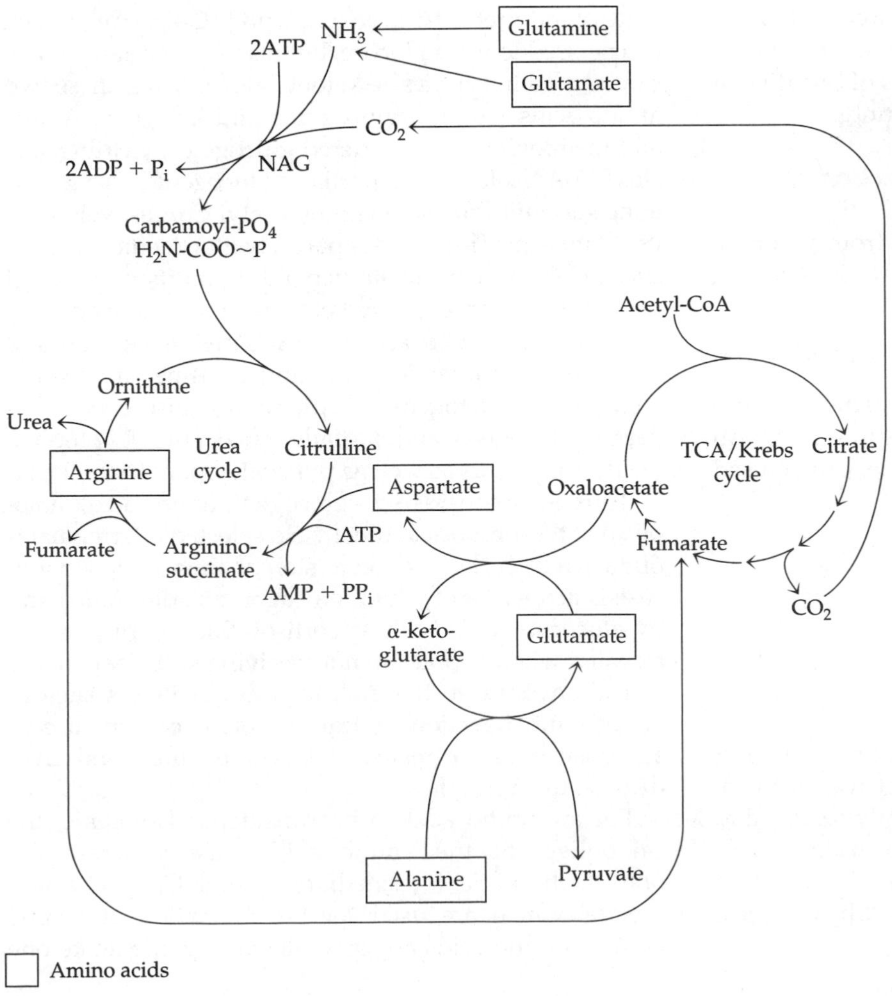

Figure 7.23 Interrelationships of amino acids and the urea and TCA/Krebs cycles in the liver.

phosphorylation through the electron transport chain can provide the ATP required for urea synthesis. The urea molecule derives one nitrogen from ammonia, a second nitrogen from aspartate, and its carbon from CO_2/HCO_3^-. Once formed, urea typically travels via the blood to the kidneys for excretion in the urine; however, up to about 25% of urea may be secreted from the blood into the intestinal lumen, where it may be degraded by bacteria to yield ammonia.

Activities of urea cycle enzymes fluctuate with diet and hormone concentrations. For example, with low-protein diets or acidosis, urea synthesis (the amount of mRNA for each of the enzymes) diminishes and urinary urea nitrogen excretion decreases significantly. Thus, substrate availability results in short-term changes in the rate of ureagenesis. In the healthy individual with a normal protein intake, blood urea nitrogen (BUN) concentrations range from about 8 to 20 mg/dL, and urinary urea nitrogen represents about 80% of total urinary nitrogen. Glucocorticoids and glucagon typically increase mRNA for the urea cycle enzymes [42].

Several urea cycle enzyme-deficient disorders have been characterized. Defects in any one of the enzymes of the urea cycle are possible. Urea cycle enzyme defects typically result in high levels of blood ammonia (hyperammonemia) and necessitate a nitrogen-restricted diet, which may be coupled with supplements of carnitine or single amino acids, among other compounds.

An Overview of Metabolism of the Carbon Skeleton or α-Keto Acid

Once an amino group has been removed from an amino acid, the remaining molecule is referred to as a carbon skeleton or α-keto acid.

$$\text{Amino acid} \longrightarrow NH_3 + \text{carbon skeleton}/\alpha\text{-keto acid}$$

Carbon skeletons of amino acids can be further metabolized with the potential for multiple uses in the cell. An amino acid's carbon skeleton, for example, can be used for the production of

- energy,
- glucose,
- ketone bodies,
- cholesterol, and
- fatty acids.

The potential use of the carbon skeleton depends in part on the original amino acid from which it was derived. Whereas all amino acids can be completely oxidized to generate energy, not all amino acids can be used for synthesis of glucose. Furthermore, the fate of the amino acid's carbon skeleton depends on the physiological nutritional state of the body.

Energy Generation. The complete oxidation of amino acids generates energy, CO_2/HCO_3^-, and ammonia/ammonium. Amino acids are used for energy in the body when diets are inadequate in energy (measured in kilocalories and abbreviated kcal).

Glucose and Ketone Body Production. The production of glucose from a noncarbohydrate source such as amino acids is known as gluconeogenesis. Gluconeogenesis occurs primarily in the liver but also in the kidney. The carbon skeletons of several amino acids can be used to synthesize glucose. Oxaloacetate, the carbon skeleton of aspartate, and pyruvate, the carbon skeleton of alanine, may be utilized to produce glucose in body cells through the process of gluconeogenesis, also discussed in Chapter 4. In addition, the carbon skeleton of asparagine can be converted into oxaloacetate, and the carbon skeletons of glycine, serine, cysteine, tryptophan, and threonine can be converted into pyruvate for glucose production in the liver.

Figure 7.24 shows the general fates of amino acid carbon skeletons with respect to key intermediates of metabolism. Some amino acids, such as phenylalanine and tyrosine, can be degraded to form fumarate (an intermediate of the Krebs/tricarboxylic acid [TCA] cycle), which can be used to form glucose, but also acetoacetate, which can be used to synthesize ketone bodies. Thus, these two amino acids are both glucogenic and ketogenic. Valine and methionine are considered glucogenic, yielding succinyl CoA. Isoleucine is partially glucogenic, also generating succinyl CoA but yielding acetyl CoA as well upon its catabolism. Threonine is partially glucogenic, yielding succinyl CoA or pyruvate depending on its pathway of degradation, and partially ketogenic when degraded by another pathway to acetyl CoA. Thus, isoleucine and threonine, like phenylalanine and tyrosine, are considered partially ketogenic. Tryptophan is also considered partially ketogenic and partially glucogenic. Tryptophan yields acetyl CoA as well as pyruvate upon catabolism.

Thus, to be considered a glucogenic amino acid, catabolism of the amino acid must yield selected intermediates of the Krebs cycle. The conversion of amino acids to glucose is accelerated by high glucagon : insulin ratios and by glucocorticoids such as cortisol. Such hormones are elevated when people are not receiving sufficient energy or carbohydrate in the diet, in times of illness such as occurs with infection or trauma, or in certain disease states such as untreated diabetes mellitus and liver disease, to name a few.

For an amino acid to be considered ketogenic, the catabolism of the amino acid must generate the non–Krebs cycle intermediates acetyl CoA or acetoacetate, which are used for the formation of ketone bodies. Amino acids are catabolized to generate ketone

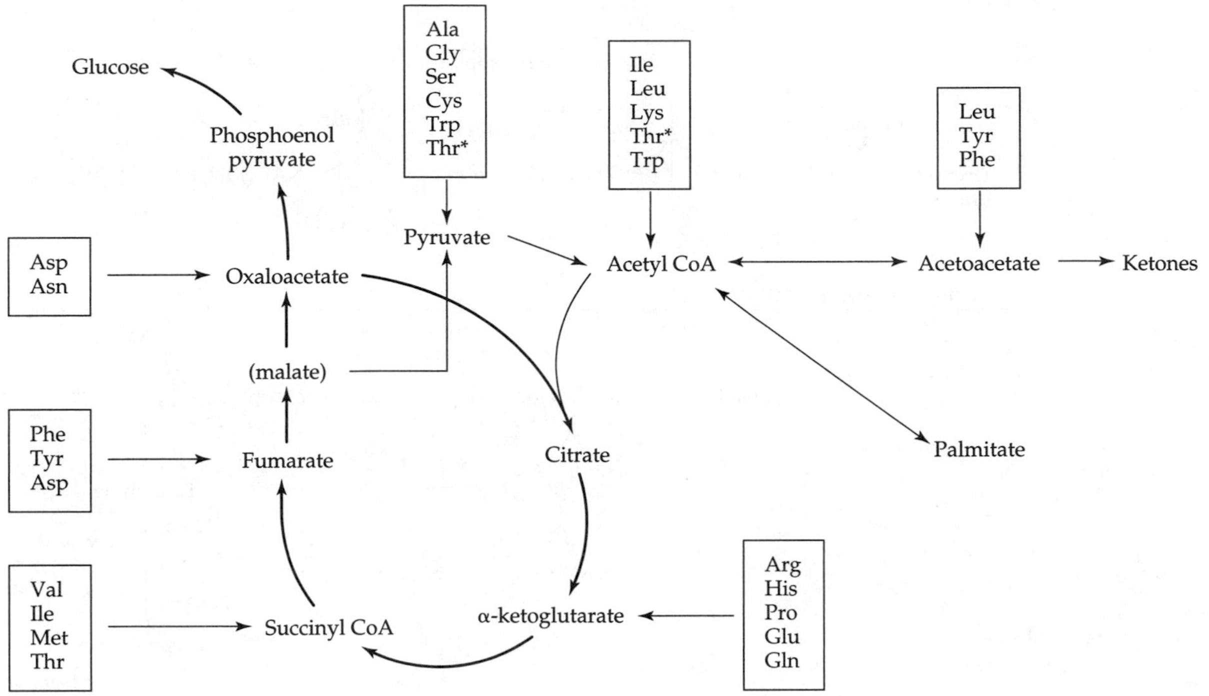

*Physiological contribution unclear

Figure 7.24 The fate of amino acid carbon skeletons. Ketogenic: Lys and Leu; partially ketogenic and glucogenic: Phe, Ile, Thr, Trp, Tyr; glucogenic: Ala, Gly, Cys, Ser, Asp, Asn, Glu, Gln, Arg, Met, Val, His, Pro.

bodies generally during times when an individual is not consuming an adequate carbohydrate intake. Leucine and lysine are the only totally ketogenic amino acids and upon catabolism generate acetyl CoA.

Cholesterol Production. Leucine is also the only amino acid whose catabolism generates HMG CoA, an important intermediate in the synthesis of cholesterol. However, other amino acids generate acetyl CoA, which can be metabolized in the liver for cholesterol production [43].

Fatty Acid Production. In times of excess energy and protein intakes coupled with adequate carbohydrate intake, the carbon skeleton of amino acids may be used to synthesize fatty acids. The details of the metabolism of selected amino acids and the formation of Krebs cycle and non–Krebs cycle intermediates will be discussed in the sections to follow. The metabolism of the amino acids is categorized according to the structural classification of amino acids.

Hepatic Metabolism of Aromatic Amino Acids

The catabolism of aromatic, along with sulfur (S)-containing, amino acids occurs primarily in the liver. In fact, in end-stage liver disease, the inability of the liver to take up and catabolize these amino acids is evidenced by the increased plasma concentrations of both the aromatic amino acids—phenylalanine, tyrosine, and tryptophan—and the S-containing amino acids methionine and cysteine.

As shown in Figure 7.25, phenylalanine and tyrosine are partially glucogenic because they are degraded to fumarate. In addition, phenylalanine and tyrosine are catabolized to acetoacetate and thus are partially ketogenic. The first step in the degradation of phenylalanine is specific to the liver and, to a smaller extent, the kidney.

- Phenylalanine is converted to tyrosine by the hepatic enzyme phenylalanine hydroxylase, also called a monooxygenase. This enzyme is iron-dependent, and vitamin C and tetrahydrobiopterin are required for the reaction. A genetic absence or deficient activity of phenylalanine hydroxylase results in the genetic disorder phenylketonuria (PKU) and necessitates a phenylalanine-restricted diet.

Further catabolism of tyrosine is not specific to the liver; however, many of the reactions for its degradation occur primarily in the liver. Other reactions, such as generation of L-dopa and the catecholamines, occur more commonly in neurons or in the adrenal medulla (Fig. 7.25).

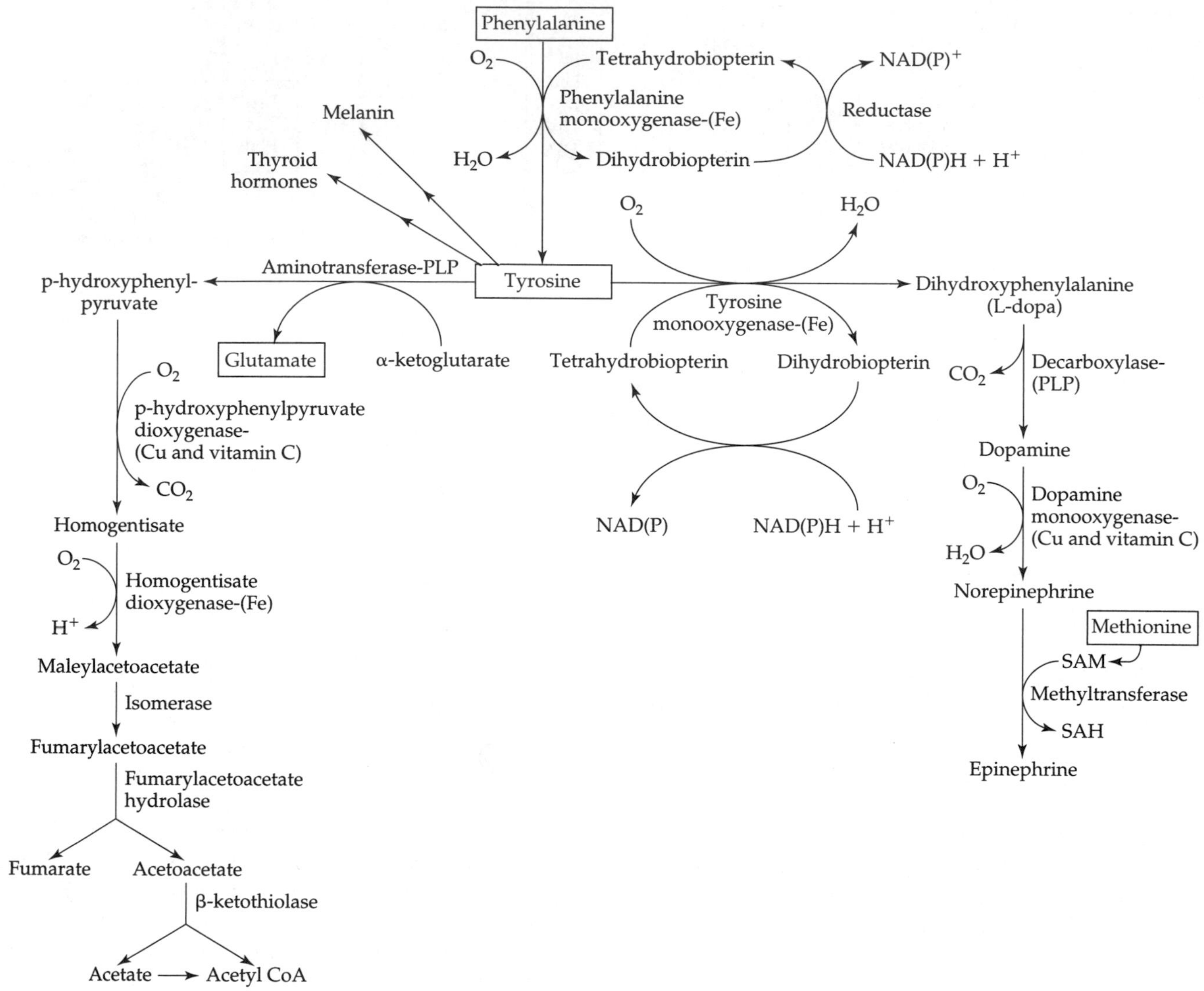

Figure 7.25 Phenylalanine and tyrosine metabolism.

• Tyrosine degradation (Fig. 7.25) begins with transamination via a vitamin B_6–dependent tyrosine aminotransferase to yield p-hydroxyphenylpyruvate. This compound is then decarboxylated by an oxidase to generate homogentisate. Homogentisate dioxidase converts homogentisate to maleylacetoacetate, which is then isomerized to fumarylacetoacetate. A hydrolase converts fumarylacetoacetate into fumarate (a TCA cycle intermediate) and acetoacetate, which may be further metabolized to acetyl CoA.

While this section of the chapter focuses on hepatic metabolism of amino acids, it is important for the reader to remember that, in addition to use for protein synthesis and for catabolism for energy, glucose, or ketone body production, tyrosine is used to synthesize other compounds.

• In other cells of the body, tyrosine is used for the synthesis of L-dopa and catecholamines. The initial reaction utilizes tyrosine hydroxylase (also called monooxygenase), an iron-dependent enzyme shown in Figure 7.25. The enzyme hydroxylates tyrosine to generate 3,4-dihydroxyphenylalanine (L-dopa). Subsequent reactions utilizing L-dopa yield the catecholamines (dopamine, norepinephrine, and epinephrine) as shown in Figure 7.25.

• In melanocytes in the skin, eye, and hair cells, tyrosine is converted into melanin. The reactions occur within melanosomes, membrane-bound organelles found in the melanocytes. Melanin is a pigment that gives color to skin, eyes, and hair.

• In the thyroid gland, tyrosine is taken up and used with iodine to synthesize thyroid hormones.

Another aromatic amino acid metabolized principally by the liver is tryptophan. Its metabolism is shown in Figure 7.26. Tryptophan is partially glucogenic, as it is metabolized to form pyruvate; it is also partially ketogenic, forming acetyl CoA.

- The first step in tryptophan metabolism yields N-formylkynurenine. The enzyme tryptophan dioxygenase, which catalyzes this first reaction, is heme iron–dependent; it is also induced by glucocorticoids and glucagon.

Figure 7.26 Tryptophan metabolism.

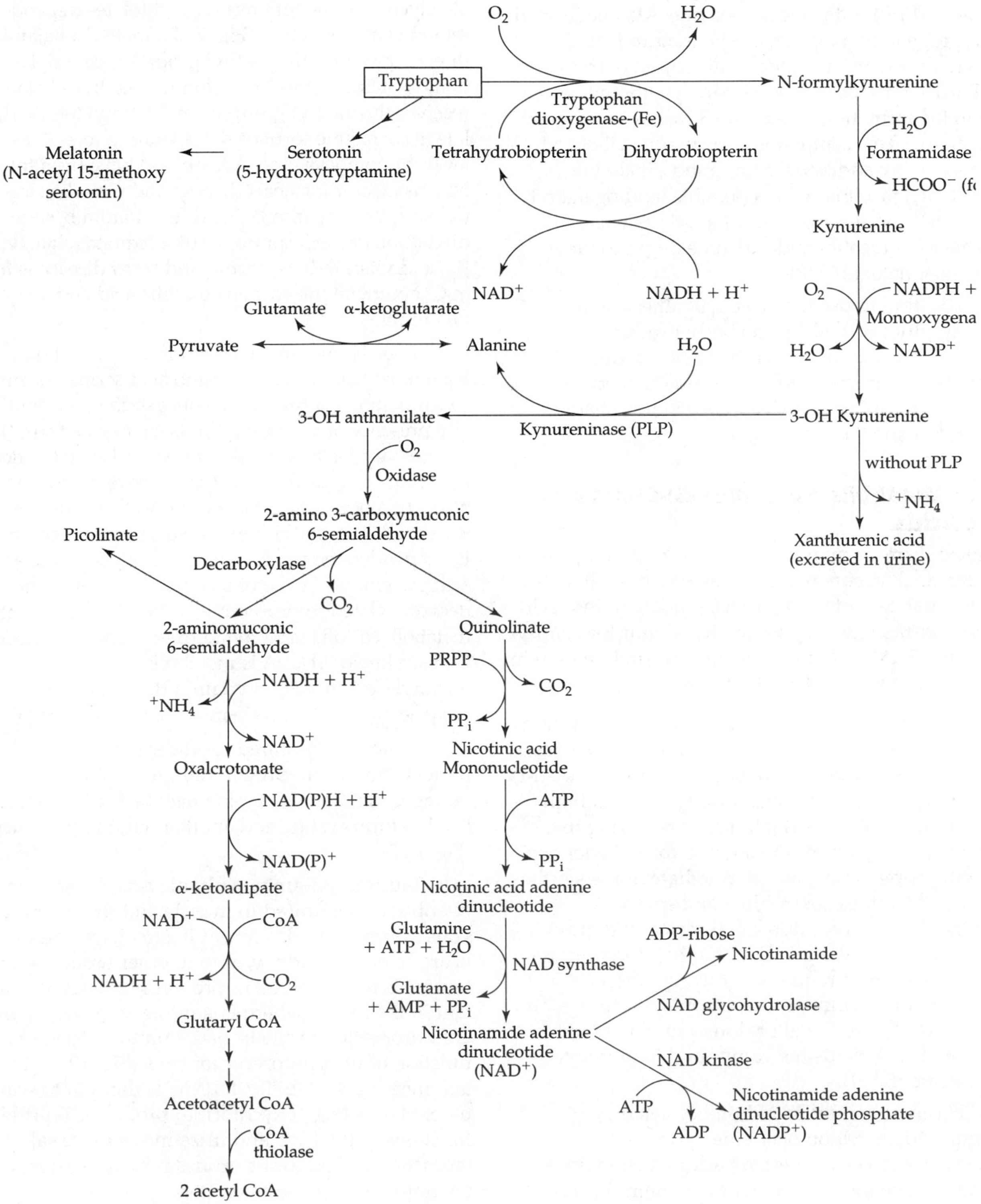

Tetrahydrobiopterin is a required cosubstrate for the reaction.

- Further metabolism of N-formylkynurenine yields formate and kynurenine. Kynurenine may be metabolized to 3-hydroxykynurenine by a monooxygenase. The 3-hydroxykynurenine may be converted to 3-hydroxyanthranilate and alanine by kynureninase, a vitamin B_6(PLP) – dependent enzyme. Alanine formed from tryptophan metabolism can be transaminated to form pyruvate, hence the glucogenic nature of tryptophan. Further metabolism of 3-hydroxyanthranilate results in the formation of 2-amino 3-carboxymuconate semialdehyde. This compound is further metabolized to produce many additional compounds, including α-ketoadipate, picolinic acid (a possible binding ligand for minerals), and niacin as nicotinamide as well as its coenzyme form nicotinamide adenine dinucleotide (NAD) phosphate (NADP).
- In addition to use for protein synthesis and for energy, glucose, and ketone body production, tryptophan is used for the synthesis of serotonin (5-hydroxytryptamine) and melatonin (N-acetyl 5-methoxyserotonin), described later in this chapter under "Brain and Accessory Tissues."

Hepatic Metabolism of Sulfur (S)-Containing Amino Acids

The metabolism of methionine, an S-containing essential amino acid, occurs to a large extent in the liver and generates the S-containing nonessential amino acids cysteine and taurine and the methyl donor S-adenosyl methionine (SAM). Methionine metabolism is shown in Figure 7.27 and briefly described here.

- The first step in methionine metabolism required for the use of methionine's methyl groups is the conversion of methionine to S-adenosyl methionine (SAM) by methionine adenosyl transferase (present in high concentrations in the liver) in an ATP-requiring reaction. SAM may be decarboxylated to form S-adenosyl methylthiopropylamine, an intermediate in the synthesis of the polyamines spermidine and spermine. Polyamines are important in cell division and growth. SAM also serves as the principal methyl donor in the body and, as such, is required for the synthesis of carnitine, creatine, epinephrine, purines, sarcosine, and nicotinamide. The removal or donation of the methyl group from SAM yields the compound S-adenosyl homocysteine (SAH).
- SAH can be converted to homocysteine by the enzyme adenosylhomocysteine hydrolase. Homocysteine can be converted back to methionine in a betaine-dependent reaction or a vitamin B_{12} (as methylcobalamin) and folate (as 5-methyl tetrahydrofolate)–dependent reaction. Betaine, generated in the liver from choline, provides a methyl group that is transferred to homocysteine by the hepatic enzyme betaine-homocysteine methyltransferase. With the loss of the methyl group, betaine becomes dimethylglycine. This latter compound can be further demethylated to generate glycine. In the vitamin B_{12} and folate–dependent remethylation reaction (Fig. 7.27), methylcobalamin directly provides the methyl group to remethylate homocysteine to form methionine. Methylcobalamin receives the methyl group from 5-methyl tetrahydrofolate (a coenzyme form of the B vitamin folate). Elevated levels of homocysteine in the blood have been found to be a risk factor for heart disease and may develop due to low folate, vitamin B_{12}, and/or vitamin B_6 status. A discussion of the importance of adequate folate, vitamin B_{12}, and vitamin B_6 nutriture and heart disease is found in Chapter 9 in the sections on folic acid and vitamin B_{12}.
- To be further metabolized in the body, homocysteine must react with the amino acid serine, forming cystathionine via the actions of cystathionine synthase. The presence of vitamin B_6 in its coenzyme form (PLP) is necessary for this reaction to occur, hence the need for adequate vitamin B_6 status to prevent elevated blood homocysteine concentrations. Cystathionine is cleaved by cystathionine lyase, another vitamin B_6–dependent enzyme, to form the dispensable amino acid cysteine and α-ketobutyrate, which is further decarboxylated to propionyl CoA and subsequently metabolized to D- and then L-methylmalonyl CoA. L-methylmalonyl CoA is metabolized by methylmalonyl CoA mutase, a vitamin B_{12}–dependent enzyme, to the TCA cycle intermediate succinyl CoA.
- Cysteine is required for the synthesis of both protein and the nonprotein nitrogen-containing compound glutathione. Cysteine may be further metabolized to form cystine and another amino acid, taurine (Fig. 7.27).
- Taurine, a β-amino sulfonic acid, is made in the liver but concentrated in muscle and the central nervous system; it is also found in smaller amounts in the heart, liver, and kidney, among other tissues. While taurine is not involved in protein synthesis, it is important in the retina, where it is thought to exhibit antioxidant properties and help maintain the structure and function of the photoreceptor cells (Fig. 10.7). To maintain membrane stability, taurine is thought to scavenge peroxidative (e.g., oxychloride) products. Taurine also functions in the liver and intestine as a bile salt taurocholate, and in the central nervous system as an inhibitory neurotransmitter.

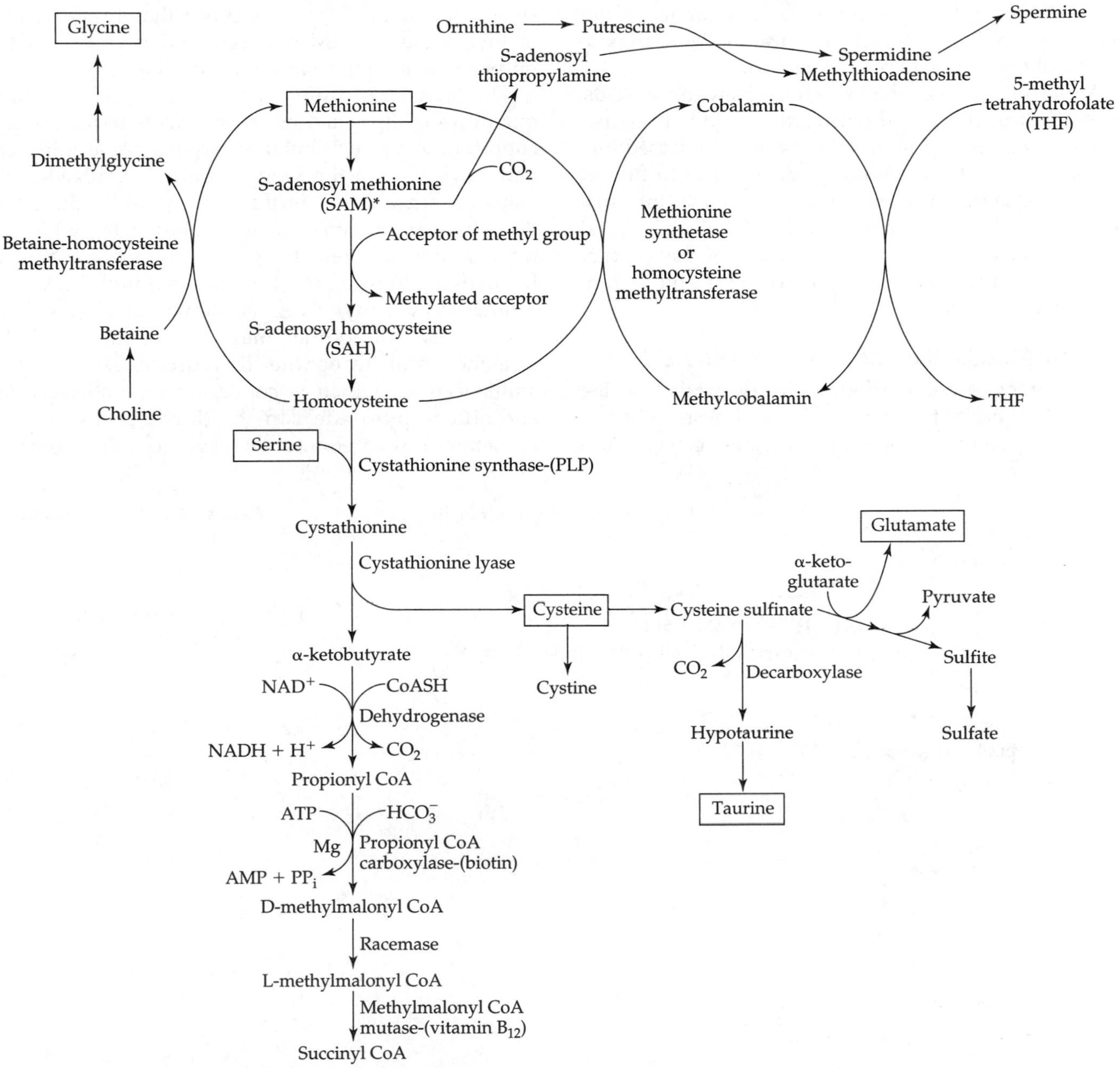

* SAM is needed for the synthesis of carnitine, creatine, epinephrine, nicotinamide, and purines.

Figure 7.27 Methionine and cysteine metabolism.

• Cysteine degradation (Fig. 7.27) yields pyruvate and sulfite. The latter compound is converted via sulfite oxidase (an iron- and molybdenum-dependent enzyme) to sulfate, which can be excreted in the urine or used in the synthesis of sulfolipids and sulfoproteins.

Genetic defects in methionine metabolism have been documented and include homocystinuria due to defects in cystathionine synthase activity and cystathioninuria due to cystathionase inactivity. Both defects necessitate a methionine-restricted diet.

Hepatic Metabolism of the Branched-Chain Amino Acids

The liver plays only a minor role in the initial metabolism of the three branched-chain amino acids, isoleucine, leucine, and valine. Transaminase activity needed to remove the amino groups is minimal in the liver, although hepatic transferases increase in response to glucocorticoid (cortisol) release, which occurs in situations such as stress, trauma, burns, and sepsis. Thus, under normal circumstances, the branched-chain amino acids typically remain in circulation and are taken up and transaminated primarily by the skeletal muscle, but also by the heart, kidney, diaphragm, and adipose, if needed.

Alpha ketoacids of the branched-chain amino acids, generated from branched-chain amino acid transamination, may be utilized within the tissues or released into circulation. The liver, among other organs, can further metabolize these alpha ketoacids. Additional information on branched-chain amino acid metabolism is found under "Skeletal Muscle" in the section of this chapter titled "Interorgan 'Flow' of Amino Acids and Organ-Specific Metabolism."

Hepatic Metabolism of Other Amino Acids

Several other reactions of amino acid metabolism are confined primarily to the liver. The catabolism of lysine, a totally ketogenic amino acid, generates acetyl CoA as shown in Figure 7.28. Remember that lysine is also methylated using SAM and used for the synthesis of the nitrogen-containing compound carnitine.

Threonine, an amino acid found in fairly high quantities relative to other amino acids in mucus glycoproteins, can be metabolized by three different pathways. One of the more commonly utilized pathways of degradation is through cytosolic threonine dehydratase to generate α-ketobutyrate, which is further metabolized to propionyl CoA, then to D-methylmalonyl CoA, L-methylmalonyl CoA, and ultimately succinyl CoA as shown in Figure 7.29. Alternately, threonine may be metabolized by mitochondrial threonine dehydrogenase to form aminoacetone, which is converted to methylglyoxal and then pyruvate. In a third pathway, the mitochondrial threonine cleavage complex converts

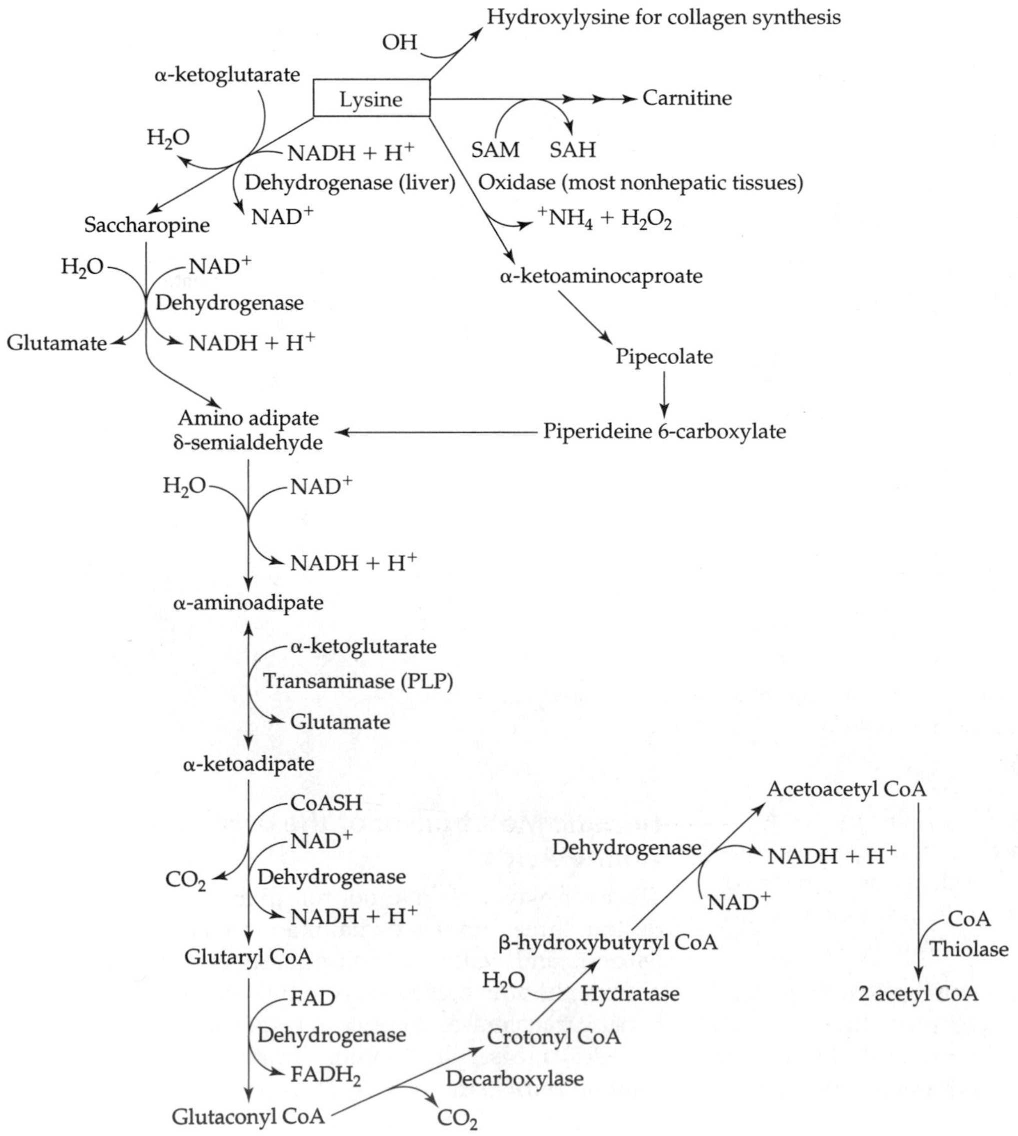

Figure 7.28 Lysine metabolism.

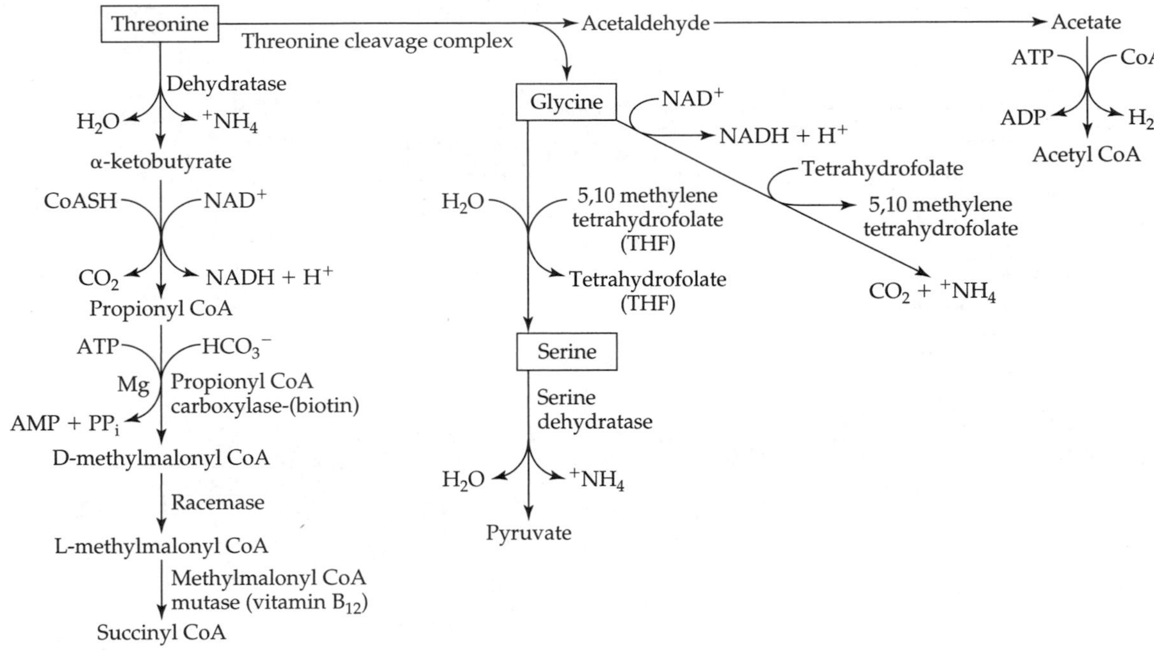

Figure 7.29 Threonine, glycine, and serine metabolism.

threonine to glycine and acetylaldehyde; the latter is further metabolized to acetate and then acetyl CoA (Fig. 7.29).

Glycine and serine are produced from one another in a reversible reaction requiring folate. Glycine, which is converted to serine mainly in the kidney (Fig. 7.29), is also needed for the synthesis of other important body compounds, including creatine, heme/**porphyrins** (nitrogen and iron-containing non-protein portions of hemoglobin; see Chap. 12), sarcosine, and the bile salt glycocholate. Serine is used for the synthesis of ethanolamine and choline for phospholipids.

Arginine catabolism occurs mostly in the liver and kidney. In the kidney, arginine is used with glycine in the first reaction of creatine synthesis. In the liver, arginine catabolism generates urea, as part of the urea cycle, and ornithine. Ornithine may be decarboxylated to form the polyamine putrescine or may be transaminated via ornithine transaminase to form glutamate γ-semialdehyde, which may then be converted to glutamate or to pyrolline 5-carboxylate. The latter may then be metabolized to form proline (Fig. 7.30), which also may be converted to glutamate. In addition, arginine is used for nitric oxide production in endothelial cells, cerebellar neurons, and neutrophils. Nitric oxide is involved in the regulation of a variety of physiological processes including regulation of blood pressure (relaxation of vascular smooth muscle) and intestinal motility, inhibition of platelet aggregation, and macrophage function. Splanchnic arginine catabolism generates some NO_3 for urinary excretion [44].

Histidine degradation is also shown in Figure 7.30. Histidine may be catabolized to form glutamate or may combine with β-alanine to generate carnosine (a nitrogen-containing compound). Through a vitamin B_6–dependent decarboxylation reaction, the amine histamine also can be formed from histidine (Fig. 7.30). Histamine is found in neurons, in cells of the gastric mucosa, and in mast cells. Histamine release causes dilation of capillaries (flushing of the skin), constriction of bronchial smooth muscle, and increased gastric secretions. Figure 7.31 provides an overview of the fates of amino acids not used for the synthesis of body proteins.

Amino Acids Not Taken Up by the Liver: Plasma Amino Acids and Amino Acid Pool(s)

Ingestion of protein-containing meals is followed by a rise in plasma amino acid concentrations, especially concentrations of the branched-chain amino acids, which are released from the liver without being metabolized. The amino acid concentrations in the plasma rise steadily for several hours, then return to basal concentrations. In basal situations or between meals, plasma amino acid concentrations are relatively stable and are species-specific; however, there is variability (large coefficients of variation) among

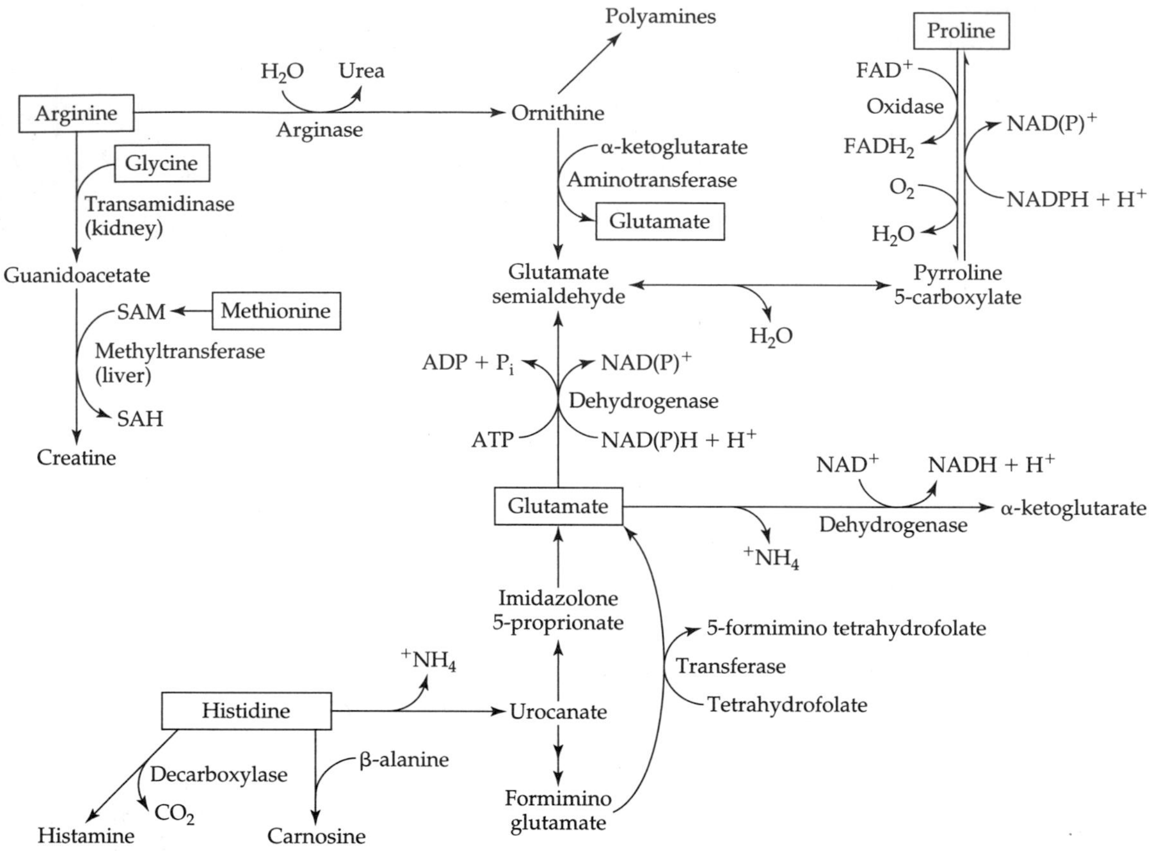

Figure 7.30 Arginine, proline, histidine, and glutamate metabolism.

people with respect to absolute concentrations of specific amino acids in the plasma.

Amino acids circulating in the plasma and found within cells arise from digestion and absorption of dietary protein as well as from the breakdown of existing body tissues. These endogenous amino acids intermingle with exogenous amino acids to form a "pool" totaling about 150 g. The pool includes amino acids in the plasma as well as amino acids in various tissues of the body. Reuse of endogenous amino acids is thought to represent the primary source of amino acids needed for protein synthesis. Despite differences in protein intake and rate of degradation of tissue protein, the pattern of the amino acids in the free amino acid pool appears to remain relatively constant, although the pattern is quite different from that found in body proteins.

The total amount of the essential amino acids found in the pool is less than that of the nonessential amino acids. The essential amino acids found in greatest concentration are lysine and threonine, both of which are totally indispensable. Of the nonessential amino acids, those found in greatest concentration are alanine, glutamate, aspartate, and glutamine. The amino acid found in greatest quantities (up to 80 g) in the pool is glutamine. The nonessential amino acids may function to conserve the essential amino acids, with the exception of histidine, lysine, and threonine, through the reamination of α-keto acids of the essential amino acid, as discussed earlier in this chapter.

Amino acids within the pool, regardless of source, are metabolized in response to various stimuli such as hormones and physiological state. Amino acids in excess of need for the synthesis of protein and/or nonprotein nitrogen-containing compounds are likely to be oxidized. Remember, if energy intake is inadequate, amino acids can be degraded to generate energy (ATP). Glucose and ketone body production from amino acids occurs when carbohydrate intake is insufficient. Cholesterol synthesis from some amino acids can also occur, and fatty acids can be made from amino acids when energy intake is in excess of the body's energy needs. The ratio of glucagon to insulin, as well as other hormones, is an important determinant of the fate of the carbon skeleton of amino acids.

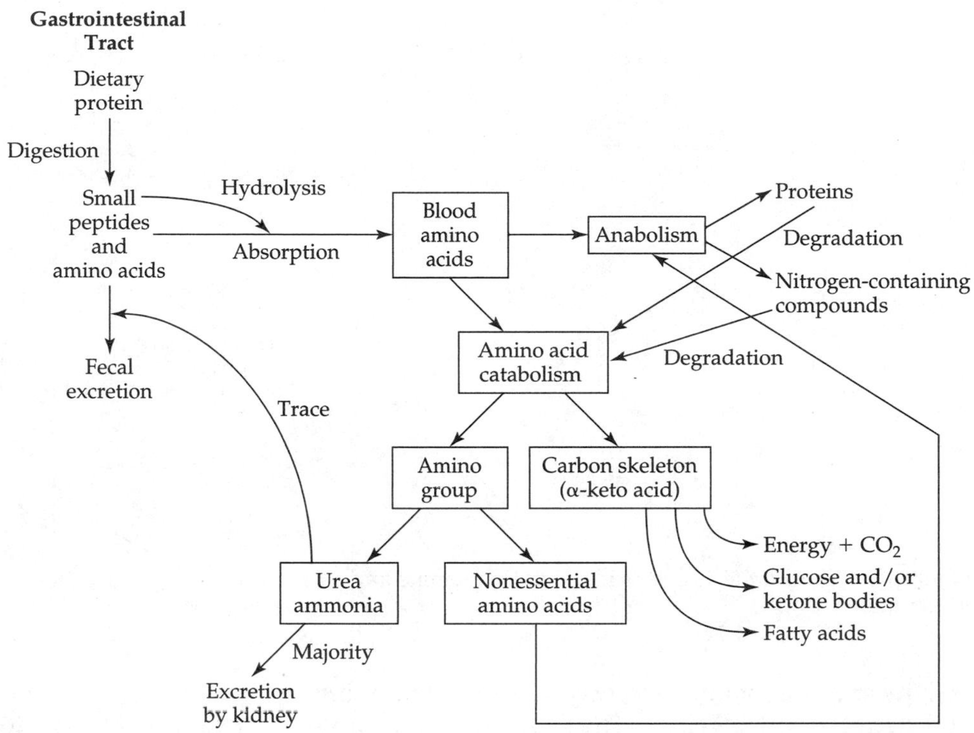

Figure 7.31 Possible fates of amino acids upon catabolism.

INTERORGAN "FLOW" OF AMINO ACIDS AND ORGAN-SPECIFIC METABOLISM

From the plasma, tissues extract amino acids for synthesis of nonessential amino acids, protein, nonprotein nitrogen-containing compounds, biogenic amines and neurotransmitters, hormones and peptides, glucose, fatty acids, or ketones or for energy production, depending on the person's nutritional status and hormonal environment. A brief review of the flow of amino acids between selected organs and organ-specific amino acid metabolism follows.

Glutamine and Alanine

Whereas ammonia arising in the liver from amino acid reactions can be readily shuttled into the urea cycle, this is not true in other tissues. In extrahepatic tissues, ammonia (NH_3) or ammonium ions (NH_4^+) generated in the cell from amino acid reactions generally combine with the amino acid glutamate to form glutamine (Fig. 7.32). This reaction is catalyzed by glutamine synthetase and requires ATP and magnesium (Mg^{2+}) or manganese (Mn^{2+}). Glutamine synthesis occurs within all tissues, including the brain and adipose [45], but especially large amounts are produced by the muscle and lungs. Glutamine functions to carry the generated ammonia safely out of the cell. Remember that too much free ammonia is toxic to cells!

Glutamine freely leaves tissues, and it travels principally to the liver, kidney, and intestine but also to organs such as the pancreas. Whereas the cells of the gastrointestinal tract, as well as the immune system (lymphocytes and macrophages), rely on glutamine catabolism for energy production, glutamine in the liver and kidney is catabolized by glutaminase, which removes the amide nitrogen to yield glutamate and ammonia (Fig. 7.32). The fate of the ammonia varies. In the absorptive state (or during periods of alkalosis), liver glutaminase activity increases, yielding ammonia for the urea cycle. In the urea cycle, ammonia reacts with HCO_3^-/CO_2 to form carbamoyl phosphate, which is made approximately in proportion to the ammonia concentration. Should the periportal hepatocytes fail to capture the ammonia for ureagenesis, the ammonia is quickly taken up by perivenous hepatocytes for glutamine synthesis. In an acidotic state, the use of glutamine for the urea cycle diminishes, and the liver releases glutamine into the blood for transport to and uptake by the kidney. Glutamine is catabolized by renal tubular glutaminase to yield ammonia and glutamate. Glutamate may be further catabolized by glutamate dehydrogenase to yield α-ketoglutarate plus another ammonia (Fig. 7.32). In the kidney, ammonium concentrations are in equilibrium with cell ammonia and H^+. Ammonia, which is lipid soluble, may diffuse into the urine and react with H^+ to form ammonium for excretion (shown later in Fig. 7.38). Renal glutaminase

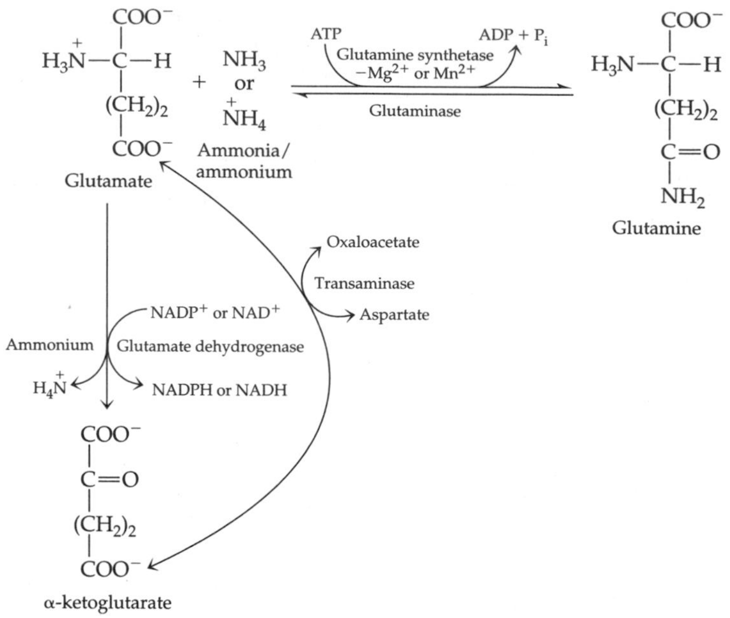

Figure 7.32 The synthesis and oxidation of glutamine and glutamate.

activity and ammonium excretion increase with acidosis and decrease with alkalosis. Thus, glutamine, by virtue of its ubiquitous synthesis in cells and its ability to diffuse out of cells for transport to tissues, is a major carrier of nitrogen between cells.

Glutamine utilization increases dramatically during hypercatabolic conditions such as sepsis and trauma. In these conditions muscle glutamine release increases but cannot meet cellular demands. Thus, glutamine stores become depleted and cell functions become compromised [15]. Remember, glutamine also promotes the synthesis of heat shock or stress proteins, is necessary for glutathione synthesis, promotes white blood cell proliferation, serves as a substrate for energy production for cells of the intestine and immune system, and, along with alanine, upon uptake into cells promotes increases in cell volume with possible associated regulatory roles in intermediary metabolism.

In addition to glutamine, another amino acid, alanine, also is important in the intertissue (between-tissue) transfer of amino groups generated from amino acid catabolism. For example, amino groups generated from branched-chain amino acid transamination in tissues such as the skeletal muscle can combine with α-ketoglutarate to form glutamate. In Figure 7.33, leucine is transaminated with α-ketoglutarate to form the α-keto acid α-ketoisocaproate and the amino acid glutamate. Glutamate may accept another amino group to form glutamine or transfer its amino group to pyruvate, generated from glucose metabolism, to form alanine (Fig. 7.33). From extrahepatic tissues, such as muscle, alanine may travel to the liver. Within the liver, alanine may undergo transamination. Alanine transamination with α-ketoglutarate produces glutamate. Glutamate may be deaminated to yield ammonia for the urea cycle, or it may be transaminated with oxaloacetate to form aspartate (Fig. 7.32). Aspartate is used in the synthesis of pyrimidines and purines and is one of the amino acids directly involved in urea generation by the urea cycle.

Alternately, alanine within the liver can be converted to glucose. These reactions, known as the glucose-alanine cycle or the alanine-glucose cycle, occur especially in situations marked by low carbohydrate stores (low liver glycogen) to maintain blood glucose or by excessive use or need for glucose. Typically, blood glucagon and possibly epinephrine and cortisol concentrations are elevated. The glucose that is generated from the alanine is subsequently released into the blood, where it is available to be taken up again and used by muscle. Muscle cells use the glucose through glycolysis and generate pyruvate. The formed pyruvate is again available for transamination with glutamate. This alanine-glucose cycle (Fig. 7.34) serves to transport nitrogen to the liver for conversion to urea while also allowing the regeneration of needed substrates.

Skeletal Muscle

The skeletal muscle mass represents about 43% of the body's mass. Uptake of amino acids by the skeletal muscles readily occurs following ingestion of a protein-containing meal. During this time, skeletal muscles typically experience a net protein synthesis. With respect to amino acid degradation, six amino acids (aspartate, asparagine, glutamate, leucine, isoleucine,

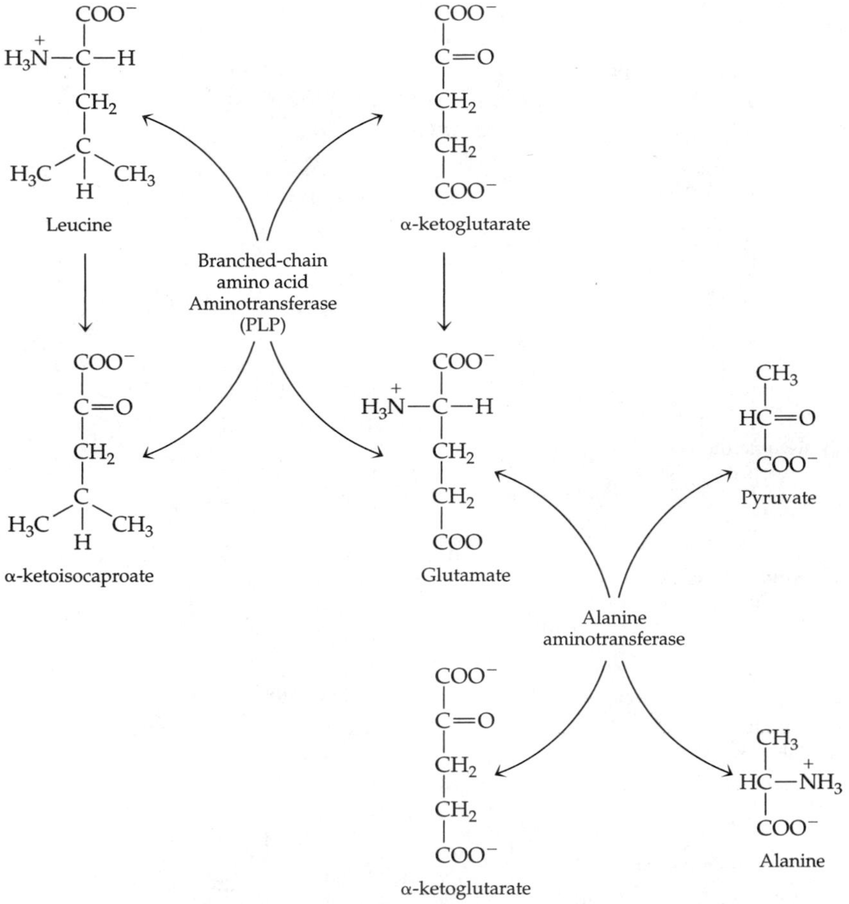

Figure 7.33 Alanine generation from leucine in body cells.

and valine) appear to be catabolized to greater extents in the skeletal muscle. The catabolism of aspartate, asparagine, and glutamate was presented earlier in the chapter. A brief review of branched-chain amino acid (isoleucine, leucine, valine) catabolism follows and is outlined in Figure 7.35.

Muscle, as well as the heart, kidney, diaphragm, adipose, and other organs (except, for the most part, the liver), possesses branched-chain aminotransferases, located in both the cytosol and mitochondria. These aminotransferases (transaminases) are needed for the transamination of the three branched-chain amino

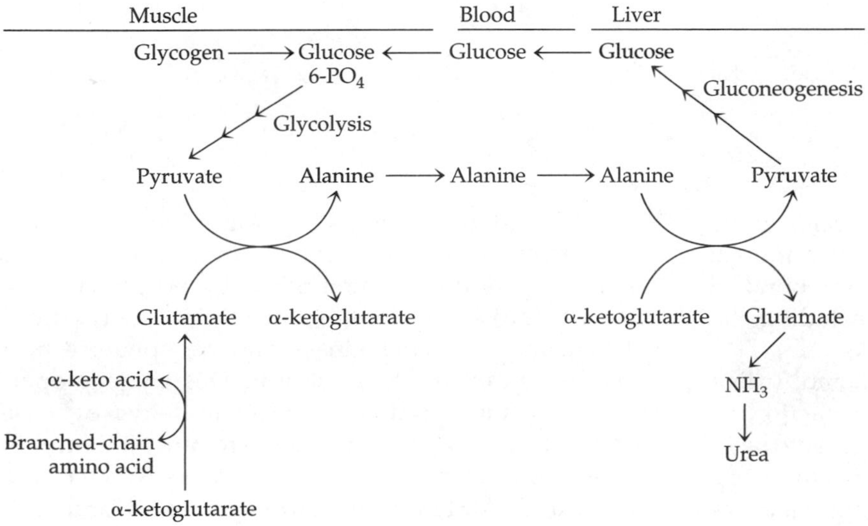

Figure 7.34 The alanine-glucose cycle: alanine generation in muscle, glucose generation in the liver.

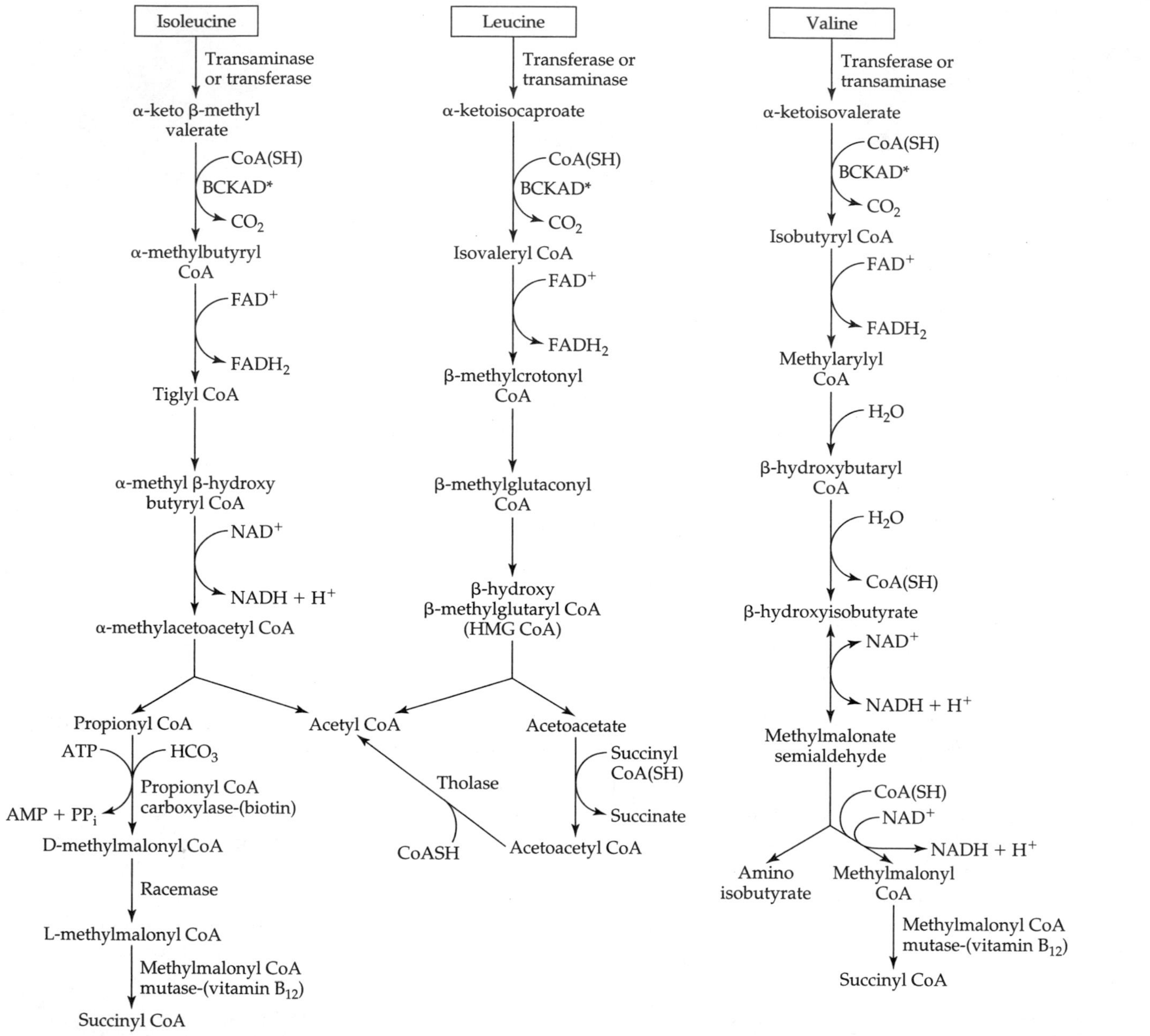

*Branched-chain α-keto acid dehydrogenase (BCKAD), requiring thiamin as TDP/TPP, niacin as NADH, and Mg^{2+} and CoA from pantothenate

Figure 7.35 Branched-chain amino acid metabolism.

acids. Following transamination, the α-keto acids of the branched-chain amino acids may remain within muscle for further oxidation or may be transported bound to albumin in the blood to other tissues (including the liver) for reamination or further catabolism.

The next step in isoleucine, leucine, and valine catabolism is decarboxylation (irreversible reaction) of the α-keto acids by the branched-chain α-keto acid dehydrogenase (BCKAD) complex, which is made up of three subunits: E1α, E1β, and E2. This enzyme complex is found in the mitochondria of many tissues, including liver, muscle, heart, kidney, intestine, and brain. It is highly regulated through phosphorylation (inactivation) and dephosphorylation (activation) mechanisms involving kinase and phosphatase proteins that act on the E1α subunit. This enzyme operates in a fashion similar to pyruvate dehydrogenase complex (see Chapter 4) in that it requires thiamin in its coenzyme form TDP/TPP, niacin as NADH, and Mg^{2+} and CoA(SH) from pantothenic acid and it is affected in some tissues by changes in dietary protein intake [46]. A genetic defect diminishing branched-chain α-keto acid dehydrogenase complex activity results in maple syrup urine disease (MSUD). MSUD necessitates a diet restricted in leucine, isoleucine, and valine intakes.

As shown in Figure 7.35, complete oxidation of valine yields succinyl CoA. Thus, valine is considered glucogenic. The end products of isoleucine catabolism are succinyl CoA and acetyl CoA, which are glucogenic and ketogenic, respectively. Complete oxidation of leucine results in acetyl CoA and acetoacetate formation, and acetoacetate may be further metabolized to form acetyl CoA. Leucine thus is totally ketogenic

Leucine is also one of the few amino acids that is completely oxidized in the muscle for energy. Leucine is oxidized in a manner similar to fatty acids, and its oxidation results in the production of 1 mol of acetyl CoA and 1 mol of acetoacetate. Complete oxidation of leucine generates more ATP molecules on a molar basis than complete oxidation of glucose. Moreover, leucine oxidation in muscles increases during certain physiological states, such as fasting. During fasting, leucine rises to high levels in the blood and muscle, while the capacity of the muscle to degrade leucine increases concurrently. By supplying the muscle with the equivalent of 3 mol of acetyl CoA per molecule of leucine oxidized, the acetyl CoA produces energy for the muscle while simultaneously inhibiting pyruvate oxidation. Pyruvate is then used for the synthesis of lactate, which is released from the muscles. Thus, the oxidation of leucine spares essential gluconeogenic precursors. Pyruvate, along with lactate, can be returned to the liver; the former is either transported as pyruvate per se or (more likely) converted to alanine for transport.

A great deal of interest in protein metabolism within the skeletal muscle was generated by the discovery that during starvation the amounts of the various amino acids released from the muscle could not reflect proteolysis alone. In particular, much more alanine and glutamine were appearing in the blood than could be attributed to muscle protein content. We now know that alanine is made in muscle from a transamination reaction with pyruvate and α-ketoglutarate. Pyruvate is generated from glucose metabolism within the muscle cells, and glutamate generates α-ketoglutarate following transamination of any of the branched-chain amino acids. The alanine then leaves the muscle for transport in the blood to the liver. During times of starvation, low carbohydrate intake (e.g., high glucagon : insulin ratio), or "stress" (e.g., high epinephrine and cortisol concentrations), the liver converts the alanine back to pyruvate, which through a series of reactions is converted back to glucose as part of gluconeogenesis. Remember, this cycling of alanine and glucose between the muscle and liver is known as the alanine-glucose cycle, as discussed in the previous section and shown in Figure 7.34.

Glutamine is generated in muscle in several pathways as shown in Figure 7.36. Initially, transamination of the branched-chain amino acids occurs primarily with α-ketoglutarate to form the branched-chain α-keto acid and glutamate, respectively. Glutamate combines with ammonia to form glutamine in an ATP-dependent reaction catalyzed by glutamine synthetase. Glutamine synthetase activity is relatively high in skeletal muscle, as well as in the lungs, brain, and adipose. Ammonia may be generated by amino acid deamination or by AMP deamination. AMP forms in the muscle with ATP degradation. The glutamine that is formed in the muscle is released into the blood and transported for use by other tissues, such as the intestine, kidneys, or liver.

Amino acids released in lesser quantities from muscle (forearm and/or leg) in a postabsorptive state include phenylalanine, methionine, lysine, arginine, histidine, tyrosine, proline, tryptophan, threonine, and glycine [47,48]. Further studies investigating the effects of meals containing all three energy nutrients on amino acid uptake and output by muscle are needed.

Creatine, a nitrogen-containing compound that is made in the kidney and liver from the amino acids arginine and glycine with methyl groups donated from the amino acid methionine, functions in skeletal muscle as an energy source. Remember from earlier in this chapter that creatine is phosphorylated in muscle by ATP to form phosphocreatine (also called creatine phosphate), which can replenish ATP in muscles that are actively contracting (as with exercise). Phosphocreatine works in muscle by reacting with ADP generated in the muscle from the hydrolysis of ATP. When phosphocreatine reacts with ADP, creatine and ATP are formed. Creatine kinase catalyzes this important reaction that enables the generation of ATP for muscle contraction. Creatine and creatine phosphate, however, do not remain indefinitely in muscle; rather, both slowly but spontaneously cyclize (Fig. 7.37) because of nonreversible, nonenzymatic dehydration. This cyclization of creatine and phosphocreatine forms creatinine. Once formed, creatinine leaves the muscle, passes across the glomerulus of the kidney, and is excreted in the urine. Small amounts of creatinine may be excreted into the gut and, like urea, metabolized by bacterial flora in the

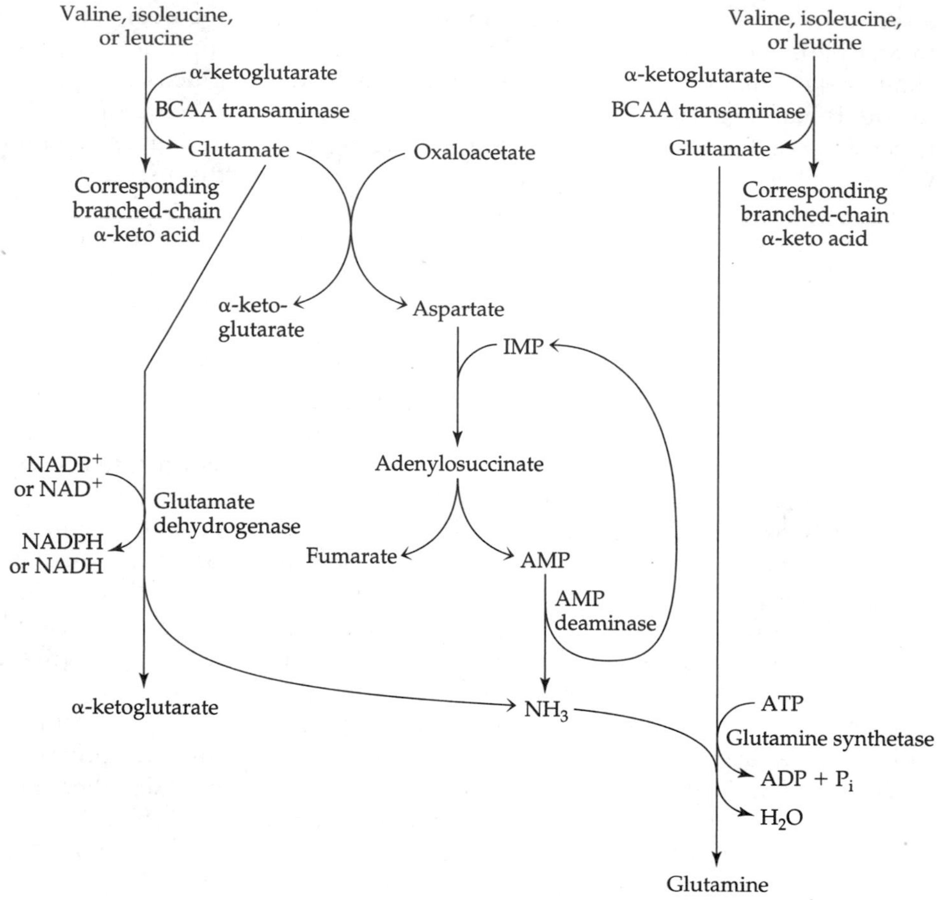

Figure 7.36 Some pathways of glutamine generation in muscle.

intestine. Creatinine clearance is frequently used as a means of estimating kidney function.

Nitrogen-Containing Compounds as Indicators of Muscle Mass and Muscle Catabolism

Urinary excretions of creatinine and 3-methylhistidine are used as indicators of the amount of existing muscle mass and the rate of muscle degradation, respectively. Urinary creatinine excretion is considered to be a reflection of muscle mass because it is the degradation product of creatine, which makes up approximately 0.3% to 0.5% of muscle mass by weight. The creatinine excreted in the urine reflects about 1.7% of the total creatine pool per day. However, urinary creatinine excretion is not considered to be a completely accurate indicator of muscle mass because of the variation in muscle creatine content.

Excretion of 3-methylhistidine provides an indicator of muscle catabolism. On proteolysis, 3-methylhistidine (shown in Table 7.1) is released and is a nonreusable amino acid because the methylation of histidine occurs posttranslationally. Because 3-methylhistidine is found primarily in actin, this compound has been used to

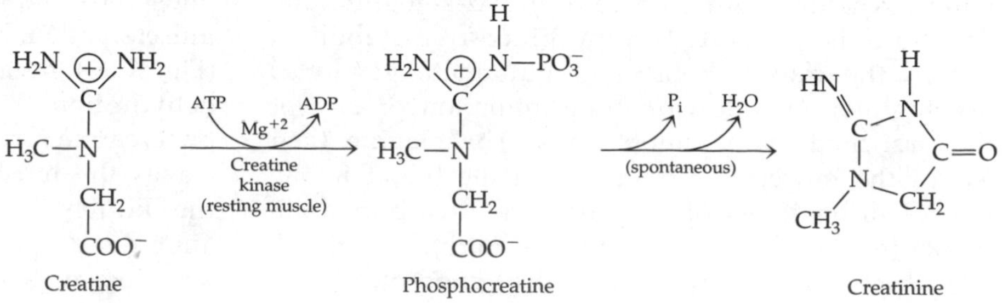

Figure 7.37 Conversion of creatine to phosphocreatine in the muscle and its spontaneous cyclization to creatinine.

estimate muscle protein degradation. Excretion of the compound is used as an index of muscle degradation. However, actin is not found only in muscle but appears to be widely distributed in the body, including in tissues such as the intestine and platelets, which have high turnover rates. Thus, urinary 3-methylhistidine excretion represents not only an index of muscle breakdown but more inclusively an index of protein breakdown for many tissues in the body.

Kidneys

Studies in humans as well as animals suggest that the kidneys preferentially take up a number of amino acids including, for example, glycine, alanine, glutamine, glutamate, phenylalanine, and aspartate. Metabolism of amino acids within the kidney (Fig. 7.38) includes

- serine synthesis from glycine,
- glycine catabolism,

Figure 7.38 Amino acid metabolism in selected organs.

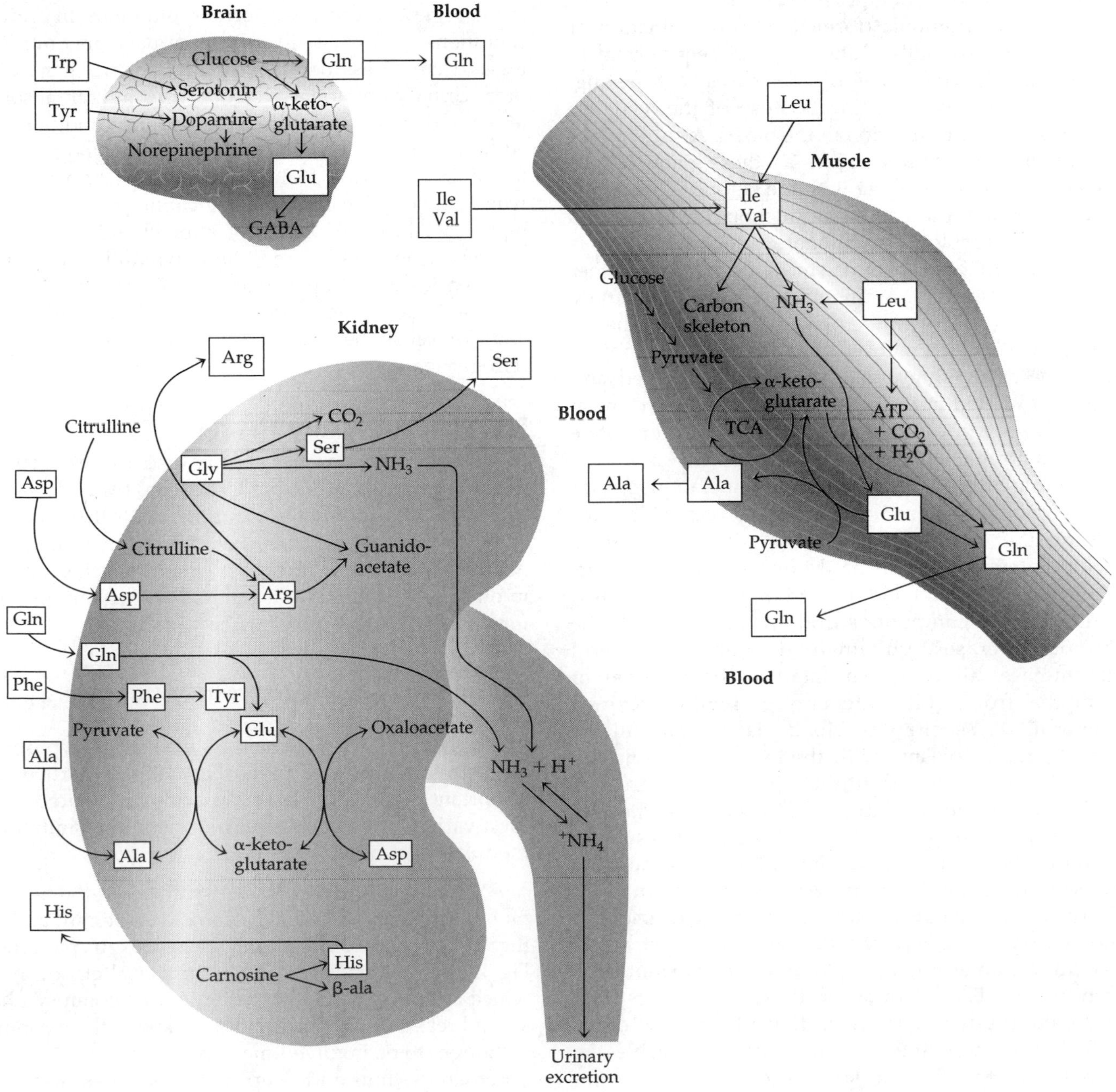

- histidine generation from carnosine degradation,
- arginine synthesis from aspartate and citrulline
- tyrosine synthesis from phenylalanine, and
- guanidoacetate formation from arginine and glycine for creatine synthesis.

The kidney is considered to be the major site for arginine, histidine, serine, and perhaps tyrosine production.

In addition, the kidney is the only organ besides the liver that has the enzymes necessary for gluconeogenesis. This renal metabolism of amino acids becomes particularly significant during fasting. Gluconeogenesis can raise the amount of glucose available to the body for energy, while ammonia (formed from deamination of amino acids, especially glutamine) can help normalize the blood pH, which typically decreases with fasting. Acidosis occurs with fasting because of the resulting rise in ketone concentration in the blood. Also, a loss of sodium and potassium occurs as these minerals are excreted in the urine along with the ketones. Renal glutamine uptake for ammonia production during periods of acidosis (or low bicarbonate concentrations) is increased, while uptake by the intestine, liver, and other organs is diminished. Ammonia generated from amino acids, especially glutamine deamination, enters the filtrate and combines with H^+ ions to form ammonium ions. The ammonium ions cannot be reabsorbed and thus are excreted in the urine. The loss of the H^+ from the body serves to increase pH from an acidotic state toward a normal value of about 7.35 to 7.45.

The role of the kidney in nitrogen metabolism cannot be overemphasized. The organ is responsible for ridding the body of nitrogenous wastes that have accumulated in the plasma. Moreover, enzymes particularly active in the kidney and involved in removal of nitrogenous compounds from the body include the aminotransferases, glutamate dehydrogenase, and glutaminase, all of which catalyze the removal of ammonia from glutamate and glutamine. Kidney glomeruli act as filters of blood plasma, and all the constituents in plasma with the exception of plasma proteins move into the filtrate. (Some albumin normally moves into the filtrate, but it is reabsorbed by the proximal tubular cells.) Essential nutrients such as sodium (Na^+), amino acids, and glucose are actively reabsorbed as the filtrate moves through the tubules. Many other substances are not actively reabsorbed and if they move into the tubular cells must either move along an electrical gradient or move osmotically with water. The amount of these substances that enters the tubular cells, then, depends on how much water moves into the cells and how permeable the cells are to the specific substances. The cell membranes are relatively impermeable to urea and uric acid, while membranes are particularly impermeable to creatinine, none of which is reabsorbed.

Table 7.5 Nitrogen-Containing Waste Products Excreted in the Urine

Compound	Approximate Amounts (g) Excreted per Day
Urea	5–20
Creatinine	1–1.8
Uric acid	0.3–1
Ammonia	0.4–1

Several forms of nitrogenous wastes are lost in the urine, as shown in Table 7.5. About 80% of nitrogen is lost in the urine as urea under normal conditions. In acidotic conditions, as occur with fasting, urinary urea nitrogen losses decrease, as does the percentage of nitrogen lost as urea. Urinary ammonia excretion rises in both absolute terms and percentage terms in acidotic conditions. In addition to urea and ammonia, usual nitrogenous wastes found in the urine include creatinine and uric acid, with lesser or trace amounts of creatine (<100 mg/day), hippuric acid (<100 mg/day), protein (<100 mg/day), and amino acids (<700 mg/day). In addition to urinary nitrogen losses, nitrogen may be lost through the skin as urea. Nitrogen also may be lost with the loss of hair and skin cells. These losses are referred to as insensible nitrogen losses.

Brain and Accessory Tissues

Because the brain has the capacity for active transport of the indispensable amino acids, neurons have access to a higher concentration of these amino acids than is found in the plasma. The brain has transport systems for neutral, dibasic, and dicarboxylic amino acids, and, as in other cells, competition occurs between amino acids for uptake by a common carrier system.

Biogenic Amines and Neurotransmitters/Hormones

The uptake of two aromatic amino acids, tryptophan and tyrosine, by the brain (Fig 7.38) is particularly important because these amino acids act as precursors for a variety of hormones and/or neurotransmitters or modulators of nerve function.

- Tryptophan is used in the synthesis of the hormone melatonin (N-acetyl 5-methoxyserotonin) and the neurotransmitter serotonin (5-hydroxytryptamine; Fig. 7.39). Melatonin is made in the pineal gland, which lies in the center of the brain. Melatonin synthesis and release correspond with darkness; the hormone is thought to be involved mainly with the regulation of circadian rhythms and sleep, and supplement use has

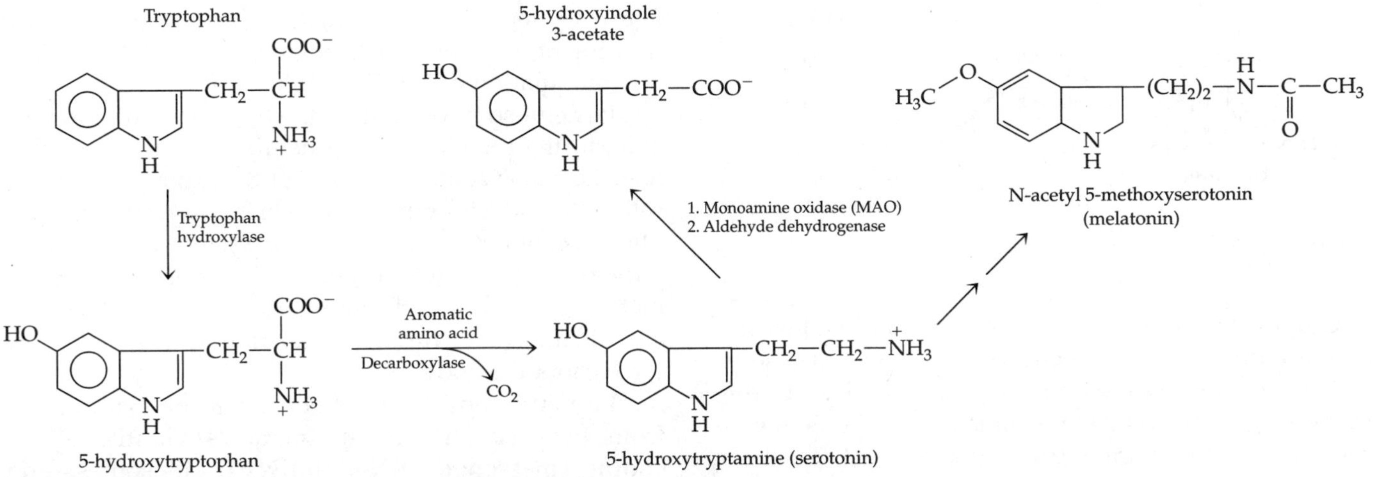

Figure 7.39 Serotonin and melatonin synthesis and degradation from tryptophan.

been helpful for some individuals with jet lag [49–51]. Serotonin functions as an excitatory neurotransmitter and as a potent vasoconstrictor and stimulator of smooth muscle contraction.

- Tyrosine is used to synthesize (mostly in the adrenal medulla) dopamine, norepinephrine, and epinephrine (Fig. 7.25), referred to as catecholamines because they are derivatives of catechol (Fig. 7.40) or amines. The actions of both epinephrine and norepinephrine have major effects on nutrient metabolism. These actions include stimulation of glycogenolysis and lipolysis (mobilization of fatty acids), and increased metabolic rate, among other effects.

Neurotransmitters are stored in the nerve axon terminal as vesicles or granules until stimuli arrive to effect their release. Following their action on the cell membranes, the neurotransmitters are inactivated. The fastest mechanism for inactivation is uptake of the neurotransmitter by adjacent cells, where mitochondrial monoamine oxidase (MAO) removes the amine group. Each of the catecholamines (dopamine, norepinephrine, epinephrine) as well as serotonin can be inactivated by MAO (Fig 7.39). A slower mechanism of inactivation requires that the catecholamines be carried by the blood to the liver, where they are methylated by catechol-O-methyltransferase (COMT). Interactions between MAO inhibitors and foods high in amines such as tyramine are discussed in the Chapter 12 perspective on nutrient drug interactions.

Other amino acids besides tryptophan and tyrosine also function as neurotransmitters in the brain:

- Glycine acts as an inhibitory neurotransmitter.
- Taurine is also thought to function as an inhibitory neurotransmitter.
- Aspartate, derived chiefly from glutamate through aspartate aminotransferase activity common in neural tissue, is thought to act as an excitatory neurotransmitter in the central nervous system.
- Glutamate acts as an excitatory neurotransmitter or may be converted into γ-amino butyric acid (GABA), an inhibitory neurotransmitter.

GABA is believed to be the neurotransmitter for cells that exert inhibitory effects on other cells in the central nervous system. The conversion of glutamate to GABA involves the removal of the α-carboxyl group of glutamate by the enzyme glutamate decarboxylase in a vitamin B_6-(PLP)–dependent reaction (Fig. 7.41). Glutamate uptake by the brain typically is low; thus, synthesis of glutamate from glucose represents the primary source of brain glutamate.

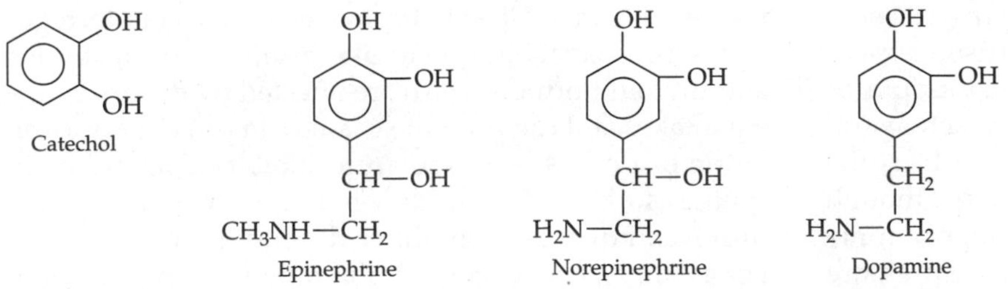

Figure 7.40 The catecholamines.

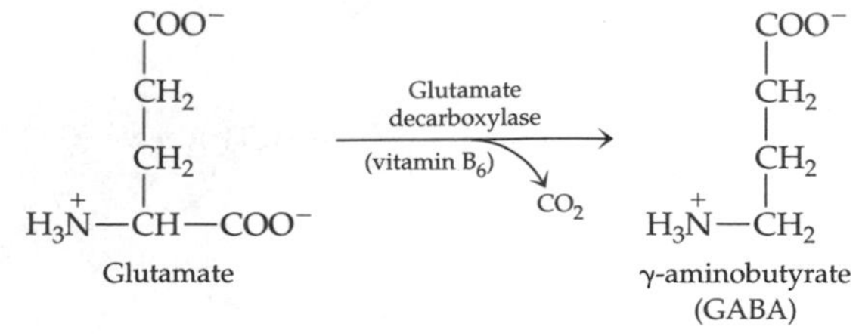

Figure 7.41 GABA synthesis.

Glutamate is of significance to the brain not just as a neuromodulator or a precursor of GABA but also as a means of ridding the brain of ammonia. The starting point for glutamate metabolism is the synthesis in neurons of α-ketoglutarate from glucose that has been transported from the blood across the blood-brain barrier. The α-ketoglutarate can be converted to glutamate via reductive amination. Whenever excessive ammonia is present in the brain, glutamine is formed through the action of glutamine synthetase, which is highly active in neural tissues (Fig. 7.32). Glutamine is freely diffusible and can move easily into the blood or cerebrospinal fluid, thereby allowing the removal of 2 mol of toxic ammonia from the brain. Any condition that causes an unusual elevation of blood ammonia can interfere with the normal handling of amino acids by the brain. Treatment of hepatic encephalopathy (dysfunction of the brain associated with liver disease, which characteristically results in elevated blood ammonia concentrations) is aimed at normalizing the effects of altered amino acid metabolism on the central nervous system.

Use of amino acid supplements has been promoted with claims that, upon ingestion, the amino acids will be utilized in the body for the synthesis of compounds necessary to evoke the desired response. For example, use of tryptophan supplements to induce sleep has been promoted. However, use of tryptophan supplements as sleep aids has not proven effective.

Neuropeptides

The central nervous system (CNS) abounds in peptides, termed neuropeptides. Many of the same peptides that were mentioned in Chapter 2 with respect to digestion and were found associated with the intestinal tract are also found associated with the CNS. These neuropeptides are of varying lengths and possess a variety of functions. Some peptides act as hormone-releasing factors, such as ACTH involved with cortisol release. Some have endocrine effects, such as somatotropin or growth hormone. Others have modulatory actions on transmitter functions, mood, or behavior, such as the enkephalins. The enkephalins and endorphins, though similar to natural opiates, possess a wide range of functions, including affecting pain sensation, blood pressure and body temperature regulation, governance of body movement, secretion of hormones, control of feeding, and modulation of learning ability.

The neurosecretory cells of the hypothalamus are foremost in the secretion of the neuropeptides. Those that have hormone action move out of the axons of the nerve cells into the pituitary, from which they are secreted. This linkage between the nervous system and the pituitary is of great significance in the overall control of metabolism because the pituitary gland is primary in coordinating the various endocrine glands scattered throughout the body.

The neuropeptides are believed to be synthesized from their constituent amino acids via the DNA-coding, messenger RNA (mRNA), ribosomes, and transfer RNA (tRNA) system. Because the nucleus and ribosomes are found in the cell body and dendrites, the peptides must travel to the end of the axon to be stored in vesicles for future release. The neuropeptides are stored as inactive precursor polypeptides, which must be cleaved to generate an active neuropeptide, as shown here:

Amino acids

Precursor peptide → Active neuropeptide

Following synthesis of the active neuropeptide, it is released by exocytosis to perform its function at the membrane. After performing its function, the neuropeptide is hydrolyzed to its constituent amino acids.

PROTEIN TURNOVER: SYNTHESIS AND CATABOLISM OF TISSUE PROTEINS

Food intake and the nutritional status of the organism affect protein turnover that is mediated through changes in the concentrations of different hormones. The secretion of insulin, glucagon, growth hormone, and glucocorticoids increases in response to elevated concentrations of selected amino acids. In general, increased protein synthesis, decreased protein degradation, and positive nitrogen balance are promoted by insulin, whereas the counterregulatory hormones, glucagon, epinephrine, and glucocorticoids have an opposite effect, promoting overall protein degradation and a negative nitrogen balance. Growth hormone, though counterregulatory, is an anabolic agent, like insulin. Prostaglandins and thyroid hormones also are affected by dietary nutrient intakes and can promote changes in protein turnover. Nitric oxide has been shown to inhibit hepatic protein synthesis [52]. The effects of a hormone on protein turnover, however, may differ depending on the tissue. For example, a glucagon : insulin ratio favoring glucagon diminishes insulin's ability to inhibit protein degradation and diminishes the overall rate of protein synthesis, yet it stimulates hepatic synthesis of proteins (enzymes) for gluconeogenesis and ureagenesis.

Each cellular protein exhibits a specific and characteristic rate of synthesis. Transcription and translation of DNA and RNA are under multiple influences, such as hormonal and nutrient. Protein synthesis is also affected by the amount and stability of mRNA, the ribosome number (amount of ribosomal RNA, or rRNA), the activity of the ribosomes (rapidity of translation, or peptide formation), the presence of both essential and nonessential amino acids in the appropriate concentrations to charge the tRNA, and the hormonal environment. Chapter 1 provides a more in-depth discussion of protein synthesis. Should amino acids not be present or be present in insufficient quantity, amino acid oxidation increases. In other words, the supply of amino acids must meet the demand. The rate of amino acid oxidation is sensitive to a surplus or deficit of specific amino acids as well as to hormonal factors and thus regulates the amino acid pool(s). Amino acid pools remain fairly constant in size and pattern in the body. Further, they serve as the connecting link between two cycles of nitrogen metabolism:

protein turnover	and	nitrogen balance
(protein synthesis vs. degradation)		(nitrogen intake vs. nitrogen output)

These two cycles operate somewhat independently, but if either cycle gets out of balance, the other is affected to some degree. For example, during growth, protein synthesis exceeds degradation, and nitrogen intake exceeds excretion, resulting in a positive nitrogen balance. The increase in protein turnover, however, is much greater than is reflected by the change in nitrogen balance. The amino acid pool(s), regulated in some manner, act as ballast between protein turnover and nitrogen balance.

When the body is considered as a whole, protein synthesis and degradation (turnover) are estimated to account for 10% to 25% of resting energy expenditure [53]. Protein degradation, for example, requires energy for proteolysis, metabolism of amino acids not reincorporated into protein, amino acid transport across membranes, and RNA metabolism [53]. Rates of protein turnover vary among tissues, as is evidenced in the more rapid turnover of visceral protein as compared with skeletal muscle. Protein synthesis and protein degradation are under independent controls. Rates of synthesis can be quite high, as with protein accretion during growth. Alternately, protein degradation can be quite high, as during fever.

Cellular Protein Degradation Systems

Degradation of proteins, either made intracellularly or brought into the cell by endocytosis, occurs primarily by the action of proteases, either lysosomal or nonlysosomal, present in the cytosol. The contributions of lysosomal and nonlysosomal cytosolic pathways in proteolysis vary depending on the cell type and the physiological status [54]. Nonetheless, the constant degradation of intracellular proteins is of prime importance to the life of the cells because it ensures a flux of proteins (amino acids) through the cytosol that can be used for cellular growth and/or maintenance.

Lysosomes, cell organelles with an internal pH of about 4 to 5 and containing a variety of digestive enzymes, represent the primary means of protein digestion. Lysosomes are found in all mammalian cell types with the exception of the erythrocyte. While skeletal muscles do not contain many lysosomes, they are particularly abundant in liver cells. Several proteases are found in lysosomes, including endopeptidases and exopeptidases known as cathepsins. Numerous cathepsins have been isolated; examples include protease cathepsins B, H, L, which are referred to as cysteine proteases, and protease cathepsin D, which is an aspartate protease. Each of the cathepsin proteases varies in specificity [55]. Lysosomal proteases appear to be responsible for degradation of extracellular proteins brought into the cell by endocytosis and for intracellular protein degradation under conditions of nutrient deprivation and some pathological conditions [54,55]. The extent to which lysosomal proteases influence muscle proteolysis is unknown, but it is believed to be fairly small [56].

The process by which lysosomal proteases digest proteins requires that the cell engulf the designated protein. Thus, for extracellular proteins being degraded, a portion of the extracellular matrix is engulfed along with the protein, and for intracellular proteins, cytoplasm and the protein are engulfed. Following engulfment, the protein designated for degradation becomes contained in a vacuole in the cytoplasm. The vacuoles containing the intracellular protein fuse with lysosomes, and the protein in turn is completely digested by the lysosomal proteases. This process, often referred to as macroautophagy, is enhanced by glucagon and suppressed by insulin as well as amino acids [57]. The high glucagon : insulin ratio is consistent with conditions in which cells would be nutritionally (amino acid) deprived.

In well-nourished cells, slow, continuous degradation of intracellular proteins by the lysosomal autophagic enzyme system typically occurs, a process referred to as basal autophagy or microautophagy [55,57]. Microautophagy needs some mechanism by which selected intracellular proteins can enter the lysosomes more rapidly than other proteins. The conformation of intracellular proteins as a determinant of intracellular degradation rates, along with regulatory control by selected amino acids, has been proposed [55,58]. In the liver, microautophagy may function in the degradation of proteins that have long half-lives and are not good substrates for other proteolytic pathways [54].

In addition to lysosome-mediated cellular protein degradation, nonlysosomal protease systems also degrade proteins. The ubiquitin proteasomal system is nonlysosomal and mediates the degradation of many cellular proteins. In the ubiquitin system, proteins that are to be degraded are ligated to **ubiquitin** (a 76-amino-acid polypeptide) in an ATP-requiring reaction. The linkage of ubiquitin to protein first necessitates activation of ubiquitin. Ubiquitin is activated by the enzyme E1. E1 is a subunit of the ubiquitin enzyme system, which hydrolyzes ATP to form a thiol ester with the carboxyl end of ubiquitin. This activated ubiquitin is transferred to another enzyme protein, E2. Next the carboxyl end of ubiquitin is ligated by E3 to the protein substrate that is ultimately to be degraded. One or more (typically five) ubiquitin proteins may bind to a protein substrate. Once ubiquitins are ligated to the protein to be degraded, proteases present as a proteasome/multienzyme complex degrade the ubiquitinated proteins in a series of reactions. Following proteolysis, ubiquitin is released for reuse.

Proteasomal degradation is thought to be responsible for the degradation of abnormal, damaged, denatured, or mislocated proteins as well as of regulatory proteins that typically have short half-lives [54,59]. Activity of ubiquitin-dependent proteasomal degradation also appears to increase during pathological conditions such as sepsis, cancer, and trauma, among others, as well as during starvation [56,60].

One signal for ubiquitin-mediated proteasomal degradation in proteins involves N-terminal (N-end rule) recognition by the E3α ubiquitin protein ligase [61]. E3 has two distinct sites that interact with specific N-terminal residues. Proteins with valine, methionine, glycine, alanine, serine, threonine, and cysteine residues at their N-terminal position are relatively stable [62]. In contrast, proteins with N-terminal basic or large hydrophobic amino acids such as lysine, arginine, histidine, leucine, isoleucine, tryptophan, phenylalanine, and tyrosine are typically susceptible to degradation by the ubiquitin proteasomal system [61,62]. Proteins with acetylated N-termini are not degraded by the ubiquitin system [61].

Other characteristics of short-lived proteins include large size, acidic net charge, hydrophobicity, and rapid inactivation by a low pH or a high temperature [55]. Rapidly degraded proteins may also possess a common amino acid sequence; the PEST hypothesis suggests that proteins with particularly short half-lives contain regions rich in proline (P), glutamic acid (E), serine (S), and threonine (T) [63]. However, neither the mechanism by which the PEST signal targets proteins for degradation nor the system that recognizes the signal has been identified [56,61].

In addition to the ubiquitin/proteasomal and the lysosomal pathways, another degradation pathway has been identified in muscle: the calpain proteolytic pathway. This pathway does not require lysosomes or energy but instead requires calcium for its function. Two proteases, μ-calpain and m-calpain, comprise the calpain proteolytic pathway and differ in their need for calcium. The overall role of the calpains in protein turnover is unclear; however, the proteases may be responsible for the initial step in degradation, the release of myofilaments from the myofibrils. The released myofilament is then thought to be ligated to ubiquitin for further degradation.

The requirement for energy for protein catabolism is a paradox that has been recognized for decades. ATP-dependent proteases have been demonstrated in the cytosolic degradation system. Based on their work with an ATP-dependent protease found in *Escherichia coli*, Waxman and Goldberg [64] have shown that this enzyme is activated both by ATP and by substrate proteins and that the two have an additive effect. When the protein is activated by ATP, it will degrade various small hydrophobic peptides that are bound to its active site, but concomitant hydrolysis of the ATP molecule does not occur. When a substrate protein activates the protease, it evidently does so by binding to two sites on the enzyme: the active site, which has a preference for specific amino acid sequences, and a regulatory site, which somehow recognizes that the protein is unfolded and vulnerable. When activated by both ATP and a substrate protein, the enzyme is believed to undergo a distinct structural change that enhances its capacity for peptide cleavage and also causes hydrolysis of ATP. A protein that binds itself to both sites of the enzyme can induce its own destruction, but other proteins that are unable to bind the enzyme at both sites will remain unaffected. Furthermore, the adenosine diphosphate (ADP) produced as a result of the proteolysis acts as an inhibitor of continued hydrolysis, thereby helping to prevent excessive proteolysis once the enzyme has been activated. Should an analogous mechanism exist in mammalian cells, this scheme could go far in explaining not only the observed heterogeneous selectivity of protein catabolism but also the function of ATP in this catabolic process [65].

PROTEIN QUALITY AND PROTEIN INTAKE

Dietary protein is required by humans because it contributes to the body's supply of indispensable amino acids and to its supply of nitrogen for the synthesis of the dispensable amino acids. The quality of a protein depends to some extent on its digestibility but primarily on its indispensable amino acid composition, both the specific amounts and the proportions of these amino acids.

Protein-containing foods can be divided into two categories:

- high-quality or complete proteins, and
- low-quality or incomplete proteins.

A **complete protein** contains all the indispensable amino acids in the approximate amounts needed by humans. Sources of complete proteins are mostly foods of animal origin such as milk, yogurt, cheese, eggs, meat, fish, and poultry. The exceptions are gelatin, which is of animal origin but does not have the indispensable amino acid tryptophan, and soy protein, which is of plant origin but is a complete protein. **Incomplete proteins** or low-quality proteins are derived from plant foods such as legumes, vegetables, cereals, and grain products. Most plant foods tend to have too little of one or more particular indispensable amino acids. The term **limiting amino acid** is used to describe the indispensable amino acid that is present in the lowest quantity in the food. Listed here are examples of incomplete protein-containing foods and their limiting amino acid(s):

Food Source of Incomplete Protein	Limiting Amino Acid(s)
Wheat, rice, corn, other grains and grain products	Lysine, threonine (sometimes), and tryptophan (sometimes)
Legumes	Methionine

Unless carefully planned, a diet containing only low-quality proteins will result in inadequate availability of selected amino acids and will inhibit the body's ability to synthesize its own body proteins. The body cannot make a protein with a missing amino acid.

To ensure that the body receives all the indispensable amino acids, certain proteins can be ingested together or combined so that their amino acid patterns become complementary. This practice or strategy is called mutual supplementation. Most, but not all, agree that the complementary proteins should be consumed at the same meal. For the vegan, this knowledge is particularly valuable. For example, legumes, with their high content of lysine but low content of sulfur-containing amino acids, complement the grains, which are more than adequate in methionine and cysteine but limited in lysine. The lacto-ovo vegetarian should have no problem with protein adequacy because when milk and eggs are combined—even in small amounts—with plant foods, the indispensable amino acids are supplied in adequate amounts. One exception is the combination of milk with legumes. Although milk contains more methionine and cysteine per gram of protein than do the legumes, it still fails to meet the standard of the ideal pattern for the sulfur-containing amino acids.

The formula for vegan protein balance is as follows: 60% of protein from grains, 35% from legumes, and 5% from leafy greens [66]. A 70-kg adult male whose RDA for protein is 56 g could obtain his needed indispensable amino acids by consuming

- 4 servings (four slices) whole-grain bread;
- 5 servings ($2\frac{1}{2}$ cups) grain from oatmeal, brown rice, cracked wheat;
- 1 serving ($\frac{1}{4}$ cup) nuts or seeds;
- $2\frac{1}{2}$ servings ($1\frac{1}{4}$ cups) beans, or 2 cups soy milk plus $\frac{1}{3}$ cup navy beans; and
- 4 servings (2 cups) vegetables, two of which are leafy greens.

Plant protein foods contribute about 65% of the per capita supply of protein worldwide but only about 32% in North America [67].

Digestibility of proteins is also important for amino acid utilization. The digestibility of a protein is a measure of the amounts of amino acids that are absorbed following ingestion of a given protein. Animal proteins have been found to be about 90% to 99% digestible, while plant proteins are about 70% to 90% digestible. Meat and cheese, for example, have a digestibility of 95%, and eggs are 97% digestible. Cooked split peas are about 70% digestible, and tofu is about 90% digestible. Both the digestibility of a protein and its amino acid content affect protein quality.

Evaluation of Protein Quality

Several methodologies are available to determine the protein quality of foods. A few of these methodologies are discussed in this section.

Chemical or Amino Acid Score

The chemical score (also called the amino acid score) involves determination of the amino acid composition of a test protein. This procedure is done in a chemical laboratory using either an amino acid analyzer or high-performance liquid chromatography techniques. Only the indispensable amino acid content of the test protein is determined. The value is then compared with that of the reference protein, for example, the amino acid pattern of egg protein (considered to have a score of 100). The amino acid/chemical score of a food protein can be calculated as follows:

$$\text{Score of test protein} = \frac{\begin{array}{c}\text{Indispensable amino}\\ \text{acid in food protein}\\ \text{(mg/g protein)}\end{array}}{\begin{array}{c}\text{Content of same amino}\\ \text{acid in reference protein}\\ \text{(mg/g protein)}\end{array}}$$

The amino acid with the lowest score on a percentage basis in relation to the reference protein (egg) becomes the first limiting amino acid, the one with the next lowest score is the second limiting amino acid, and so on. For example, if after testing all amino acids lysine was found to be present in the lowest amount relative to the reference protein (e.g., 85%), then the test protein's chemical score would be 85. The amino acid present in the lowest amount is the limiting amino acid and determines the amino acid or chemical score for the protein. Table 7.6 gives the amino acid pattern in whole egg. Comparison of the quality of different food proteins against the standard of whole-egg protein can be valuable but probably is not nearly as important to adequate protein nutriture as comparison with reference patterns for the various population groups.

Protein Digestibility Corrected Amino Acid Score

The protein digestibility corrected amino acid score (PDCAAS) is another measure of protein quality. This method involves dividing the amount (mg) of the limiting amino acid for a test protein by the amount (mg) of the same amino acid in 1 g of a reference protein (usually egg or milk) and then multiplying this value by the digestibility of the test protein, as shown in the formula below.

$$\text{PDCAAS (\%)} = \frac{\text{Amount (mg) of limiting amino acid in 1 g test protein}}{\text{Amount (mg) of same amino acid in 1 g reference protein}} \times \text{True digestibility (\%)}$$

Examples of foods with a PDCAAS of 100 include milk protein (casein), egg white, ground beef, and tuna, along with some other animal products. Soybean protein has a PDCAAS of 94, while the values for various lentils, peas, and legumes range from <50 to about 70.

Table 7.6 Amino Acid Scoring/Reference Patterns and Whole-Egg Pattern [68]

Amino Acid	Infants (mg/g protein)	Children and Adults (mg/g protein)	Whole Egg (mg/g protein)
Histidine	23	18	22
Isoleucine	57	25	54
Leucine	101	55	86
Lysine	69	51	70
Methionine + cysteine	38	25	57
Phenylalanine + tyrosine	87	47	93
Threonine	47	27	47
Tryptophan	18	7	17
Valine	56	32	66

Another approach involves a comparison of the amino acid composition of a test protein with a reference *pattern*. The reference pattern (shown in Table 7.6) that has been selected for use for all individuals (except infants) is the amino acid requirements of preschool children age 1 to 3 years. The requirements of preschool children, which include needs for growth and development, are higher for each amino acid than are those of adults (who are not undergoing growth and development) and thus should meet or exceed the needs of older individuals. This overall approach permits evaluation of the protein's ability to meet the nitrogen and indispensable amino acid requirements of individuals [68].

The scoring pattern, expressed as (mg amino acid)/(g protein), is calculated by dividing the requirements of individual indispensable amino acids (in milligrams) for children by the protein requirements (in grams). The scoring pattern for foods intended for children age 1 year or older and for older age groups is shown in Table 7.6, along with the recommended amino acid scoring pattern for infant formulas and foods, which is based on the amino acid composition of human milk [68]. Table 7.6 also shows the whole-egg pattern.

Protein Efficiency Ratio

The protein efficiency ratio (PER) represents body weight gained on a test protein divided by the grams of protein consumed. To calculate the PER of proteins, young growing animals are typically placed on a standard diet with about 10% (by weight) of the diet as test protein. Weight gain is measured for a specific time period and compared to the amount of the protein consumed. The PER for the protein is then calculated using the following formula:

$$\text{PER} = \frac{\text{Gain in body weight (g)}}{\text{Grams of protein consumed}}$$

To illustrate, the PER for casein (a protein found in milk) is 2.5; thus, rats gain 2.5 g of weight for every 1 g of casein consumed. However, a food with a PER of 5 does not have double the protein quality of casein, with a PER of 2.5. Furthermore, although the PER allows determination of which proteins promote weight gain (per gram of protein ingested) in growing animals, no distinction is made regarding the composition (fat versus muscle/organ) of the weight gain.

In addition to chemical/amino acid score, protein digestibility corrected amino acid score, and protein efficiency ratio, two additional methods—biological value and net protein utilization—are used to determine protein quality. These methods, however, involve nitrogen balance studies. Thus, a brief review of nitrogen balance will precede our discussion of biological value and net protein utilization.

Nitrogen Balance

Nitrogen balance studies involve the measurement and summation of nitrogen losses from the body. Protein contains approximately 16% nitrogen. Thus, to calculate grams of protein from grams of nitrogen, we can do the following calculation:

$$\underset{\text{(measured in grams)}}{0.16 \times \text{Protein}} = \underset{\text{(measured in grams)}}{\text{Nitrogen}}$$

Expressed alternately,

$$\text{Protein (g)} = \text{Nitrogen (g)} \times 100/16, \text{ or}$$

$$\text{Protein (g)} = \text{Nitrogen (g)} \times 6.25$$

Nitrogen balance studies are conducted when subjects consume a diet with a protein (nitrogen) intake that is

- at or near a predicted adequate amount,
- less than (including protein-free nitrogen) a predicted adequate amount, or
- greater than a predicted adequate amount.

Nitrogen losses are measured in the urine (U), feces (F), and skin (S). For example, in the urine, nitrogen is found mainly as urea but also as creatinine, amino acids, ammonia, and uric acid. In the feces, nitrogen may be found as amino acids and ammonia. The calculation of nitrogen balance is shown in this formula; stated simply, nitrogen losses are summed and then subtracted from nitrogen intake (I_n):

$$\text{Nitrogen balance} = I_n - [(U - U_e) + (F - F_e) + S]$$

The subscript *e* (in U_e and F_e) in the equation stands for *endogenous* (also called obligatory) and refers to losses of nitrogen that occur when the subject is on a nitrogen-free diet.

Unfortunately, nitrogen balance studies have been criticized for overestimating true nitrogen retention rates in the body due to incomplete collection and/or measurement of losses. In addition, nitrogen balance does not necessarily mean amino acid balance; that is, a person may be in nitrogen balance but in amino acid imbalance.

Biological Value

The biological value (BV) of proteins is another method used to assess protein quality. BV is a measure of how much nitrogen is retained in the body for maintenance and/or growth versus the amount of nitrogen absorbed. BV is most often determined in experimental animals, but it can be determined in humans. Subjects are fed a nitrogen-free diet for a period of about 7 to 10 days, then fed a diet containing the test protein in an amount equal to their protein requirement for a similar time period. Nitrogen that is excreted in the feces and in the urine is analyzed and compared during the time period when subjects consumed the nitrogen-free diet versus when the subjects consumed the test protein. In other words, the change in urinary and fecal nitrogen excretion between the two diets is calculated. The BV of the test protein is determined through the use of the following equation:

$$\text{BV of test protein} = \frac{I - (F - F_0) - (U - U_0)}{I - (F - F_0)} \times 100$$

$$= \frac{\text{Nitrogen retained}}{\text{Nitrogen absorbed}} \times 100$$

where I is intake of nitrogen, F is fecal nitrogen while subjects are consuming a test protein, F_0 is endogenous fecal nitrogen when subjects are maintained on a nitrogen-free diet, U is urinary nitrogen while subjects are consuming a test protein, and U_0 is endogenous urinary nitrogen when subjects are maintained on a nitrogen-free diet.

Foods with a high BV are those that provide the amino acids in amounts consistent with body amino acid needs. The body will retain much of the absorbed nitrogen if the protein is of high BV. Eggs, for example, have a BV of 100, meaning that 100% of the nitrogen absorbed from egg protein is retained. Although the BV provides useful information, the equation fails to account for losses of nitrogen through insensible routes such as the hair and nails. This criticism is true of any method involving nitrogen balance studies. A further consideration is that proteins will exhibit a higher BV when fed at levels below the amount necessary for nitrogen equilibrium and retention will decrease as protein intake approaches or exceeds adequacy.

Net Protein Utilization

Another measure of protein quality involving nitrogen balance studies is net protein utilization (NPU). NPU measures retention of food nitrogen consumed rather than retention of food nitrogen absorbed. NPU is calculated from the following equation:

$$\text{NPU of test protein} = \frac{I - (F - F_0) - (U - U_0)}{I} \times 100$$

$$= \frac{\text{Nitrogen retained}}{\text{Nitrogen consumed}} \times 100$$

where I is intake of nitrogen, F is fecal nitrogen while subjects are consuming a test protein, F_0 is endogenous fecal nitrogen when subjects are maintained on a nitrogen-free diet, U is urinary nitrogen while subjects are consuming a test protein, and U_0 is endogenous urinary nitrogen when subjects are maintained on a nitrogen-free diet.

Although NPU can be measured in humans through nitrogen balance studies in which two groups of well-matched experimental subjects are used, a more nearly accurate measurement is made on experimental animals through direct analysis of the animal carcasses. In either case, one experimental group is fed the test protein, while the other group receives an isocaloric, protein-free diet. When experimental animals are used as subjects, their carcasses can be analyzed for nitrogen directly (total carcass nitrogen, or TCN) or indirectly at the end of the feeding period. The indirect measurement of nitrogen is made by water analysis. Given the amount of water removed from the carcasses, an approximate nitrogen content can be calculated. NPU involving animal studies is calculated from the following equation:

$$\text{NPU} = \frac{\text{TCN on test protein} - \text{TCN on protein-free diet}}{\text{Nitrogen consumed}}$$

Proteins of higher quality typically cause a greater retention of nitrogen in the carcass than poor-quality proteins and thus would have a higher NPU.

Net Dietary Protein Calories Percentage

The net dietary protein calories percentage (NDpCal%) can be helpful in the evaluation of human diets in which the protein : calorie ratio varies greatly. The formula is as follows:

$$\text{NDpCal\%} = \text{Protein kcal/Total kcal intake} \times 100 \times \text{NPU}_{op}$$

where NPU_{op} is NPU when protein is fed above the minimum requirement for nitrogen equilibrium.

Protein Information on Food Labels

Food labels are required to indicate the amount (quantity) of protein in a food in grams. The % Daily Value for protein also must be specified if the food is intended for consumption by children under 4 years of age or if a health claim is made. To calculate the % Daily Value, the protein quality of the food must be assessed using the protein digestibility corrected amino acid score methodology if the food is intended for individuals older than 1 year of age or using the protein efficiency ratio if the food is an infant formula or a baby food.

The Food and Drug Administration specifies the use of the milk protein casein as a standard for comparison of protein quality based on the protein efficiency ratio (PER). Specifically, for infant formulas and baby foods, if a test protein has a protein quality equal to or better than that of casein—that is, if the PER is ≥2.5—then 45 g of protein is considered to meet 100% Daily Value. If a test protein is lower in quality than casein—that is, if the PER is <2.5—then 65 g of protein is needed to meet 100% Daily Value. To establish the protein quality of foods (except foods for infants) for % Daily Value on food labels, a protein digestibility corrected amino acid score (PDCAAS) is used. Specifically, 50 g protein is considered sufficient if the food protein has a PDCAAS equal to or higher than that of milk protein (casein). However, 65 g protein is needed if the protein is of lower quality than milk protein.

Recommended Protein and Amino Acid Intakes

Protein and amino acid requirements of humans are influenced by age, body size, and physiological state, as well as by the level of energy intake. Multiple studies using multiple methods, especially nitrogen balance studies and the factorial method, have been used to determine protein and amino acid needs of adults. Recent meta-analyses of nitrogen balance studies were considered in the latest recommendations for protein needs for adults. The estimated average requirement for protein for adults (men and women age 19 years and older) was 0.66 g protein per kg body weight or 105 mg nitrogen per kg body weight per day [68]. This value represents the lowest continuing dietary protein intake necessary to achieve nitrogen equilibrium or a zero nitrogen balance in a healthy adult [68]. The recommended dietary allowance (RDA) for protein for adults is 0.8 g protein per kg body weight per day [68]. This RDA value is identical to the 1989 RDA value for protein for adults.

The protein RDAs for children, adolescents, and adults, including women during pregnancy and lactation, are provided on the inside cover of this book. Instead of RDA, the recommendations for protein for infants from birth to 6 months of age are given as an adequate intake (AI). The AI was derived based on data from infants fed human milk as the primary nutrient source for the first 6 months [68].

In addition to recommendations for protein intake, RDAs for the indispensable amino acids have also

Table 7.7 Recommended Dietary Allowances for Indispensable Amino Acids for Adults [68]

Amino Acid	RDA (mg/kg/day)
Histidine	14
Isoleucine	19
Leucine	42
Lysine	38
Methionine + cysteine	19
Phenylalanine + tyrosine	33
Threonine	20
Tryptophan	5
Valine	24

been established. These recommendations, based on a variety of methodologies including amino acid balance and oxidation studies and indicators of amino acid oxidation, are listed in Table 7.7. The reader is directed to the Dietary Reference Intakes for Energy, Carbohydrate, Fiber, Fat, Protein and Amino Acids [68] for in-depth information on the methodologies used in determining the recommendations for the amino acids and protein.

No tolerable upper intake level for protein or any of the amino acids has been established. An upper level of recommended protein intake based on percentage of total energy (kcal) in the diet supplied by protein has been established at 30% [68]. Long-term effects from ingestion of a diet supplying >30% of kilocalories from protein have not been investigated. Moreover, data are sparse from studies or reports of individuals consuming relatively high amounts of dietary protein.

summary

Proteins in foods become available for use by the body after they have been broken down into their component amino acids. Nine of these amino acids are considered essential; therefore, the quality of dietary proteins correlates with their content of these indispensable amino acids.

An important concept in protein metabolism is that of amino acid pools, which contain amino acids of dietary origin plus those contributed by the breakdown of body tissue. The amino acids comprising the pool(s) are used in a variety of ways: (1) for synthesis of new proteins for growth and/or replacement of existing body proteins; (2) for production of important nonprotein nitrogen-containing molecules; (3) for oxidation as a source of energy; and (4) for synthesis of glucose, ketones, or fatty acids.

The liver is the primary site of amino acid metabolism, but no clear picture of the body's overall handling of nitrogen can emerge without consideration of amino acid metabolism in a variety of tissues and organs. Of particular significance is the metabolism of the branched-chain amino acids in the skeletal muscle and the production of the ammonium ion in the kidney. In addition, current research on neuropeptides spotlights the importance of amino acid metabolism in neural tissue.

Of the nonessential amino acids, glutamine, glutamate, and alanine assume particular importance because of the versatility in the overall metabolism of these amino acids. Glutamate and its α-keto acid make possible many crucial reactions in various metabolic pathways for amino acids. An appreciation for the functions performed by glutamine and glutamate makes one realize that the term "dispensable" as applied to these amino acids may be misleading.

Protein metabolism is particularly responsive to hormonal action, and this action can vary according to the tissue effect. Protein metabolism as regulated by hormonal action is particularly significant during periods of stress (see the perspective).

Protein plays many roles in the body: it provides structure, it can be used as a source of energy, and many protein molecules including enzymes and neuropeptides serve in a regulatory capacity. Because of its contribution to both energy production and synthesis of regulatory molecules, protein provides an excellent transition from the energy-producing nutrients to nutrients with regulatory functions.

References Cited

1. Rose W. The amino acid requirements of adult man. Nutr Abstr Rev 1957;27:631–43.

2. Mahe S, Roos N, Benamouzig R, Sick H, Baglieri A, Huneau J, Tome D. True exogenous and endogenous nitrogen fractions in the human jejunum after ingestion of small amounts of ^{15}N-labeled casein. J Nutr 1994;124:548–55.

3. Kilberg M, Stevens B, Novak D. Recent advances in mammalian amino acid transport. Ann Rev Nutr 1993;13:137–65.

4. Souba W, Pacitti A. How amino acids get into cells: mechanisms, models, menus, and mediators. JPEN 1992;16:569–78.

5. Christensen H. Naming plan for membrane transport systems for amino acids. Neurochem Res 1984;9:1757–58.

6. Adibi S, Gray S, Menden E. The kinetics of amino acid absorption and alteration of plasma composition of free amino acids after intestinal perfusion of amino acid mixtures. Am J Clin Nutr 1967;20:24–33.

7. Thwaites D, Hirst B, Simmons N. Substrate specificity of the di/tripeptide transporter in human intestinal epithelia (Caco-2): identification of substrates that undergo H^+-coupled absorption. Br J Pharmacol 1994;113:1050–56.

8. Ganapathy V, Leibach F. Is intestinal peptide transport energized by a proton gradient? Am J Physiol 1995;249:G153–60.

9. Vazquez J, Daniel H, Adibi S. Dipeptides in parenteral nutrition: from basic science to clinical applications. Nutr Clin Prac 1993; 8:95–105.

10. Grimble G, Rees R, Keohane P, Cartwright T, Desreumaux M, Silk D. Effect of peptide chain length on absorption of egg protein hydrolysates in the normal human jejunum. Gastroenterology 1987;92:136–42.

11. Zaloga GP. Physiological effects of peptide-based enteral formulas. Nutr Clin Prac 1990; 5:231–37.

12. Scheppach W, Loges C, Bartram P, Christl SU, Richter F, Dusel G, Stehle P, Fuerst P, Kasper H. Effect of free glutamine and alanyl-glutamine dipeptide on mucosal proliferation of the human ileum and colon. Gastroenterology 1994;107:429–34.

13. Matthews DE, Marano MA, Campbell RG. Splanchnic bed utilization of glutamine and glutamic acid in humans. Am J Physiol 1993;264:E848–54.

14. Watford M. Glutamine metabolism in rat small intestine: synthesis of three-carbon products in isolated enterocytes. Biochim Biophys Acta 1994;1200:73–78.

15. Welbourne T, King A, Horton K. Enteral glutamine supports hepatic glutathione efflux during inflammation. J Nutr Biochem 1993;4:236–42.

16. Morris S. Regulation of enzymes of the urea cycle and arginine metabolism. Ann Rev Nutr 2002;22:87–105.

17. Gardner M. Gastrointestinal absorption of intact proteins. Ann Rev Nutr 1988;8:329–50.

18. Backwell F. Peptide utilization by tissues: current status and applications of stable isotope procedures. Proc Nutr Soc 1994; 53:457–64.

19. Daniel H, Morse E, Adibi S. Determinants of substrate affinity for the oligopeptide/H^+ symporter in the renal brush border membrane. J Biol Chem 1992;267:9565–73.

20. Minami H, Daniel H, Morse E, Adibi S. Oligopeptides: mechanism of renal clearance depends on molecular structure. Am J Physiol 1992;263:F109–15.

21. Berthold H, Jahoor F, Klein PD, Reeds PJ. Estimates of the effect of feeding on whole-body protein degradation in women vary with the amino acid used as tracer. J Nutr 1995;125:2516–27.

22. Jahoor F, Wykes L, Reeds P, Henry J, Del Rosario M, Frazer M. Protein-deficient pigs cannot maintain reduced glutathione homeostasis when subjected to the stress of inflammation. J Nutr 1995;125:1462–72.

23. Tanphaichitr V, Leelahagul P. Carnitine metabolism and carnitine deficiency. Nutr 1993;9:246–54.

24. Colombani P, Wenk C, Kunz I, Krahenbuhl S, Kuhnt M, Arnold M, Frey-Rindova P, Frey W, Langhans W. Effects of L-carnitine supplementation on physical performance and energy metabolism of endurance-trained athletes: a double blind crossover field study. Eur J Physiol 1996;73:434–39.

25. Marconi C, Sassi G, Carpinelli A, Cerretelli P. Effects of L-carnitine loading on the aerobic and anaerobic performance of endurance athletes. Eur J Appl Physiol 1985;54:131–35.

26. Cerretelli P, Marconi C. L-carnitine supplementation in humans: the effects on physical performance. Int J Sports Med 1990;11:1–14.

27. Vukovich M, Costill D, Fink WJ. Carnitine supplementation: effect on muscle carnitine and glycogen content during exercise. Med Sci Sports Exerc 1994;26:1122–29.

28. Brass E. Supplemental carnitine and exercise. Am J Clin Nutr 2000;72(suppl):618S–23S.

29. Harris R, Soderlund K, Hultman E. Elevation of creatine in resting and exercised muscle of normal subjects by creatine supplementation. Clin Sci 1992;83:367–74.

30. Birch R, Noble D, Greenhaff P. The influence of dietary creatine supplementation on performance during repeated bouts of maximal isokinetic cycling in man. Eur J Appl Physiol 1994;69:268–70.

31. Balsom P, Harridge S. Creatine supplementation per se does not enhance endurance exercise performance. Acta Physiol Scan 1993;149:521–23.

32. Hultman E, Soderlund K, Timmons J, Cederblad G, Greenhaff P. Muscle creatine loading in men. J Appl Physiol 1996;81:232–37.

33. Green A, Hultman E, Macdonald I, Sewell D, Greenhaff P. Carbohydrate ingestion augments skeletal muscle creatine accumulation during creatine supplementation in humans. Am J Physiol 1996; 271:E821–26.

34. Greenhaff P, Casey A, Short A, Harris R, Soderlund K, Hultman E. Influence of oral creatine supplementation on muscle torque during repeated bouts of maximal voluntary exercise in man. Clin Sci Lond 1993;84:565–71.

35. Cooke W, Grandjean P, Barnes W. Effect of oral creatine supplementation on power output and fatigue during bicycle ergometry. J Appl Physiol 1995; 78:670–73.

36. Mujika I, Chatard JC, Lacoste L, Barale F, Geyssant A. Creatine supplementation does not improve sprint performance in competitive swimmers. Med Sci Sports Exerc 1996;28:1435–41.

37. Gariballa S, Sinclair A. Carnosine: physiological properties and therapeutic potential. Age and Ageing 2000;29:207–10.

38. Hipkiss A. Carnosine, a protective, anti-ageing peptide? Int J Biochem Cell Biol 1998;30:863–68.

39. Zaloga G, Roberts P, Nelson T. Carnosine: a novel peptide regulator of intracellular calcium and contractility in cardiac muscle. New Horizons 1996;4:26–35.

40. Food and Nutrition Board. Dietary Reference Intakes for Thiamin, Riboflavin, Niacin, Vitamin B_6, Folate, Vitamin B_{12}, Pantothenic Acid, Biotin, and Choline. Washington, DC: National Academy Press, 1998, pp. 390–422.

41. Watford M. The urea cycle: a two-compartment system. Essays in Biochemistry 1991;26:49–58.

42. Morris S. Regulation of enzymes of urea and arginine synthesis. Ann Rev Nutr 1992;12:81–101.

43. Kurowska E, Carroll K. Hypercholesterolemic responses in rabbits to selected groups of dietary essential amino acids. J Nutr 1994; 124:364–70.

44. Castillo L, deRojas T, Chapman T, Vogt J, Burke J, Tannenbaum S. Splanchnic metabolism of dietary arginine in relation to nitric oxide synthesis in normal adult man. Proc Natl Acad Sci USA 1993; 90:193–97.

45. Kowalski T, Watford M. Production of glutamine and utilization of glutamate of rat subcutaneous adipose tissue in vivo. Am J Physiol 1994;266:E151–54.

46. Chinsky J, Bohlen L, Costeas P. Noncoordinated responses of branched-chain α-ketoacid dehydrogenase subunit genes to dietary protein. FASEB J 1994;8:11–20.

47. Abumrad N, Rabin D, Wise K, Lacy W. The disposal of an intravenously administered amino acid load across the human forearm. Metabolism 1982; 31:463–70.

48. Wahren J, Felig P, Hagenfeldt L. Effect of protein ingestion on splanchnic and leg metabolism in normal man and in patients with diabetes mellitus. J Clin Invest 1976;57:987–99.

49. Pevet P. Melatonin: from seasonal to circadian signal. J Neuroendocrin 2003;15:422–26.

50. Cajochen C, Krauchi K, Wirz-Justice A. Role of melatonin in the regulation of human circadian rhythms and sleep. J Neuroendocrin 2003;15:432–37.

51. Parry B. Jet lag: minimizing its effects with critically timed bright light and melatonin administration. J Mol Microbiol Biotech 2002;4:463–66.

52. Curran R, Ferrari F, Kispert P, Stadler J, Stuehr D, Simmons R, Billiar T. Nitric oxide and nitric oxide–generating compounds inhibit hepatocyte protein synthesis. FASEB J 1991;5:2085–92.

53. Welle S, Nair K. Relationship of resting metabolic rate to body composition and protein turnover. Am J Physiol 1990; 258:E990–98.

54. Dice J. Peptide sequences that target cytosolic proteins for lysosomal proteolysis. Trends Biol Sci 1990;15:305–9.

55. Beynon R, Bond J. Catabolism of intracellular protein: molecular aspects. Am J Physiol 1986;251:C141–52.

56. Attaix D, Taillandier D, Temparis S, Larbaid D, Aurousseau E, Combaret L, Voisin L. Regulation of ATP ubiquitin-dependent proteolysis in muscle wasting. Reprod Nutr Dev 1994;34:583–97.

57. Mortimore G, Poso A. Intracellular protein catabolism and its control during nutrient deprivation and supply. Ann Rev Nutr 1987;7:539–64.

58. Kadowaki M, Kanazawa T. Amino acids as regulators of proteolysis. J Nutr 2003;133:2052S-56S.

59. Rechsteiner M. Natural substrates of the ubiquitin proteolytic pathway. Cell 1991;66:615–18.

60. Tiao G, Fagan J, Samuels N, James J, Hudson K, Lieberman M, Fischer J, Hasselgren P. Sepsis stimulates nonlysosomal, energy dependent proteolysis and increases ubiquitin mRNA levels in rat skeletal muscle. J Clin Invest 1994;94:2255–64.

61. Hershko A, Ciechanover A. The ubiquitin system for protein degradation. Ann Rev Biochem 1992;61:761–807.

62. Bachmair A, Finley D, Varshavsky A. In vivo half-life of a protein is a function of its amino-terminal residue. Science 1986;234:179–86.

63. Rogers S, Wells R, Rechsteiner M. Amino acid sequences common to rapidly degraded proteins: the PEST hypothesis. Science 1986;234:364–68.

64. Waxman L, Goldberg A. Selectivity of proteolysis: protein substrates activate the ATP-dependent protease (La). Science 1986;232:500–503.

65. Goldberg A. The mechanism and functions of ATP-dependent proteases in bacterial and animal cells. Eur J Biochem 1992;203:9–23.

66. Robertson L, Flinder C, Godfrey B. Laurel's Kitchen—a Handbook for Vegetarian Cookery and Nutrition. Petaluma, CA: Nilgiri Press, 1984.

67. Young V, Pellett P. Plant proteins in relation to human protein and amino acid nutrition. Am J Clin Nutr 1994;59(suppl):1203S-12S.

68. Food and Nutrition Board. Dietary Reference Intakes for Energy, Carbohydrate, Fiber, Fat, Protein and Amino Acids. Washington, DC: National Academy Press, 2002.

Protein Turnover: Starvation versus "Stress"

Starve a cold, feed a fever? Or feed a cold, starve a fever? In the healthy adult, protein synthesis approximately balances protein degradation. Together, protein synthesis and degradation make up what is referred to as protein turnover. Protein turnover in humans is correlated to a person's mass ($W^{0.75}$), where W is body weight in kilograms. Daily protein turnover in humans is calculated to be approximately 4.6 g/kg body weight. Thus, for a 70-kg male, protein turnover would approximate 320 g daily [1]. However, such calculations only approximate reality in a healthy adult. With illness, such as infection or sepsis (the presence of pathogenic micro-organisms or their toxins in the blood and/or body tissues), or during starvation, protein synthesis and protein degradation are not in balance. An imbalance between protein synthesis and protein degradation is also found with injury, including surgery, trauma, and burns; however, this imbalance exceeds that found in fasting (starvation) conditions. Conditions of illness or injury comprise what is referred to as "stress" in the title of this perspective. This perspective will compare and contrast what happens to a person's protein status during starvation and illness or injury (i.e., stress).

In starvation, protein synthesis decreases. This decrease occurs because of a reduction in mRNA needed for the translation of proteins and because of a decreased rate of peptide bond formation (or RNA "activity"). Even proteins with very rapid turnover, such as plasma proteins, are synthesized at a rate 30% to 40% below normal. In muscle, protein synthesis rates drop even lower. However, protein degradation rates decrease concurrently so that in chronic starvation daily losses of nitrogen become quite small. For example, a person fully adapted to starvation can survive at a cost of 3 to 4 g of his or her body protein per day [2]; however, differences in the extent of nutrient metabolism between lean and obese individuals have been reported [3].

The principal mechanism of adjustment to starvation is a change in hormone balance. In particular, there is a sharp decrease in insulin production. In addition, the muscle and adipocytes become somewhat resistant to the action of insulin so that whatever insulin is circulating is ineffective in promoting cellular nutrient uptake for protein synthesis and lipogenesis. Decreased insulin activity, coupled with increased synthesis of counterregulatory hormones such as glucagon, promotes fatty acid mobilization from adipose tissue, production of ketones, and the availability of amino acids for gluconeogenesis. The glucocorticoids are important in gluconeogenesis because they promote catabolism of muscle protein to provide substrates for gluconeogenesis. However, an increased adjustment to starvation is characterized by a decrease in the secretion of glucocorticoids. An additional hormonal change facilitating adjustment to starvation is decreased synthesis of tri-iodothyronine (T_3, a thyroid hormone), which results in a lowered metabolic rate.

In the initial stages or first few days of fasting or starvation, glycogen in the liver is depleted. Muscles undergo proteolysis. Urinary 3-methylhistidine excretion increases to reflect myofibrillar protein catabolism. Muscles undergoing proteolysis also release a mixture of amino acids containing relatively high alanine and glutamine concentrations. Alanine is a preferred substrate for gluconeogenesis and serves to stimulate the secretion of the gluconeogenic hormone glucagon. Alanine released from muscle is taken up by the liver, where the nitrogen is removed and converted to urea for excretion by the kidney and where the pyruvate formed can enter the gluconeogenic pathway. Glucose formed in the liver may be released into the blood for cellular uptake and metabolism. Glutamine released from muscles circulates in the blood for uptake and metabolism primarily by the gastrointestinal tract and kidney, and not the liver. Within the liver, glutamine synthesis is increased and urea synthesis diminishes. These hepatic changes help direct glutamine to the kidneys for maintenance of acid-base balance.

As fasting or starvation continues, tissues continue to use fatty acids and glucose for energy but also begin to use ketones formed in the liver from fatty acid oxidation. A decrease in protein catabolism and gluconeogenesis occurs concurrently with the brain's and other tissues' adaptation to ketones as a source of energy. Glutamine metabolism in the kidney increases as starvation continues and acidosis occurs. Within the kidney, glutamine catabolism generates ammonia, which is able to combine with hydrogen ions and be excreted in the urine to help correct the acidosis.

Figure 1a illustrates how adaptation to starvation allows the conservation of body protein. Fatty acids are shown generating ketones that are then used for energy by muscle. The utilization of the ketones means that less glucose is needed and allows the sparing of lean body mass for glucose production. In other words, because less carbohydrate is required by the body, less protein must be broken down to supply amino acids for gluconeogenesis. Amino acids resulting from proteolysis of muscle tissue can be used for the synthesis of crucial visceral proteins such as plasma proteins, which have more rapid turnover rates than muscle. It is estimated that under normal conditions visceral protein has a turnover rate three times greater than that of muscle protein [4].

Figure 1b depicts the substrate utilization in sepsis. With sepsis (an example of "stress"), as with starvation, adipose tissue undergoes lipolysis. Although the body can partially defend itself against starvation through conservation of energy and adaptation to ketosis, it has no such defense against injury, trauma, surgery, and/or infection. Unlike during starvation, ketogenesis is inhibited by insulin during sepsis, burns, injury or trauma, and surgery. Without the utilization of ketones, body protein must continue to be degraded to supply amino acids for glucose synthesis (gluconeogenesis). Degradation of muscle protein provides the majority of the amino acids needed by other organs. In "stress" situations, muscles experience decreased amino acid uptake and protein synthesis with larger increases in protein breakdown. Degradation of white fast-twitch skeletal muscle is more pronounced than that of red slow-twitch skeletal muscle [5]. Urinary 3-methylhistidine excretion increases, reflecting increased catabolism of myofibrillar protein. Muscle cachexia, characterized by muscle wasting and weakness, results. Thus, protein degradation in sepsis, as well as in injury, trauma,

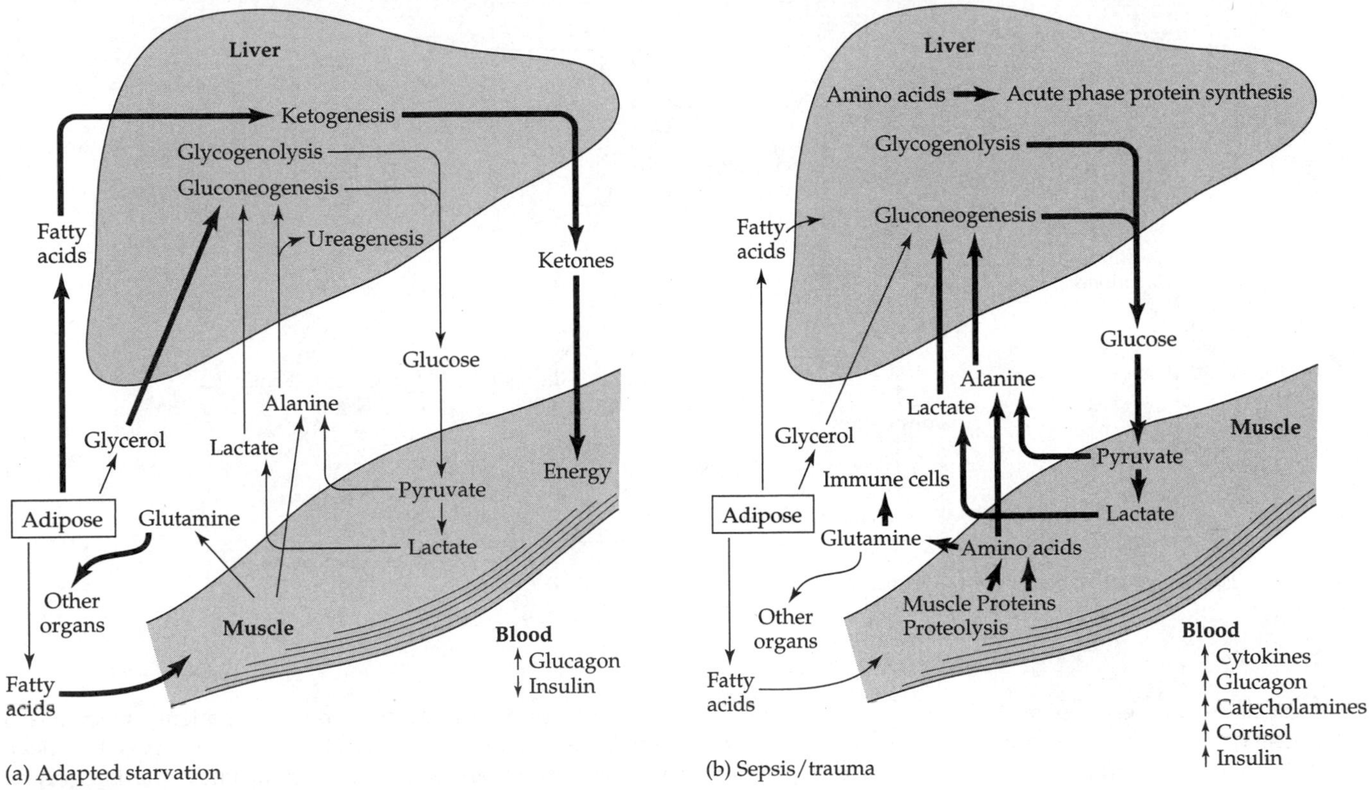

Figure 1 Substrate utilization during (a) adapted starvation and (b) sepsis/trauma. Note: Increased responses are shown by heavy blue arrows.

and burns, exceeds that in starvation. Each gram of nitrogen lost can be translated into the breakdown of approximately 30 g of hydrated lean tissue [6].

The differences in substrate utilization between starvation and stress result in part from differences in hormone concentrations. Figure 2 demonstrates the metabolic stress response. As shown in this diagram, with stress (including sepsis, trauma, surgery, and burns), glucocorticoids (primarily cortisol), catecholamines (e.g., epinephrine), insulin, and glucagon release increase. However, the glucagon : insulin ratio favors glucagon. Consequently, tissues become resistant to insulin action, and hyperglycemia (high blood glucose concentration) persists. In addition, cortisol concentrations may remain elevated in the blood for prolonged periods following severe trauma or stress events. High blood cortisol promotes proteolysis and hyperglycemia. Besides hormone release, cytokines contribute to differences in substrate utilization during stress. Cytokines are low-molecular-weight peptides that evoke a number of varied reactions in the body and are used primarily by immune cells to communicate with each other. Cytokines such as interleukin-1 (IL-1) and tumor necrosis factor (TNF)-α produced from macrophages in part mediate proteolysis and the hormonal response. Inflammation involves similar cytokines, such as IL-1 and TNF-α, but also interleukin (IL)-6, interleukin (IL)-8, and interferon (IFN)-γ.

Additional hormonal changes associated with "stress," illustrated in Figure 2, include the release of aldosterone and antidiuretic hormone. Aldosterone promotes renal sodium and fluid reabsorption, thus increasing blood volume. Antidiuretic hormone (ADH) inhibits diuresis (urination), also effecting an increase in blood volume. Both aldosterone and ADH help restore circulation if it has been depressed by shock or loss of blood fluids by hemorrhage associated with injury or surgery. These hormones thus help diminish total fluid losses, which may be high with skin loss from burns or with increased dermal losses from fever.

While surgery, sepsis, burns, and trauma are associated with continued protein degradation to supply amino acids for glucose synthesis, protein turnover also occurs because of the immune response and the acute phase response. The acute phase response is characterized by fever, hormonal changes, and blood cell count changes, as well as by changes in protein turnover. During the acute phase response, certain body proteins such as muscle protein are preferentially degraded by ubiquitin/ proteasomal and calpain/calcium systems; however, in the liver, protein synthesis predominates. Glucocorticoids, in part, are thought to stimulate the increase in the synthesis of some proteins in the liver. Proteins that are synthesized in the liver during these stress situations include primarily a group of proteins referred to as acute phase reactant (APR) proteins or acute phase response proteins (APRPs). In contrast, synthesis of some proteins, such as the plasma proteins albumin and transferrin, diminishes with "stress" situations. Some examples of APR proteins and their functions include

- haptoglobin, a protein that binds free hemoglobin (hemoglobin not in the red blood cell) that has been released by hemolysis of the red blood cell;

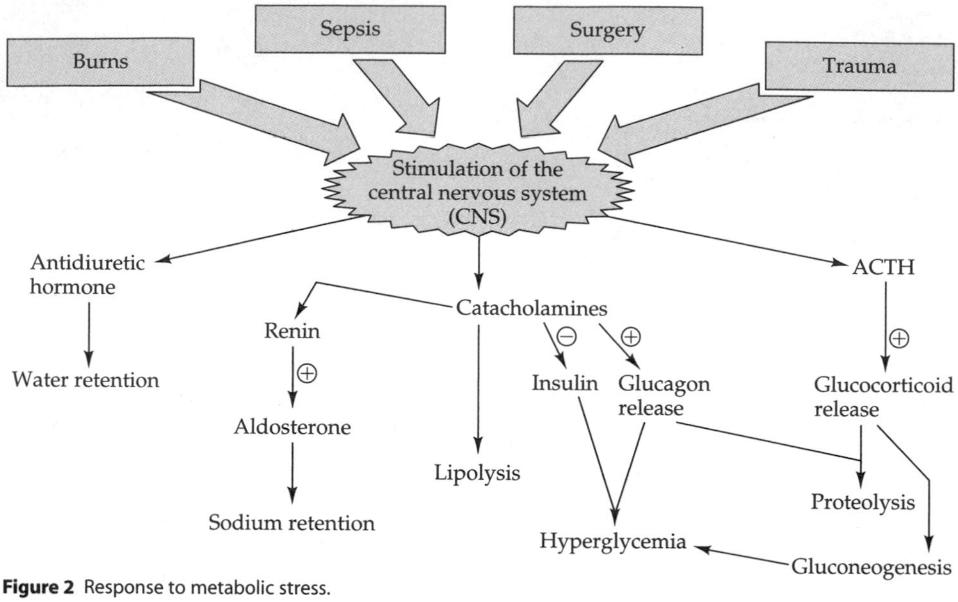

Figure 2 Response to metabolic stress.

- ceruloplasmin, a copper-containing protein with oxidase activity and the ability to scavenge radicals;
- alpha 2 macroglobulin, a protease inhibitor that functions to effect changes in tissue damage and restructuring;
- alpha 1 antitrypsin, a protease inhibitor that minimizes further tissue damage associated with phagocytosis of micro-organisms;
- fibrinogen, a protein required for blood coagulation;
- C-reactive protein, a protein that stimulates phagocytosis by white blood cells and activates complement proteins, which are needed for antibody-induced destruction of microorganisms;
- orosomucoid (alpha 1 acid glycoprotein), a protein necessary for wound healing; and
- serum amyloid A, a protein involved in the oxidative burst.

In addition to the synthesis of these proteins, more metallothionein (a zinc-containing protein; see Chap. 12) is made in the liver with sepsis and inflammation. Consequently, hepatic zinc concentrations increase while plasma zinc concentrations decrease. Similarly, in sepsis the concentrations of iron and iron-containing proteins in the blood diminish while hepatic iron stores as ferritin rise.

However, when whole-body protein turnover is considered, the increased rate of hepatic synthesis of protein with sepsis and other stress situations is insignificant compared to the rate of protein degradation. Whole-body protein catabolism predominates over synthesis. Moreover, protein deficiency can diminish the magnitude and pattern of the acute phase response as well as the ability of the body to synthesize antioxidant defense compounds such as glutathione [7–9]. Even a delay in or the lack of enteral (meaning by way of or into the gastrointestinal tract) nutrition, which may accompany severe illness, can result in the atrophy of intestinal mucosa. When enterocytes atrophy, bacteria or toxins can more easily translocate from the lumen of the intestinal tract through the enterocytes and into the blood. Such bacterial translocation further increases the risk of sepsis, especially gram-negative sepsis. Glutamine has been shown to be a vital fuel for enterocytes. Moreover, glutamine needs by the cells of the immune system also are increased with sepsis and other "stress" conditions. Yet, during illness, the rate of glutamine production and release from body sites does not meet the intestinal cells' need for glutamine. Further, lack of sufficient glutamine may contribute to inadequate glutathione production observed in stress [10,11]. Glutathione, remember, is an important antioxidant. A glutamine-enriched diet for patients hospitalized with such catabolic illnesses has been shown to help maintain the integrity of the intestine, decrease intestinal permeability, help preserve skeletal muscle, decrease infectious complication rates, and decrease the length of hospital stay [12]. Thus, glutamine becomes a conditionally indispensable amino acid during times of sepsis or injury.

It has been suggested [6] that the body places a high priority on wound repair and host defense, gambling that convalescence will occur before depletion of tissues becomes a threat to survival. To improve recovery, feed a cold and feed a fever!

References Cited

1. Waterlow JC. Protein turnover with special reference to man. Q J Exp Physiol 1984;69:409–38.
2. Tepperman J, Tepperman HM. Metabolic and Endocrine Physiology, 5th ed. Chicago: Year Book Medical, 1987.
3. Elia M, Stubbs R, Henry C. Differences in fat, carbohydrate, and protein metabolism between lean and obese subjects undergoing total starvation. Obes Res 1999;7:597–604.
4. Anon. Measuring human muscle protein synthesis. Nutr Rev 1989;47:77–79.
5. Wray C, Mammen J, Hasselgren P. Catabolic response to stress and potential benefits of nutrition support. Nutr 2002;18:971–77.
6. Kinney JM, Elwyn DH. Protein metabolism and injury. Ann Rev Nutr 1983;3:433–66.
7. Doherty JF, Golden MNH, Raynes JG, Griffin GE. Acute phase protein response is impaired in severely malnourished children. Clin Sci 1993;84:169–75.

8. Jennings G, Bourgeois C, Elia M. The magnitude of the acute phase protein response is attenuated by protein deficiency in rats. J Nutr 1992;122:1325–31.

9. Grimble RF, Jackson AA, Persaud C, Wriede MJ, Delers F, Engler R. Cysteine and glycine supplementation modulate the metabolic response to tumor necrosis factor in rats fed a low protein diet. J Nutr 1992;122:2066–73.

10. Welbourne TC, King AB, Horton K. Enteral glutamine supports hepatic glutathione efflux during inflammation. J Nutr Biochem 1993;4:236–42.

11. Roth E, Oehler R, Manhart N, Exner R, Wessner B, Strasser E, Spittler A. Regulative potential of glutamine—relation to glutathione metabolism. Nutr 2002;18:217–21.

12. Novak F, Heyland D, Avenell A, Drover J, Su X. Glutamine supplementation in serious illness: a systemic review of the evidence. Crit Care Med 2002;30:2022–29.

Additional Readings

2nd Amino Acid Assessment Workshop. J Nutr 2003;133:2015S-2107S.

Argiles J, Busquets S, Lopez-Soriano F. Metabolic interrelationships between liver and skeletal muscle in pathological states. Life Sci 2001;69:1345–61.

Hasselgren P, Fischer J. Counter-regulatory hormones and mechanisms in amino acid metabolism with special reference to the catabolic response in skeletal muscle. Curr Opin Clin Nutr Metab Care 1999;2:9–14.

Hasselgren P, Fischer J. Muscle cachexia: current concepts of intracellular mechanisms and molecular regulation. Ann Surg 2001;233:9–17.

Romijn J. Substrate metabolism in the metabolic response to injury. Proc Nutr Soc 2000;59:447–49.

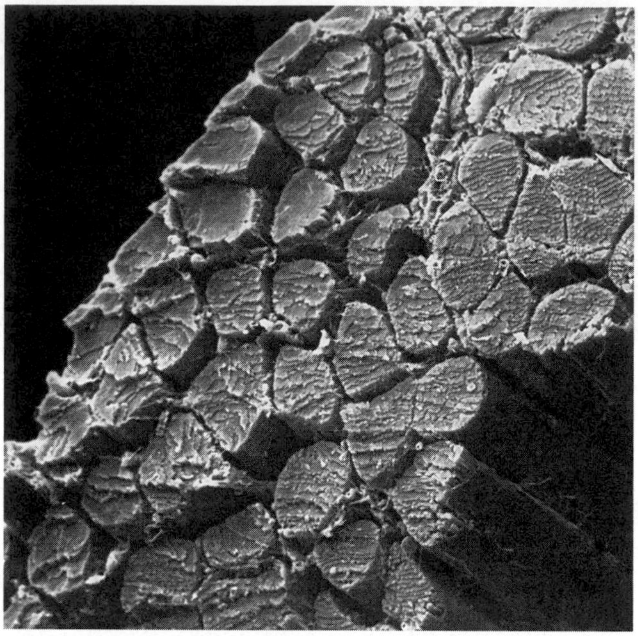

© Dr. Fred Hossler/Visuals Unlimited

Human skeletal muscle tissue

chapter 8

Integration and Regulation of Metabolism and the Impact of Exercise and Sport

CHAPTERS 4, 6, AND 7 FEATURED carbohydrate, lipid, and protein metabolism at the level of the individual cell, with emphasis on metabolic pathways common to nearly all eukaryotic cells. Those chapters also discussed how the pathways are regulated at the level of certain regulatory enzymes by substrate availability, allosteric mechanisms, and covalent modifications such as phosphorylation.

For their significance to be fully appreciated, metabolic pathways—and the specific metabolic roles of different organs and tissues—must be viewed in the context of the whole organism. Therefore, in this chapter we will examine (1) how the major organs and tissues interact through integration of their metabolic pathways, (2) hormonal regulation of these metabolic processes in maintaining homeostasis, and (3) examples of the body's ability to maintain homeostasis under special circumstances of fasting and intense exercise. The pathways themselves are not reproduced again in this chapter. When appropriate, the reader will be referred to pertinent sections in previous chapters where the pathways are described. A section on the currently attractive field of sports nutrition is included at the end of this chapter. This topic is presented at this point in the text because the dynamics of substrate utilization in supplying energy for physical exercise provide a practical example of how the various metabolic pathways interrelate. Skeletal muscle represents 43% of body mass by weight. During strenuous exercise, skeletal muscle utilizes a disproportionate amount of the body's energy reserves.

The interrelationship among carbohydrates, lipids, and proteins has been alluded to in the previous chapters. Each of these macronutrients is involved in both anabolic and catabolic reactions. Generally, anabolic reactions require energy and catabolic reactions produce energy. Much of the interrelationship among the macronutrients centers around the flux of energy and the availability of substrates. This interrelationship is discussed in more detail in this chapter.

INTERRELATIONSHIP OF CARBOHYDRATE, LIPID, AND PROTEIN METABOLISM

If ingested in sufficient amounts, any of the three energy-producing nutrients—carbohydrate, fat, and protein (amino acids)—can provide the body with its needed energy on a short-term basis. Within certain limitations, anabolic interconversion among the nutrients also occurs. For example, as explained in Chapter 7, certain amino acids can be synthesized in the body from carbohydrate or fat, and, conversely, most amino acids can serve as precursors for carbohydrate or fat synthesis. An overview of the considerable metabolic interconversion among the nutrients is given in Figure 8.1. Not evident from the figure, but very important to recall, is that the Krebs cycle is an **amphibolic pathway,** meaning that it

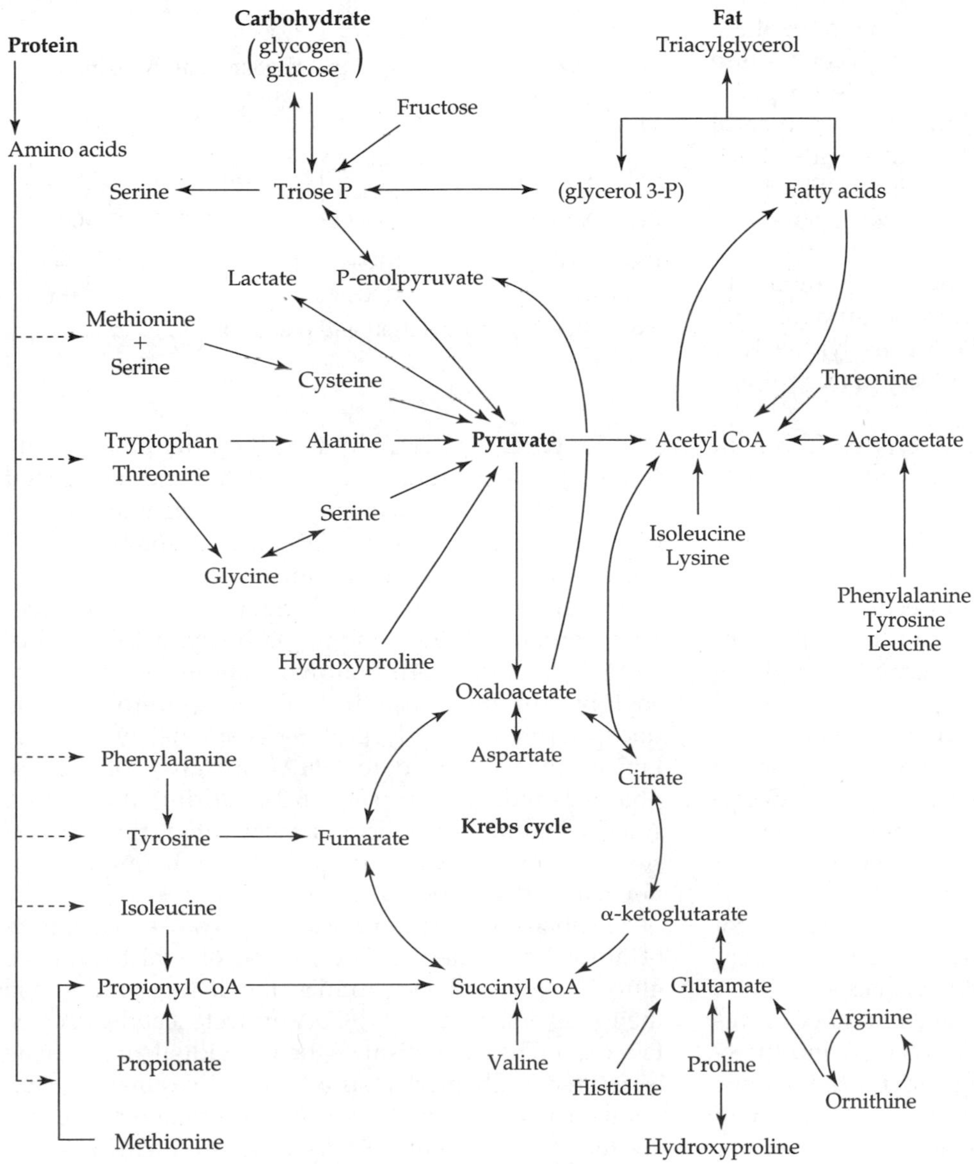

Figure 8.1 Interconversion of the macronutrients.

not only functions in the oxidative catabolism of carbohydrates, fatty acids, and amino acids, but also provides precursors for many biosynthetic pathways, particularly gluconeogenesis (Fig. 4.14). Along with pyruvate, several Krebs cycle intermediates—including α-ketoglutarate, succinate, fumarate, and oxaloacetate—can be formed from the carbon skeletons of certain amino acids and can function as gluconeogenic precursors.

The fact that animals can be fattened on a predominantly carbohydrate diet is evidence of the apparent ease by which carbohydrate can be converted to fat. However, it is believed that, in the human, lipogenesis from glucose may be much less efficient than previously proposed [1] and that weight gain from carbohydrate is probably due to a sparing of lipolysis rather than direct carbohydrate lipogenesis [2]. Glucose is the precursor for both the glycerol and the fatty acid components of triacylglycerols. The glycerol portion can be formed from dihydroxyacetone phosphate (DHAP), a three-carbon intermediate in glycolysis (see Fig. 4.14). Reduction of DHAP by glycerol 3-phosphate dehydrogenase and NADH produces glycerol 3-phosphate, to which CoA-activated fatty acids attach in the course of triacylglycerol synthesis (see Fig. 6.33). A most significant reaction linking glucose metabolism to fatty acid synthesis is the reaction of the pyruvate dehydrogenase complex, which converts pyruvate to acetyl CoA by dehydrogenation and decarboxylation. Acetyl CoA is the starting material for the synthesis of long-chain fatty acids as well as a variety of other lipids (Fig. 6.30 and Fig. 8.2).

Although carbohydrate can be converted into both the glycerol and the fatty acid components of fat, only the glycerol portion of fat can be converted to carbohydrate. The conversion of fatty acids into carbohydrate is not possible because *the pyruvate dehydrogenase reaction is not reversible.* This prevents the direct conversion of acetyl CoA, the sole catabolic product of even-numbered-carbon fatty acids, into pyruvate for gluconeogenesis. In addition, gluconeogenesis from acetyl CoA as a Krebs cycle intermediate cannot occur, because for every two carbons in the form of acetyl CoA entering the cycle, two carbons are lost by decarboxylation in early reactions of the Krebs cycle (see Fig. 4.15). Therefore, there can be no net conversion of acetyl CoA to pyruvate or to the gluconeogenic intermediates of the cycle. Consequently, acetyl CoA produced from whatever source must be used for energy, lipogenesis, cholesterogenesis, or ketogenesis.

Although fatty acids having an even number of carbons are degraded exclusively to acetyl CoA and therefore are not glucogenic (gluconeogenic) for the reasons mentioned, fatty acids possessing an odd number of carbon atoms are partially glucogenic. This is because

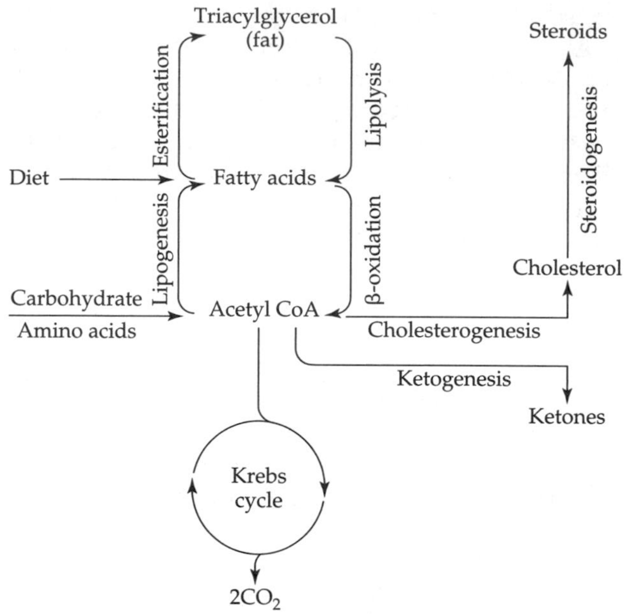

Figure 8.2 Overview of lipid metabolism, emphasizing the central role of acetyl CoA.

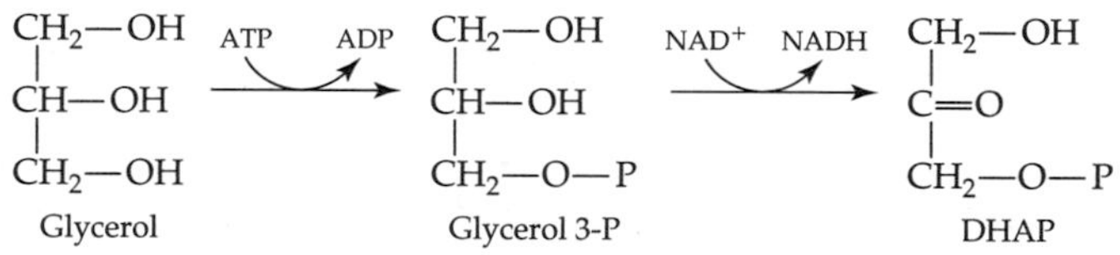

Figure 8.3 Phosphorylation and oxidation of glycerol.

propionyl CoA (CH_3—CH_2—COSCoA), ultimately formed by β-oxidation, is carboxylated and rearranged to succinyl CoA, a glucogenic Krebs cycle intermediate (see Fig. 6.26). Fatty acids with an odd number of carbon atoms are not common in the diet.

The glycerol portion of all triacylglycerols is glucogenic, entering the glycolytic pathway at the level of DHAP (see Fig. 4.14). Following its release from triacylglycerol by lipase hydrolysis, glycerol can be phosphorylated to glycerol 3-phosphate by glycerokinase, then oxidized to DHAP by glycerol 3-phosphate dehydrogenase (Fig. 8.3). During the fasting state, when fat catabolism is accelerated, this conversion assumes greater importance in maintaining a normal level of blood glucose.

Metabolism of the amino acids gives rise to a variety of amphibolic intermediates, some of which produce glucose while others produce the ketone bodies via their conversion to acetyl CoA or acetoacetyl CoA (see Fig. 6.27). The catabolism of the individual amino acids is covered in Chapter 7. It is important to remember that amino acids that can be used for production of glucose are termed glucogenic, while those producing ketones are called ketogenic. Only the amino acids leucine and lysine are purely ketogenic. The dispensable (nonessential) glucogenic amino acids are usually interconverted with carbohydrate, but like the ketogenic amino acids they can be converted (indirectly, however) into fatty acids via acetyl CoA. The fatty acids, however, cannot be converted into the glucogenic amino acids for the same reason that fatty acids cannot form glucose—namely, the irreversibility of the pyruvate dehydrogenase reaction. Although entirely possible, the conversion of the glucogenic amino acids into fat is rather uncommon. Only when protein is supplying a high percentage of calories would glucogenic amino acids be expected to be used in fat synthesis. All the amino acids producing acetyl CoA directly—isoleucine, threonine, phenylalanine, tyrosine,* lysine, and leucine—are indispensable.

The interconversion of the energy-producing nutrients appears to be skewed toward providing the organism with an energy source that can be easily stored (fat), thereby providing for times when food is not readily available. Energy released by the catabolic processes of the major nutrients must be shared by the energy-requiring synthetic pathways discussed earlier. On reaching the cells, the energy-producing nutrients can be catabolized to produce phosphorylative energy (ATP) and/or reductive energy (NADH, NADPH, $FADH_2$). Alternatively, the energy-producing nutrients may be synthesized into more complex organic compounds and/or macromolecules that become cellular components. For synthesis of a cellular component to occur, however, chemical energy must be provided. Therefore, when the cell placespriority on the synthesis of a particular component, another energy-producing material must be catabolized. The common energy pool within a cell is finite, and all anabolic and endergonic processes compete for this energy. For example, when the liver is producing more glucose by reversing glycolysis (i.e., gluconeogenesis), it cannot be synthesizing lipids and proteins at the same time. Instead, some of the existing cellular proteins or lipids are hydrolyzed, and the resulting amino acids or fatty acids are oxidized to generate the NADH and ATP needed for gluconeogenesis. Likewise, when hepatic lipogenesis occurs, glucose must be used to produce the NADPH and ATP necessary for the conversion of acetyl CoA to fatty acids.

The final common catabolic pathway for carbohydrate, fat, and protein is the Krebs cycle and oxidative phosphorylation via the electron transport chain (Figs. 4.15 and 3.16). In addition to releasing energy, these mitochondrial processes are crucial for many other metabolic sequences:

- CO_2 produced by oxidation of acetyl CoA is a source of cellular carbon dioxide for carboxylation reactions that initiate fatty acid synthesis and gluconeogenesis. This CO_2 also supplies the carbon of urea and certain portions of the purine and pyrimidine rings (Figs. 7.16, 7.17, 7.23).
- The Krebs cycle provides common intermediates that provide the cross-linkages between lipid, carbohydrate, and protein metabolism, as illustrated in Figure 8.1. Particularly notable intermediates are α-ketoglutarate and oxaloacetate. Another interrelationship, not shown in Figure 8.1, is that between heme and an intermediate of the Krebs cycle, succinyl CoA. The initial step in heme biosynthesis is the formation of α-aminolevulinic acid from "active" succinate and glycine.
- Krebs cycle intermediates—citrate and malate—intermesh with lipogenesis. Citrate can move from the mitochondria into the cytoplast, where citrate lyase cleaves it into oxaloacetate and acetyl CoA, the initiator of fatty acid synthesis. Malate, in the presence of $NADP^+$-linked malic enzyme, may provide a portion of the $NADPH^+$ required for reductive stages of fatty acid synthesis.

THE CENTRAL ROLE OF THE LIVER IN METABOLISM

Each tissue and organ of the human body has a specific function that is reflected in its anatomy and its metabolic activity. For example, skeletal muscle uses metabolic energy to perform mechanical work, the brain uses energy to pump ions against concentration gradients in the transfer of electrical impulses, and adipose tissue serves as a depot for stored fat, which on release provides fuel for the rest of the body. Central to all these processes is the liver. It plays the key role of processor and distributor in metabolism, furnishing by way of the bloodstream a proper combination of nutrients to all other organs and tissues. The liver thus warrants special attention in a discussion of tissue-specific metabolism.

Figures 8.4, 8.5, and 8.6 illustrate the fate of glucose 6-phosphate, amino acids, and fatty acids, respectively, in the liver. In these figures, anabolic pathways are shown pointing upward; catabolic pathways, pointing down; and distribution to other tissues, running horizontally.

*Tyrosine is formed by hydroxylation of phenylalanine; therefore, its carbon skeleton cannot be synthesized in the body but must be obtained from food.

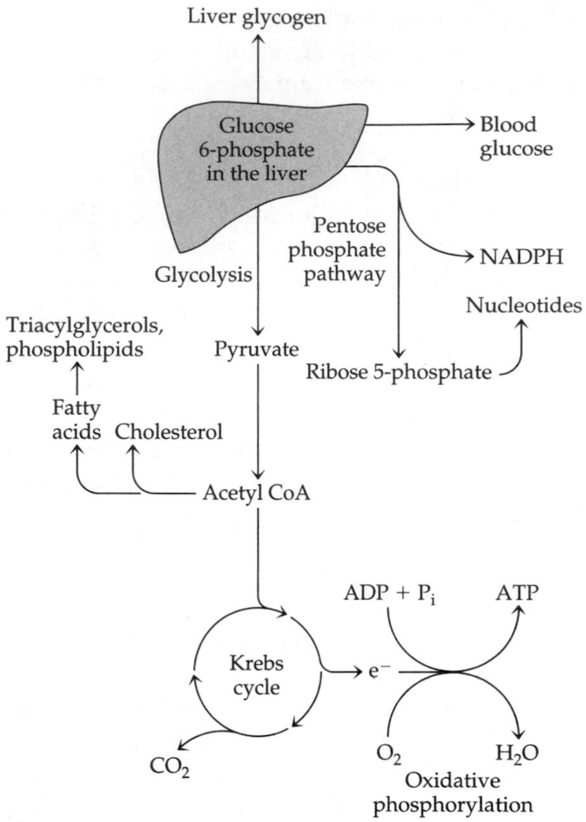

Figure 8.4 Metabolic pathways for glucose 6-phosphate in the liver. Here and in Figures 8.5 and 8.6, anabolic pathways are shown pointing upward; catabolic pathways, downward; and distribution to other tissues, horizontally.

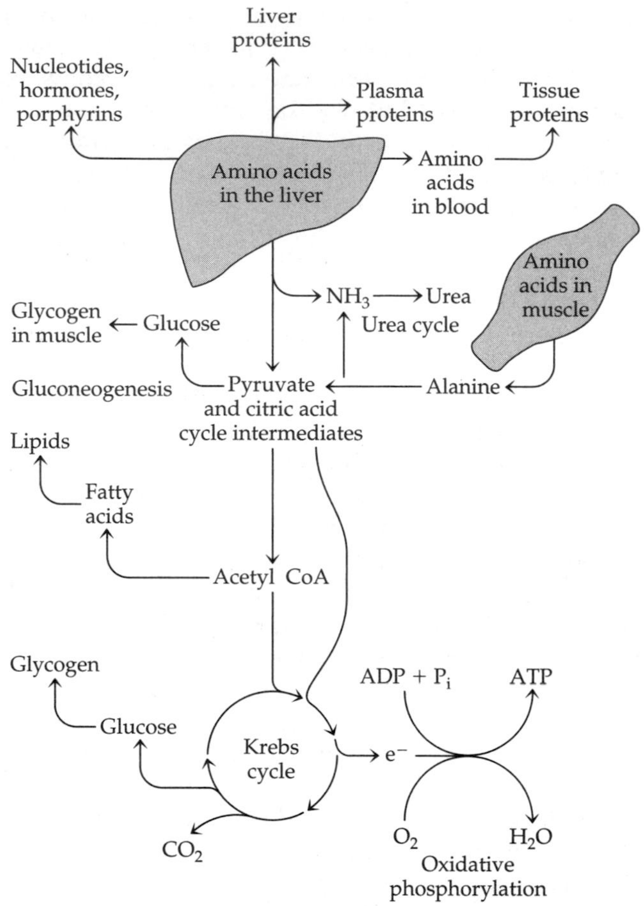

Figure 8.5 Pathways of amino acid metabolism in the liver.

The pathways indicated are described in detail in Chapters 4, 6, and 7, which deal with carbohydrate, lipid, and protein metabolism, respectively.

Glucose entering the hepatocytes is phosphorylated by glucokinase to glucose 6-phosphate. Other dietary monosaccharides (fructose, galactose, and mannose) are also phosphorylated and rearranged to glucose 6-phosphate. Figure 8.4 shows the possible metabolic routes available to glucose 6-phosphate. Liver glycogenesis likely occurs primarily from newly synthesized glucose derived from gluconeogenic precursors delivered to the hepatocytes from peripheral tissues rather than through preformed glucose directly [3] (see also Fig. 4.11). This finding is referred to again in the following section.

Figure 8.5 reviews the particularly active role of the liver in amino acid metabolism. The liver is the site of synthesis of many different proteins, both structural and plasma-borne, from amino acids. Amino acids also can be converted in the liver into nonprotein products such as nucleotides, hormones, and porphyrins. Catabolism of amino acids can take place in the liver, where most are transaminated and degraded to acetyl CoA and other Krebs cycle intermediates. These in turn can be oxidized for energy or converted to glucose or fat. Glucose formed from gluconeogenesis can be transported to muscle for use by that tissue. Newly synthesized fatty acids can be mobilized to adipose tissue for storage or used as fuel by muscle. Hepatocytes are the exclusive site for the formation of urea, the major excretory form of amino acid nitrogen.

The fate of fatty acids entering the liver is outlined in Figure 8.6. Fatty acids can be assembled into liver triacylglycerols or released into the circulation as plasma lipoproteins. In humans, most fatty acid synthesis takes place in the liver rather than in adipocytes. Adipocytes store triacylglycerols arriving from the liver, primarily in the form of plasma VLDLs, and from the lipoprotein lipase action on chylomicrons. Under most circumstances, fatty acids are the major fuel supplying energy to the liver by oxidation. Acetyl CoA not used for energy can be used for the formation of the ketone bodies, which are very important fuels for certain peripheral tissues such as the brain and heart muscle, particularly during periods of prolonged fasting.

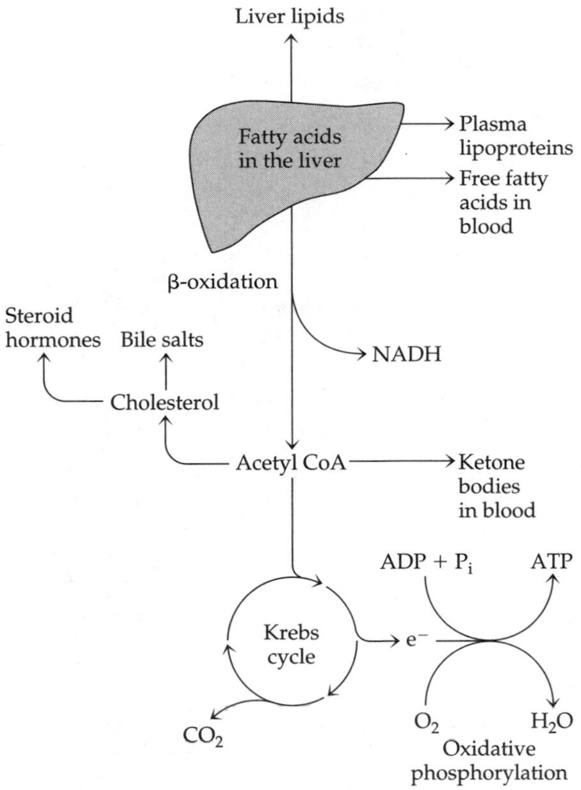

Figure 8.6 Pathways of fatty acid metabolism in the liver.

TISSUE-SPECIFIC METABOLISM DURING THE FED-FAST CYCLE

Carbohydrate and Lipid Metabolism

The best way to appreciate the interrelationship of metabolic pathways and the involvement of different organs and tissues in metabolism is to gain an understanding of the fed-fast cycle. The human typically eats specific meals followed by a period of not eating. Food consumption is often 100 times greater than basic caloric needs during the short period of time the meal is consumed, allowing humans to survive from meal to meal without nibbling continuously. Because glucose is a major fuel for tissues, it is very important that glucose homeostasis be maintained whether food has just been consumed or a state of fasting exists. If the period since the last meal is short (less than 18 hours), the mechanisms used to maintain glucose homeostasis are different from those used if the fasting state is prolonged. During prolonged fasts, other fuels gain importance. The extent to which different organs are involved in carbohydrate and fat metabolism varies within the fed-fast cycles that underlie the eating habits of the human being. When energy consumption exceeds expenditures, the excess calories are stored as glycogen and fat, which can be used as needed. A fed-fast cycle can be divided into four states, or phases:

1. The fed state, lasting about 3 hours after the ingestion of a meal
2. The postabsorptive or early fasting state, occurring during a time span of from 3 hours to about 12 to 18 hours following the meal
3. The fasting state, lasting from about 18 hours up to about 2 days without additional intake of food
4. The starvation state or long-term fast, a fully adapted state of food deprivation lasting as long as several weeks

Clearly, in a normal eating routine only the fed and early fasting states apply. The time frames of the phases cited are only approximate and are strongly influenced by factors such as activity level, the caloric value and nutrient composition of the meal, and the subject's metabolic rate.

The Fed State

Figure 8.7 illustrates the disposition of glucose, fat, and amino acids among the various tissues during the fed state. The red blood cells (RBCs) do not have mitochondria and can burn glucose only anaerobically. The central nervous system (CNS) has no metabolic mechanisms by which glucose can be converted to energy stores, nor can it make glycogen or store triacylglycerols. Glucose available to these tissues is oxidized immediately to produce energy. In the liver, in contrast, some glucose can be converted directly to glycogen. Contrary to the conventional view of liver glycogenesis, however, research indicates that most liver glycogen is synthesized indirectly from gluconeogenic precursors (pyruvate, alanine, and lactate) returning to the liver from the periphery rather than directly from glucose entering the liver via the portal vein [3]. A likely source of lactate for the liver is the red blood cells, as indicated in Figure 8.7. The reason why glucose is not used well as a direct precursor of glycogen has been attributed to the low phosphorylating activity of the liver at physiological concentrations of glucose [4].

The liver is the first tissue to have the opportunity to use dietary glucose. In the liver, glucose can be converted to glycogen. When available glucose or its gluconeogenic precursors exceed the glycogen storage capacity of the liver, the excess glucose can be metabolized in a variety of ways, as shown in Figure 8.4 and in somewhat more detail in Figure 8.7. The conversion of glucose to fatty acids and glycogen is important because both represent the storage of glucose carbon. The conversion of glucose to fatty acids appears to occur only if energy intake exceeds energy expenditure. The potential conversion of excess glucose to fatty acids is particularly crucial because these fatty acids, along with

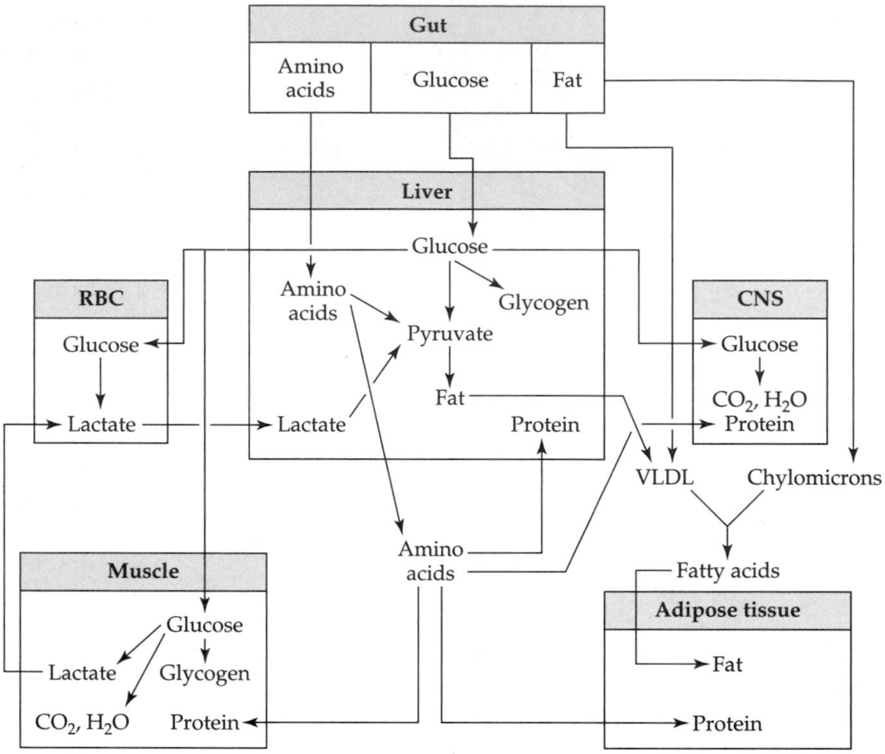

Figure 8.7 Disposition of dietary glucose, amino acids, and fat in the fed state.

those removed from the chylomicrons and VLDL by lipoprotein lipase, can be stored in the adipose tissue, thereby providing a ready source of fuel for most body tissues during the postabsorptive and fasting states.

Some exogenous glucose—that coming from the intestine—bypasses the liver and circulates to other tissues. The brain and other tissues of the central nervous system are almost solely dependent on glucose as an energy source during the fed and postabsorptive states. Other major users of glucose include

- the RBCs, which, lacking mitochondria, convert it via the glycolytic pathway to lactate for the small amount of energy the cell requires and also use it as a source of NADPH via the hexosemonophosphate shunt;
- adipose tissue, which can use glucose to some extent as a precursor for both the glycerol and the fatty acid components of triacylglycerols (although, in the human, most triacylglycerols are synthesized by the liver and transported to the adipose tissue); and
- muscle, which uses glucose for the synthesis of glycogen and for the production of energy.

With the exception of the RBCs, all the tissues included in Figure 8.7 actively catabolize glucose for energy via the Krebs cycle.

In considering fat delivery to the tissues, it is necessary to differentiate between exogenous and endogenous fat. Dietary fat, except for short-chain fatty acids, enters the bloodstream as chylomicrons, which are promptly acted on by lipoprotein lipase from the vascular endothelium, releasing free fatty acids and glycerol (Chapter 6). Chylomicron remnants remaining from this hydrolysis are taken up by the liver, and their lipid contents are transferred to the very low density lipoprotein fraction. Endogenous fatty acids of the serum are taken up by the adipocytes, reesterified with glycerol to form triacylglycerols, and stored as such as large fat droplets within the cells.

The Postabsorptive or Early Fasting State

With the onset of the postabsorptive state, tissues can no longer derive their energy directly from ingested glucose and other macronutrients but instead must begin to depend on other sources of fuel (Fig. 8.8). During the short period of time marking this phase (a few hours after eating), hepatic glycogenolysis is the major provider of glucose to the blood, which serves to deliver it to other tissues for use as fuel. When glycogenolysis is occurring, the synthesis of glycogen and triacylglycerols in the liver is diminished, and the de novo synthesis of glucose (gluconeogenesis) begins to help maintain blood glucose levels.

Lactate, formed in and released by RBCs and muscle tissue, becomes an important carbon source for hepatic gluconeogenesis. The glucose-alanine cycle, in which

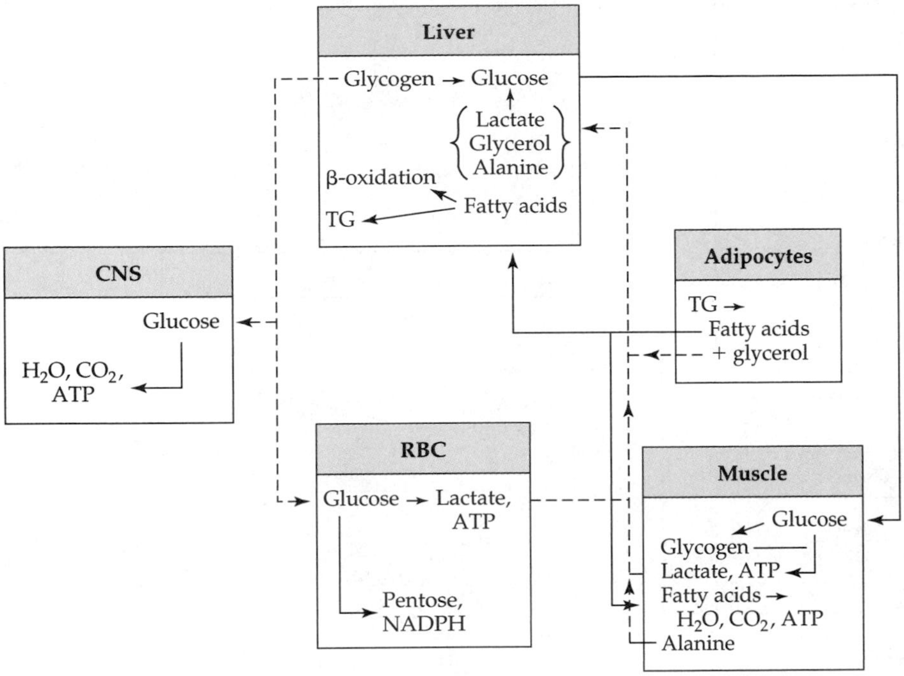

Figure 8.8 The primary postabsorption flow of substrates among the liver, CNS, adipose tissue, muscle, and red blood cells. *Source:* Modified from Zakim D, Boyer T. eds. *Hepatology: A Textbook of Liver Disease,* 4th ed. Philadelphia: WB Saunders, 2003.

carbon in the form of alanine returns to the liver from muscle cells, also becomes important. The alanine is then converted to pyruvate as the first step in the gluconeogenic conversion of alanine in the liver. The alanine cannot be converted to glucose in the muscle. In the postabsorptive state, glucose provided to the muscle by the liver comes primarily from the recycling of lactate and alanine and to a lesser extent from hepatic glycogenolysis. Muscle glycogenolysis provides glucose as fuel only for muscle cells in which the glycogen is stored, because muscle lacks the enzyme glucose 6-phosphatase. Once phosphorylated in the muscle, glucose is trapped there and cannot leave except as three-carbon units of lactate or alanine.

The brain and other tissues of the CNS are extravagant consumers of glucose, oxidizing it for energy and releasing no gluconeogenic precursors in return. The rate of glucose use is greater than the rate of glucose production by gluconeogenesis, and the stores of liver glycogen begin to diminish rapidly. In the course of an overnight fast, nearly all reserves of liver glycogen and most muscle glycogen have been depleted. Figure 8.8 shows the shifts of metabolic pathways that occur in the tissues during the postabsorptive state.

The Fasting State

The postabsorptive state evolves into the early fasting state after 18 to 48 hours of no food intake. Particularly notable in the liver is the de novo glucose synthesis (gluconeogenesis) occurring in the wake of glycogen depletion (Fig. 8.9). Amino acids from muscle protein breakdown provide the chief substrate for gluconeogenesis, although the glycerol from lipolysis and the lactate from anaerobic metabolism of glucose also are used to some extent.

The shift to gluconeogenesis during prolonged fasting is signaled by the secretion of the hormone glucagon and the glucocorticosteroid hormones in response to low levels of blood glucose. Proteins are hydrolyzed in muscle cells at an accelerated rate to provide the glucogenic amino acids. Of all the amino acids, only leucine and lysine cannot contribute at all to gluconeogenesis because, as noted previously, these amino acids are totally ketogenic. However, ketogenic amino acids released by muscle protein hydrolysis serve a purpose as well. Because they are converted into ketones—that is, acetyl CoA, acetoacetyl CoA, or acetoacetate—they allow the brain, heart, and skeletal muscle to adapt to the use of these substrates should the nutritive state continue to deteriorate into a state of long-term fast or starvation.

The early fasting state is accompanied by large daily losses of urinary nitrogen, in keeping with the high rate of breakdown of muscle protein and the synthesis of glucose through hepatic gluconeogenesis.

The Starvation State

If the fasting state persists and progresses into a starvation state (often referred to as a long-term fast), a metabolic fuel shift occurs again, this time in an effort to spare body protein. This new priority is justified by the vital physiological importance of body proteins. Proteins that

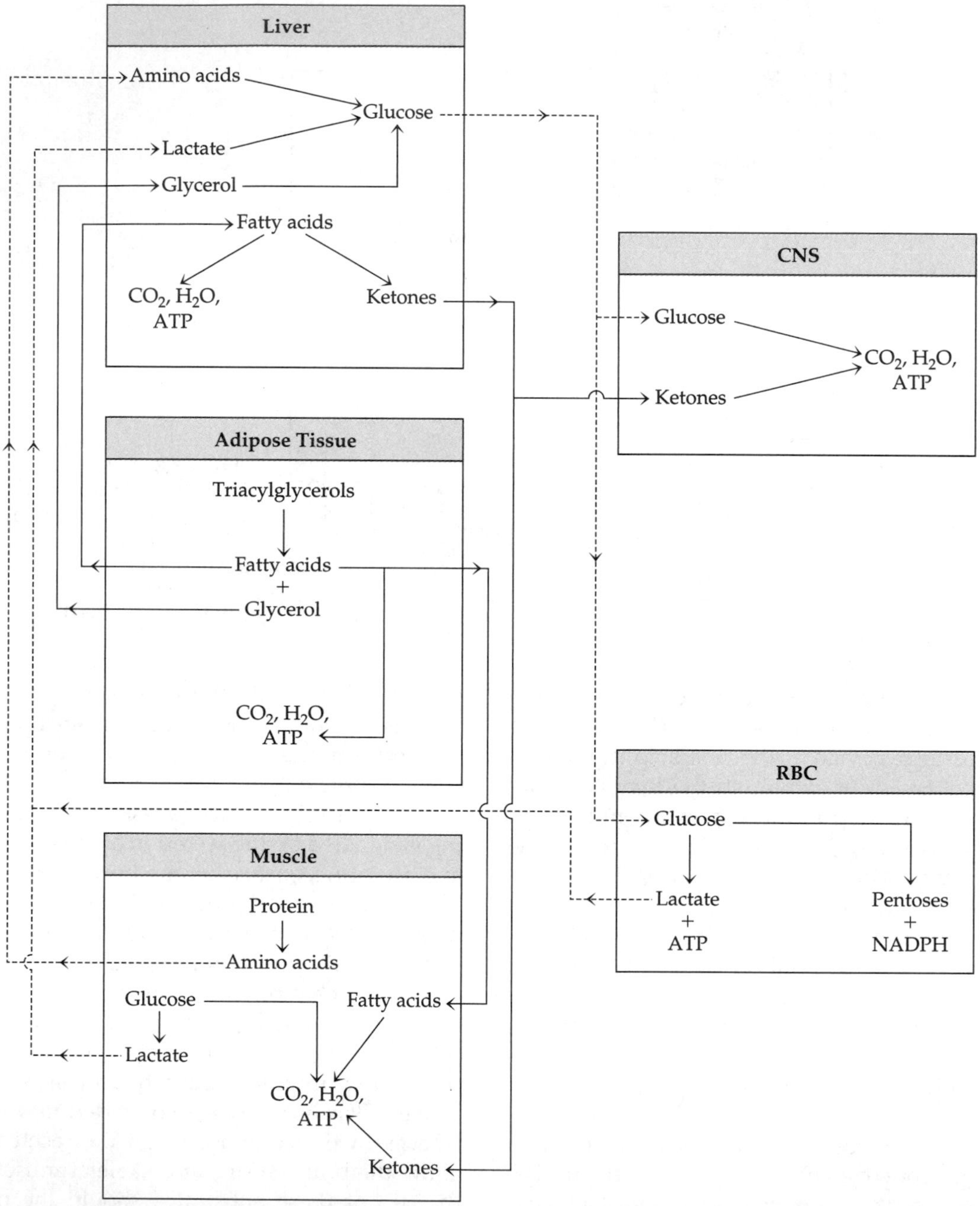

Figure 8.9 Flow of substrates among the liver, CNS, adipose tissue, muscle, and red blood cells during fasting and starvation states. Broken lines indicate major substrate flow during fasting lasting about 2 days. Solid lines reflect predominant substrate flow during the starvation state. Notice the shift during starvation to fatty acid and glycerol export from adipose tissue and the increased use of fatty acids and ketones as fuel by CNS and muscle.

must be conserved for life to continue include antibodies, needed to fight infection; enzymes, which catalyze life-sustaining reactions; and hemoglobin, necessary for the transport of oxygen to tissues. The protein-sparing shift at this point is from gluconeogenesis to lipolysis, as the fat stores become the major supplier of energy. Fat stores, deposited when more calories were consumed than expended, are large in most individuals. The blood level of fatty acids increases sharply, and fatty acids become the primary fuel for heart, liver, and skeletal muscle tissues that oxidize them for energy. The brain cannot use fatty acids for energy because fatty acids cannot cross the blood-brain barrier. However, the shift to fat breakdown also releases a large amount of glycerol, which replaces amino acids as the major gluconeogenic precursor, assuring a continued supply of glucose as fuel for the brain. The brain and skeletal muscle also adapt to use ketone bodies for energy.

Eventually, the use of Krebs cycle intermediates for gluconeogenesis depletes the supply of oxaloacetate. Low levels of oxaloacetate, coupled with the rapid production of acetyl CoA from fatty acid catabolism, cause acetyl CoA to accumulate, favoring the formation of acetoacetyl CoA and the ketone bodies. Ketone body concentration in the blood then rises (ketosis) as these fuels are exported from the liver, which cannot use them. They are delivered through the bloodstream to the skeletal muscle, heart, and brain, which oxidize them instead of glucose. As long as ketone bodies are maintained at a high level by hepatic fatty acid oxidation, the need for glucose and gluconeogenesis is reduced, thereby sparing valuable protein. Figure 8.9 illustrates the changes in energy metabolism that occur in various tissues during the fasting and starvation states.

Survival time in starvation depends mostly on the quantity of fat stored before starvation. Stored triacylglycerols in the adipose tissue of an individual of normal weight and adiposity can provide enough fuel to sustain basal metabolism for about 3 months. A very obese adult probably has enough fat calories stored to endure a fast of more than a year, but physiological damage and even death could result from the accompanying extreme ketosis. When fat reserves are gone, the degradation of essential protein begins, leading to loss of liver and muscle function and, ultimately, death [5].

Amino Acid Metabolism

Organ interactions in amino acid metabolism, illustrated in Figure 8.10, are largely coordinated by the liver. The pathways shown undergo regulatory adjustments after consumption of a meal containing protein.

In the fed state, absorbed amino acids pass into the liver, where the fate of most of them is determined in relation to needs of the body. Amounts in excess of need are degraded. Only the branched-chain amino acids (BCAAs) are not regulated by the liver according to the body's needs. Instead, the BCAAs pass to the periphery, primarily to the muscles and adipose tissue, where they may be metabolized. Of particular interest is the fate of the BCAAs that reach the muscle. These amino acids are usually greatly in excess of the need for muscle protein synthesis. The excess is believed to be used for synthesis of the dispensable amino acids needed for the increase in protein synthesis that occurs after a protein meal.

The liver is the site of urea synthesis, the primary mechanism for disposing of the excess nitrogen derived from amino acids used for energy or gluconeogenesis. (Chap. 7 describes how urea is formed.) The liver is active in removing the nitrogen from amino acids and uses the α-keto acids (amino acids from which the amine group has been removed) as the chief substrate. During fasting, gluconeogenesis becomes a very important metabolic pathway in the regulation of plasma glucose levels, and even more nitrogen is available for excretion. Kidney gluconeogenesis is accompanied by the formation and excretion of ammonia.

The importance of the liver to the functioning of muscle during the fasting state or during very vigorous exercise is exemplified in the alanine-glucose cycle (Fig. 7.34). During periods of fasting or strenuous exercise, the muscle breaks down protein to amino acids. The nitrogen from the amino acids is transaminated to α-ketoglutarate (formed in the Krebs cycle) to make glutamic acid. The glutamic acid then transaminates its α amino group to pyruvate (formed from glycolysis) to make alanine. The alanine enters the bloodstream and is transported to the liver, where it again undergoes transamination. Alanine is converted to pyruvate, and α-ketoglutarate is converted to glutamic acid. This cycle serves several functions. It removes the nitrogen from muscle during a period of high proteolysis and transports it to the liver in the form of alanine. The carbon structure of pyruvate also is transported to the liver, where it can be made into glucose through gluconeogenesis. The synthesized glucose can be transported back to the muscle and used for energy by that tissue. The glucose-alanine cycle also acts as a carrier of amino-nitrogen from intestinal mucosal cells to the liver during periods of amino acid absorption.

Glutamine also plays a central role in the transport and excretion of amino acid nitrogen. Many tissues, including the brain, combine ammonia, released primarily by the glutamate dehydrogenase reaction, with glutamate to form glutamine. The reaction is catalyzed by glutamine synthetase. In the form of glutamine, ammonia can then be carried to the liver or kidneys for excretion as urea or ammonium ion, respectively. In those tissues, glutamine is acted on by the enzyme glutaminase, releasing the ammonia for excretion and re-forming glutamate. Figure 8.10 gives an overview of organ cooperation in these and other aspects of amino acid metabolism. See Chapter 7 for a more detailed discussion of amino acid metabolism in general.

SYSTEM INTEGRATION AND HOMEOSTASIS

Integration of the metabolic processes, as outlined in the preceding sections, allows the "constancy of the internal milieu" of humans and other multicellular organisms that was described by the French physiologist Claude

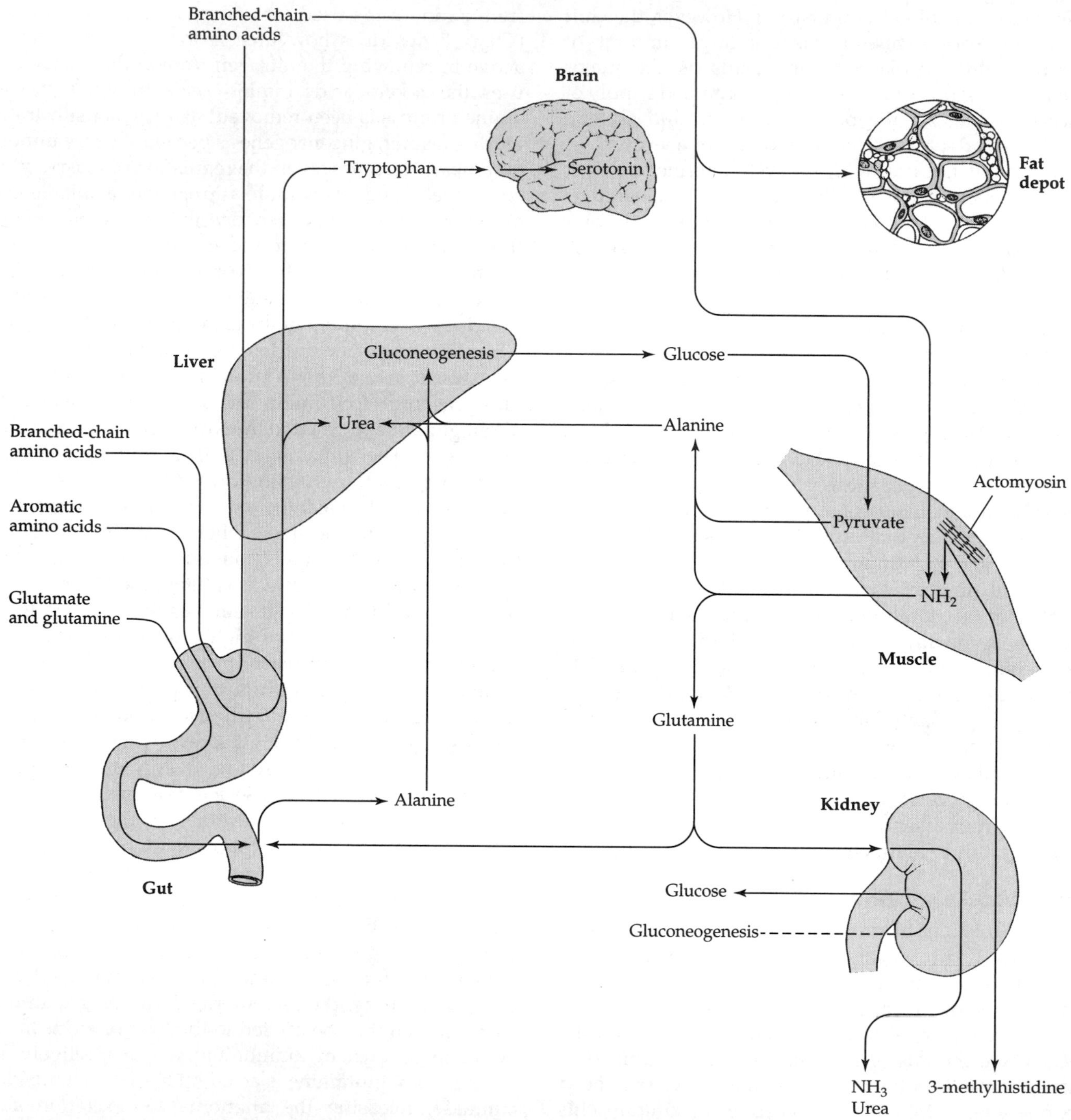

Figure 8.10 Interchanges of selected amino acids and their metabolites among body organs and tissue. *Source:* Modified from Munro HN. Metabolic integration of organs in health and diseases. J Parent Enter Nutr 1982;6:271–79. © American Society of Parenteral and Enteral Nutrition. Used with permission.

Bernard about a century ago. This integration of metabolism at the cellular and the organ and tissue levels, which is essential for the survival of the entire organism, receives its direction via body systems. The integration of body systems makes possible communication among all parts of the body.

Three major systems direct activities of the cells, tissues, and organs to ensure their harmony with the whole organism: the nervous, endocrine, and vascular systems.

The **nervous system** is considered the primary communication system because it not only has receiving mechanisms to assess the body's status in relation to its environment but also has transmitting processes to relay appropriate commands to various tissues and organs. The nervous system can inform the body of conditions such as hunger, thirst, pain, and lack of oxygen. This information allows organs to adjust to external changes and may initiate appropriate behavior by the whole organism. Tepperman and Tepperman [6] compare the nervous system to an elaborate system of telegraphy that has a "wire" connection from the source of message initiation to the place where message reception has its needed effect.

The **endocrine system** [6] is compared to a wireless system that transmits messages via highly specialized substances called hormones. The endocrine system depends on the vascular system to carry messages to target tissues.

The **vascular system** is comparable to a plumbing system with flexible pipes. It is the primary transport mechanism for the body, not only delivering specialized chemical substances but also carrying oxygen, organic nutrients, and minerals from the external environment to cells throughout the body. It also transports the waste products of metabolism from the cells, carrying them to the lungs and/or kidneys for elimination.

The concentration of solutes in the blood must be regulated within a narrow range. Among the most prominent sentinel cells that monitor and regulate solute concentration are those that synthesize and secrete hormones. Although hormone synthesis and secretion occur primarily in the endocrine system, considerable overlap exists between the endocrine system and the CNS. With the recent discovery of a variety of neuropeptides and recognition of the hormonal action of many of these peptides, it has become apparent that the CNS and the endocrine system are functionally interdependent [6,7].

Tissues and cells that respond to hormones are called the target tissues and cells of the hormones. These hormone-responsive cells have been preprogrammed by the process of differentiation to respond to the presence of hormones by acting in a predictable way. Not only do hormone-responsive cells respond to hormones via specific receptors, but their metabolic pathways also can be affected by the concentration of available substrates. Hormone-responsive cells live in a complex and continually changing environment of fuels and ions. Their ultimate response to these changes is the net result of both hormonal and nonhormonal information brought to them by the extracellular fluids in which they are bathed [6]. The response of the endocrine system to this information is discussed next.

Endocrine Function in Fed State

Endocrine organs are distributed throughout the body, and most are involved primarily with nutrient ingestion—that is, the gastrointestinal (GI) tract. Interspersed among the absorptive and exocrine secretory cells of the upper GI tract are the highly specialized endocrine cells. These cells present a sensor face to the lumen and secrete granule-stored hormones into the bloodstream. Each of these cells is stimulated to secrete hormones by a different combination of chemical messages. Chemical messages include, for example, glucose, amino acids, fatty acids, and alkaline or acid pH. Hormones secreted by these stimulated GI cells (GIP, CCK, gastrin, secretin) (Table 2.1) then enter the bloodstream and sensitize appropriate cells of the endocrine pancreas for response to the approaching nutrients. The primary action of the GI hormones, secreted in response to a mixed diet, is to amplify the response of the pancreatic islet β-cells to glucose [6].

Insulin, secreted by the β-cells, is the hormone primarily responsible for the direction of energy metabolism during the fed state (Fig. 8.7). Its effects can be categorized, based on the time of action, as (1) very fast, occurring in a matter of seconds; (2) fast, occurring in minutes; (3) slower, occurring in minutes to several hours; (4) slowest, occurring only after several hours or even days.

An example of a very fast action of insulin is membrane changes stimulated by the hormone. These changes occur in specific cells where glucose entry depends on membrane transport (see the section "Glucose Transporters" in Chap. 4). The fast action of insulin involves the activation or inhibition of many enzymes, with anabolic actions accentuated. For example, insulin stimulates glycogenesis, lipogenesis, and protein synthesis while it inhibits opposing catabolic actions. Several metabolic effects of insulin and the corresponding target enzymes involved are listed in Table 8.1. Insulin favors glycogenesis through the activation of a phosphatase that dephosphorylates phosphorylase and glycogen synthase. This dephosphorylation activates glycogen synthetase while inhibiting the phosphorylase

Table 8.1 Metabolic Effects of Insulin and Its Action on Specific Enzymes

Metabolic Effect	Target Enzyme
↑ Glucose uptake (muscle)	↑ Glucose transporter
↑ Glucose uptake (liver)	↑ Glucokinase
↑ Glycogen synthesis (liver, muscle)	↑ Glycogen synthase
↓ Glycogen breakdown (liver, muscle)	↓ Glycogen phosphorylase
↑ Glycolysis, acetyl CoA production (liver, muscle)	↑ Phosphofructokinase-1 ↑ Pyruvate dehydrogenase complex
↑ Fatty acid synthesis (liver)	↑ Acetyl CoA carboxylase
↑ Triacylglycerol synthesis (adipose tissue)	↑ Lipoprotein lipase

that initiates glycogenolysis. The fast effect of insulin on protein synthesis is not as clear-cut as its influence on lipogenesis and glycogenesis. Nevertheless, protein synthesis is promoted and appears to be related to stimulation of the translation process [6].

One slower action of insulin involves a further regulation of enzyme activity. This regulation is accomplished through the selective induction or repression of enzyme synthesis. The induced enzymes are the key rate-limiting enzymes for anabolic reaction sequences, while the repressed enzymes are crucial to the control of opposing catabolic reactions. An example of selective induction is the effect of insulin on glucokinase activity. Insulin increases the synthesis of glucokinase by promoting transcription of the glucokinase gene. Another, slower action of insulin is its stimulation of cellular amino acid influx. The slowest effect of insulin is its promotion of growth through mitogenesis and cell replication. The passage of a cell through its various phases before it can replicate is a relatively slow process that requires 18 to 24 hours for completion.

Endocrine Function in Postabsorptive or Fasting State

Metabolic adjustments that occur in response to food deprivation operate on two time scales: acutely, measured in minutes (such as adjustments operating in a postabsorptive state), and chronically, measured in hours and days (adjustments occurring during fasting or starvation). In contrast to the fed state, in which insulin is the hormone primarily responsible for the direction of energy metabolism, the body deprived of food requires a variety of hormones to regulate its fuel supply.

Figure 8.8 depicts the postabsorptive state in which hepatic glycogenolysis is providing some glucose to the body while increased use of fatty acids for energy is decreasing the glucose requirement of cells. Also, gluconeogenesis is being initiated, with lactate, glycerol, and alanine serving as substrates.

Hepatic glycogenolysis is initiated through the action of glucagon, which is secreted by the α-cells of the endocrine pancreas, and of epinephrine (adrenaline) and norepinephrine, which are synthesized primarily in the adrenal medulla and the sympathetic nerve endings, respectively. Epinephrine is considerably more potent in stimulating glycogenolysis than is norepinephrine, which functions mainly as a neurotransmitter. Epinephrine and norepinephrine are called the catecholamine hormones because they are derivatives of the aromatic alcohol catechol. Although they influence hepatic glycogenolysis somewhat, the catecholamines exert their effect primarily on the muscles. The action of glucagon and the catecholamines is mediated through cAMP and protein kinase phosphorylation. (This mechanism is described in the section on glycogenolysis in Chap. 4; see also Fig. 4.13.) Through the action of glucagon on the liver, phosphorylase and glycogen synthetase are phosphorylated, in direct opposition to the action of insulin. Consequently, phosphorylase is activated and glycogen synthetase is inhibited. As a result, glycogen is broken down, giving rise to glucose 6-phosphate, which then can be hydrolyzed by the specific liver phosphatase (glucose 6-phosphatase) to produce free glucose. The free glucose can then enter the bloodstream to maintain blood glucose levels.

Muscle glycogenolysis, in contrast, stimulated by the catecholamines, provides glucose only for use by the particular muscle in which the glycogen has been stored. Phosphorylated glucose cannot cross the cell membrane. Muscle tissue lacks glucose 6-phosphatase and cannot release free glucose into the circulation. The catecholamines, however, raise blood glucose levels indirectly by stimulating the secretion of glucagon and inhibiting the uptake of blood glucose by the muscles.

Glycogenolysis can occur within minutes and thus meets an acute need for raising the blood glucose level. However, because so little glycogen is stored in the liver (~60–100 g), blood glucose cannot be maintained over a prolonged period. The content of total muscle glycogen is ~350 g. Twelve to 18 hours following a meal, liver glycogen levels are very low. As mentioned previously, gluconeogenesis in the liver is a major supplier of glucose during fasting. Lactate, glycerol, alanine, and other amino acids are the primary precursors. Gluconeogenesis is fostered by the same hormones that initiate glycogenolysis (glucagon and epinephrine), but the amino acids needed as substrates are made available through the action of the glucocorticoids secreted by the adrenal cortex. Glucocorticoid hormones stimulate gluconeogenesis. Alanine, generated in the muscle from other amino acids and from pyruvate by transamination, not only serves as the principal gluconeogenic substrate but also acts as a stimulant of gluconeogenesis via its effect on the secretion of glucagon. In fact, alanine is the prime stimulator of glucagon secretion by β-cells that have been sensitized to the action of alanine by the glucocorticoids.

Low levels of circulating insulin not only decrease the use of glucose but also promote lipolysis and a rise in free fatty acids. Contributing to this effect is the increase in glucagon during the fasting period. Glucagon raises the level of cAMP in adipose cells, and the cAMP then activates a lipase that hydrolyzes stored triacylglycerols. The muscles, inhibited from taking up glucose by the catecholamines, begin to use fatty acids as the major source of energy. This increased use of fatty acids by the

Table 8.2 Fuel Metabolism in Starvation

Fuel Exchanges and Consumption	Amount Formed or Consumedin 24 Hours (g)	
	Day 3	Day 40
Fuel use by the brain		
Glucose	100	40
Ketones	50	100
Fuel mobilization		
Adipose tissue lipolysis	180	180
Muscle protein degradation	75	20
Fuel output of the liver		
Glucose	150	80
Ketones	150	150

Source: Adapted from Stryer L. *Biochemistry.* 3rd ed. New York: Freeman 1988 p. 640.

muscles represents an important adaptation to fasting. Growth hormone and the glucocorticoids foster this adaptation because they, like the catecholamines, inhibit in some manner the use of glucose by the muscles.

As starvation is prolonged, less and less glucose is used, thereby reducing the amount of protein that must be catabolized to provide substrate for gluconeogenesis. As glucose use decreases, hepatic ketogenesis increases and the brain adapts to the use of ketones (primarily β-hydroxybutyrate) as a partial source of energy. After 3 days of starvation, about one-third of the energy needs of the brain are met by ketones. With prolonged starvation, ketones become the major fuel source for the brain. Under conditions of continued carbohydrate shortage, ketones are oxidized by the muscles in preference not only to glucose but also to fatty acids. During starvation, the use of ketones by the muscles as the preferred source of energy spares protein, thereby prolonging life. Although Figure 8.9 depicts fuel metabolism during starvation, it does not show some of the adjustments in energy substrates that occur when starvation is prolonged. These adjustments are shown in Table 8.2. As mentioned previously, the duration of starvation compatible with life depends to a large degree on depot fat status.

SPORTS NUTRITION

Humans have courted the challenge of athletic performance and competition since the days of the early Greeks. The science of nutrition emerged much later, spurred by the expanding knowledge of metabolism and the biochemistry on which it is based. Because the energy for physical performance must be derived from nutrient intake, it was only a matter of time before these areas of interest would be linked. The heavy emphasis on the enhancement of health and physical performance in today's society has led to the emergence of sports nutrition as an important science. Nutrition, as a means of positive impact on physical performance, has become a topic of great interest to all those involved in human performance, the scientist as well as the athlete and athletic trainer.

The human body converts the potential energy of nutrients to usable energy, part of which drives the contraction of muscle, a process fundamental to athletic prowess. Fluctuations in the body's demand for energy—for example, changes in exertion level among resting, mild exercise, and strenuous exercise—are accompanied by shifts in the rate of catabolism of the different stored forms of nutrients. It follows that an understanding of sports nutrition requires an understanding of the integration of the metabolic pathways that furnish the needed energy. In this respect, therefore, the energy demands of sport resemble the fed-fast cycle described earlier in this chapter, so a discussion of sports nutrition at this point in the text seems appropriate.

Biochemical Assessment of Physical Exertion

To fully understand sports nutrition, we need to examine different types of skeletal muscle. A more detailed discussion of this topic can be found in an exercise physiology text (such as [8]). Muscle generally is classified as one of three distinct types, each emphasizing a different metabolic pathway: Type I, Type IIa, and Type IIb. Type I muscle, sometimes called red muscle, is oxidative and red in color. It has a large number of mitochondria and therefore is capable of oxidizing glucose to CO_2 and H_2O and carrying out β-oxidation of fatty acids. This muscle typically is used for aerobic endurance events. Type IIa muscle and Type IIb muscle have been called white muscle. Type IIb has fewer mitochondria, has a very active glycolytic pathway, and is white in appearance. This type of muscle is used primarily for short-duration anaerobic events and power events. Type IIa muscle can be considered a hybrid of Type I and Type IIb muscle, with some characteristics of each. Endurance training can make Type IIa muscle act more like Type I muscle, while strength training or sprint training can make it look more like Type IIb. Much more could be said about the muscle types and their response to nervous system stimulation and training, but this brief description provides sufficient information to foster an understanding of the resemblance of sports nutrition to the fed-fast cycle.

To understand how the muscle types relate to physical exercise at the cellular level, we need to examine two common measurements used by the exercise physiologist [8]: the **respiratory quotient (RQ)** and the maximal oxygen consumption **(VO_2 max).** Typical RQs for carbohydrate, fat, and protein are 1.0, 0.70, and 0.82, respectively (values are explained below). A newer generation of procedures (e.g., the **isotope infusion** method) has been developed to measure the relative contribution of substrates to energy supply during exercise. These measurements will be described briefly here. Further details of how the duration and intensity of physical conditioning influence which muscle cell type is used and which metabolic pathways are active are discussed in the perspective "Nutrient Usage during Strenuous Exercise" at the end of this chapter.

The respiratory quotient (RQ) is the ratio of the volume of CO_2 expired to the volume of O_2 consumed. It has served for nearly a century as the basis for determining the relative participation of carbohydrates and fats in exercise [9,10].

$$RQ = CO_2/O_2$$

For carbohydrate catabolism, the RQ is 1:

$$C_6H_{12}O_6 \text{ (glucose)} + 6\ O_2 \longrightarrow 6\ CO_2 + 6\ H_2O$$

For fat catabolism, the RQ is approximately 0.7:

$$C_{16}H_{32}O_2 \text{ (palmitic acid)} + 23\ O_2 \longrightarrow 16\ CO_2 + 16\ H_2O$$

The RQ for protein is about 0.82:

$$C_{72}H_{112}N_2O_{22}S + 77\ O_2 \longrightarrow 63\ CO_2 + 38\ H_2O + SO_3 + 9\ CO(NH_2)_2$$

The amount of protein being oxidized can be estimated from the amount of urinary nitrogen produced, and the remainder of the metabolic energy must be a combination of carbohydrate and fat. Should the principal fuel source shift from mainly fat to carbohydrate, the RQ correspondingly increases, while a shift from carbohydrate to fat lowers the RQ. Tables exist that permit the estimation of the relative percentage of either carbohydrate or lipid being used as a metabolic fuel based on the RQ at any given time (for short-term exercise activities, it is often assumed that no amino acids are used for energy). During the past 20 years, however, such knowledge has been advanced by invasive techniques such as arteriovenous measurements and the use of needle biopsies to quantify tissue stores of the energy nutrients. These measurements are used clinically to evaluate elevated rates of metabolism. For examples, see the perspective "Nutrient Usage during Strenuous Exercise" at the end of Chapter 7.

The concept of maximum oxygen uptake is fundamental. As work increases in intensity, the volume of oxygen taken up by the body also increases. The VO_2 max is defined as the point at which an increase in the intensity of the exercise no longer results in an increase in the volume of oxygen uptake. The intensity level of a particular workload is most commonly expressed in terms of the percentage of the VO_2 max that it induces. As we discuss later, the metabolic pathway that supplies energy for work is determined by the availability of metabolic energy (carbohydrate or lipid) and oxygen as well as by the duration of the activity and the conditioned state of the individual performing the work.

Isotope infusion can be used to quantify the contribution of the major energy substrates, plasma glucose and fatty acids, and muscle triacylglycerols and glycogen to energy expenditure during exercise. It involves the intravenous infusion of stable isotope (e.g., ^{2}H (deuterium))-labeled glucose, palmitate, and glycerol during periods of rest and exercise. By monitoring the uptake of infused labeled glucose and palmitate and knowing whole-body substrate oxidation, the contribution of muscle triacylglycerol and glycogen to overall energy supply can be estimated [8].

Energy Sources during Exercise

The hydrolysis of the terminal phosphate group of ATP ultimately provides the energy for conducting biological work. In terms of physical performance, the form of work that is of greatest interest is the mechanical contraction of skeletal muscles. It is obvious, therefore, that physical exertion depends on a reservoir of ATP, which is in an ever-changing state of metabolic turnover. Whereas ATP is consumed by physical exertion, its stores are supplemented by the metabolic pathway discussed next and are repleted during periods of rest. The key to optimizing physical performance lies in nutritional strategies that maximize cellular levels of stored nutrients as fuels for ATP production. Three energy systems supply ATP during different forms of exercise [10]:

- the ATP-CP (creatine phosphate) system,
- the lactic acid system (anaerobic), and
- the aerobic system.

The ATP-CP (Phosphagen) System

The ATP-CP system is a cooperative system in muscle cells utilizing the high-energy phosphate bond of creatine phosphate (CP) together with ATP. When the body is at rest, energy needs are fulfilled by aerobic catabolism (see the section "The Aerobic System," below) because the low demand for oxygen can easily be met by oxygen exchange in the lungs and by the oxygen carried to the muscle by the cardiovascular system. (The ATP-CP system also operates continuously during this time, though at a slow pace). If physical activity is initiated, the energy requirements of contracting muscle are met by existing ATP. However, stores of ATP in muscle are limited, providing enough energy for only a few seconds of maximal exercise. As ATP levels diminish, they are replenished by the transfer of high-energy phosphate from creatine phosphate (CP) to form ATP in the ATP-CP system. The muscle cell concentration of CP is only four to five times greater than that of ATP, and therefore all energy furnished by this system is expended after approximately 10 to 25 seconds of strenuous exercise. When the ATP-CP is expended, the lactic acid system kicks in to produce more ATP. Performance demands of high intensity and short duration such as weightlifting, 100-m sprinting, some positions in football, and various short-duration field events benefit most from the ATP-CP system. Lower-intensity activity may allow a person to use this system for up to 3 minutes.

The Lactic Acid System

This system involves the glycolytic pathway by which ATP is produced in skeletal muscle by the incomplete breakdown of glucose anaerobically into 2 mol of lactate. The source of glucose is primarily muscle glycogen and, to a lesser extent, circulating glucose, and the lactic acid system can generate ATP quickly for high-intensity exercise. The lactate system is not efficient from the standpoint of the quantity of ATP produced. However, because the process is so rapid, the small amount of ATP is produced quickly and absolutely by substrate-level phosphorylation of ADP (Chap. 3). The lactate produced by this system quickly crosses the muscle cell membrane into the bloodstream, from which it can be cleared by other tissues (primarily the liver) for aerobic production of ATP or gluconeogenesis. In the event that the rate of production of lactate exceeds its clearance rate, blood lactic acid accumulates. This lowers the pH of the blood and is one cause of fatigue. Other factors of fatigue include a combination of lactate build-up and the lowering of pH. Under such circumstances, exercise cannot be continued for long periods. The lactic acid system is engaged to provide a rapid source of energy. When an inadequate supply of oxygen prevents the aerobic system from furnishing sufficient ATP to meet the demands of exercise, the lactic acid system will continue to function. Although the system is operative upon the onset of strenuous exercise, it becomes the primary supplier of energy only after the depletion of CP stores in the muscle. As a back-up to the ATP-CP system, the lactic acid system becomes very important in high-intensity anaerobic power events lasting from 20 seconds to a few minutes, for example, longer sprints of up to 800 m and swimming events of 100 or 200 m.

The Aerobic System

This system involves the Krebs cycle, through which carbohydrates, fats, and possibly amino acids are completely oxidized to CO_2 and H_2O. The system, which requires oxygen, is highly efficient from the standpoint of the quantity of ATP produced. Because oxygen is necessary for the system to function, an individual's VO_2 max becomes an important factor in his or her performance capacity. Contributing to the VO_2 max are the cardiovascular system's ability to deliver blood (which carries the oxygen) to exercising muscle, pulmonary ventilation, oxygenation of blood, and the utilization of the oxygen by skeletal muscle mitochondria. Matching these contributors to the cellular need for oxygen in exercising muscle is complex because a low efficiency of any of them becomes rate limiting for the entire process. In terms of cellular metabolism, the aerobic pathway is slow to become activated and begins to dominate the course of activity only after about 5 minutes of continuous activity. The aerobic system is an important supplier of energy for forms of exercise lasting longer than 3 or 4 minutes, depending on the intensity of the exercise. Both intracellular triacylglycerols and plasma fatty acids also contribute to the overall energy supply. Many types of exercise or sports meet these criteria, for example, distance running and swimming and cross-country skiing, just a few of the so-called endurance feats.

Current thinking is that the three energy systems do not simply take turns serially and that a particular system is not skipped in meeting the demands of exercise. Rather, all systems function at all times, and as one predominates the others participate to varying degrees (see the perspective "Nutrient Usage during Strenuous Exercise"). The interaction of the three systems over the course of the first 2 minutes of exercise is complex but appears to involve the following energy contributions:

- ATP-CP decreasing from most contributory to least contributory during the period;
- lactic acid steady, with high contribution; and
- aerobic progressing from least to highest contribution during the period.

Energy contributions to long-term activity from aerobic and anaerobic systems are shown in Figure 8.11.

Fuel Sources during Exercise

Carbohydrate, fat, and protein are the dietary sources that provide the fuel for energy transformation in the muscle. At rest, and during normal daily activities, fats are the primary source of energy, providing 80% to 90% of the energy. Carbohydrates provide 5% to 18% and protein 2% to 5% of energy during the resting state [11].

During exercise, the oxidation of amino acids contributes only minimally to the total amount of ATP used by working muscles. Significant breakdown of amino acids occurs only toward the end of a long endurance event, when carbohydrate (glycogen) stores are somewhat depleted. Amino acids can be transaminated to form alanine from pyruvate. The alanine is transported to the liver and is a primary substrate for gluconeogenesis.

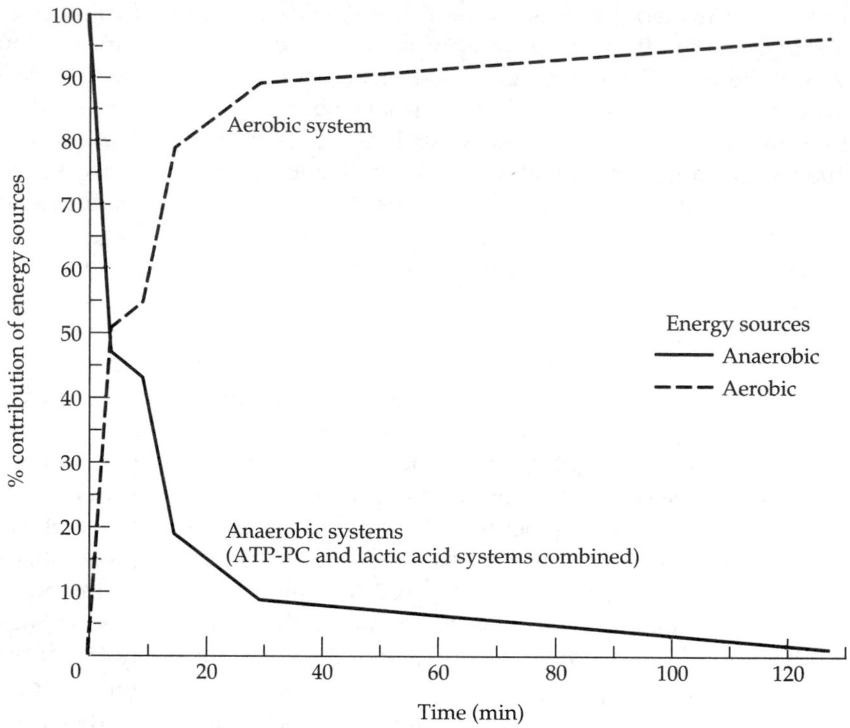

Figure 8.11 Primary energy sources for long-duration activity. *Source:* Adapted from Fox EL, Bowers RW, Foss ML. *The Physiological Basis for Exercise and Sports,* 3rd ed. Dubuque, IA: Brown and Benchmark, 1989, p. 37. Reproduced with permission of The McGraw-Hill Companies.

The carbon skeleton of some amino acids can be oxidized directly in the muscle. The four major endogenous sources of energy during exercise are

- muscle glycogen,
- plasma glucose,
- plasma fatty acids, and
- intramuscular triacylglycerols.

The extent to which each of these substrates contributes energy for exercise depends on several factors, including

- the intensity and duration of exercise,
- the level of exercise training,
- initial muscle glycogen levels, and
- supplementation with carbohydrates through the intestinal tract during exercise.

We will discuss the relationship between these factors and the "substrate of choice" for energy supply. A graphical representation of the contribution of these substrates at 25%, 65%, and 85% VO_2 max is shown in Figure 8.12.

Exercise Intensity and Duration

In the fasting state, much of the energy required for low-intensity levels of exercise (25%–30% VO_2 max) is derived from muscle triacylglycerols and plasma fatty acid oxidation, with a small contribution from plasma glucose. The pattern does not change significantly over a period of up to 2 hours at this exercise level, which is equivalent to walking. During this time, the consumed plasma fatty acids are replaced by mobilization of fatty acids from the large triacylglycerol stores in adipocytes throughout the body. However, as exercise intensity

Figure 8.12 Contribution of the four major substrates to energy expenditure after 30 minutes of exercise at 25%, 65%, and 85% VO_2 max.

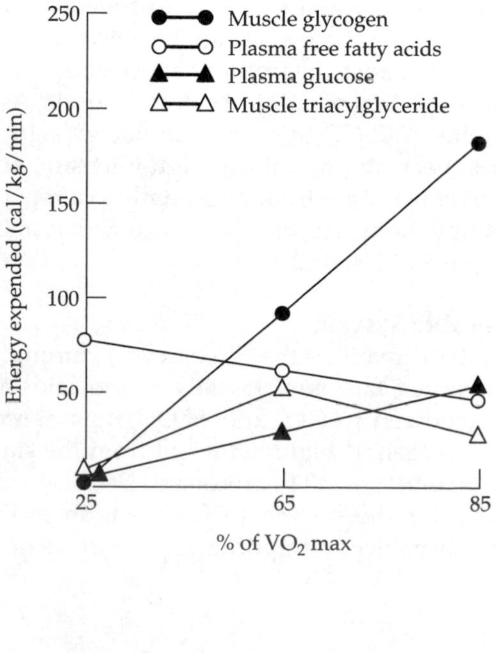

increases to 65% and on up to 85% VO_2 max, the release of adipocyte fatty acids into the plasma is reduced, resulting in a decrease in the concentration of plasma fatty acids. This decrease occurs despite a continuing high rate of lipolysis in adipocytes. The decreased replacement of plasma fatty acids from fat stores at higher levels of exercise has been attributed to insufficient blood flow and albumin delivery of fatty acids from adipose tissue into the systemic circulation [12]. Therefore, we would predict that fatty acids become trapped in adipose tissue and accumulate there during high levels of exercise, a theory supported by research [8].

With moderate-intensity exercise (~65% VO_2 max) equivalent to running for 1 to 3 hours, total fat oxidation increases despite the reduced rate of return of adipose fatty acids into the circulation. This is attributed to an increase in the oxidation of muscle triacylglycerols. In fact, as shown in Figure 8.12, plasma fatty acids and muscle triacylglycerols contribute equally to energy expenditure at this level of exertion in endurance-trained athletes. Within the exertion range of 60% to 75% VO_2 max, however, fat cannot be oxidized at a rate sufficiently high to provide needed energy, and therefore nearly half of the required energy must be furnished by carbohydrate oxidation. Note that fatty acids have only two oxygen molecules compared to an equal number of oxygen and carbon molecules in carbohydrates. This means that fatty acids require more oxygen to be delivered by the cardiovascular system. Also, the transfer of fatty acids into mitochondria is slow, and this may be a rate-limiting event. The result is that when tissue oxygen levels begin to be low and/or high-intensity exercise calls for a large quantity of energy, carbohydrate becomes a more favored substrate. Fatty acids are the favored substrates for intensities of up to about 50% VO_2 max.

As exercise intensity increases to 85% VO_2 max, the relative contribution of carbohydrate oxidation to total metabolism increases sharply (see Fig. 8.12). At VO_2 max, carbohydrate in the form of blood glucose (derived from glycogenolysis of hepatic glycogen stores) and muscle glycogen essentially become the sole suppliers of energy. Like muscle glycogen, the concentration of blood glucose falls progressively during prolonged, strenuous exercise. This is due to the fact that glucose uptake by working muscle (independent of insulin) may increase to as much as 20-fold or more above resting levels, while hepatic glucose output decreases with exercise duration. Interestingly, however, hypoglycemia is not always observed at exhaustion, particularly at exercise intensities >70% VO_2 max. Hypoglycemia following liver glycogen depletion apparently can be postponed by an inhibition of glucose uptake and accelerated gluconeogenesis in the liver, using the glycerol produced in lipolysis, and by lactate and pyruvate produced by the glycolytic activity of the working muscles.

Accompanying high rates of carbohydrate catabolism is a rise in the production of lactic acid, which accumulates in muscle and blood. This is particularly evident in situations of oxygen debt, in which insufficient oxygen to complete the oxidation of pyruvate to CO_2 and H_2O instead favors its reduction to lactate.

The essentiality of carbohydrate as an energy substrate at moderate to high levels of exercise is due to the need for Krebs cycle intermediates from carbohydrates to oxidize the fatty acids, the slow rate of fat oxidation, and the limited ability of muscle to oxidize fat. Muscle fatigue occurs when the supply of glucose is inadequate, such as occurs with muscle glycogen depletion or hypoglycemia. To prevent this from happening, the individual must reduce workload intensity to a level that matches his or her ability to oxidize fat predominantly, possibly as low as 30% VO_2 max. The reason for this limitation, and thus the dependence of muscle on carbohydrate as an energy source, is not fully understood. However, traditional thinking is that the limitation may be based on two factors: (1) oxidation of fatty acids is limited by the enzyme carnitine acyltransferase (CAT), which catalyzes the transport of fatty acids across the mitochondrial membrane; (2) CAT is known to be inhibited by malonyl CoA. When availability of carbohydrate to the muscle is high, fatty acid oxidation may be reduced by the inhibition of CAT by glucose-derived malonyl CoA [13].

Level of Exercise Training

Endurance training increases an athlete's ability to perform more aerobically at the same absolute exercise intensity. Several factors aid in this. Endurance-trained muscle exhibits an increase in the number and size of mitochondria as well as an increase in cardiovascular capacity, lung capacity, and hypertrophy of the Type I muscle. The activity of oxidative enzymes in endurance-trained subjects has been shown to be 100% greater than in untrained subjects at 65% VO_2 max. Endurance training also results in an increased utilization of fat as an energy source during submaximal exercise. In skeletal muscle, fatty acid oxidation has an inhibitory effect on glucose uptake and glycolysis. For this reason, the trained athlete benefits from the carbohydrate-sparing effect of enhanced fatty acid oxidation during competition because of slower depletion of muscle glycogen and plasma glucose. This largely accounts for the training-induced increase in endurance for exercise over a prolonged period.

It has been reported that trained individuals have a lower plasma fatty acid concentration and reduced adipose tissue lipolysis compared to untrained counterparts at similar exercise intensity. This suggests that the primary source of fatty acids used by the trained individual is intramuscular triacylglycerol stores rather than adipocyte triacylglycerols. After a period of exercise, the intramuscular triacylglycerols are replaced with the fatty acids coming from plasma. Lipolysis from adipocytes increases the free fatty acid levels in plasma.

Endurance training appears to result in an increased capacity for muscle glycogen storage. Therefore, the trained athlete benefits not only from a slower utilization of muscle glycogen (as explained earlier) but also from the capacity to have higher glycogen stores at the onset of competition.

Initial Muscle Glycogen Levels

The ability to sustain prolonged moderate to heavy exercise is largely dependent on the initial content of skeletal muscle glycogen, and the depletion of muscle glycogen is the single most consistently observed factor contributing to fatigue. High muscle glycogen levels allow exercise to continue longer at a submaximal workload. Even in the absence of carbohydrate loading (see the following section), a strong positive correlation exists between initial glycogen level and time to exhaustion and/or level of performance during exercise periods lasting more than 1 hour. The correlation does not apply at low levels of exertion (25%–35% VO_2 max) or at high levels of exertion for short time periods because glycogen depletion is not a limiting factor under these conditions. It has been suggested that the importance of initial muscle glycogen stores is related to the inability of glucose and fatty acids to cross the cell membrane rapidly enough to provide adequate substrate for mitochondrial respiration [14].

Carbohydrate Supplementation (Supercompensation)

When muscle glycogen was identified as the limiting factor for the capacity to exercise at intensities requiring 70% to 85% VO_2 max, dietary manipulation to maximize glycogen stores followed naturally. The most popular subject for research of this nature has been the marathon runner or cross-country skier because of the prolonged physical taxation of these events and the fact that the athlete's performance is readily measurable by the time required to complete the course. The major dietary concern to emerge in the endurance training of marathon runners was how to elevate muscle glycogen to above-normal (supercompensated) levels. In sporting vernacular, maximizing glycogen content by dietary manipulation is referred to as "carbohydrate loading."

The so-called classical regimen for carbohydrate loading resulted from investigations in the late 1960s by Scandinavian scientists [15]. This regimen involved two sessions of intense exercise to exhaustion to deplete muscle glycogen stores separated by 2 days of low-carbohydrate diet (<10%) to "starve" the muscle of carbohydrate. This was followed by 3 days of high-carbohydrate diet (>90%) and rest. The event would be performed on day 7 of the regimen. On completion of this regimen, muscle glycogen levels approached 220 mmol/kg wet weight (expressed as glucose residues), more than double the athlete's resting level. However, because of various undesirable side effects of the classical regimen, such as irritability, dizziness, and a diminished exercise capacity, a less stringent regimen of diet and exercise has evolved that produces comparably high muscle glycogen levels.

In the modified regimen, runners perform "tapered-down" exercise sessions over the course of 5 days, followed by 1 day of rest. During this time, 3 days of a 50% carbohydrate diet are followed by 3 days of a 70% carbohydrate diet, generally achieved by consuming large quantities of pasta and rice or bread. The modified regimen, which can increase muscle glycogen stores 20% to 40% above normal, has been shown to be as effective as the classical approach with fewer adverse side effects.

Figure 8.13 illustrates graphically the amount of muscle glycogen formed as a result of each regimen. Predictably, the supercompensation of muscle glycogen by either approach has been shown to improve performance in trained runners during races of 30 km and longer. It did not improve performance in shorter races (<21 km) owing to the fact that glycogen depletion is not the limiting factor in such events. Other nutritional factors involving carbohydrate intake may enhance performance, as discussed next.

Preevent Meal. The timing of the final meal before intense exercise is crucial, because fasting results in a reduction of the labile glycogen stores of liver, while carbohydrate meals consumed too close in time to the event may cause **hyperinsulinemia.** Stimulation of insulin release just before an event results in a rapid reduction in plasma glucose, significantly impairing work capacity. Exercise permits a rapid uptake of glucose by the muscle in addition to the insulin-stimulated uptake. Elevated plasma insulin also inhibits liver glucose output and the normal rise of plasma free fatty acids. Under such conditions, excessive muscle glycogen degradation occurs, resulting in early fatigue. The final meal before intense exercise should be consumed several hours before the event so that the stomach is empty and allows for rapid water absorption. For long endurance events, the meal generally should be high in complex carbohydrates and low in fat, conditions that

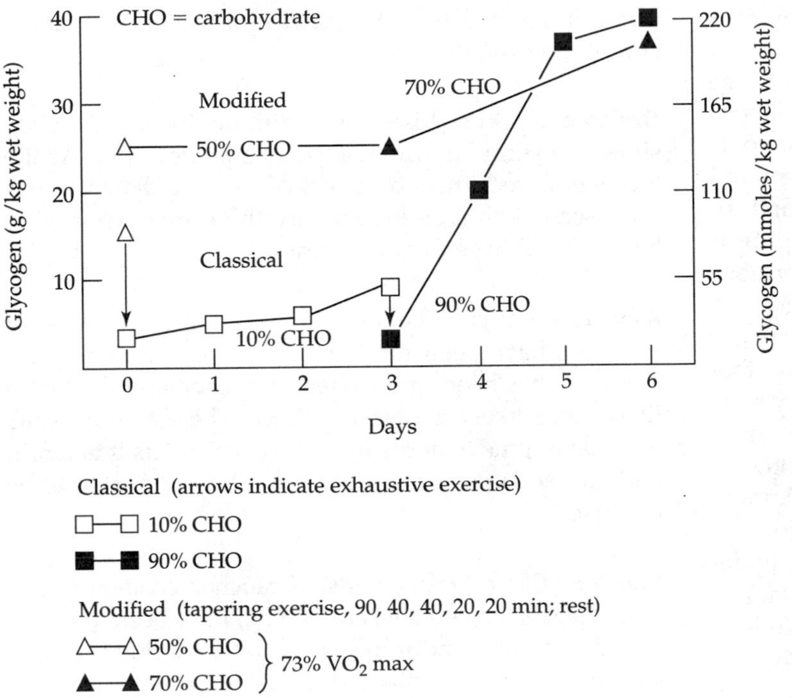

Figure 8.13 Schematic representation of the "classical" regimen of muscle glycogen supercompensation described by Scandinavian investigators and the "modified" regimen of muscle glycogen supercompensation, which has been shown to elevate muscle glycogen stores to comparably high levels with "normal" diets and a "tapering-down" sequence of exercise. *Source:* From Sherman WM. Carbohydrate, muscle glycogen, and muscle glycogen supercompensation. In: *Ergogenic Aids in Sport.* by Williams MH, Champaign, IL: Human Kinetics Publishers, 1983, p. 14. Reprinted by permission.

promote rapid emptying of the stomach. The nature of the food consumed is up to the athlete.

An isotonic or hypotonic beverage containing carbohydrate 15 to 20 minutes prior to the event provides extra dietary glucose without stimulating insulin release. For prolonged events (longer than 90 minutes), the consumption of fluid containing some carbohydrate helps with fluid balance as well as with maintaining blood glucose (see Chap. 14). Balance must be maintained to allow the liquid to empty rapidly from the stomach and the carbohydrate to be rapidly absorbed. A full discussion of these factors is beyond the scope of this text. In brief, the beverage should be cool, not cold, be isotonic or hypotonic, and contain glucose or polyglucose. Large amounts of fructose should not be included because of its slow absorption rate.

Glycemic Index. The form of carbohydrate ingested is also an important consideration in optimizing endurance performance. The principal factor in this regard is the glycemic index (GI) of the food (see Chap. 4 for a full explanation of glycemic index). Potato starch is considered to have a relatively high GI, though not as high as the simple sugars. Generally, low to moderate GI carbohydrate loading prior to the performance is preferred to high GI carbohydrate intake because the hyperinsulinemic effect of the high GI food, as mentioned earlier, results in a rapid reduction in blood glucose, suppressed release of fatty acids from store, and inhibition of hepatic glycogenolysis.

After a prolonged event, the reverse is true with respect to the GI of foods consumed. Immediately after a glycogen-depleting event, liver and muscle glycogen levels are very low, and glycogen levels will recover faster if a high GI food or beverage is consumed. These foods can be as simple as wedges of orange or apple or one of the sports drinks containing glucose, sucrose, or polyglucose. Recovery depends on replacing lost body water, rebuilding glycogen levels, rebuilding lost muscle protein, and, for very long events, restoring electrolyte balance. This last topic will be covered in more detail in Chapter 14.

Nutritional Ergogenic Aids

The word *ergogenic* is derived from the Greek word *ergon*, meaning "work," and is defined as increasing work or the potential to do work. An ergogenic aid does not need to be nutritional; it can also be mechanical. For example, a running shoe or body suit to improve aerodynamics can be a mechanical ergogenic aid. We will limit this discussion to nutritional ergogenic supplements, or ergogenic aids. Often these are substances that are part of a normal diet, or they may be cellular metabolites that are ingested in an effort to enhance the capacity for sport, exercise, and physical performance. Several nutritional practices have ergogenic properties that are not necessarily considered ergogenic supplementation, for example, carbohydrate loading and fat loading. Fat loading has been purported to "spare" the more limited carbohydrates. As mentioned previously, fats are the major fuel source for exercise below 50% VO_2 max.

Nutritional ergogenic supplements are also to be distinguished from ergogenic drugs such as anabolic steroids or stimulants. The risks of using anabolic steroids are so great that they have prompted the enactment and enforcement of laws prohibiting their use in strength or endurance competitions. The compulsion for improved performance among athletes has led to an enormous increase in the testing and use of nutritional ergogenic aids. As expected, the literature dealing with the subject has expanded with equal zeal. Many supplements that have not been fully tested for either safety or efficacy have been recommended through the lay press. The information presented here will be restricted to the theoretical basis for their use and a brief overview of what is known about the effectiveness of ergogenic supplementation.

There appears to be a dichotomy between the widespread public use of certain supplements and the lack of scientific support for such use. A problem for researchers is the common perception of subjects under study that they simply "feel better" as a result of supplementation, even though actual physiological changes may not be documented by the research. In other words, psychological effects are adding a new dimension to the testing of ergogenic aids. These must be considered along with true physiological effects, because as mood and mental outlook improve, so does physical performance. This is the bottom line for using supplements in the first place. For all nutritional ergogenic aids, the placebo effect is significant. The level of athletic performance is influenced by psychological factors. By "believing" that a certain supplement will make you perform better, you may actually perform better. Often there is a theoretical "rationale" for supplement use, but it does not necessarily translate into enhancement of performance.

Following is a listing of micronutrient ergogenic supplements that have been consumed on a broad basis. The supplements chosen for citing were selected on the basis of their reputed efficacy from a much longer list of hit-or-miss trial substances. In most instances, research results neither totally support nor totally refute supplement efficacy but instead are divided in their findings. Reference occasionally will be made to the number of "pro and con" study conclusions to help the reader evaluate a substance's efficacy. Although specific references will not be included, they, along with many more pertinent sources of information, are available to the interested reader [16,17].

Amino Acids

Arginine. Arginine has been shown to elicit the release of somatotropin with large oral doses. Somatotropin, which has been referred to as insulin-like growth factor, stimulates protein synthesis.

Ornithine. Oral doses of ornithine have also been shown to stimulate the release of somatotropin. At the levels required, the side effect of osmotic diarrhea was often seen. Both arginine and ornithine are purported to be beneficial in resistance training.

Aspartate Salts. The potassium-magnesium salts of aspartate have been marketed as an antifatigue agent. Their use has been questioned, however, and the benefit is more likely a placebo effect. The aspartate salts may have some benefits in endurance events if taken in high doses. Time to exhaustion has been reported to be increased.

Branched-Chain Amino Acids. Branched-chained amino acids (isoleucine, leucine, and valine) have been hypothesized to benefit endurance activities by influencing the level of serum tryptophan. BCAAs compete with tryptophan for entry into the brain. One theory on fatigue is that brain tryptophan is converted to serotonin, which causes fatigue. This may be one of several factors bringing about fatigue. BCAAs are also used by muscle for energy near the end of very long endurance events. It has been suggested that consuming BCAAs prior to an event will provide energy toward the end of the event and thereby reduce the amount of muscle breakdown.

Antioxidants

Endurance exercise increases the amount of oxygen moving into the muscle. Increased exposure to large volumes of oxygen in turn increases the generation of free radicals, which have been shown to be involved with fatigue and damage to the muscle cell membrane. This information provides the rationale for the use of antioxidants to prevent muscle damage and delay fatigue. Many antioxidants have been used, including vitamin C, vitamin E, and selenium. Coenzyme Q_{10} also has antioxidant activity, though its use as an ergogenic aid is based on other properties.

Herbs

Much interest has recently been directed toward herbal preparations. It is difficult to evaluate and compare studies on these preparations because their collection, processing, and agricultural growing conditions influence the active components. One class of herbals, ephedra, was previously used for its ephedrine content. The risk of harmful side effects or death has discouraged its use and caused it to be banned from use by athletes in most sports.

The Ginsengs. The most widely used and studied herbs are the ginsengs. Some purported ergogenic benefits of *Panax* (Chinese/Korean) ginseng include

- increased run time to exhaustion (three out of seven studies),
- increased muscle strength (one out of two studies),
- improved recovery from exercise (three out of four studies),
- improved oxygen metabolism during exercise (seven out of nine studies),
- reduced exercise-induced lactate (five out of nine studies),
- improved auditory and visual reaction times (six out of seven studies), and
- improved vitality and feelings of well-being (six out of nine studies).

These benefits have more consistently been reported following supplementation over more than 8 weeks [18].

Caffeine

Ergogenic effects of caffeine are seen in endurance events. It is generally recognized that the largest impact is seen in individuals who do not consume caffeine on a regular basis. Caffeine is a CNS stimulant, increasing blood flow to the kidneys (thus acting as a diuretic) and stimulating the release of fatty acids from adipose. Sport regulatory bodies have set an upper limit for the permissible level of caffeine consumption.

Intermediary Metabolites

Bicarbonate. Bicarbonate is a primary buffering agent in the body. Athletes competing in short anaerobic events (lasting only a few minutes) build up lactic acid. The lowering of blood pH is one factor leading to fatigue. Theoretically, loading with sodium bicarbonate would delay the drop in pH and thereby delay fatigue. Studies have supported this benefit, and it is often mentioned in reviews of ergogenic aids. In conversations with many sprint athletes and coaches, however, none reported having used sodium bicarbonate, nor did they know of anyone who did.

Carnitine. L-carnitine is used by the body to transfer acyl CoA from the cytoplasm of a cell into the mitochondria. This is the theoretical basis for the use of carnitine as a nutritional ergogenic aid. In individuals fed parenterally for long periods of time, it has been shown that fatty acid utilization can be enhanced by supplementation with carnitine. Individuals with chronic cardiovascular disease have also been shown to benefit from carnitine. For the athlete, studies that show benefit and those that do not are about even.

Coenzyme Q_{10}. The theoretical basis for coenzyme Q_{10} as an ergogenic aid stems from its pivotal role in electron transport and production of ATP in the mitochondrion. Clinical studies have shown its safety and use in cardiovascular disease. Supplementation with coenzyme Q_{10} longer than 4 weeks has been purported to provide benefits for the long-term endurance athlete. This benefit has not been shown conclusively, however.

Creatine. Muscle creatine is part of the ATP-CP energy system that supplies the initial energy during the first few seconds to minutes of exercise. The theoretical basis for using creatine as a nutritional ergogenic aid is that the saturation of muscle with creatine increases the amount of creatine phosphate in the muscle. Creatine has been shown to be effective for short, intense exercise. However, there are associated risks in taking it. Individuals taking creatine appear to add 1 to 2 kg of water weight. Those taking creatine in hot, humid environments have become dehydrated and more susceptible to heat stress. Deaths have been reported.

Other. Many other nutritional materials have been recommended in the lay literature as possessing ergogenic properties, including minerals such as calcium, magnesium, zinc, iron, phosphates, chromium, boron, and vanadium and most vitamins. Reviews of mineral supplements [16] suggest that performance enhancement is not well established and that the major benefit of mineral supplementation lies in the correction of deficiencies should they exist.

General problems of research design remain as the popularity of nutritional ergogenic supplements surges forward. As indicated previously, many ergogenic effects may be attributed to mental and psychological changes, and it behooves future researchers to rule these out in an effort to establish strictly physiological effects. The fact that the number of studies finding "for" performance enhancement is nearly equaled by the number of those finding "against" enhancement testifies to the difficulty involved in researching this important field.

summary

Animal survival depends on a constant internal environment maintained through specific control mechanisms. Controls, operative at all levels (cellular, organ, and system), integrate energy metabolism and allow the body to adapt to a wide variety of environmental conditions. Primary among the mechanisms of adaptation is the regulation of metabolism through the cooperative input of the nervous, endocrine, and vascular systems. In the normal operation of these systems, metabolic pathways may be stimulated, maintained, or inhibited, depending on the conditions imposed on the body. A pointed example of metabolic adaptation is the shift that occurs in substrate utilization and metabolic pathways in answer to changes in the body's nourishment status (i.e., fed, fasting, and starvation states).

The physical stress of exercise and sport presents an interesting challenge to the regulatory capacity of the body to provide the additional energy needed by the exercising muscles. Substrates fueling this energy include plasma free fatty acids, plasma glucose, muscle glycogen, and muscle triacylglycerols, and their utilization varies according to the intensity and duration of the exercise. Many substances have been tested for their ergogenic properties in attempts to improve performance in high-intensity and endurance sports. In most cases, test results remain controversial, and more research is needed to establish which of the reputed ergogenic aids produce true physiological improvement.

References Cited

1. Role of fat and fatty acids in modulation of energy exchange. Nutr Rev 1988;46:382–84.

2. Hellerstein M, Schwarz J-M, Neese R. Regulation of hepatic de novo lipogenesis in humans. Ann Rev Nutr 1996;16:523–57.

3. McGarry JD, Kuwajima M, Newgard CB, et al. From dietary glucose to liver glycogen: the full circle round. Ann Rev Nutr 1987;7:51–73.

4. Foster DW. From glycogen to ketones and back. Banting Lecture, 1984. Diabetes 1984;33:1188–99.

5. Lehninger AL, Nelson DL, Cox MM. Principles of Biochemistry, 2nd ed. New York: Worth, 1993, pp. 757–58.

6. Tepperman J, Tepperman HM. Metabolic and Endocrine Physiology, 5th ed. Chicago: Year Book, 1987.

7. Turner AJ, ed. Neuropeptides and Their Peptidases. New York: VCH, 1987.

8. Romijn J, Coyle E, Sidossis L, et al. Regulation of endogenous fat and carbohydrate metabolism in relation to exercise intensity. Am J Physiol 1993;265:E380–91.

9. Hermansen L, Hultman E, Saltin B. Muscle glycogen during prolonged severe exercise. Acta Physiol Scand 1967;71:129–39.

10. McArdle W, Katch F, and Katch V. Exercise Physiology: Energy, Nutrition, and Human Performance, 3rd ed. Philadelphia: Lea and Febiger, 1991, chaps. 1, 6, 11.

11. Wolinsky I. Nutrition in Exercise and Sport, 3rd ed. Boca Raton: CRC Press, 1998, chaps. 6, 13.

12. Hodgetts A, Coppack SW, Frayn KN, and Hockaday TDR. Factors controlling fat mobilization from human subcutaneous adipose tissue during exercise. J Appl Physiol 1991;71:445–51.

13. Elayan I, Winder W. Effect of glucose infusion on muscle malonyl CoA during exercise. J Appl Physiol 1991;70:1495–99.

14. Saltin B, Gollnick P. Fuel for muscular exercise: role of carbohydrate. In: Horton E, Terjung R, eds. Exercise, Nutrition, and Energy Metabolism. New York: MacMillan, 1988, chap. 4.

15. Bergstrom J, Hultman E. A study of the glycogen metabolism during exercise in man. Scand J Clin Lab Invest 1967;19:218–28.

16. Wolinsky I. Nutrition in Exercise and Sport, 3rd ed. Boca Raton: CRC Press, 1998.

17. Green GA, Catlin DH, Starcevic B. Analysis of over-the-counter dietary supplements. Clin J Sport Med 2001;11:254–59.

18. Mahady G, Gyllenhall C, Fong H. Ginsengs: a review of safety and efficacy. Nutr Clin Care 2000;3:90–101.

Suggested Readings

Coyle EF. Substrate utilization during exercise in active people. Am J Clin Nutr 1995;61(suppl):968S–79S. A very useful review of the hierarchy of substrates as they are used for energy release in exercise.

Harris RA, Crabb DW. Metabolic interrelationships. In: Devlin TM, ed. Textbook of Biochemistry with Clinical Correlations, 3rd ed. New York: Wiley, 1992, pp. 576–606. This integration of human metabolic pathways is written primarily for the medical student. Information is presented so as to be relevant for the health practitioner.

Tepperman J, Tepperman HM. Metabolic and Endocrine Physiology, 5th ed. Chicago: Year Book, 1987. This is a well-illustrated, easy-to-read explanation of the regulatory role of the endocrine system in human metabolism.

Wolinsky I. Nutrition in Exercise and Sport, 3rd ed. Boca Raton: CRC Press, 1998. A thorough treatment of what is known and what is not in sports nutrition.

Web Sites

www.nal.usda.gov/fnic/pubs/bibs/gen/97-sp-hp.htm
National Agricultural Library: Sports Nutrition Resource List for Health Professionals

www.umass.edu/cnshp/index.html
Center for Nutrition in Sport and Human Performance at the University of Massachusetts

www.faseb.org/ajcn
American Journal of Clinical Nutrition

www.gssiweb.com/
Gatorade Sports Science Institute

Diabetes: Metabolism Out of Control

Diabetes mellitus, the disease characterized by the body's inability to metabolize glucose, manifests as one of two types: type 1, or insulin-dependent diabetes mellitus, ketosis prone (IDDM); and type 2, non-insulin-dependent diabetes mellitus (NIDDM). The long-term consequences of diabetes demonstrate that lipid metabolism is also involved. The two types are mechanistically very different and will be discussed separately. Current theories on the etiology and characteristics of these two classifications of diabetes are shown in Figure 1.

Non-Insulin-Dependent Diabetes Mellitus (Type 2)

Type 2 diabetes accounts for 80% to 90% of all reported cases of the disease. The cause of type 2 diabetes has not been completely resolved, but it appears to be associated with insulin resistance in peripheral target tissue. This condition is caused not by a failure of target cells to bind insulin but by a postbinding abnormality, arising somewhere in the sequence of events that follows the binding of insulin to its receptor and leads to the cell's normal response to that signal. Experimental evidence suggests that a primary cause for the interrupted insulin signal may be compromised synthesis or mobilization of the cell's glucose transporters (refer to the section "Glucose Transporters," Chap. 4).

In skeletal muscle cells, insulin resistance associated with NIDDM has been shown to be caused by a reduction in glucose transporter activity, specifically the failure of the vesicles to translocate in response to insulin (see Fig. 4.8). The error can be thought of as a block or short-circuit in the insulin signal that normally initiates the translocation process. The result is a reduced concentration of transporters at the cell surface and a consequent reduction in the rate of glucose uptake. Although a similar defect was found in adipocytes of NIDDM patients, it is not the major cause of the insulin resistance in these cells. Rather, the consequence of NIDDM in adipocytes is a marked depletion of mRNA encoding the GLUT4 transporter, resulting in depleted intracellular stores of the protein [1]. This describes a pretranslational defect, meaning that it interferes with protein synthesis at a level before the translation process, the step that requires mRNA as template. Therefore, even if the vesicle translocation process were not compromised, an inadequate number of surface receptors would still be expressed upon insulin stimulation.

Insulin resistance has also been described in obesity as well as in NIDDM. Insulin resistance in obesity is mechanistically similar to the NIDDM effect on adipocytes. Reduction in GLUT4 mRNA in obese subjects results in a decrease in de novo synthesis of the transporter. Furthermore, the extent to which mRNA expression is suppressed appears to relate directly to increasing adiposity.

Figure 1 Overview of present theories of diabetes mellitus etiology. (a) depicts the factors impinging on the development of diabetes mellitus that requires exogenous insulin. This type of diabetes presently is most commonly designated as insulin-dependent diabetes mellitus (IDDM). (b) illustrates the interaction of factors that may result in non-insulin-dependent diabetes mellitus (NIDDM).

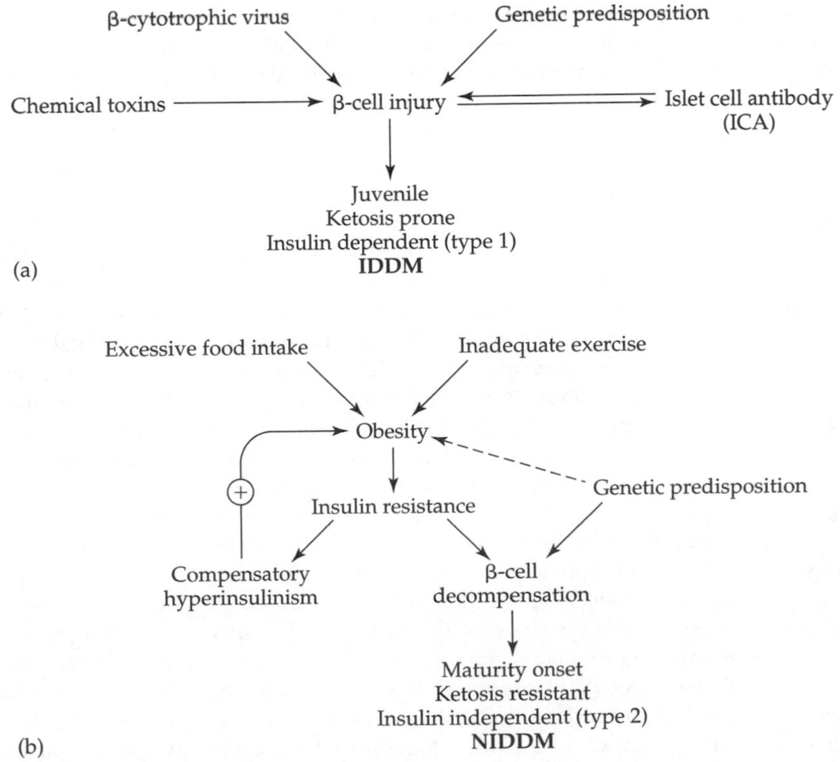

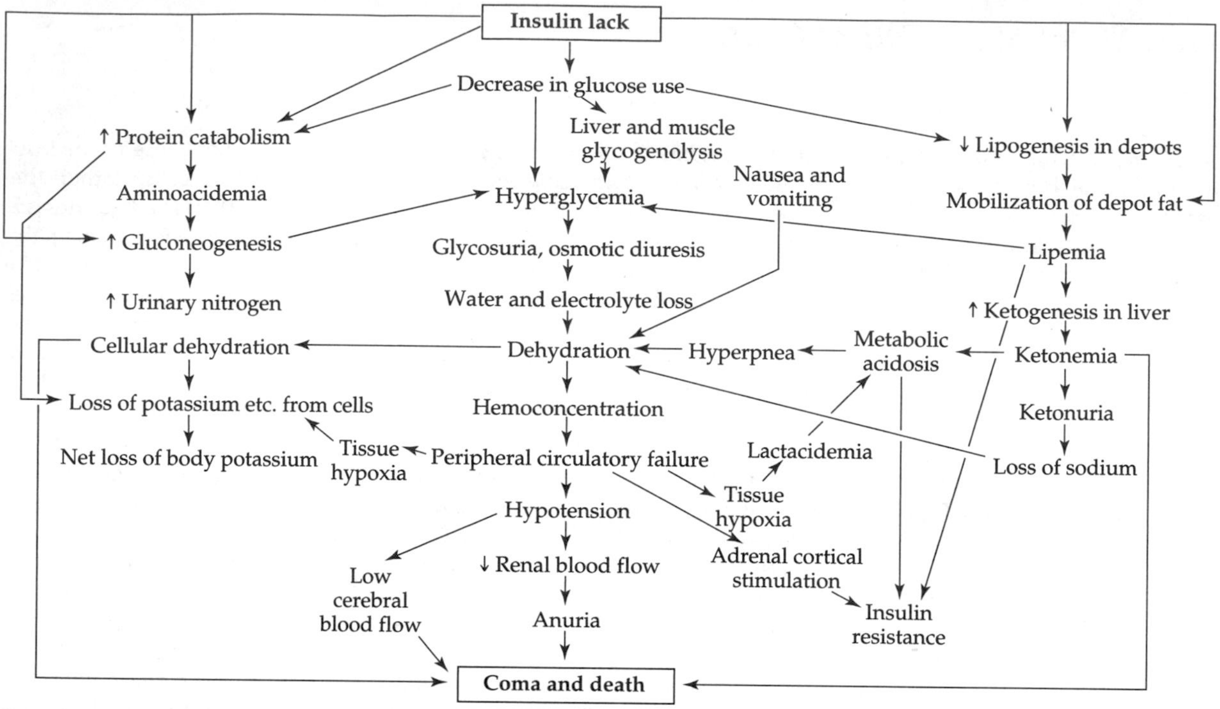

Figure 2 Composite summary of pathophysiology of diabetic acidosis. Particularly striking are the aberrations in the metabolism of carbohydrates, lipids, and protein caused by an insulin lack and the interconnections among these altered metabolic pathways. *Source:* Tepperman D., Tepperman H. *Metabolic and Endocrine Physiology,* 5th ed. Chicago: Year Book, 1987, p. 284.

In summary, NIDDM is characterized by insulin resistance in peripheral target tissues because of a diminished population of functional glucose transporters. In muscle cells, the defect appears to arise from a failure, on insulin stimulation, of vesicle-bound transporters to translocate to the plasma membrane. In adipocytes, translocation is also compromised, but the major mechanism for insulin resistance in these cells, in both NIDDM and obesity, is a pretranslational depletion of GLUT4 mRNA. In the latter stages of NIDDM, the pancreas loses its ability to produce insulin. Insulin therapy is more likely to be used at this stage.

Insulin-Dependent Diabetes Mellitus (Type 1)

The hyperglycemia of type 1 diabetes can be attributed to a primary failure of the β-cells of the pancreas to produce and secrete insulin. IDDM is regarded as an autoimmune disease in which the pancreatic islet cells, which are composed largely of β-cells, become targets of an immune response. This ultimately causes cellular dysfunction of the β-cells, with an inability of the cells to produce insulin. Factors that trigger the immune attack remain unknown.

Figure 2 emphasizes the crucial role of insulin in the regulation of metabolism and the metabolic events set in motion by lack of insulin. An absence of insulin not only inhibits the use of glucose by muscles and adipose tissue but also sets in motion a sequence of events that, without effective intervention, will result in coma and death of the affected animal or human. Insulin acts on metabolism in various ways, most of which have the effect of lowering blood glucose. These actions include decreasing hepatic glucose output while increasing glucose oxidation, glycogen deposition, lipogenesis, protein synthesis, and cell replication. In the absence of insulin, all the hormones favoring catabolism and the raising of blood glucose operate without opposition. The direction of metabolism in response to these catabolic hormones is shown in Figure 8.9, which depicts the body's adaptation to fasting. In diabetes, however, the responses are much more violent than those occurring in the body's adaptation to fasting or starvation. In the latter case, the purpose is maintenance of a blood glucose level sufficient to meet the crucial demands of the CNS and RBCs. The unrestrained action of the catabolic hormones in the absence of insulin, along with the dramatically decreased use of glucose caused by an insulin lack, results in aberrations in metabolism. Not only is metabolism of carbohydrate, fat, and protein affected, but water and electrolyte imbalance also occurs.

Hyperglycemia, the hallmark of diabetes, is due to decreased glucose uptake by the cells and increased hepatic glucose output and results in an osmotic diuresis that proves fatal if uninterrupted (Fig. 2). The water and electrolytes lost through this diuresis lead to a dehydration compounded by increased insensible water loss due to the **hyperpnea** (abnormally rapid breathing) of metabolic acidosis. Metabolic acidosis results from the excessive ketogenesis occurring in the liver.

Peripheral circulatory failure, a consequence of severe hemoconcentration, leads to tissue hypoxia with a consequent shift of the tissues to anaerobic metabolism. Anaerobic metabolism raises the concentration of lactic acid in the blood, thereby worsening the metabolic acidosis.

The ketonuria along with glucosuria associated with acidosis causes an excessive loss of sodium from the body, and loss of this extracellular cation further compromises body water balance. A net loss of potassium, the chief intracellular cation, accompanies increased protein catabolism and cellular dehydration, both of which characterize uncontrolled diabetes.

The normal flow of substrates following food intake, as depicted in Figure 8.7, is largely dependent on the secretion of insulin. Insulin exerts a potent, positive effect on anabolism, emphasized in the figure, while inhibiting catabolic pathways. Figure 2, in contrast, shows metabolism out of control when the inhibiting effect of insulin is lacking and conservation of energy is impossible. Diabetes is a vivid negative example of the integration of metabolism and the importance of metabolic regulation (homeostasis) to continuance of life.

Reference Cited

1. Garvey WT, Maianu L, Huecksteadt TP, et al. Pretranslational suppression of a glucose transporter protein causes insulin resistance in adipocytes from patients with non-insulin-dependent diabetes mellitus. J Clin Invest 1991;87:1072–81.

Web Sites

www.diabetes.org
American Diabetes Association

www.jdfcure.org
Juvenile Diabetes Foundation

perspective

Nutrient Usage during Strenuous Exercise

Nutrient use during anaerobic exercise is straightforward. The ATP-CP system provides the initial energy. If the exercise goes beyond a few seconds, intramuscular glucose and then intramuscular glycogen serve as substrates for anaerobic glycolysis, producing lactic acid. After the exercise is over, the lactic acid is carried to the liver to be used as a substrate for gluconeogenesis, and the muscular ATP/creatine phosphate is replenished through aerobic glycolysis. For most anaerobic, sprint power activities, Type IIb muscle is used. Type IIb is rich in the glycolytic pathway enzymes.

It is much harder to clearly define the energy-producing substrates, pathways, or muscle types used in long-term endurance events. The purpose of this perspective is to develop a logical scenario that is consistent with what is likely to be happening to a well-trained long-term endurance athlete running a marathon. Chapter 8 has provided the basis for describing the events, but the modifying conditions cloud the picture. We can discuss the nature of factors that influence energy production, but we cannot accurately assess their quantitative contribution to whatever nutrients or pathways are being used at any given moment. There is simply too much biological variation. Factors that need to be considered include genetics, state of training, initial muscle and liver glycogen levels, the availability of energy nutrients (which is influenced by insulin and glucagon levels and their ratio), recent intake of fat and carbohydrate, and the use of ergogenic aids such as caffeine. Several of these factors are discussed briefly in this perspective.

Genetics

Every individual is born with a predetermined percentage of muscle types. Some individuals have more Type I muscle, others have more Type IIb muscle, and so on. In other words, some people are more adapted to aerobic events and others to sprint and power events. The age-old question is why an athlete selects a specific sport or a particular position. Is it because of coaching, or because of genetic makeup? There is no doubt that training and conditioning can modify muscle types to better adapt to a particular sport, but the relative percentage of each muscle type does not change. In becoming a world-class athlete, genetics play a major role. An interesting new development is the growing body of research showing that women have more Type I muscle than men. Under usual conditions of long-term aerobic exercise, women will burn lipid at a higher percentage of VO_2 max than men [1].

State of Training

The state of training and conditioning for a particular athletic event has a profound effect on metabolism. Aerobic training increases the size of the muscle (**hypertrophy**) and the number and size of the muscle mitochondria, thereby increasing the oxidative capacity of the trained muscle. Training increases the ability of the lungs to transfer oxygen to the blood and the ability of the cardiovascular system to deliver the oxygen to the muscle. All of these factors increase the percentage of VO_2 max at which aerobic oxidation can occur. The storage of triacylglycerols intramuscularly is increased with training, as is the ability to store glycogen in the muscle. The synthesis of many enzymes induced by training permits the changes listed above to occur.

Availability of Energy Nutrients

Muscle metabolism is greatly influenced by the ready availability of substrates. Recall from Chapter 3 that the energy of a reaction is influenced by the concentration of the reactants. The availability of carbohydrate and fatty acids depends on the storage levels of glycogen and triacylglycerols and the blood level of each. Conditions that stimulate lipolysis in adipose tissue and cause the release of fatty acids into the serum, such as low insulin levels and elevated epinephrine levels, stimulate the uptake of fatty acids by the muscle and promote the oxidation of fatty acids. The availability of additional serum glucose by either gluconeogenesis or the consumption of carbohydrate during the event promotes the use of glucose. Insulin and glucagon levels either stimulate the uptake of glucose or stimulate gluconeogenesis. These factors are variable and are heavily influenced by conditioning.

The discussion is not intended to be comprehensive but rather is meant to give the reader an idea of the many factors involved in nutrient use. Let us assume we are examining a single athlete who is running a marathon. The athlete is well trained, ate a pregame meal 4 to 5 hours prior to the event, and had a carbohydrate snack 15 minutes before the event started. We will look at several specific times (shown in Fig. 1) and discuss what is happening at each of those times. Keep in mind that there is a transition from one time to the next and it is difficult to quantify just what is happening at any given moment.

- *10 seconds:* As stated earlier, during the first 10 seconds or so energy is being supplied by the ATP-CP system.
- *30 seconds:* As the creatine phosphate is used up, anaerobic glycolysis kicks in and supplies the energy. The glucose comes from intramuscular glucose.
- *1–2 minutes:* Aerobic glycolysis starts to phase in shortly after anaerobic glycolysis. The glucose is supplied by intramuscular glucose and intramuscular glycogen.
- *5 minutes:* By this time a major portion of the energy is being supplied by aerobic glycolysis. The glucose, mostly muscle glycogen and blood glucose, is being absorbed into the muscle cells. This absorption is insulin independent. The β-oxidation of fatty acids is just starting. Fatty acid oxidation is not an efficient

Figure 1 Time line of the running of a marathon.

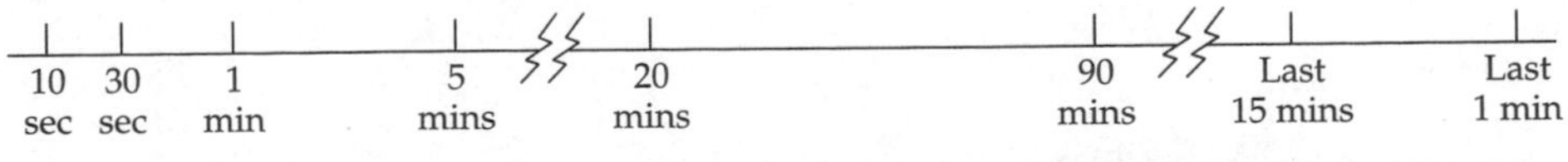

pathway to get started. The triacylglycerols stored in the muscle must be hydrolyzed, the activated fatty acid must be transferred into the mitochondria, and the Krebs cycle must start.

- *20 minutes:* At this time, fatty acid oxidation is fully activated and is supplying a major portion of the energy. Aerobic glycolysis is also active at this time. Just how much each process contributes depends on the level of conditioning and the intensity of the effort. One reason why advice is given to exercise at least 20 minutes for weight loss is that it takes that long for fat oxidation to be in full operation. The fatty acids come from intramuscular triacylglycerols and blood fatty acids. Other factors must be considered in order to determine how much of the blood fatty acid is coming from lipolysis of the fats in adipose. Note that adipose fatty acids will replenish the fat stored in the muscle after the exercise is completed.
- *90 minutes:* During the middle part of the race, most of the energy is supplied by a combination of glycolysis and fatty acid oxidation. A small amount of anaerobic glycolysis is going on. The amount is controlled by the delivery of oxygen to the muscle. Ongoing consumption of carbohydrate during the race will favor glycolysis. The mix is 40/60 and could be either lipid or carbohydrate predominating depending on the availability of the substrate. Muscle glycogen will begin to be low by this time, and active gluconeogenesis will be occurring. The muscle will be getting its glucose from the blood.
- *Last 15 minutes:* At this point, much of the available glycogen has been used. Muscle protein is breaking down, and the amino acids are being transaminated to pyruvate to form alanine. The glucose-alanine cycle is active, and the liver is supplying glucose through gluconeogenesis. The carbon skeleton of the amino acids is being broken down for energy either by their entering the Krebs cycle or by their entering glycolysis.
- *Last 1 minute:* Normally, an athlete trying to win a race will give a final kick and go all out for the last distance. Anaerobic glycolysis will be used to provide the last amount of energy. When the available glucose and oxygen are used up, the athlete will be completely exhausted.

Until that last kick, it is important that the athlete maintain an intensity that permits an adequate supply of oxygen, maintain body temperature by drinking enough liquid, and maintain sufficient glucose intake to supply energy. Generally, for a race lasting only 3 to 4 hours a well-conditioned athlete need not replenish electrolytes during the race. In the case of a longer event, a lower level of conditioning, or high heat or humidity, some athletes may benefit from consuming electrolytes. Electrolytes, along with carbohydrate and some protein, will speed up recovery from the event.

These examples of how the major energy systems work are intended to provide a dynamic view of the changing physiological environment during a long endurance event for a well-trained athlete. Not everyone will follow the same pattern.

Reference Cited

1. Tarnopolsky M, ed. Gender Differences in Metabolism. Boca Raton: CRC Press, 1999.

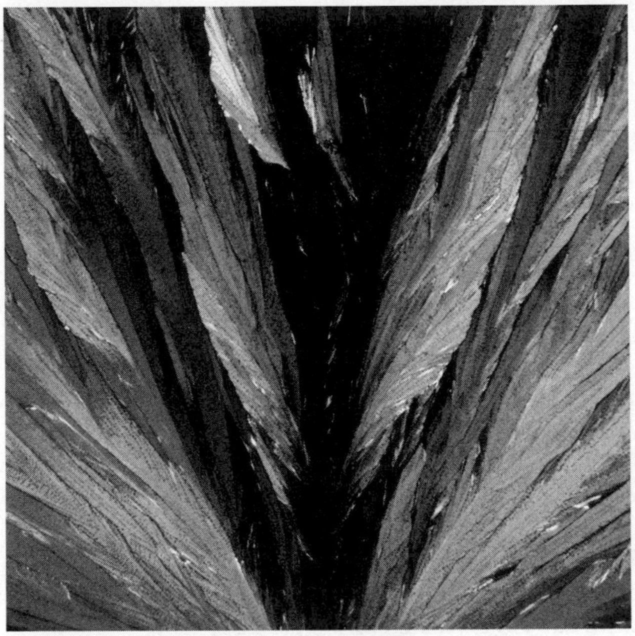

© Michael W. Davidson/Photo Researchers, Inc.

Photomicrograph of crystalized vitamin B_6

Vitamin C (Ascorbic Acid)
Thiamin (Vitamin B_1)
Riboflavin (Vitamin B_2)
Niacin (Vitamin B_3)
Pantothenic Acid
Biotin
Folic Acid
Vitamin B_{12} (Cobalamin)
Vitamin B_6

For each vitamin, the following subtopics (when applicable) are discussed:
Sources
Digestion, Absorption, Transport, and Storage
Functions and Mechanisms of Action
Interactions with Other Nutrients
Metabolism and Excretion
Recommended Dietary Allowances or Adequate Intakes
Deficiency
Toxicity
Assessment of Nutriture

perspective

Genetics and Nutrition: Human Folate Needs and Chronic Disease Risk

chapter 9

The Water-Soluble Vitamins

THE EARLY PART OF THE 20TH CENTURY marks the most exciting era in the history of nutrition science. It was during this time that the discovery of vitamins, or "accessory growth factors," began. Researchers found that for life and growth, animals required something more than a chemically defined diet consisting of purified carbohydrate, protein, fat, minerals, and water. The first of these dietary essentials to be discovered was an antiberiberi substance isolated from rice polishings by Casimir Funk, a Polish biochemist. Funk gave it the name *vitamine* because the substance was an amine and necessary for life. Very shortly thereafter McCollum and Davis extracted a factor from butter fat that they called fat-soluble A to distinguish it from the water-soluble antiberiberi substance. These two essential factors became known as vitamine A and vitamine B.

As each additional vitamin was discovered, it was assigned a letter. The *e* on *vitamine* was dropped to give the general name *vitamin* because only a few of the essential substances were found to be amines. As the chemical structure of a vitamin became known through its isolation and synthesis, it was given a chemical name. When the chemical name was assigned, it was assumed that the name applied to one substance with one specific activity. It is now evident that a vitamin may have a variety of functions and that vitamin activity may be found in several closely related compounds known as vitamers. An excellent example of this is vitamin A, which has several seemingly unrelated functions and encompasses not only retinol but also retinal and retinoic acid.

Vitamins can be defined as essential organic compounds required in very small amounts (micronutrients) that are involved in fundamental functions of the body, such as growth, maintenance of health, and metabolism. Because these substances must be supplied wholly or partially by the diet, their discovery came about because of their absence in the diet. Although in the case of a deficiency the clinician should be able to recognize the syndrome caused by a lack of the particular vitamin, in this country of abundant and varied food supply it is more relevant for the nutrition professional to think in terms of what a specific vitamin does rather than what disease it prevents. Unfortunately, it is often impossible to relate the function of the vitamin directly to its deficiency syndrome.

Vitamins, for the most part, are not related chemically and differ in their physiological roles. The broad classifications of water-soluble vitamins and fat-soluble vitamins are made because of certain properties common to each group. The fat-soluble vitamins are discussed in Chapter 10. The body handles the water-soluble vitamins differently from the way it handles the fat-soluble vitamins. They are absorbed into portal blood, in contrast to fat-soluble vitamins, and, with the exception of cobalamin (vitamin B_{12}), they cannot be retained for long periods by the body. Any storage that occurs results from their binding to enzymes and transport proteins. Water-soluble vitamins are excreted in the urine whenever plasma levels exceed renal thresholds.

With the exception of vitamin C (ascorbic acid), water-soluble vitamins are members of the B complex. Most of the B-complex group can be further divided according to general function: energy releasing or hematopoietic. Other vitamins cannot be classified this narrowly because of their wide range of functions. Figure 9.1 shows the classification of water-soluble vitamins.

In this chapter, discussions of the various vitamins are grouped similarly. For each vitamin, consideration is given (when precise information is available) to structure, sources, absorption (also digestion where applicable), transport, storage, functions and mechanisms of action, metabolism and excretion, recommended dietary allowance or adequate intake, deficiency, toxicity, and assessment of nutriture. Specific interrelationships with other nutrients are also noted for selected vitamins. Table 9.1 contains a summary of the discovery, coenzyme

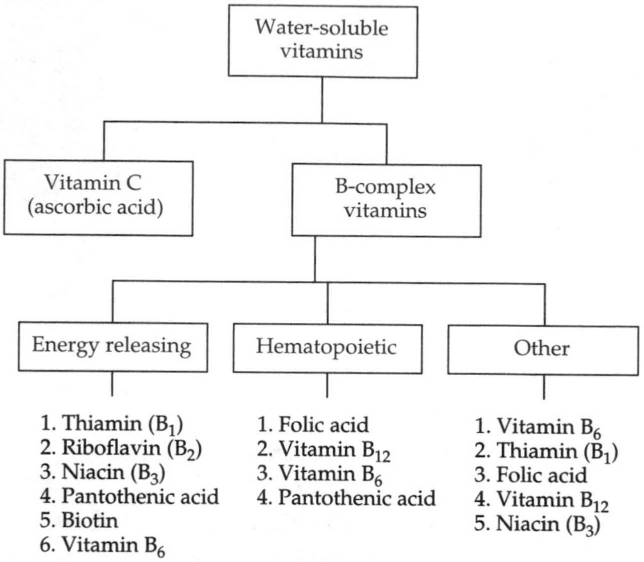

Figure 9.1 The water-soluble vitamins.

form, functions, deficiency syndrome, sources, and recommended dietary allowance (RDA) or adequate intake (AI) of each of the water-soluble vitamins. The inside book covers provide the dietary reference intakes (DRIs), when available, for all nutrients and for all age groups. DRIs represent quantitative approximations of nutrient intakes for the purpose of planning and assessing the diets of healthy people. DRIs include RDAs as well as AIs, tolerable upper intake levels (ULs), and **estimated average requirements (EARs). RDAs** represent the average daily dietary intake level that is sufficient to meet the nutrient requirements of about 97% of healthy individuals. They are based on EARs, which are the amounts of nutrients thought to meet the nutrient requirements of 50% of the healthy individuals in a specified age and gender group. RDAs are set higher than EARs by either two standard deviations or a coefficient of variation for the EAR. AIs are provided for nutrients instead of RDAs when scientific data are insufficient to calculate the EAR for the given nutrients. ULs provide the highest intake level for a nutrient that is unlikely to cause any risk of adverse health to almost all individuals in the age- or gender-specified groups.

Suggested Reading

McCollum EV. A History of Nutrition. Boston: Houghton Mifflin, 1957.

VITAMIN C (ASCORBIC ACID)

The human being is one of the few mammals unable to synthesize vitamin C, also known as ascorbic acid or ascorbate. Other animals unable to synthesize vitamin C include primates, fruit bats, guinea pigs, and some

Table 9.1 The Water-Soluble Vitamins: Discovery, Functions, Human Deficiency Syndromes, Food Sources, and Recommended Intake

Water-Soluble Vitamins						
Vitamin	**Discovery**	**Main Coenzymes**	**Biochemical or Physiological Function**	**Deficiency Syndrome or Symptoms**	**Good Food Sources**	**RDA* or AI†**
Thiamin (vitamin B_1)	Casimir Funk (1912)	Thiamin diphosphate (TDP) or thiamin pyrophosphate (TPP)	Oxidative decarboxylation of α-keto acids and 2-keto sugars	*Beriberi*, muscle weakness, anorexia, tachycardia, enlarged heart, edema	Yeast, pork, sunflower seeds, legumes	1.1 mg* 1.2 mg
Riboflavin (vitamin B_2)	Kuhn, Szent-György, and Wagner-Jaunergy (1933)	Flavin adenine dinucleotide (FAD); flavin mononucleotide (FMN)	Electron (hydrogen) transfer reactions	*Ariboflavinosis*, cheilosis, glossitis, hyperemia and edema of pharyngeal and oral mucous membranes, angular stomatitis, photophobia	Beef liver, braunschweiger sausage, steak, mushrooms, ricotta cheese, nonfat milk, oysters	1.1 mg* 1.3 mg
Niacin (vitamin B_3) (nicotinic acid, nicotinamide)	Elvehjem et al. (1937)	Nicotinamide adenine dinucleotide (NAD); nicotinamide adenine dinucleotide phosphate (NADP)	Electron (hydrogen) transfer reactions	*Pellagra*, diarrhea, dermatitis, mental confusion, or dementia	Tuna, beef liver, chicken breast, beef, halibut, mushrooms	14 mg* 16 mg
Pantothenic acid	R. J. Williams (1933)	Coenzyme A (CoA)	Acyl transfer reactions	Deficiency very rare; numbness and tingling of hands and feet, vomiting, fatigue	Widespread in foods; exceptionally high amounts in egg yolk, liver, kidney, yeast	5 mg†
Biotin	Szent-György (1940)	N-carboxybiotinyl lysine	CO_2 transfer/ carboxylation reactions	Deficiency very rare, anorexia, nausea, glossitis, depression, dry scaly dermatitis	Synthesized by microflora of digestive tract; yeast, liver, kidney	30 μg†
Vitamin B_6 (pyridoxine, pyridoxal, pyridoxamine)	Szent-György, Kuhn (1938)	Pyridoxal phosphate (PLP)	Transamination and decarboxylation reactions	Dermatitis, glossitis, convulsions	Steak, navy beans, potato, salmon, banana, whole grains	1.3 mg*
Folic acid (folacin)	Mitchell et al. (1941)	Derivatives of tetrahydrofolic acid: 5,10-methylidyne THF, 10-formyl THF, 5-formimino THF, 5,10-methylene THF, 5-methyl THF	One-carbon transfer reactions	*Megaloblastic anemia*, diarrhea, fatigue, depression, confusion	Brewer's yeast, spinach, asparagus, turnip greens, lima beans, beef liver	400 μg*
Vitamin B_{12} (cobalamin)	Riches, Folkers, et al. (1948)	Methyl cobalamin, adenosyl cobalamin (cobalamides)	Methylation of homocysteine to methionine; conversion of methylmalonyl CoA to succinyl CoA	*Megaloblastic anemia*, degeneration of peripheral nerves, skin hypersensitivity, glossitis	Meat, fish, shellfish, poultry, milk	2.4 μg*
Ascorbic acid (vitamin C)	Szent-György‡ (1928) King‡ (1932)	None	Antioxidant, cofactor of hydroxylating enzymes involved in synthesis of collagen, carnitine, norepinephrine	*Scurvy*, loss of appetite, fatigue, retarded wound healing, bleeding gums, spontaneous rupture of capillaries	Papaya, orange juice, cantaloupe, broccoli, brussels sprouts, green peppers, grapefruit juice, strawberries	75 mg* 90 mg

*Adults age 19 to 50 years, females and males respectively.
†Adequate intake.
‡Szent-György and King are considered to be codiscoverers of vitamin C.

birds. The inability to synthesize vitamin C results from the lack of gulonolactone oxidase, the last enzyme in the vitamin C synthetic pathway. The synthetic pathway and structure of the vitamin are shown in Figure 9.2, which indicates that vitamin C is a six-carbon compound. It is the L-isomer of the vitamin that is biologically active in man.

Sources

The best food sources of vitamin C include asparagus, papaya, oranges, orange juice, cantaloupe, cauliflower, broccoli, brussels sprouts, green peppers, grapefruit, grapefruit juice, kale, lemons, and strawberries. Of these foods, citrus products are most commonly cited as significant sources of the vitamin. Supplements supply vitamin C typically as free ascorbic acid, calcium ascorbate, sodium ascorbate, and ascorbyl palmitate. Rose hip (*Rosa*), a seed capsule found in roses, also contains vitamin C and is used commercially in vitamin C supplements; vitamin C from rose hips does not appear to be superior to other vitamin C sources such as orange juice.

Absorption, Transport, and Storage

Absorption of ascorbate across the brush border occurs throughout the small intestine, including the ileum, primarily by sodium-dependent active transport [1]. Simple diffusion, which may occur throughout the stomach and small intestine, provides for vitamin C absorption with ingestion of higher amounts of the vitamin. Transport of vitamin C across the basolateral membrane of the intestinal cell occurs by carrier-mediated transport systems.

Prior to absorption, ascorbate may be oxidized (two electrons and two protons removed) to form dehydroascorbate (Fig. 9.3), which may be absorbed by passive diffusion or by use of glucose (GLUT) transporters [1]. Absorption of dehydroascorbate is thought to occur

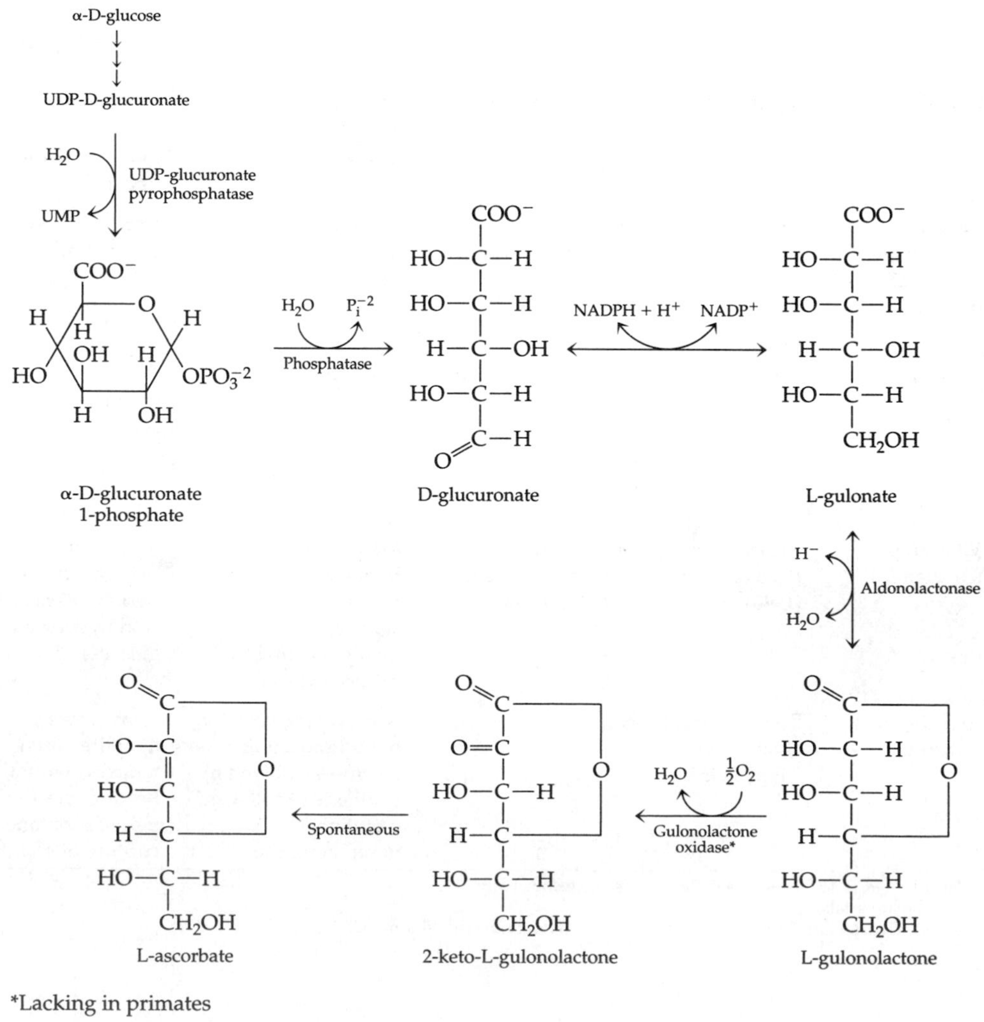

Figure 9.2 Synthesis of ascorbic acid. Primates lack the gulonolactone oxidase that catalyzes the final enzymatic reaction.

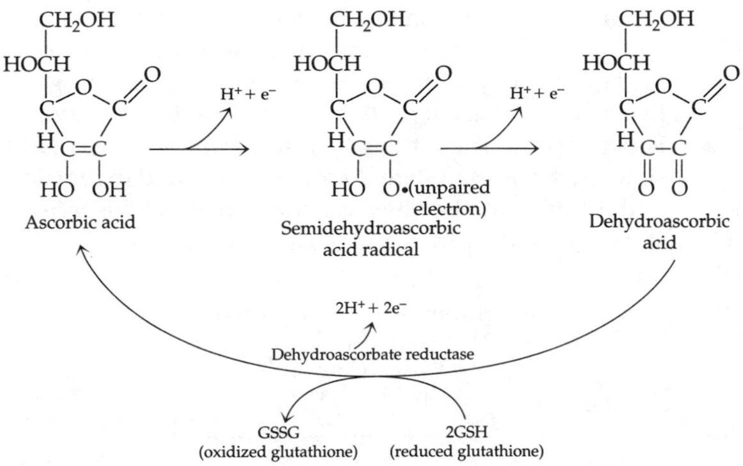

Figure 9.3 The interconversion of ascorbate and dehydroascorbate.

to a greater extent than absorption of ascorbate [1,2]. Yet within the intestinal cells (but also other cells) dehydroascorbic acid is rapidly reduced back (recycled) to ascorbic acid (Fig. 9.3) by the enzyme dehydroascorbate reductase and the protein glutaredoxin, which exhibits reductase activity. Glutathione (GSH), which is required for the reduction of dehydroascorbate, is oxidized (GSSG) in the process shown here:

$$\text{Dehydroascorbate} + 2\text{GSH} \longrightarrow \text{Ascorbate} + \text{GSSG}$$

Glutathione spares vitamin C and, in general, improves the antioxidant protection capacity of blood [3,4].

Notice in Figure 9.3 that during the oxidation of ascorbate, a free radical called semidehydroascorbate (also called ascorbate free radical, ascorbyl, monodehydroascorbate radical, or a 1-electron oxidation product) is formed. The ascorbate free radical is thought to have a short half-life and reacts poorly with oxygen (and thus does not typically generate reactive oxygen species such as superoxides). Instead, the ascorbate free radical either is oxidized to dehydroascorbate or reacts with another semidehydroascorbate radical to form ascorbate and dehydroascorbate (2 semidehydroascorbate radicals $\longrightarrow$ ascorbate + dehydroascorbate). Other reactions that provide for the regeneration of ascorbate from dehydroascorbate and from semidehydroascorbate are shown under "Antioxidant Activity" in the functions and mechanisms of action section of vitamin C.

The degree of vitamin C absorption decreases with increased vitamin intake. Absorption can vary from 16% at high intakes (~12 g) to 98% at low intakes (<20 mg) [5]. Over a range of usual intakes from food (30–180 mg/day), the average overall absorption is about 70% to 95% [6,7]. Unabsorbed vitamin C may be metabolized by intestinal flora. Ingestion of large amounts of iron present with vitamin C in the digestive tract may result in the oxidative destruction of the vitamin, yielding diketogulonic acid and other products without vitamin C activity [6].

Absorbed ascorbic acid is transported in the plasma primarily in free form, with any dehydroascorbate appearing in small concentrations due to rapid cellular uptake via GLUT transporters [1,8]. Normal plasma concentrations of ascorbate range from about 0.4 to 1.7 mg/dL. Uptake of ascorbate into body cells requires sodium and a carrier, and into some cells, such as leukocytes (also called white blood cells), uptake is also energy dependent. Tissue concentrations of vitamin C usually exceed plasma concentrations, with the magnitude dependent on the specific tissue. The vitamin C content of white blood cells, for example, can be as high as 80 times greater than plasma concentrations.

Ascorbate and dehydroascorbate concentrations are much greater in some tissues than in others. The highest concentrations of vitamin C are found in the adrenal and pituitary glands (with each possessing ~30–50 mg/100 g of wet tissue) [9]. Intermediate levels of vitamin C are found in the liver, spleen, heart, kidneys, lungs, pancreas, and leukocytes, while smaller amounts occur in the muscles and red blood cells [9]. In absolute terms based on total weight, the liver contains the most vitamin C [1]. The maximal vitamin C pool is estimated at about 1,500 mg [7]. Intakes of 100 mg vitamin C per day by men have been shown to produce plasma concentrations of about 1.0 mg/dL and to maximize the body pool [7].

Functions and Mechanisms of Action

Despite its uncomplicated structure, vitamin C has very complex functional roles in the body. Ascorbic acid is required in several reactions involved in body processes, including collagen synthesis, carnitine synthesis, tyrosine synthesis and catabolism, and neurotransmitter synthesis. In these reactions, vitamin C functions to maintain the iron and copper atoms in the metalloenzymes in the reduced state. In addition to its cofactor-like role, vitamin C functions as an important antioxidant in the body. Each of these processes, as well as some additional roles of vitamin C, will be reviewed.

Collagen Synthesis

Ascorbate functions in a number of hydroxylation reactions. Three hydroxylation reactions requiring vitamin C are necessary for collagen synthesis. Remember that collagen is a structural protein found in skin, bones, tendons, and cartilage. After the collagen chains are made, the vitamin C–dependent hydroxylation reactions occur posttranslationally. These reactions are important in order for the collagen molecule to aggregate and cross-link into its triple-helix configuration. Prolyl 4-hydroxylase and prolyl 3-hydroxylase (also called dioxygenases) catalyze the hydroxylations of specific proline residues on newly synthesized collagen α chains. Proline and hydroxyproline provide more rigidity to the collagen. Lysine hydroxylation by lysyl hydroxylase (also called dioxygenase) results in the formation of hydroxylysyl residues. These hydroxylysyl residues may undergo additional posttranslational modifications, such as glycosylation and phosphorylation. The lysine and hydroxylysyl residues also are further acted upon by lysyl oxidase, a copper-dependent enzyme that facilitates cross-linking between collagen molecules to provide added strength.

The role of vitamin C in the hydroxylation reactions relates to the iron cofactor. Prolyl hydroxylases and lysyl hydroxylase both require iron bound as a cofactor, although silicon also may be needed for maximal prolyl hydroxylase activity (see Fig. 13.2). During the reactions, the dioxygenase enzymes catalyze reactions in which one of two atoms of O_2 becomes incorporated into the product and the second of the two atoms of O_2 becomes incorporated into the cosubstrate α-ketoglutarate to form the new carboxyl group of succinate (Fig. 9.4). During the hydroxylation reactions, the iron cofactor in the enzymes is oxidized; that is, it is converted from a ferrous (2+) state to a ferric (3+) state. Ascorbate is needed to function as the reductant, thereby reducing iron back to its ferrous state (2+) in the prolyl and lysyl hydroxylases.

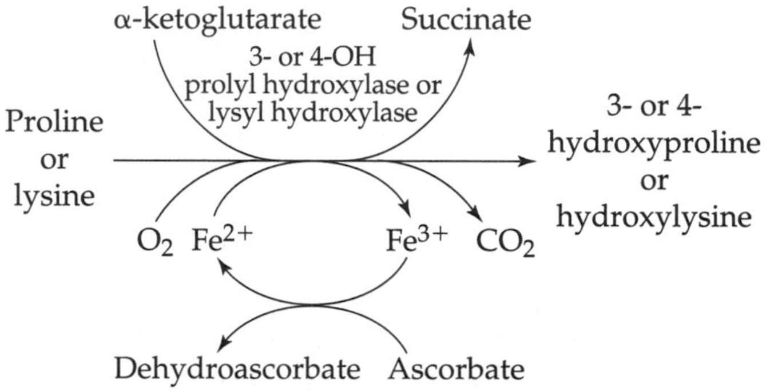

Although these reactions may seem simple, normal development and maintenance of skin, tendons, cartilage, bone, and dentine depend on an adequate supply of vitamin C. Also, the basement membrane lining the capillaries, the "intracellular cement" holding together the endothelial cells, and the scar tissue responsible for wound healing all require the presence of vitamin C for their formation and maintenance.

Carnitine Synthesis

Ascorbate is involved in two reactions required for the synthesis of carnitine (Fig. 9.5) [10]. Carnitine synthesis begins with the substrate trimethyllysine.

Figure 9.4 Ascorbate functions in the hydroxylation of peptide-bound proline and lysine in procollagen. The reaction is driven by α-ketoglutarate decarboxylation. One atom of oxygen (*) appears in the hydroxyl group of the product and the other in succinate.

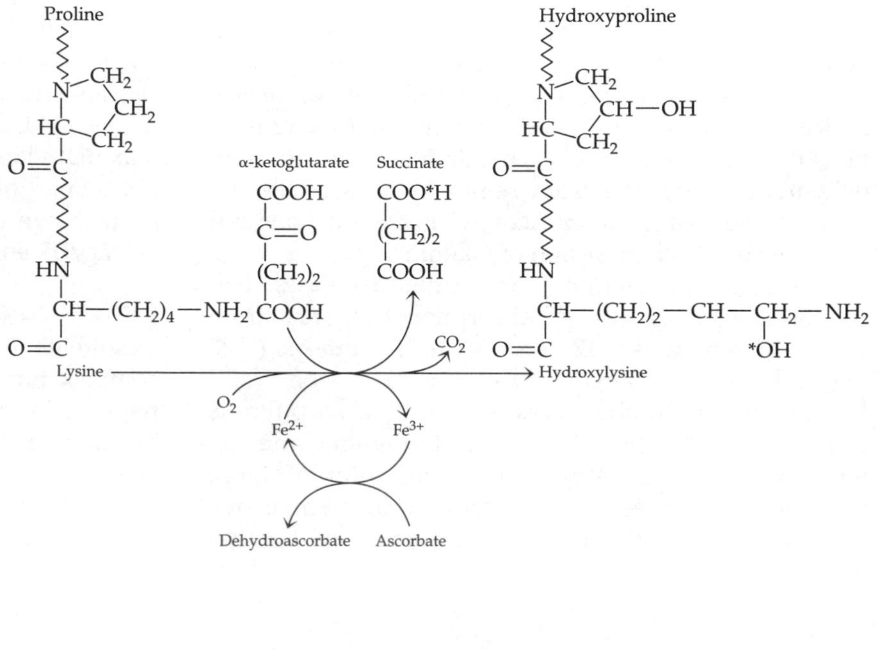

- The first reaction involving vitamin C requires the iron-containing enzyme trimethyllysine dioxygenase (also called hydroxylase), which catalyzes the conversion of trimethyllysine to 3-hydroxy trimethyllysine.

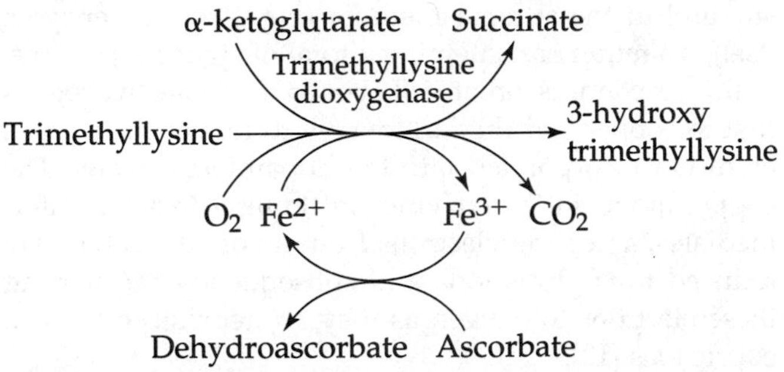

- Next, in the last step of carnitine synthesis, the iron-containing enzyme 4(γ)-butyrobetaine dioxygenase (also called hydroxylase) catalyzes the conversion of 4(γ)-butyrobetaine to carnitine.

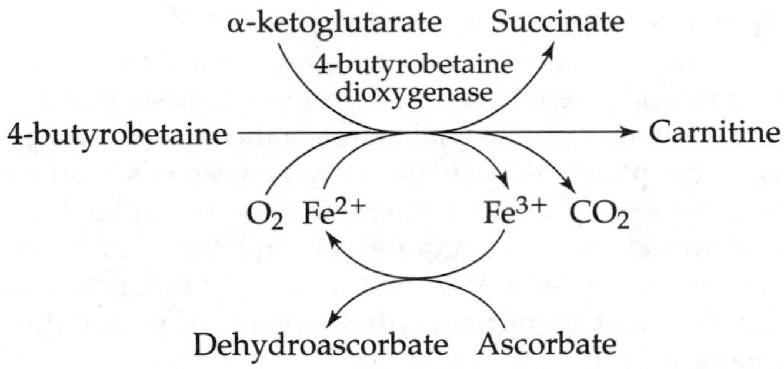

These reactions involving ascorbate are hydroxylations that require α-ketoglutarate and are almost identical to those for proline and lysine hydroxylation. Vitamin C is the preferred reducing agent in carnitine synthesis; however, other substances may be able to replace the ascorbate [10]. Sufficient production of carnitine is of significance in fat metabolism because carnitine is essential for the transport of long-chain fatty acids from the cell cytoplasm into the mitochondrial matrix where β-oxidation occurs.

Figure 9.5 The function of vitamin C (ascorbate) in carnitine synthesis.

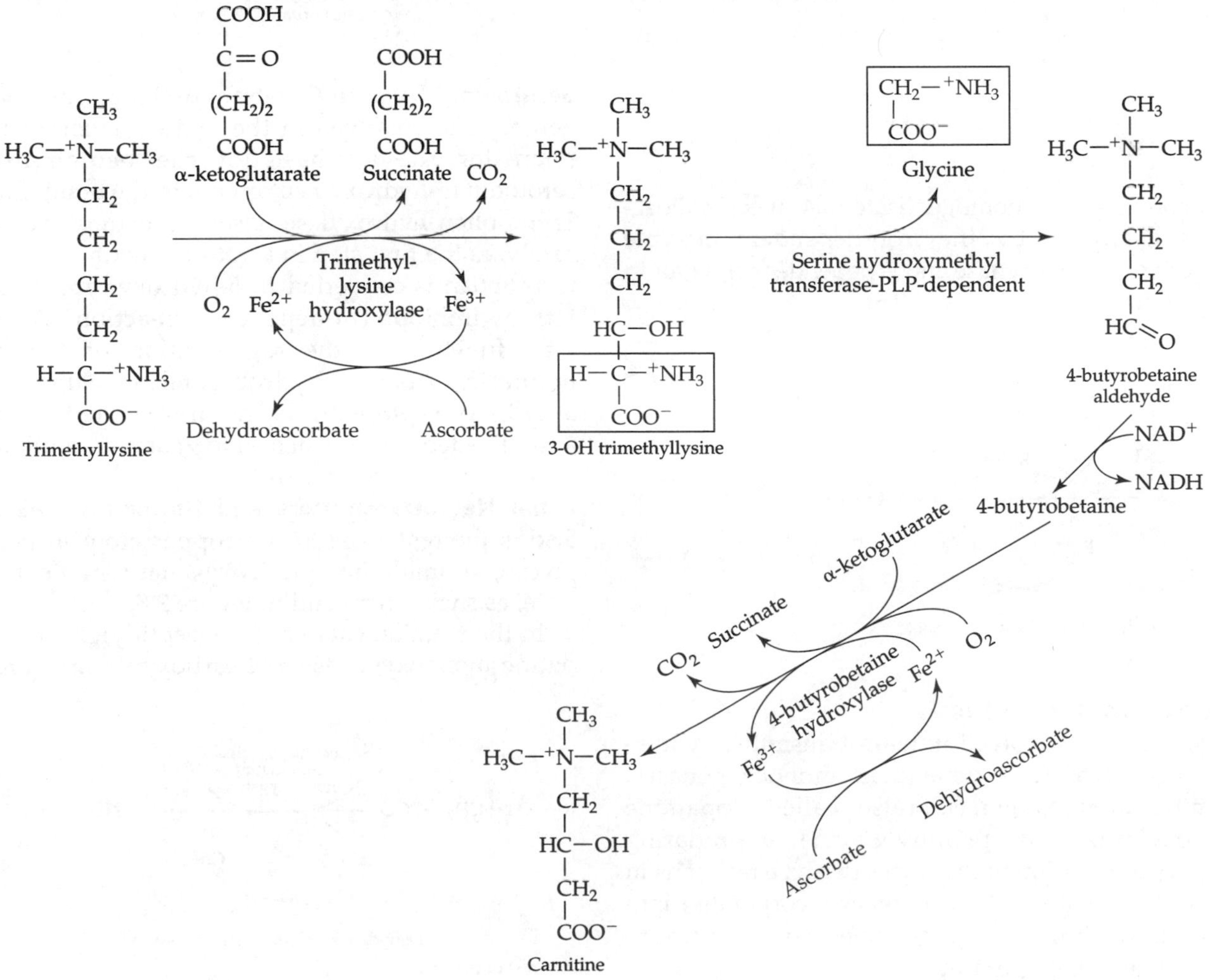

Tyrosine Synthesis and Catabolism

Tyrosine is synthesized in the body from the essential amino acid phenylalanine. Tyrosine synthesis requires hydroxylation of phenylalanine via the iron-dependent enzyme phenylalanine monooxygenase (also called hydroxylase). The reaction (Fig. 9.6) occurs in the liver and the kidney and requires O_2 and the cosubstrate tetrahydrobiopterin. Vitamin C is thought to function in the regeneration of tetrahydrobiopterin from dihydrobiopterin [11].

Also involved in tyrosine catabolism is another hydroxylation in which ascorbate participates. Ascorbate is a preferred reductant for the copper-dependent enzyme para (p)-hydroxyphenylpyruvate hydroxylase (also called dioxygenase), the enzyme necessary for conversion of para (p)-hydroxyphenylpyruvate to homogentisate.

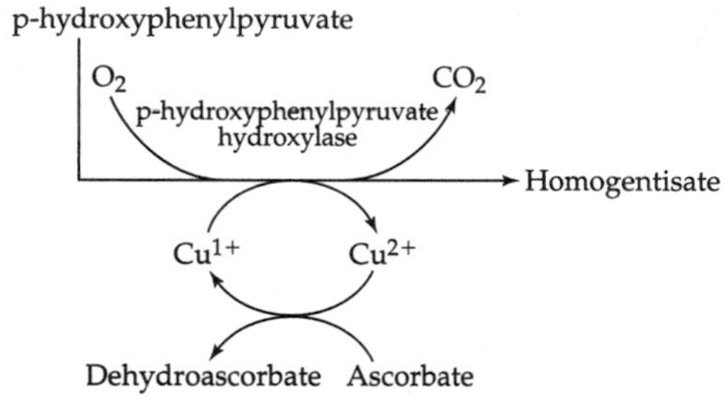

The conversion of homogentisate to 4-maleylacetoacetate is catalyzed by the iron-dependent enzyme homogentisate dioxygenase and is dependent on vitamin C as a reductant (Figs. 7.25 and 9.6).

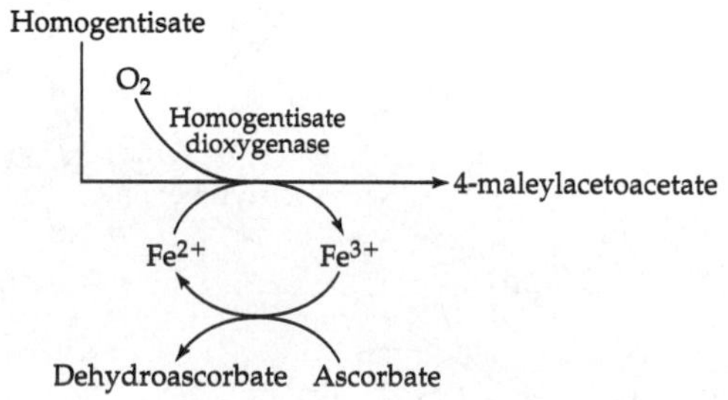

Neurotransmitter Synthesis

Ascorbate is also involved in neurotransmitter synthesis through two Cu^{1+}-dependent monooxygenases, dopamine monooxygenase (also called dopamine β-hydroxylase) and peptidylglycine α-amidating monooxygenase. Monooxygenases catalyze reactions in which only one atom of O_2 becomes incorporated into the product. Neither of these enzymes requires a cosubstrate such as α-ketoglutarate.

Norepinephrine. Norepinephrine (a catecholamine) is generated from the hydroxylation of the side chain of dopamine in a vitamin C–dependent reaction. The reaction is catalyzed by the copper-dependent enzyme dopamine monooxygenase, which is found in nervous tissue and in the adrenal medulla (Fig. 9.6). The enzyme itself is a tetramer containing a total of eight copper ions. In this reaction, ascorbate is believed to donate hydrogens first to copper and then ultimately to reduce the oxygen atom not incorporated into the dopamine to water. The copper atoms in the enzyme are thought to act as intermediates, accepting electrons from ascorbate as they are reduced to cuprous ions and subsequently transferring these electrons to oxygen as they are reoxidized back to cupric ions [12].

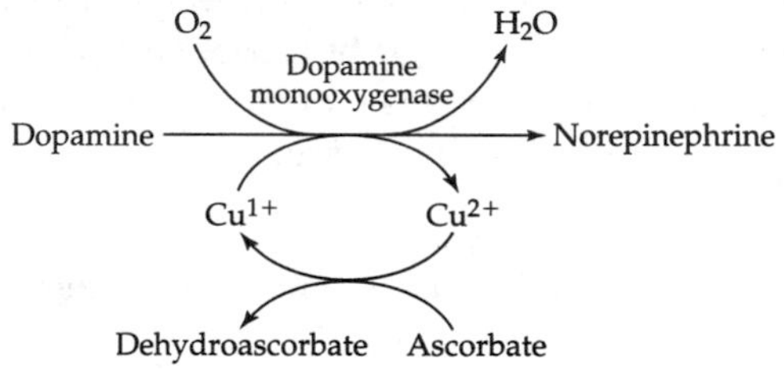

Serotonin. Vitamin C, tetrahydrobiopterin, and oxygen are also involved in the hydroxylation of tryptophan for the synthesis of the neurotransmitter serotonin (5-hydroxytryptamine) in the brain (Fig. 9.7). Tryptophan hydroxylase, also called monooxygenase, catalyzes the first step in serotonin synthesis, whereby tryptophan is converted to 5-hydroxytryptophan in a tetrahydrobiopterin-dependent reaction. Ascorbate may function in the regeneration of tetrahydrobiopterin from dihydrobiopterin. Subsequently, 5-hydroxytryptophan is decarboxylated in a vitamin B_6–dependent reaction to generate serotonin.

Other Neurotransmitters and Hormones. Ascorbate also is thought to keep the copper atom in peptidylglycine α-amidating monooxygenase in its reduced state, as shown here and in Figure 9.8:

In the reaction catalyzed by peptidylglycine α-amidating monooxygenase, the carboxyl-terminal residue

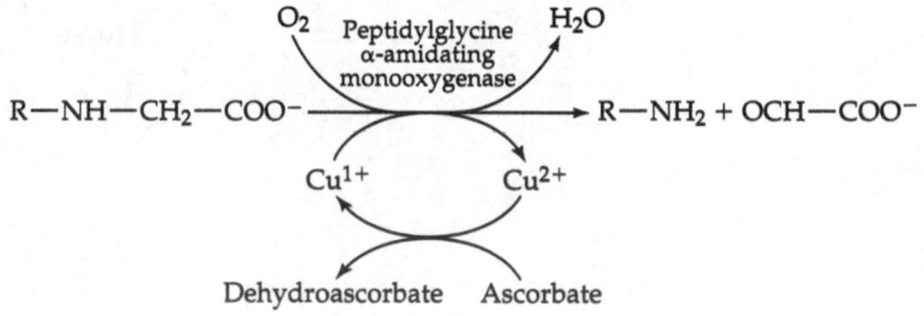

R = rest of peptide

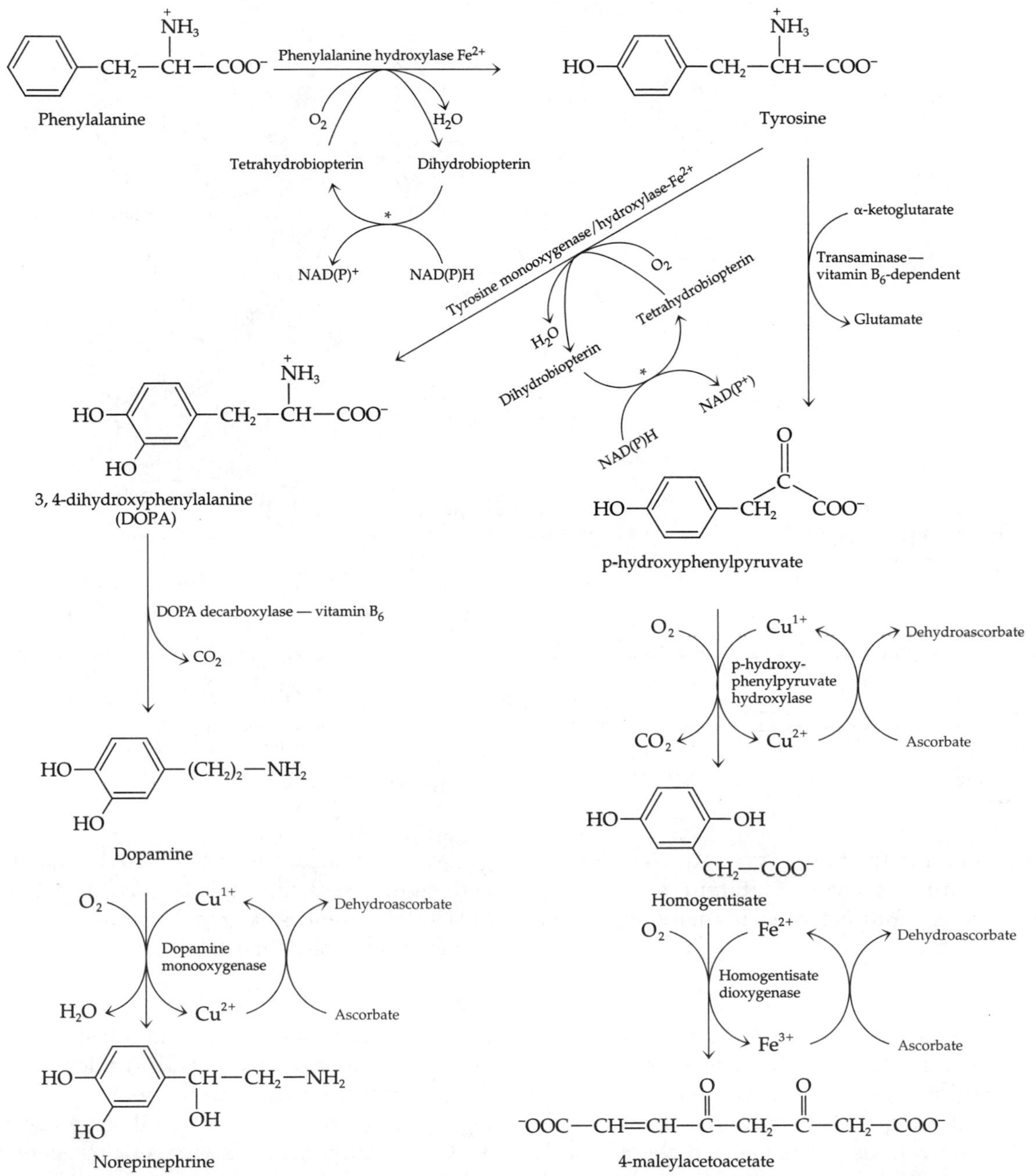

*Vitamin C may function in tetrahydrobiopterin regeneration.

Figure 9.6 The roles of vitamin C (ascorbate) in phenylalanine and tyrosine metabolism, including norepinephrine synthesis.

is oxidatively cleaved through use of molecular oxygen. The cleavage is not a simple hydrolytic cleavage of a peptide bond because the amino group is retained as a terminal amide while the rest of the oxidized residue is released as glyoxylate (Fig. 9.8). Although most of the substrate peptides for this enzyme have a terminal glycine residue, the enzyme is also active with peptides terminating in other amino acids. Many of the amidated peptides resulting from this reaction are active as hormones, hormone-releasing factors, or neurotransmitters. Examples include bombesin or gastrin-releasing peptide (GRP), calcitonin, cholecystokinin (CCK), thyrotropin, corticotropin-releasing factor, gastrin, growth hormone–releasing factor, oxytocin, and vasopressin [11]. The enzyme is found in neuroendocrine cells of the pituitary, adrenal, and

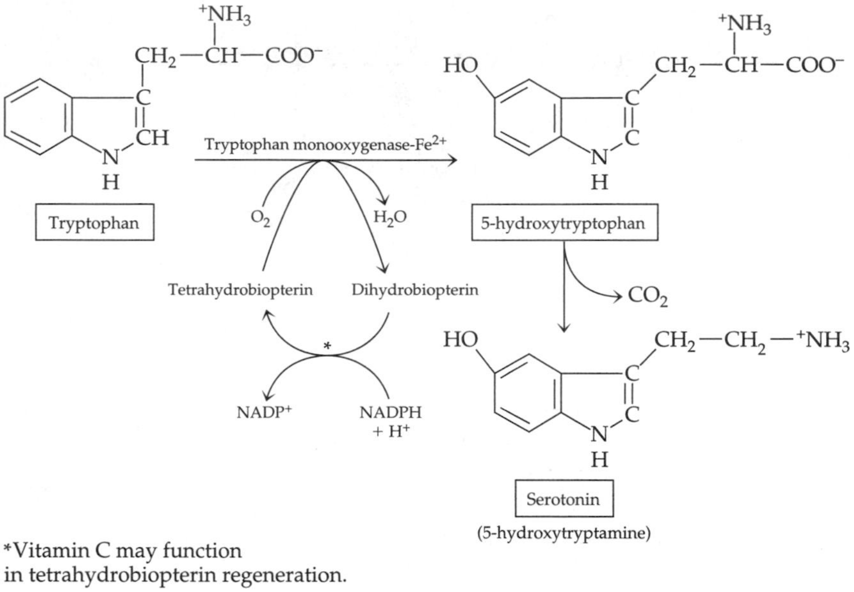

Figure 9.7 Serotonin synthesis.

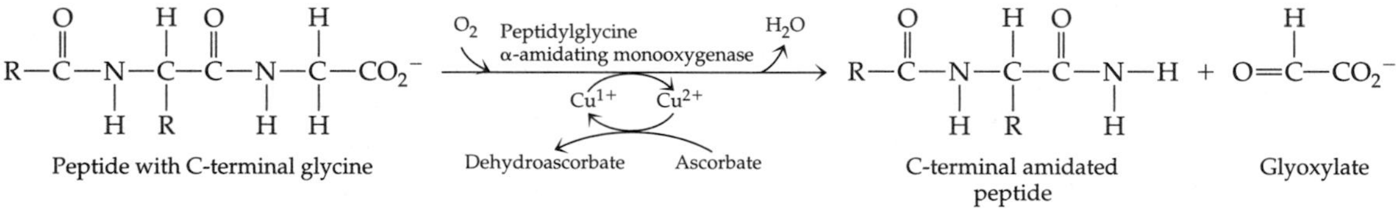

Figure 9.8 Amidation of peptides with C-terminal glycine requires vitamin C.

thyroid glands and in the brain. As a reductant for the required amidating enzyme, vitamin C assumes important, although indirect, roles in many regulatory processes.

Microsomal Metabolism

A group of enzymes makes up a microsomal metabolizing system that functions mostly in liver microsomes and reticuloendothelial tissues to inactivate both endogenous and exogenous substances. Endogenous substrates include various hormones and steroids such as cholesterol. For example, cholesterol 7α-hydroxylase, found in the microsomes of the liver, is required for the initial step in the synthesis of bile acids from cholesterol. Vitamin C plays an undefined role in this hydroxylation. Vitamin C also participates in aldosterone and cortisol synthesis. Exogenous substrates for the microsomal metabolizing system are usually xenobiotics. *Xenos* means "stranger" in Greek, and **xenobiotics** are foreign chemicals such as drugs, carcinogens, pesticides, food additives, pollutants, or other noxious compounds. The reactions needed to metabolize these substances usually involve hydroxylations followed by conjugations or methylations to produce polar metabolites for excretion. The hydroxylation reactions are catalyzed by monooxygenases or cytochrome P450 mixed function oxidases and require reducing agents such as vitamin C and NAD(P)H as well as oxygen. The exact role of vitamin C, however, has not been established.

Antioxidant Activity

In addition to ascorbate's roles in collagen, carnitine, and neurotransmitter synthesis and in microsomal metabolism, vitamin C functions in a general capacity as a reducing agent or electron donor and thereby has antioxidant activity. Ascorbic acid acts as a reducing agent in aqueous solutions such as the blood and within cells. Stated slightly differently, ascorbate is an antioxidant in that it reverses oxidation. Reducing agents or antioxidants such as ascorbate may reverse oxidation by donating electrons and hydrogen ions. The reduction potential of ascorbate is such that it readily donates electrons/hydrogen ions to regenerate other antioxidants such as vitamin E, glutathione, and urate as well as to reduce numerous reactive oxygen and nitrogen species [4,13–15].

As an antioxidant, ascorbate may react in blood or intracellularly with a variety of reactive oxygen and nitrogen species and give the radicals an electron in the form of a hydrogen ion. Free radicals exist independently and contain one or more unpaired electrons in an outer orbital surrounding the nucleus of the atom. Remember from chemistry that electrons are usually found in pairs in an orbital. Free radicals and other reactive oxygen species are formed during normal cellular metabolism, a process discussed in more detail in the perspective at the end of Chapter 10. Examples of reactive oxygen species that vitamin C may reduce include

- hydroxyl radical ($OH\cdot$), a very reactive oxygen-centered radical;
- hydroperoxyl radical ($HO_2\cdot$), an oxygen-centered radical;
- superoxide radical (O_2^-), an oxygen-centered radical;
- alkoxyl radical ($RO\cdot$), an oxygen-centered radical; and
- peroxyl radical ($RO_2\cdot$), an oxygen-centered radical.

Hydrogen peroxide, H_2O_2, a nonradical because it has no unpaired electrons in its orbital, is an example of a reactive oxygen species that, like hypochlorous acid (HOCl) and singlet oxygen ($^1O_2$), is scavenged by vitamin C. Two reactive nitrogen species, peroxynitrite radicals and nitric oxide radicals, also may be reduced by vitamin C.

Once formed, free radicals and reactive species attack nucleic acids in DNA, polyunsaturated fatty acids in phospholipids, and proteins in cells. Ascorbic acid has been shown to interact with oxidants in the aqueous phase before they initiate damage, especially to cell lipids [16–20]. Furthermore, ascorbic acid appears to be superior to other water-soluble antioxidants such as bilirubin, uric acid, and protein thiols. The order of use of plasma antioxidants in the protection of lipids against peroxidation has been shown to be ascorbate = thiols > bilirubin > uric acid > vitamin E [17,20–22].

Some examples of reactions involving ascorbate as an antioxidant include these [21]:

$$\text{Ascorbate} + OH\cdot \longrightarrow \text{Semidehydroascorbate radical} + H_2O$$

$$\text{Ascorbate} + O_2\cdot \longrightarrow \text{Dehydroascorbate} + H_2O_2$$

$$\text{Ascorbate} + H_2O_2 \longrightarrow \text{Dehydroascorbate} + 2H_2O$$

The role of vitamin C and other antioxidants as a defense against oxidative damage to the cell is discussed in the perspective at the end of Chapter 10.

As an antioxidant, ascorbate provides electrons and becomes oxidized in the process. Regeneration of ascorbic acid from semidehydroascorbate radical and from dehydroascorbate is crucial. To regenerate ascorbic acid, two semidehydroascorbate radicals may react as follows:

$$2\ \text{semidehydroascorbate radicals} \longrightarrow \text{Ascorbate} + \text{dehydroascorbate}$$

Alternately, reductases are found in most tissues to reduce the semidehydroascorbate radical to ascorbate. Niacin and thiols such as dihydrolipoic acid, glutathione, and thioredoxin assist in vitamin C regeneration [12,21,23,24]. Niacin in its coenzyme forms NADH and NADPH allows the regeneration of vitamin C as follows:

$$2\ \text{semidehydroascorbate radicals} + \text{NAD(P)H} + H^+ \longrightarrow \text{Ascorbate} + \text{NAD(P)}^+$$

Dihydrolipoic acid provides hydrogens to the dehydroascorbate form of vitamin C to recycle ascorbate, as shown here:

$$\text{Dehydroascorbate} + \text{dihydrolipoic acid} \longrightarrow \text{Ascorbate} + \text{lipoic acid}$$

Glutathione in its reduced state (GSH) functions as shown:

$$2\ \text{semidehydroascorbate radicals} + 2\text{GSH} \longrightarrow 2\ \text{ascorbate} + \text{GSSG}$$

$$\text{Dehydroascorbate} + 2\text{GSH} \longrightarrow \text{Ascorbate} + \text{GSSG}$$

Thioredoxin (Trx-(SH)_2) a dithiol, also provides reducing equivalents to dehydroascorbate, as shown here:

$$\text{Dehydroascorbate} + \text{Trx-(SH)}_2 \longrightarrow \text{Ascorbate} + \text{Trx-S}_2$$

Pro-oxidant

Paradoxically, vitamin C also may act as a pro-oxidant. Vitamin C can reduce transition metals, such as cupric ions (Cu^{2+}) to cuprous (Cu^{1+}) and ferric ions (Fe^{3+}) to ferrous (Fe^{2+}), while itself becoming oxidized to semidehydroascorbate:

$$\text{Ascorbate } (AH_2) + Fe^{3+} \text{ or } Cu^{2+} \longrightarrow \text{Semidehydroascorbate radical } (AH^-) + Fe^{2+} \text{ or } Cu^{1+}$$

The products—Fe^{2+} and Cu^{1+}—generated from these reactions can proceed to cause cell damage through the generation of reactive oxygen species and free radicals. Examples of some of these reactions include:

$$Fe^{2+} \text{ or } Cu^{1+} + H_2O_2 \longrightarrow Fe^{3+} \text{ or } Cu^{2+} + OH_2 + OH\cdot$$

$$Fe^{2+} \text{ or } Cu^{1+} + O_2 \longrightarrow Fe^{3+} \text{ or } Cu^{2+} + O_2^-$$

It is noteworthy that vitamin C reacts with *free* ferric or cupric ions. In the body, iron and copper are both *bound* to various proteins (i.e., not free) to minimize the likelihood of such interactions.

Other Functions

Many other diverse biochemical functions for vitamin C have been proposed. Experimental evidence supporting these functions varies considerably. Experimental results often conflict, and the mechanism by which ascorbate may be involved is generally unclear. Possible functions for vitamin C include roles in collagen gene expression; synthesis of bone matrix, proteoglycans, fibronectin, and elastin; regulation of cellular nucleotide (cAMP and cGMP) concentrations; and immune function, including complement synthesis [12,25,26]. Ascorbic acid also appears to be necessary for folate metabolism; specifically, vitamin C is thought to be needed to maintain folate in a reduced state either as tetrahydrofolate, the active form of the vitamin, or as dihydrofolate.

Much attention also has been directed toward vitamin C and its possible effect on diseases ranging from the common cold to cancer and heart disease, among others.

Colds. The possible pharmacological effects of vitamin C on the incidence, severity, and duration of the common cold have been almost totally refuted by some investigators [27]. High doses of ascorbate appear to be only weakly prophylactic, if at all, and to be of little or no use in the treatment of colds [27]. Vitamin C (1 g/day) had no more effect in protection against or in combating the common cold than 50 mg/day. Further, no significant differences between the groups were evident with regard to the number of colds, their severity, or their duration [27]. Other reports, however, conflict and suggest a decrease in the duration of cold episodes and the severity of symptoms [28,29]. Vitamin C is thought to moderate colds by enhancing many immune cell (such as some leukocyte) functions while also destroying histamine, which causes many of a cold's symptoms [30].

Cancer. Epidemiological studies provide evidence that increased intakes of fruits and vegetables are associated with a decreased risk of some cancers [31–35]. The association between high vitamin C intake and a protective effect against cancer is generally stronger with cancers of the oral cavity, pharynx, esophagus, and stomach than with other cancers, such as of the lung, colon, pancreas, and cervix [31,35]. Other studies [33–36] both support some and negate some of these associations. In clinical trials, some researchers have shown that the survival time in cancer patients could be prolonged through massive doses of vitamin C, whereas others have demonstrated no such success [31,32,37–39].

Possible mechanisms of ascorbate action against cancer development include roles in immunocompetence and as an antioxidant and an ability to detoxify carcinogens or block carcinogenic processes [31,33,34,39]. The fact that vitamin C in amounts of about 1 g when ingested with nitrates and/or nitrites can prevent formation of carcinogenic nitrosamines supports this latter theory and has lent credence to the vitamin's being somewhat protective against stomach and/or esophageal cancers [38,40,41]. Vitamin C is not unique in this regard, as other reducing agents and some food components are also effective in preventing nitrosocarcinogens [39].

Cardiovascular Disease. Many (but not all) epidemiological and prospective studies report the association of increased vitamin C intakes or plasma vitamin C concentrations with decreased risk of heart disease [42–53]. Low vitamin C status also has been found to be related to increased blood total cholesterol concentrations, while high plasma vitamin C concentrations have been associated with lower blood pressure and with higher plasma high-density lipoprotein cholesterol concentrations, both of which are protective against heart disease [54].

The mechanisms by which vitamin C may protect against heart disease in humans are not clearly identified. Animal studies suggest that vitamin C deficiency alters cholesterol metabolism for the generation of bile salts [12]. Vitamin C decreases monocyte adhesion to endothelial cells lining blood vessels, and adhesion represents one of the first steps in atherogenesis. Following adhesion, monocytes typically can migrate into the arterial intima (the innermost layer of blood vessels), where they become macrophages and take up oxidized cholesterol in low-density lipoproteins (LDL). Impaired vitamin C status, as well as activation of leukocytes, results in increased LDL oxidation [55–57]. Macrophages take up oxidized LDL. With continued accumulation of oxidized LDL, macrophages develop into foam cells, and over time fatty streaks develop. This sequence represents the initial steps in atherosclerosis. Vitamin C, alone and with vitamin E, may help prevent heart disease through its ability to scavenge reactive species/free radicals before they reach and initiate oxidation of LDL. Vitamin C deficiency in guinea pigs is associated with myocardial lipid peroxidative damage [14,25,55,58]. The addition of vitamin C to LDL undergoing oxidation in vitro mediated by aqueous peroxyl radicals (ROO•) results in diminished utilization of vitamin E and diminished LDL oxidation [58]. Vitamin C concentrations >0.8 mg/dL in vitro inhibit metal-induced LDL oxidation [18,59]. Urinary isoprostane concentrations (an indicator of free radical damage) were diminished in smokers receiving vitamin C supplementation [60].

Cataracts. High vitamin C intakes also are thought to be beneficial in regard to cataracts and possibly age-related macular degeneration, both of which are major causes of blindness, especially in older individuals. Cataracts result in part from oxidative damage to proteins in the lens of the eye. The damaged proteins aggregate and precipitate, causing the lens to become cloudy. Oxygen and oxyradicals are thought to contribute to the development of cataracts. Poor antioxidant status or intake, especially of vitamins E and C, has been shown in many but not all studies to be associated with development of cataracts [61–69]. While some epidemiological studies suggest a protective effect of vitamin C against cataracts, the effect cannot be attributed solely to vitamin C because subjects in many of the studies were consuming a multivitamin preparation [61–63].

Interactions with Other Nutrients

Vitamin C interacts mainly with two minerals, iron and copper. The interaction between iron and vitamin C is related not only to the vitamin's effect on intestinal absorption of nonheme iron but also to the distribution of iron in the body. Specifically, ascorbate enhances the intestinal absorption of nonheme iron either by reducing iron to a ferrous (Fe^{2+}) form from a ferric (Fe^{3+}) form or by forming a soluble complex with the iron in the alkaline pH of the small intestine, thereby enhancing iron's absorption. Excessive iron in the presence of vitamin C, however, may accelerate the oxidative catabolism of vitamin C, negating the enhancing effects of vitamin C on iron absorption. Incorporation of iron into ferritin, the storage form of iron, and stabilization of ferritin by ascorbate have also been demonstrated [70]. The effect of the vitamin in the distribution and mobilization of storage iron is uncertain. Ascorbic acid supplements can cause a change in the distribution of iron in patients suffering from iron overload, but not necessarily in other individuals [71]. Vitamin C–initiated free radical generation from mobilization of storage iron has been suggested but also refuted [17,63,72,73].

With respect to copper, vitamin C intakes of 1.5 g daily for about 2 months resulted in decreased serum copper and ceruloplasmin, a copper-containing protein with oxidase activity; however, despite the decrease, serum copper levels remained within normal range [74]. Dietary vitamin C intakes in excess of 600 mg daily have also been shown to decrease the oxidase activity of ceruloplasmin. Ascorbate may cause copper dissociation from ceruloplasmin or may influence the binding of copper to enzymes [38,75]. Human cells treated with vitamin C have exhibited enhanced copper uptake from ceruloplasmin [38]. Decreased intestinal absorption of copper by ascorbic acid has been observed in several animal species. A proposed mechanism of interaction for this effect suggests that vitamin C stimulated iron mobilization and the mobilized iron in turn inhibited copper absorption [75]. In addition, vitamin C may inhibit the binding of copper to metallothionein, a protein found in the intestinal cells and other body cells. It has been proposed that the delayed binding may inhibit copper transport across the intestinal cell [75].

Metabolism and Excretion

As vitamin C intakes increase, plasma vitamin C concentrations increase but reach an upper limit as renal handling of the vitamin shifts from active saturable reabsorption in the renal tubules to a renal threshold in which the maximum reabsorption of the vitamin is achieved. The renal reabsorption threshold occurs with plasma vitamin C concentrations of about 1.2 mg/dL.

Vitamin C may be excreted intact or may be oxidized to dehydroascorbate. Oxidation occurs primarily in the liver but also to some extent in the kidney. Oxidation of dehydroascorbate begins with hydrolysis (opening) of the ring structure to yield 2,3-diketogulonic acid, which possesses no vitamin C activity and can be excreted in the urine or further hydrolyzed (Fig. 9.9). Diketogulonate is cleaved by separate pathways either into oxalic acid and the four-carbon sugar threonic acid or into a variety of five-carbon sugars (xylose, xylonate, and lyxonate). The oxalic acid is excreted in the urine, and its concentration does not appear to vary with intakes up to about 200 mg of the vitamin [5]. The four- and five-carbon sugars can be converted into cellular compounds or be oxidized and excreted as CO_2 and water. Other urinary vitamin C metabolites include 2-O-methyl ascorbate, ascorbate 2-sulfate, and 2-ketoascorbitol.

Recommended Dietary Allowances

Current (2000) requirements for vitamin C intake are based on nearly maximizing tissue concentrations and minimizing urinary excretion of the vitamin [76]. The RDA for adult men and women is 90 mg and 75 mg, respectively, with requirements estimated at 75 mg and 60 mg, respectively [76]. During pregnancy and lactation, recommendations for vitamin C increase to 100 mg and 120 mg, respectively [76]. The 1989 RDA for the first time singled out cigarette smokers for an increased vitamin C requirement based on studies showing that smoking accelerates depletion of the body's ascorbate pool [77]. Current recommendations for smokers suggest an added 35 mg vitamin C daily [76].

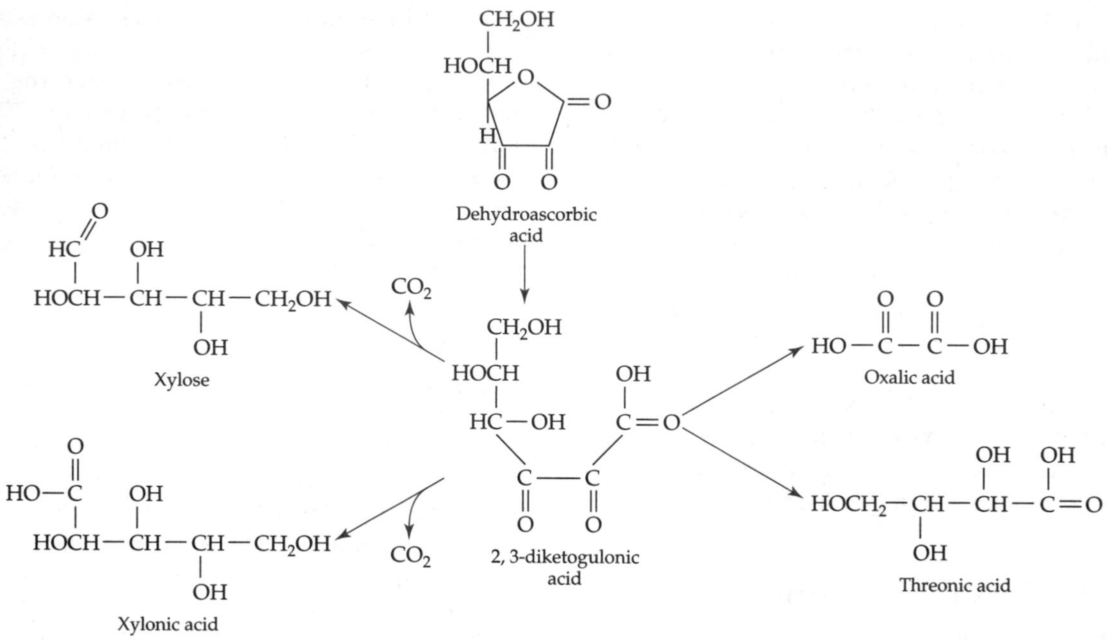

Figure 9.9 Vitamin C metabolism.

Deficiency: Scurvy

Deficient vitamin C intakes result in the deficiency condition known as **scurvy.** Scurvy is typically manifested when the total body vitamin C pools fall below about 300 mg and plasma vitamin C concentrations drop to <0.2 mg/dL [7,11]. Scurvy may be characterized by a multitude of signs and symptoms, many of which are thought to result from impaired hydroxyproline and hydroxylysine synthesis needed for collagen formation. The most notable signs and symptoms include bleeding gums, small skin discolorations due to ruptured small blood vessels (**petechiae**), sublingual hemorrhages, easy bruising (ecchymoses and purpurae), impaired wound and fracture healing, joint pain (arthralgia), loose and decaying teeth, and hyperkeratosis of hair follicles, especially on the arms, legs, and buttocks [78]. Scurvy is fatal if untreated. The four Hs—*hemorrhagic* signs, *hyperkeratosis* of hair follicles, *hypochondriasis* (psychological manifestation), and *hematologic* abnormalities (associated with impaired iron absorption)—are often used as a mnemonic device for remembering scurvy signs [11].

Although scurvy is rare in the United States, low plasma vitamin C levels have been observed in the elderly, especially if institutionalized. People who have poor diets, especially if coupled with alcoholism or drug abuse, are likely to be deficient, as are people with diseases such as diabetes mellitus and some cancers that increase the turnover rate of the vitamin.

Toxicity

Daily intakes of up to 2 g vitamin C are routinely consumed without adverse effects [5,73,79]. Because vitamin C absorption is saturable and dose dependent, more vitamin C is absorbed, and thus toxicity is theoretically more likely, with ingestion of several large (>1 g) doses of the vitamin throughout the day than with ingestion of the same amount as one single dose. The most common side effect with ingestion of large amounts (>2 g) of the vitamin is gastrointestinal problems characterized by abdominal pain and osmotic diarrhea. The unabsorbed vitamin C in the intestinal tract that is metabolized by bacteria within the colon is what promotes the osmotic diarrhea [2,6,38,79,80]. Based on this side effect, a tolerable upper intake level of 2 g vitamin C has been recommended [76].

Two other side effects reported from the use of large amounts of vitamin C are thought to affect (if at all) only selected populations. These side effects include increased risk of kidney stones and iron toxicity for those with renal disease and disorders of iron metabolism, respectively. The possible development of kidney stones (nephrolithiasis), either oxalic acid or uric acid in content, is based on vitamin C's metabolism. Because vitamin C is metabolized in the body to oxalate and because calcium oxalate is a common constituent of kidney stones, ingestion of large doses of vitamin C has been purported as an etiologic factor in nephrolithiasis. However, although doses of up to 10 g of vitamin C have been shown to increase oxalate excretion, the amount of oxalate excreted (generally <50 mg) typically has remained within a normal and safe range [80–83]. Nevertheless, some suggest that people predisposed to calcium oxalate kidney stones avoid high doses (≥500 mg) of vitamin C [79–83]. Furthermore, because of interactions in the kidney between vitamin C and uric acid, which also is a constituent of kidney stones, ingestion of large doses of ascorbic acid should be avoided by individuals with uric acid kidney stones [84]. Specifically, vitamin C competitively inhibits renal reabsorption of uric acid, thereby increasing uric acid excretion. The resulting urine acidification, along with the excessive amount of uric acid being excreted, could cause precipitation of urate crystals and urate kidney stones [79,84]. The actual clinical importance of uricosuria (high levels of uric acid in the urine) with regard to stone formation is unknown [79].

In addition to increasing the probability of kidney stones, chronic high doses of vitamin C are also purported to be unsafe for people with disorders involving iron metabolism, including individuals with **hemochromatosis, thalassemia,** and **sideroblastic anemia** [72,79]. However, others contend that pro-oxidant effects of vitamin C on mobilization of iron stores do not occur in vivo [17,37,73].

The issue of systemic conditioning to high intakes of vitamin C is currently deemed doubtful. Although scurvylike symptoms were reported in a few individuals on abrupt withdrawal of large intakes of vitamin C, the reports are anecdotal. Further substantiation of conditioned (also called rebound) scurvy is needed before recommendations can be made [73,76].

Excessive ascorbate excretion can interfere with some clinical laboratory tests. Vitamin C in the urine, for example, may act as a reductive agent and thus interfere with diagnostic tests using redox chemistry. For example, tests for glucose in the urine can be rendered invalid, false-negative tests for fecal occult blood may be generated, and occult blood in the urine may not be detected [38,79].

Assessment of Nutriture

Plasma and serum vitamin C concentrations respond to changes in dietary vitamin C intakes and thus are used to assess recent vitamin C intake. White blood cell (wbc) content of the vitamin better reflects body stores, but this measurement is technically more difficult to perform. Plasma concentrations of vitamin C below 0.2 mg/dL are considered to be deficient. Concentrations associated with tissue saturation are about 1.0 mg/dL, and those typically found with recommended intakes range from about 0.6 to 0.8 mg/dL [5]. Leukocyte vitamin C concentrations of 10 μg/10^8 wbc or less are considered deficient [85].

References Cited for Vitamin C

1. Rumsey S, Levine M. Absorption, transport, and disposition of ascorbic acid in humans. J Nutr Biochem 1998;9:116–30.

2. Goldenberg H, Schweinzer E. Transport of vitamin C in animal and human cells. J Bioenergetics Biomembranes 1994;26:359–67.

3. Johnston C, Meyer C, Srilakshmi J. Vitamin C elevates red blood cell glutathione in healthy adults. Am J Clin Nutr 1993; 58:103–5.

4. Martensson J, Han J, Griffith O, Meister A. Glutathione ester delays the onset of scurvy in ascorbate-deficient guinea pigs. Proc Natl Acad Sci 1993;90:317–21.

5. Levine M, Cantilena-Conry C, Wang Y, Welch R, Washko P, Dhariwal K, Park J, Lazarev A, Graumlich J, King J, Cantilena L. Vitamin C pharmocokinetics in healthy volunteers: evidence for a recommended requirement. Proc Natl Acad Sci USA 1996;93:3704–9.

6. Sauberlich H. Bioavailability of vitamins. Prog Food Nutr Sci 1985;9:1–33.

7. Kallner A, Hartmann D, Hornig D. Steady-state turnover and body pool of ascorbic acid in man. Am J Clin Nutr 1979;32:530–39.

8. Levine M, Dhariwal K, Wang Y, Park J, Welch R. Ascorbic acid in neutrophils. In: Frei B, ed. Natural Antioxidants in Health and Disease. San Diego: Academic Press, 1994, pp. 469–88.

9. Hornig D. Distribution of ascorbic acid, metabolites and analogues in man and animals. Ann NY Acad Sci 1975;258:103–18.

10. Rebouche C. Ascorbic acid and carnitine biosynthesis. Am J Clin Nutr 1991;54:1147S–52S.

11. Levine M. New concepts in the biology and biochemistry of ascorbic acid. N Engl J Med 1986;314:892–902.

12. Basu T, Schorah C. Vitamin C in Health and Disease. Westport, CT: AVI, 1982.

13. Halpner A, Handelman G, Belmont C, Harris J, Blumberg J. Protection by vitamin C of oxidant induced loss of vitamin E in rat hepatocytes. J Nutr Biochem 1998;9:355–59.

14. Niki E, Noguchi N, Tsuchihashi H, Gotoh N. Interaction among vitamin C, vitamin E and β-carotene. Am J Clin Nutr 1995; 62:1322S–26S.

15. Jacob R. The integrated antioxidant system. Nutr Res 1995; 15:755–66.

16. Niki E. Action of ascorbic acid as a scavenger of active and stable oxygen radicals. Am J Clin Nutr 1991;54:1119S–24S.

17. Frei B. Ascorbic acid protects lipids in human plasma and low density lipoprotein against oxidative damage. Am J Clin Nutr 1991;54:1113S–18S.

18. Jialal I, Vega G, Grundy S. Physiologic levels of ascorbate inhibit the oxidative modification of low density lipoprotein. Atherosclerosis 1990;82:185–91.

19. Heller R, Munscher-Paulig F, Grabner R, Till U. L-ascorbic acid potentiates nitric oxide synthesis in endothelial cells. J Biol Chem 1999;274:8254–60.

20. Frei B, Stocker R, Ames B. Antioxidant defenses and lipid peroxidation in human blood plasma. Proc Natl Acad Sci USA 1988;85:9748–52.

21. Stadtman E. Ascorbic acid and oxidative inactivation of proteins. Am J Clin Nutr 1991;54:1125S–28S.

22. Frei B, England L, Ames B. Ascorbate is an outstanding antioxidant in human blood plasma. Proc Natl Acad Sci USA 1989;86:6377–81.

23. Park J, Levine M. Purification, cloning and expression of dehydroascorbic acid reducing activity from human neutrophils: identification as glutaredoxin. Biochem J 1996;315:931–38.

24. May J, Cobb C, Mendiratta S, Hill K, Burk R. Reduction of the ascorbyl free radical to ascorbate by thioredoxin reductase. J Biol Chem 1998;273:23039–45.

25. Levine M, Morita K. Ascorbic acid in endocrine systems. Vitamins & Hormones 1985;42:2–64.

26. Englard S, Seifter S. The biochemical functions of ascorbic acid. Ann Rev Nutr 1986;6:365–406.

27. Briggs M. Vitamin C and infectious disease: a review of the literature and the results of a randomized, double-blind, prospective study over 8 years. In: Briggs MH, ed. Recent Vitamin Research. Boca Raton, FL: CRC Press, 1984, pp. 39–81.

28. Hemila H. Vitamin C and the common cold. Br J Nutr 1992;67:3–16.

29. Jariwalla R, Harakeh S. Antiviral and immunomodulatory activities of ascorbic acid. Subcell Biochem 1996;25:213–31.

30. Johnston C, Martin L, Cai X. Antihistamine effect of supplemental ascorbic acid and neutrophil chemotaxis. J Am Coll Nutr 1992;11:172–76.

31. Block G. Vitamin C status and cancer: epidemiologic evidence of reduced risk. Ann NY Acad Sci 1992;669:280–90.

32. Block G. Vitamin C and cancer prevention: the epidemiologic evidence. Am J Clin Nutr 1991;53:270S–82S.

33. Block G, Patterson B, Subar A. Fruit, vegetables, and cancer prevention: a review of the epidemiological evidence. Nutr Cancer 1992;18:1–29.

34. Block G. The data support a role for antioxidants in reducing cancer risk. Nutr Rev 1992;50:207–13.

35. Byers T, Guerrero N. Epidemiologic evidence for vitamin C and vitamin E in cancer prevention. Am J Clin Nutr 1995;62(suppl):1385S–92S.

36. Gershoff S. Vitamin C (ascorbic acid): new roles, new requirements? Nutr Rev 1993;51:313–26.

37. Bendich A, Langseth L. The health effects of vitamin C supplementation: a review. J Am Coll Nutr 1995;14:124–36.

38. Davies M, Austin J, Partridge D. Vitamin C. Its Chemistry and Biochemistry. Cambridge, England: Royal Society of Chemistry, 1991.

39. Carpenter M. Roles of vitamins E and C in cancer. In: Laidlaw SA, Swendseid ME. Contemporary Issues in Clinical Nutrition. New York: Wiley-Liss, 1991, pp. 61–90.

40. Tannenbaum S, Wishnok J, Leaf C. Inhibition of nitrosamine formation by ascorbic acid. Am J Clin Nutr 1991;53:247S–50S.

41. Schorah C, Sobala G, Sanderson M, Collis N, Primrose J. Gastric juice ascorbic acid: effects of disease and implications for gastric carcinogenesis. Am J Clin Nutr 91;53:287S–93S.

42. Schwartz J, Weiss S. Relationship between dietary vitamin C intake and pulmonary function in the First National Health and Nutrition Examination Survey (NHANES I). Am J Clin Nutr 1994;59:110–14.

43. Enstrom J, Kanim L, Klein M. Vitamin C intake and mortality among a sample of the United States population. Epidemiol 1992;3:194–202.

44. Simon J, Hudes E, Browner W. Serum ascorbic acid and cardiovascular disease prevalence in US adults. Epidemiol 1998;9:316–21.

45. Kushi L, Folsom A, Prineas R, Mink P, Wu Y, Bostick R. Dietary antioxidant vitamins and death from coronary heart disease in postmenopausal women. N Engl J Med 1996;334:1156–62.

46. Losonczy K, Harris T, Havlik R. Vitamin E and vitamin C supplement use and risk of all-cause and coronary heart disease mortality in older persons: the established populations for epidemiologic studies of the elderly. Am J Clin Nutr 1996;64:190–96.

47. Knekt P, Reunanen A, Jarvinen R, Seppanen R, Heliovaara M, Aromaa A. Antioxidant vitamin intake and coronary mortality in a longitudinal population study. Am J Epidemiol 1994; 139:1180–89.

48. Nyyssonen K, Parviainen M, Salonen R, Tuomilehto J, Salonen J. Vitamin C deficiency and risk of myocardial infarction: prospective population study of men from eastern Finland. Br Med J 1997; 314:634–38.

49. Singh R, Ghosh S, Niaz M, Singh R, Beegum R, Chibo H, Shoumin Z, Postiglione A. Dietary intake, plasma levels of antioxidant vitamins, and oxidative stress in relation to coronary artery disease in elderly subjects. Am J Cardiol 1995;76:1233–38.

50. Gey K, Moser U, Jordan P, Stahelin H, Eichholzer M, Ludin E. Increased risk of cardiovascular disease at suboptimal plasma concentrations of essential antioxidants: an epidemiological update with special attention to carotene and vitamin C. Am J Clin Nutr 1993;57(suppl):787S–97S.

51. Sahyoun N, Jacques P, Russell R. Carotenoids, vitamins C and E, and mortality in an elderly population. Am J Epidemiol 1996;144: 501–11.

52. Gale C, Martyn C, Winter P, Cooper C. Vitamin C and risk of death from stroke and coronary heart disease in cohort of elderly people. Br Med J 1995;310:1563–66.

53. Pandey D, Shekelle R, Selwyn B, Tangney C, Stamler J. Dietary vitamin C and beta-carotene and risk of death in middle-aged men. The Western Electric study. Am J Epidemiol 1995;142:1269–78.

54. Simon J. Vitamin C and cardiovascular disease: a review. J Am Coll Nutr 1992;11:107–25.

55. Chakrabarty S, Nandi A, Mukhopadhyay C, Chatterjee I. Protective role of ascorbic acid against lipid peroxidation and myocardial injury. Molec Cell Biochem 1992;111:41–47.

56. Jialal I, Grundy S. Effect of combined supplementation with alpha-tocopherol, ascorbate, and beta carotene on low-density lipoprotein oxidation. Circulation 1993;88:2780–86.

57. Scaccini C, Jialal I. LDL modification by activated polymorphonuclear leukocytes: a cellular model of mild oxidative stress. Free Radical Biol Med 1994;16:49–55.

58. Thomas S, Neuzil J, Mohr D, Stocker R. Coantioxidants make α-tocopherol an efficient antioxidant for low-density lipoprotein. Am J Clin Nutr 1995;62(suppl):1357S–64S.

59. Jialal I, Grundy S. Preservation of the endogenous antioxidants in low density lipoprotein by ascorbate but not probucol during oxidative modification. J Clin Invest 1991;87:597–601.

60. Reilly M, Delanty N, Lawson J, Fitzgerald G. Modulation of oxidant stress in vivo in chronic cigarette smokers. Circulation 1996;94:19–25.

61. Taylor A, Jacques P, Epstein E. Relations among aging, antioxidant status, and cataract. Am J Clin Nutr 1995;62(suppl):1439S–47S.

62. Jacques P, Taylor A, Hankinson S. Long term vitamin C supplement use and prevalence of early age-related lens opacities. Am J Clin Nutr 1997;66:911–16.

63. Bendich A, Langseth L. The health effects of vitamin C supplementation: a review. J Am Coll Nutr 1995;14:124–36.

64. Varma S. Scientific basis for medical therapy of cataracts by antioxidants. Am J Clin Nutr 1991;53:335S–45S.

65. Robertson J, Donner A, Trevithick J. A possible role for vitamins C and E in cataract prevention. Am J Clin Nutr 1991;53:346S–51S.

66. Vitale S, West S, Hallfrisch J, Alston C, Wang F, Moorman C, Muller D, Singh V, Taylor H. Plasma antioxidants and risk of cortical and nuclear cataract. Epidemiol 1993;4:195–203.

67. Knekt P, Heliovaara M, Rissanen A, Aromaa A, Aaran R. Serum antioxidant vitamins and risk of cataract. Br Med J 1992;305: 1392–94.

68. Leske M, Chylack L, Wu S. The Lens Opacities Case-Control Study. Risk factors for cataract. Arch Ophthalmol 1991;109:244–51.

69. Jacques P, Chylack L. Epidemiologic evidence of a role for the antioxidant vitamins and carotenoids in cataract prevention. Am J Clin Nutr 1991;53:352S–55S.

70. Hoffman K, Yanelli K, Bridges K. Ascorbic acid and iron metabolism: alterations in lysosomal function. Am J Clin Nutr 1991;54: 1188S–92S.

71. Cook J, Watson S, Simpson K, Lipschitz D, Skikne B. The effect of high ascorbic acid supplementation on body iron stores. Blood 1984;64:721–26.

72. Herbert V, Shaw S, Jayatilleke E. Vitamin C–driven free radical generation from iron. J Nutr 1996;126:1213S–20S.

73. Hathcock J. Vitamins and minerals: efficacy and safety. Am J Clin Nutr 1997;66:427–37.

74. Finley E, Cerklewski F. Influence of ascorbic acid supplementation on copper status in young adult men. Am J Clin Nutr 1983;37:553–56.

75. Harris E, Percival S. A role of ascorbic acid in copper transport. Am J Clin Nutr 1991;54:1193S–97S.

76. Food and Nutrition Board. Dietary Reference Intakes for Vitamin C, Vitamin E, Selenium, and Carotenoids. Washington, DC: National Academy Press, 2000, pp. 95–185.

77. Lykkesfeldt J, Loft S, Nielsen J, Poulsen H. Ascorbic acid and dehydroascorbic acid as biomarkers of oxidative stress caused by smoking. Am J Clin Nutr 1997;65:959–63.

78. Hodges R, Baker E, Hood J, Sauberlich H, March S. Experimental scurvy in man. Am J Clin Nutr 1969;22:535–48.

79. Alhadeff L, Gualtieri C, Lipton M. Toxic effects of water-soluble vitamins. Nutr Rev 1984;42:33–40.

80. Johnston C. Biomarkers for establishing a tolerable upper intake level for vitamin C. Nutr Rev 1999;57:71–77.

81. Tsao C, Salimi S. Effect of large intake of ascorbic acid on urinary and plasma oxalic acid levels. Internatl J Vit Nutr Res 1984; 54:245–49.

82. Hughes C, Dutton S, Truswell A. High intakes of ascorbic acid and urinary oxalate. J Hum Nutr 1981;35:274–80.

83. Urivetzky M, Kessaris D, Smith A. Ascorbic acid overdosing: a risk factor for calcium oxalate nephrolithiasis. J Urol 1992; 147:1215–18.

84. Sutton J, Basu T, Dickerson J. Effect of large doses of ascorbic acid in man on some nitrogenous components of urine. Human Nutr Appl Nutr 1983;37A:136–40.

85. Jacob R. Assessment of human vitamin C status. J Nutr 1990;120:1480–85.

THIAMIN (VITAMIN B_1)

Thiamin (vitamin B_1), the structural formula of which is shown in Figure 9.10, consists of a pyrimidine ring and a thiazole moiety (meaning one of two parts) linked by a methylene (CH_2) bridge.

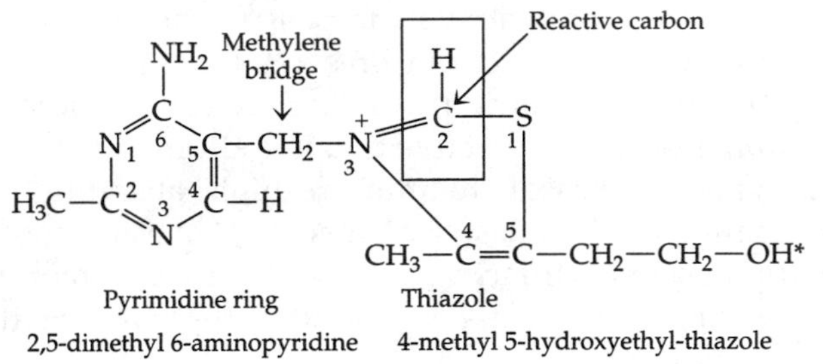

*Diphosphate addition occurs here to form the active coenzyme thiamin diphosphate (TDP).

Figure 9.10 Structure of thiamin.

Sources

Thiamin is widely distributed in foods, including meat (especially pork), legumes, and whole, fortified, or enriched grain products, cereals, and breads. Yeast and wheat germ also contain significant amounts of the vitamin. In supplements, thiamin is found mainly as thiamin hydrochloride or as thiamin mononitrate salt.

Digestion, Absorption, Transport, and Storage

In plants, thiamin exists in a free (nonphosphorylated) form. However, in animal products, >95% of thiamin occurs in a phosphorylated form, primarily thiamin diphosphate (TDP), also called thiamin pyrophosphate (TPP). Intestinal phosphatases hydrolyze the phosphates from the thiamin diphosphate prior to absorption.

Absorption of thiamin from foods is thought to be high. Occasionally, however, antithiamin factors may be present in the diet. For example, thiaminases present in raw fish catalyze the cleavage of thiamin, destroying the vitamin. These thiaminases are thermolabile, so cooking fish renders the enzymes inactive. Other antithiamin factors include polyhydroxyphenols such as tannic and caffeic acids. Polyhydroxyphenols, which are thermostable, are found in coffee, tea, betel nuts, and certain fruits and vegetables such as blueberries, black currants, brussels sprouts, and red cabbage. These polyhydroxyphenols inactivate thiamin by an oxyreductive process; the destructive process can be facilitated by the presence of divalent minerals such as calcium and magnesium. Thiamin destruction may be prevented, however, by the presence of reducing compounds such as vitamin C and citric acid.

Free thiamin, not phosphorylated thiamin, is absorbed into the intestinal cells. Absorption of thiamin can be both active and passive, depending on the amount of the vitamin presented in the intestine for absorption. At low physiological concentrations, thiamin absorption is active and is sodium-dependent [1]. When intakes of thiamin are high, absorption is predominantly by passive diffusion [1]. Absorption of thiamin occurs primarily in the jejunum but can occur in the ileum with lesser amounts absorbed in the duodenum.

Within the mucosal cells, thiamin may be phosphorylated (i.e., converted into a phosphate ester). Thiamin transport across the basolateral membrane is sodium- and energy-dependent. Ethanol ingestion, however, interferes with active transport of thiamin from the mucosal cell across the basolateral membrane, but not the brush border membrane. Thiamin appearing on the serosal side of the enterocyte is not initially bound to phosphates.

Thiamin in the blood is typically either in its free form, bound to albumin, or found as thiamin monophosphate (TMP). Most (~90%) of the thiamin in the blood, however, is present not in the plasma but within the blood cells. Transport of thiamin into red blood cells is thought to occur by facilitated diffusion, whereas transport into other tissues requires energy. Only free thiamin or TMP is thought to be able to cross cell membranes. In red blood cells, most thiamin exists as TDP, with smaller amounts of free thiamin and TMP.

The human body contains approximately 30 mg of thiamin, with relatively high but still small concentrations found (stored) in the liver, skeletal muscles, heart, kidney, and brain. In fact, skeletal muscles are thought to contain about half of the body's thiamin.

Following absorption, most free thiamin is taken up by the liver and phosphorylated, such that thiamin is converted to its coenzyme phosphorylated form, thiamin diphosphate (TDP). Conversion of thiamin to TDP requires adenosine triphosphate (ATP) and thiamin pyrophosphokinase, an enzyme found in the liver, brain, and other tissues. About 80% of the total thiamin in the body exists as TDP.

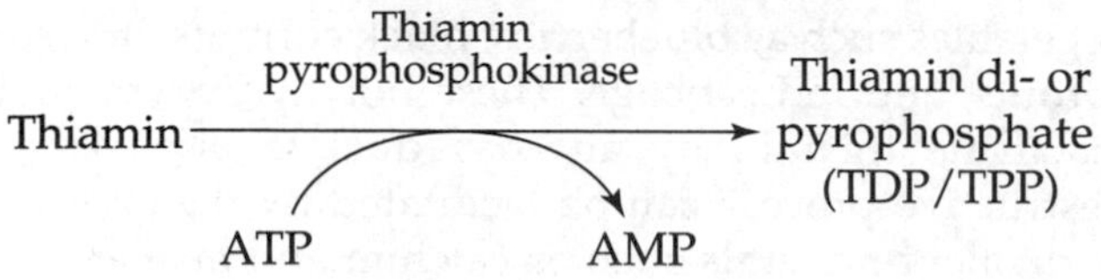

Another form of thiamin, thiamin triphosphate (TTP), represents about 10% of total body thiamin. TTP is synthesized by action of a TDP-ATP phosphoryl transferase that phosphorylates TDP.

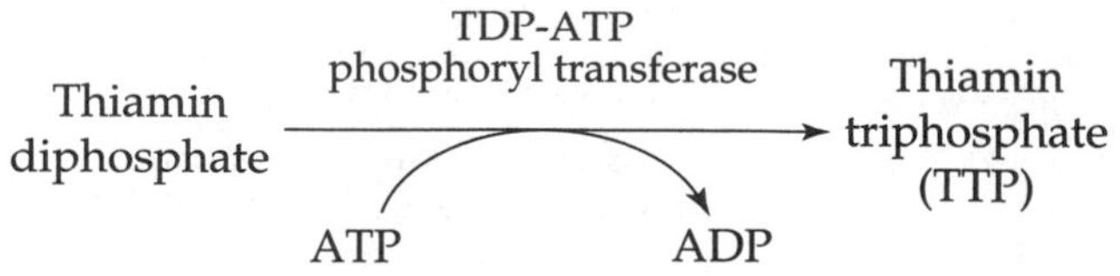

The terminal phosphate on TTP may be hydrolyzed by thiamin triphosphatase to yield TDP.

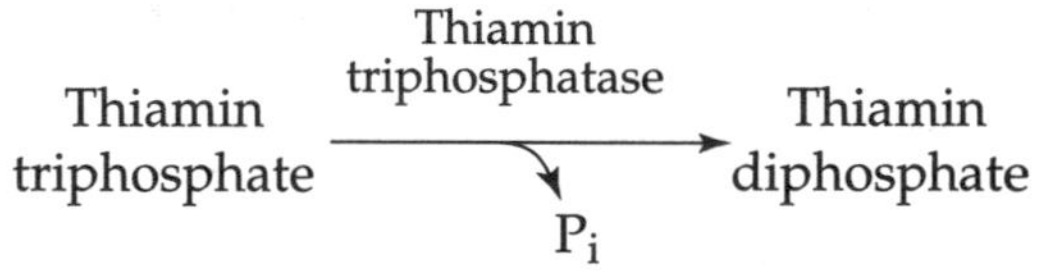

TTP, as well as TDP and TMP, can be found in small amounts in several tissues, including the brain, heart, liver, muscles, and kidney. TMP is thought to be derived from the catabolism of the terminal phosphate on TDP and is believed to be inactive.

Functions and Mechanisms of Action

Thiamin plays essential roles in the body, including these:

- energy transformation (a coenzyme),
- synthesis of pentoses and nicotinamide adenine dinucleotide phosphate (NADPH) (also as a coenzyme), and
- membrane and nerve conduction (in a noncoenzyme capacity).

We will discuss each of these three roles.

Coenzyme Roles

As TDP, thiamin functions in energy transformation as a coenzyme of the pyruvate dehydrogenase complex, the α-ketoglutarate dehydrogenase complex, and the branched-chain α-keto acid dehydrogenase complex. In addition, TDP serves as a coenzyme for transketolase needed for the synthesis of NADPH and pentoses.

Energy Transformation. Thiamin as TDP functions as a coenzyme necessary for the oxidative decarboxylation of pyruvate, α-ketoglutarate, and the three branched-chain amino acids isoleucine, leucine, and valine. These reactions (Figs. 9.11 and 7.35) are instrumental in generating energy (ATP). Inhibition of the decarboxylation reactions of, especially, pyruvate and α-ketoglutarate prevents synthesis of ATP and of the acetyl CoA needed for the synthesis of, for example, fatty acids, cholesterol, and other important compounds. The inhibition also results in the accumulation of pyruvate, lactate, and α-ketoglutarate in the blood.

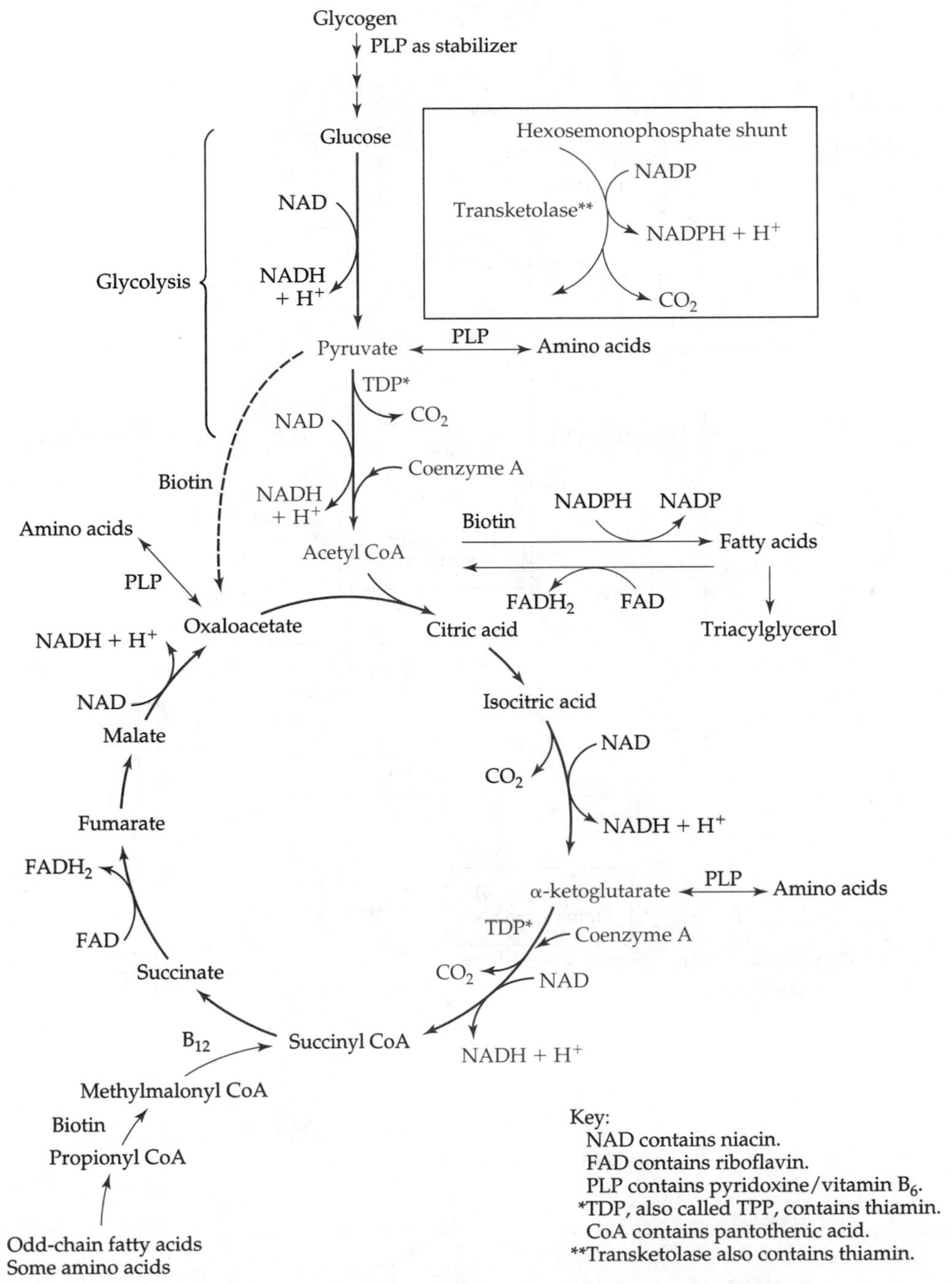

Figure 9.11 Various vitamin cofactors and their action sites in energy metabolism. The role of thiamin as TDP is shown by an asterisk.

The steps that occur in the oxidative decarboxylation of pyruvate, shown in Figure 9.12, require a multienzyme complex known as the pyruvate dehydrogenase complex, which is bound to the mitochondrial membrane. Three enzymes make up the pyruvate dehydrogenase complex: enzyme 1, a TDP-dependent pyruvate decarboxylase; enzyme 2, a lipoic acid–dependent dihydrolipoyl transacetylase; and enzyme 3, an FAD-dependent dihydrolipoyl dehydrogenase. The roles of four vitamins—thiamin (TDP), riboflavin (FAD), niacin (NAD^+), and pantothenic acid (CoA)—in this decarboxylation process can be identified in the steps outlined here and in Figure 9.12.

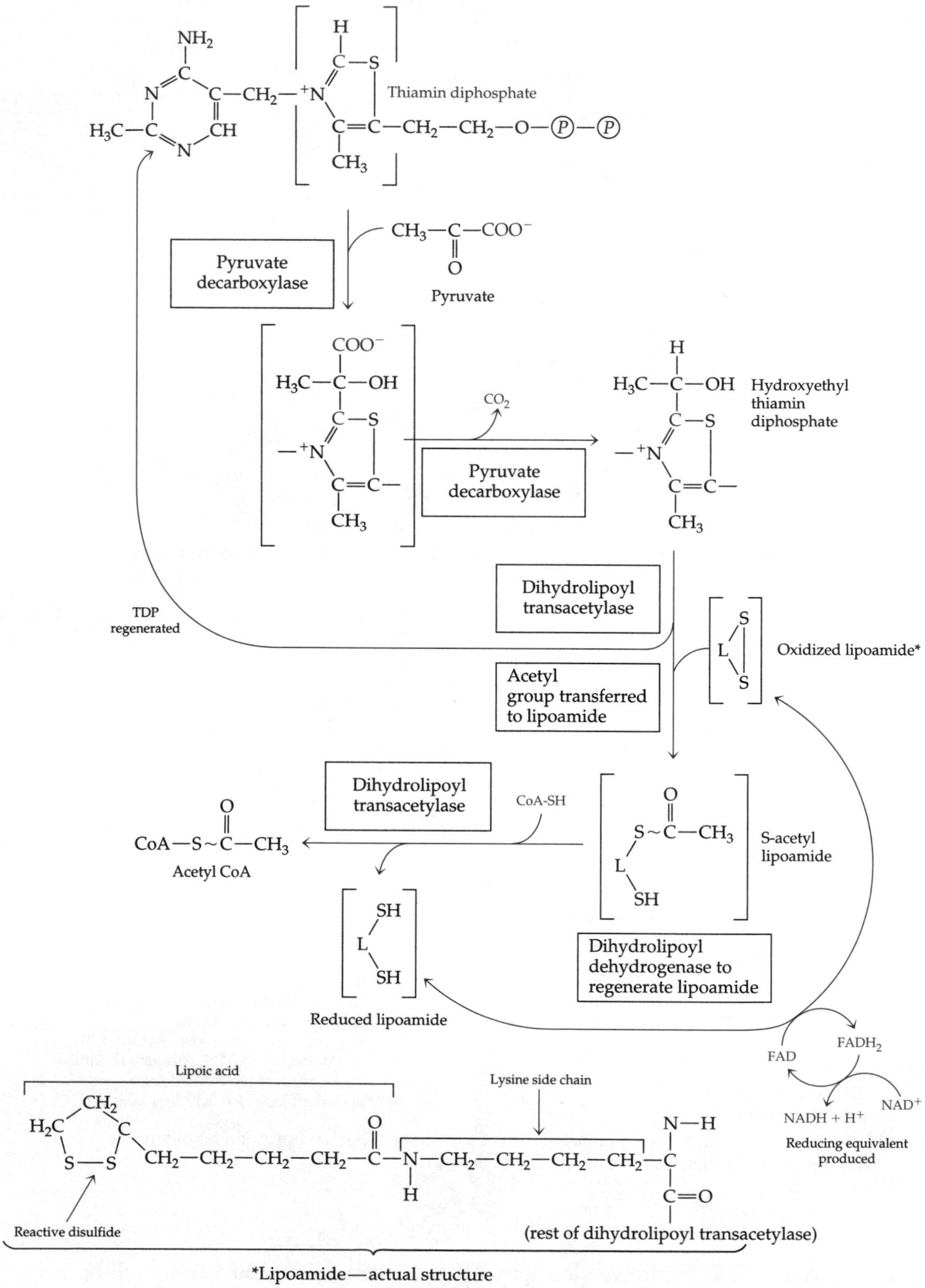

Figure 9.12 Oxidative decarboxylation of pyruvate by pyruvate dehydrogenase complex.

Five basic steps (see also Figs. 4.15 and 9.12) are involved in the oxidative decarboxylation of α-keto acids such as pyruvate and α-ketoglutarate:

Step 1: The pyruvate decarboxylase enzyme 1–TDP complex reacts with the keto acid (R–CO–COOH).

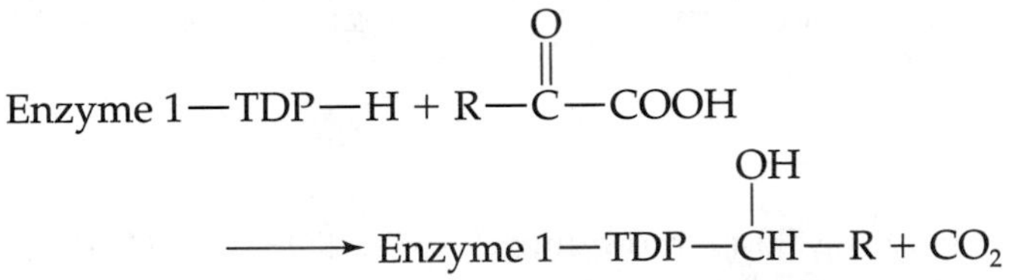

During the reaction, the enzyme 1–TDP complex covalently binds to the decarboxylated keto acid, forming hydroxyethyl TDP; carbon dioxide (CO_2) is released in the process.

Step 2: The enzyme 1–TDP–decarboxylated complex is acted on by enzyme 2–lipoic acid (LA)–dependent dihydrolipoyl transacetylase, which transfers an acetyl group from enzyme 1–TDP to a sulfur atom in lipoic acid.

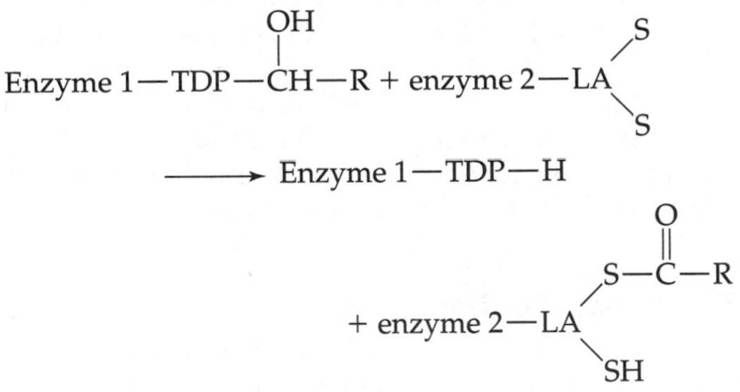

Although lipoic acid functions as a prosthetic group, it is not considered a vitamin. Lipoic acid is classified as a sulfur-containing fatty acid; uncertainty exists as to whether it is synthesized in the body or obtained by diet. Lipoate functions similarly to biotin at the end of the long flexible side chain of the enzyme; specifically, it rotates from one active site to another site on the multisubunit enzyme. Lipoamide picks up the acetyl group from enzyme 1–TDP to form acetyl lipoamide.

Step 3: The acetyl group is transferred from acetyl lipoamide to CoA with the formation of acetyl CoA and dihydrolipoamide.

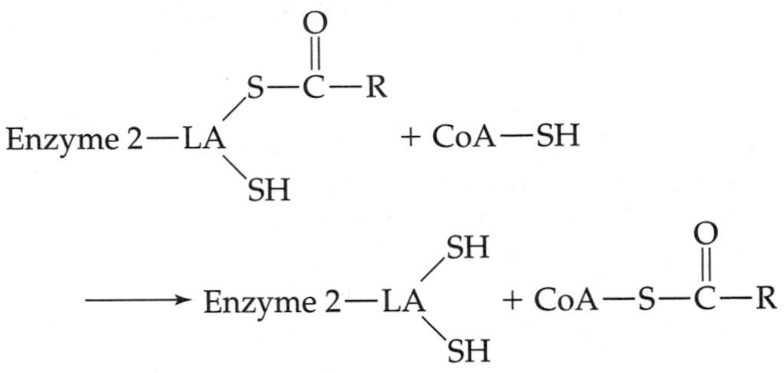

Step 4: The dehydrolipoamide is then oxidized back to the original lipoamide by an enzyme 3–FAD–dependent dihydrolipoyl dehydrogenase.

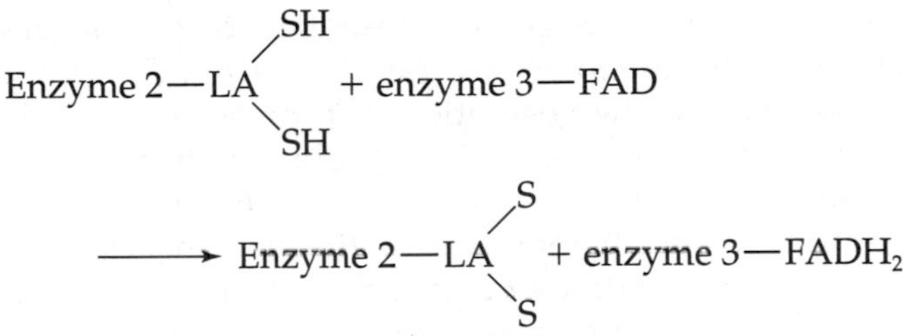

Step 5: $FADH_2$ is oxidized by NAD^+.

$$\text{Enzyme 3—FADH}_2 + \text{NAD}^+ \longrightarrow \text{Enzyme 3—FAD} + \text{NADH} + \text{H}^+$$

The decarboxylation of α-ketoglutarate by the α-ketoglutarate dehydrogenase complex is similar to that for pyruvate. The α-ketoglutarate dehydrogenase complex serves to decarboxylate α-ketoglutarate and forms succinyl CoA.

A key feature of TDP (Fig. 9.13) is that the carbon atom between the nitrogen and sulfur atoms in the thiazole ring is more acidic than most CH groups [2]. It ionizes (deprotonizes) to form a carbanion at carbon 2 of the thiazole ring. The carbanion is stabilized by the positively charged nitrogen in the thiazole ring [2]. The carbanion combines with the 2-carbonyl group of pyruvate, α-ketoglutarate, and other α-keto acids to form a covalent bond [2].

Decarboxylation of the branched-chain α-keto acids, which arise from the transamination of valine, isoleucine, and leucine, is an oxidative process that also requires thiamin as TDP/TPP (see Fig 7.35). Failure to oxidize the α-keto acids α-ketoisocaproic, α-keto β-methyl valeric, and α-ketoisovaleric acids from leucine, isoleucine, and valine, respectively, results in the accumulation of both the branched-chain amino acids and their α-keto acids in blood and other body fluids. Such findings are characteristic of maple syrup urine disease (MSUD), which results

Figure 9.13 Combination of TDP carbanion with substrate pyruvate.

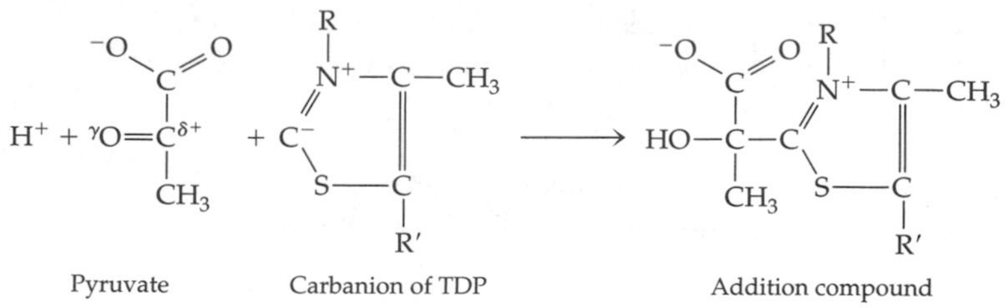

from a genetic (inborn error of metabolism) absence or insufficient activity of the branched-chain α-keto acid dehydrogenase enzyme complex. People with MSUD must limit intakes of protein-containing foods to limit intakes of leucine, isoleucine, and valine. Medical foods devoid of these three amino acids provide the majority of nutrient intake for such people.

Synthesis of Pentoses and NADPH. Thiamin as TDP also functions as a loosely bound prosthetic group of transketolase, a key cytosolic enzyme in the hexose monophosphate shunt. The hexose monophosphate shunt is the pathway in which sugars of varying chain lengths are interconverted (Fig. 4.19). The shunt is essential for the generation of pentoses for nucleic acid synthesis and of NADPH, which is needed, for example, for fatty acid synthesis. TDP forms a carbanion (Fig. 9.13) that acts to transfer an activated aldehyde from a donor ketose substrate to an acceptor. The acceptor in the hexose monophosphate shunt is xylulose. Transketolase hydrolyzes the carbon-to-carbon bond in xylose 5-P, sedoheptulose 7-P, and fructose 6-P (i.e., ketoses) and transfers the two-carbon fragment (carbons 1 and 2 of the ketoses) to an aldose receptor [2]. The transketolase-activated reaction that requires Mg^{2+} can be written as follows:

$$\text{Xylulose 5-P} + \text{ribose 5-P} \xrightleftharpoons{\text{Transketolase}} \text{Sedoheptulose 7-P} + \text{glyceraldehyde 3-P}$$

$$\text{Xylulose 5-P} + \text{erythrose 4-P} \xrightleftharpoons{\text{Transketolase}} \text{Glyceraldehyde 3-P} + \text{fructose 6-P}$$

Noncoenzyme Roles: Membrane and Nerve Conduction

In addition to its coenzyme roles, thiamin, as TTP, is thought to function in a manner other than as a coenzyme. In nerve membranes, TTP is thought to activate ion (specifically chloride) transport [3–5]. Thiamin also may be involved in nerve impulse transmission via regulation of sodium channels [3–5].

Metabolism and Excretion

Thiamin in excess of tissue needs and storage capacity is excreted intact, as well as metabolized for urinary excretion. Degradation of thiamin begins with the cleavage of the molecule into its pyrimidine and thiazole moieties. The two rings are then further metabolized, generating 20 or more metabolites. TDP and TMP are also excreted intact.

Recommended Dietary Allowances

As with the 1989 RDA for thiamin, the basis for the 1998 RDA relies on the results of numerous metabolic studies examining urinary excretion of thiamin, changes in erythrocyte transketolase activity, and thiamin intake data. The 1998 Dietary Reference Intakes RDA for individual intake for thiamin for adult men is 1.2 mg/day and for adult women is 1.1 mg daily; the requirements for adult men and women are 1.0 and 0.9 mg/day, respectively [6]. Differences in thiamin needs between men and women are based on differences in body size and energy needs. Thiamin intakes with pregnancy and lactation increase to 1.4 and 1.5 mg/day, respectively [6]. The inside covers of the book provide additional RDAs for thiamin for other age groups.

Deficiency: Beriberi

Despite the known functional roles of thiamin at the cellular level, it has as yet been impossible to explain all the pathophysiological manifestations in animals or humans that are associated with thiamin deficiency, or **beriberi** (*beri* means "weakness"). One of the first symptoms of thiamin deficiency is a loss of appetite (anorexia) and thus weight loss. As deficiency worsens, cardiovascular system involvement (such as hypertrophy and altered heart rate) and neurological symptoms such as apathy, confusion, decreased short-term memory, and irritability appear.

Three types of beriberi have been identified. Dry beriberi, found predominantly in older adults, is thought to result from a chronic low thiamin intake, especially if coupled with a high carbohydrate intake; it is characterized by muscle weakness and wasting, especially in the lower extremities. Wet beriberi results in more extensive cardiovascular system involvement than dry beriberi; right-side heart failure leads to respiratory involvement with edema. Acute beriberi, seen mostly in infants, has been documented in countries including Japan.

In the United States and in Western countries, thiamin deficiency associated with alcoholism is common. Such a deficiency is referred to as Wernicke's encephalopathy or Wernicke-Korsakoff syndrome. Individuals with alcohol dependency are particularly prone to thiamin deficiency because of

- decreased intake of the vitamin due to decreased food consumption,
- an increased requirement in the case of liver damage (decreased liver function impairs TDP formation and, consequently, vitamin use), and
- decreased thiamin absorption [7].

Wernicke's encephalopathy, often manifested in those with a history of alcohol abuse, is characterized by **ophthalmoplegia** (paralysis of the ocular muscles), **nystagmus** (constant, involuntary eyeball movement), **ataxia** (impaired muscle coordination), loss of recent memory, and confusion [7]. Treatment consists of therapeutic doses (~100 mg) of thiamin. Typically, some aspects of confusion and ophthalmoplegia begin to improve with the massive thiamin doses [7].

Elderly populations are also at risk for thiamin deficiency. People with diseases that impair absorption of the vitamin (e.g., some cancers, biliary disease, inflammatory bowel diseases) are also at greater risk of developing deficiency. Excess glucose infusion intravenously and ingestion of diets that are made up primarily of refined, unenriched grain products necessitate increased thiamin intake.

Toxicity

There appears to be little danger of thiamin toxicity associated with oral intake of large amounts (500 mg daily for 1 month) of thiamin [8,9]. Excessive thiamin (100 times recommendations) administered parenterally (intravenous or intramuscular), however, has been associated with headache, convulsions, cardiac arrhythmia, and anaphylactic shock, among other signs [6]. No tolerable upper intake level has been established [6].

Pharmacological levels of thiamin are used in the treatment of certain inborn errors of metabolism. For example, one variant form of maple syrup urine disease has been shown to respond to oral thiamin supplements (up to 500 mg daily). Other metabolic diseases that may respond to large doses of the vitamin are thiamin-responsive megaloblastic anemia and thiamin-responsive lactic acidosis. While the role of thiamin in the correction of anemia is not clear, in lactic acidosis large doses of thiamin increase hepatic pyruvate dehydrogenase activity, thereby decreasing lactic acid concentrations as more pyruvate is decarboxylated for entry into the Krebs cycle.

Assessment of Nutriture

Adequacy of thiamin nutriture may be assessed by measurement of erythrocyte transketolase activity in hemolyzed whole blood or by measurement of thiamin in the blood or urine [10,11]. Urinary thiamin excretion decreases with decreased thiamin status; excretion also is correlated with intake [12]. Urinary thiamin excretion <40 μg suggests thiamin deficiency. Transketolase is the thiamin-dependent enzyme of the hexose monophosphate shunt. In cases of thiamin deficiency, the enzyme increases activity with the addition of thiamin to the incubation medium. An increase in transketolase activity of >25% is indicative of thiamin deficiency, while an increase in activity of 15% to 25% suggests marginal status and an increase of <15% suggests adequate status.

References Cited for Thiamin

1. Laforenza U, Patrini C, Alvisi C, Faelli A, Licandro A, Rindi G. Thiamine uptake in human biopsy specimens, including observations from a patient with acute thiamine deficiency. Am J Clin Nutr 1997;66:320–26.
2. Tanphaichtr V. Thiamin. In: Machlin LJ, ed. Handbook of Vitamins, 3rd ed. New York: Dekker, 2001, pp. 275–316.
3. Haas R. Thiamin and the brain. Ann Rev Nutr 1988;8:483–515.
4. Bettendorff L. Thiamine in excitable tissues: reflections on a non-cofactor role. Metab Brain Dis 1994;9:183–209.
5. Bettendorff L, Kolb H, Schoffeniels E. Thiamine triphosphate activates an anion channel of large unit conductance in neuroblastoma cells. J Membr Biol 1993;136:281–88.
6. Food and Nutrition Board. Dietary Reference Intakes for Thiamin, Riboflavin, Niacin, Vitamin B_6, Folate, Vitamin B_{12}, Pantothenic Acid, Biotin, and Choline. Washington, DC: National Academy Press, 1998, pp. 58–86.
7. Wood B, Currie J. Presentation of acute Wernicke's encephalopathy and treatment with thiamine. Metab Brain Dis 1995;10:57–71.
8. Council on Scientific Affairs, American Medical Association. Vitamin preparations as dietary supplements and as therapeutic agents. JAMA 1987;257:1929–36.
9. Alhadeff L, Gualtieri C, Lipton M. Toxic effects of water-soluble vitamins. Nutr Rev 1984;42:33–40.
10. Finglass P. Thiamin. Int J Vitam Nutr Res 1994;63:270–74.
11. Warnock L, Prudhonme C, Wagner C. The determination of thiamin pyrophosphate in blood and other tissues, and its correlation with erythrocyte transketolase activity. J Nutr 1979;108:421–27.
12. Bayliss R, Brookes R, McCulloch J, Kuyl J, Metz J. Urinary thiamine excretion after oral physiological doses of the vitamin. Internl J Vitam Nutr Res 1984;54:161–64.

RIBOFLAVIN (VITAMIN B_2)

Riboflavin consists of flavin (isoalloxazine ring), to which is attached a ribitol (sugar alcohol) side chain. The structures of riboflavin and its two coenzyme

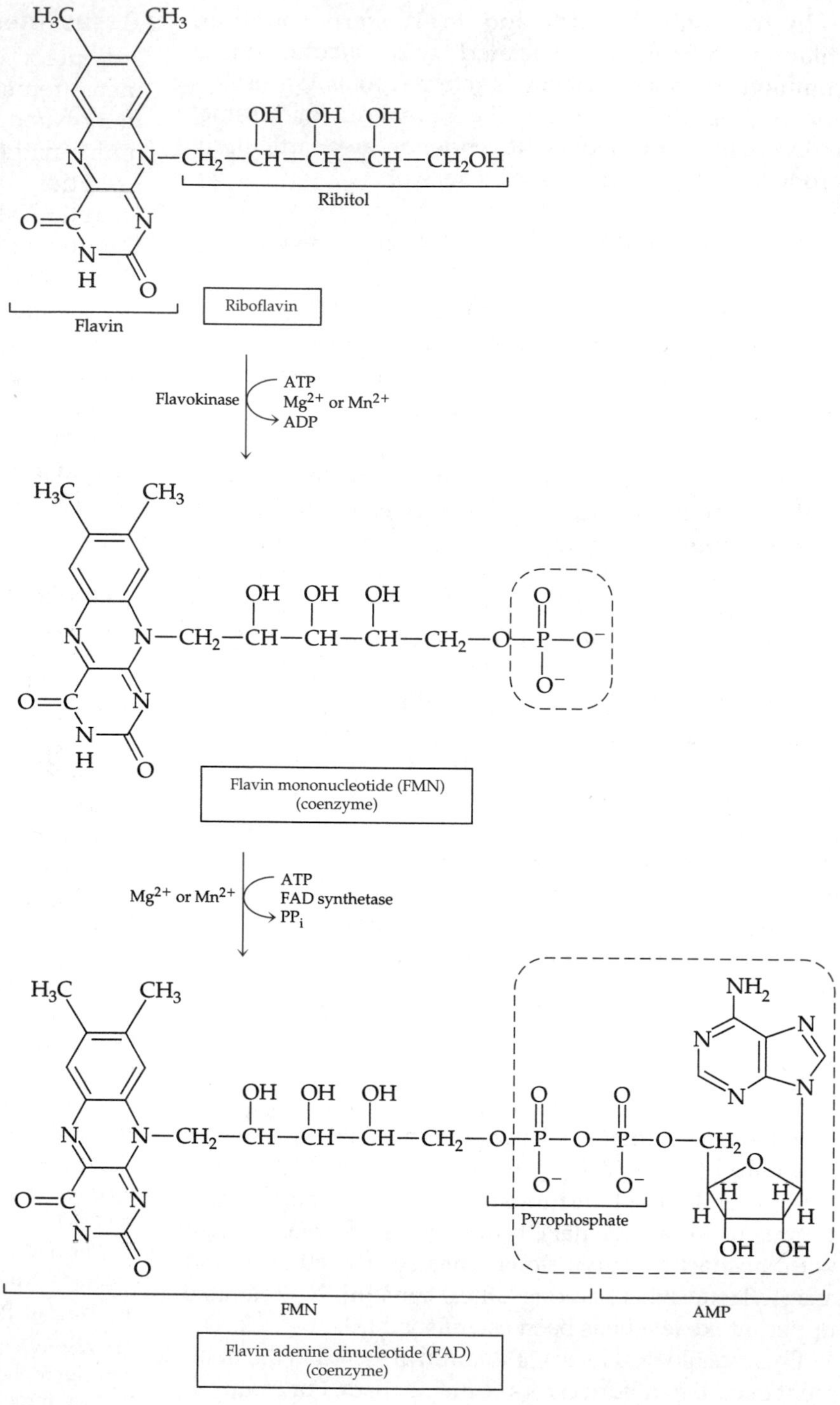

Figure 9.14 Structures of riboflavin and its coenzyme forms.

derivatives, FMN (flavin mononucleotide) and FAD (flavin adenine dinucleotide), are given in Figure 9.14.

Sources

Riboflavin is found in a wide variety of foods, but especially those of animal origin. Milk and milk products such as cheeses are thought to contribute the majority of dietary riboflavin. Eggs, meat, and legumes also provide riboflavin in significant quantities. Green vegetables provide fairly good riboflavin content. Fruits and cereal grains are minor contributors of dietary riboflavin.

The form of riboflavin in food varies. Free or protein-bound riboflavin is found in milk, eggs, and enriched breads and cereals. In most other foods the vitamin occurs as one or the other of its coenzyme derivatives, FMN or FAD, although phosphorus-bound riboflavin is also found in some foods.

Digestion, Absorption, Transport, and Storage

Riboflavin attached noncovalently to proteins may be freed by the action of hydrochloric acid secreted within the stomach and by gastric and intestinal enzymatic hydrolysis of the protein. Riboflavin in foods as FAD, FMN, and riboflavin phosphate must also be freed prior to absorption. Within the intestinal lumen, FAD pyrophosphatase converts FAD to FMN; FMN in turn is converted to free riboflavin by FMN phosphatase.

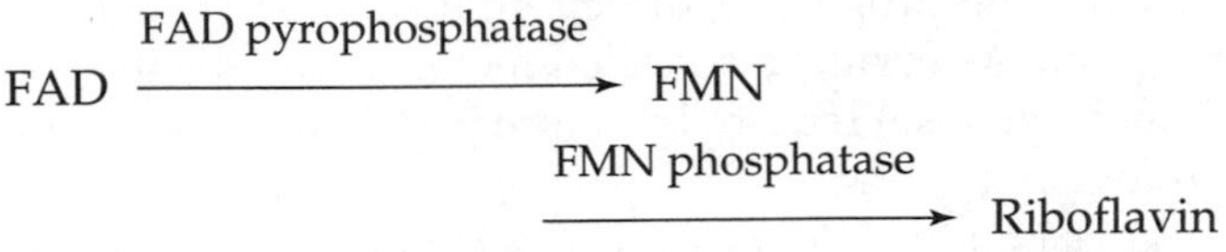

Other intestinal phosphatases, such as nucleotide diphosphatase and alkaline phosphatase, may also hydrolyze riboflavin from riboflavin phosphate.

Not all bound riboflavin is hydrolyzed and available for absorption. A small amount (~7%) of FAD is covalently bound to either of two amino acids, histidine or cysteine. For example, following consumption of foods containing succinate dehydrogenase or monoamine oxidase, these proteins are degraded; however, the riboflavin remains bound, typically to histidine or cysteine residues, and cannot function in the body [1]. Should absorption of the histidine- and cysteine-bound riboflavin occur, the complex is excreted unchanged in the urine.

Generally, animal sources of riboflavin are thought to be better absorbed than plant sources. Divalent metals such as copper, zinc, iron, and manganese have been shown to chelate riboflavin and FMN and to inhibit riboflavin absorption. Ingestion of alcohol also impairs riboflavin digestion and absorption [2].

Free riboflavin is absorbed via a saturable, energy-dependent carrier mechanism primarily in the proximal small intestine [3]. When large amounts of the vitamin are ingested, riboflavin may be absorbed by diffusion. Absorption rate is proportional to dose. About 95% of riboflavin intake from foods is absorbed, up to a maximum of about 25 mg [1,4]. Peak concentrations of the vitamin in the plasma correlate with intakes of 15 to 20 mg [5].

On absorption into the mucosal cells, riboflavin is phosphorylated to form FMN, a reaction catalyzed by flavokinase and requiring ATP, as shown here and in Figure 9.14.

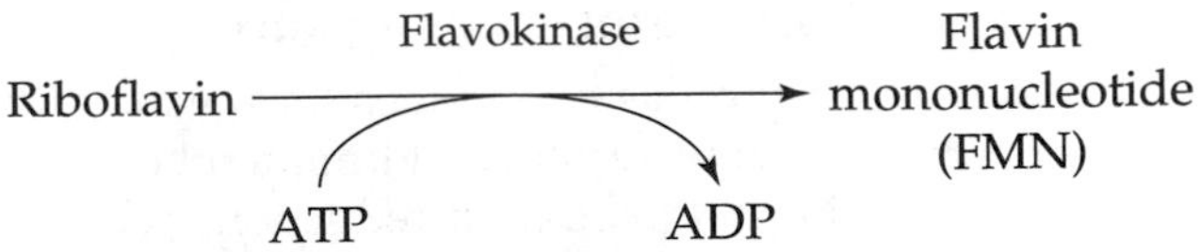

At the serosal surface, most of the FMN is probably dephosphorylated to riboflavin, which enters the portal system. The vitamin is carried to the liver, where it is converted again to FMN by flavokinase and to its other coenzyme derivative, FAD, by FAD synthetase (Fig. 9.14). FAD is the predominant flavoenzyme in tissues.

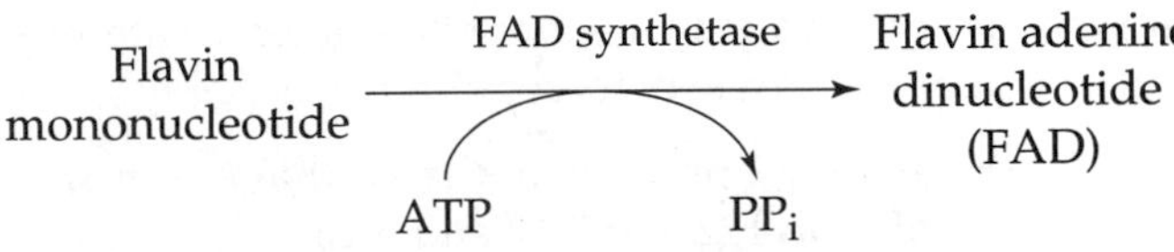

Most flavins in systemic plasma are found as riboflavin rather than as one of its coenzyme forms, although all three may be present. Riboflavin, FMN, and FAD are transported in the plasma by a variety of proteins, including albumin, fibrinogen, and globulins (principally immunoglobulins) [6]. Albumin appears to be the primary transport protein.

Regardless of the form in which the vitamin reaches the tissues, it is free riboflavin that traverses most cell membranes by a carrier-mediated process. An exception to this is riboflavin uptake by the brain, which is thought to occur by a high-affinity transport system for riboflavin as its coenzyme FAD.

Riboflavin is found in small quantities in a variety of tissues. The greatest concentrations of riboflavin are found in the liver, kidney, and heart.

While it is free riboflavin that is transported into and out of cells, within cells riboflavin is typically converted to its coenzyme forms by flavokinase and FAD synthetase, both of which are widely distributed in tissues [7]. Synthesis of FMN and FAD appears to be under hormonal regulation. Hormones shown to be particularly important in this regulation are ACTH, aldosterone, and the thyroid hormones, all of which accelerate the conversion of riboflavin into its coenzyme forms, apparently by increasing the activity of flavokinase [8,9]. Synthesis of the coenzymes is also regulated by product inhibition in the case of FAD synthesis [10]. Following synthesis of the flavin coenzymes, the coenzyme forms of the vitamin become bound to apoenzymes. FMN and FAD function as prosthetic groups for enzymes involved in oxidation-reduction reactions. These enzymes are referred to as flavoproteins.

Functions and Mechanisms of Action

FMN and FAD function as coenzymes for a wide variety of oxidative enzyme systems and remain bound to the enzymes during the oxidation-reduction reactions. Flavins can act as oxidizing agents because of their ability to accept a pair of hydrogen atoms. The isoalloxazine ring is reduced by two successive one-electron transfers with the intermediate formation of a semiquinone free radical, as shown in Figure 9.15. Reduction of the isoalloxazine ring yields the reduced forms of the flavoprotein, which can be found in $FMNH_2$ and $FADH_2$.

Flavoproteins

Flavoproteins exhibit a wide range of redox potentials and therefore can play a wide variety of roles in intermediary metabolism. Some of these roles are discussed here.

- The role of flavoproteins in the *electron transport chain* is provided in Figures 3.12 and 3.16.
- In the *oxidative decarboxylation of pyruvate* (Fig. 9.12) and α-ketoglutarate, FAD serves as an intermediate electron carrier, with NADH being the final reduced product.
- *Succinate dehydrogenase* is an FAD flavoprotein that removes electrons from succinate to form fumarate and that forms $FADH_2$ from FAD (Fig. 9.11). The electrons are then passed into the electron transport chain via coenzyme Q (Fig. 3.12).
- In fatty acid oxidation, *fatty acyl CoA* dehydrogenase requires FAD (Fig 6.24).
- *Sphinganine oxidase,* in sphingosine synthesis, requires FAD.
- As a coenzyme for an oxidase such as *xanthine oxidase,* FAD transfers electrons directly to oxygen with the formation of hydrogen peroxide. Xanthine oxidase, which contains both iron and molybdenum, is necessary for purine catabolism in the liver. The enzyme converts hypoxanthine to xanthine and then xanthine to uric acid (see Fig. 7.18; also see molybdenum, Chap. 12).
- Similarly, *aldehyde oxidase* using FAD converts aldehydes, such as pyridoxal (vitamin B_6) to pyridoxic acid, an excretory product, and retinal (vitamin A) to retinoic acid (Fig. 10.4), while also passing electrons to oxygen and generating hydrogen peroxide.
- Also in vitamin B_6 metabolism (Fig. 9.39), *pyridoxine phosphate oxidase*—which converts pyridoxamine phosphate (PMP) and pyridoxine phosphate (PNP) to pyridoxal phosphate (PLP), the primary coenzyme form of vitamin B_6—is dependent on FMN.
- Synthesis of an *active form of folate,* 5-methyl THF, requires $FADH_2$ (Fig. 9.31).
- A step in *the synthesis of niacin from tryptophan* that is catalyzed by kynureninase monooxygenase requires FAD (Fig. 9.18).
- In *choline catabolism,* several enzymes (such as choline dehydrogenase, dimethylglycine dehydrogenase, and sarcosine, also called monomethylglycine dehydrogenase) require FAD (see p. 305 in the section on folate).
- *Thioredoxin reductase* is a flavo(FAD)enzyme that contains selenocysteine at its active site and functions to transfer reducing equivalents from NADPH through its bound FAD to reduce disulfide bonds within the oxidized form of thioredoxin (see also selenium, Chap. 12).
- Some neurotransmitters (such as dopamine) and other amines (tyramine and histamine) require FAD-dependent *monoamine oxidase* for metabolism.
- Reduction of the oxidized form of glutathione (GSSG) to its reduced form (GSH) is also dependent on FAD-dependent *glutathione reductase.* This reaction forms the basis of one assay used to assess riboflavin status (see the section "Assessment of Nutriture").

Metabolism and Excretion

Riboflavin and its metabolites are excreted primarily in the urine, with only small amounts lost via the feces. Fecal riboflavin metabolites may also arise from the metabolism of riboflavin by intestinal flora [1]. It is believed that some of these metabolites formed in the intestinal tract by bacteria also can be absorbed but then are excreted in the urine [1].

Figure 9.15 Oxidation and reduction of isoalloxazine ring.

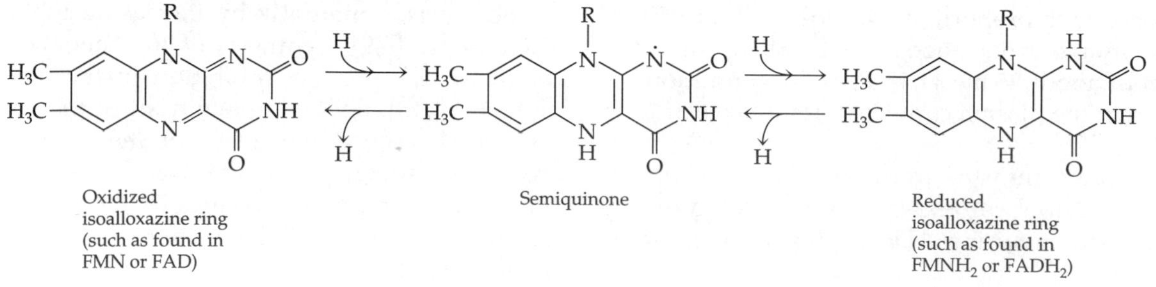

The riboflavin that is not bound to proteins in the plasma is filtered by the glomerulus and excreted. Most riboflavin (~60%–70%) is excreted intact in the urine. Metabolites arise from tissue degradation of covalently bound flavins as well as from degradation of the vitamin. Metabolites present in the greatest concentrations in the urine include 7-α- and 8-α-hydroxymethyl riboflavin, 8-α-sulfonyl riboflavin, 10-hydroxyethyl flavin, and riboflavinyl peptide ester. Riboflavin bound to cysteine and histidine is also found in the urine if absorbed in such form from the gastrointestinal tract or if generated in body cells from the degradation of flavoenzymes such as succinate dehydrogenase and monoamine oxidase [1].

Urinary excretion of riboflavin may be noticeable a couple of hours following oral ingestion of the vitamin. Riboflavin is a fluorescent yellow compound. Thus, following riboflavin intake in a quantity such as 1.7 mg (similar to that found in a vitamin pill), a color change of the urine occurs whereby the urine will deepen in color from a typical light yellow to a brighter orangish yellow.

Recommended Dietary Allowances

The RDAs for riboflavin have been estimated through various studies involving urinary excretion of riboflavin, the relationship of dietary intake to clinical signs of deficiency, and the activity of erythrocyte glutathione reductase. The latest (1998) recommendations for riboflavin are similar to the 1989 RDA, which, for adults, suggested a minimum intake of 1.2 mg for persons whose caloric intake may be <2,000 kcal [11]. The current RDAs for riboflavin for adult men and women are 1.3 and 1.1 mg/day, respectively; the estimated average requirements for adult men and women are 1.1 and 0.9 mg, respectively [1]. With pregnancy and lactation, recommendations for daily riboflavin intake increase to 1.4 and 1.6 mg, respectively [1]. The inside covers of the book provide additional RDAs for riboflavin for other age groups.

Deficiency: Ariboflavinosis

A deficiency of riboflavin, known as ariboflavinosis, rarely occurs in isolation but most often is accompanied by other nutrient deficits. No clear riboflavin deficiency disease has been characterized; however, clinical symptoms of deficiency after almost 4 months of inadequate intake include lesions on the outside of the lips (cheilosis) and corners of the mouth (angular stomatitis), inflammation of the tongue (glossitis), redness or bloody (hyperemia) and swollen (edema) mouth/oral cavity, an inflammatory skin condition seborrheic dermatitis, anemia, and peripheral nerve dysfunction (neuropathy), among other signs. Severe deficiency of riboflavin may diminish the synthesis of the coenzyme form of vitamin B_6 and the synthesis of niacin (NAD) from tryptophan.

Because of limited dietary intake, people with congenital heart disease, some cancers, and excess alcohol intake may develop deficiency. The deficiency condition also remains fairly common in developing countries such as India [12]. Riboflavin metabolism is altered with thyroid disease. Excretion of riboflavin is enhanced with diabetes mellitus, trauma, and stress. Women on oral contraceptives are more likely to develop deficiency than women not taking these drugs.

Toxicity

Toxicity associated with large oral doses of riboflavin has not been reported, and no tolerable upper intake level for riboflavin has been established [1]. Trials have shown use of large amounts (400 mg) of the vitamin to be effective in the treatment of migraine headaches without side effects [13,14].

Assessment of Nutriture

The most sensitive method for determining riboflavin nutriture is the measurement of the activity of erythrocyte glutathione reductase, an enzyme requiring FAD as a coenzyme. The method is based on the following reaction:

$$\text{NADPH} + \text{H}^+ + \text{GSSG} \xrightarrow{\text{Glutathione reductase–FAD}} \text{NADP}^+ + 2\,\text{GSH}$$

Glutathione in its oxidized form is designated GSSG, and in its reduced form GSH. In cases of a riboflavin deficiency or marginal riboflavin status, the activity of glutathione reductase is limited, and less NADPH is used to reduce the oxidized glutathione. In vitro enzyme activity in terms of "activity coefficients" (AC) is determined both with and without the addition of FAD to the medium. Activity coefficients represent a ratio of the enzyme's activity with FAD to the enzyme's activity without FAD. When addition of FAD stimulates enzyme activity to generate an AC of 1.2 to 1.4, riboflavin status is considered low; an AC > 1.4 suggests riboflavin deficiency.

Cellular riboflavin concentrations and urinary riboflavin excretion also are used to assess status. Cellular riboflavin concentrations <10 μg/dL and urinary riboflavin excretion <19 μg/g creatinine (without recent riboflavin intake) are indicative of deficiency.

References Cited for Riboflavin

1. Food and Nutrition Board. Dietary Reference Intakes for Thiamin, Riboflavin, Niacin, Vitamin B_6, Folate, Vitamin B_{12}, Pantothenic Acid, Biotin, and Choline. Washington, DC: National Academy Press, 1998, pp. 87–122.

2. Pinto J, Huang Y, Rivlin R. Mechanisms underlying the differential effects of ethanol upon the bioavailability of riboflavin and flavin adenine dinucleotide. J Clin Invest 1987;79:1343–48.

3. Said H, Ma T. Mechanism of riboflavin uptake by Caco-2 human intestinal epithelial cells. Am J Physiol 1994;266:G15–21.

4. Zempleni J, Galloway J, McCormick D. Pharmacokinetics of orally and intravenously administered riboflavin in healthy humans. Am J Clin Nutr 1996;63:54–66.

5. Bender D. Nutritional Biochemistry of the Vitamins. New York: Cambridge University Press, 1992, pp. 156–83.

6. White H, Merrill A. Riboflavin-binding proteins. Ann Rev Nutr 1988; 8:279–99.

7. Merrill A, Lambeth J, Edmondson D, McCormick D. Formation and mode of action of flavoproteins. Ann Rev Nutr 1981;1:281–317.

8. Lee S, McCormick D. Thyroid hormone regulation of flavocoenzyme biosynthesis. Arch Biochem Biophys 1985;237:197–201.

9. Rivlin R. Hormones, drugs, and riboflavin. Nutr Rev 1979; 37:241–45.

10. Yamada Y, Merrill A, McCormick D. Probable reaction mechanisms of flavokinase and FAD synthetase from rat liver. Arch Biochem Biophys 1990;278:125–30.

11. National Research Council. Recommended Dietary Allowances, 10th ed. Washington, DC: National Academy Press, 1989, pp. 132–37.

12. Lakshmi A. Riboflavin metabolism—relevance to human metabolism. Ind J Med Res 1998;108:182–90.

13. Schoenen J, Lenaerts M, Basting E. High-dose riboflavin as a prophylactic treatment of migraine: results of an open pilot study. Cephalalgia 1994;14:328–29.

14. Schoenen J, Jacquy J, Lenaerts M. Effectiveness of high-dose riboflavin in migraine prophylaxis. A randomized controlled trial. Neurology 1998;50:466–70.

NIACIN (VITAMIN B_3)

The term *niacin* (vitamin B_3) is considered a generic term for nicotinic acid and nicotinamide (also called niacinamide). The vitamin was once referred to as the anti–black tongue factor in dogs. The vitamin activity of niacin is provided by both nicotinic acid and nicotinamide. Structurally, nicotinic acid is pyridine 3-carboxylic acid, while nicotinamide is nicotinic acid amide (Fig. 9.16).

Sources

The best sources of niacin include fish such as tuna and halibut, and meats such as beef, chicken, turkey, and pork, among others. Enriched cereals and bread products, whole grains, fortified cereals, seeds, and legumes also contain appreciable amounts of niacin. Niacin is also found in coffee and tea, and in lesser amounts in green vegetables and milk. In supplements, niacin is generally found as nicotinamide (niacinamide).

Figure 9.16 Nicotinic acid and nicotinamide.

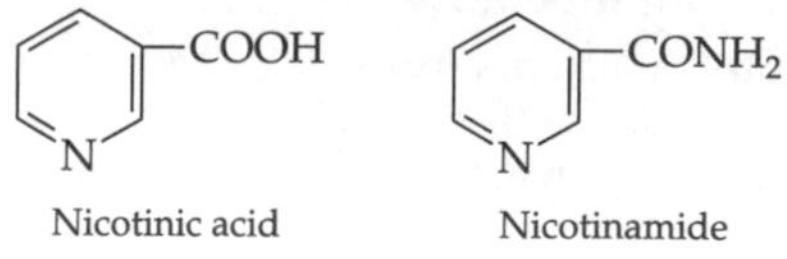

In animals, niacin occurs mainly as the nicotinamide nucleotides, that is, nicotinamide adenine dinucleotide (NAD) and nicotinamide adenine dinucleotide phosphate (NADP). However, following the slaughter of animals, NAD and NADP are thought to undergo hydrolysis; thus, meats provide niacin as free nicotinamide. Figure 9.17 shows the structures of NAD and NADP. In their oxidized forms, NAD and NADP possess a positive charge and therefore may alternatively be written NAD^+ and $NADP^+$.

In some foods, niacin may be bound covalently to complex carbohydrates and called niacytin, or it may be bound to small peptides and called niacinogens. This bound form of niacin is found primarily in corn but also in wheat and some other cereal products. Chemical treatment with bases such as lime water can improve availability of some bound niacin. Some niacin also may be released from niacytin on exposure to gastric acid. However, only about 10% of the niacin from maize is thought to be available for absorption.

In addition to dietary sources of niacin, NAD may be synthesized in the liver from the amino acid tryptophan.

Figure 9.17 The structures of NAD and NADP.

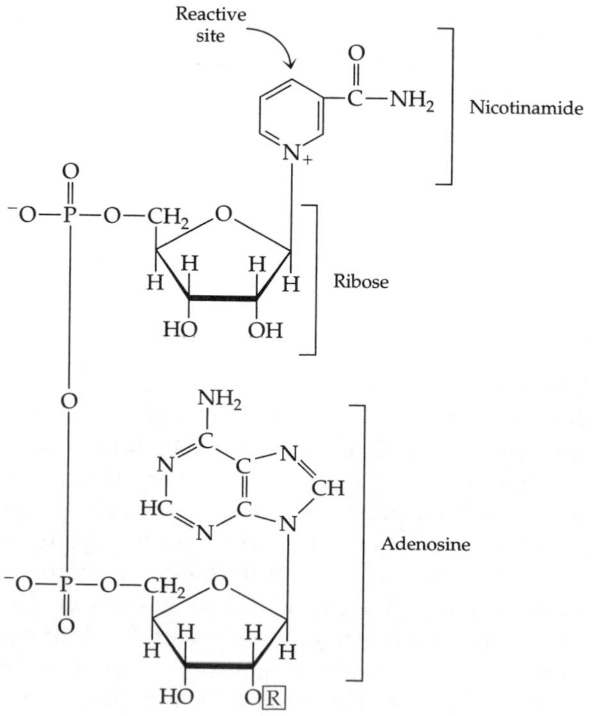

R = H for NAD^+ nicotinamide adenine dinucleotide

R = PO_3^{-2} for $NADP^+$ nicotinamide adenine dinucleotide phosphate

This biosynthetic pathway, which provides an important contribution to the niacin needs of the body, is depicted in Figure 9.18. Only about 3% of the tryptophan that is metabolized follows the pathway to NAD synthesis. It is estimated that 1 mg niacin is produced from the ingestion of 60 mg dietary tryptophan (see the RDA section for niacin to understand how this synthesis is accounted for in niacin recommendations). Riboflavin (FAD), vitamin B_6 (PLP), and iron are required in some of the reactions involved in the conversion of tryptophan to NAD. In fact, deficiency of these nutrients, along with other dietary factors such as poor tryptophan and energy intakes, can impair NAD synthesis.

Digestion, Absorption, Transport, and Storage

NAD and NADP may be hydrolyzed within the intestinal tract or enterocyte by glycohydrolase to release free nicotinamide. A pyrophosphatase also is involved in phosphate hydrolysis.

$$\text{NAD and NADP} \xrightarrow{\text{Glycohydrolase}} \text{Nicotinamide}$$

Nicotinamide and nicotinic acid can be absorbed in the stomach, but they are more readily absorbed in the small intestine [1].

The absorption of niacin in the small intestine occurs primarily by a sodium-dependent, saturable system. Concentration of the vitamin in the lumen of the intestine, however, appears to determine its mode of absorption. At low concentrations niacin is absorbed via sodium-dependent, carrier-mediated (facilitated) diffusion, while at high concentrations (as with 3–4 g pharmacological doses) it is absorbed almost completely by passive diffusion.

In the plasma, niacin is found primarily as nicotinamide, but nicotinic acid also may be found. Up to about one-third of nicotinic acid in the plasma is bound to plasma proteins. From the blood, nicotinamide and nicotinic acid move across cell membranes

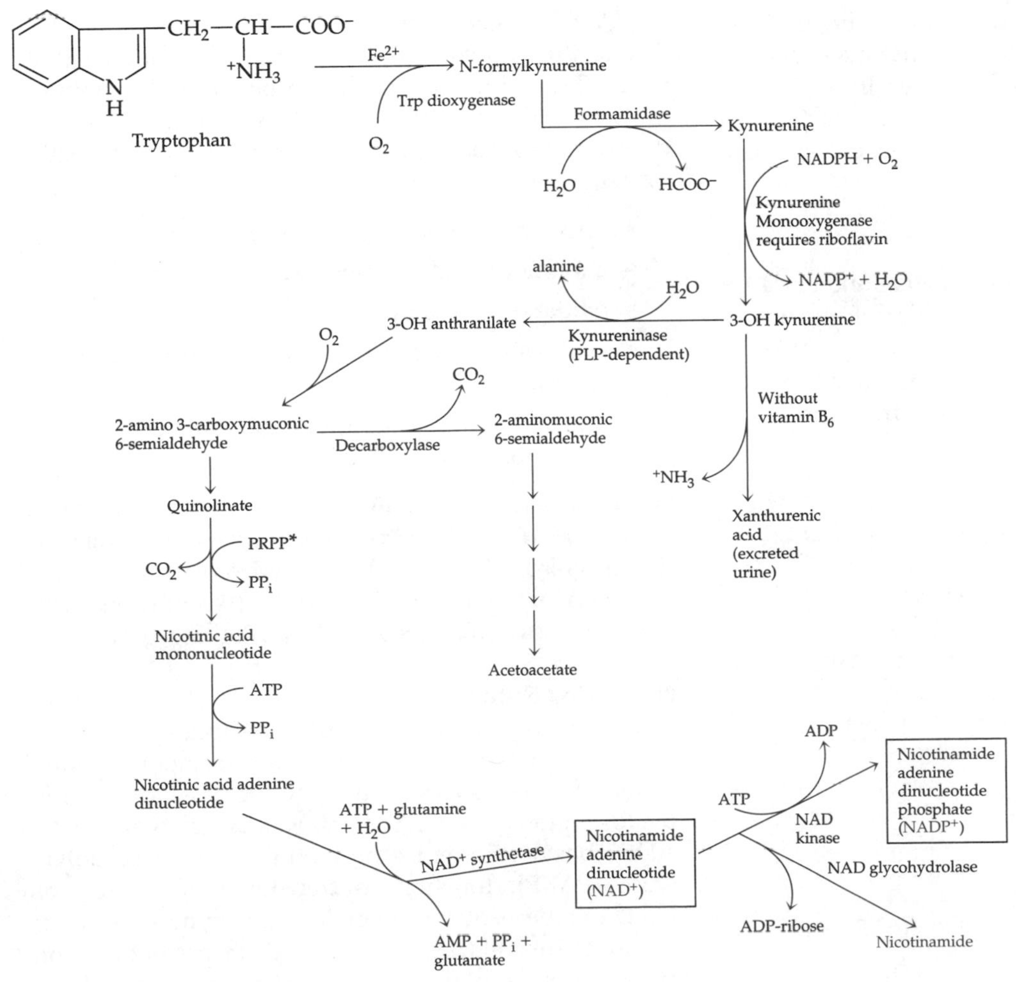

*PRPP = 5-phosphoribosyl pyrophosphate

Figure 9.18 NAD^+ and $NADP^+$ synthesis from tryptophan.

by simple diffusion; however, nicotinic acid transport into the kidney tubules and red blood cells requires a carrier.

Nicotinamide serves as the primary precursor of NAD, which is synthesized in all tissues. In the liver, NAD synthesis from nicotinamide appears to be influenced by various hormones. However, nicotinic acid in the liver also may be used to synthesize NAD.

As NAD or NADP, the vitamin is trapped within the cell. Intracellular concentrations of NAD typically predominate over those of NADP. In the liver, excess niacin and tryptophan are converted to NAD, which is stored in small amounts not bound to enzymes. NAD may be degraded to yield nicotinamide, which then is available for transport to other tissues. It is primarily as NAD and NADP that niacin functions in the body. NAD is found primarily in its oxidized form (NAD), while NADP is found in cells mainly in its reduced form (NADPH).

Functions and Mechanisms of Action

Approximately 200 enzymes, primarily dehydrogenases, require the coenzymes NAD and NADP, which act as a hydrogen donor or electron acceptor. Figure 9.19 demonstrates the oxidation-reduction that may occur in the nicotinamide moiety of the coenzymes. In addition to its coenzyme roles, niacin functions as a substrate in nonredox roles as a donor of adenosine diphosphate ribose (ADP-ribose).

Coenzymes

Although NAD and NADP are very similar and undergo reversible reduction in the same way, their functions in the cell are quite different. The major role of NADH, formed from NAD, is to transfer its electrons from metabolic intermediates through the electron transport chain (Fig. 3.16), thereby producing adenosine triphosphate (ATP). NADPH, in contrast, acts as a reducing agent in many biosynthetic pathways such as fatty acid, cholesterol, and steroid hormone synthesis and also in other pathways. NAD and NADP coenzymes are tightly bound to their apoenzymes and can easily transport hydrogen atoms from one part of the cell to another. Reactions in which they participate occur both in the mitochondria and in the cytoplasm.

Figure 9.19 (a) The oxidation and reduction in the nicotinamide moiety. (b) The role of NAD in dehydrogenation reactions. One H of the substrate goes to NAD.

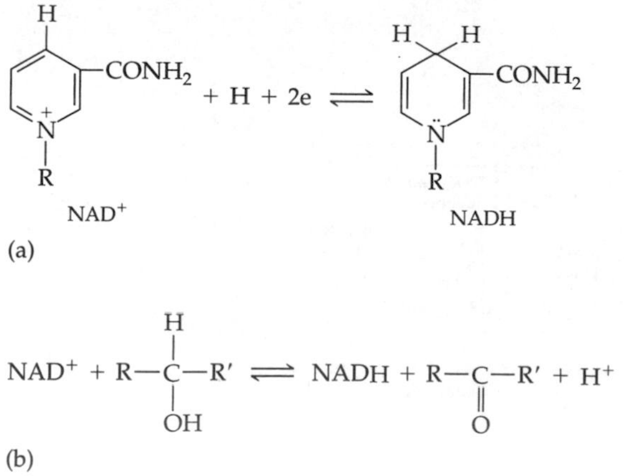

Oxidative reactions in which NAD participates and is reduced to NADH include

- glycolysis (Fig. 4.14),
- oxidative decarboxylation of pyruvate (Fig. 9.12),
- oxidation of acetyl CoA via the Krebs cycle (Fig. 4.15),
- β-oxidation of fatty acids (Fig. 6.24), and
- oxidation of ethanol (Fig. 4.23).

NAD is also required by aldehyde dehydrogenase for catabolism of vitamin B_6 as pyridoxal to its excretory product, pyridoxic acid.

NADPH is generated from NADP by reduction. This reaction occurs as part of the hexosemonophosphate shunt (Fig. 4.19) and via the mitochondrial membrane malate pyruvate shuttle (Fig. 4.18). The NADPH produced in these reactions is used in a variety of reductive biosyntheses, including

- fatty acid synthesis (Fig. 6.30),
- cholesterol and steroid hormone synthesis,
- oxidation of glutamate (Fig. 7.32),
- synthesis of deoxyribonucleotides (precursors of DNA), and
- regeneration of glutathione, vitamin C, and thioredoxin (pp. 285, 269, and 460).

Several reactions in folate metabolism also are dependent on NADPH. For example, conversion of folate to dihydrofolate (DHF) and tetrahydrofolate (THF) and synthesis of 5-methyl THF and 5,10-methylene THF, active forms of folate, require NADPH (Fig. 9.31).

Nonredox Roles

NAD acts as a donor of adenosine diphosphate ribose (ADP-ribose) (Fig. 9.18) for the posttranslational modification of proteins as well as a donor of ADP-ribose for the formation of cyclic ADP-ribose. Two enzymes, mono ADP-ribosyl transferase and poly ADP-ribose polymerase (PARP), function to transfer ADP-ribose from NAD to an acceptor protein. These enzymes attach one (*mono*) or several (*poly*, > 200) ADP-riboses onto various chromosomal proteins, including both histone and nonhistone proteins. The proteins are thought to function in the nucleus in DNA repair and replication as well as in cell differentiation [2,3]. Cylic ADP-ribose, generated by NAD glycohydrolases, is thought to function in certain cells as a second messenger involved in control of ryanodine receptors and in mobilization of calcium from intracellular stores [4–6].

Another possible nonredox function of niacin is as a suspected component of glucose tolerance factor (GTF). The exact function of niacin in GTF is not clear; however, GTF is thought to potentiate the action of insulin (see chromium, Chap. 12 and Fig. 12.18).

Metabolism and Excretion

NAD, generated from nicotinamide or produced in the liver from tryptophan, and NADP can be degraded by glycohydrolase into nicotinamide and ADP-ribose (Fig. 9.18). The released nicotinamide is methylated and is then oxidized in the liver into a variety of products that are excreted in the urine. There is typically little excretion of nicotinic acid or nicotinamide because both compounds may be actively reabsorbed from glomerular filtrate.

The primary metabolites of nicotinamide are N′ methyl nicotinamide (sometimes abbreviated NMN and representing ~20% to 30% of niacin metabolites) and N′ methyl 2-pyridone 5-carboxamide (also called 2-pyridone and representing ~40% to 60%). Small amounts of N′ methyl 4-pyridone carboxamide (referred to as 4-pyridone) also may be present. Nicotinic acid is metabolized mainly to N′ methylnicotinic acid.

Recommended Dietary Allowances

Recommendations for niacin intake include calculations of niacin derived from the amino acid tryptophan, with 60 mg of tryptophan thought to generate 1 mg of niacin. Total niacin thus is provided to the body as nicotinic acid and nicotinamide and from 1/60 mg of tryptophan. The term *niacin equivalent* (NE) is used to account for the provision by tryptophan.

Although recommendations are given in niacin equivalents, food composition tables report only preformed niacin. A rough estimate of niacin equivalents from a protein can be made by assuming that 10 mg of tryptophan are provided for every 1 g of high-quality (complete) protein in the diet; that is, 1 g of complete, high-quality protein = 10 mg of tryptophan. This means that an intake of 60 g of complete protein, for example, would provide 600 mg of tryptophan: 10 mg of tryptophan/1 g of protein × 60 g of protein = 600 mg of tryptophan. Then, because it takes 60 mg of tryptophan to generate 1 mg of NE, 60 g of protein would generate about 10 NEs: 600 mg of tryptophan × 1 mg of NE/60 mg of tryptophan = 10 NEs. The average U.S. diet usually contains about 900 mg of tryptophan daily [7].

Information used in estimating niacin requirements and recommendations has come from several studies, including human depletion and repletion studies as well as other studies with primarily urinary metabolites of niacin serving as indicators to base requirements and recommendations. The RDAs for individual intake of niacin (as niacin equivalents) for adult men and women are 16 and 14 mg/day, respectively [8]. Estimated requirements are 12 mg and 11 mg niacin for adult men and women, respectively. With pregnancy and lactation, the RDA for niacin increases to 18 and 17 mg niacin equivalents, respectively [8]. The inside covers of the book provide additional RDAs for niacin for other age groups.

Deficiency: Pellagra

Classical deficiency of niacin results in a condition known as **pellagra.** The four Ds—dermatitis, dementia, diarrhea, and death—are often used as a mnemonic device for remembering signs of pellagra [9]. The dermatitis is similar to sunburn at first and appears on areas exposed to sun, such as the face and neck, and on extremities such as the back of the hands, wrists, elbows, knees, and feet. Neurological manifestations include headache, apathy, loss of memory, peripheral neuritis, paralysis of extremities, and dementia or delirium. Gastrointestinal manifestations include glossitis, cheilosis, stomatitis, nausea, vomiting, and diarrhea or constipation. If untreated, death occurs.

A niacin deficiency or diminished niacin status also can result from the use of some medications and from some disorders such as malabsorptive conditions. The antituberculosis drug isoniazid, for example, binds with vitamin B_6 as PLP and thereby reduces PLP-dependent kynureninase activity required for niacin synthesis. Malabsorptive disorders (chronic diarrhea, inflammatory bowel diseases, some cancers) may impair niacin and tryptophan absorption and result in the increased likelihood of niacin deficiency. Hartnup disease results in impaired tryptophan absorption, thus decreasing concentrations of the precursor tryptophan needed for niacin synthesis. Individuals with poor nutrient intakes, such as those who consume excessive amounts of alcohol, are at risk for deficiency.

Toxicity

Large doses of nicotinic acid (up to 4 g/day, but given in divided doses such as 1 g four times a day) are used in the treatment of hypercholesterolemia (high blood cholesterol). These pharmacological doses have been shown to significantly lower total serum cholesterol and low-density lipoproteins (LDLs) and increase high-density lipoproteins (HDLs), although the mechanism of action is unclear [10].

Despite the therapeutic benefits of nicotinic acid, many undesirable side effects are associated with its use as a drug, especially in doses of 1 g or more per day and of (but not limited to) the time-released form of nicotinic acid. Some of these side effects include

- vasodilatory effects, mediated in part by release of histamine, including uncomfortable flushing and redness along with burning, itching (pruritus), tingling, and headaches;
- gastrointestinal problems such as heartburn, nausea, and possibly vomiting;
- liver injury (hepatic toxicity), indicated by elevated serum levels of enzymes of hepatic origin (e.g., transaminases and alkaline phosphatases), jaundice secondary to obstruction of normal bile flow from the liver to the small intestine, hepatitis, and liver failure;
- hyperuricemia and possibly gout due to competition of niacin with uric acid for excretion, thus raising serum uric acid levels; and
- elevation of plasma glucose concentrations (i.e., glucose intolerance) [10–16].

Nicotinamide in large doses does not exhibit toxic effects, but neither does it reduce blood lipids.

Because of the vasodilatory effects associated with nicotinic acid consumption from supplements, a tolerable upper intake level for adults for niacin (both nicotinic acid and nicotinamide) from supplements (including immediate, slow-release, and sustained-release forms) and from fortified foods [8] has been set at 35 mg/day. Use of nicotinic acid as a cholesterol-lowering agent must be weighed against its toxic effects for those using the vitamin to treat hyperlipidemia.

Assessment of Nutriture

Several methods have been employed to assess niacin status. Most methods involve the measurement of one or more urinary metabolites of the vitamin. Urinary excretion of <0.8 mg/day of N′ methyl nicotinamide is considered suggestive of niacin deficiency. Urinary excretion of <0.5 mg N′ methyl nicotinamide/1 g creatinine also has been suggested as indicative of poor (deficient) niacin status [17]. This ratio, however, has been criticized as being difficult to interpret due to multiple influences on urinary creatinine excretion. It usually is employed during a period of 4 to 5 hours after a 50-mg test dose of nicotinamide. Marginal niacin status is suggested by urinary amounts in the range of 0.5 to 1.59 mg N′ methyl nicotinamide/1 g creatinine, while levels in excess of 1.69 suggest adequate status [17]. Another ratio employed to assess niacin status is that of urinary N′ methyl 2-pyridone 5-carboxamide (2-pyridone) to N′ methyl nicotinamide (NMN). This ratio, however, is not thought to be sensitive enough to detect marginal intakes of niacin and may better reflect dietary protein adequacy as opposed to niacin status [18]. Ratios of other urinary metabolites, such as 6-pyridone to N′ methyl nicotinamide, are being investigated for possible use in niacin assessment [19].

In addition to measurement of urinary metabolites, erythrocyte NAD concentrations and the ratio of NAD to NADP (<1.0) have been used to assess niacin status [20,21]. Plasma concentrations of 2-pyridone have been shown to drop below the level of detection with low niacin intakes and thus may be used as an index of niacin status [20].

References Cited for Niacin

1. Bechgaard H, Jespersen S. GI absorption of niacin in humans. J Pharm Sci 1977;66:871–72.
2. Lautier D, Lagueux J, Thibodeau J, Menard L, Poirier G. Molecular and biochemical features of poly (ADP-ribose) metabolism. Mol Cell Biochem 1993;122:171–93.
3. Stierum R, Van Herwijnen M, Hageman G, Kleinjans J. Increased poly (ADP-ribose) polymerase activity during repair of (±) anti-benzo[a]pyrene diolepoxide-induced DNA damage in human peripheral blood lymphocytes in vitro. Carcinogenesis 1994;15:745–51.
4. Kim H, Jacobson E, Jacobson M. NAD glycohydrolases: a possible function in calcium homeostasis. Mol Cell Biochem 1994;138:237–43.
5. Adebanjo O, Anandatheerthavarada H, Koval A, et al. A new function for CD38/ADP-ribosyl cyclase in nuclear Ca^{2+} homeostasis. Nat Cell Biol 1999;1:409–14.
6. Lee H, Walseth T, Bratt G, Hayes R, Clapper D. Structural determination of a cyclic metabolite of NAD^+ with intracellular Ca^{2+} mobilizing activity. J Biol Chem 1989;264:1608–15.
7. Food and Nutrition Board. Dietary Reference Intakes for Energy, Carbohydrates, Fiber, Fat, Protein and Amino Acids. Washington, DC: National Academy Press, 2002.
8. Food and Nutrition Board. Dietary Reference Intakes for Thiamin, Riboflavin, Niacin, Vitamin B_6, Folate, Vitamin B_{12}, Pantothenic Acid, Biotin, and Choline. Washington, DC: National Academy Press, 1998, pp. 123–49.
9. Combs G. The Vitamins. San Diego, CA: Academic Press, 1992, pp. 289–309.
10. McKenney J, Proctor J, Harris S, Chinchili V. A comparison of the efficacy and toxic effects of sustained vs immediate release niacin in hypercholesterolemic patients. JAMA 1994;271:672–77.
11. Gibbons L, Gonzalez V, Gordon N, Gundy S. The prevalence of side effects with regular and sustained-release nicotinic acid. Am J Med 1995;99:378–85.
12. Gray D, Morgan T, Chretien S, Kashyap M. Efficacy and safety of controlled-release niacin in dyslipoproteinemic veterans. Ann Intern Med 1994;121:252–58.
13. Rader J, Calvert R, Hathcock J. Hepatic toxicity of unmodified and time-release preparations of niacin. Am J Med 1992;92:77–81.
14. Schwartz M. Severe reversible hyperglycemia as a consequence of niacin therapy. Arch Intern Med 1993;153:2050–52.
15. Alhadeff L, Gualtieri C, Lipton M. Toxic effects of water-soluble vitamins. Nutr Rev 1984;42:33–40.

16. Robinson A, Sloan H, Arnold G. Use of niacin in the prevention and management of hyperlipidemia. Prog Cardiovasc Nurs 2001;16:14–20.

17. Gibson RS. Principles of Nutrition Assessment. New York: Oxford University Press, 1990, pp. 437–44.

18. Shibata K, Matsuo H. Effect of supplementing low protein diets with the limiting amino acids on the excretion of N′ methylnicotinamide and its pyridones in the rat. J Nutr 1989;119:896–901.

19. Dillion J, Malfait P, Demaux G, Foldi-Hope C. Urinary metabolites of niacin during the course of pellagra. Ann Nutr Metab 1992;36:181–85.

20. Jacob R, Swendseid M, McKee R. Biochemical markers for assessment of niacin status in young men: urinary and blood levels of niacin metabolites. J Nutr 1989;119:591–98.

21. Fu C, Swendseid M, Jacob R, McKee R. Biochemical markers for assessment of niacin status in young men: levels of erythrocyte niacin coenzymes and plasma tryptophan. J Nutr 1989;119:1949–55.

PANTOTHENIC ACID

Pantothenic acid (pantothenate) consists of β-alanine and pantoic acid joined by a peptide bond/amide linkage. The structure of pantothenate is shown at the top of Figure 9.20 and as part of coenzyme A in Figure 9.21.

Sources

The Greek word *pantos* means "everywhere," and the vitamin pantothenic acid, as its name implies, is found widely distributed in nature. Because this vitamin is present in virtually all plant and animal foods, a deficiency is quite unlikely. Meats (particularly liver), egg yolk, legumes, whole-grain cereals, potatoes, mushrooms, broccoli, and avocados, among other foods, are good sources of the vitamin. Royal jelly from bees also provides large amounts of pantothenate. In supplements, pantothenate is usually found as calcium pantothenate or as panthenol, an alcohol form of the vitamin.

Digestion, Absorption, Transport, and Storage

Pantothenic acid occurs in foods in free and bound forms. About 85% of the pantothenic acid in food occurs bound as a component of coenzyme A, abbreviated CoA (Fig. 9.21). During the digestive process, CoA is hydrolyzed in several steps to pantetheine and then to pantothenic acid by phosphatases and pyrophosphatases.

Pantothenic acid is thought to be absorbed principally in the jejunum by passive diffusion when present in high concentrations and by a sodium-dependent active multivitamin carrier when present in low concentrations. Pantothenic acid shares a common intestinal multivitamin transporter/carrier with biotin (another B vitamin) and lipoic acid [1]. Approximately 40% to 61%, mean 50%, of the ingested pantothenic acid is absorbed [2,3]. Panthenol, the alcohol form of the vitamin used in multivitamins, is also absorbed and converted to pantothenate. However, pantothenate absorption has been shown to decrease to about 10% when pantothenate ingestion approaches 10 times the recommended intakes in pill form.

From the intestinal cell, pantothenate enters portal blood for transport to body cells. Pantothenic acid is found free in blood plasma/serum; however, higher concentrations are found intracellularly (specifically within red blood cells) than extracellularly (in plasma/serum) [4].

Uptake of pantothenate by tissues differs. The uptake of pantothenic acid by tissues such as the heart, muscle, brain, and liver cells occurs by sodium-dependent active transport, while uptake by other tissues occurs by facilitated diffusion [4–7]. Within cells, pantothenate along with 4-phosphopantothenate and pantetheine may be found. Most pantothenate is used to synthesize or resynthesize CoA [4], which is found in fairly high concentrations in the liver, adrenal gland, kidney, brain, and heart [5–7].

Functions and Mechanisms of Action

Pantothenic acid functions in the body as a component of CoA and 4′-phosphopantetheine. The synthesis of 4′-phosphopantetheine and CoA from pantothenate is depicted in Figure 9.20. Overall, the synthesis requires pantothenic acid, the amino acid cysteine, and ATP.

- The synthesis of coenzyme A starts with the rate-limiting phosphorylation of pantothenic acid by pantothenate kinase and the formation of 4′-phosphopantothenate. ATP and Mg^{2+} are required for this reaction.
- Next, in another ATP- and Mg^{2+}-requiring reaction, cysteine reacts with the 4′-phosphopantothenate. A peptide bond is formed between the carboxyl group of the 4′-phosphopantothenate and the amino group of cysteine.
- Third, a carboxyl group from the cysteine moiety is removed to generate 4′-phosphopantetheine.
- Next, an adenylation occurs whereby ATP reacts with the 4′-phosphopantetheine; adenosine monophosphate (AMP) is added to the 4′-phosphopantotheine to form dephosphocoenzyme A with the release of pyrophosphate.
- Last, phosphorylation with ATP of the 3′-hydroxyl group of the dephosphocoenzyme A produces CoA.

The synthesis of CoA is inhibited by acetyl CoA, malonyl CoA, and propionyl CoA as well as by other, longer-chain acyl CoAs. CoA metabolism has been

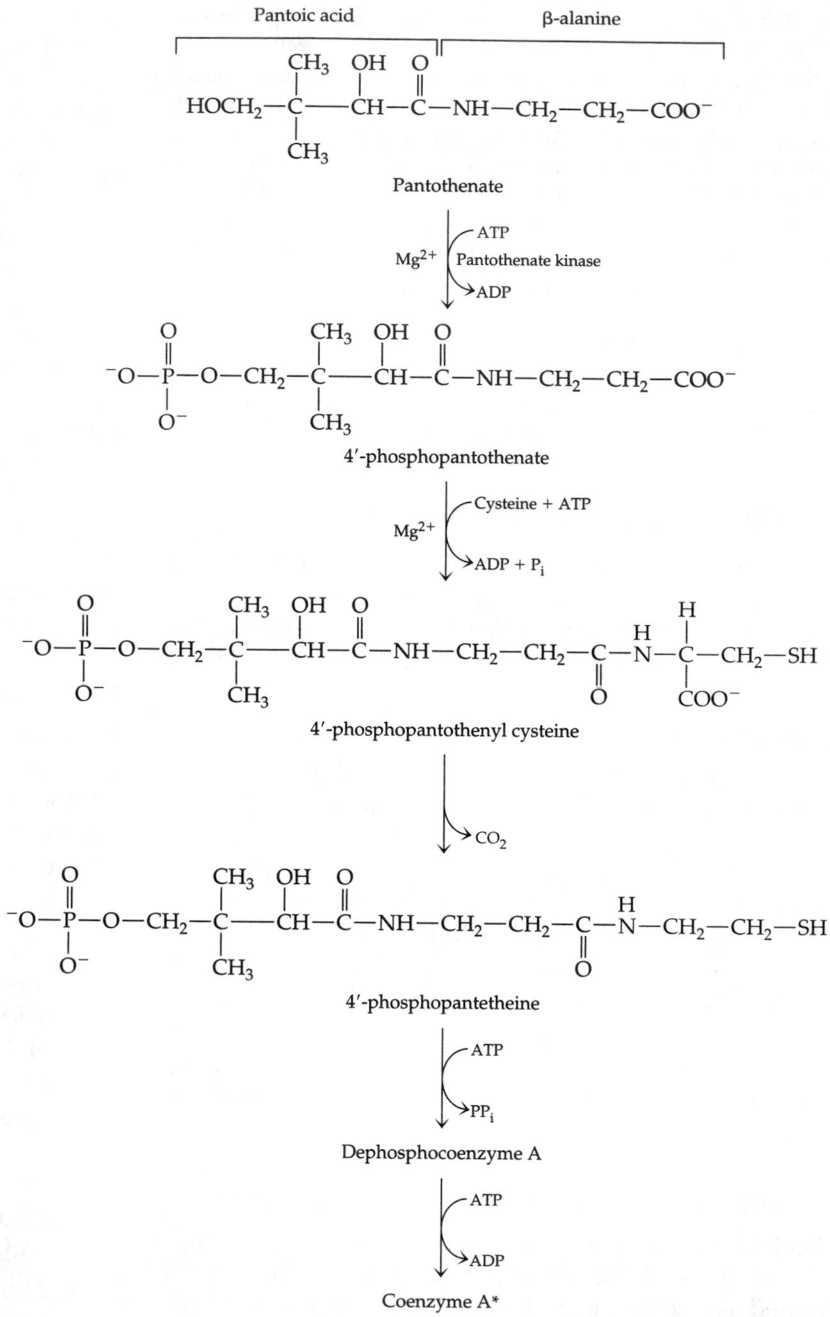

Figure 9.20 Synthesis of coenzyme A from pantothenate.

*Structure shown in Fig. 9.21

reviewed in depth by Robishaw and Neely [8]. Figure 9.21 shows the structure of CoA. Note from this figure that CoA contains several components, including phosphopantetheine and adenosine 3′,5′-bisphosphate. The figure also identifies the active site where CoA binds to acyl groups.

The compound 4′-phosphopantetheine, as part of the acyl carrier protein complex, and CoA function as carriers or transporters of acetyl and acyl groups. The vitamin forms thio esters ($-S-\overset{O}{\overset{\|}{C}}-R$) with carboxylic acids and can transfer the acetyl or acyl groups, typically 2 to 13 carbons, as needed for various cellular reactions. Examples of carboxylic acids carried by CoA include

- acetic (two carbons),
- malonic (three carbons),

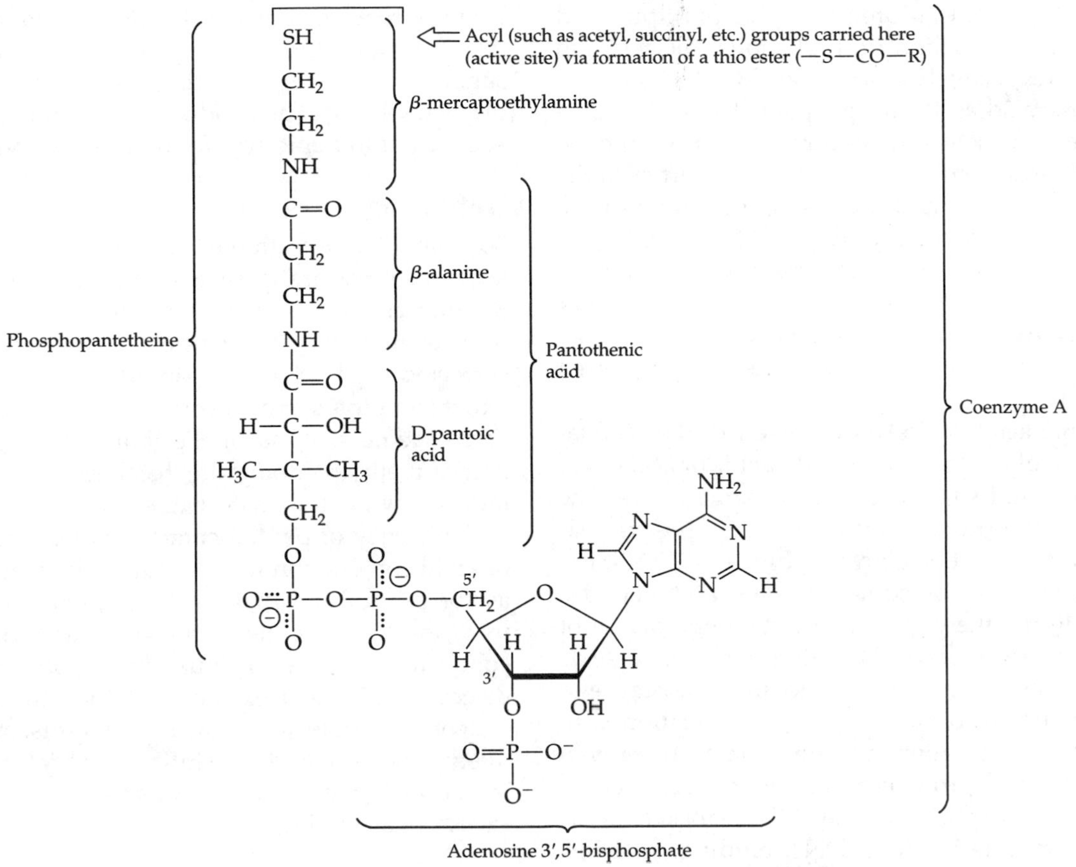

Figure 9.21 Structure of coenzyme A and identification of components.

- propionic (three carbons),
- methylmalonic (four carbons), and
- succinic (four carbons).

These carboxylic acids arise in the body during metabolism, and some can be obtained exogenously with the ingestion of food. For example, propionic acid is found naturally in some fish and also is derived from the catabolism of several amino acids, including methionine, threonine, valine, and isoleucine, and from the catabolism of odd-chain fatty acids. As another example, succinate is found as an intermediate in the Krebs cycle.

Pantothenic acid, as part of CoA and 4′-phosphopantetheine, participates extensively in nutrient metabolism, including degradation reactions resulting in energy production and synthetic reactions for the production of many vital compounds. In addition to its role in nutrient metabolism, CoA serves to acetylate nutrients including sugars and proteins among others. Some of the specific reactions and/or processes involving CoA and 4′-phosphopantetheine are presented next.

The metabolism of carbohydrate, lipids, and protein (energy-producing nutrients) relies to varying degrees on CoA. For example, a crucial reaction in nutrient metabolism is the conversion of pyruvate to acetyl CoA, which condenses with oxaloacetate to introduce acetate for oxidation via the Krebs cycle (Fig. 9.11). Acetyl CoA, the common compound formed from the three energy-producing nutrients, holds the central position in the transformation of energy. Pantothenic acid thus joins the B vitamins thiamin, riboflavin, and niacin in the oxidative decarboxylation of pyruvate (Fig. 9.11). These same vitamins also participate in the oxidative decarboxylation of α-ketoglutarate to succinyl CoA, which is involved in energy production as part of the Krebs cycle and also is involved with the amino acid glycine in the first step of heme synthesis (Fig. 12.5).

In lipid metabolism, CoA is important in the synthesis of cholesterol, bile salts, ketone bodies, fatty acids, and steroid hormones. For example, in cholesterol and ketone body synthesis, acetyl CoA and acetoacetyl CoA react to form the key intermediate HMG CoA (Fig. 6.34). Condensation of acetyl CoA with activated CO_2 to form malonyl CoA represents the first step in fatty acid synthesis (Fig. 6.28). Moreover, phospholipid and sphingomyelin production from phosphatidic acid and sphingosine, respectively, also use acyl CoA.

Pantothenic acid as 4′-phosphopantetheine also functions as the prosthetic group for acyl carrier protein (ACP). Acyl carrier protein acts as the acyl carrier in the synthesis of fatty acids and is a necessary component of the fatty acid synthase complex (Fig. 6.30). The sulfhydryl group in the 4′-phosphopantetheine and a sulfhydryl group in the protein are the active sites in the acyl carrier protein. These two groups are located close to each other so the acyl chain being synthesized can be transferred between them.

Pantothenic acid as CoA is involved in the acetylation (donation of the long-chain fatty acids or acetate) of some proteins and sugars as well as some drugs. The acetylation of the proteins by CoA occurs posttranslationally and in turn affects protein functions [9,10]. For example, acetylation of some proteins and peptides prolongs half-life, thereby delaying the degradation of the protein. Acetylation of the N-terminal amino acids of some proteins has been shown to affect resistance to ubiquitin-mediated proteolysis [9]. Acetylation also affects the activity, location, and function of the protein in cells [9,10]. Other proteins that may undergo acetylation include microtubules of the cell's cytoskeleton as well as histones and other DNA-binding proteins. Choline is acetylated to form the neurotransmitter acetylcholine. Also, aminosugars such as glucosamine and galactosamine are acetylated by CoA to form N-acetyl glucosamine and N-acetyl galactosamine, respectively. These acetylated aminosugars in turn may function structurally in the cell, for example, to provide recognition sites on cell surfaces or to direct proteins for membrane functions, among other functions.

A yet unidentified role of pantothenic acid, based on animal studies, involves healing. The vitamin appears to accelerate the normal healing process following surgery [11]. The exact mechanism by which pantothenate improves healing is unclear; however, an increase in cellular multiplication during the first postoperative period has been proposed [11].

Excretion

Pantothenate is excreted intact primarily in the urine, with only small amounts excreted via the feces. No metabolites of the vitamin have been identified in the urine or feces.

Adequate Intakes

The adequate intake (AI) recommendation for adults age 19 years and older for pantothenate has been set at 5 mg [3]. Adequate intake is used instead of RDA when insufficient data are available to establish an estimated average requirement (EAR) and subsequent RDA [3]. AIs for pantothenic acid of 6 and 7 mg/day are suggested for women during pregnancy and lactation, respectively [3]. The inside covers of this book provide AIs for pantothenic acid for other age groups.

Deficiency

"Burning feet syndrome," characterized by abnormal skin sensations of the feet and lower legs, exacerbated by warmth and diminished with cold, is thought to result from pantothenic acid deficiency. The syndrome can be corrected with calcium pantothenate administration. Other symptoms of deficiency include vomiting, fatigue, and weakness. A metabolic inhibitor of pantothenate, omega methylpantothenate, has been used in studies to induce low pantothenate status in humans.

Deficiency of pantothenate is thought to occur more often in conjunction with multiple nutrient deficiencies, as for example in malnutrition. Some conditions that may increase the need for the vitamin include alcoholism, diabetes mellitus, and inflammatory bowel diseases. Increased excretion of the vitamin has been shown in people with diabetes mellitus. Absorption is likely to be impaired with inflammatory bowel diseases. Intake of the vitamin typically is low in people with excessive alcohol intake.

Toxicity

Pantothenate toxicity has not been reported to date in humans. Intakes of about 10 g pantothenate as calcium pantothenate daily for up to 6 weeks have resulted in no problems [3]. However, intakes of up to 20 g have been associated with mild intestinal distress and diarrhea, and lower intakes of 100 mg may increase niacin excretion [3,12].

Assessment of Nutriture

Plasma pantothenic acid concentrations <100 mg/dL are thought to reflect low dietary pantothenate intakes; however, plasma concentrations do not correlate well with changes in dietary pantothenate intake and status [13,14]. Urinary pantothenate excretion is considered to be a better indicator of status, with excretion of <1 mg/day considered indicative of poor status.

References Cited for Pantothenic Acid

1. Prasad P, Ganapathy V. Structure and function of mammalian sodium-dependent multivitamin transporter. Curr Opin Nutr Metab Care 2000;3:263–66.

2. Tarr J, Tamura T, Stokstad E. Availability of vitamin B_6 and pantothenate in an average American diet in man. Am J Clin Nutr 1981; 34:1328–37.

3. Food and Nutrition Board. Dietary Reference Intakes for Thiamin, Riboflavin, Niacin, Vitamin B_6, Folate, Vitamin B_{12}, Pantothenic Acid,

Biotin, and Choline. Washington, DC: National Academy Press, 1998, pp. 357–73.

4. Annous K, Song W. Pantothenic acid uptake and metabolism by red blood cells of rats. J Nutr 1995;125:2586–93.

5. Smith C, Milner R. The mechanism of pantothenate transport by rat liver parenchymal cells in primary culture. J Biol Chem 1985; 260:4823–31.

6. Beinlich C, Robishaw J, Neely J. Metabolism of pantothenic acid in hearts of diabetic rats. J Mol Cell Cardiol 1989;21:641–50.

7. Lopaschukf G, Michalak M, Tsang H. Regulation of pantothenic acid transport in the heart: involvement of a Na+ cotransport system. J Biol Chem 1987;262:3615–19.

8. Robishaw J, Neely J. Coenzyme A metabolism. Am J Physiol 1985;248:E1–E9.

9. Plesofsky-Vig N. Pantothenic acid and coenzyme A. In: Shils ME, Olson JA, Shike M, eds. Modern Nutrition in Health and Disease, 8th ed. Philadelphia: Lea and Febiger, 1994, pp. 395–401.

10. Plesofsky-Vig N, Brambl R. Pantothenic acid and coenzyme A in cellular modification of proteins. Ann Rev Nutr 1988;8:461–82.

11. Aprahamian M, Dentinger A, Stock-Damge C, Kouassi J, Grenier J. Effects of supplemental pantothenic acid on wound healing: experimental study in rabbits. Am J Clin Nutr 1985;41:578–89.

12. Clarke J, Kies C. Niacin nutritional status of adolescent humans fed high dosage pantothenic acid supplements. Nutr Rep Internl 1985;31:1271–79.

13. Cohenour S, Calloway D. Blood, urine, and dietary pantothenic acid levels of pregnant teenagers. Am J Clin Nutr 1972;25:512–17.

14. Sauberlich H. Pantothenic acid. In: Laboratory Tests for the Assessment of Nutritional Status, 2nd ed. Boca Raton, FL: CRC Press, 1999, pp. 175–83.

BIOTIN

Biotin's structure consists of two rings—a ureido ring joined to a thiophene ring—with an additional valeric acid side chain (Fig. 9.22). The vitamin was previously referred to as vitamin H as well as vitamin B_7.

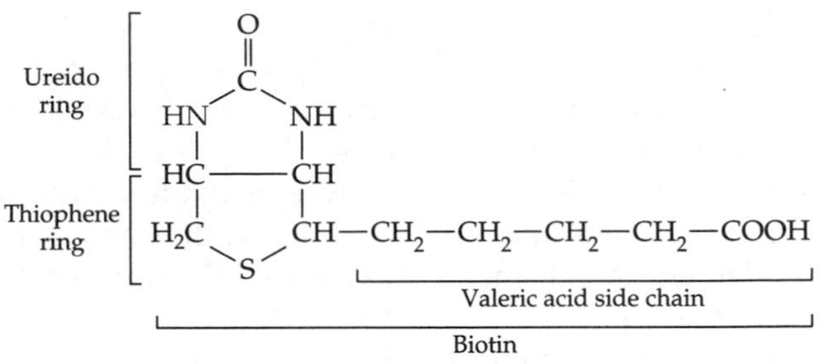

Figure 9.22 The structure of biotin.

Sources

Sources of biotin for humans include biotin in dietary foods as well as biotin made by intestinal bacteria living within the large intestine. Biotin is found widely distributed in foods. Good food sources of the vitamin include liver, soybeans, and egg yolk, as well as cereals, legumes, and nuts. Within many foods, biotin is found either bound covalently to protein or as biocytin, which consists of biotin bound to the amino acid lysine and is sometimes called biotinyllysine (Fig. 9.23).

One substance in foods, avidin, has been found to bind biotin and prevent its absorption and utilization by the body. A glycoprotein in raw egg whites, avidin irreversibly binds biotin in a noncovalent bond and prevents biotin absorption. Because avidin is heat-labile (unstable with heat), ingestion of cooked egg whites does not compromise biotin absorption.

Digestion, Absorption, Transport, and Storage

Protein-bound biotin requires digestion by proteolytic enzymes prior to absorption. Proteolysis by proteases yields free biotin, biocytin, or biotinyl peptides. Biotinyl peptides can be further hydrolyzed by other proteases or peptidases within the small intestine, while biocytin can be further hydrolyzed by biotinidase. Biotinidase is found on the intestinal brush border as well as in pancreatic and/or intestinal juice secreted into the small intestine. The enzyme hydrolyzes the biocytin to release free biotin and lysine. Some undigested biocytin may be absorbed intact by peptide carriers and subsequently hydrolyzed by biotinidase present in plasma or in most other body tissues. Any absorbed biocytin not metabolized by biotinidase is excreted in the urine.

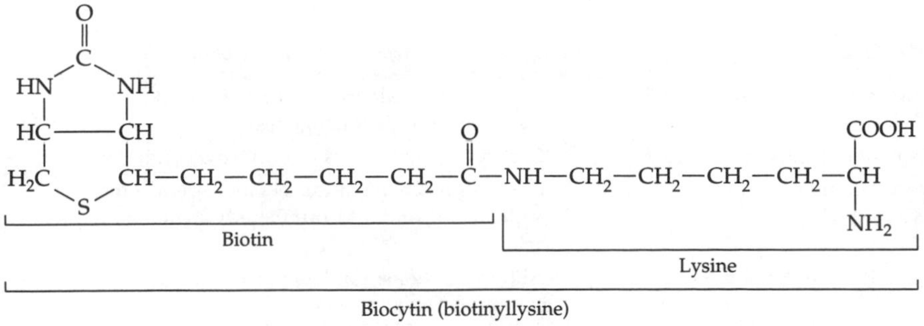

Figure 9.23 The structure of biocytin, also called biotinyllysine.

Biotinidase is active over a wide pH range and is specific for the biotinyl moiety [1–4]. It is found in most body cells, and its activity is expressed in multiple cellular locations including the nucleus [3,4]. While at more acidic pH the enzyme cleaves biocytin to produce biotin and lysine, at a more alkaline pH the enzyme has been shown to become biotinyated while also generating free lysine; in other words, the biotinidase enzyme becomes attached to the biotin that was previously part of biocytin. Biotinidase deficiency (first discovered in 1983) is due to an autosomal recessive inborn error of metabolism. Should infants and children with the disorder go untreated, a biotin deficiency, among other problems, develops. Some clinical features associated with the genetic disorder include seizures, ataxia, skin rash, alopecia (hair loss), and acidosis [1,2].

Free biotin is absorbed primarily in the jejunum followed by the ileum due to differences in carrier concentrations [5]. Dietary biotin is thought to be nearly completely absorbed [6]. Biotin that is synthesized by colonic bacteria is absorbed in the proximal and midtransverse colon; however, bacterially made biotin cannot totally meet the biotin needs of humans [5].

The mechanism of biotin absorption varies with intake. Biotin absorption occurs by passive diffusion with consumption of pharmacologic doses. With physiological biotin intakes, biotin absorption across the brush border membrane of the small intestine and across the colonocytes is carrier mediated and sodium dependent. The small intestine's carrier for biotin also transports pantothenic acid and lipoic acid [5,7]. Transport of biotin across the basolateral membrane of the enterocyte is carrier mediated but not sodium dependent [5]. Alcohol has been shown to inhibit intestinal biotin absorption.

Biotin is found in the plasma mostly in a free, unbound state, with lesser amounts bound to protein. Albumin and α- and β-globulins bind biotin, as does plasma biotinidase, which has two binding sites for biotin and arises from hepatic secretion [8]. Biotin is stored in small quantities in the muscle, liver, and brain [9]. Uptake of biotin into tissues is via active, sodium-dependent carriers.

Functions and Mechanisms of Action

Biotin functions in cells covalently bound to enzymes and thus is referred to as a coenzyme. In addition, biotin functions in non-coenzyme roles including possible roles in gene expression and the cell cycle.

Coenzyme Roles

For coenzyme functions within cells, biotin is attached (covalently bound) to four apocarboxylases. The attachment of biotin to these apoenzymes occurs in two steps and is catalyzed by the enzyme holocarboxylase synthetase, which is found in the cytosol and mitochondria. In the first step of the synthesis of the apocarboxylases, biotin reacts with ATP in a Mg^{2+}-dependent reaction to form biotinyl adenosine monophosphate (also referred to as activated biotin) and pyrophosphate. In the second step, the activated biotin reacts with the apocarboxylase to form a holoenzyme carboxylase with the release of AMP.

Holocarboxylase synthetase is essential for the formation of the holoenzyme carboxylases (sometimes called holocarboxylases), which are the coenzyme forms of biotin. Multiple holoenzyme carboxylase deficiencies can arise due to a mutation in holocarboxylase synthetase, as was first discovered in 1981, or due to a mutation in any of the four holocarboxylases. Propionic acidemia, for example, results from mutations in the enzyme propionyl CoA carboxylase.

The four biotin-dependent carboxylases, which are synthesized by holocarboxylase synthetase, are acetyl CoA carboxylase, pyruvate carboxylase, propionyl CoA carboxylase, and β-methylcrotonyl CoA carboxylase. Table 9.2 lists these enzymes and their roles in metabolism. Knowles [10] provides detailed information on the mechanism of action of the biotin-dependent enzymes.

Each holoenzyme carboxylase is a multisubunit enzyme to which biotin is attached by an amide linkage. Specifically, the carboxyl terminus of biotin's valeric acid side chain is linked to the epsilon amino group of a specified lysine residue in the apoenzyme [11]. The chain connecting biotin and the apoenzyme is long and

Table 9.2 Biotin-Dependent Enzymes

Enzyme	Role	Significance
Pyruvate carboxylase	Converts pyruvate to oxaloacetate	Replenishes oxaloacetate for Krebs cycle. Necessary for gluconeogenesis
Acetyl CoA carboxylase	Forms malonyl CoA from acetate	Commits acetate units to fatty acid synthesis
Propionyl CoA carboxylase	Converts propionyl CoA to methylmalonyl CoA	Provides mechanism for metabolism of some amino acids and odd-numbered–chain fatty acids.
β-methylcrotonyl CoA carboxylase	Converts β-methylcrotonyl CoA to β-methylglutaconyl CoA	Allows catabolism of leucine and certain isoprenoid compounds

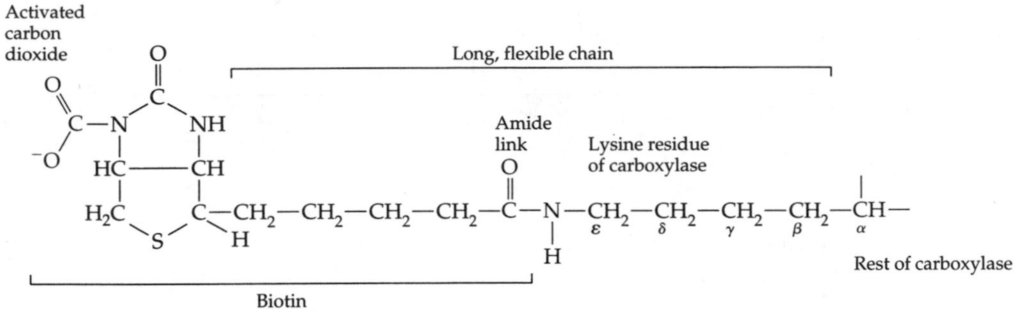

Figure 9.24 Biotin bound to the lysine residue of carboxylase and functioning as a carrier of activated CO_2.

flexible, allowing the biotin to move from one active site of the carboxylase to another. Figure 9.24 depicts the attachment of biotin to the enzyme, emphasizing the long, flexible chain and the amide linkage between the vitamin and the lysine residue of the enzyme. One active site on the apoenzyme generates the carboxybiotin enzyme, while the other transfers the activated carbon dioxide to a reactive carbon on the substrate. Figure 9.25 illustrates the formation of the CO_2-biotin-enzyme complex.

Pyruvate Carboxylase. Pyruvate carboxylase is a particularly interesting and important enzyme because of its regulatory function. Specifically, pyruvate carboxylase (a mitochondrial enzyme) catalyzes the carboxylation of pyruvate to form oxaloacetate (Fig. 9.26). For its activation, pyruvate carboxylase requires the presence of acetyl CoA as well as ATP and Mg^{2+}. Acetyl CoA serves as an allosteric activator, and its presence indicates the need for increased amounts of oxaloacetate. If there is a surplus of ATP in the cell, the oxaloacetate is then used for gluconeogenesis. However, if there is a deficiency of ATP, the oxaloacetate will enter the Krebs cycle on condensation with acetyl CoA.

Acetyl CoA Carboxylase. The importance of biotin in energy metabolism is further exemplified by its role in the initiation of fatty acid synthesis, that is, the formation of malonyl CoA from acetyl CoA by the regulatory and rate-limiting enzyme acetyl CoA carboxylase. This enzyme (found in both the mitochondria and cytosol) is allosterically activated by citrate and isocitrate and inhibited by long-chain fatty acyl CoA derivatives. ATP and Mg^{2+} are required for the reaction (see Fig. 6.28).

Propionyl CoA Carboxylase. Propionyl CoA carboxylase (a mitochondrial enzyme) is important for the catabolism of the amino acids isoleucine, threonine, and methionine, each of which generates propionyl CoA. Propionyl CoA also arises from the catabolism of odd-number–chain fatty acids found, for example, in some fish. Propionyl CoA carboxylase catalyzes the carboxylation of propionyl CoA to D-methylmalonyl CoA (Fig. 9.27). The reaction requires ATP and Mg^{2+}. D-methylmalonyl CoA, after being acted on by racemase, generates succinyl CoA in a vitamin B_{12}–dependent reaction catalyzed by methylmalonyl CoA mutase (Fig. 9.27). Deficient propionyl CoA carboxylase activity causes accumulation of propionyl CoA, which is then shifted into an alternate metabolic pathway. This alternate pathway results in increased production and urinary excretion of 3-hydroxypropionic acid and methylcitrate.

β-methylcrotonyl CoA Carboxylase. β-methylcrotonyl CoA carboxylase is important in the catabolism of the amino acid leucine. During leucine catabolism (Figs. 9.28

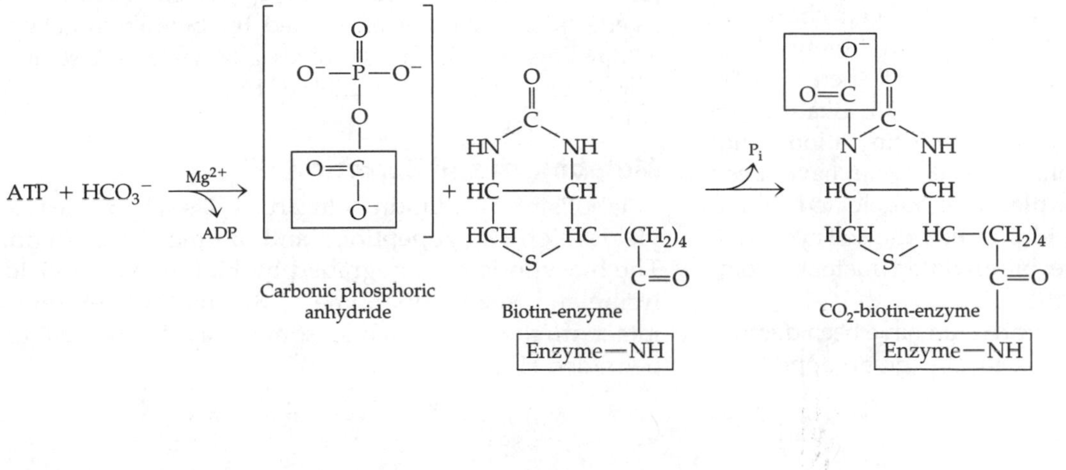

Figure 9.25 The formation of the CO_2-biotin-enzyme complex.

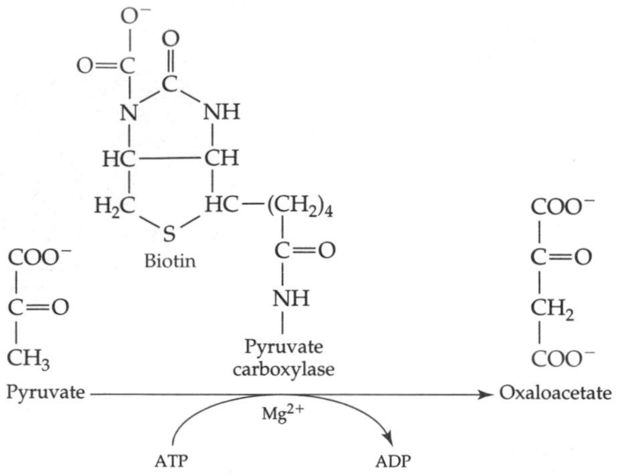

Figure 9.26 The role of biotin in the synthesis of oxaloacetate from pyruvate.

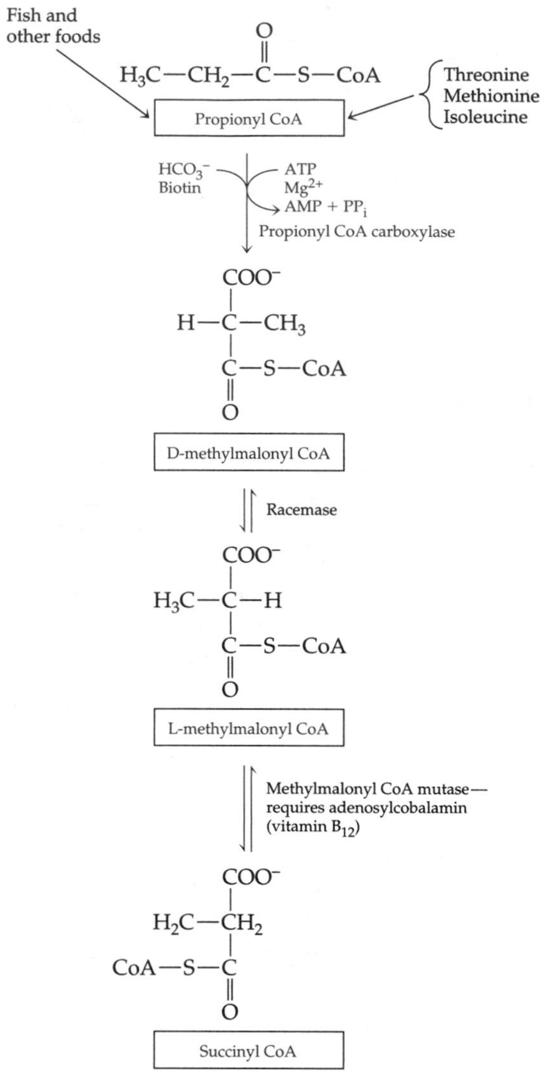

Figure 9.27 The oxidation of propionyl CoA and the role of biotin.

and 7.35), β-methylcrotonyl CoA is formed. This compound is carboxylated in an ATP-, Mg^{2+}-, and biotin-dependent reaction by β-methylcrotonyl CoA carboxylase to form β-methylglutaconyl CoA, which is further catabolized to generate acetoacetate and acetyl CoA. Deficient β-methylcrotonyl CoA carboxylase activity causes accumulation of β-methylcrotonyl CoA, which is then shunted to an alternate metabolic pathway. This alternate pathway results in increased production and urinary excretion of 3-hydroxy isovaleric acid (3-HIA) and 3-methylcrotonylglycine [11,12]. Increased 3-HIA and decreased biotin concentrations in the urine are indicative of biotin deficiency [13].

Non-Coenzyme Roles

While the coenzyme role of biotin is well characterized, other possible roles of biotin are less known and investigated. These roles include possible effects of biotin on DNA, gene expression, and cell development and growth. Biotin is hypothesized to exert effects on DNA (replication and/or transcription, or other) through its attachment to histones in the nucleus of cells. Histones bind to DNA to influence multiple processes. The attachment of biotin to histones is mediated by biotinidase, which has been shown to become biotinylated (i.e., to form biotinyl biotinidase) from the biotin moiety of biocytin and then transfer the biotin moiety to the histones at an alkaline pH [3,4,14,15]. The significance of the biotinylation is not clear, although effects on the cell cycle have been demonstrated. For example, mononucleated blood cells at the G1, S, G2, and M phase of the cell cycle displayed significantly more biotinylated histones compared to quiescent cells [16].

Effects of biotin on gene expression have been demonstrated in animal studies. Specifically, biotin appears to be necessary for the transcription of some genes and/or the translation of some mRNAs, including, for example, glucokinase, ornithine transcarbamylase, 6-phosphofructokinase, and phosphoenolpyruvate carboxykinase [15,17–19]. Possible mechanisms by which biotin exerts its effects have not been elucidated, but biotin may act via a signaling cascade that involves guanylate cyclase and cGMP-dependent protein kinase [15].

Metabolism and Excretion

Catabolism of the biotin holocarboxylases by proteases yields biotin oligopeptides and ultimately biocytin. The biocytin is then degraded by biotinidase to yield lysine and free biotin. Some of this biotin is excreted intact in the urine, while some may be reused or degraded [17].

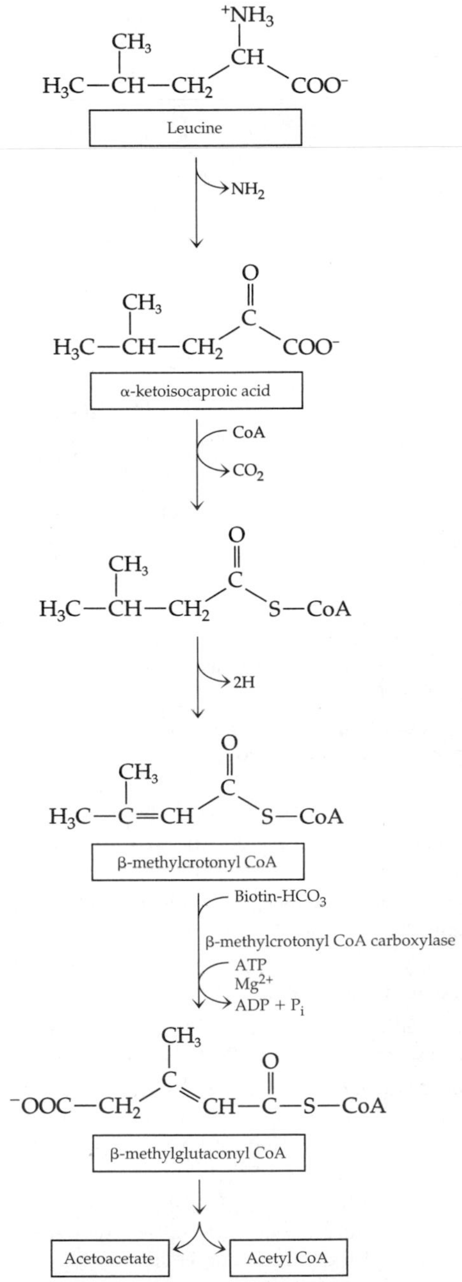

Figure 9.28 The role of biotin in leucine catabolism.

In the catabolism of biotin, little degradation of the ring system of the vitamin occurs in humans. Most of the metabolites arise from degradation of the valeric acid side chain of biotin by β-oxidation. The main metabolites following catabolism of this side chain are bisnorbiotin and tetranorbiotin (Fig. 9.29) and, to a lesser degree, other derived metabolites such as bisnorbiotin methyl ketone and tetranorbiotin methyl ketone [6,20]. Bisnorbiotin and tetranorbiotin, along with the other metabolites, are excreted in the urine. Small amounts of other biotin metabolites are formed from oxidation of the sulfur in biotin's ring. These metabolites, which also are excreted in the urine, include biotin sulfoxide and biotin sulfone (Fig. 9.29) [6,20,21].

Biotin that has been synthesized by intestinal bacteria but not absorbed is excreted in the feces. Very little dietary biotin that is absorbed is found excreted via the feces [5].

Adequate Intakes

Because intestinally synthesized biotin is not sufficient to maintain normal biotin status, humans need to obtain biotin from the diet. An adequate intake (AI) recommendation for adults age 19 years and older of 30 μg biotin per day has been suggested [13]. As discussed earlier in this chapter under panthothenic acid, an AI is used instead of an RDA when insufficient data are available to establish an estimated average requirement (EAR) and subsequent RDA [13]. AIs for biotin of 30 and 35 μg per day are suggested for women during pregnancy and lactation, respectively [13]. The inside covers of this book provide additional AIs for biotin for other age groups.

Deficiency

Biotin deficiency in humans is characterized by lethargy, depression, hallucinations, muscle pain, paresthesia in extremities, anorexia, nausea, alopecia (hair loss), and scaly, red dermatitis. In addition, changes in some biotin-dependent enzyme activities and alterations in the urinary excretion of biotin and some of its metabolites occur [6,12,22].

Biotin deficiency or poor biotin status, though fairly rare, occurs in various populations. People ingesting raw eggs in excess amounts are likely to develop biotin deficiency due to impaired biotin absorption. Impaired biotin absorption also may occur with gastrointestinal disorders such as inflammatory bowel disease and achlorhydria (lack of hydrochloric acid in gastric juices), or in people on anticonvulsant drug therapy or chronic consumers of excessive amounts of alcohol. Biotin status has been shown to decline in some women during pregnancy [12]. Biotin deficiency is known to be teratogenic in animals [23]. Individuals with genetic defects involving biotinidase and holocarboxylase synthetase activities develop biotin deficiency unless treated with pharmacologic doses of biotin. Biotin supplements in amounts of 5 to 10 mg daily are used to treat biotinidase deficiency, while doses of 40 to 100 mg biotin daily are effective in people with holocarboxylase synthetase deficiency [2].

Toxicity

Toxicity of biotin has not been reported, and thus no tolerable upper intake level has been established [13]. For

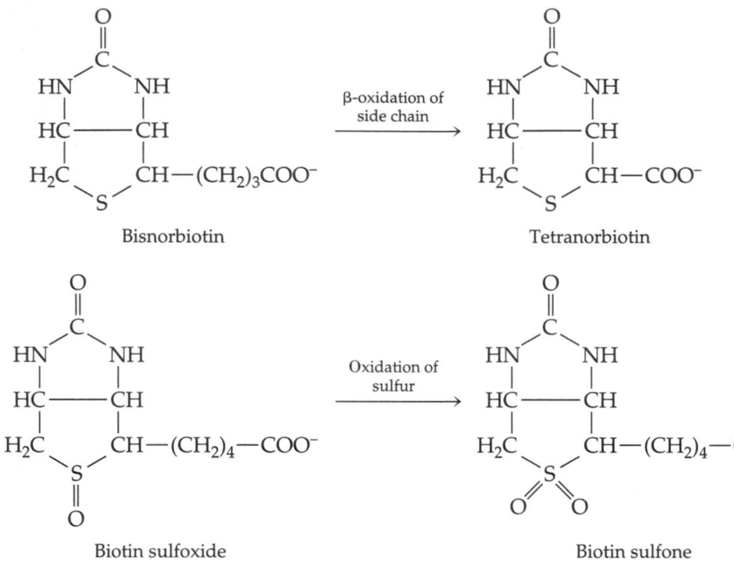

Figure 9.29 Selected metabolites from biotin degradation.

example, fairly large doses (100 mg or more) of biotin have been given daily to individuals with inherited disorders of biotin metabolism without side effects [13]. Use of biotin as hair and skin conditioning agents in cosmetics has also been shown to be safe [24].

Assessment of Nutriture

Evaluation of biotin in blood as well as in urine has most often been used to assess biotin status. Low plasma concentrations of biotin, however, have not been shown to accurately reflect intake or status [13]. Decreased urinary biotin excretion coupled with increased urinary excretion of 3-hydroxy isovaleric acid generated from altered metabolism of β-methylcrotonyl CoA has been shown to be a sensitive indicator of biotin deficiency [12,13]. Alterations in urinary 3-hydroxy isovaleric acid excretion, which can be detected within about 2 weeks of consumption of a biotin-deficient diet, are thought to be a more sensitive indicator than urinary biotin excretion [25,26].

References Cited for Biotin

1. Wolf B, Heard G, McVoy J, Grier R. Biotinidase deficiency. Ann NY Acad Sci 1985;447:252–62.

2. Baumgartner E, Suormala T. Inherited defects of biotin metabolism. BioFactors 1999;10:287–90.

3. Hymes J, Wolf B. Biotinidase and its roles in biotin metabolism. Clin Chim Acta 1996;255:1–11.

4. Hymes J, Wolf B. Human biotinidase isn't just for recycling biotin. J Nutr 1999;129:485S–89S.

5. Said H. Cellular uptake of biotin: mechanisms and regulation. J Nutr 1999;129:490S–93S.

6. Zempleni J, Mock D. Advanced analysis of biotin metabolites in body fluids allows a more accurate measurement of biotin bioavailability and metabolism in humans. J Nutr 1999;129:494S–97S.

7. Prasad P, Ganapathy V. Structure and function of mammalian sodium-dependent multivitamin transporter. Curr Opin Nutr Metab Care 2000;3:263–66.

8. Mock D, Malik M. Distribution of biotin in human plasma: most of the biotin is not bound to protein. Am J Clin Nutr 1992; 56:427–32.

9. Shriver B, Roman-Shriver C, Allred J. Depletion and repletion of biotinyl enzymes in liver of biotin deficient rats: evidence of a biotin storage system. J Nutr 1993;123:1140–49.

10. Knowles J. The mechanism of biotin-dependent enzymes. Ann Rev Biochem 1989;58:195–221.

11. Chapman-Smith A, Cronan J. Molecular biology of biotin attachment to proteins. J Nutr 1999;129:477S–84S.

12. Mock D, Stadler D, Stratton S, Mock N. Biotin status assessed longitudinally in pregnant women. J Nutr 1997;127:710–16.

13. Food and Nutrition Board. Dietary Reference Intakes for Thiamin, Riboflavin, Niacin, Vitamin B_6, Folate, Vitamin B_{12}, Pantothenic Acid, Biotin, and Choline. Washington, DC: National Academy Press, 1998, pp. 374–89.

14. Hymes J, Fleischhauer K, Wolf B. Biotinylation of histones by human serum biotinidase: assessment of biotinyl transferase activity in sera from normal individuals and children with biotinidase deficiency. Biochem Molec Med 1995;56:76–83.

15. Pacheo-Alvarez D, Solorzano-Vargas R, Del Rio A. Biotin in metabolism and its relationship to human disease. Arch Med Res 2002;33:439–47.

16. Stanley J, Griffin J, Zempleni J. Biotinylation of histone in human cells. Effects of cell proliferation. Eur J Biochem 2001;268:5424–29.

17. Dakshinamurti K, Litvak S. Biotin and protein synthesis in rat liver. J Biol Chem 1970;245:5600–5605.

18. Dakshinamurti K, Cheah-Tan C. Liver glucokinase of the biotin deficient rat. Can J Biochem 1968;46:75–80.

19. Maeda Y, Kawata S, Inui Y, Fukuda K, Igura T, Matsuzawa Y. Biotin deficiency decreases ornithine transcarbamylase activity and mRNA in rat liver. J Nutr 1996;126:61–66.

20. Mock D, Lankford G, Cazin J. Biotin and biotin analogs in human urine: biotin accounts for only half of the total. J Nutr 1993;123: 1844–51.

21. Zempleni J, McCormick D, Mock D. Identification of biotin sulfone, bisnorbiotin methyl ketone, and tetranorbiotin-1-sulfoxide in human urine. Am J Clin Nutr 1997;65:508–11.

22. Baez-Saldana A, Diaz G, Espinoza B, Ortega E. Biotin deficiency induces changes in subpopulations of spleen lymphocytes in mice. Am J Clin Nutr 1998;67:431–77.

23. Watanabe T, Dakshinamurti K, Persaud T. Biotin influences palatal development of mouse embryos in organ culture. J Nutr 1995;125:2114–21.

24. Fiume M. Final report on the safety assessment of biotin. Internl J Toxicology 2001;20(suppl4):1–12.

25. Mock N, Mock D. Biotin deficiency in rats: disturbances of leucine metabolism are detectable early. J Nutr 1992;122:1493–99.

26. McMahon R. Biotin metabolism and molecular biology. Ann Rev Nutr 2002;22:221–39.

FOLIC ACID

Folacin is a generic term for compounds that have chemical structures and nutritional properties similar to those of folic acid (folate), which is also called pteroylglutamate or pteroylmonoglutamate [1]. Folic acid is made up of three distinct parts, all of which must be present for vitamin activity. Figure 9.30 shows the structure of folic acid. As shown in the figure, 2-amino-4-hydroxypteridine, also called pteridine or pterin, is conjugated via a methylene group (—CH_2—) to para-aminobenzoic acid (PABA) to form pteroic acid. The carboxy group of PABA is peptide-bound to the amino group of glutamic acid to form folic acid. In the body, metabolically active folate has multiple glutamic acid residues attached. Although mammals can synthesize all the component parts of the vitamin, they do not have the enzyme necessary for the coupling of the pterin molecule to PABA to form pteroic acid [1].

Figure 9.30 Structural formula of folic acid.

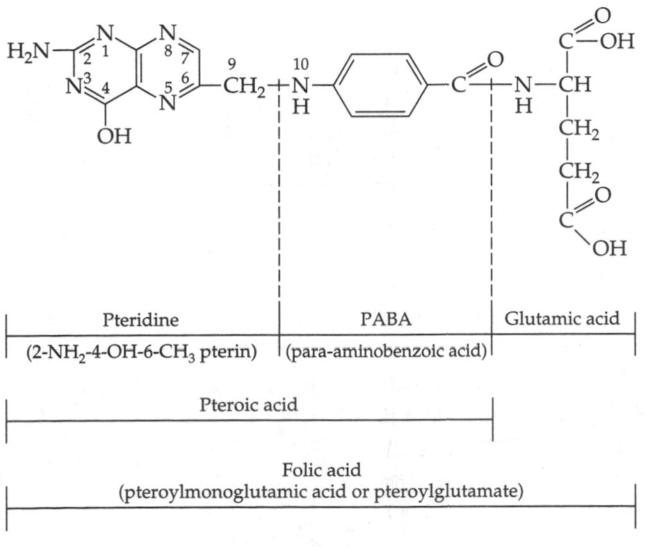

Sources

Good food sources of folate include mushrooms and green vegetables such as spinach, brussels sprouts, broccoli, asparagus, and turnip greens, among others, as well as peanuts, legumes (especially lima and kidney beans), citrus fruits (especially strawberries and oranges) and their juices, and liver. Raw foods typically are higher in folate than cooked foods because of folate losses incurred with cooking. Fortification of flours, grains, and cereals with folate (140 μg folate per 100 g of product) was initiated in 1998. Thus, fortified cereals, breads, and grain products now represent major sources of the vitamin.

Folate in foods exists primarily in the form of pteroylpolyglutamates containing up to nine glutamate residues instead of the one glutamate shown in Figure 9.30. The principal pteroylpolyglutamates in foods are 5-methyl tetrahydrofolate (THF) and 10-formyl THF, although over 150 different forms of folate have been reported [2,3]. In supplements and in fortified foods, folate is provided as pteroylmonoglutamate, the most oxidized and stable form of the vitamin.

Folate bioavailability in individual foods varies from as high as 96% in cooked lima beans to as low as 25% in romaine lettuce [2]. Moreover, reduced forms of pteroylpolyglutamates in foods are labile and easily oxidized. It is estimated that in food preparation or processing 50% to 95% of the folates originally present can be lost [2,3]. The effect of thermal processing on folate bioavailability depends to a great extent on the form of folate present in food.

Digestion, Absorption, Transport, and Storage

Before the polyglutamate forms of folate in foods can be absorbed, they must be hydrolyzed to the monoglutamate form. This hydrolysis is performed by pteroylpolyglutamate hydrolases, also called conjugases or glutamate carboxypeptidases. The group of conjugases exhibits separate activities in the human jejunal mucosa, one soluble and the other membrane-bound in the intestinal brush border [2,4]. The conjugases are also found in the pancreatic juice and bile. The brush border conjugase is a zinc-dependent exopeptidase that stepwise cleaves the polyglutamate into monoglutamate. Zinc deficiency impairs conjugase activity and diminishes digestion and thus absorption of folate [5]. Chronic alcohol ingestion and conjugase inhibitors in foods such as legumes, lentils, cabbage, and oranges also diminish conjugase activity to impair digestion of polyglutamate forms of folate and thus inhibit folate absorption.

The carrier system responsible for transporting folate across the intestinal cell membrane is saturable and pH, energy, and sodium dependent [2,4]. Folate-binding proteins (FBPs), also called folate carriers or folate receptors, are found in the intestinal brush border [3,6,7]. Absorption occurs throughout the small intestine but is most efficient in the jejunum. The folate in milk, which is bound to a high-affinity folate-binding protein, however, appears to be absorbed more avidly in the ileum. Diffusion also accounts for some folate absorption, especially when pharmacological doses of the vitamin are consumed. Efficiency of folate absorption from foods is estimated to be about 50%, while folate absorption from supplements (especially if consumed on an empty stomach) and fortified grain products is higher [1,5,8]. The difference in absorbability has led to the use of folate equivalents in recommendations for dietary folate intakes (see the section on RDA under folate) [1].

Within the intestinal cell, folate and subsequently dihydrofolate (DHF) are reduced to generate THF (Fig. 9.31). The reduction of various folate forms to THF occurs stepwise through the action of NADPH-dependent dihydrofolate reductase, a cytosolic enzyme (Fig. 9.31). Four additional hydrogens are added at positions 5, 6, 7, and 8. THF is then either methylated in a two-step reaction to 5-methyl THF or formylated (Fig. 9.31).

Figure 9.31 Interconversions of coenzyme forms of THF.

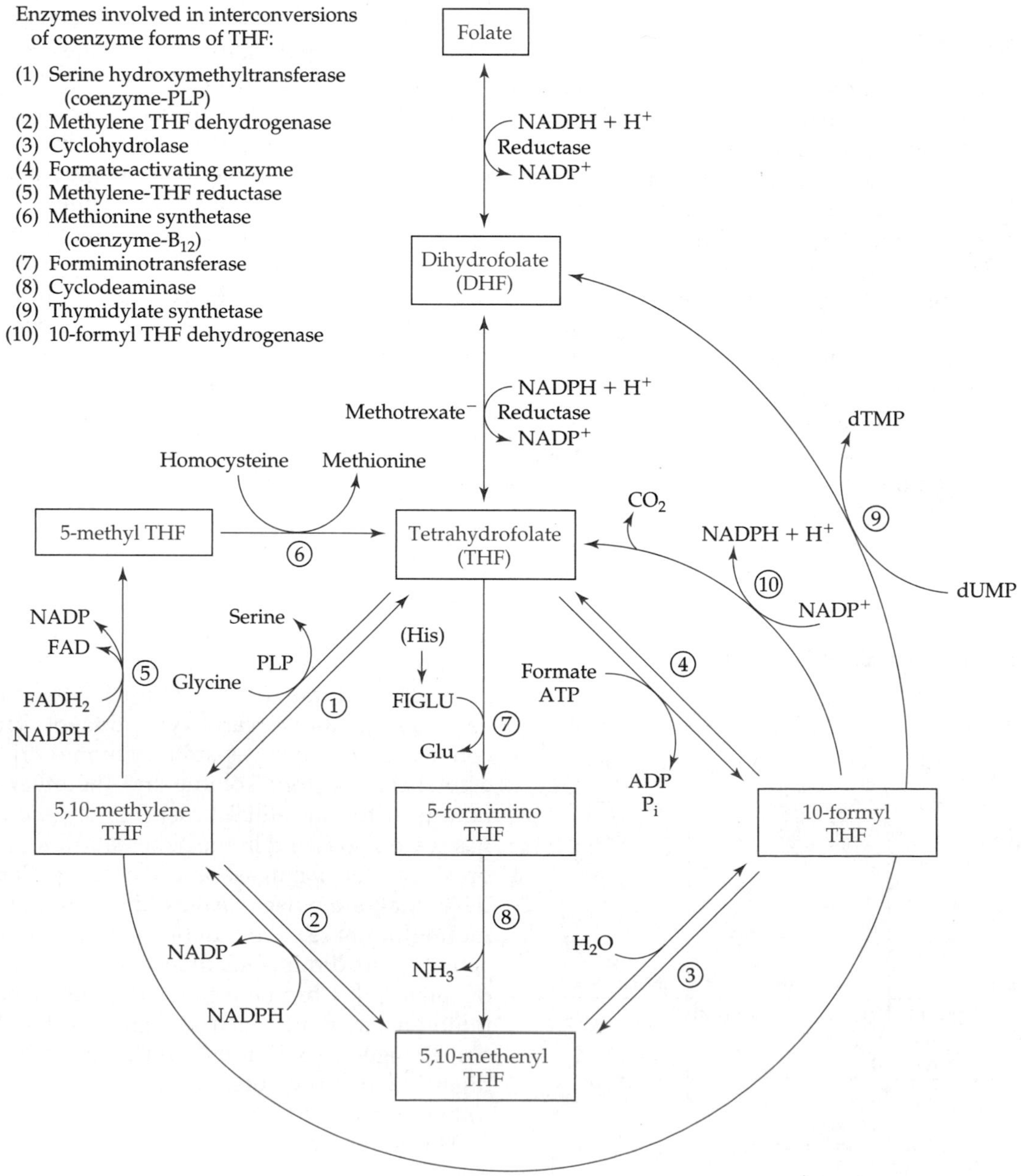

Folate-binding proteins are thought to transport folate within cells. Folate is found in portal circulation as 5-methyl THF, although dihydrofolate and formylated forms are also present; all forms are as mono- and not polyglutamates.

Uptake of folate into the liver is carrier mediated by folate receptors. Dihydrofolate is typically reduced to THF in the liver and conjugated to glutamates either for storage or for conversion to 5-methyl THF [2]. Within the liver, about 33% of folate is present as THF, 37% as 5-methyl THF, 23% as 10-formyl THF, and 7% as 5-formyl THF [9]. Bound to the various folates, especially to 5-methyl THF and 10-formyl THF, are glutamates typically varying in length from 3 to 9. Folylpolyglutamate synthetase catalyzes the ATP-dependent additions of the glutamates. Polyglutamate forms of folate are better substrates for folate-dependent enzymes than monoglutamate forms. Before release into systemic blood, however, glutamate residues are removed from folate polyglutamates by hydrolases.

In the blood, folate is found as a monoglutamate. Almost two-thirds of the folate in systemic blood plasma is bound to proteins; free folate accounts for the other one-third [4,6]. In the blood, folate-binding proteins bind folate with high affinity; albumin and α-2 macroglobulin also bind folate, but with relatively low affinity. Monoglutamate forms of folate in the blood include THF, 5-methyl THF, and 10-formyl THF, among other forms [2]. Red blood cells contain more folate than does plasma; however, red blood cell folate is attained during erythropoiesis. In other words, folate is not taken up by mature red blood cells. Thus, red blood cell folate concentrations represent an index of longer-term (2 to 3 months) folate status than does plasma.

Folate transport into most tissue cells occurs by folate receptors. Receptors have been identified in several tissues, including the liver, renal tubule, and hematopoietic cells [6,7,10]. Within the kidney, for example, folate-binding proteins present in the renal brush border and coupled with tubular reabsorption of folate help the body retain needed folate. As within the liver, THF is converted by folylpolyglutamate synthetase in extrahepatic cells into a polyglutamate form to become a functional coenzyme. Glutamate residues are usually added one at a time to the monoglutamate in ATP-requiring reactions. Addition of these glutamate residues not only allows the production of the various folate coenzyme forms but also traps the folate in the cell.

Total body folate levels are estimated to be 11 to 28 mg [1]. The liver stores about one-half of the body's folate. The main storage forms are the polyglutamate forms of THF and 5-methyl THF. Storage may occur in association with intracellular folate-binding proteins [6].

Folate is found in both the cytosol and mitochondria of cells, where it functions as a coenzyme (or cosubstrate) to accept and donate one-carbon units. Availability of folate to crucial tissues where rapid cell division is occurring appears to be carefully regulated when the supply of dietary folate is limited. The mechanisms of regulation are unclear, but regulation seems to occur through changes in the rate of synthesis of polyglutamates. The less metabolically active tissues return folate monoglutamates to the liver, which then redistributes the folate to the actively proliferating cells. How circulating folates are directed to specific tissues is uncertain, but folate-binding proteins (folate receptors) may provide tissue-specific uptake [4,10].

Functions and Mechanisms of Action

THF functions in the body as a coenzyme in both the mitochondria and cytosol to accept one-carbon groups typically generated from amino acid metabolism. These THF derivatives then serve as donors of one-carbon units in a variety of synthetic reactions, such as dispensable amino acid synthesis and purine and pyrimidine synthesis. The one-carbon group accepted by THF is bonded to its nitrogen in position 5 or 10 or to both (Fig. 9.31). The coenzyme forms are interconvertible, except that 5-methyl THF cannot be converted back to 5,10-methylene (Fig. 9.31). Genetic polymorphisms in some of the folate-dependent enzymes have been identified. Several mutations in methylene THF reductase (sometimes abbreviated MTHFR) have been demonstrated. MTHFR converts 5,10-methylene THF to 5-methyl THF. The enzyme requires riboflavin as FAD as a prosthetic group. Mutations in MTHFR impair 5-methyl folate formation and thus prevent remethylation of homocysteine, resulting in hyperhomocysteinemia, a risk factor for heart disease [11].

The THF derivatives, which participate in a variety of reactions, are illustrated as follows.

5-and 10-formyl THF	O=CH
5-formimino THF	—HC=NH—
5,10-methenyl THF	=CH—
5,10-methylene THF	$—CH_2—$
5-methyl THF	$—CH_3$

The formyl derivatives represent the most oxidized forms of folate, while 5-methyl THF is the most reduced form.

Amino Acid Metabolism

Folate is involved in the metabolism of several amino acids, including histidine, serine, glycine, and methionine.

Histidine. Histidine metabolism requires THF. Deamination of histidine generates urocanic acid, which can undergo further metabolism to yield formiminoglutamate (FIGLU). The formimino group is removed from FIGLU with the help of formiminotransferase to generate glutamate. THF receives the formimino group to yield 5-formimino THF, as shown below and in Figures 7.30 and 9.32.

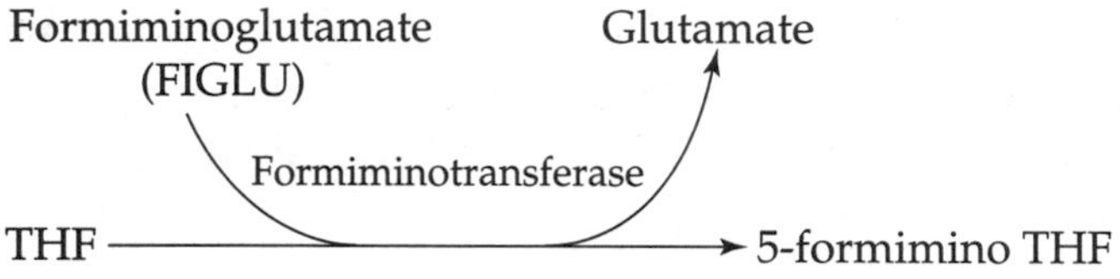

This reaction can be used as a basis for determination of folate deficiency. In the medical procedure, subjects are given an oral histidine load, and FIGLU excretion is measured in the urine. With folate deficiency, FIGLU accumulates in the blood and is excreted in higher concentrations in the urine, because if THF were available FIGLU would be converted into glutamate.

Serine and Glycine. Folate as 5,10-methylene THF is required for serine synthesis from glycine (Fig. 9.31). The 5,10-methylene THF contributes a hydroxymethyl group to glycine to produce serine. Serine represents a major source of one-carbon units for use in folate reactions. Vitamin B_6 as pyridoxal phosphate (PLP) is required for serine hydroxymethyltransferase activity. This enzyme is found in all tissues, especially the liver and kidney, in both the cytosol and mitochondria.

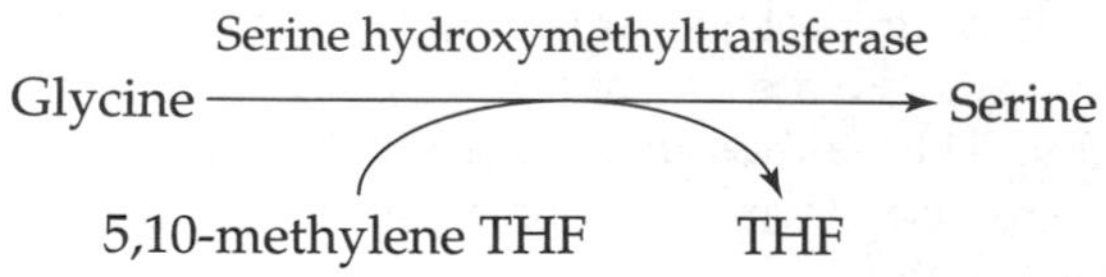

The conversion of glycine to serine is reversible such that glycine may be synthesized from serine in a THF-dependent reaction. However, the direction of the reaction varies between tissues; some tissues, such as the kidney, generate more serine, while others generate more glycine.

Some other reactions involving glycine metabolism also require folate. Glycine degradation, for example, requires THF as shown below and in Figure 7.29.

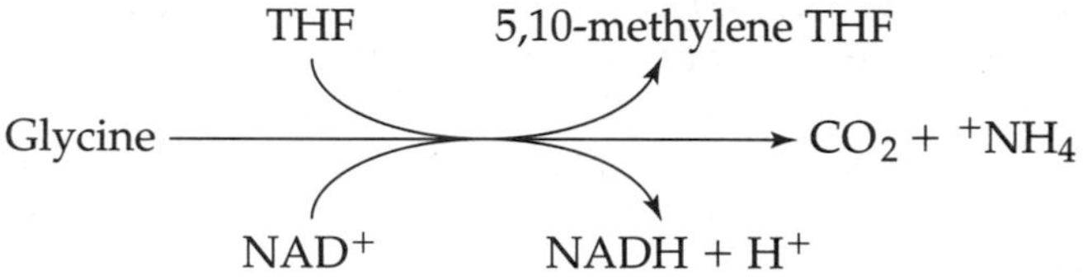

Glycine synthesis from choline degradation also involves folate. Choline is catabolized in the liver in an NAD^+-dependent reaction to form betaine and $NADH + H^+$. Betaine functions as a methyl donor providing methyl groups to other compounds, such as homocysteine, via a methyltransferase and generating dimethylglycine. The dimethylglycine resulting from demethylation of betaine undergoes further metabolism to generate sarcosine in a reaction catalyzed by dimethylglycine dehydrogenase. In that reaction and the subsequent reaction catalyzed by sarcosine dehydrogenase (in which sarcosine, also called monomethylglycine, is converted to glycine), THF functions as the carbon acceptor, forming 5,10-methylene THF. Riboflavin as FAD also is required.

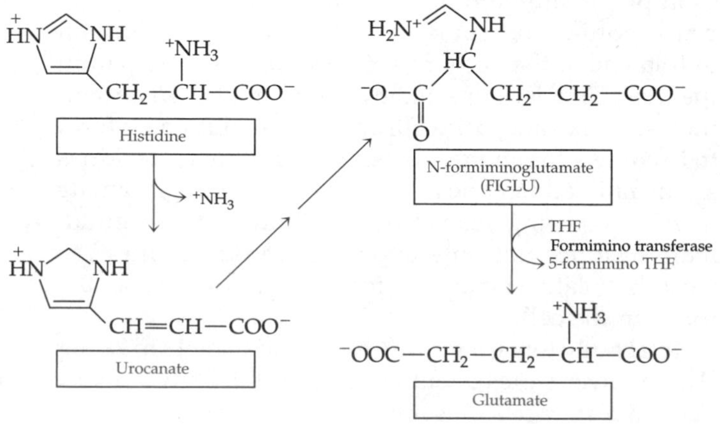

Figure 9.32 The role of folic acid in histidine catabolism.

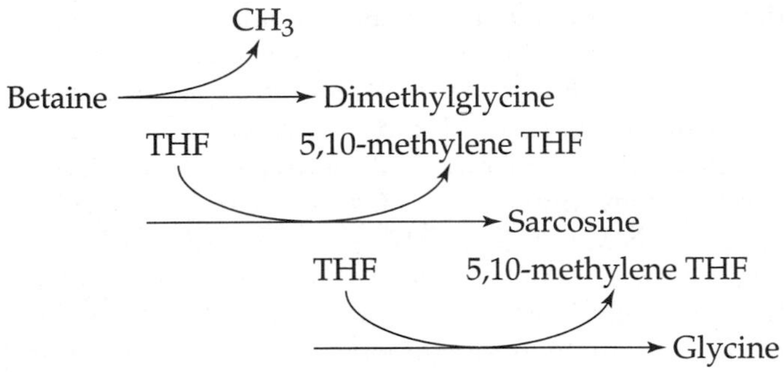

Methionine. Methionine regeneration from homocysteine also involves folate as 5-methyl THF. Before addressing this regeneration, we will give a brief overview of the conversion of methionine to homocysteine. As shown in Figure 9.33, methionine is converted to S-adenosyl methionine (SAM) in an ATP-requiring reaction catalyzed by methionine adenosyl transferase. The removal of the methyl group from SAM results in the formation of S-adenosyl homocysteine (SAH). Removal of the adenosyl group from SAH yields homocysteine.

Folate is needed for the remethylation of homocysteine to form methionine. This reaction, which occurs when SAM concentrations are low, requires folate as 5-methyl THF as a methyl donor and vitamin B_{12} in the form of methylcobalamin as a prosthetic group for homocysteine methyltransferase (also called methionine synthase). For methionine synthase to transfer a methyl group from 5-methyl THF to homocysteine, cobalamin must be tightly bound to the enzyme. While bound to methionine synthase, cobalamin picks up the methyl group from 5-methyl THF to generate methylcobalamin and THF. Methylcobalamin then serves as the methyl donor for converting homocysteine to methionine. These reactions are shown in Figure 9.33 and are broken down into steps to facilitate understanding in the "Functions and Mechanisms of Action" section under vitamin B_{12} (p. 312).

SAM is an important compound, serving as a methyl donor in many reactions in the body. For example, DNA and RNA methylation, myelin maintenance, neural function, and polyamine, carnitine, and catecholamine synthesis, among other processes, are dependent on methylation reactions using SAM. SAM concentrations in part regulate methionine metabolism, including the remethylation of homocysteine to methionine. SAM

Figure 9.33 The resynthesis of methionine from homocysteine, showing the roles of folate and vitamin B_{12}.

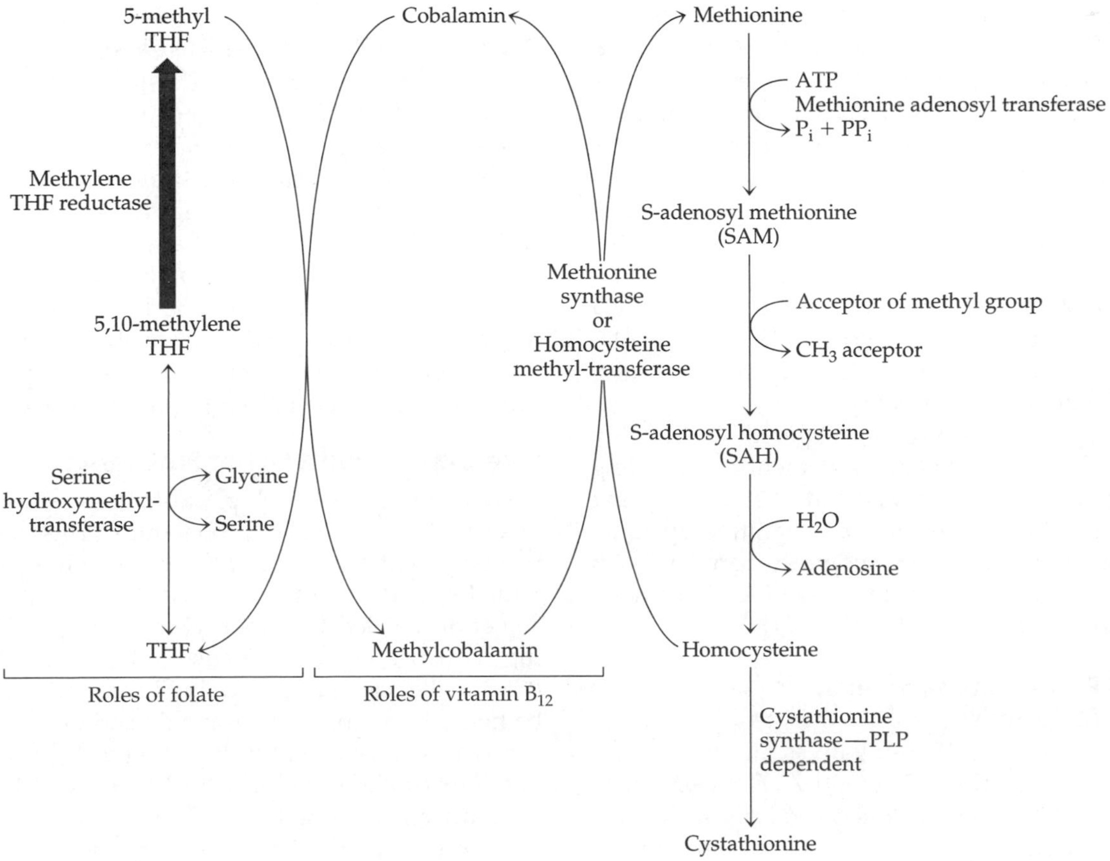

concentrations increase with increased methionine. Higher SAM concentrations stimulate the transsulfuration pathway in which homocysteine is converted, in an irreversible reaction, to cystathionine via vitamin B_6–dependent cystathionine synthase (Fig. 9.33) and ultimately is converted to cysteine. Higher SAM concentrations inhibit methylene THF reductase, which converts 5,10-methylene THF to 5-methyl THF. This inhibition decreases 5-methyl THF availability to decrease remethylation of homocysteine.

Possible Relationships with Diseases. The roles of folate and vitamin B_{12} in the conversion of homocysteine to methionine, along with the role of vitamin B_6 in the conversion of homocysteine to cystathionine (see Figs. 9.33 and 9.42), continue to receive considerable attention because intakes of these three vitamins are inversely associated with plasma homocysteine concentrations, and elevated plasma homocysteine concentrations (>15 μM) are associated with premature coronary artery disease, as well as with premature occlusive vascular disease and cerebral or peripheral vascular disease [12–15]. The mechanisms by which hyperhomocysteinemia increases vascular disease risk have not been elucidated, but it may act by impairing endothelial function, promoting the growth of smooth muscle cells leading to vascular lesions, and/or promoting platelet adhesiveness and clotting, among other hypotheses [11,16,17]. Research suggests that an increase of 5 μmol/L in plasma homocysteine concentrations increases the risk for heart disease as much as an increase of 0.5 mmol/L (20 mg/dL) in plasma cholesterol concentrations [13]. Supplementation of folic acid, vitamin B_{12}, and vitamin B_6 in individuals (both healthy and with heart disease) with hyperhomocysteinemia (high blood homocysteine concentrations) has been shown to normalize or reduce blood homocysteine concentrations and thus decrease a risk factor for heart disease [18,19]. Folate supplementation in individuals with hyperhomocysteinemia also improves endothelial function [14].

Another condition being investigated as possibly linked to poor folate status is dementia, including Alzheimer's dementia. Memory and abstract thinking appear to be influenced by folate. Cognitive dysfunction and dementia have been shown to correlate with plasma homocysteine concentrations, which in turn are influenced in part by folate status [20,21].

Purine and Pyrimidine Synthesis/ Nucleotide Metabolism

The involvement of THF derivatives in purine and pyrimidine synthesis (Figs. 7.16 and 7.17) makes folate essential for cell division. Synthesis of cells with short life spans, such as enterocytes, is particularly dependent on adequate levels of folate. In pyrimidine synthesis (Fig. 7.16), thymidylate synthetase uses 5,10-methylene THF to convert dUMP to dTMP and dihydrofolate (DHF) (Fig. 9.31). dTMP is required for DNA synthesis. To regenerate 5,10-methylene THF, DHF is converted by dihydroreductase to THF in a reaction requiring NADPH. The THF is converted to 5,10-methylene THF as serine is converted to glycine by serine hydroxymethyl transferase, a vitamin B_6–dependent enzyme. Both thymidylate synthetase and dihydrofolate reductase are active enzymes in cells undergoing cell division. Inhibitors of dihydrofolate reductase, such as the therapeutic drug Methotrexate, which binds to the enzyme's active site, have been employed in the treatment of cancer, rheumatoid arthritis, and psoriasis, among other conditions, to prevent synthesis of THF needed for actively dividing cells.

Folate as 10-formyl THF is needed for purine (adenine and guanine) ring formation (Fig. 7.17). C8 atom of the purine involves the formylation of glycinamide ribotide (GAR) to form formylglycinamidine ribotide (FGAR). 10-formyl THF donates the formyl group in this reaction. Purine-ring atom C2 is acquired by formylation of 5-aminoimidazole 4-carboxamide ribonucleotide (AICAR). 10-formyl THF formylates AICAR to generate 5-formaminoimidazole 4-carboxamide ribotide (FAICAR).

Other Relationships with Diseases

Folate deficiency or poor folate status is also suspected in the development (initiation) of some cancers, especially colon cancer. Folate deficiency in cells and tissues is thought to increase the potential for neoplastic changes in normal cells during the early stages of cancer [22,23]. Some evidence suggests that decreased methylation of DNA, especially tumor suppression genes, or increased DNA strand breaks associated with misincorporation of uridylate for thymidylate in DNA due to folate deficiency may alter gene expression and thus promote cancer [24–26]. (See Chap. 9, Perspective.)

Interactions with Other Nutrients

A synergistic relationship exists between folate and vitamin B_{12}, also called cobalamin. This relationship, whereby without vitamin B_{12} the methyl group from 5-methyl THF can't be removed and thus is trapped, is sometimes called the "methyl-folate trap." The following sequence of events leads to the methyl-folate trap (tracing the reactions shown in Figures 9.31 and 9.33 will be helpful). Serine donates single carbons through conversion to glycine, and in the process THF is converted to 5,10-methylene THF. The 5,10-methylene THF is readily reduced to 5-methyl THF by a reductase (whose activity is inhibited by its end product, 5-methyl THF, and by SAM). 5-methyl THF is required for methionine synthesis from homocysteine. Methyl groups are transferred by the enzyme methionine synthase from 5-methyl THF to vitamin B_{12}. Adequate vitamin B_{12} must be present for the activity of methionine synthase. The addition of the methyl group to cobalamin generates methylcobalamin, which serves as the methyl donor for converting homocysteine to methionine. Without cobalamin to accept the methyl group from 5-methyl THF, the 5-methyl THF accumulates and is trapped, and THF is not regenerated. With adequate vitamin B_{12} status, the THF resulting from the synthesis of methionine is needed as a substrate for conversion into its various other coenzyme forms. For example, 10-formyl THF is needed for purine synthesis, and 5,10-methylene THF is needed for thymidylate synthesis, which in turn must be present for DNA synthesis. Thus, the synergism between folate and vitamin B_{12} is very important for support of rapidly proliferating cells. See the section "Toxicity" under folate for a discussion on the ability of folate supplements to mask vitamin B_{12} deficiency.

Metabolism and Excretion

Folate is excreted from the body in both the urine and the feces. In the urine, some folate is excreted intact, while some is metabolized in the liver prior to excretion. Oxidative cleavage of folate is thought to occur between C9 and N10 of polyglutamate forms of the vitamin. This cleavage generates para-aminobenzoyl polyglutamate. Glutamate residues (except for one) are then hydrolyzed, and usually the compound is acetylated to form the major urinary metabolite N-acetyl para-aminobenzoyl glutamate. Smaller amounts of para-aminobenzoyl glutamate also are found in the urine.

In addition to urinary losses, folate is secreted by the liver into the bile. Most of this folate, however, is reabsorbed via enterohepatic recirculation, so losses in the stool are minimal [1,4,27]. Folate of microbial origin, however, may appear in the feces in relatively high amounts.

Recommended Dietary Allowances

The 1998 RDA for folate considers its bioavailability as well as several indices of nutriture. The requirement and RDA for adults for folate are 320 μg dietary folate equivalents (DFE) and 400 μg DFE per day, respectively [1]. These recommendations are consistent with those from the Centers for Disease Control and Prevention [28], which suggest 400 μg folate/day for women capable of becoming pregnant because of evidence that folate supplementation during the periconceptional period of pregnancy may reduce the incidence of neural tube defects. Foods that are good sources of folate (that is, the food provides either ≥10% of the Daily Value or at least 40 μg/serving) are permitted by the Food and Drug Administration to make the health claim "Healthful diets with adequate folate may reduce a woman's risk of having a child with a neural tube (brain or spinal cord) defect" [29]. RDAs for folate of 600 μg and 500 μg of DFE per day are suggested for pregnancy and lactation, respectively [1]. One DFE is equal to 1 μg of food folate, which is equal to 0.6 μg of folate from a supplement or fortified food consumed with a meal, which is equal to 0.5 μg of folate from a supplement taken without food (empty stomach) [1]. Additional RDAs for folate for other age groups are provided on the inside covers of the book.

Deficiency: Megaloblastic, Macrocytic Anemia

Marginal folate deficiency results in megaloblastic macrocytic anemia. The deficiency is characterized initially (within a month if the diet is devoid of folate) by low plasma folate. Red blood cell folate concentrations diminish after about 3 to 4 months of low folate intake [22]. After approximately 4 to 5 months, bone marrow cells and other rapidly dividing cells become megaloblastic [22]. Mean cell volumes (MCV) increase, and hypersegmentation (increased lobes) of white blood cells (neutrophils) occurs, along with decreased blood cell counts. Individuals with folate deficiency may exhibit fatigue, weakness, headaches, irritability, difficulty concentrating, shortness of breath, and palpitations, among other symptoms.

Megaloblastic anemia—the release into circulation of red blood cells that are fewer than normal and large and immature—due to folate deficiency is relatively common in the United States. However, megaloblastic anemia also occurs with deficiency of vitamin B_{12}. The anemia results from abnormal DNA synthesis and failure of blood cells to divide properly, coupled with the continued formation of RNA. The quantity of RNA becomes greater than normal, leading to excess production of other cytoplasmic constituents, including hemoglobin. The result is immature, enlarged macrocytic cells often containing excessive hemoglobin.

Figure 9.34 reviews the formation and maturation of erythrocytes and may better illustrate the effects of a folate and vitamin B_{12} deficiency. Briefly, the proerythroblast develops from stem cells in bone marrow under the stimulation of hypoxia (low blood oxygen) via erythropoietin (a hormone produced in the kidney). In the proerythroblast, active DNA and RNA synthesis occurs and cell division begins. Cells resulting from the first division are given the name basophilic erythroblasts because they stain blue with basic dyes due to the many organelles present within the cell. During this stage, hemoglobin synthesis begins. The next generation of cells consists of the polychromatophil erythroblasts, in which hemoglobin

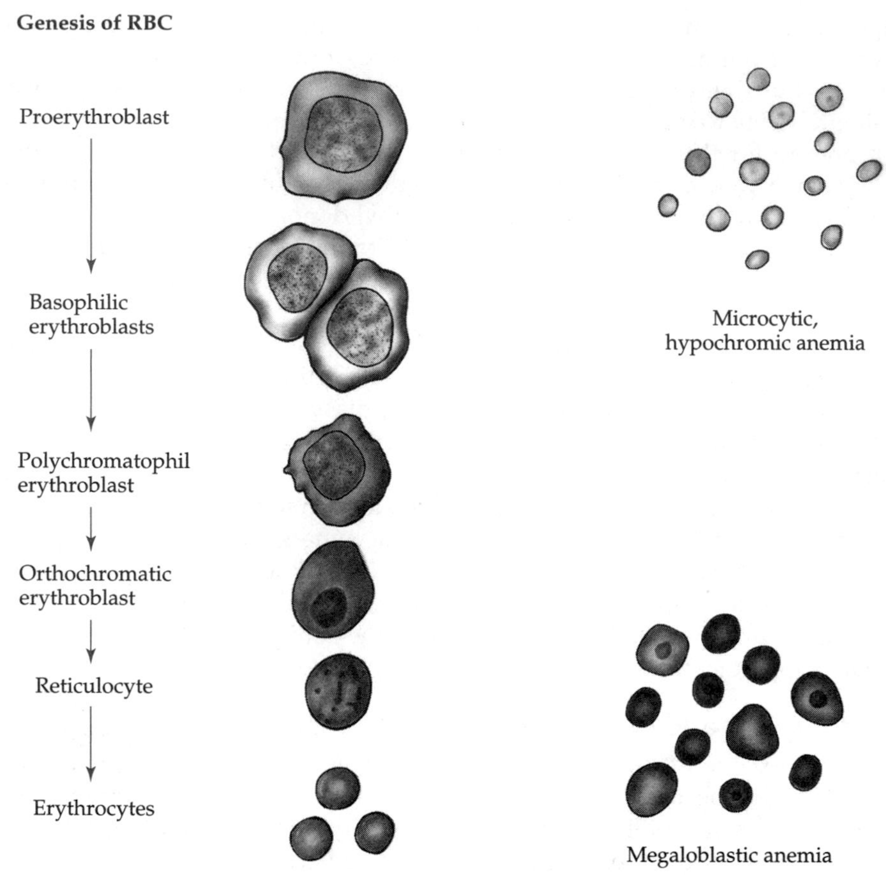

Figure 9.34 Genesis and maturation of the red blood cells (left); red blood cells characteristic of microcytic and megaloblastic anemias (right).

synthesis intensifies. The concentration of hemoglobin influences DNA synthesis and cell division. Cell division usually continues into the orthochromatic stage. The orthochromatic erythroblasts are characterized by continued hemoglobin synthesis, discontinuation of DNA synthesis, a slowing of RNA synthesis, and migration of the nucleus to the cell wall in preparation for extrusion. The cell now becomes the reticulocyte, in which hemoglobin synthesis continues up to a concentration of approximately 34%. Once this concentration is reached, the ribosomes disappear and the cells pass into blood capillaries by squeezing through pores of the membrane. In about 2 to 3 days, when the rest of the cell organelles have disappeared, the reticulocytes become erythrocytes. The erythrocyte, or mature red blood cell, is all cytoplasm packed with hemoglobin. Glycolysis and hexosemonophosphate shunt are the only metabolic pathways occurring in the erythrocyte.

A deficiency of folate and/or vitamin B_{12} interferes with normal cell division. With folate deficiency, increased strand breaks occur within the DNA, and imbalances in DNA bases occur with decreased conversion of deoxyuridylate to thymidylate, which is required for normal cell division. Problems are theorized to arise in part, and among other reasons, because uracil may be misincorporated for thymidylate into DNA; while enzymes will remove the uracil, lack of thymidine triphosphate (TTP) inhibits repair of the DNA [24–26]. Without appropriate repair, double strand breaks and fragmentation occur in the DNA [26,30,31]. Over time, cell division diminishes. Large, malformed, and sometimes nucleated red blood cells result.

Some conditions and populations associated with increased need for folate intake include people with excessive alcohol ingestion, those with malabsorption disorders such as inflammatory bowel diseases, and individuals taking certain medications. Folate deficiency has been observed in people treated with diphenylhydantoin or phenytoin, anticonvulsants used in the treatment of epilepsy. Folate and phenytoin each inhibit the cellular uptake of the other in the gastrointestinal tract and possibly in the brain [1,32]. Methotrexate, used to treat rheumatoid arthritis, among other conditions, antagonizes folate by binding to dihydrofolate reductase, preventing THF synthesis (Fig. 9.31). Other drugs, including cholestyramine (used to treat high cholesterol concentrations) and sulfasalazine (used to treat inflammatory bowel diseases), have also been shown to interact with folate to create folate deficiency. Conditions such as inflammatory bowel diseases (e.g., Crohn's and ulcerative colitis) and excessive alcohol ingestion are known to cause malabsorption of folate.

Toxicity

Toxicity of oral folic acid in moderate doses reportedly is virtually nonexistent [1,33]. Other studies, however, indicate that folate intakes of up to 15 mg daily are problematic. Problems include insomnia, malaise, irritability, and gastrointestinal distress [32,34]. Folate supplementation also is problematic if it masks a vitamin B_{12} deficiency [35,36]. Folate supplements can alleviate the megaloblastic anemia due to a vitamin B_{12} deficiency while the neurological damage due to the deficiency progresses undetected. A tolerable upper intake level for adults of 1,000 μg (1 mg) for synthetic folate in supplements or from fortified foods (not natural foods) has been suggested based on the ability of folate to mask the neurological manifestations of vitamin B_{12} deficiency [1].

Assessment of Nutriture

Folate status is most often assessed through measurement of folate concentrations in the plasma, serum, or red blood cells. Serum or plasma folate levels reflect recent dietary intake; thus, true deficiency must be interpreted through repeated measures of serum or plasma folate. Serum folate concentrations <3 ng/mL suggest deficiency [1,37,38]. Red blood cell folate concentrations are more reflective of folate tissue status than is serum folate and represent vitamin status at the time the red blood cells were synthesized [1,39]. Red blood cell folate concentrations <140 ng/mL suggest folate deficiency; however, concentrations are also lowered with a vitamin B_{12} deficiency [1,39].

N-formiminoglutamate (FIGLU) excretion may also be used to measure folate nutriture, because folate as THF must be available for the formimino group to be removed from FIGLU and glutamate to be formed (see Fig. 9.32). FIGLU excretion is measured in a 6-hour urine collection after ingestion of 2 to 5 g of oral L-histidine. Normal FIGLU excretion is about 5 to 20 mg, whereas with folate deficiency it is 5 to 10 times higher. A deficiency of vitamin B_{12}, however, will also cause an elevated FIGLU excretion.

The deoxyuridine suppression test, another method for assessing folate status, measures the availability of folate for de novo thymidine synthesis. In this test, the activity of thymidylate synthetase is measured in cultured lymphocytes or bone marrow cells. The reaction catalyzed by thymidylate synthetase is dependent on folate and, indirectly, on vitamin B_{12}; therefore, the change in activity elicited by the addition of one or the other vitamin allows identification of the deficiency. In other words, if a person were folate deficient, the addition of folate—but not vitamin B_{12}—would normalize enzyme activity. Likewise, if a person were vitamin B_{12} deficient, the addition of vitamin B_{12}—and not folate—would normalize thymidylate synthetase activity. In the case of a deficiency of both vitamins, normalization of enzyme activity would be possible only after the addition of both vitamins [39,40].

A functional marker of folate and vitamin B_{12} deficiencies is elevated plasma homocysteine concentrations. Remember, both vitamins are required for the remethylation of homocysteine to methionine. With deficiency of either vitamin, plasma homocysteine concentrations become elevated [41].

References Cited for Folic Acid

1. Food and Nutrition Board. Dietary Reference Intakes for Thiamin, Riboflavin, Niacin, Vitamin B_6, Folate, Vitamin B_{12}, Pantothenic Acid, Biotin, and Choline. Washington, DC: National Academy Press, 1998, pp. 196–305.

2. Sauberlich H. Bioavailability of vitamins. Prog Food Nutr Sci 1985;9:1–33.

3. Sauberlich H. Vitamins—how much is for keeps? Nutr Today 1987;22:20–28.

4. Steinberg S. Mechanisms of folate homeostasis. Am J Physiol 1984;246:G319–24.

5. Pfeffer C, Rogers L, Bailey L, Gregory J. Absorption of folate from fortified cereal grain products and of supplemental folate consumed with or without food determined using a dual label stable isotope protocol. Am J Clin Nutr 1997;66:1388–97.

6. Wagner C. Cellular folate binding proteins: function and significance. Ann Rev Nutr 1982;2:229–48.

7. Geller J, Kronn D, Jayabose S, Sandoval C. Hereditary folate malabsorption. Medicine 2002;81:51–68.

8. Gregory J. Bioavailability of folate. Eur J Clin Nutr 1997;51:S54–59.

9. Bender D. Nutritional Biochemistry of the Vitamins. New York: Cambridge University Press, 1992, pp. 269–317.

10. Wang H, Ross J, Ratnam M. Structure and regulation of a polymorphic gene encoding folate receptor type γ/γ. Nucleic Acids Res 1998;26:2132–42.

11. Cortese C, Motti C. MTHFR gene polymorphism, homocysteine and cardiovascular disease. Pub Hlth Nutr 2001;4:493–97.

12. Shimakawa T, Nieto F, Malinow M, Chambless L, Schreiner P, Szklo M. Vitamin intake: a possible determinant of plasma homocyst(e)ine among middle-aged adults. Ann Epidemiol 1997; 7:285–93.

13. Boushey C, Beresford S, Omenn G, Motulsky A. A quantitative assessment of plasma homocysteine as a risk factor for vascular disease: probable benefits of increasing folic acid intakes. JAMA 1995;274:1049–57.

14. Verhaar M, Stroes E, Rabelink T. Folates and cardiovascular disease. Atheroscler Thromb Vas Biol 2002;22:6–13.

15. Refsum H, Ueland P, Nygard I, Vollset S. Homocysteine and cardiovascular disease. Ann Rev Med 1998;49:31–62.

16. Tsai J, Perrella M, Yoshizumi M, Hsieh C, Haber E, Schlegel R, Lee M. Promotion of vascular smooth muscle cell growth by homocysteine: a link to atherosclerosis. Proc Natl Acad Sci USA 1994; 91:6369–73.

17. Mayer E, Jacobsen D, Robinson K. Homocysteine and coronary atherosclerosis. J Am Coll Cardiol 1996;27:517–27.

18. Ubbink J. Vitamin B_{12}, vitamin B_6, and folate nutritional status in men with hyperhomocysteinemia. Am J Clin Nutr 1993;57:47–53.

19. Ubbink J, Vermaak W, Merwe A, Becker P, Delport AR, Potgieter H. Vitamin requirements for the treatment of hyperhomocysteinemia in humans. J Nutr 1994;124:1927–33.

20. Selhub J. Folate, vitamin B_{12} and vitamin B_6 and one carbon metabolism. J Nutr Hlth Aging 2002;6:39–42.

21. Clarke R, Smith A, Jobst K, Refsum H, Sutton L, Ueland P. Folate, vitamin B_{12} and serum total homocysteine in confirmed Alzheimer's disease. Arch Neurol 1998;55:1449–55.

22. Hine R. Folic acid: contemporary clinical perspective. Persp Appl Nutr 1993;1:3–14.

23. Folate, alcohol, methionine, and colon cancer risk: is there a unifying theme? Nutr Rev 1994;2:18–20.

24. Kim Y, Pogribny I, Basnakian A, Miller J, Selhub J, James S, Mason J. Folate deficiency in rats induces DNA strand breaks and hypomethylation with the p52 tumor suppressor gene. Am J Clin Nutr 1997;65:46–52.

25. Duthie S, Narayanan S, Brand G, Pirie L, Grant G. Impact of folate deficiency on DNA stability. J Nutr 2002;132:2444S–49S.

26. Mason J, Levesque T. Folate: effects on carcinogenesis and the potential for cancer chemoprevention. Oncology 1996;10:1727–36.

27. Weir D, McGing P, Scott J. Commentary: folate metabolism, the enterohepatic circulation and alcohol. Biochem Pharmacol 1985; 34:1–7.

28. Centers for Disease Control and Prevention. Recommendations for the use of folic acid to reduce the number of cases of spina bifida and other neural tube defects. MMWSR 1992;41:1–7.

29. www.cfsan.fda.gov

30. Friso S, Choi S-W. Gene-nutrient interactions and DNA methylation. J Nutr 2002;132:2382S–87S.

31. Beck W. Neuropsychiatric consequences of cobalamin deficiency. Adv Intern Med 1991;36:33–56.

32. Alhadeff L, Gualtieri C, Lipton M. Toxic effects of water-soluble vitamins. Nutr Rev 1984;42:33–40.

33. Butterworth C, Tamura T. Folic acid safety and toxicity: a brief review. Am J Clin Nutr 1989;50:353–58.

34. Zimmerman M, Shane B. Supplemental folic acid. Am J Clin Nutr 1993;58:127–28.

35. Hathcock J. Vitamins and minerals: efficacy and safety. Am J Clin Nutr 1997;66:427–37.

36. Drazkowski J, Sirven J, Blum D. Symptoms of B_{12} deficiency can occur in women of child-bearing age supplemented with folate. Neurology 2002;58:1572–73.

37. Lindenbaum J, Healton E, Savage D, Brust J, Garrett T, Podell E, Marcell P, Stabler S, Allen R. Neuropsychiatric disorders caused by cobalamin deficiency in the absence of anemia or macrocytosis. N Engl J Med 1988;318:1720–28.

38. Jacques P, Sulsky S, Sadowski J, Phillips J, Rush D, Willett W. Comparison of micronutrient intake measured by a dietary questionnaire and biochemical indicators of micronutrient status. Am J Clin Nutr 1993;57:182–89.

39. Bailey L. Folate status assessment. J Nutr 1990;120:1508–11.

40. Simko M, Cowell C, Gilbride J. Nutrition Assessment. Rockville, MD: Aspen, 1995.

41. Kuzminski A, Del Glacco E, Allen R, Stabler S, Lindenbaum J. Effective treatment of cobalamin deficiency with oral cobalamin. Blood 1998;92:1191–98.

VITAMIN B_{12} (COBALAMIN)

Vitamin B_{12}, also called cobalamin, is considered a generic term for a group of compounds called corrinoids because of their corrin nucleus. The corrin is a macrocyclic ring made of four reduced pyrrole rings linked together. The corrin of vitamin B_{12} has an atom of cobalt in its center to which is attached, at almost right angles, the nucleotide 5,6-dimethylbenzimidazole. Also attached to the cobalt atom in vitamin B_{12} is one of the following:

Group Attached	Resulting Compound
–CN	Cyanocobalamin
–OH	Hydroxocobalamin
$-H_2O$	Aquocobalamin
$-NO_2$	Nitritocobalamin
5′-deoxyadenosyl	5′-deoxyadenosylcobalamin
$-CH_3$	Methylcobalamin

The structure of cyanocobalamin is shown in Figure 9.35. Only two cobalamins, 5′-deoxyadenosylcobalamin (subsequently called adenosylcobalamin) and methylcobalamin, are active as coenzymes. The human body has the biochemical ability to convert most of the other cobalamins into an active coenzyme form of the vitamin.

Sources

The only dietary sources of vitamin B_{12} for humans are animal products, which have derived their cobalamins from microorganisms. All naturally occurring vitamin B_{12} is produced by microorganisms. Any vitamin B_{12} found in plant foods probably could be traced either to contamination with microorganisms contained in manure or, in the case of legumes, to the presence of nitrogen-fixing bacteria in the plant root nodules [1]. Contaminated hands taking foods to the mouth may also provide vitamin B_{12}.

The best sources of the cobalamins are meat and meat products, poultry, fish, shellfish (especially clams and oysters), and eggs (especially the yolk); the cobalamins in these products are predominantly adenosyl- and hydroxocobalamin. Milk and milk products such as cheese and yogurt contain less of the vitamin, mainly as methyl- and hydroxocobalamins [2,3]. Cyanocobalamin may be found in a few foods as well as in tobacco. Cyanocobalamin and hydroxocobalamin are the forms commercially available in, for example, vitamin preparations. Within the body, cyanocobalamin is converted to aquo- or hydroxocobalamin, among other forms.

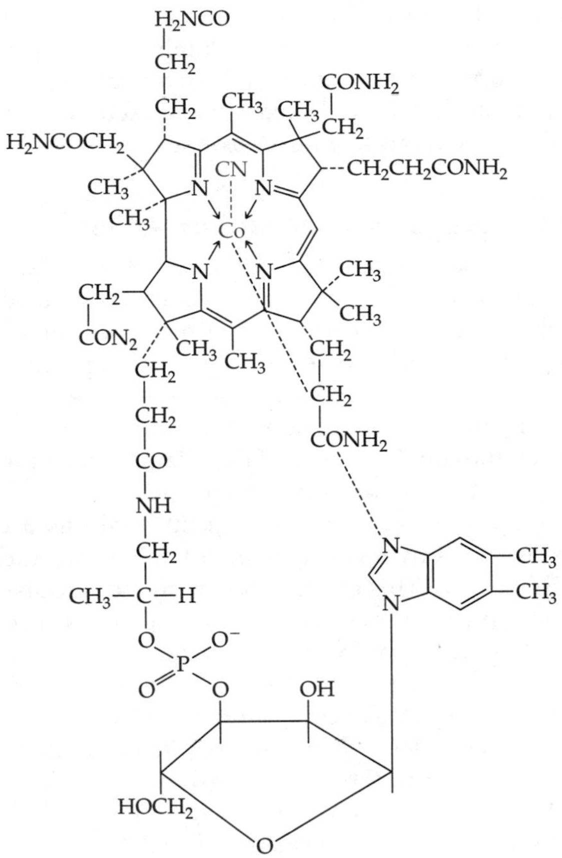

Figure 9.35 Structural formula of vitamin B_{12} (cyanocobalamin).

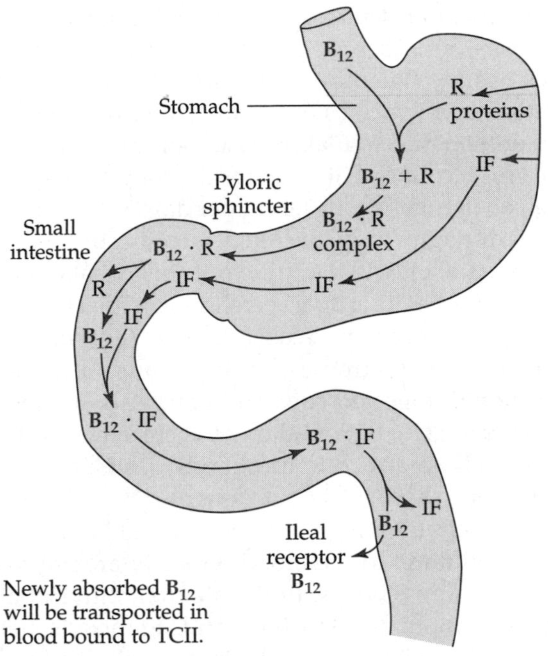

Figure 9.36 Vitamin B_{12} absorption.

Digestion, Absorption, Transport, and Storage

The digestion and absorption of vitamin B_{12} are believed to proceed according to the scheme depicted in Figure 9.36. Ingested cobalamins must be released from the polypeptides to which they are linked in foods. This release usually occurs through the actions of the gastric proteolytic enzyme pepsin and hydrochloric acid in the stomach.

Two nonenzymatic proteins made within the gastrointestinal tract also play important roles in vitamin B_{12} digestion and absorption: R protein and intrinsic factor (IF) protein. A cobalamin-binding R protein, found in saliva and gastric juice, may bind to the vitamin prior to its release from food protein. R proteins, known collectively as **cobalophilins** or **haptocorrins** (HCs), have a high affinity for cobalamins. Intrinsic factor (IF) is a glycoprotein synthesized by gastric parietal cells. Although made in the stomach, IF functions in the small intestine in the binding of vitamin B_{12} for absorption.

Once released from foods in the stomach, vitamin B_{12} remains bound to the R protein as the vitamin is emptied from the stomach into the duodenum, the proximal or upper region of the small intestine. Within the duodenum, the R protein is hydrolyzed by pancreatic proteases, and free cobalamin is released. Pancreatic insufficiency is known to interfere with the release of cobalamin from the R protein and thus reduce the amount of the vitamin available for absorption. R proteins or other factors secreted by pancreatic juice may also serve to protect vitamin B_{12} from bacterial use [4].

In the proximal small intestine, IF, which escapes the catabolic action of the proteases, binds the cobalamin (any of the forms) once it is released from the R proteins. The cobalamin-IF complex travels to the ileum, where receptors (called cubilins) for vitamin B_{12} are present [5]. Absorption of the vitamin occurs throughout the ileum, especially the distal third [1].

The cobalamin absorption process is complex and poorly understood. The absorption of the cubilin-IF–vitamin B_{12} complex into the enterocyte is thought to occur by receptor-mediated endocytosis; however, it may be that only the vitamin, and not the complex, is absorbed. A protein, megalin, is also thought to bind to the complex and to play a role in its transport into the cell.

While most vitamin B_{12} is absorbed by a receptor-mediated process, about 1% to 3% of intake (physiological) can be absorbed by passive diffusion. When pharmacological doses of vitamin B_{12} are ingested, however-passive diffusion accounts for much of the vitamin's absorption throughout the intestinal tract. Overall absorption of vitamin B_{12} from the diet ranges from about

11% to 65%; in calculating recommendations for dietary B_{12} intakes, 50% absorption was assumed [6]. Absorption of free cyanocobalamin in individuals with healthy gastrointestinal tracts does not diminish with aging [7–10].

Enterohepatic circulation is important in vitamin B_{12} nutriture, accounting in part for the long biological half-life of cobalamin. About 1.4 μg per day (1.85 nmol) cobalamin is thought to be secreted into the bile [11]. With enterohepatic circulation, much of this cobalamin in the bile and in other intestinal secretions can bind to IF in the small intestine and be reabsorbed in the ileum. Thus, malabsorption syndromes not only cause a decrease in absorption of ingested cobalamin but also interfere with enterohepatic circulation, thereby increasing the amount of vitamin B_{12} required to meet body needs.

Following absorption of vitamin B_{12}, the vitamin appears in circulation about 3 to 4 hours later. Peak levels of the vitamin in the blood typically are not reached for another 4 to 8 hours. In the blood, methylcobalamin comprises about 60% to 80% and adenosylcobalamin perhaps up to 20% of total plasma cobalamin. Other forms of cobalamin in the blood include cyanocobalamin and hydroxocobalamin.

Vitamin B_{12} is found in the blood bound to one of three transcobalamins (TC), designated TCI, TCII, or TCIII. Whether attachment to TC occurs within the enterocyte or at the serosal surface is not known. The transcobalamins are considered R proteins. TCII is the main protein that carries newly absorbed cobalamin, in a one-to-one ratio, to the tissues. About 20% of cobalamin is transported on TCII. The exact functions of TCI and TCIII are unknown. TCIII may function in the delivery of cobalamin from peripheral tissues back to the liver. Up to about 80% of vitamin B_{12} is bound to TCI, which may function as a circulating storage form of the vitamin.

Uptake of vitamin B_{12} into tissues is receptor dependent. All tissues appear to have receptors for TCII. The TCII-cobalamin complex is thought to bind to TCII receptors on cells and to be taken into cells by endocytosis and fused to lysosomes that provide for the degradation of TCII and release of the vitamin within the cell cytosol.

Metabolism of the various forms of the vitamin occurs within cells. Hydroxocobalamin, for example, may undergo cytosolic methylation to generate methylcobalamin or may undergo reduction and subsequent reaction with ATP in the mitochondria to yield adenosylcobalamin [1].

Vitamin B_{12}, unlike other water-soluble vitamins, can be stored and retained in the body for long periods of time, even years. About 2 to 4 mg of the vitamin is stored in the body, mainly in the liver, but with small amounts also found in the muscle, bone, kidneys, heart, brain, and spleen and circulating in the blood as transcobalamins. Adenosylcobalamin is the primary storage form of the vitamin in the liver, and possibly in other organs. Hydroxocobalamin and methylcobalamin are also stored, but to a lesser extent.

Functions and Mechanisms of Action

Two enzymatic reactions requiring vitamin B_{12} have been recognized in humans. One of these reactions requires methylcobalamin, while the other must have adenosylcobalamin. Adenosyl- and methylcobalamin are formed by a complex reaction sequence (see [12]) resulting in the production of a carbon-cobalt bond between the cobalt nucleus of the vitamin and either the methyl or the 5′-deoxyadenosyl ligand.

The reaction requiring methylcobalamin as a coenzyme is the conversion of homocysteine into methionine (Fig. 9.33). This reaction occurs in the cytoplasm of the cell and is shown below in a two-step process to facilitate understanding of the sequential nature of the reaction. First, to form the methylcobalamin needed in methionine synthesis, cobalamin bound to the methionine synthase (also called homocysteine methyltransferase) picks up the methyl group from 5-methyl tetrahydrofolate (THF), forming methylcobalamin bound to methionine synthase and THF.

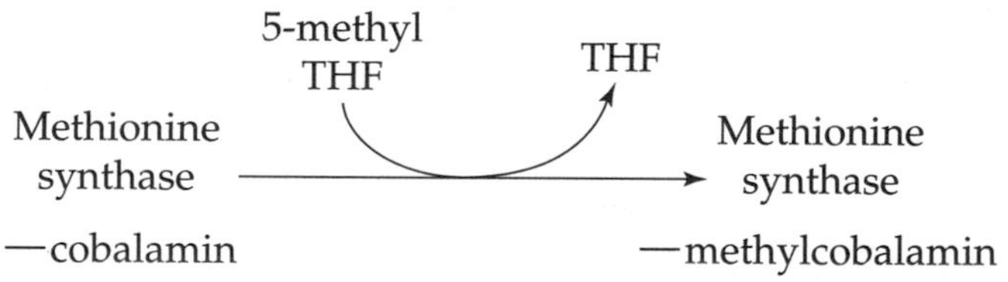

Next, the methylcobalamin bound to methionine synthase releases the methyl group for transfer to homocysteine, producing methionine and cobalamin.

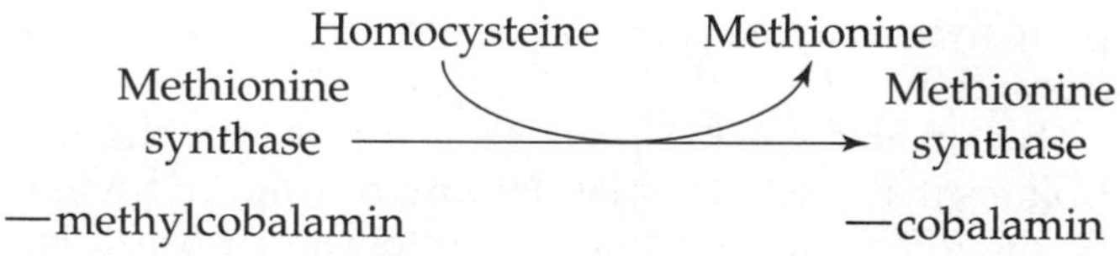

Because the formation of 5-methyl THF is irreversible, a vitamin B_{12} deficiency traps body folate in the 5-methyl form, in what is known as the methyl-folate trap hypothesis. This hypothesis helps explain in part the synergism between folate and vitamin B_{12} (see p. 306).

The second of the vitamin B_{12}-dependent reactions requires adenosylcobalamin. This reaction is catalyzed by a mutase and occurs in the mitochondria. Specifically, adenosylcobalamin is needed for methylmalonyl CoA mutase, which converts L-methylmalonyl CoA to succinyl CoA (Fig. 9.37). L-methylmalonyl CoA is made from D-methylmalonyl CoA, which in turn is generated from propionyl CoA. Propionyl CoA arises from the oxidation of methionine, isoleucine, and threonine and of odd-chain fatty acids. The conversion of propionyl CoA to D-methylmalonyl CoA is an ATP-, Mg^{2+}-, and biotin-dependent reaction (previously discussed on p. 297 in the section on biotin) (Fig. 9.37). Methylmalonyl CoA mutase (a dimer) requires two adenosylcobalamin molecules (one per subunit) to convert L-methylmalonyl CoA to succinyl CoA, the Krebs cycle intermediate (Fig. 9.37). With a deficiency of vitamin B_{12}, mutase activity is impaired and methylmalonyl CoA and methylmalonic acid, formed from hydrolysis of methylmalonyl CoA, accumulate in body fluids. Genetic defects in methylmalonyl CoA mutase and adenosylcobalamin synthesis have also been demonstrated and result in the accumulation of methylmalonyl CoA and methylmalonic acid. The response of serum methylmalonic acid to vitamin B_{12} depletion and repletion is useful in the diagnosis of vitamin B_{12} deficiency and response to treatment.

Figure 9.37 Role of vitamin B_{12} in oxidation of L-methylmalonyl CoA.

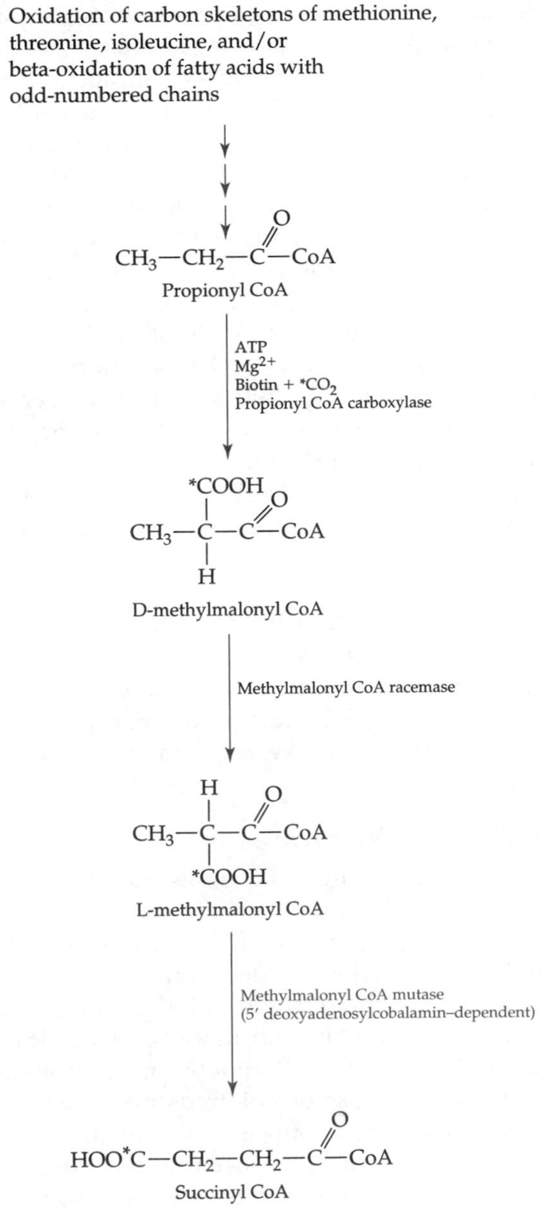

Metabolism and Excretion

Vitamin B_{12} is not extensively (if at all) degraded prior to excretion. Turnover of the vitamin is approximately 0.1% per day, with most of the vitamin excreted bound to R protein via the bile. Little urinary excretion occurs; there are trace dermal losses of vitamin B_{12}.

Recommended Dietary Allowances

Recommendations for vitamin B_{12} intake are based on estimates of vitamin intake and turnover and on amounts of the vitamin needed for the maintenance of normal serum indices of the vitamin and hematological status. The RDA for adults for vitamin B_{12} is 2.4 µg per day, with increases of 0.2 and 0.4 µg per day suggested for women during pregnancy and lactation, respectively [6]. The requirement for the vitamin for adults is 2.0 µg/day [6]. It is further suggested that individuals age 51 years and older consume foods fortified with the vitamin or consume vitamin B_{12} supplements, because 10% to 30% of older individuals have changes to the gastrointestinal tract that limit their ability to absorb food-bound forms of the vitamin [6]. The inside cover of the book provides additional recommendations for vitamin B_{12} intake for other age groups.

Deficiency: Megaloblastic, Macrocytic Anemia

Deficiency of vitamin B_{12}, like that of folate, results in megaloblastic macrocytic anemia. Manifestations of vitamin B_{12} deficiency occur in stages. Initially, serum concentrations diminish, as indicated by low holotranscobalamin II. Second, cell concentrations of the vitamin diminish. Third, biochemical deficiency occurs, as evidenced by decreased DNA synthesis and by elevated homocysteine and methylmalonic acid concentrations in the serum. Finally, a macrocytic megaloblastic (large immature cell) anemia occurs [13]. Some signs and symptoms of deficiency include skin pallor, fatigue, shortness of breath, palpitations, insomnia, tingling and numbness (paresthesia) in extremities, abnormal gait, loss of concentration, memory loss, disorientation, swelling of myelinated fibers, and possibly dementia. Neurological problems occur in about 75% to 90% of deficient individuals [6,14].

The megaloblastic macrocytic anemia associated with a vitamin B_{12} deficiency is detailed under folic acid deficiency (p. 307), because deficiencies of both vitamins result in megaloblastic macrocytic anemia. In fact, the megaloblastic anemia due to a vitamin deficiency can be corrected with large doses of folate. However, the neuropathy, characterized by demyelination of nerves, caused by a lack of vitamin B_{12} is not responsive to folate therapy. The neuropathy is usually found in vitamin B_{12}–deficient individuals with decreased activity of both vitamin B_{12}–dependent enzymes. Its cause may be related to the availability of methionine [15,16]. The neuropathy can be ameliorated through increased exogenous methionine or an accelerated production of methionine from homocysteine, a reaction that requires vitamin B_{12}. An inadequate amount of methionine caused by a deficiency of vitamin B_{12} decreases the availability of S-adenosyl methionine (SAM). Remember that SAM is required for methylation reactions, which are essential to myelin maintenance and thus neural function. SAM deficiency in the nervous system (i.e., cerebrospinal fluid) has been implicated in the pathogenesis of cobalamin neuropathy [17].

In addition to anemia, plasma vitamin B_{12} concentrations are inversely associated with plasma homocysteine concentrations [18–23]. Elevated plasma homocysteine concentrations are considered a risk factor for coronary heart disease, and concentrations may be lowered with vitamin B_{12}, folate, and vitamin B_6 supplements [18, 22–24]. This relationship among vitamin B_{12}, folate, vitamin B_6, plasma homocysteine concentrations, and heart disease is discussed in further detail under folic acid, page 306.

Inadequate absorption of the vitamin, rather than inadequate dietary intake, is responsible for the majority of the vitamin B_{12} deficiency seen in the United States. However, a strict vegetarian diet can produce a deficiency of the vitamin fairly quickly in an infant or a young child with minimal stores of the vitamin. In contrast to children, adults consuming animal-based diets who switch to strict vegetarian diets without consuming vitamin-fortified foods may not develop clinical symptoms of deficiency for decades due to fairly large stores of the vitamin. Inadequate vitamin B_{12} absorption can result from any of several problems and is especially prevalent in older individuals. Malabsorption can result from pernicious anemia, an autoimmune condition in which the body produces antibodies that attack gastric parietal cells and thereby diminish IF production. Remember, IF is required for the absorption of the vitamin. Other conditions that can impair absorption of the vitamin include those causing a lack of IF, such as atrophic gastritis (loss and inflammation of gastric cells) or gastrectomy (removal of all or a portion of the stomach). In some forms of atrophic gastritis, antibodies are made against the proton pump in gastric parietal cells [25]. Diminished hydrochloric acid release **(achlorhydria)** also decreases release of the vitamin bound to food, causing malabsorption of the vitamin. People with a decreased absorptive surface in the ileum, such as occurs with ileal resection, celiac and tropical sprue, ileitis (inflammation of the ileum), or Zollinger-Ellison syndrome, also will malabsorb the vitamin and be at risk for deficiency. In addition, people with parasitic infections such as tapeworms may develop a vitamin B_{12} deficiency due to use of the vitamin by the parasite and a consequent limited availability to the infected person. Prolonged use of some medications, such as H_2 blockers and proton pump inhibitors used to treat individuals with ulcers or gastroesophageal reflux disease (GERD), also is associated with diminished absorption of vitamin B_{12}. Finally, individuals who have poor vitamin B_{12} status may exhibit deterioration of nervous system function, especially demyelinating problems, following nitrous oxide anesthesia [26–28]. Nitrous oxide (an anesthetic agent) has been shown to inhibit the activity of methionine synthase by reacting with methylcobalamin and possibly altering the oxidation state of the cobalt (from +1 to +3) [1].

The incidence of vitamin B_{12} deficiency in the elderly may be as high as 15%, and the vitamin B_{12} content of multivitamin preparations is not sufficient to adequately raise serum vitamin B_{12} concentrations [9,29]. Oral vitamin B_{12} in amounts of at least 6 to 9 μg and possibly up to 300 μg appears to be necessary to correct deficiency in the elderly [29]. Treatment of pernicious anemia or deficiency secondary to malabsorption often requires monthly intramuscular injection of the vitamin in amounts of 500 to 1,000 μg [6] or oral ingestion of pharmacologic amounts (2 mg) of the vitamin [30].

Toxicity

Although no clear toxicity from massive doses of vitamin B_{12} has ever been recorded, neither has any benefit been noted from an excessive intake of the vitamin by people with adequate vitamin status [6]. No tolerable upper intake level for vitamin B_{12} has been established [6].

Assessment of Nutriture

Vitamin B_{12} status may be assessed using several indices. Serum vitamin B_{12} concentrations, which include cobalamin bound to TCI, TCII, and TCII, are commonly measured and reflect both intake and status. Concentrations in the serum of $<$200 pg/mL (based on a radioassay method) are considered deficient [6]. Only cobalamin bound to TCII, however, is provided to tissues for uptake. Use of holotranscobalamin II as an indicator of status has not been accepted at present [6]. Because serum vitamin B_{12} concentrations can be maintained at the expense of tissues, a person may exhibit normal serum concentrations but have low tissue concentrations [14]. Thus, assessment that includes measurement of indices in addition to serum concentrations is beneficial.

Measurements of serum methylmalonyl CoA or methylmalonic acid and of homocysteine also are used to assess vitamin B_{12} status. Increased concentrations of methylmalonyl CoA (or methylmalonic acid) and of homocysteine, substrates normally metabolized by vitamin B_{12}–dependent enzymes, occur with diminished enzyme activity resulting from insufficient vitamin B_{12}. Increased blood or urinary excretion of methylmalonic acid with deficient vitamin B_{12} status and response (decreases) of blood methylmalonic acid concentrations to vitamin B_{12} supplementation are helpful indicators of vitamin status [30]. Normally, no or only trace amounts of methylmalonic acid are excreted in the urine; however, with vitamin B_{12} deficiency, methylmalonic acid excretion may exceed 300 mg per day [14]. Reticulocyte counts also increase within 48 hours following vitamin B_{12} supplementation of deficient individuals.

Other tests used to assess vitamin B_{12} nutriture include the deoxyuridine suppression test, discussed previously under "Assessment of Nutriture" in the folic acid section (p. 309), and the Schilling test, which is used to determine problems of vitamin B_{12} absorption related to IF insufficiency. The Schilling test involves oral administration of radioactive vitamin B_{12} and measurement of urinary excretion of the vitamin over various times. Below-normal urinary excretion of the vitamin suggests impaired absorption.

References Cited for Vitamin B_{12}

1. Seatharam B, Alpers D. Absorption and transport of cobalamin (vitamin B_{12}). Ann Rev Nutr 1982;2:343–69.

2. National Research Council. Recommended Dietary Allowances, 10th ed. Washington, DC: National Academy Press, 1989, pp. 158–65.

3. Sandberg D, Begley J, Hall C. The content, binding and forms of vitamin B_{12} in milk. Am J Clin Nutr 1981;34:1717–24.

4. Toskes P, Hansell J, Cerda J, Deren J. Vitamin B_{12} malabsorption in chronic pancreatic insufficiency. N Engl J Med 1971;284:627–32.

5. Moestrup S, Verroust P. Mammalian receptors of vitamin B_{12} binding proteins. In: Banerjee R, ed. Chemistry and Biochemistry of B_{12}. New York: Wiley Interscience, 1999, pp. 475–88.

6. Food and Nutrition Board. Dietary Reference Intakes for Thiamin, Riboflavin, Niacin, Vitamin B_6, Folate, Vitamin B_{12}, Pantothenic Acid, Biotin, and Choline. Washington, DC: National Academy Press, 1998, pp. 306–56.

7. McEvoy A, Fenwick J, Boddy K, James O. Vitamin B_{12} absorption from the gut does not decline with age in normal elderly humans. Age Ageing 1982;11:180–83.

8. Nilsson-Ehle H, Jagenburg R, Landahl S, Lindstedt G, Swolin B, Westin J. Cyanocobalamin absorption in the elderly: results for healthy subjects and for subjects with low serum cobalamin concentration. Clin Chem 1986;32:1368–71.

9. Carmel R. Cobalamin, the stomach and aging. Am J Clin Nutr 1997;66:750–59.

10. Van Asselt D, van den Broek W, Lamers C, Corstens F, Hoefnagels W. Free and protein-bound cobalamin absorption in healthy middle-aged and older subjects. J Am Geriatr Soc 1996;44:949–53.

11. El-Kholty S, Gueant J, Bressler L, Djalali M, Boissel P, Gerard P, Nicolas J. Portal and biliary phases of enterohepatic circulation of corrinoids in humans. Gastroenterology 1991;101:1399–1408.

12. Ludwig M, Mathews R. Structure-based perspectives on B_{12} dependent enzymes. Ann Rev Biochem 1997;66:269–313.

13. Herbert V. Staging of vitamin B_{12} (cobalamin) status in vegetarians. Am J Clin Nutr 1994;59(suppl):1213S–22S.

14. Beck W. Neuropsychiatric consequences of cobalamin deficiency. Adv Intern Med 1991;36:33–56.

15. Metz J. Pathogenesis of cobalamin neuropathy: deficiency of nervous system S-adenosylmethionine. Nutr Rev 1993;51:12–15.

16. Davis R. Clinical chemistry of vitamin B_{12}. Adv Clin Chem 1984;24:163–216.

17. Council on Scientific Affairs, American Medical Association. Vitamin preparations as dietary supplements and as therapeutic agents. JAMA 1987;257:1929–36.

18. Pancharuniti N, Lewis C, Sauberlich H, Perkins L, Go R, Alvarez J, Masaluso M, Acton R, Copeland R, Cousins A, Gore T, Cornwell P, Roseman J. Plasma homocyst(e)ine, folate, and vitamin B_{12} concentrations and risk for early-onset coronary artery disease. Am J Clin Nutr 1994;59:940–48.

19. Mansoor M, Ueland P, Svardal A. Redox status and protein binding of plasma homocysteine and other aminothiols in patients with hyperhomocysteinemia due to cobalamin deficiency. Am J Clin Nutr 1994;59:631–35.

20. Ubbink J. Vitamin B_{12}, vitamin B_6, and folate nutritional status in men with hyperhomocysteinemia. Am J Clin Nutr 1993;57:47–53.

21. Shimakawa T, Nieto F, Malinow M, Chambess L, Schreiner P, Szklo M. Vitamin intake: possible determinant of plasma homocyst(e)ine among middle-aged adults. Ann Epidemiol 1997; 7:285–93.

22. Boushey C, Beresford S, Omenn G, Motulsky A. A quantitative assessment of plasma homocysteine as a risk factor for vascular disease: probable benefits of increasing folic acid intakes. JAMA 1995;274:1049–57.

23. Ubbink J, Vermaak W, Merwe A, Becker P, Delport A, Potgieter H. Vitamin requirements for the treatment of hyperhomocysteinemia in humans. J Nutr 1994;124:1927–33.

24. Refsum H, Ueland P, Nygard O, Vollset SE. Homocysteine and cardiovascular disease. Ann Rev Med 1998;49:31–62.

25. Ban-Hock T, van Driel I, Gleeson P. Pernicious anemia. N Engl J Med 1997;337:1441–48.

26. Metz J. Cobalamin deficiency and the pathogenesis of nervous system disease. Ann Rev Nutr 1992;12:59–79.

27. Flippo T, Holder W. Neurologic degeneration associated with nitrous oxide anesthesia in patients with vitamin B_{12} deficiency. Archives Surg 1993;128:1391–95.

28. Guttormsen A, Refsum H, Ueland P. The interaction between nitrous oxide and cobalamin biochemical effects and clinical consequences. Acta Anaesthesiol Scand 1994;38:753–56.

29. Stabler S, Lindenbaum J, Allen R. Vitamin B_{12} deficiency in the elderly: current dilemmas. Am J Clin Nutr 1997;66:741–49.

30. Kuzminski A, Del Glacco E, Allen R, Stabler S, Lindenbaum J. Effective treatment of cobalamin deficiency with oral cobalamin. Blood 1998;92:1191–98.

Suggested Reading

Banerjee R, ed. Chemistry and Biochemistry of B_{12}. New York: Wiley Interscience, 1999.

VITAMIN B_6

Vitamin B_6 exists as several vitamers, the structural formulas of which are given in Figure 9.38. These vitamers are interchangeable and comparably active (Fig. 9.39). Pyridoxine represents the alcohol form, pyridoxal the aldehyde form, and pyridoxamine the amine form. Each has a 5′-phosphate derivative.

Sources

All B_6 vitamers are found in food. Pyridoxine, the stablest of the compounds, and its phosphorylated form are found almost exclusively in plant foods. In some plants, vitamin B_6 is found in a conjugated form, pyridoxine β-glucoside. Pyridoxal phosphate and pyridoxamine phosphate are found primarily in animal products, with sirloin steak, salmon, and the light meat of chicken being rich sources [1,2]. Excellent sources of vitamin B_6 in commonly consumed foods include meats, whole-grain products, vegetables, some fruits (e.g., bananas), and nuts. Fortified cereals also represent a major contributor of vitamin B_6 in the diet. Vitamin B_6 in supplements is generally found as pyridoxine hydrochloride.

The bioavailability of vitamin B_6 from different food sources is influenced by the extent and type of processing to which the foods are subjected. Much of the vitamin originally present in foods can be lost through processing, including, for example, heating, canning, milling of wheat, sterilization, and freezing [1–3].

Digestion, Absorption, Transport, and Storage

For absorption of vitamin B_6 to occur, the phosphorylated vitamers must be dephosphorylated. Alkaline phosphatase, a zinc-dependent enzyme found at the intestinal brush border, or other intestinal phosphatases hydrolyze the phosphate to yield either pyridoxine (PN), pyridoxal (PL), or pyridoxamine (PM).

Absorption of PL, PN, and PM occurs primarily in the jejunum by passive diffusion. At physiological

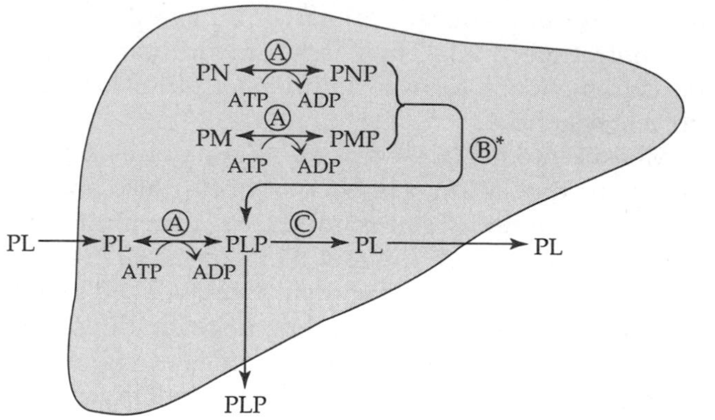

Enzymes
Ⓐ Kinase (ATP dependent)
Ⓑ PMP and PNP oxidase* (FMN dependent)
Ⓒ Phosphatase

*Oxidase is found mainly in the liver and enterocytes.

Figure 9.39 Vitamin B_6 metabolism in the liver.

Figure 9.38 Vitamin B_6 structures.

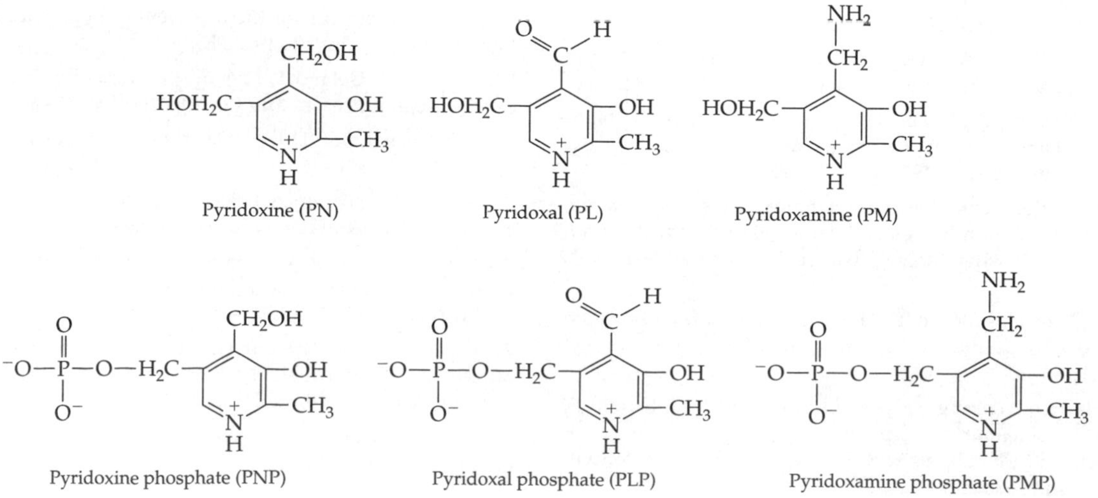

intakes, the vitamin is absorbed rapidly in its free form; however, when the phosphorylated vitamers are ingested in high concentrations, some of these compounds may be absorbed per se [3]. Absorption of some pyridoxine glucosides may also occur by passive diffusion; mucosal glucosidase can hydrolyze the glucosides to varying degrees [4]. Overall absorption of vitamin B_6 furnished by the average U.S. diet is about 75%, with a range of about 61% to 92% [5,6].

Little metabolism of the vitamin occurs within the intestinal cell. Most PN, PL, and PM is released unchanged into portal blood and taken up by the liver, where it is converted primarily to PLP. PLP is the main (60% to 90% of the total) form of the vitamin found in systemic blood. Most PLP is bound to albumin. Other forms of the vitamin present in blood include PL, PN, PM, and PMP. From the plasma, the unphosphorylated vitamers may be taken up by red blood cells, converted to PLP, and bound to hemoglobin.

The liver is the main organ that takes up (by passive diffusion) and metabolizes newly absorbed vitamin B_6. The liver stores about 5% to 10% of the vitamin [7]. Muscles represent the major (75%–80%) storage site for the vitamin, which is found in the body in amounts totaling about 165 mg [8]. Most vitamin B_6 occurs in muscle as PLP bound to glycogen phosphorylase [5,8,9]. Phosphorylation of the vitamin prevents its diffusion out of the cell, and the binding of the vitamin to protein prevents hydrolysis by phosphatases.

Most vitamin B_6 metabolism occurs in the liver. Unphosphorylated forms of the vitamin typically are phosphorylated by a kinase using ATP within the cytoplasm of the hepatocyte (liver cell), as shown in Figure 9.39. PNP and PMP are then generally converted by the action of an FMN-dependent oxidase to PLP. Thus, vitamin B_6 metabolism is dependent on normal riboflavin status.

Pyridoxine or pyridoxamine phosphate —(FMN-dependent oxidase)→ Pyridoxal phosphate

Figure 9.39 depicts the interconversion of the B_6 vitamers. Intracellular PLP concentrations are dependent, in part, on the availability of binding proteins. With saturation of binding proteins, unbound PLP is hydrolyzed to PL, which then is released into the blood for use by other tissues. From the liver, mostly PLP and PL, with smaller amounts of the other vitamers, are released for transport to extrahepatic tissues.

Only unphosphorylated forms of the vitamin are taken up by tissues; thus, PLP in the blood is hydrolyzed by alkaline phosphatase prior to cellular uptake. Within the cell, PL is phosphorylated by pyridoxine kinase in an ATP-dependent reaction. Pyridoxine kinase is found in almost all tissues, and phosphorylation traps the vitamin in the cells. Most tissues, however, lack sufficient oxidase to convert PNP and PMP into the coenzyme form PLP. PNP/PMP oxidase is found mainly in the liver and intestine and to lesser extents in the muscle, kidney, brain, and red blood cells.

Functions and Mechanisms of Action

The coenzyme form of vitamin B_6, PLP, is associated with a vast number (>100) of enzymes, the majority of which are involved in amino acid metabolism. Some non-coenzyme roles of the vitamin impact the action of steroid hormones and gene expression.

Coenzymes

As a coenzyme in reactions involving amino acids, PLP, through the formation of a Schiff base (the product formed by an amino group and an aldehyde), labilizes all the bonds around the α-carbon of the amino acid. The specific bond that is broken is determined by the catalytic groups of the particular enzyme to which PLP is attached. The covalent bonds of an α-amino acid that can be made labile by its binding to specific PLP-containing enzymes are shown in Figure 9.40.

Some of the reactions involving amino acids that are catalyzed by PLP include transamination (which can also be catalyzed by PMP), decarboxylation, transulfhydration and desulfhydration, cleavage, racemization, and synthesis. In addition to its participation in reactions involving amino acids, vitamin B_6 functions via a different mechanism in the initial step of glycogen metabolism. Each of these reactions is discussed briefly.

Transamination. Of particular importance are the transamination reactions in which PMP as well as PLP can serve as a coenzyme. The most common aminotransferases for which PLP (or PMP) is a coenzyme are

Figure 9.40 The covalent bonds of an α-amino acid that can be made labile by its binding to PLP-containing enzymes.

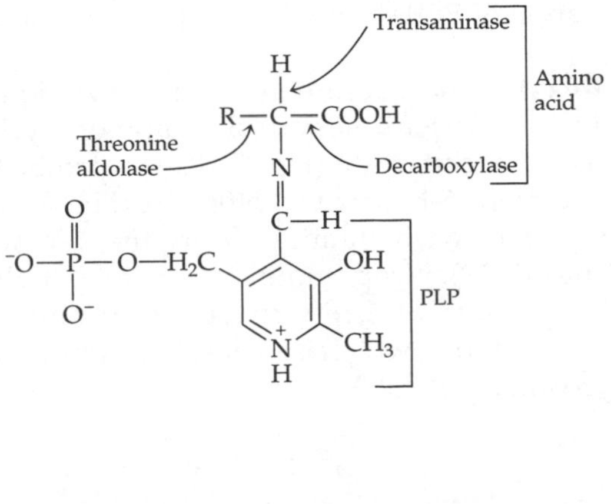

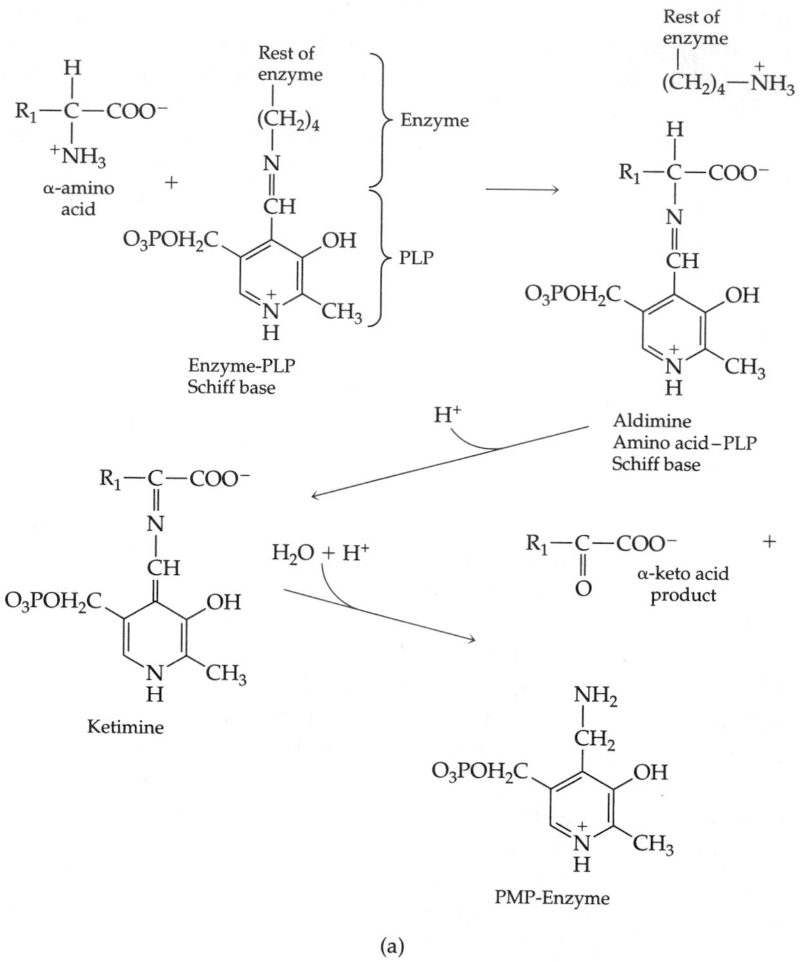

Figure 9.41 (a) The role of vitamin B_6 in transamination, phase 1. (b) The role of vitamin B_6 in transamination, phase 2.

glutamate oxaloacetate transaminase (GOT, also called aspartic amino transferase or AST) and glutamate pyruvate transaminase (GPT, also called alanine aminotransferase or ALT) (Fig. 7.22). Figures 9.41a and b show the two phases of transamination and demonstrate how PLP forms a Schiff base. In the first phase, the corresponding α-keto acid of the amino acid is produced along with PMP. In the second phase, the transamination cycle is completed as a new α-keto acid substrate receives the amino group from the PMP. The corresponding amino acid is generated, along with regeneration of PLP.

Decarboxylation. Common decarboxylation reactions include the formation of γ-aminobutyric acid (GABA) from glutamate (Fig. 7.41), the production of serotonin from 5-hydroxytryptophan (Fig. 7.39), and the synthesis of histamine from the amino acid histidine (7.30). Dopamine is formed following decarboxylation of dihydroxyphenylalanine (also known as L-dopa), which is generated from the amino acid tyrosine (Fig. 7.25).

Transulfhydration and Desulfhydration. PLP is required for transulfhydration reactions in which cysteine is synthesized from methionine (Figs. 7.27 and 9.42). Both cystathionine synthase and cystathionine lyase require PLP. Cysteine undergoes desulfhydration followed by transamination to generate pyruvate.

Cleavage. An example of a cleavage reaction requiring PLP is the removal of the hydroxymethyl group from serine. In this reaction, PLP is the coenzyme for a transferase that transfers the hydroxymethyl group of serine to tetrahydrofolate (THF) so that glycine is formed (Fig. 9.31).

Racemization. PLP is required by racemases that catalyze the interconversion of D- and L-amino acids. Although such reactions are more prevalent in bacterial metabolism, some occur in humans.

Other Synthetic Reactions. Vitamin B_6 is also necessary as a coenzyme in the first step in the synthesis of

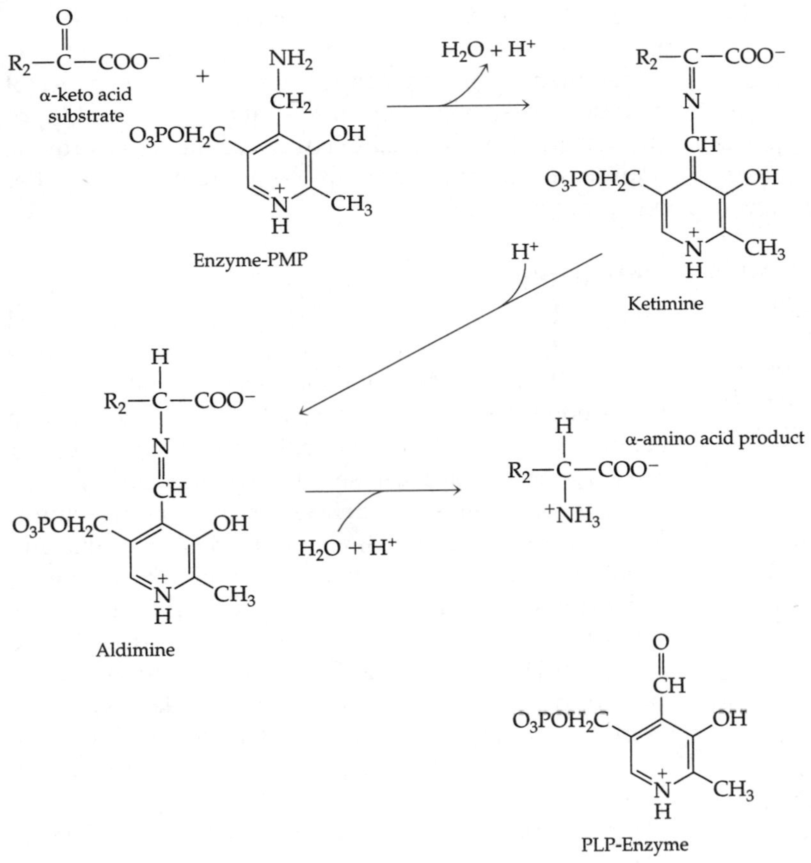

(b)

heme (Fig. 12.5). PLP is required for δ-aminolevulinic acid synthetase, which catalyzes the condensation, followed by decarboxylation, of glycine with succinyl CoA to form δ-aminolevulinic acid (ALA) in the mitochondria of the cell. ALA moves into the cytosol of the cell, where it is used to synthesize porphobilinogen (PBG), the parent pyrrole compound in porphyrin synthesis. Through a series of reactions, PBG is converted into protoporphyrin IX, which with the addition of Fe^{2+} by ferrocheletase forms heme.

Figure 9.42 Cysteine synthesis from methionine requires vitamin B_6 as PLP.

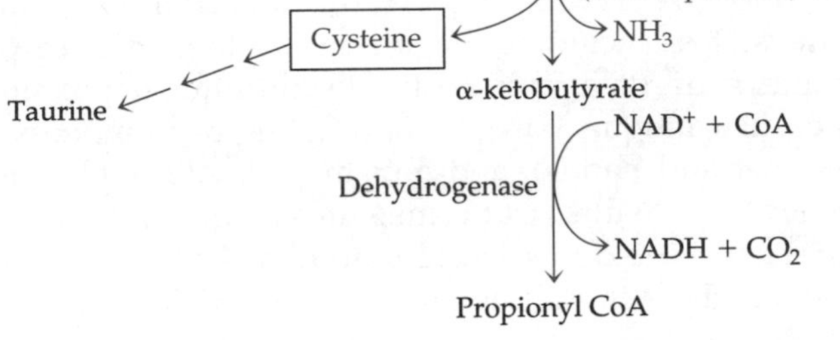

PLP functions as a cofactor for another condensation reaction necessary for sphingolipid synthesis. Specifically, the amino acid serine condenses with palmitoyl CoA in a reaction catalyzed by a PLP-dependent transferase to form 3-dehydrosphinganine. This latter compound serves as a precursor for sphingolipids.

Niacin (NAD) synthesis from tryptophan also requires an important PLP-dependent reaction. Specifically, kynureninase required for the conversion of 3-hydroxykynurenine to 3-hydroxyanthranilate requires vitamin B_6 (PLP) as a coenzyme (Figs. 7.26 and 9.18).

Other compounds synthesized in the body in vitamin B_6-dependent reactions include carnitine, a nonprotein nitrogen-containing compound required for fatty acid oxidation, and taurine, a neuromodulatory compound generated from cysteine metabolism (Fig. 7.27).

Glycogen Degradation. The function of PLP in glycogen degradation is poorly understood. Glycogen is catabolized by glycogen phosphorylase to form glucose 1-PO_4 (Fig. 4.13); vitamin B_6 is required for glycogen phosphorylase activity. The mechanism of action of the coenzyme appears to be different from that exerted with other enzymes. The phosphate of the coenzyme is believed to be involved as a proton buffer to stabilize the compound and permit covalent bonding of the phosphate to form glucose 1-PO_4 [10]. Most vitamin B_6 found in muscle is present as PLP, which in turn is bound to glycogen phosphorylase.

Non-Coenzyme Roles: Steroid Hormone Action

While the coenzyme roles of vitamin B_6 have been more thoroughly investigated, the vitamin also appears to moderate the effects of some steroid hormones. Vitamin B_6 as PLP has been shown to react with lysine residues in steroid hormone receptor proteins to prevent or interfere with hormone binding. These receptor proteins mediate nuclear uptake of steroid hormones and the interaction of the nucleoproteins with the DNA [7]. Thus, vitamin B_6 appears to be able to diminish the actions of steroids. Diminishing the action of, for example, glucocorticoid hormones can in turn influence metabolism of protein, carbohydrate, and lipid.

Metabolism and Excretion

Little vitamin B_6 is excreted in the feces [5,11]. 4-pyridoxic acid (PIC) is the major metabolite of the vitamin and results from the oxidation of PL by either NAD-dependent aldehyde dehydrogenase, found in all tissues, or FAD-dependent aldehyde oxidases, found in the liver and kidneys. 4-pyridoxic acid is excreted via the urine and is indicative of recent vitamin intake, not vitamin stores [5]. Ingestion of large doses (100 mg) of the vitamin as PN results in the urinary excretion of PN intact and 5-pyridoxic acid and lower urinary 4-pyridoxic acid excretion. It appears that when PN is administered at high levels, the kidney tubules reduce plasma content of the vitamer by excreting some of it into the urine [5,11].

Recommended Dietary Allowances

The 1998 RDA for vitamin B_6 for adult men age 19 to 50 years is 1.3 mg per day (requirement 1.1 mg) and for men age 51 years and older is higher, at 1.7 mg per day (requirement 1.4 mg) [5]. For adult women age 19 to 50 years, the RDA for vitamin B_6 is also 1.3 mg per day (requirement 1.1 mg), and for women age 51 years and older it is 1.5 mg daily (requirement 1.3 mg) [5]. With pregnancy and lactation, recommendations for vitamin intake increase to 1.9 and 2.0 mg, respectively [5]. Recommendations are based largely on maintenance of adequate plasma concentrations (at least 20 nmol/L) of the vitamin [5]. The inside covers of the book provide additional recommendations for vitamin B_6 for other age groups.

Deficiency

Vitamin B_6 deficiency is relatively rare in the United States. In the 1950s, deficiency occurred in infants because of severe heat treatment of infant milk. The heat processing resulted in a reaction between the PLP and the epsilon amino group of lysine in the milk proteins to form pyridoxyl-lysine, which possesses little vitamin activity.

Signs of vitamin B_6 deficiency include sleepiness, fatigue, cheilosis, glossitis, and stomatitis in adults, and neurological problems such as abnormal EEGs, seizures, and convulsions in infants. A hypochromic, microcytic anemia may also result from a vitamin B_6 deficiency due to impaired heme synthesis. Deficiency also alters calcium and magnesium metabolism, impairs niacin synthesis from tryptophan, and inhibits metabolism of homocysteine. The last results in hyperhomocysteinemia, a risk factor for heart disease (see p. 306) [12].

Groups particularly at risk for vitamin B_6 deficiency are

- the elderly, who have a poor intake of the vitamin and may also have accelerated hydrolysis of PLP and oxidation of PL to PIC;
- people who consume excessive amounts of alcohol (alcohol can impair conversion of PN and PM to PLP, and the presence of acetaldehyde formed from ethanol metabolism may enhance hydrolysis of PLP to PL with subsequent formation of the excretory product pyridoxic acid);
- renal patients on maintenance dialysis, which causes an abnormal loss of vitamin B_6; and
- people on a variety of drug therapies, including isoniazid, penicillamine, corticosteroids, and anticonvulsants [1,2].

Toxicity

Pharmacological doses of vitamin B_6 have been advocated for the prevention or treatment of a variety of disease states, including hyperhomocysteinemia, carpal tunnel syndrome, premenstrual syndrome, depression, muscular fatigue, paresthesia (tingling or numbness of the feet and hands), and autism [13]. Although some beneficial results from megadoses of the vitamin have been noted in selected individuals, indiscriminate use of the vitamin is not without risk. Excessive pyridoxine use causes sensory and peripheral neuropathy [14]. Some symptoms include unsteady gait, paresthesia, and impaired tendon reflexes [15]. High intakes of pyridoxine also appear to cause degeneration of dorsal root ganglia in the spinal cord, loss of myelination, and degeneration of sensory fibers in peripheral nerves [13,15]. The tolerable upper intake level for vitamin B_6 is 100 mg per day for adults to minimize the development of neuropathy [5].

Assessment of Nutriture

Plasma PLP concentrations are thought to be the best indicator of vitamin B_6 tissue stores, with plasma PLP <10 nmol/L suggestive of vitamin deficiency [5,11]. Several other indices may be used in combination with plasma PLP concentration to assess vitamin B_6 nutriture.

A commonly used functional test measures xanthurenic acid excretion following tryptophan loading (2 g or 100 mg of tryptophan/kg body weight). Abnormally high xanthurenic acid excretion (>25 mg in 6 hours) is found in vitamin B_6 deficiency because 3-hydroxykynurenine, an intermediate in tryptophan metabolism, cannot lose its alanine moiety and be converted to 3-hydroxyanthranilate, as should occur in the liver (Fig. 9.18). Instead, 3-hydroxykynurenine is converted to xanthurenic acid, which is excreted in the urine. Interpretation of this test is sometimes difficult owing to factors other than vitamin B_6 in tryptophan metabolism. Acceptable xanthurenic acid excretion following the tryptophan load is <25 mg/6 hours.

Urinary vitamin B_6 and 4-pyridoxic acid also have been used to assess the status of vitamin B_6. Urinary vitamin B_6 excretion measured over several 24-hour urine collections for a period of 1 to 3 weeks is recommended to more accurately assess vitamin B_6. Urinary 4-pyridoxic acid concentrations of <3.0 mmol per day are thought to be indicative of deficiency [16]. Urinary vitamin B_6 excretion in comparison to creatinine excretion is also used: urinary levels of <20 mg/g creatinine suggest B_6 deficiency, while excretion >20 mg/g creatinine suggests acceptable vitamin B_6 status. Urinary 4-pyridoxic acid excretion is considered to be a short-term indicator of vitamin B_6 status; however, cutoff values are controversial [5,11,16].

Measurement of erythrocyte transaminase activity before and after the addition of vitamin B_6 is also useful in determining vitamin B_6 nutriture. However, because of a variety of limitations with the assays, these tests are better used as an adjunct to other tests. Erythrocyte transaminase index examines activity of erythrocyte glutamic oxaloacetic transaminase (EGOT, also called aspartic amino transferase or EAST) after the addition of vitamin B_6. This assay and the assay discussed next are thought to represent long-term vitamin status. Deficient vitamin B_6 status is suggested by activity of >1.8 following the addition of the vitamin [16]. Similarly, activity of erythrocyte glutamic pyruvic transaminase (EGPT, also called alanine aminotransferase or EALT) of >1.25 suggests B_6 deficiency, whereas activity of <1.25 indicates adequate status [16,17].

References Cited for Vitamin B_6

1. Sauberlich H. Bioavailability of vitamins. Prog Food Nutr Sci 1985;9:1–33.

2. Sauberlich H. Vitamins—how much is for keeps? Nutr Today 1987;22:20–28.

3. Ink S, Henderson L. Vitamin B_6 metabolism. Ann Rev Nutr 1984;4:455–70.

4. Nakano H, Gregory J. Pyridoxine and pyridoxine 5′-β-D-glucoside exert different effects on tissue B_6 vitamers but similar effects on β-glucosidase activity in rats. J Nutr 1995;125:2751–62.

5. Food and Nutrition Board. Dietary Reference Intakes for Thiamin, Riboflavin, Niacin, Vitamin B_6, Folate, Vitamin B_{12}, Pantothenic Acid, Biotin, and Choline. Washington, DC: National Academy Press, 1998, pp. 150–95.

6. Tarr J, Tamura T, Stokstad E. Availability of vitamin B_6 and pantothenate in an average diet in man. Am J Clin Nutr 1981;34:1328–37.

7. Allgood V, Cidlowski J. Novel role for vitamin B_6 in steroid hormone action: a link between nutrition and the endocrine system. J Nutr Biochem 1991;2:523–34.

8. Coburn S, Lewis D, Fink W, Mahuren J, Schaltenbrand W, Costill D. Human vitamin B_6 pools estimated through muscle biopsies. Am J Clin Nutr 1988;48:291–94.

9. Coburn S. Location and turnover of vitamin B_6 pools and vitamin B_6 requirements of humans. Ann NY Acad Sci 1990;585:75–85.

10. Palm D, Klein H, Schinzel R, et al. The role of pyridoxal 5′phosphate in glycogen phosphorylase catalysis. Biochemistry 1990; 29:1099–1107.

11. Lui A, Lumeng L, Aronoff G, Li T-K. Relationship between body store of vitamin B_6 and plasma pyridoxal-P clearance; metabolic balance studies in humans. J Lab Clin Med 1985;106:491–97.

12. Turlund J, Betschart A, Liebman M, Kretsch M, Sauberlich H. Vitamin B_6 depletion followed by repletion with animal or plant source diets and calcium and magnesium metabolism in young women. Am J Clin Nutr 1992;56:905–10.

13. Alhadeff L, Gualtieri C, Lipton M. Toxic effects of water-soluble vitamins. Nutr Rev 1984;42:33–40.

14. Council on Scientific Affairs, American Medical Association. Vitamin preparations as dietary supplements and as therapeutic agents. JAMA 1987;257:1929–36.

15. Berger A, Schaumburg H, Schroeder C, Apfel S, Reynolds R. Dose response, coasting and differential fiber vulnerability in human toxic neuropathy: a prospective study of pyridoxine neurotoxicity. Neurology 1992;42:1367–70.

16. Leklem J. Vitamin B_6: a status report. J Nutr 1990;120:1503–7.

17. Simko M, Cowell C, Gilbride J. Nutrition Assessment. Rockville, MD: Aspen, 1995.

Genetics and Nutrition: Human Folate Needs and Chronic Disease Risk, by Rita M. Johnson, Ph.D., R.D., F.A.D.A.

"Genomic medicine holds the ultimate promise of revolutionizing the diagnosis and treatment of many illnesses." [1]

The results of the Human Genome Project have spawned a huge number of articles—both peer-reviewed and in the mass media—about the implications for individuals, families, and society [2,3]. While the current results are most applicable to medicine, it is likely that nutrigenomics will grow and provide insight into individual nutrient needs [2,4,5]. Nutrigenomics studies the interaction and influence of nutrients on gene expression and resulting health outcomes. DeBusk summarizes that there are three effects of nutrients on the expression of our genes [2]:

1. Nutrients can complete gaps in our DNA.
2. Nutrients can interact with DNA, causing the synthesis of necessary proteins for the body.
3. Nutrients can interfere with the expression of genes that could produce harmful effects.

Nutrition professionals in the near future may need to both understand and practice nutrigenomics in order to provide individualized nutrition advice designed for their clients' and patients' unique genetic traits [5,6]. Recently, the Commission on the Accreditation of Dietetic Education added genetics and nutrition to its list of required knowledge for the education of dietetic professionals [7]. By increasing our study and understanding of nutrigenomics, nutrition professionals will continue to be able to provide high-quality, science-based care.

Discoveries about folate metabolism provide an often-used example of nutrigenomics [8]. The identification of genetic variations in folate metabolism have been linked to neural tube defects, fetal malformations, coronary heart disease, colorectal cancer, dementia, and other health problems. The purpose of this perspective is to

- describe the most common types of genetic variants in 5,10-methylenetetrahydrofolate reductase,
- review the prevalence of genetic variation among different ethnic groups, and
- provide an overview of the research that links these variants to alterations in disease risk.

5,10-methylenetetrahydrofolate Reductase and Its Genetic Variants

Under normal circumstances, as shown in Figure 9.31, 5,10-methylenetetrahydrofolate reductase (methylene-THF reductase, or MTHFR) catalyzes the unidirectional conversion of 5,10-methylene THF to 5-methyl THF. The activity of MTHFR, along with adequate amounts of NADPH and $FADH_2$, is essential to maintain appropriate levels of 5-methyl THF in the cell.

In circumstances where MTHFR activity is low, intracellular 5-methyl THF decreases, and the conversion of homocysteine to methionine is impaired. The lack of methionine results in a lack of methyl groups, which are necessary for methylation reactions such as the synthesis of DNA, carnitine, creatine, epinephrine, purines, and nicotinamide. Thus, when the formation of 5-methyl THF is impaired, the body's ability to synthesize methylated products and remove homocysteine is affected. An accumulation of homocysteine is widely believed to increase risk of cardiovascular disease and dementias.

Several genetic variations of MTHFR have been reported. These variants are caused by substitutions in the DNA sequence that codes for the enzyme, and because they are shared by >1% of the population they are termed genetic polymorphisms [8]. The genetic polymorphisms of MTHFR cause a decrease in its activity and in the subsequent formation of 5-methyl THF. Two MTHFR polymorphisms have been reported [9]: a substitution of a thymine (abnormal) for a cytosine (normal) base at position 677 (called C677T), and a substitution of a cytosine base (abnormal) for an adenine (normal) base at position 1298 (called A1298C). These substitutions cause a molecule of valine to be inserted into MTHFR instead of alanine (C677T), or alanine instead of glutamate (A1298C) [9,10]. The polymorphism that is the most studied is the C677T (thymine for cytosine), but characterizations of the A1298C have also occurred.

The C677T variant can be heterozygous or homozygous. An individual with the heterozygous genotype (abbreviated CT) received one normal and one abnormal allele, while an individual with the homozygous genotype received two abnormal alleles (abbreviated TT) or two normal alleles, (abbreviated CC) [2,9]. The homozygous individual with two abnormal alleles (TT) has a lower MTHFR activity. The homozygous CC individual does not have an altered genotype and is considered to have a normal MTHFR activity.

The individual with the TT genotype may have an increased plasma homocysteine level and a decrease in the methylation reactions that were described. Research has identified that these individuals have increased hypomethylation of DNA, lower serum and red blood cell folate levels, and an increased risk of neural tube defects [11]. This increased risk of disease is less associated with the CT heterozygous genotype, and thus most research occurs in the TT homozygous genotype.

Like the C677T polymorphism, the A1298C (cytosine for adenine) variant occurs as homozygote normal-activity (AA), heterozygote (AC), and homozygote low-activity (CC).

Since these polymorphisms in MTHFR were identified, many researchers have questioned the folate needs of individuals who do not have normal MTHFR activity and the effect on their individualized risk of chronic diseases. The identification of MTHFR polymorphisms has implications related to the individualization of nutrition care.

Ethnic Differences in Genetic Variations in MTHFR

Research reports indicate that these polymorphisms are distributed differently in different ethnic groups. Esfahani, Cogger, and Caudill [10] reported that among a convenience sample of 433 women living in California, 18.1% of Mexican women had the C677T TT genotype, compared to only 7.2% of Caucasian, 3.8% of Asian, and 0% of African American women. The A1298C CC genotype was found in 7.9% of white women but was present in much lower percentages for all other ethnic groups. Further characterization found that 17.6% of Mexican women and 15.1% of white women had the homozygous low-activity genotype for both C677T and A1298C MTHFR. These findings differ from those reported by Botto and Yang [12], who reported that less than 10% of African Americans, over 40% of Italians and California Hispanics, and 22% of Norwegians had the C677T MTHFR genotype. Therefore, it is not clear exactly how these polymorphisms are distributed, but some ethnic groups are at greater risk than others.

While the literature often reports a differing risk of disease in individuals with the C677T TT homozygote genotype, it is not clear that these individuals have greater folate needs. Using a depletion/repletion design with Mexican women, Guinotte et al. [13] measured serum folate, RBC folate, plasma homocysteine, and urinary folate excretion. The subjects had the CC (normal), CT (heterozygote), or TT (homozygote) genotype for MTHFR. The subjects all showed moderate folate deficiency after the 7-week depletion phase and returned to folate sufficiency with 7 weeks of repletion with 400 μg DFE. There were no differences among plasma homocysteine levels. Guinotte et al. [13] stated that their data support the RDA of 400 μg DFE to meet the needs of these subjects.

Not all research matches these findings. In a study of 126 healthy subjects with different MTHFR genotypes, the C677T TT subjects had similar plasma folate but higher plasma homocysteine levels than the CT or CC subjects when consuming a folate-rich diet that contained an average of 660 DFEs [14]. The differences in plasma homocysteine levels disappeared when a supplement was added, boosting folate intake to an average of 814 DFEs. However, even with the consumption of 660 DFEs, the plasma homocysteine level of the TT subjects was not above 12 μmol/L, a level that reflects folate sufficiency [14].

These findings can be compared to those of de Bree and coauthors [15], who studied data collected on 2,051 Dutch subjects and found that at a similar intake subjects with the TT genotype for the C677T MTHFR had the lowest plasma folate and highest plasma homocysteine. However, these subjects were consuming only ~200 μg folate per day, and the Dutch do not fortify grain products with folic acid [16].

The MTHFR polymorphisms appear to have their greatest impact on folate status when folate intake is low. The fortification policies of the United States and Canada ensure that folate intake has increased.

MTHFR Variations and Risk of Chronic Disease

Since the identification of the MTHFR polymorphisms, a great deal of research has investigated and reported risks of neural tube defects, cardiovascular disease, colorectal cancer, and dementias in people with poor folate status [11,17]. The following overview limits its discussion of chronic disease risk to comparison of subjects with the C677T MTHFR low-activity (TT) genotype to those with the normal-activity (CC) genotype, because most research is about this genetic variant.

Neural Tube Defects (NTDs)

Bailey, Rampersaud, and Kauwell [16] reviewed the impact of folate fortification on the improving folate status of Americans and Canadians and the decline in neural tube defects (NTDs) in both countries. The decline of NTDs is estimated to be between 15% and 30% in the United States and greater in Canada, but it may be due to factors in addition to positive effects of fortification, such as more prenatal screening for NTDs, more research about the nutritional risk factors for NTDs, and increased use of folic acid supplementation due to public education programs [18].

Botto and Yang [12] reviewed the relationship between NTD risk and the C677T mutation in several studies and reported no significantly increased risk for an NTD. A recent study of 175 American Caucasians with NTDs who had the TT genotype for the C677T mutation reported a nonsignificant relationship to the parents' genotype. While prenatal folate is credited for a reduction in NTDs, the relationship appears to be more complicated than it originally appeared [19].

Cardiovascular Disease

While the increased risk of cardiovascular disease in individuals with hyperhomocysteinemia is well documented in case control studies, some large prospective trials have not found the same relationship. Some argue that increases in plasma homocysteine are the outcome of renal atherosclerosis and decreased homocysteine excretion, not the cause of cardiovascular disease. This argument is reinforced by the general finding that individuals with the C677T TT genotype have higher plasma homocysteine levels but do not have a greater risk of cardiovascular disease [20]. Others believe that the relationship of the TT genotype to cardiovascular disease cannot be evaluated because the studies are too small to establish causality [20]. A recently published meta-analysis of 40 studies stated that individuals with the C677T TT genotype had a 16% higher odds ratio for cardiovascular disease than those with the CC genotype [21]. This was particularly true when the subjects had low folate status. Low dietary folate intake may be the explanatory factor in the manifestation of the effect of the MTHFR polymorphism on cardiovascular disease risk.

Dementias

If homocysteine accumulates inside cells, the cells will evict this metabolic oxidant into the bloodstream. Homocysteine crosses the blood-brain barrier and is theorized to be neurotoxic [22]. Because research indicates that high plasma homocysteine is a risk factor for dementias and other cognitive problems (depression, psychosis), it follows logically that individuals with MTHFR genetic polymorphisms are at a greater risk. However, this relationship has not been verified [17,22]. A recent review concluded that there was no effect of folic acid supplementation, with or without vitamin B_{12}, in treating mild or moderate problems with cognition, dementia, or Alzheimer's disease [23].

Colorectal Cancer

Poor folate status is positively correlated to risk of colorectal cancer. This can be explained theoretically because a decrease in folate leads to DNA hypomethylation and increased uracil (instead of thymine) incorporation into DNA. The presence of uracil increases the activity of DNA repair mechanisms, but the repair may not be totally effective. Thus, DNA is more prone to damage, causing an increased risk of invasion by a cancer virus. The combination of DNA hypomethylation and increased uracil incorporation, caused by poor folate status, explains the folate-cancer relationship [11]. Unlike other disease risks that we have discussed, the MTHFR polymorphism may protect individuals from colorectal cancer. While studies generally report no difference in risk for the heterozygous (CT) or homozygous (TT) individual, a trend in some studies indicates that as long as folate intake is high and alcohol intake is low, the TT homozygote may have a lower risk. This may be due to the shunting of 5,10-methylenetetrahydrofolate toward the formation of nucleotides (because MTHFR activity is low). Consequently, malformed DNA would not occur [11]. This possible protective relationship of the MTHFR polymorphism is preliminary, and more research is needed.

Summary

As with most scientific research, a variety of research and opinions surround the topic of health implications for individuals with an MTHFR polymorphism. Some ethnic groups have a greater susceptibility to this condition, which causes an increase in dietary folate needs. However, it is not clear that once those dietary needs are met the individual has an increased risk of NTDs, cardiovascular disease, or dementias. The interaction of the genotype, dietary intake, other genetic factors, and the environment may explain the relationship.

This brief discussion about the possible impact of MTHFR polymorphisms and the impact of nutrigenomics currently has limited application to the general public, for two reasons. First, there is currently little individualized genetic mapping. Second, the impact of having an MTHFR polymorphism on health is not clear. Both of these limitations are likely to decline with enhanced technology and continued research. Future nutrition professionals may consider MTHFR, along with many other genetic traits, in their nutrition assessment and subsequent recommendations. Understanding how slight alterations in the human genome might affect nutrient needs and disease risk sheds light on the future of nutrition care.

References Cited

1. Collins F, McKusick VA. Implications of the human genome project for medical science. JAMA 2001;285: 540–44.
2. DeBusk R. Genetics: The Nutrition Connection. Chicago: American Dietetic Association, 2003.
3. **www.nhgri.nih.gov**
4. Muller M, Kersten S. Nutrigenomics: goals and strategies. Nature Reviews, Genetics, 2003;4:315–22.
5. Shattuck D. Nutritional genomics. J Am Diet Assoc 2003;103:16–18.
6. Stover PJ, Garza C. Bringing individuality to public health recommendations. J Nutr 2002;132:2476S–80S.
7. Bruening KS, Mitchell BE, Pfeiffer MM. Accreditation standards for dietetics education. J Am Diet Assoc 2002; 102:566–77.
8. Nussbaum RL, McInnes RR, Willard HF. Genetics in Medicine, 6th ed. Philadelphia: W. B. Saunders, 2001, p. 87.
9. Moyers S, Bailey LB. Fetal malformation and folate metabolism: review of recent evidence. Nutr Rev 2001;7: 215–24.
10. Esfahani S, Cogger EA, Caudill MA. Heterogeneity in the prevalence of methylenetetrahydrofolate reductase gene polymorphisms in women of different ethnic groups. J Am Diet Assoc, 2003;103:200–207.
11. Rampersaud GC, Bailey LB, Kauwell GP. Relationship of folate to colorectal and cervical cancer: review and recommendations for practitioners. J Am Diet Assoc 2002;102:1273–82.
12. Botto LD, Yang Q. Methylene-tetrahydrofolate reductase (MTHFR) and birth defects. Am J Epidem 2000;151:862–77.
13. Guinotte CL, Burns MG, Asume JA, Hata H, Urrutia TF, Alamilla A, et al. Methylenetetrahydrofolate reductase 677C ⟶ T variant modulated folate status response to controlled folate intakes in young women. J Nutr 2003;133:1272–80.
14. Ashfield-Watt PA, Pullin CH, Whiting JM, Clark ZE, Moat SJ, Newcombe RG, et al. Methylenetetrahydrofolate reductase 677C ⟶ T genotype modulates homocysteine responses to a folate-rich diet or a low-dose folic acid supplement: a randomized controlled trial. Am J Clin Nutr 2002;76:180–86.
15. De Bree A, Verschuren WM, Bjorke-Monsen A, van der Put N, Heil SG, Trijbels F, et al. Effect of methylenetetrahydrofolate reductase 677C ⟶ T mutation on the relations among folate intake and plasma folate and homocysteine concentrations in a general population sample. Am J Clin Nutr 2003;77:687–93.
16. Bailey LB, Rampersaud GC, Kauwell, GP. Folic acid supplements and fortification affect the risk for neural tube defects, vascular disease and cancer: evolving science. J Nutr 2003;133:1961S–68S.
17. Ames BN, Elson-Schwab I, Silver EA. High-dose vitamin therapy stimulates variant enzymes with decreased coenzyme binding affinity (increased K_m): relevance to genetic disease and polymorphisms. Am J Clin Nutr 2002;75:616–58.
18. Olney RS, Mulinare J. Trends in neural tube defect prevalence, folic acid fortification, and vitamin supplement use. Sem Perinatology 2002;26:2777–85.
19. Rampersaud E, Melvin EC, Siegel D, Mehltretter L, Dickerson ME, George TM, et al. Updated investigations of the role of methylenetetrahydrofolate reductase in human neural tube defects [Abstract]. Clin Genet 63: 210–14.
20. Scott JM. Homocysteine and cardiovascular risk. Am J Clin Nutr 2000;72: 333–34.
21. Kerk M, Verhoef P, Clarke R, Blom HJ, Kok FJ, Schouten EG. MTHFR 677 C to T polymorphism and risk of coronary heart disease: a meta analysis [Abstract]. JAMA 2002;288:2023–31.
22. Shea TB, Lyons-Weiler J, Rogers E. Homocysteine, folate deprivation and Alzheimer neuropathology. J Alzheimer's Dis 2002;4:261–67.
23. Malouf M, Grimley EJ, Areosa SA. Folic acid with or without vitamin B_{12} for cognition and dementia [Abstract]. Cochrane Database Systematic Reviews 2003; 4:CD004514.

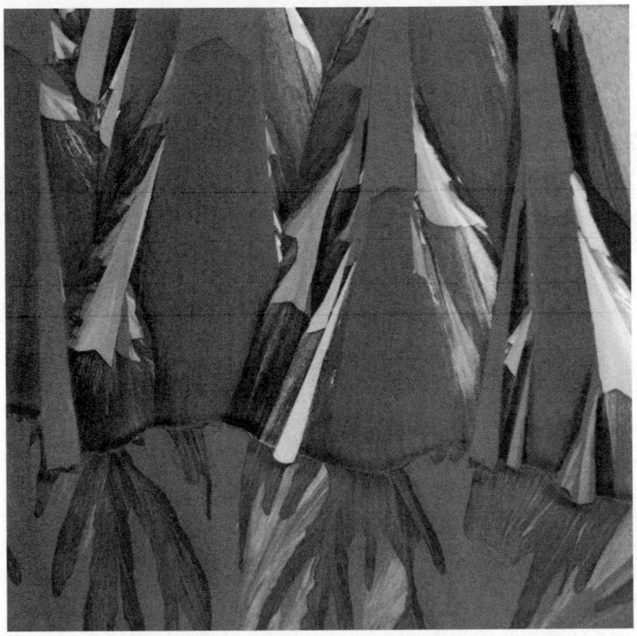

© Michael W. Davidson/Photo Researchers, Inc.

Photomicrograph of crystalized vitamin E

Vitamin A and Carotenoids
Vitamin D
Vitamin E
Vitamin K

For each vitamin, the following subtopics (when applicable) are discussed:

Sources
Digestion, Absorption, Transport, and Storage
Functions and Mechanisms of Action
Interactions with Other Nutrients
Metabolism and Excretion
Recommended Dietary Allowances or Adequate Intakes
Deficiency
Toxicity
Assessment of Nutriture

perspective

The Antioxidant Nutrients, Reactive Species, and Disease

chapter 10 The Fat-Soluble Vitamins

THIS CHAPTER ADDRESSES EACH of the four fat-soluble vitamins—A, D, E, and K—and the carotenoids. The reader is referred to Chapter 9 for an overview of vitamins and information pertaining to the water-soluble vitamins. The absorption and transport of the fat-soluble vitamins, in contrast to those of the water-soluble vitamins, are closely associated with the absorption and transport of lipids. As with dietary lipids, optimal fat-soluble vitamin absorption requires the presence of bile salts. Similarly, the transport of the fat-soluble vitamins in the body occurs initially by chylomicrons. Moreover, the fat-soluble vitamins are stored in body lipids, although the amount stored varies widely among the four fat-soluble vitamins. Table 10.1 provides an overview of the discovery, function, deficiency syndrome, food sources, and recommended dietary allowance (RDA) or adequate intake (AI) of each of the fat-soluble vitamins. The RDAs and AIs for all nutrients and for all age groups are provided on the inside cover of the book.

Table 10.1 The Fat-Soluble Vitamins: Discovery, Function, Deficiency Syndrome, Food Sources, and Recommended Dietary Allowance (RDA) or Adequate Intake (AI)

Vitamin	Discovery	Biochemical or Physiological Function	Deficiency Syndrome or Symptoms	Good Sources in Rank Order	RDA or AI
Vitamin A (retinol, retinal, retinoic acid) Provitamins Carotenoids, particularly β-carotene	McCollum (1916)	Synthesis of rhodopsin and other light receptor pigments; metabolites involved in growth, cell differentiation, bone development, and immune function	Poor dark adaptation, night blindness, xerosis, keratomalacia, xeroderma, Bitot's spots	Beef liver, dairy products, sweet potato, carrots, spinach, butternut squash, greens, broccoli, cantaloupe	900 μg RAE[a] 700 μg RAE[b]
Vitamin D Provitamins Ergosterol 7-dehydrocholesterol Vitamin D_2 (ergocalciferol) Vitamin D_3 (cholecalciferol)	McCollum (1922)	Regulator of bone mineral metabolism, blood calcium homeostasis, and cell differentiation, proliferation, and growth	Children: rickets Adults: osteomalacia	Synthesized in skin exposed to ultraviolet light; fortified milk	5–15 μg[c,d,e]
Vitamin E Tocopherols Tocotrienols	Evans and Bishop (1922)	Antioxidant	Infants: anemia Children and adults: neuropathy and myopathy	Vegetable seed oils	15 mg α-tocopherol[c]
Vitamin K Phylloquinones Menaquinones Menadione	Dam (1935)	Activates blood-clotting factors II, VII, IX, X by γ-carboxylating glutamic acid residues; carboxylates bone and kidney proteins	Children: hemorrhagic disease of newborns Adults: defective blood clotting	Synthesized by intestinal bacteria; green leafy vegetables, soy beans, beef liver	120 μg[a,e] 90 μg[b,e]

[a] Adult males.
[b] Adult females.
[c] Both males and females.
[d] Varies with age for adults, see text.
[e] Adequate intake.

VITAMIN A AND CAROTENOIDS

The term *vitamin A* is generally used to refer to a group of compounds that possess the biological activity of all-*trans* retinol. The retinoids are structurally similar and include retinol, retinal, retinoic acid, and retinyl ester, as well as synthetic analogues. Structurally, retinoids contain a β-ionone ring and a polyunsaturated side chain, with either an alcohol group (retinol, Fig. 10.1a), an aldehyde group (retinal, Fig. 10.1b), a carboxylic acid group (retinoic acid, Fig. 10.1c), or an ester group (retinyl ester, Fig. 10.1d). The side chain is made up of four isoprenoid units with a series of conjugated double bonds.

Provitamin A carotenoids represent a group of compounds that are precursors of vitamin A. While there are over 600 carotenoids (lipid-soluble red, orange, and yellow pigments produced by plants), fewer than 10% are thought to exhibit vitamin A activity. In other words, fewer than 60 can be converted to retinol. Structurally, carotenoids have an expanded carbon chain containing conjugated double bonds usually, but not always, with an unsubstituted β-ionone ring at one or both ends of the chain. Three dietary provitamin A carotenoids, which are found most often in the all-*trans* form, are β-carotene (Fig. 10.1e), α-carotene (Fig. 10.1f), and β-cryptoxanthin (Fig. 10.1g). While not all carotenoids are vitamin A precursors, many carotenoids, such as lycopene (an open-chain analog of β-carotene; Fig. 10.1h), and many oxycarotenoids (also called oxygenated carotenoids), such as canthaxanthin (Fig. 10.1i), lutein (Fig. 10.1j), and zeaxanthin, are thought to be of physiological importance to the body.

Sources

Both retinoids (often called preformed vitamin A or simply vitamin A) and carotenoids are found naturally in foods. Vitamin A is found primarily in selected foods of animal origin, especially liver and dairy products (including whole milk, cheese, and butter) as well as

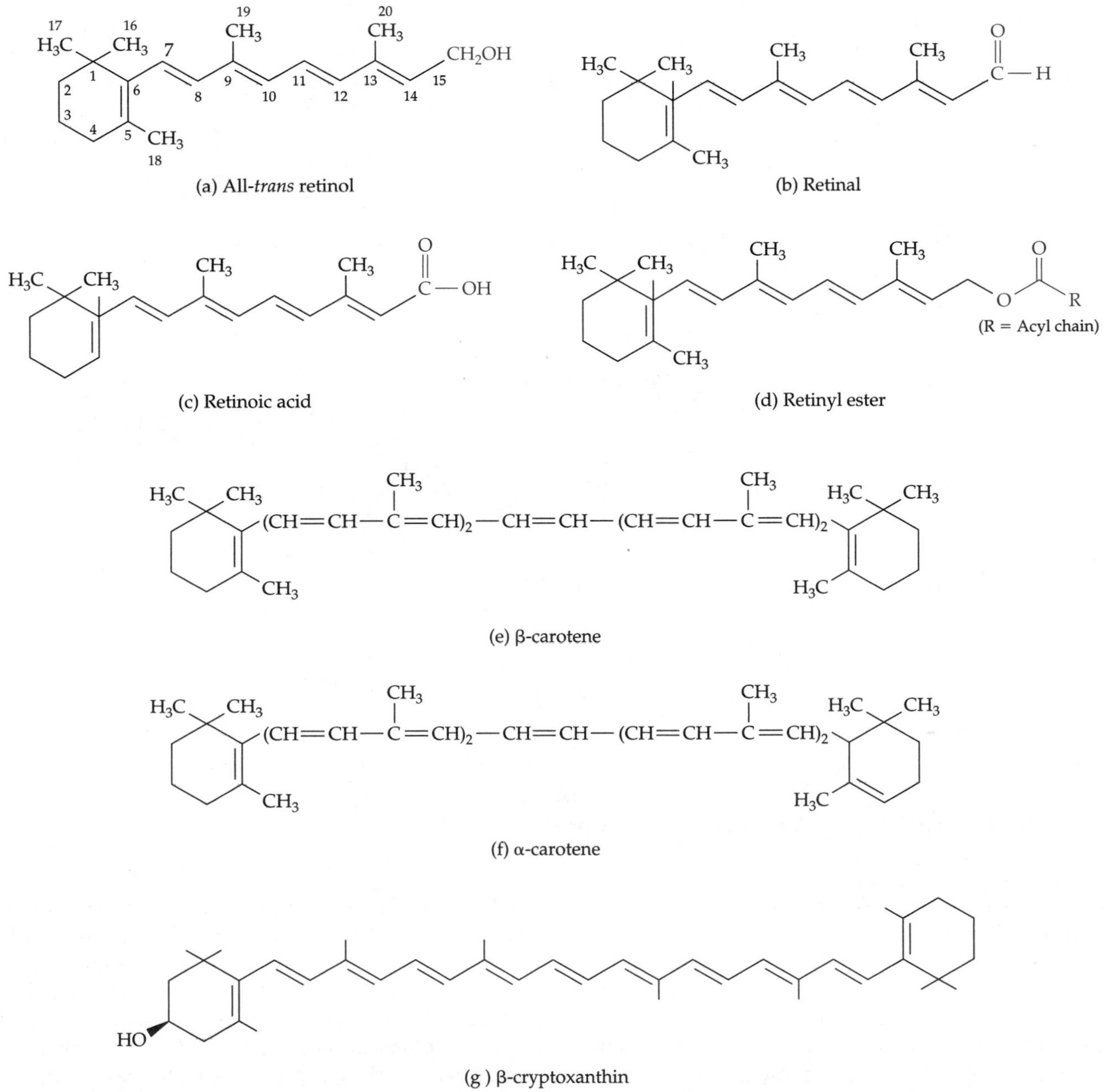

Figure 10.1 Vitamin A and carotenoid structures *(continued on next page).*

fish such as tuna, sardines, and herring. Some products, such as margarine, also may be fortified with vitamin A. Liver oils of fish (such as cod liver oil) are also high in vitamin A. The main form of vitamin A in foods is as retinyl esters such as retinyl palmitate, shown in Figure 10.1k. Retinoids are lipid soluble and can undergo oxidation if exposed to varying degrees of, for example, oxygen, light, heat, and some metals. In pharmaceutical vitamin preparations, all-*trans* retinyl acetate and all-*trans* retinyl palmitate are commonly used. Aquasol A, a water-miscible form of the vitamin, is available for individuals with a fat malabsorptive disorder.

Carotenoids are synthesized by a wide variety of plants and thus are found naturally in many fruits and vegetables. One of the most abundant carotenoids is β-carotene, which exhibits the greatest amount of provitamin A activity. Other common dietary carotenoids include α-carotene and β-cryptoxanthin (both provitamin A carotenoids) along with lycopene, lutein, and zeaxanthin. In general, yellow, orange, and red (brightly colored) fruits and vegetables such as carrots, papayas, tomatoes, squash, and pumpkins provide significant amounts of carotenoids. Green vegetables also contain some carotenoids, although the pigment cannot be seen

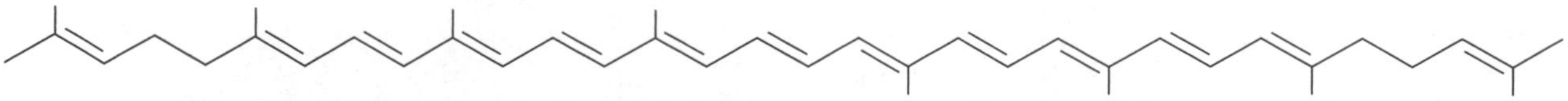

(h) Lycopene

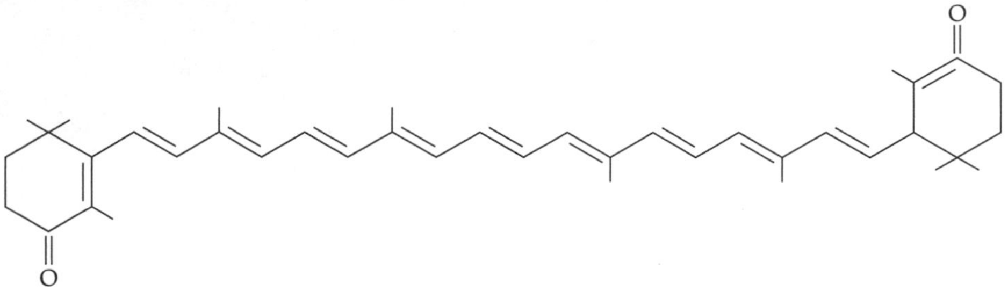

(i) Canthaxanthin

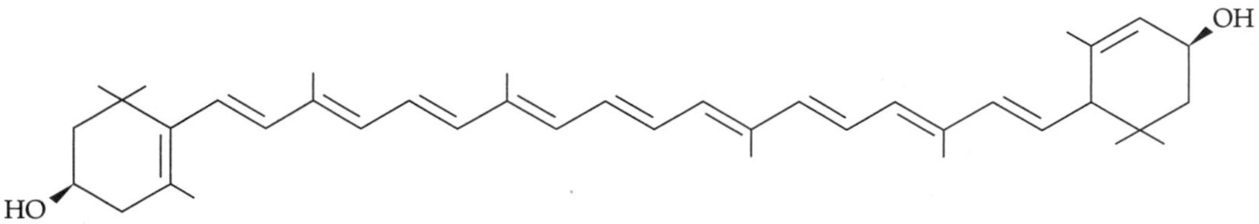

(j) Lutein

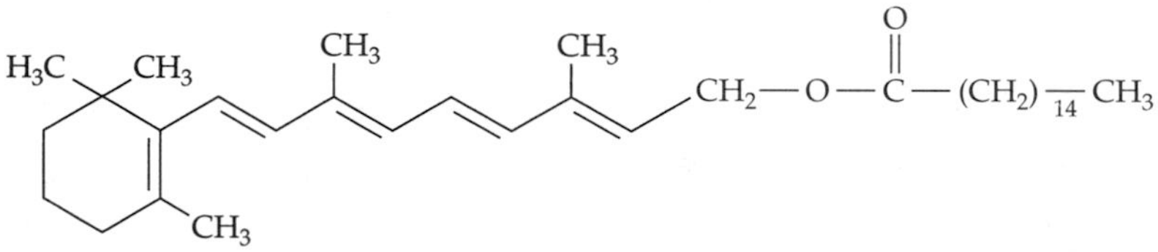

(k) Retinyl palmitate

Figure 10.1 *(continued)* Vitamin A and carotenoid structures.

because it is masked by chlorophyll. Carrots typically represent a major source of both α- and β-carotene in American diets. Other major dietary contributors of β-carotene include broccoli, cantaloupe, squash, peas, and spinach. Fruits provide much of the dietary β-cryptoxanthin, and tomatoes, along with tomato sauces and watermelon, are good sources of dietary lycopene, a carotenoid that is red in color. Good sources of zeaxanthin include peppers (orange), corn, and potatoes. Broccoli, beets, and kiwi fruit provide some lutein. Canthaxanthin, a red-orange carotenoid, is found in plants as well as in fish and seafood such as sea trout and crustaceans. While meat and fish are not major sources of carotenoids, because animals and fish feed on plants they can accumulate some carotenoids. Carotenoids also may be added to foods. β-carotene and canthaxanthin, for example, are approved by the Food and Drug Administration for use as a food color additive.

Digestion and Absorption

Vitamin A, because it is bound to other food components, requires some digestion prior to its absorption into the body. Retinol, for example, is typically bound to fatty acid esters, the most commonly occurring of which is retinyl palmitate (Fig. 10.1k). Furthermore, retinyl esters and carotenes in foods are often complexed with protein from which they must be released. Although the heating of plant foods has been shown to weaken some complexes, such as protein-carotenoid complexes, enzymatic digestion is still required. Hydrolysis of carotenoids and retinyl esters from protein occurs initially by the action of pepsin in the stomach. Because of their fat solubility, the freed (i.e., no longer bound to protein) retinyl esters and carotenoids typically coalesce to form fat globules in the stomach. These fat globules containing the vitamin are emptied into the duodenum, where they are emulsified (broken up into smaller droplets) by bile. Proteolytic enzymes in the proximal small intestine also can hydrolyze any protein-bound retinyl esters or carotenoids not freed in the stomach.

Micelles form within the lumen of the small intestine from bile salts, phospholipids, triglycerides, and retinyl and carotenoid esters. Hydrolysis of retinyl and carotenoid esters by various hydrolases and esterases occurs at the same time that triacylglycerols, phospholipids, and cholesteryl esters are being hydrolyzed by pancreatic enzymes. Pancreatic lipase and pancreatic cholesterol ester hydrolase are secreted into the lumen of the small intestine to facilitate vitamin A digestion, while enzymes such as retinyl ester hydrolase function on the intestinal brush border [1–4]. Pancreatic hydrolases cleave shorter-chain retinyl esters, while intestinal brush border hydrolases act on longer-chain retinyl esters.

The released or now free carotenoids and retinols in the small intestine remain solubilized in micellar solutions along with the other fat-soluble food components. The micellar solutions containing the carotenoids and preformed vitamin A are absorbed across the microvilli brush border membrane of the duodenum and jejunum and into the enterocyte. When retinol is ingested in physiological amounts, absorption is thought to occur by a specific protein carrier in the brush border of the enterocyte [3]. Absorption of preformed vitamin A following ingestion of pharmacological doses of the vitamin is thought to be nonsaturable [3]. Carotenoids also are absorbed by passive diffusion.

The efficiency of absorption differs between preformed vitamin A and carotenoids. Approximately 70% to 90% of dietary preformed vitamin A is absorbed as long as the meal contains some (~10 g or more) fat [5]. Dietary carotenoid absorption varies considerably depending on food processing and typically is less than that of the retinoids. Carotenoid absorption ranges from about <5% for carotenoids from uncooked vegetables or non–heat processed vegetable juices to about 60% if present as a pure oil or as part of an aqueous dispersion supplement [2,5–10]. Fiber intake as well as excessive vitamin E consumption can diminish carotenoid absorption. In addition, various carotenoids appear to interact to influence (enhance or inhibit) individual carotenoid absorption. Figure 10.2 depicts the digestion and absorption of preformed vitamin A and carotenoids.

Within the intestinal mucosal cell/enterocyte (and to some extent in the liver, adipose tissue, and lungs, among other organs), some carotenoids, including α- and β-carotene and cryptoxanthin, undergo metabolism. The extent to which provitamin A carotenoids are converted to retinoids is influenced by several factors, such as the vitamin A status of the individual and the amounts and forms of the carotenoids consumed. Within the enterocyte, for example, β-carotene is hydrolyzed by noncentral cleavage or by β-carotene 15,15′-dioxygenase. Other enzymes involved in carotenoid metabolism have also been identified in various species, as reviewed by Yeum and Russell [11]. Noncentral cleavage generates several metabolites (alcohols, aldehydes, etc.) [12,13], whereas dioxygenase converts one molecule of β-carotene into two molecules of retinaldehyde/retinal (Fig. 10.3). However, because the activity of β-carotene 15,15′-dioxygenase is relatively low, only about 60% to 75% of the β-carotene is hydrolyzed [14]. The presence of vitamin E is thought to protect β-carotene and its product from oxidation; large doses of vitamin E, however, may inhibit β-carotene absorption or its conversion to retinol in the intestine [5]. Up to about 15% of β-carotene may leave the intestine intact (i.e., without oxidation) for transport via chylomicrons to tissues. It

Figure 10.2 Digestion and absorption of carotenoids and vitamin A, and reesterification of retinol in the intestinal cell.

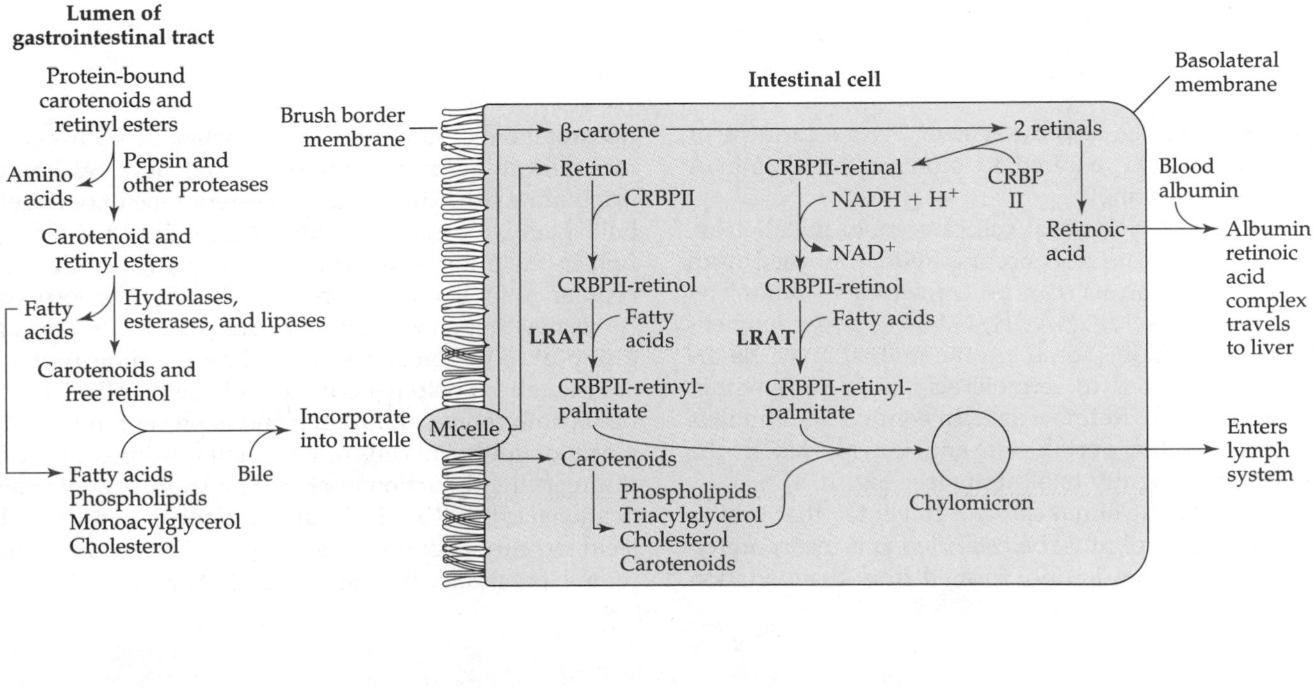

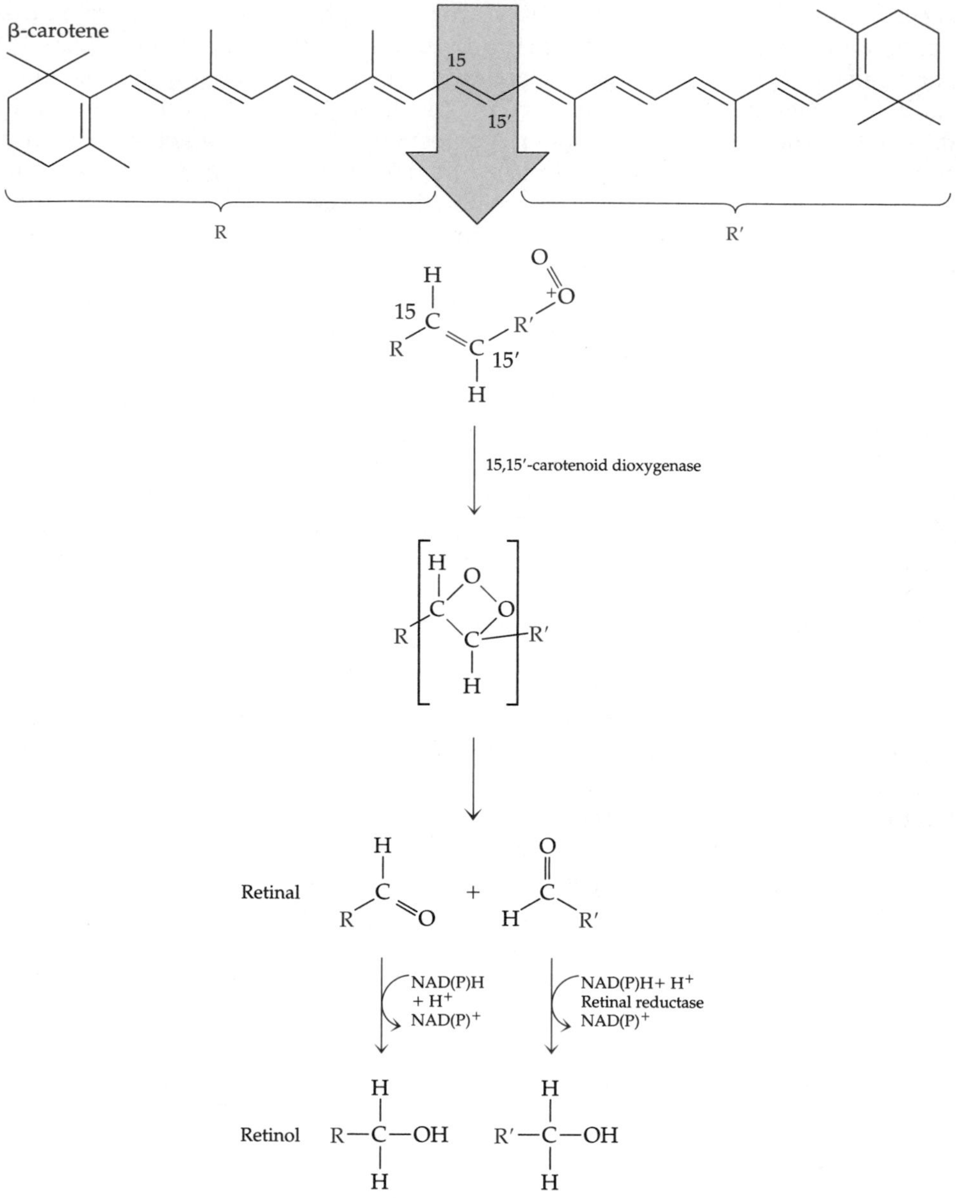

Figure 10.3 Cleavage of carotene to retinal and its reduction to retinol.

is estimated that 12 μg β-carotene or 24 μg α-carotene or β-cryptoxanthin is required to produce the vitamin A activity of 1 μg retinol.

In addition to intestinal cell carotenoid metabolism, retinoid metabolism also occurs. Retinal, formed from β-carotene hydrolysis, can be converted to retinol by retinal reductase, an NADH/NADPH-dependent enzyme. In addition, some of the retinal may be irreversibly oxidized to retinoic acid (Fig. 10.4) within the intestinal cell. Retinoic acid, in contrast to retinol, is picked up by the portal vein and transported in the plasma bound tightly to albumin (see Fig. 10.2).

To leave the intestinal cell and travel to other tissues in the body, retinol must be esterified and incorporated into a chylomicron. Retinol formed from the oxidation of carotenoids follows the same metabolic pathways of reesterification in the intestinal cell as does retinol originating from dietary retinyl esters. One of two metabolic pathways may be followed for retinol reesterification in the enterocyte. The primary pathway involves cellular retinol binding protein (CRBP) II, whose synthesis may depend on retinoic acid [2]. CRBPs, part of a group of low-molecular-weight lipid-binding proteins, are thought to help regulate retinol use in cells. CRBP II binds both retinol and retinal and is present in the cytoplasm of epithelial cells of the small intestine [1]. CRBP II directs the reduction of retinal and subsequent esterification [15]. CRBP II–bound retinol is esterified by lecithin retinol acyl transferase (LRAT) to form mainly retinyl palmitate, but also retinyl stearate and retinyl

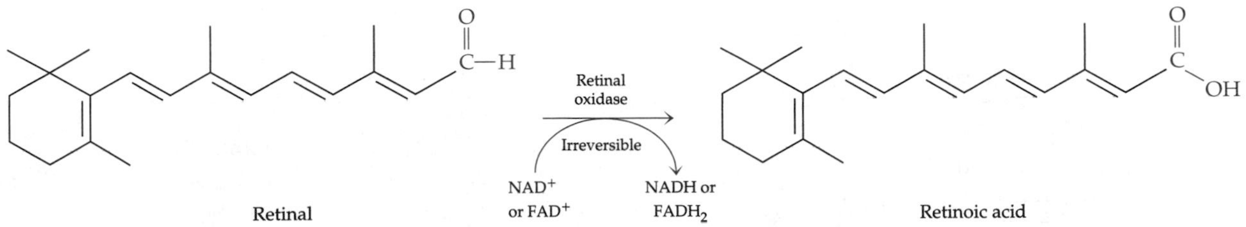

Figure 10.4 The irreversible oxidation of retinal to retinoic acid.

oleate, among others. The minor second pathway for reesterification involves binding of retinol to a cellular protein that is nonspecific, with subsequent reesterification by acyl CoA retinol acyl transferase (ARAT) [1]. ARAT may serve to esterify retinol when large doses of the vitamin are ingested [16].

Transport, Metabolism, and Storage

Within the intestinal cell, the newly formed retinyl esters, along with a small amount of unesterified retinol and any carotenoids that have been absorbed unchanged, are incorporated into chylomicrons containing cholesterol esters, phospholipid, triacylglycerols, and apoproteins. These chylomicrons are then carried first into the lymphatic system and then into general circulation (i.e., the blood). Chylomicrons deliver retinyl esters, some unesterified retinol, and carotenoids to many extrahepatic tissues, including bone marrow, blood cells, spleen, adipose tissue, muscle, lungs, and kidneys [17]. Retinyl esters and carotenoids not taken up by peripheral tissue are transported to the liver as part of the chylomicron remnant.

Carotenoids and vitamin A reaching the liver typically undergo additional metabolism. For example, carotenoids reaching the liver can follow three routes: cleavage to form retinol, incorporation into and release as part of very low density lipoproteins (VLDLs) for transport to other tissues, and/or storage in the liver (or adipose tissue).

The handling of retinyl esters reaching the liver is shown in Figure 10.5. However, most cells of the body are able to metabolize retinol generated from the retinyl esters through a number of metabolic pathways. Hydrolysis of the retinyl esters by a retinyl ester hydrolase occurs following their uptake by the hepatic **parenchymal cells** (functional cells of an organ). Within the cell, retinol binds with a cellular retinol-binding protein (CRBP). CRBPs have been found in many body cells, especially in the intestine (CRBP II), the liver, and the kidneys. CRBP is thought to function both to help control concentrations of free retinol within the cell cytoplasm and thus prevent its oxidation and to direct the vitamin, through a series of protein-protein interactions, to specific enzymes of metabolism [15,18,19]. CRBP may also assist in the transfer of retinal across organelles for metabolism [18]. Enzymatic metabolism of retinol as shown in Figure 10.5 includes possible esterification by enzymes such as LRAT, if retinol is bound to CRBP, or ARAT, if retinol is unbound. Unbound CRBP concentrations are thought to inhibit LRAT and thereby prevent esterification for storage. CRBP-bound retinol also may be oxidized to retinal by NAD(P)H-dependent retinol dehydrogenase and/or phosphorylated to retinyl phosphate by ATP for glycoprotein functions [19].

Retinol that has been esterified may be stored in the liver. Some storage of retinol occurs in the parenchymal cells, but about 80% to 95% of the retinol is stored in the liver in small perisinusoidal cells called **stellate cells** (also known as Ito cells). Note that retinoic acid does not accumulate in appreciable amounts in the liver or other tissues [20]. In the stellate cells, vitamin A (retinol) is stored as retinyl esters (primarily retinyl palmitate, but also retinyl stearate, oleate, and linoleate) with lipid droplets. Hydrolases can release the retinol from its stores as needed for use. With adequate liver stores of vitamin A (minimum 20 μg vitamin A per g liver) [5], plasma vitamin A concentrations remain fairly constant over a wide range of dietary intakes. Only after the hepatic stellate cells can accept no more retinol for storage does hypervitaminosis A occur (see p. 340).

Retinol transport in the blood requires two specific proteins, retinol binding protein (RBP) and transthyretin (TTR), formerly known as prealbumin. Both proteins are synthesized by hepatic parenchymal cells. Initially, for hepatic release into the blood, each mol of retinol released by a hydrolase from its ester storage form combines with 1 mol of RBP to form holo-RBP (Fig. 10.5). Synthesis of RBP is dependent on a person's protein, retinol, and zinc status. Holo-RBP (which contains the vitamin A bound in an interior portion or hydrophobic region of the complex) then interacts with 1 mol of TTR, a tetrameric protein (Fig. 10.5). In the plasma, the holo-RBP-TTR complex circulates bound to thyroxine (T_4) as part of a trimolecular complex (Fig. 10.5), with a half-life of about 11 to 15 hours.

Uptake of retinol from the complex by tissues is not completely understood, but it is thought to be mediated by cellular RBP receptors and by a receptor-independent mode depending on the specific tissue [21–24]. Factors

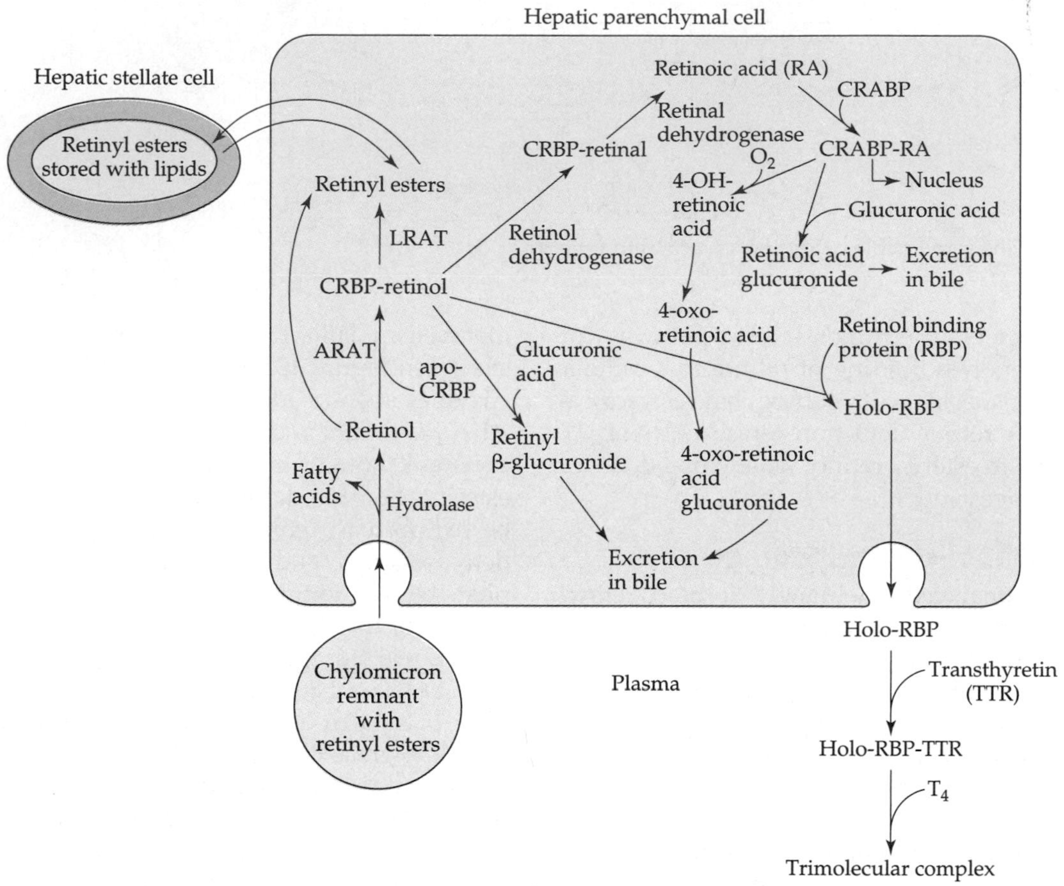

Figure 10.5 Vitamin A metabolism in the liver.

influencing uptake are not known but may involve CRBP concentrations and/or saturation and the extent of intracellular retinol metabolism, among others. For receptor-dependent uptake, TTR is thought to dissociate from the complex while holo-RBP binds to the cellular RBP receptor. The complex is then endocytosed with cytosolic release of vitamin A and apo-RBP. Apo-RBP is thought to be secreted back into the blood for reuse or degradation by the kidney. Some of the many tissues utilizing vitamin A from the complex include adipose tissue, skeletal muscle, lungs, kidneys, eyes, white blood cells, and bone marrow [2,3]. In rats, extensive recycling of retinol (7 to 13 times prior to degradation) occurs among plasma, extrahepatic tissues, and the liver [2,3,16].

Carotenoids are also found in the blood, with transport occurring as part of lipoproteins. Carotenoids such as β-carotene and lycopene are thought to concentrate in the hydrophobic core of lipoproteins for serum transport, while carotenoids with polar groups are found partly on the lipoprotein surface [9,12]. β-carotene, α-carotene, and lycopene distribution among lipoproteins is similar: Low-density lipoproteins (LDLs) carry 58% to 73%, high-density lipoproteins (HDLs) carry 17% to 26%, and very low density lipoproteins (VLDLs) carry 10% to 16% [12]. In contrast, lutein and zeaxanthin (polar carotenoids) are carried predominantly (53%) by HDLs, but also by LDLs (31%) and VLDLs (16%) in a fasting state [12]. Serum carotene concentrations reflect recent intake and not body stores. The most common serum carotenoids are β-carotene, α-carotene, lycopene, lutein, zeaxanthin, and cryptoxanthin.

Uptake of carotenoids into target tissues differs from that of retinol. Carotenoids are taken up as part of the lipoprotein, with uptake mediated by specific apoprotein receptors found in a variety of tissues. Storage of carotenoids occurs mainly in the liver and adipose tissue, but some specific tissues concentrate selected carotenoids. For example, the retina of the eye is relatively rich in lutein and zeaxanthin.

In contrast to retinol, which is mobilized from the liver for transport to other tissues, retinoic acid is thought to be produced in small amounts by individual cells. Whether central production of retinoic acid occurs by the intestine or the liver for transport to other tissues is unclear. Retinoic acid is usually bound to albumin for transport in the blood, but plasma retinoic acid concentrations typically are low. Within the cell cytoplasm, retinoic acid binds to cellular retinoic acid-binding proteins (CRABPs). CRABPs are thought to function in a capacity similar to that described for CRBPs. While both CRBPs and CRABPs are often found in the same tissues, their relative distribution in the tissues differs. CRABP, like CRBP, functions to help solubilize retinoic acid, regulate metabolism of retinoic acid within the cell, and direct the usage of retinoic acid intracellularly.

Functions and Mechanisms of Action

Vitamin A

Vitamin A is recognized as being essential for vision as well as for cellular differentiation, growth, reproduction, bone development, and immune system actions. We will review each of these functions before addressing the functions of the carotenoids.

Visual Cycle. One of the most well-known roles of vitamin A in the body is its role in vision. In basic terms, when a flash of light hits the dark-adapted retina, **rhodopsin** (a vitamin A–containing protein) is cleaved, vitamin A is released, and signals are sent to the part of the brain involved with eyesight. To regain vision in the dark, the rhodopsin molecule must be remade using vitamin A. Failure or delayed recovery of vision in the dark following a light flash, referred to as night blindness, may be due to inadequate vitamin A.

For the visual cycle (Fig. 10.6) to occur, vitamin A must first be transported into the retina and metabolized. This section focuses on how the vitamin is metabolized as part of the visual cycle. Retinol is transported to the retina via the blood as part of the holo-RBP-TTR complex. Retinol appears to move into the pigment epithelium of photoreceptor rod cells (Figs. 10.6 and 10.7). Within the pigment epithelium, much of the retinol is converted by LRAT to all-*trans* retinyl esters and some into 11-*cis* retinyl esters. The all-*trans* retinyl esters in turn may be stored in the pigment epithelium and metabolized, by an all-*trans* retinyl ester isomerohydrolase, as needed, to generate 11-*cis* retinol plus a fatty acid. Similarly, the 11-*cis* retinyl esters may be hydrolyzed, as needed, to 11-*cis* retinol and a fatty acid by retinyl ester hydrolase.

For the visual cycle to operate effectively, conversion of 11-*cis* retinol to 11-*cis* retinal is necessary. The 11-*cis* retinal must then be transported into the photoreceptor cells. The synthesis of 11-*cis* retinal occurs within the pigment epithelium by the action of 11-*cis* retinol dehydrogenase, which utilizes either NAD^+ or $NADP^+$. Transport of 11-*cis* retinol and 11-*cis* retinal is accomplished in the pigment epithelium by cellular retinal binding protein (CRALBP), and transport of all-*trans* retinol and 11-*cis* retinal between the pigment epithelium and the photoreceptor (rod) cells (and thus across the interphotoreceptor matrix/space) is accomplished by interstitial or interphotoreceptor retinol-binding protein (IRBP) [25,26]. Specifically, IRBP, a glycolipoprotein, resides within the retinal interphotoreceptor space that lies between the pigment epithelium and the photoreceptor cells [26]. CRBP and CRABP are also found in the retina.

Figure 10.6 The visual cycle.

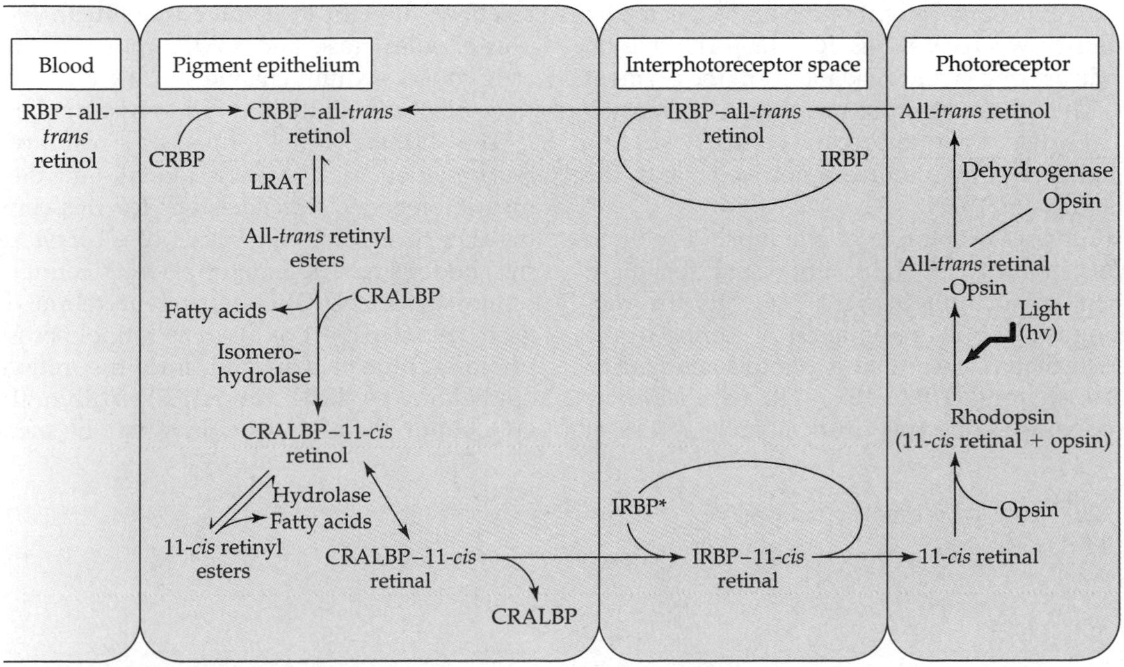

* IRBP-Interphotoreceptor retinol-binding protein.

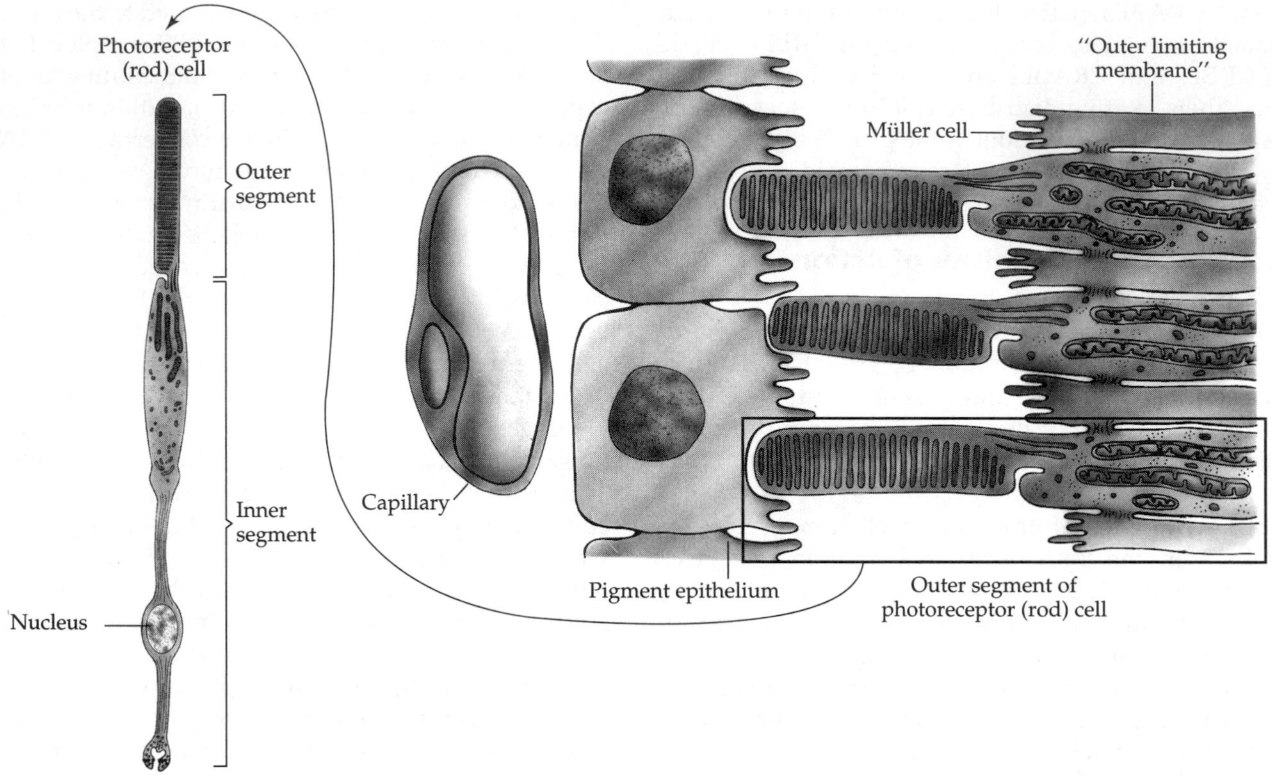

Figure 10.7 Photoreceptor (rod) cells, their structure, and their surroundings.

Within the photoreceptor cells, 11-*cis* retinal binds as a protonated Schiff base to a lysine amino acid residue in the protein opsin (Fig. 10.8) to produce the compound rhodopsin. Rhodopsin is embedded in disks located in the rod's outer segment, which is enclosed within a restricted compartment of the retina created by tight junctions between cells (Fig. 10.7) [25]. The cells on the blood side are one layer thick and form the pigment epithelium. The "outer limiting membrane" is formed on the vitreal side of the photoreceptor cells by specific junctions between the photoreceptor cells and the Müller cells (Fig. 10.7) [25].

Within the photoreceptor cells, rhodopsin is able to detect small amounts of light, important for night vision. When a quantum of light (hv) hits the rhodopsin, changes occur in the vitamin A portion of the molecule such that 11-*cis* retinal is photoisomerized to generate all-*trans* retinal (Fig. 10.6). The term *bleaching* is often used to describe this event because a loss of color occurs. A chain of events triggered by the absorption of light by 11-*cis* retinal results in an electrical signal or impulse to and along the optic nerve to the brain. To transmit through the cell to the plasma membrane the message that light has hit the rhodopsin, a cascade of reactions thought to involve **transducin** (a G protein), phosphodiesterase, and cGMP occurs. This reaction cascade causes sodium channels in the plasma membrane to be blocked and the rod cell to hyperpolarize.

The all-*trans* retinal formed as a result of light must be converted back to 11-*cis* retinal, and the rhodopsin must be regenerated. The steps for this conversion are thought to involve hydrolysis of all-*trans* retinal from the rhodopsin, reduction of all-*trans* retinal to all-*trans* retinol by an NADPH-dependent retinol dehydrogenase, and transport of all-*trans* retinol across the interphotoreceptor matrix and into the retinal pigment epithelium by IRBP (Fig. 10.6). Within the pigment epithelium, the all-*trans* retinol may be metabolized to

Figure 10.8 Rhodopsin 11-*cis* retinal bound to the protein opsin.

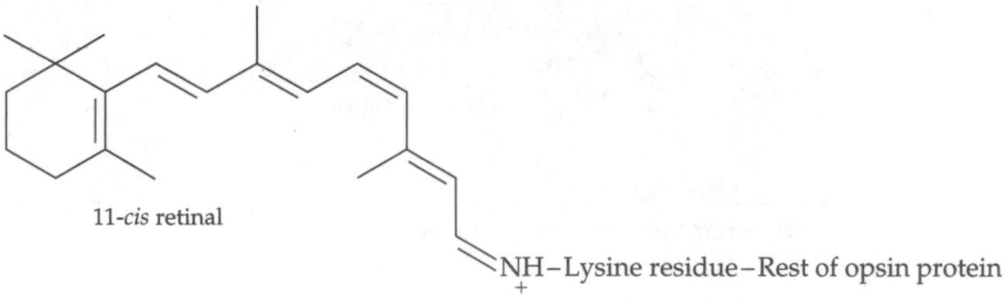

all-*trans* retinyl esters, which may be directly isomerized to 11-*cis* retinol and subsequently oxidized to 11-*cis* retinal. Stored all-*trans* retinyl esters also may be mobilized from the pigment epithelium for isomerization and oxidation to yield 11-*cis* retinal. The latter may undergo transport back into the photoreceptor cells to bind again with opsin and complete the visual cycle.

Cellular Differentiation. Vitamin A, especially as retinoic acid, is needed by epithelial cells for cell differentiation. Epithelial cells are found as part of our skin and in all internal body tracts, such as the respiratory, gastrointestinal, and urogenital tracts. Retinoic acid helps maintain both the normal structure and the functions of the epithelial cells [19]. For example, retinoic acid directs the differentiation of **keratinocytes** (immature skin cells) into mature epidermal cells. Retinoic acid is thought to act as a signal to "switch on" the genes for keratin proteins [19]. Vitamin A appears to direct the synthesis of keratins, with genes for smaller (vs. larger) keratin molecules transcribed and translated in the presence of vitamin A [24,27]. Vitamin A, in vitro, directs differentiation of squamous epithelial keratinizing cells into mucus-secreting cells [27]. With vitamin A deficiency, keratin-producing cells replace mucus-secreting cells in many body tissues.

The mechanism by which retinoic acid is thought to affect cell differentiation, at least in part, is through its effects on gene expression (Fig. 10.9). A series of events occurs to move the retinoic acid into the nucleus, where it can interact with the DNA. First, all-*trans* retinoic acid or 9-*cis* retinoic acid (generated from 9-*cis* retinol) is transported into the nucleus, likely bound to CRABP. Within the nucleus, all-*trans* retinoic acid and/or 9-*cis* retinoic acid binds to retinoic acid receptors. These nuclear retinoic acid receptors are part of a family of receptors that also includes receptors for vitamin D, specifically calcitriol/1,25-$(OH)_2$ D_3; for thyroid hormones; and for steroid hormones. Within the nucleus, all-*trans* retinoic acid (and possibly 9-*cis* retinoic acid) binds to one or more of three (α,β,γ) retinoic acid receptors (RAR), while 9-*cis* retinoic acid binds to one or more of three (α,β,γ) retinoid X receptors (RXR). RAR may require release from a corepressor prior to binding by all-*trans* retinoic acid. Once formed, the vitamin A–receptor complexes typically interact with other receptors, transcription factors, or coactivator proteins (which may include vitamin D receptors, thyroid hormone receptors, or orphan receptors with no known ligand) to form various **homodimers** or **heterodimers.** A homodimer is formed when two of the same receptors interact, such as RAR-RAR or RXR-RXR. A heterodimer is formed between two or more different receptors, such as RXR-RAR or VDR (vitamin D receptor)-RXR. The resulting homodimer or heterodimer complexes bind to specific DNA nucleotide sequences, referred to as retinoic acid response elements (RARE), in promoter regions of specific genes. The roles and effects on gene expression of these vitamin A–containing complexes are mostly unknown, but the complexes are thought to affect

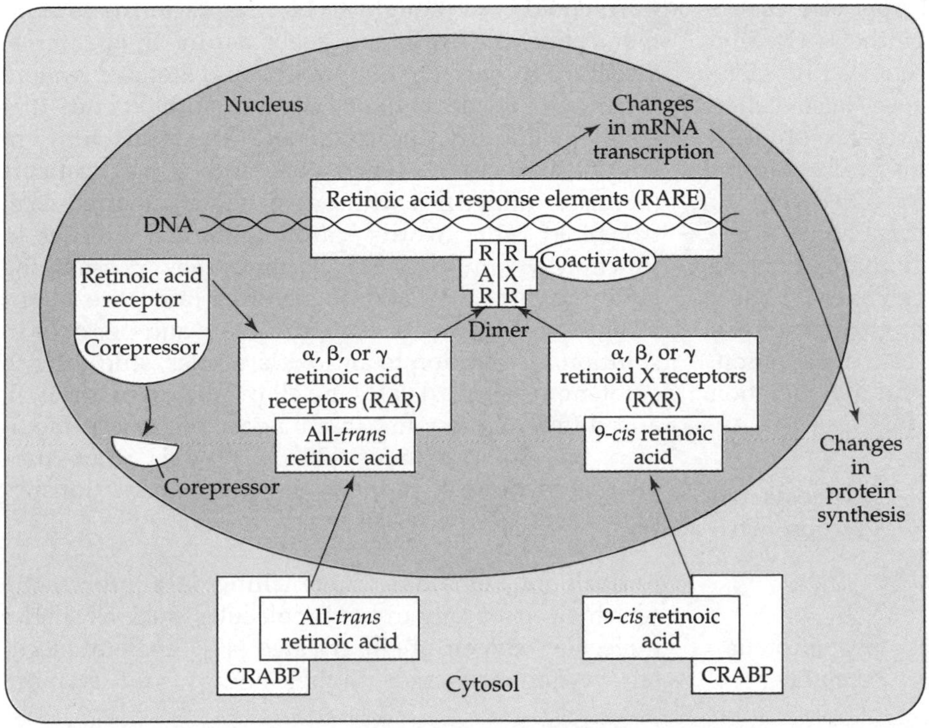

Figure 10.9 Hypothesized mode of action for retinoic acid.

a wide variety of cellular processes (including cell death, or apoptosis) and body processes through effects on genes that code for enzymes and for growth and transcription factors, among others.

Growth. Vitamin A deficiency has long been characterized in animals by impaired growth that can be stimulated with replacement by either retinol or retinoic acid. Specifically, vitamin A has been shown to stimulate the growth of epithelial cells. Retinyl β-glucuronide, formed in a variety of tissues from retinol and UDP-glucuronic acid, has been shown to actively support growth and differentiation [27,28].

The exact mechanism by which vitamin A affects growth is unclear. Cell growth is stimulated, in part, by growth factors that bind to specific receptors on cell surfaces. Retinoic acid appears to increase the number of specific receptors for growth factors [27]. Retinoic acid and 4-oxoretinoic acid generated from carotenoid metabolism also have been shown to increase synthesis of a specific gap junction protein known as connexin 43 by stabilizing connexin 43 mRNA [29–32]. **Gap junctions,** cell-to-cell channels formed from connexin proteins, are important for the exchange of small signaling compounds and thus for cell-to-cell communication. A lack of gap junction communication results in uncontrolled cell growth, as can occur with cancer cells. Thus, vitamin A, in preserving this communication, plays a role in the control of cell growth. Retinoic acid also may be able to modify cell surfaces, possibly by increasing glycoprotein synthesis at the gene level or by improving the attachment of glycoproteins to cell surfaces to induce cell adhesion [27,28]. Retinol may also play a more direct role in glycoprotein synthesis. Retinyl phosphate (generated from retinol plus ATP) can be converted to retinyl phosphomannose (also called mannosyl retinyl phosphate) in the presence of GDP-mannose. Retinyl phosphomannose can in turn transfer the mannose to glycoprotein acceptors. On receipt of the mannose, the glycoprotein acceptors become mannosylated glycoproteins [27,28]. Such changes in the glycan portion of the glycoprotein can greatly affect differentiation of cells or tissues through their effects on cell recognition, adhesion, and cell aggregation. These reactions involving vitamin A and glycosylation are shown here.

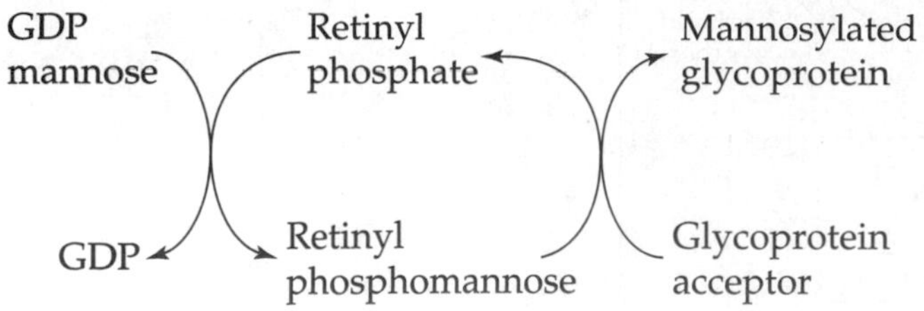

Other Functions. Vitamin A, as retinol but not as retinoic acid, is essential for reproductive processes in both males and females, although the mechanism(s) of its action(s) are unclear [33]. Bone development and maintenance also require vitamin A. Vitamin A is necessary for bone metabolism through involvement with **osteoblasts** (bone-forming cells) and **osteoclasts** (cells involved in bone resorption). Although the mechanism of action is unclear, vitamin A deficiency results in excessive deposition of bone by osteoblasts and reduced bone degradation by osteoclasts. Excess vitamin A, in contrast, stimulates osteoclasts and inhibits osteoblasts. Vitamin A appears to be involved in hematopoiesis and iron distribution among tissues, also via an unknown mechanism of action. Several aspects of immune system function, both humoral and cell-mediated, also are influenced by vitamin A. Retinoic acid, for example, stimulates phagocytic activity and cytokine production and maintains natural killer cell concentrations [34–38]. Depletion studies suggest that vitamin A appears to be needed for T-lymphocyte function and for antibody response to viral, parasitic, and bacterial infections [34,38]. Another role of vitamin A, likely mediated by effects on cell differentiation and growth, is in morphogenesis/embryogenesis. Specifically, retinoic acid is thought to act as a morphogen in embryonic developments, and nuclear retinoic acid receptors have been found in different cells during different times of development in the embryo.

Carotenoids

Carotenoids are thought to be present in the interior membranes of cells as well as in lipoproteins. Structurally, carotenoids possess an extended system (often nine or more) of conjugated double bonds that enable solubility in lipids and the quenching of **singlet molecular oxygen** ($^1O_2$) and of **free radicals** (atoms or molecules with one or more unpaired electrons). In other words, carotenoids are thought to function as antioxidants, because they possess the ability to react with and quench free-radical reactions in lipid membranes or compartments and possibly in solution. In addition to antioxidant roles, studies with carotenoids suggest roles in cell proliferation, growth, and differentiation and in enhancement of cell-mediated immune functions [29–32,39–41]. Some proposed functions of carotenoids and their relationship to diseases are discussed next.

Antioxidant Functions. **Quenching** is a process by which electronically excited molecules, such as singlet molecular oxygen, are inactivated [42]. Singlet molecular oxygen possesses higher energy and is more reactive than ground state molecular oxygen, which typically exists in triplet ($^3O_2$) versus singlet ($^1O_2$) form. Singlet oxygen is generated from lipid peroxidation of membranes, transfer of energy from light (photochemical reactions), or the respiratory burst occurring in neutrophils, for example (enzymatic reactions). Singlet molecular oxygen readily reacts with organic molecules such as protein, lipids, and DNA and thus can damage cellular components unless removed. Carotenoids such as β-carotene or lycopene can react with (quench) singlet oxygen, and it is the conjugated double-bond systems within the carotenoids that permit the quenching. For example, β-carotene bound to lymphocytes taken from human blood has been shown to directly quench singlet molecular oxygen in vitro [43]. Lycopene appears to have the highest rate constant (i.e., ability to react or complex) and is a more effective quencher of singlet oxygen than other carotenoids [44]. The singlet oxygen ($^1O_2$) transfers its excitation energy and returns to the ground state ($^3O_2$), while the carotenoid receiving the energy enters an excited state. Resonance states in the excited carotenoid allow some stabilization. Carotenoids then release the energy in the form of heat and thus do not need to be regenerated.

$$^1O_2 + \beta\text{-carotene} \longrightarrow {}^3O_2 + \text{excited } \beta\text{-carotene}$$
$$\longrightarrow \beta\text{-carotene} + \text{heat}$$

In addition to quenching singlet oxygen, β-carotene and other carotenoids have the ability to react directly with **peroxyl radicals** (O_2^{2-}) involved in lipid peroxidation [45]. This ability has been demonstrated in the range of partial pressures of oxygen that exist under physiological conditions. Studies suggest that β-carotene works synergistically with vitamin E in scavenging radicals and inhibiting lipid peroxidation, although vitamin E has higher reactivity toward peroxyl radicals than does β-carotene [46,47]. β-carotene is thought to function in the interior of the membrane, whereas α-tocopherol functions on or at the surface of the membrane [46]. Lipid peroxidation has been significantly reduced in smokers (who have chronic oxidative damage due to the effects of smoking) receiving only 20 mg β-carotene for 4 weeks [48]. β-carotene supplementation (50–100 mg daily for 3 weeks) has been shown to shorten the lag phase of metal (copper)-dependent lipid peroxidation of LDLs. In other words, β-carotene supplementation helps make LDL more resistant to metal-induced lipid oxidation [49]. Lipid peroxidation is an indicator of free radical activity and reflects damage to membranes and possibly other organelles or DNA. Supplements providing 120 mg β-carotene also significantly reduced lipid peroxidation in humans [50]. Carotene depletion in humans results in significantly lower serum carotene concentrations and higher concentrations of **thiobarbituric acid–reactive substances,** such as hexanal, pentanal, and pentane (compounds indicative of oxidative damage) [51]. Repletion studies providing β-carotene (15 or 120 mg) have been shown to decrease the concentrations of circulating peroxides [51,52].

While most studies have focused on β-carotene, lycopene (in chemical assays) has been shown to be the strongest antioxidant [53]. In these in vitro assays, lycopene is followed in descending order by α-tocopherol (vitamin E), α-carotene, β-cryptoxanthin, zeaxanthin and β-carotene, and lutein [53]. Combinations of the carotenoids, however, especially lycopene and lutein, have been shown to work synergistically and thus are more effective than any one of the carotenoids by itself.

Because of the ability of carotenoids to react with free radicals and quench singlet oxygen, carotenoids are thought to be protective against several diseases. Epidemiological studies have shown that individuals with high intakes of fruits and vegetables, which are also rich in carotenoids, or individuals with higher serum carotenoid concentrations have a lower incidence of diseases such as cardiovascular disease, cancer, and age-related macular degeneration [54–60]. Age-related macular degeneration is a common cause of blindness in older individuals. The macula, found in the center of the retina, maintains central vision. Lutein and zeaxanthin, which are found in the eye, can inhibit oxidation of cell membranes and thus may be protective against UV-induced eye damage. Studies have demonstrated that individuals in the highest quintile of intake of dietary carotenoids, especially lutein and zeaxanthin, have significantly lower risk of macular degeneration [60].

In the mechanism(s) thought to lead to the development of atherosclerosis, oxidation of cholesterol in LDLs increases the likelihood of monocyte or macrophage uptake in comparison with native (unoxidized) cholesterol. Oxidized cholesterol also impairs arterial nitric oxide release, which may contribute to vasospasms and platelet adhesion associated with heart disease [61]. Oxidized LDL cholesterol stimulates the binding of monocytes to blood vessel endothelium. These monocytes become embedded in the endothelium, as do native LDLs, which have the potential to become oxidized within the subendothelial space. Macrophages in the blood vessel endothelia continue to take up oxidized LDL cholesterol via a specific cell surface scavenger receptor and when filled with cholesterol become foam cells. Fatty streaks (an accumulation of foam cells) lead to atherosclerotic plaque in blood vessels. Carotenoids, including β-carotene, lycopene, lutein, and α-carotene, among others, are thought to prevent the oxidation of LDL cholesterol and other cell membrane lipids and thus prevent or slow the development of atherosclerosis [62–64]. However, α-tocopherol (vitamin E) may be more effective than β-carotene in inhibiting LDL oxidation [65]. Supplementation with 800 IU vitamin E, 1,000 mg vitamin C, and 24 mg β-carotene in individuals with coronary artery disease has been shown to effectively reduce LDL susceptibility to oxidation [66].

Cell Proliferation, Growth, and Differentiation. Carotenoids inhibit cell proliferation and stimulate cell differentiation while also affecting growth. Lycopene, for example, has been shown to inhibit the growth and proliferation of various cancer cells and to induce cell differentiation [67,68]. In vitro, canthaxanthin and β-carotene have been shown to inhibit carcinogen-induced neoplastic transformation as well as to inhibit lipid oxidation in plasma membranes [69]. As in their antioxidant roles, carotenoids appear to vary in their abilities to inhibit cell transformation. For example, canthaxanthin appears to be more effective than β-carotene, followed by α-carotene and then lycopene, in inhibiting chemically induced neoplastic transformation [70].

The mechanisms by which carotenoids carry out these roles are not clear, but in their capacities they may be similar to the retinoids. For example, carotenoid-induced enhancement or induction of gap junction communication similar to that of retinoic acid has been proposed. Some carotenoids up-regulate the gene expression of connexin 43 [69]. Connexin proteins enable connections (bridges) to form between cells, and these connections in turn affect cell proliferation and growth [29–32]. Gap junction communications are inhibited in some cancer cells. Thus, the ability of carotenoids to protect this activity may be of significance in cancer prevention [71].

Intervention trials using β-carotene have failed to show protective effects. Intervention trials with 20 mg of β-carotene (BC) along with α-tocopherol (AT) in Finland (referred to as the ATBC trial) as well as intervention with 30 mg of β-carotene and 25,000 IU of vitamin A (CARET trial) showed no benefit versus placebo in disease prevention in asbestos-exposed workers and in individuals with a long history of smoking [72,73]. β-carotene taken with the vitamin A even appeared to increase the risk of lung cancer and increase the risk of mortality from cancer and heart disease in the high-risk populations (smokers and asbestos-exposed) [73]. These two intervention trials appear to suggest that β-carotene supplementation increases the risk of cancer; however, others suggest that the populations were at high risk for disease, with a long history of smoking (one pack or more cigarettes daily) or asbestos exposure along with alcohol consumption, and that only with these cofactors does β-carotene supplementation increase cancer risk [74,75].

Health claims that are approved by the U.S. Food and Drug Administration are targeted at carotenoid-rich foods (fruits and vegetables) as well as grain products. These claims require the food to be low in fat and a good source of dietary fiber without fortification. An example model claim is "Low fat diets rich in fiber-containing grain products, fruits and vegetables may reduce the risk of some types of cancer, a disease associated with many factors" [76]. Another sample claim for fruits, vegetables, or grain products that are low in (saturated and total) fat and cholesterol and contain at least 0.6 g soluble fiber per reference amount without fortification is "Diets low in saturated fat and cholesterol and rich in fruits and vegetables and grain products that contain some types of dietary fiber, particularly soluble fiber, may reduce the risk of heart disease, a disease associated with many factors" [76]. Another model claim—"Low fat diets rich in fruits and vegetables (foods that are low in fat and may contain dietary fiber, vitamin A, or vitamin C) may reduce the risk of some types of cancer, a disease associated with many factors"—has also been approved for fruits and vegetables that are a good source of vitamin A or C or dietary fiber [76].

Interactions with Other Nutrients

Vitamin A or carotenoids interact with vitamins E and K. Excess dietary vitamin A intakes interfere with vitamin K absorption. High β-carotene, in turn, may decrease plasma vitamin E concentrations.

Protein and zinc influence vitamin A status and transport. First, the activity of the enzyme carotenoid dioxygenase that cleaves β-carotene is depressed by inadequate protein intake. Second, overall vitamin A metabolism is closely related to protein and zinc status because transport and use of the vitamin depend on several vitamin A–binding proteins and because zinc is required for protein synthesis. Impairments in the synthesis of proteins, including retinol-binding protein and transthyretin, diminish retinol mobilization from the liver. In addition, in peripheral tissue, alcohol dehydrogenase, which converts retinol into retinal, is directly dependent on zinc.

Iron status and vitamin A are also interrelated. The effects may be mediated through a role played by vitamin A in hematopoiesis. Vitamin A deficiency diminishes the mobilization of iron from stores, often leading to microcytic anemia. Vitamin A supplementation, in turn, corrects the anemia, with observed improvements in indices of iron status [77–80]. Vitamin A may be directly acting on iron metabolism or storage or may be affecting differentiation of blood cells.

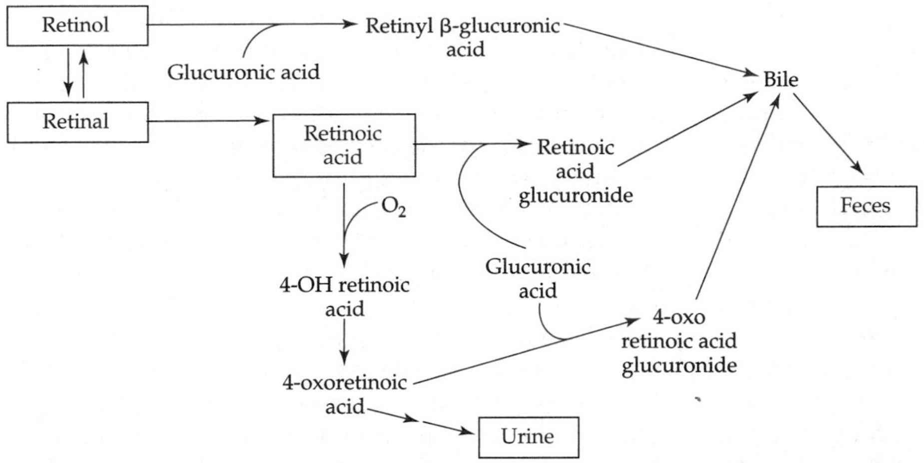

Figure 10.10 Metabolism of vitamin A, showing some excretory products.

Metabolism and Excretion

Urinary excretion of vitamin A metabolites accounts for up to about 60% of vitamin A excretion. Many of the urinary products are metabolites derived from 4-oxoretinoic acid. In addition, small amounts of vitamin A have been found expired by the lungs as CO_2, while up to about 40% of vitamin A metabolites are excreted in the feces [5]. Fecal vitamin A metabolites are typically those oxidized products of vitamin A that contain intact chains and have been conjugated to glucuronic acid (Fig. 10.10) or taurine and excreted into the bile. Some examples of fecal vitamin A metabolites are retinoic acid glucuronide and 4-oxoretinoic acid glucuronide. However, some polar products such as 4-oxoretinoic acid glucuronide can be absorbed and returned to the liver via enterohepatic circulation. This recycling mechanism helps conserve the body's supply of vitamin A when necessary.

Carotenoids newly absorbed and not stored or converted to retinal or retinol may be metabolized into a variety of compounds depending on the individual carotenoid. Carotenoid metabolites are excreted into the bile for elimination in the feces [28].

Recommended Dietary Allowances

In 2001, the Institute of Medicine's Food and Nutrition Board published new recommendations for vitamin A; however, no recommendations were established for carotenoids because the carotenoids are not considered essential nutrients [5]. Recommendations for vitamin A intake are expressed as retinol activity equivalents (RAE). Older units of measure include international units (IU) and retinol equivalents (RE). The RAE equivalencies of retinol, β-carotene, and other provitamin A carotenoids are as follows [5]: 1 RAE = 1 μg retinol = 12 μg β-carotene = 24 μg α-carotene or β-cryptoxanthin.

The requirements for vitamin A for adult men and women are 625 and 500 μg RAE, respectively [5]. The recommended dietary allowance (RDA) for vitamin A is based on the requirement plus twice the coefficient of variation (20%) with the value rounded to the nearest 100 μg [5]. The RDAs for vitamin A for adult men and women are 900 and 700 μg RAE, respectively [5]. During pregnancy and lactation, the RDAs for vitamin A for adult women are higher at 770 and 1,300 μg RAE, respectively [5]. A daily tolerable upper intake level (UL) for adults of 3,000 μg has been established for preformed vitamin A [5].

Deficiency

Vitamin A deficiency is less common in the United States than in developing countries, where inadequate intake is fairly common in children under 5 years of age. In developing countries, increased mortality is associated both with clinically evident vitamin A deficiency in children and with inadequate vitamin A stores in children with no clinical signs of deficiency [81]. Increased infectious morbidity also is associated with vitamin A deficiency [38].

Selected signs and symptoms of deficiency include **xerophthalmia,** anorexia, retarded growth, increased susceptibility to infections, obstruction and enlargement of hair follicles, and keratinization of epithelial (mucous) cells of the skin with accompanying failure of normal differentiation. Xerophthalmia is characterized by dryness of the eye and abnormalities of the conjunctiva and cornea of the eye; it includes conjunctival and corneal xerosis, Bitot's spots, corneal scarring and ulcerations, and night blindness. Conjunctival changes include the disappearance of goblet cells in the conjunctiva, the enlargement and keratinization of epithelial cells, and the appearance of Bitot's spots overlying the keratinized epithelia of the conjunctiva. Bitot's spots are white accumulations of sloughed cells and secretions.

Keratomalacia may occur if the changes in the cornea become severe and irreversible (such as with corneal perforation and loss of aqueous humor). Night blindness, which may be one of the first symptoms of vitamin A deficiency related to vision, results from impaired production of rhodopsin in the outer segments of the rods.

Conditions and populations associated with increased need for vitamin A include individuals with malabsorptive disorders such as **steatorrhea** (excessive fat in the feces) or pancreatic, liver, or gallbladder diseases. People with chronic nephritis, acute protein deficiency, intestinal parasites, or acute infections may also become vitamin A–deficient. Measles infections in developing countries are associated with high mortality. Measles is thought to depress vitamin A status (which may already be low in children in developing countries) by diminishing vitamin A intake, absorption, and utilization and by increasing urinary vitamin A excretion [38,82]. Vitamin A supplements are recommended by WHO and UNICEF for children with measles living in a country with measles fatality rates of 1% or greater [31].

Toxicity: Hypervitaminosis A

Ingestion of a large amount of vitamin A for a short time period (even a single dose) may result in acute hypervitaminosis A. Symptoms of acute hypervitaminosis A include nausea, vomiting, double vision, headache, dizziness, and general desquamation of the skin. Chronic intakes (daily for months or years) of lower doses (but still in excess of recommendations) also can lead to hypervitaminosis A. In adults, chronic oral intakes of vitamin A (retinol) in amounts as little as 3 to 4 times greater than the RDA can result in hypervitaminosis A, although generally it is higher intakes (about 10 or more times the RDA) that result in toxicity. Chronic vitamin A toxicity is manifested by a variety of maladies, including anorexia; dry, itchy, and desquamating skin; alopecia (hair loss) and coarsening of the hair; ataxia; headache; bone and muscle pain; conjunctivitis; and ocular pain, among others. Most manifestations of toxicity appear to subside gradually once excessive intake of the vitamin is discontinued [83]. The tolerable upper intake level for preformed vitamin A is 3,000 μg (10,000 IU) per day [5].

Excess vitamin A also has been shown to be **teratogenic** (causing birth defects). For example, an oral intake of more than 7,500 μg of vitamin A by pregnant women has been associated with increased risk of malformations in infants born to the women [84–86]. Moreover, the topical medication Accutane (for treatment of acne), which contains a modified form of vitamin A (13-*cis* retinoic acid) also has been shown to be teratogenic. Use of this compound by women in the early months of their pregnancy resulted in a number of birth defects among the infants born to these women. Consequently, dermatologists advise against Accutane usage for women who are or may become pregnant and thus prescribe contraceptives for patients in their childbearing years taking the drug.

One mechanism by which excess vitamin A is thought to exert toxic effects is related to its transport in the blood. When vitamin A intake is in excess, serum retinol levels rise above 200 μg/dL (normal is 45–65 μg/dL), and retinol is no longer transported exclusively by RBP but instead can be carried to the tissues by plasma lipoproteins. It has been suggested that when retinol is presented to the cell membranes in a form other than in an RBP complex, the released retinol produces toxic effects [5,24]. Effects on the liver, the primary storage site for vitamin A, are multiple. They include fat-storing cell **hyperplasia** (excessive cell proliferation) and hypertrophy, fibrogenesis, sclerosis of veins, portal hypertension, and congestion in perisinusoid cells, which leads to hepatocellular damage and cirrhosis or a cirrhosis-like hepatic disorder [83,87,88]. Other toxic effects of excess vitamin A intakes are thought to be mediated by changes in the regulation of vitamin A (retinoid) receptors in the nucleus and by effects on cell differentiation and growth, among other means.

Carotenoids, in contrast to vitamin A, appear to have few side effects. In fact, β-carotene is listed on the generally recognized as safe (GRAS) list with the FDA for use as a dietary and nutrient supplement as well as for use as a colorant in foods, drugs, and cosmetics [89]. Ingestion by adults in amounts as high as 180 mg of β-carotene daily for several months has been shown to pose no serious side effects [90]. Hypercarotenosis in individuals ingesting about 30 mg or more of β-carotene daily can, however, cause a yellow discoloration of the skin, especially in the fat pads or fatty areas of the palms of the hands and soles of the feet [91]. The condition usually disappears following removal of the carotenoids from the diet. While no tolerable upper intake level has been established for β-carotene or other carotenoids [9], excessive consumption of carotenoids may be detrimental to smokers [73–75] and possibly to nonsmokers with effects, to date, unknown. Carotenoid supplements are not advised for the general public; instead, the public is encouraged to consume at least five servings of fruits and vegetables per day [9].

Assessment of Nutriture

Vitamin A status may be assessed in a variety of ways, including histological tests, biochemical measures, and functional tests. The last includes assessment of night blindness or dark adaptation threshold.

Electrophysiological measurements made via electroretinograms measure the level of rhodopsin and its rate of regeneration [92].

Conjunctival impression cytology (CIC), a histological method of assessment, involves the examination of the eye. The conjunctiva is examined for changes, specifically a reduction in goblet cells and the derangement of epithelial cells, that occur with impaired vitamin A status [93].

Plasma retinol concentrations are frequently measured as a biochemical indicator of vitamin A status. Plasma retinol levels reflect status best if the individual has exhausted his or her stores of the vitamin, as with deficiency, or if the stores are filled to capacity, as with toxicity. Use of plasma retinol concentrations, however, also depends on the adequacy of dietary energy, protein, and zinc due to their roles in the synthesis of retinol-binding protein. Moreover, use of plasma retinol is unreliable as an indicator of vitamin A status in individuals with infection or inflammation, both of which depress plasma concentrations of the vitamin [93]. Plasma retinol concentrations less than ~20 μg/dL are usually considered an indication of inadequate stores of vitamin A [5,94–96].

Adequacy of vitamin A stores in the liver can be assessed via other biochemical tests: the relative dose response (RDR) test or the modified relative dose response (MRDR) test. The RDR test involves measurement of changes in plasma retinol concentration before and 5 hours after oral administration of retinyl esters (usually as acetate or palmitate). Blood is taken initially, then vitamin A is ingested, and 5 hours later blood is taken again. Retinol concentrations of the blood are determined, and the difference in concentration is calculated and divided by the 5-hour concentration. RDR is then expressed as a percentage.

$$\text{RDR (\%)} = \frac{\text{5-hour plasma retinol} - \text{initial plasma retinol}}{\text{5-hour plasma retinol concentration}} \times 100$$

A % RDR equal to or greater than 20% suggests inadequate liver vitamin A stores [5,97,98].

References Cited for Vitamin A

1. Ong D. Retinoid metabolism during intestinal absorption. J Nutr 1993;123:351–55.

2. Blomhoff R, Green M, Norum K. Vitamin A: physiological and biochemical processing. Ann Rev Nutr 1992;12:37–57.

3. Harrison E, Hussain M. Mechanisms involved in the intestinal digestion and absorption of dietary vitamin A. J Nutr 2001;131:1405–8.

4. Rigtrup K, McEwen L, Said H, Ong D. Retinyl ester hydrolytic activity associated with human intestinal brush border membranes. Am J Clin Nutr 1994;60:111–16.

5. Food and Nutrition Board, Institute of Medicine. Dietary Reference Intakes. Washington, DC: National Academy Press, 2001, pp. 82–161.

6. Novotny J, Dueker S, Zech L, Clifford A. Compartmental analysis of dynamics of β-carotene metabolism in an adult volunteer. J Lipid Res 1995;36:1825–38.

7. Rodreguez M, Irwin M. A conspectus of research on vitamin A requirements of man. J Nutr 1972;102:909–68.

8. Brubacher G, Weiser H. The vitamin A activity of beta-carotene. Internatl J Vitam Nutr Res 1985;55:5–15.

9. Food and Nutrition Board, Institute of Medicine. Dietary Reference Intakes. Washington, DC: National Academy Press, 2000, pp. 325–82.

10. Stahl W, Sies H. Uptake of lycopene and its geometrical isomers is greater from heat-processed than from unprocessed tomato juice in humans. J Nutr 1992;122:2161–66.

11. Yeum K, Russell R. Carotenoid bioavailability and bioconversion. Ann Rev Nutr 2002;22:483–504.

12. Parker R. Absorption, metabolism, and transport of carotenoids. FASEB J 1996;10:542–51.

13. Wang X. Absorption and metabolism of beta-carotene. J Am Coll Nutr 1994;13:314–25.

14. Boileau T, Moore A, Erdman J, Jr. Carotenoids and vitamin A. In: Papas AM, ed. Antioxidant Status, Diet, Nutrition, and Health. Boca Raton, FL: CRC Press, 1999, pp. 133–58.

15. Ong D. Cellular transport and metabolism of vitamin A: roles of the cellular retinoid-binding proteins. Nutr Rev 1994;52: S24–S31.

16. Blomhoff R. Transport and metabolism of vitamin A. Nutr Rev 1994;52:S13–S23.

17. Schmitz H, Poor C, Wellman R, Erdman J. Concentrations of selected carotenoids and vitamin A in human liver, kidney and lung tissue. J Nutr 1991;121:1613–21.

18. Napoli J. Biosynthesis and metabolism of retinoic acid: roles of CRBP and CRABP in retinoic acid: roles of CRBP and CRABP in retinoic acid homeostasis. J Nutr 1993;123:362–66.

19. Ross A, Ternus M. Vitamin A as a hormone: recent advances in understanding the actions of retinol, retinoic acid, and beta carotene. J Am Diet Assoc 1993;93:1285–90.

20. Goodman D. Vitamin A and retinoids in health and disease. N Engl J Med 1984;310:1023–31.

21. Soprano D, Blaner W. Plasma retinol binding protein. In: Sporn M, Robers A, and Goodman D, eds. Retinoids: Biology, Chemistry, and Medicine. New York: Raven Press, 1994, pp. 257–81.

22. Noy N, Xu ZJ. The interactions of retinol with binding proteins: implications for the mechanism of uptake by cells. Biochem 1990;29:3878–83.

23. Noy N, Blaner W. Interactions of retinol with binding proteins: studies with rat cellular retinol-binding proteins and with rat retinol-binding protein. Biochem 1991;30:6380–86.

24. Creek K, St. Hilaire P, Hodam J. A comparison of the uptake, metabolism and biologic effects of retinol delivered to human keratinocytes either free or bound to serum retinol-binding protein. J Nutr 1993;123:356–61.

25. Ong D. Vitamin A–binding proteins. Nutr Rev 1985;43:225–32.

26. Wolf G. The intracellular vitamin A–binding proteins: an overview of their functions. Nutr Rev 1991;49:1–12.

27. Wolf G. Multiple functions of vitamin A. Physiol Rev 1984;64:873–937.

28. Olson J. 1992 Atwater Lecture: the irresistible fascination of carotenoids and vitamin A. Am J Clin Nutr 1993;57:833–39.

29. Bertram J. Cancer prevention by carotenoids: mechanistic studies in cultured cells. Ann NY Acad Sci 1993;691:177–91.

30. Hanusch M, Stahl W, Schulz W, Sies H. Induction of gap junctional communication by 4-oxoretinoic acid generated from its precursor canthaxanthin. Arch Biochem Biophys 1995;317:423–28.

31. Sies H, Stahl W. Carotenoids and intercellular communication via gap junctions. Int J Vit Nutr Res 1997;67:364–67.

32. Zhang L, Cooney R, Bertram J. Carotenoids enhance gap junctional communication and inhibit lipid peroxidation in C3H/10T1/2 cells: relationship to their cancer chemopreventive action. Carcinogenesis 1991;12:2109–14.

33. Clagett-Dame M, DeLuca H. The role of vitamin A in mammalian reproduction and embryonic development. Ann Rev Nutr 2002;22:347–82.

34. Ross A. Vitamin A and protective immunity. Nutr Today 1992;27 (July–Aug):18–26.

35. Zhao Z, Ross A. Retinoic acid repletion restores the number of leukocytes and their subsets and stimulates natural cytotoxicity in vitamin A–deficient rats. J Nutr 1995;125:2064–73.

36. Katz D, Drzymala M, Turton J, Hicks R, Hunt R, Palmer L, Malkovsky M. Regulation of accessory cell function by retinoids in murine immune responses. Br J Exp Pathol 1987;68:343–50.

37. Trechsel U, Evequoz V, Fleisch H. Stimulation of interleukin 1 and 3 production by retinoic acid in vitro. Biochem J 1985;230:339–44.

38. Stephensen C. Vitamin A, infection, and immune function. Ann Rev Nutr 2001;21:167–92.

39. Hughes D, Wright A, Finglas P, Peerless A, Bailey A, Astley S, Pinder A, Southon S. The effect of beta-carotene supplementation on the immune function of blood monocytes from healthy male nonsmokers. J Lab Clin Med 1997;129:309–17.

40. Kramer T, Burri B. Modulated mitogenic proliferative responsiveness of lymphocytes in whole-blood cultures after a low-carotene diet and mixed carotenoid supplementation in women. Am J Clin Nutr 1997;65:871–75.

41. Santos M, Meydani SN, Leka L, Wu D, Fotouhi N, Meydani M, Hennekens C, Gaziano J. Natural killer cell activity in elderly men is enhanced by beta-carotene supplementation. Am J Clin Nutr 1996;64:772–77.

42. Mascio P, Murphy M, Sies H. Antioxidant defense systems: the role of carotenoids, tocopherols, and thiols. Am J Clin Nutr 1991;53:194S–200S.

43. Bohm F, Haley J, Truscott T, Schalch W. Cellular-bound β-carotene quenches singlet oxygen in man. J Photochem Photobiol B Biol 1993;21:219–21.

44. Conn P, Schalch W, Truscott T. The singlet oxygen and carotenoid interaction. J Photochem Photobiol B 1991;11:41–47.

45. Burton G, Ingold K. β-carotene: an unusual type of lipid antioxidant. Science 1984;224:569–73.

46. Niki E, Noguchi N, Tsuchihashi H, Gotoh N. Interaction among vitamin C, vitamin E, and β-carotene. Am J Clin Nutr 1995;62(suppl):1322S–26S.

47. Palozza P, Krinsky N. β-carotene and α-tocopherol are synergistic antioxidants. Arch Biochem Biophys 1992;297:184–87.

48. Allard J, Royall D, Kurian R, Muggli R, Jeejeebhoy K. Effects of β-carotene supplementation on lipid peroxidation in humans. Am J Clin Nutr 1994;59:884–90.

49. Gaziano J, Hatta A, Flynn M, Johnson E, Krinsky N, Ridker P, Hennekens C, Frei B. Supplementation with β-carotene in vivo and in vitro does not inhibit low density lipoprotein oxidation. Atherosclerosis 1995;112:187–95.

50. Gottlieb K, Zarling E, Mobarhan S, Bowen P, Sugerman S. β-carotene decreases markers of lipid peroxidation in healthy volunteers. Nutr Cancer 1993;19:207–12.

51. Dixon Z, Burri B, Clifford A, Frankel E, Schneeman B, Parks E, Keim N, Barbieri T, Wu M, Fong A, Kretsch M, Sowell A, Erdman J. Effects of a carotene-deficient diet on measures of oxidative susceptibility and superoxide dismutase activity in adult women. Free Radic Biol Med 1994;17:537–44.

52. Mobarhan S, Bowen P, Andersen B, Evans M, Sapuntzakis M, Sugerman S, Simms P, Lucchesi D, Friedman H. Effects of β-carotene repletion on β-carotene absorption, lipid peroxidation, and neutrophil superoxide formation in young men. Nutr Cancer 1990;14:195–206.

53. DiMascio P, Kaiser S, Sies H. Lycopene as the most efficient biological carotenoid singlet oxygen quencher. Arch Biochem Biophys 1989;274:532–38.

54. Block G, Patterson B, Subar A. Fruit, vegetables, and cancer prevention: a review of the epidemiological evidence. Nutr Cancer 1992; 18:1–29.

55. Ziegler R. Vegetables, fruits and carotenoids and risk of cancer. Am J Clin Nutr 1991;53(suppl):251S–59S.

56. Gaziano J, Hennekens C. The role of beta carotene in the prevention of cardiovascular disease. Ann NY Acad Sci 1993;69:148–54.

57. Morris D, Kritchevsky S, Davis C. Serum carotenoids and coronary heart disease. JAMA 1994;272:1439–41.

58. Poppel G, Goldbolm R. Epidemiologic evidence for β-carotene and cancer prevention. Am J Clin Invest 1995;62(suppl):1393S–1402S.

59. Seddon J, Ajani U, Sperduto F, Hiller R, Blair N, Burton T, Farber M, Gragoudas E, Haller J, Miller D, Yannuzzi L, Willett W. Dietary carotenoids, vitamins A, C, and E, and advanced age-related macular degeneration. JAMA 1994;272:1413–20.

60. Snodderly D. Evidence for protection against age-related macular degeneration by carotenoids and antioxidant vitamins. Am J Clin Nutr 1995;62:1448S–61S.

61. Levine G, Keaney J, Vita J. Cholesterol reduction in cardiovascular disease. N Eng J Med 1995;332:512–21.

62. Luc G, Fruchart J-C. Oxidation of lipoproteins and atherosclerosis. Am J Clin Nutr 1991;53:206S–9S.

63. Prince M, Frisoli J. Beta-carotene accumulation in serum and skin. Am J Clin Nutr 1993;57:175–81.

64. Krinsky N. Actions of carotenoids in biological systems. Ann Rev Nutr 1993;13:561–87.

65. Abbey M, Nestel P, Baghurst P. Antioxidant vitamins and low-density-lipoprotein oxidation. Am J Clin Nutr 1993;58:525–32.

66. Mosca L, Rubenfire M, Mandel C, Rock C, Tarshis T, Tsai A, Pearson T. Antioxidant nutrient supplementation reduces the susceptibility of low density lipoprotein to oxidation in patients with coronary artery disease. J Am Coll Cardiol 1997;30:392–99.

67. Amir H, Karas M, Giat J, Danilenko M, Levy R, Yermiahu T, Levy J, Sharoni Y. Lycopene and 1,25 dihydroxy vitamin D3 cooperate in the inhibition of cell cycle progression and induction of differentiation in HL-60 leukemic cells. Nutr Cancer 1999;33:105–12.

68. Karas M, Amir H, Fishman D, Danilenko M, Segal S, Nahum A, Koifmann A, Giat Y, Levy J, Sharoni Y. Lycopene interferes with cell cycle progression and insulin-like growth factor 1 signaling in mammary cancer cells. Nutr Cancer 2000;36:101–11.

69. Bertram J, Bortkiewicz H. Dietary carotenoids inhibit neoplastic transformation and modulate gene expression in mouse and human cells. Am J Clin Nutr 1995;62(suppl):1327S–36S.

70. Bertram J, Pung A, Churley M, Kappock T, Wilkins L, Cooney R. Diverse carotenoids protect against chemically induced neoplastic transformation. Carcinogenesis 1991;12:671–78.

71. Acevedo P, Bertram J. Liarozole potentiates the cancer chemopreventive activity of and the up-regulation of gap junctional communication and connexin 43 expression by retinoic acid and beta-carotene in 10T1/2 cells. Carcinogenesis 1995;16:2215–22.

72. Alpha-tocopherol, Beta-carotene (ATBC) Cancer Prevention Study Group. The effect of vitamin E and beta carotene on the incidence of lung cancer and other cancers in male smokers. N Engl J Med 1994;330:1029–35.

73. Omenn G, Goodman G, Thomquist M, Balmes J, Cullen M, Glass A, Keogh J, Meyskens F, Valanis B, Williams J, Barnhart S, Hammar S. Effects of a combination of beta carotene and vitamin A on lung cancer and cardiovascular disease. N Engl J Med 1996;334:1150–55.

74. Omenn G, Goodman G, Thornquist M, Balmes J, Cullen M, Glass A, Keogh J, Meyskens F, Valanis B, Williams J, Barnhart S, Cherniack M, Brodkin C, Hammar S. Risk factors for lung cancer and for intervention effects in CARET, the beta-carotene and retinol efficacy trial. J Natl Cancer Inst 1996;88:1550–59.

75. Mayne S, Handelman G, Beecher G. β-carotene and lung cancer promotion in heavy smokers—a plausible relationship? J Natl Cancer Inst 1996;88:1513–15.

76. www.cfsan.fda.gov.

77. Lynch S. Interaction of iron with other nutrients. Nutr Rev 1997;55:102–10.

78. Suharno D, West C, Muhilal K, Hautvast J. Supplementation with vitamin A and irons for nutritional anaemia in pregnant women in West Java, Indonesia. Lancet 1993;342:1325–28.

79. Mejia L, Hodges R, Rucker R. Role of vitamin A in the absorption, retention, and distribution of iron in the rat. J Nutr 1979;109:129–37.

80. Goldberg L, Smith J. Vitamin A deficiencies in relation to iron overload in the rat. J Pathol Bacteriol 1960;8:173–80.

81. Olson J. Hypovitaminosis A: contemporary scientific issues. J Nutr 1994;124:1461S–66S.

82. Stephensen C, Alvarez J, Kohatsu J, Hardmeier R, Kennedy J, Gammon RB. Vitamin A is excreted in the urine during acute infection. Am J Clin Nutr 1994;60:388–92.

83. Stimson W. Vitamin A intoxication in adults. Report of a case with a summary of the literature. N Engl J Med 1961;265:369–73.

84. Bauernfeind J. The Safe Use of Vitamin A. A Report of the International Vitamin A Consultative Group. Washington, DC: The Nutrition Foundation, 1980.

85. Bernhardt I, Dorsey D. Hypervitaminosis A and congenital renal anomalies in a human infant. Obstet Gynecol 1974;43:750–55.

86. Rothman K, Moore L, Singer M, Nguyen U, Mannino S, Milunsky A. Teratogenicity of high vitamin A intake. N Engl J Med 1995; 333:1369–73.

87. Russell R, Boyer J, Bagheri S, Hruban Z. Hepatic injury from chronic hypervitaminosis A resulting in portal hypertension and ascites. N Engl J Med 1974;291:435–40.

88. Geubel A, Galocsy C, Alves N, Rahier J, Dive C. Liver damage caused by therapeutic vitamin A administration: estimate of dose-related toxicity in 41 cases. Gastroenterology 1991;100:1701–9.

89. Life Sciences Research Office FDA Contract No. 223-75-2004. Evaluation of the Health Aspects of Carotene (β-carotene) as a Food Ingredient. Bethesda, MD: Federation of American Societies for Experimental Biology, 1979.

90. Matthews-Roth M. Beta-carotene therapy for erythropoietic protoporphyria and other photosensitivity diseases. Biochim 1986;68:875–84.

91. Diplock A. Safety of antioxidant vitamins and β-carotene. Am J Clin Nutr 1995;62(suppl):1510S–16S.

92. Underwood B. Methods for assessment of vitamin A status. J Nutr 1990;120:1459–63.

93. Olson J. Needs and sources of carotenoids and vitamin A. Nutr Rev 1994;52:S67–S73.

94. Craft N. Innovative approaches to vitamin A assessment. J Nutr 2001;131:1626S–30S.

95. Flores H. Frequency distributions of serum vitamin A levels in cross-sectional surveys and in surveys before and after vitamin A supplementation. In: A Brief Guide to Current Methods of Assessing Vitamin A Status. A report of the International Vitamin A Consultative Group. Washington, DC: The Nutrition Foundation, 1993, pp. 9–11.

96. Underwood B. Hypovitaminosis A: international programmatic issues. J Nutr 1994;124:1467S–72S.

97. Tanumihardjo S. The modified relative dose-response assay. In: A Brief Guide to Current Methods of Assessing Vitamin A Status. A report of the International Vitamin A Consultative Group. Washington, DC: The Nutrition Foundation, 1993 pp. 14–15.

98. Russell R. The vitamin A spectrum: from deficiency to toxicity. Am J Clin Nutr 2000;71:878–84.

Web Sites

www.nal.usda.gov/fnic/foodcomp
Food composition data.

www.cfsan.fda.gov
Health claims.

VITAMIN D

Through the years vitamin D has been associated with skeletal growth and strong bones. This association arose because early in the 20th century it was shown that rickets, a childhood disease characterized by improper development of bones, could be prevented by a fat-soluble factor D in the diet or by body exposure to ultraviolet light. Emphasis was placed on the dietary factor; therefore, any compound with curative action on rickets was designated as vitamin D.

Structurally, vitamin D is derived from a steroid and is considered to be a seco-steroid because one of its four rings is broken. Vitamin D contains three intact rings (A, C, and D) with a break between carbon 9 and 10 in the B ring (Fig. 10.11). The vitamin and its metabolites exhibit an unusual conformational flexibility that allows them to effectively interact with binding proteins [1,2].

Sources

Dietary vitamin D is provided primarily by foods of animal origin, especially liver, beef, veal, and eggs; dairy

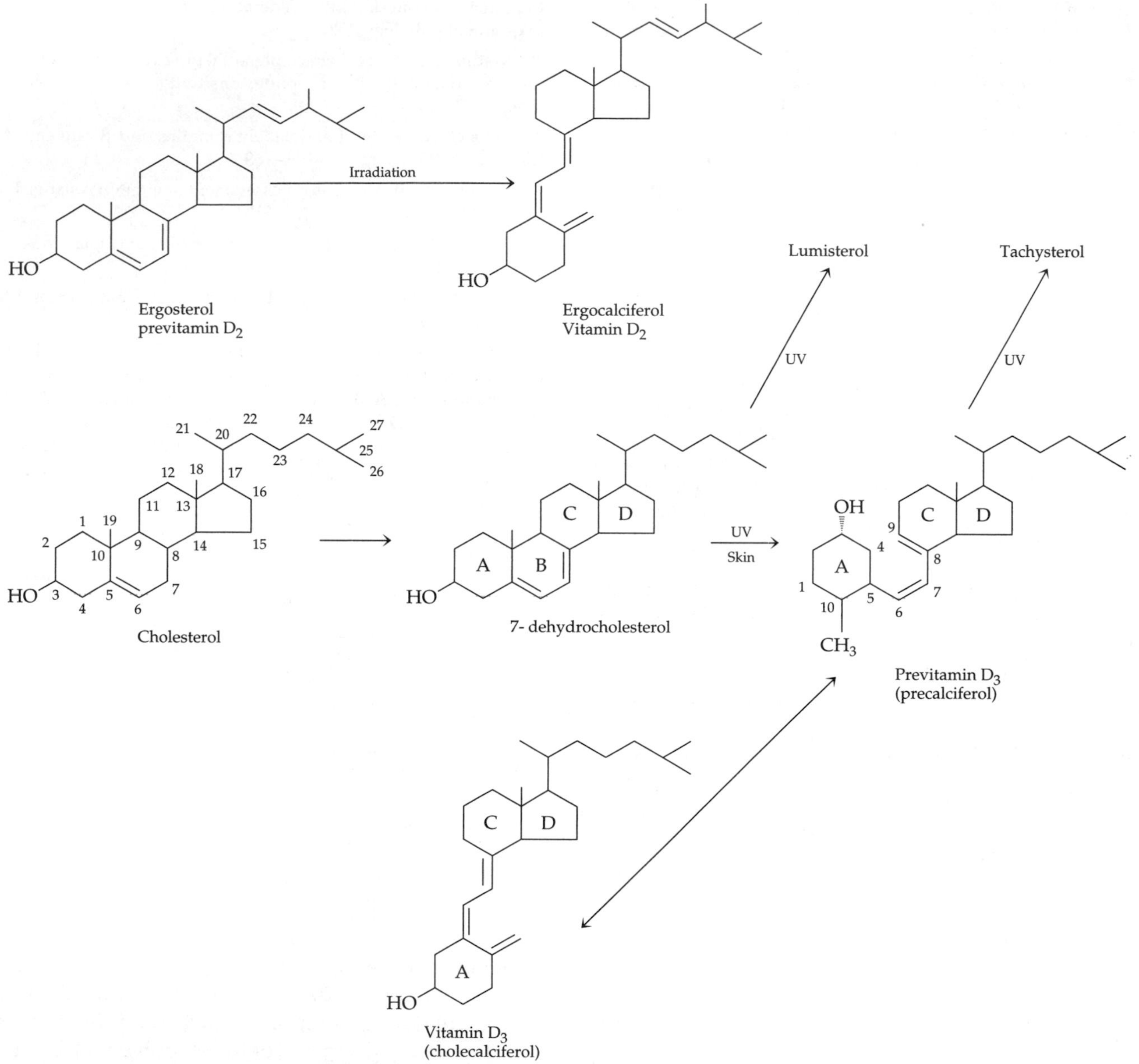

Figure 10.11 Production of ergocalciferol and vitamin D_3.

products such as milk, cheese, and butter; and some saltwater fish, including herring, salmon, tuna, and sardines. In the United States, selected foods, such as milk and margarine as well as some breads and cereals, are fortified with vitamin D. Milk, for example, is fortified with 10 μg (400 IU) vitamin D/qt in the United States. Table 10.2 provides information on major food sources of the vitamin. Dietary vitamin D is a stable compound not prone to cooking, storage, or processing losses.

In plants, a commonly occurring steroid, ergosterol, can be activated by irradiation to form ergocalciferol (also called vitamin D_2 or ercalciol; see Fig. 10.11). This is the form of the vitamin that is commonly sold commercially. No ergosterol occurs in animals, but another steroid, 5,7-cholestradienol, commonly called 7-dehydrocholesterol, is found in animals and humans. The steroid 7-dehydrocholesterol is synthesized in the sebaceous glands of the skin and secreted onto the skin's surface, and may be reabsorbed into the various layers of the skin. It appears to be uniformly distributed throughout the epidermis and dermis. The conjugated set of double bonds (five to seven) in ring B of 7-dehydrocholesterol allows the absorption of specific wavelengths of light found in the ultraviolet range. Thus,

Table 10.2 Major Food Sources of Vitamin D

Food	Approximate Vitamin D Content (μg/100 g)
Fortified	
Milk	0.8–1.3
Margarine	8.0–10.0
Nonfortified	
Butter	0.3–2.0
Milk	<1.0
Cheese	<1.0
Liver	0.5–4.0
Fish*	5.0–40.0

*Fatty fish such as herring, salmon, sardines, and tuna.

during exposure to sunlight, some of the epidermal cutaneous reservoir of 7-dehydrocholesterol is converted to previtamin D_3 (also called precalciferol; see Fig. 10.11). Lumisterol is also produced from 7-dehydrocholesterol in the presence of ultraviolet light, while tachysterol is generated by further irradiation of previtamin D_3 [3]. Much of the previtamin D_3 is thermally isomerized within 2 to 3 days into vitamin D_3, also called cholecalciferol or calciol.

Cholecalciferol diffuses from the skin into the blood, with transport in the blood occurring via a transport α-2 globulin vitamin D–binding protein (DBP), also called transcalciferin, that is synthesized in the liver. Because neither lumisterol, tachysterol, nor previtamin D_3 has much affinity for the DBP, these compounds typically are lost with the sloughing off of the skin.

Absorption, Transport, and Storage

Vitamin D_3 (cholecalciferol) from the diet is absorbed from a micelle, in association with fat and with the aid of bile salts, by passive diffusion into the intestinal cell. About 50% of dietary vitamin D_3 is absorbed. Although the rate of absorption is most rapid in the duodenum, the largest amount of vitamin D is absorbed in the distal small intestine.

Within the intestinal cell, vitamin D is incorporated primarily into chylomicrons, which then enter the lymphatic system with subsequent entry into the blood. Chylomicrons transport about 40% of the cholecalciferol in the blood, although some vitamin D may be transferred from the chylomicron to DBP for delivery to extrahepatic tissues. Chylomicron remnants deliver the vitamin to the liver.

Cholecalciferol, which slowly diffuses from the skin into the blood, is picked up for transport by DBP. About 60% of plasma cholecalciferol is bound to DBP for transport. The vitamin D bound to DBP travels primarily to the liver but may be picked up by other tissues, especially muscle and adipose tissue, prior to hepatic uptake. Thus, the difference in the transport mechanism for cholecalciferol formed in the skin and that absorbed from the digestive tract impacts the distribution of the vitamin in the body.

Cholecalciferol reaching the liver either by way of chylomicron remnants or by DBP typically is metabolized by a couple of different hydroxylases to generate the active form of the vitamin. Detailed reviews of these cytochrome P_{450} hydroxylases, which are collectively referred to as mixed-function oxidases (the enzymes reduce one atom of molecular oxygen to water and one to the hydroxyl group), are available [4]. In the liver, 25-hydroxylase functions in the mitochondria to hydroxylate cholecalciferol at carbon 25 to form 25-OH D_3, also called calcidiol (Fig. 10.12). The efficiency of the liver 25-hydroxylase in converting cholecalciferol to 25-OH D_3 appears to be related to the concentrations of vitamin D and its metabolites. The NADPH-dependent 25-hydroxylase enzyme is more efficient during periods of vitamin D deprivation than when normal amounts of the cholecalciferol are available. While the liver is the major tissue expressing the 25-hydroxylase, the enzyme is found in other organs, including the lungs, intestine, and kidneys. Once generated, 25-OH D_3 is most often released into the blood, where it represents the main form of vitamin D.

Circulating concentrations of 25-OH D_3 are considered to reflect vitamin D status and will vary depending on both dietary vitamin D intake and exposure to sunlight. Lower calcidiol concentrations, for example, are reported among many healthy individuals in the winter months because of diminished exposure to the sun and are inversely associated with parathyroid hormone (PTH) concentrations [5,6]. Serum calcidiol concentrations have shown significant correlation with vitamin D intake [6].

Most of the 25-OH D_3 synthesized in the liver is secreted into the blood and transported by DBP. Because little 25-OH D_3 remains in the liver and very little of this metabolite is taken up by the extrahepatic tissues, the blood is the largest single pool (storage site) of 25-OH D_3, which has a half-life of about 10 days to 3 weeks [7]. When the 25-OH D_3 pool has been depleted during vitamin D deprivation, maintenance of vitamin D activity is made possible for variable time periods through the release of cholecalciferol from its skin reservoir and from other sites in adipose tissues. Storage sites for the vitamin are considered to include the blood and muscle (for 25-OH D_3) and adipose tissue (for cholecalciferol).

Following hydroxylation in the liver, 25-OH D_3 bound to DBP is released into the blood and taken up mainly by the kidney. In the kidney, a second hydroxylation of 25-OH D_3 occurs at position 1, resulting in 1,25-$(OH)_2$ D_3 (also called calcitriol; see Fig. 10.12),

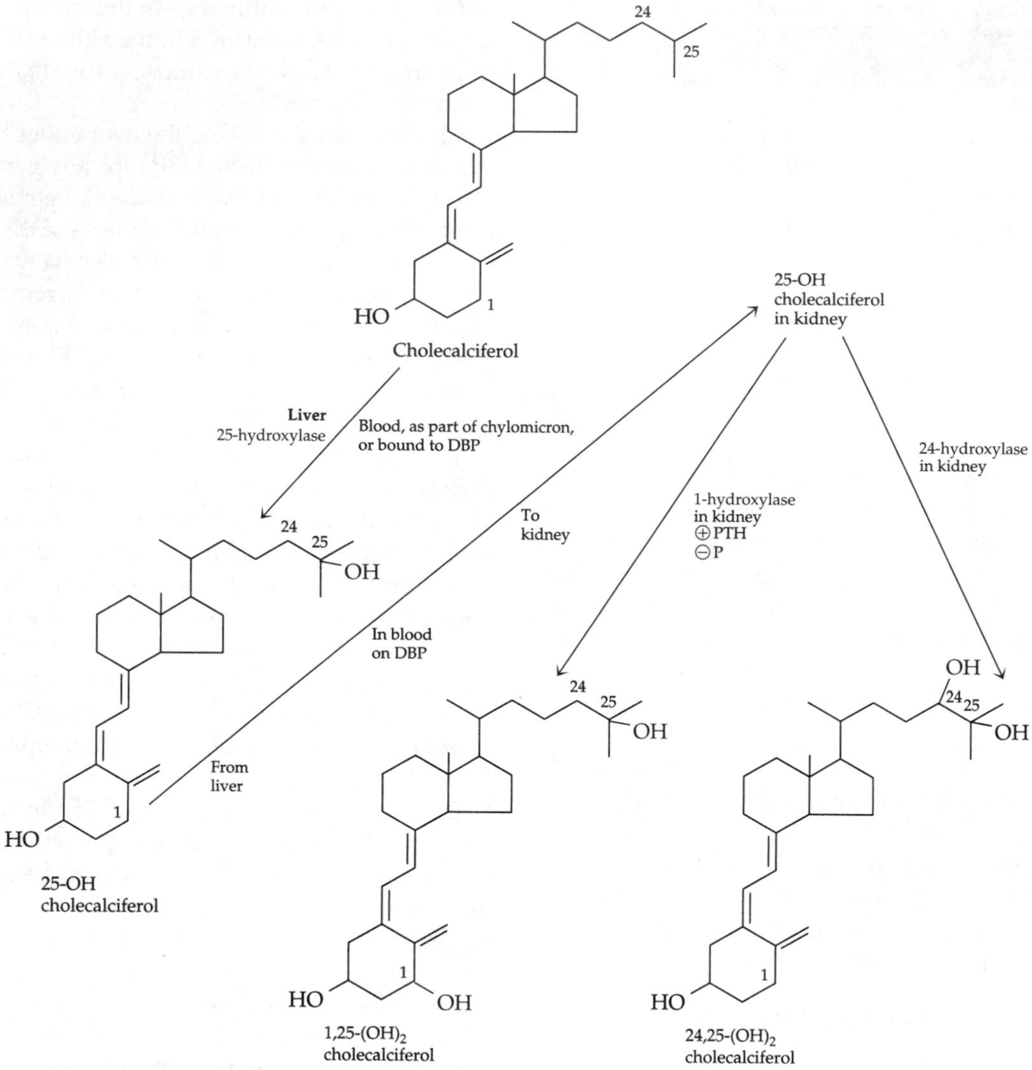

Figure 10.12 Hydroxylation of vitamin D.

which is considered the active vitamin. Calcitriol formation in the kidney tubules occurs through the action of an NADPH-dependent mitochondrial enzyme, 1-hydroxylase. This enzyme is expressed in highest concentrations in the kidney but is also present in macrophages, skin, intestine, and bone.

The activity of 1-hydroxylase is influenced by a variety of factors. Parathyroid hormone (PTH) and low plasma calcium concentrations stimulate 1-hydroxylase activity. The concentration of the enzyme's end product, 1,25-$(OH)_2$ D_3 (calcitriol), also influences the enzyme's activity: high concentrations inhibit 1-hydroxylase activity, and low concentrations stimulate it. Dietary phosphorus intake impairs calcitriol production by 1-hydroxylase. A high intake of phosphorus causes a decrease in serum 1,25-$(OH)_2$ D_3, whereas a low phosphorus intake stimulates its production [8]. When sufficient amounts of calcitriol are present, the activity of 1-hydroxylase in the kidney is decreased significantly, and the activity of another mixed-function oxidase, 24-hydroxylase, is increased in the kidney and possibly in other tissues such as cartilage and the intestine. The vitamin D metabolites 24R,25-$(OH)_2$ D_3 and 1,24,25-$(OH)_3$ D_3 are formed from hydroxylation of 25-OH D_3 and 1,25-$(OH)_2$ D_3, respectively, by 24-hydroxylase (Fig. 10.12). Production of 24R,25-$(OH)_2$ D_3 appears to increase during periods of adequate vitamin D status and calcium homeostasis. The 24R,25-$(OH)_2$ D_3 form of the vitamin is released into the blood bound to vitamin D–binding protein for functioning at various tissues.

Once synthesized, calcitriol is released from the kidney and bound to DBP for transport in the blood. DBP is one of the major proteins in the blood; the protein loosely binds 1,25-$(OH)_2$ D_3, in contrast to its tight binding of 25-OH D_3. Calcitriol in the blood has a half-life of about 4 to 6 hours. On reaching its target tissues, calcitriol is easily released from the DBP and quickly bound by a vitamin D receptor (VDR). DBP also transports other vitamin D metabolites, including 24R,25-$(OH)_2$ D_3, to various target tissues.

Functions and Mechanisms of Action

Calcitriol (1,25-$(OH)_2$ D_3), the main active form of vitamin D, functions like a steroid hormone. Remember that hormones are synthesized in one organ and act on a target organ or organs. The target tissues of the vitamin initially were believed to be limited to intestine, bone, and kidney. The presence of specific cell membrane receptors for the hormone in many other tissues, however, supports the present belief that calcitriol acts in a wide variety of tissues—not just intestine, kidney, and bone, but also cardiac, muscle, pancreas (β-cells), brain, skin, hematopoietic, and immune system tissues, among others [7]. Expression of the cell receptors in some tissues is thought to represent a need for the vitamin for cell differentiation. For example, vitamin D may affect immune function through promotion of differentiation of stem cells to macrophages and monocytes. Alternately, it has been suggested—and in some cases demonstrated—that vitamin D functions in other capacities, playing roles in ATP-dependent calcium uptake by sarcoplasmic reticulum in muscle and in β-cell function for insulin secretion.

Two main mechanisms (genomic and nongenomic) by which calcitriol exerts its functions are known, although the details of the mechanisms have not been clearly elucidated. In some cases, vitamin D is thought to function through signal transduction pathways linked to cell membrane VDR. In other cases, calcitriol is known to promote genomic actions via interaction with nuclear VDR to influence gene transcription. We will describe both mechanisms of action.

The binding of calcitriol to cell membrane VDR in selected tissues (especially intestine, bone, parathyroid, liver, and pancreatic β-cells) triggers a series of events through intracellular signaling pathways to evoke relatively rapid changes in some body processes. The many actions initiated with this binding include increased intestinal calcium absorption via **transcaltachia** (*trans* means "across," *cal* refers to calcium, and *tachia* means "rapidly") and the opening of gated calcium channels, and increased calcium uptake into osteoblasts and skeletal muscle cells. These cellular events are thought to be mediated by phosphorylation/dephosphorylation of a number of enzymes and/or by second messengers such as MAP kinase, protein kinase C, cAMP, tyrosine kinase, phospholipase C, diacylglycerol, inositol phosphate, and arachidonic acid, among others.

Nuclear receptors for the vitamin have been found in over 30 organs, including bone, intestine, kidney, lung, muscle, and skin. These vitamin D nuclear receptors are part of a so-called superfamily of receptors that also includes receptors for retinoic acid and thyroid and steroid hormones. In target tissues, calcitriol binds to nuclear VDR, and this interaction in turn initiates a conformational change in the newly formed complex. The 1,25-$(OH)_2$ D_3–VDR complex is phosphorylated and then thought to bind with retinoid X or retinoic acid receptors (RXR or RAR) to form a heterodimeric complex. The VDR portion of the heterodimeric complex contains regions with zinc fingers (see p. 442) that can interact with specific vitamin D response elements, or VDRE, found in the promoter regions of specific target genes (Fig. 10.13). Once the heterodimeric complex is bound to the VDRE, additional comodulatory (either

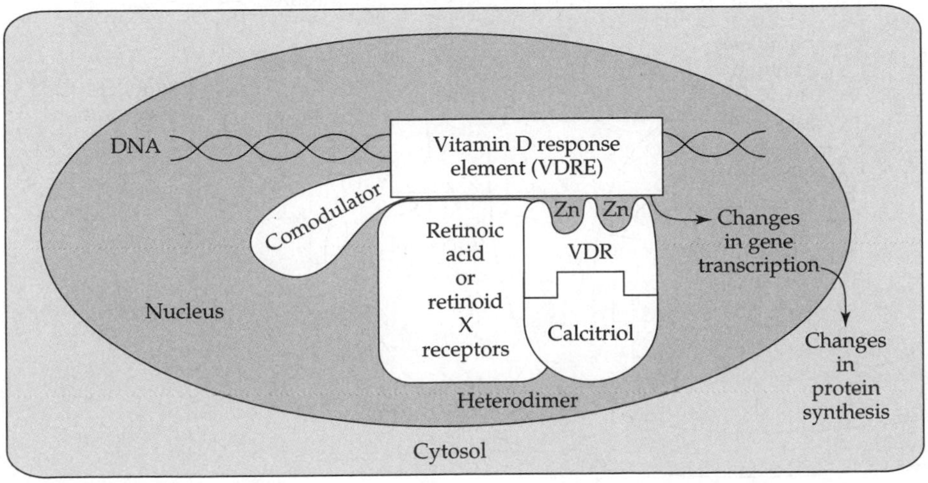

Figure 10.13 Proposed role of calcitriol in gene expression.

coactivator or corepressor) proteins may further interact with the heterodimeric complex to influence (enhance or inhibit) the transcription of genes coding for proteins. The mechanisms by which these comodulatory proteins function are mostly unknown, but they may help link the receptor to enzymes, such as RNA polymerase II, or to other components such as transcription factors necessary for transcription [9]. The comodulatory proteins are thought to include SRC-1, SRC-2, and SRC-3 (the SRC family) as well as NCoA-62 [9].

As a hormone, one of calcitriol's main functions in the body is acting with parathyroid hormone (PTH) in the homeostasis of blood calcium concentrations. In performing this function, calcitriol and PTH impact several tissues, including intestine, bone, and kidney (Fig. 10.14). The effects of calcitriol and PTH on these tissues are discussed next, along with calcitriol's role in cell differentiation, proliferation, and growth.

Calcium Homeostasis

Calcitriol synthesis is stimulated in response to changes in blood calcium concentrations and the release of another hormone, PTH. **Hypocalcemia** (low blood calcium) initially stimulates secretion of PTH from the parathyroid gland. The PTH, in turn, stimulates 1-hydroxylase in the kidney such that 25-OH D_3 is converted to calcitriol. Calcitriol then acts alone or with PTH on its target tissues, causing serum calcium concentrations to rise. The three main target tissues are the intestine, kidney, and bone, as discussed below and shown in Figure 10.14.

Calcitriol and the Intestine. A more thoroughly investigated target tissue of calcitriol is the intestine (Figs. 10.14 and 10.15). The primary function of calcitriol in the intestine is increased absorption of calcium and phosphorus. The vitamin is believed to function through interactions with both cell membrane receptors and nuclear receptors to impact gene expression.

With respect to calcium absorption, calcitriol, as a hormone, interacts with high-affinity receptors in the enterocyte and is carried to the nucleus, where it interacts with specific genes encoding for proteins involved in calcium transport. As the result of this interaction, a selective DNA transcription occurs that results in biosynthesis of

Figure 10.14 Calcitriol, 1,25 $(OH)_2$ D_3, synthesis and actions with parathyroid hormone (PTH).

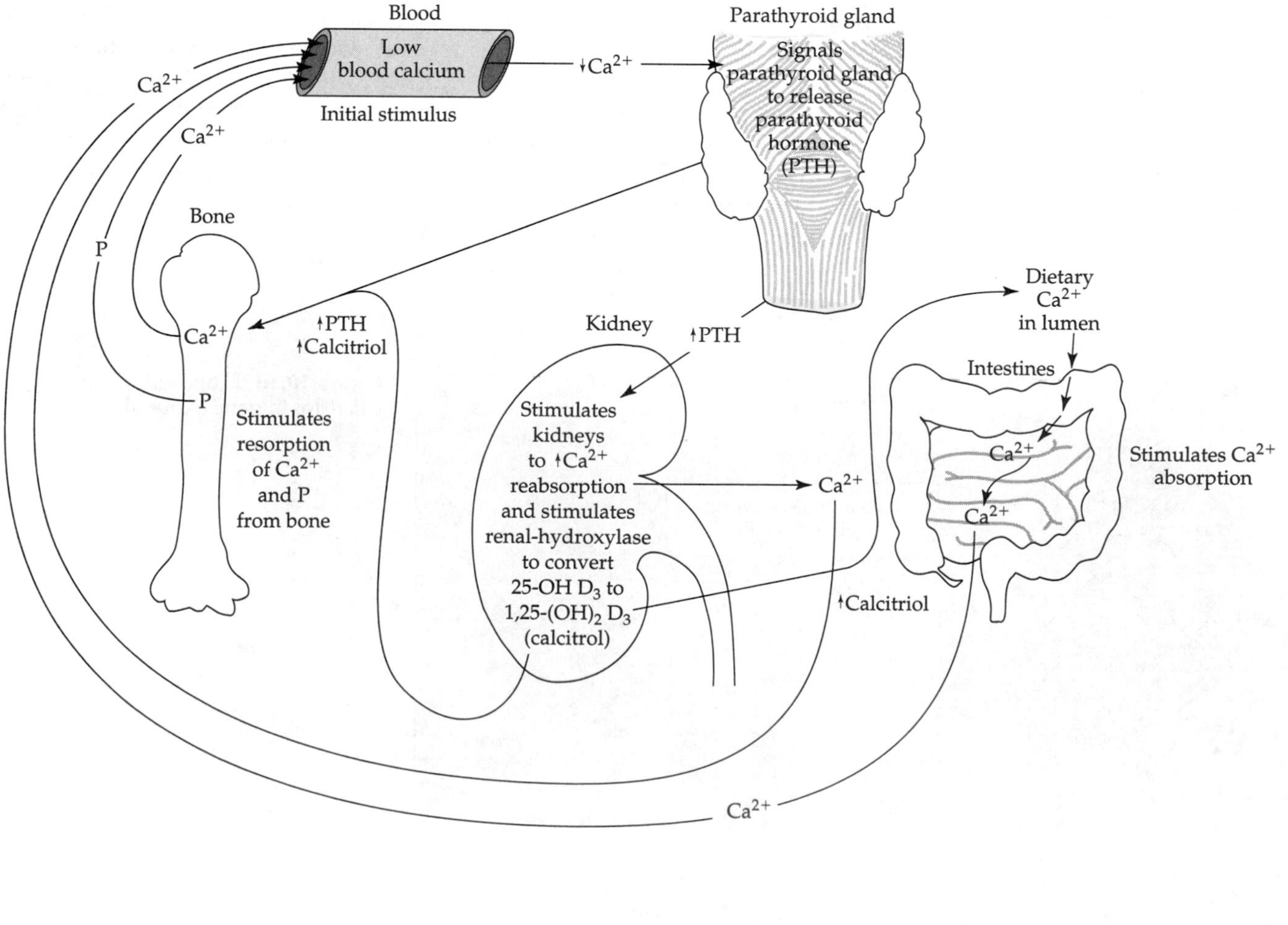

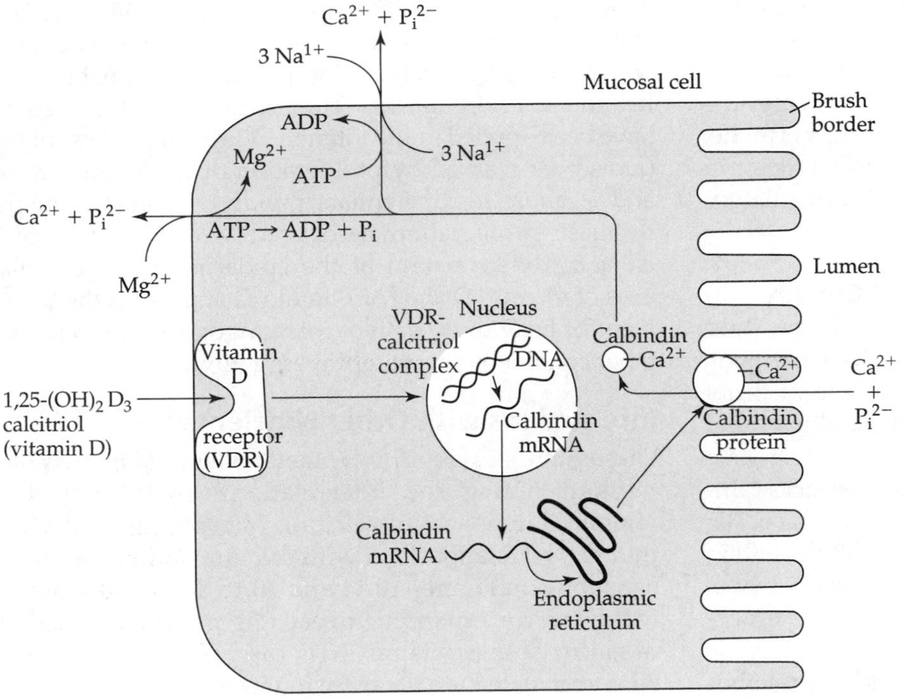

Figure 10.15 The actions of vitamin D on the intestinal absorption of calcium.

new messenger RNA (mRNA) molecules. These mRNA molecules are then translated on the endoplasmic reticulum into selected proteins. The proteins may act at the brush border, in the cytoplasm, and/or at the basolateral membrane of the intestinal cells, especially in the duodenum and jejunum, to promote calcium absorption. Calbindin D_{9k}, a calcium-binding protein in the intestinal mucosa, has been shown to be synthesized in response to the action of calcitriol. Although the amount of this calcium-binding protein is positively correlated with calcium absorption and transport, its exact role in the process is not yet defined. Also with respect to calcium absorption, calcitriol exhibits additional actions by nongenomic methods. Calcitriol is thought to induce changes in brush border composition and topology to increase calcium absorption. Vitamin D rapidly initiates intestinal calcium absorption via a process referred to as transcaltachia. The transcaltachic response is thought to involve endocytosis of calcium across the brush border membrane, followed by lysosome-mediated release of calcium within the cytosol and finally calcium release across the basolateral membrane via exocytosis. Rapid absorption of calcium into the intestine is also thought to result from the calcitriol-induced (along with second messengers) opening of voltage-gated calcium channels [10].

With respect to phosphorus, calcitriol is thought to increase the activity of brush border alkaline phosphatase, which hydrolyzes phosphate ester bonds, thereby allowing phosphorus absorption. Calcitriol is also thought to modulate the number of carriers available for sodium-dependent phosphorus absorption at the intestinal (especially jejunum and ileum) brush border membrane.

Calcitriol and the Kidney. Calcitriol appears to be involved in the parathyroid hormone–induced stimulation of calcium and especially phosphorus reabsorption in the distal renal tubule (Fig. 10.14). Calbindin D_{28k}, a larger form of the protein calbindin D_{9k} found in the intestine, is thought to be synthesized in response to genomic effects of calcitriol and to play a role in renal calcium reabsorption.

Calcitriol, 24R,25-$(OH)_2$ D_3, and the Bone. With respect to bone, PTH, alone or with calcitriol (which has been found to be produced directly within bone), directs the mobilization of calcium and phosphorus from bone to help achieve a normal blood calcium concentration (Fig. 10.14). This process may be mediated by calcitriol-induced cell differentiation of hemopoietic cells to ultimately influence osteoblast-directed production of osteoclasts and/or osteoblast activity. Osteoclasts mediate bone resorption.

Should blood calcium levels begin to rise above normal concentrations, calcitonin (a hormone produced by endocrine cells located in the connective tissue of the thyroid gland) is released and promotes the deposition (mineralization) of calcium and phosphorus in bones. Calcitriol or the metabolite 24R,25-$(OH)_2$ D_3 also may be involved in bone mineralization. Elevated serum calcitriol and elevated ionized serum calcium in turn cause a decrease in PTH production through feedback loops. The long feedback loop is indirect due to the inhibitory effect of elevated ionized serum calcium on PTH secretion. The short feedback loop is direct: The calcitriol decreases the transcription of the gene for preparathyroid hormone, presumably by interacting with the vitamin D receptor in the parathyroid tissue and influencing the regulatory region of the PTH gene [8].

Cell Differentiation, Proliferation, and Growth

Calcitriol affects cell differentiation, proliferation, and growth in a variety of different tissues. The hormone generally promotes differentiation. For example, calcitriol stimulates differentiation of hematopoietic and intestinal epithelial cells, among others. In response to genomic effects, osteoblasts are triggered to produce osteoclast differentiation factor, which in turn promotes osteoclast differentiation [11]. Calcitriol-induced cell differentiation of stem cells in the bone marrow to osteoclasts increases the number of osteoclasts, thus promoting bone resorption and increased serum calcium concentration.

During various differentiation and possibly proliferation stages of bone cells, 1,25-$(OH)_2$ D_3 stimulates synthesis of a variety of proteins involved in the modeling and remodeling of bone. In osteoblasts, calcitriol stimulates the synthesis of type I collagen and noncollagenous proteins, including osteopontin and osteocalcin, as well as plasminogen activators, collagenase, and alkaline phosphatase [12]. See pages 365 and 385 for further information on some of these proteins in bone.

Whereas differentiation in many instances appears to be stimulated by calcitriol, calcitriol reduces proliferation of cells such as fibroblasts, keratinocytes, and lymphocytes. Proliferation of abnormal intestinal, lymphatic, mammary, and skeletal cells (to name a few) is diminished by vitamin D. Calcitriol appears to be able to inhibit cancer cell proliferation and growth. Vitamin D's ability to stimulate skin epidermal cell differentiation while preventing proliferation provides potential for the treatment of skin diseases. These functions of the vitamin have been applied in the vitamin D treatment of psoriasis (a disorder marked by proliferation of the keratinocytes and a failure to differentiate rapidly). Vitamin D helps decrease proliferation associated with psoriasis and enhance differentiation of the epidermis [13]. Potential uses of vitamin D and/or vitamin D analogs in the treatment of bone disease, hyperparathyroidism, cancer, and other conditions are under investigation.

Interactions with Other Nutrients

Discussion of vitamin D metabolism is impossible without noting the interrelationships among this vitamin/hormone and calcium, phosphorus, and vitamin K. The relationships with calcium and phosphorus are shown in Figures 10.14 and 10.15 and are discussed in the text corresponding to each figure. The interaction of calcitriol and vitamin K is discussed on page 365. Also speculated is a decrease in vitamin D absorption as a result of iron deficiency [14].

Metabolism and Excretion

Calcitriol hydroxylation at carbon 24 generates the metabolite 1,24,25-$(OH)_3$ D_3 (Fig. 10.16), which may be further oxidized to 1,25-$(OH)_2$ 24-oxo D_3. Subsequent reactions, including side-chain cleavage, yield calcitroic acid (Fig. 10.16). Other vitamin D metabolites are also formed after hydroxylation and oxidation. These other vitamin D metabolites may be conjugated and then excreted primarily in the bile. The majority (over 70%) of vitamin D metabolites are excreted via the feces, with lesser amounts excreted in the urine.

Figure 10.16 Some metabolites of vitamin D.

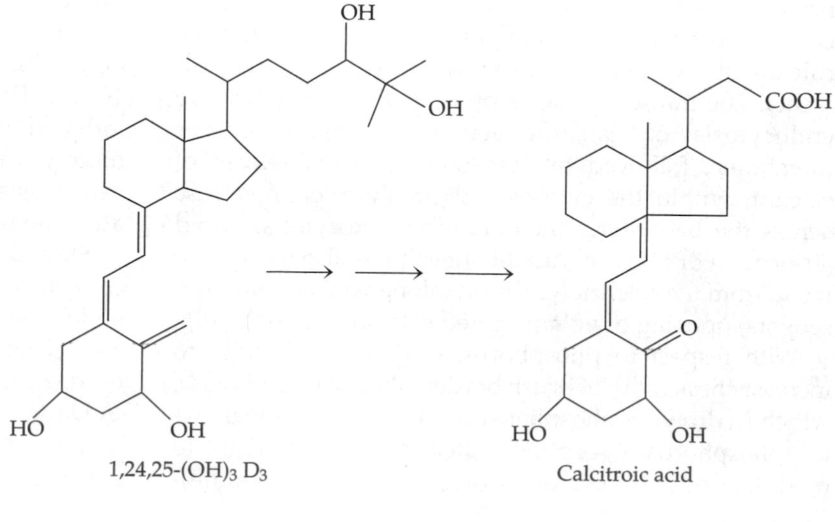

1,24,25-(OH)3 D3

Calcitroic acid

Adequate Intakes

The requirement for vitamin D is unknown. Adequate intakes (AIs) for the vitamin were last published in 1997 [15]. These latest recommendations suggest an AI for vitamin D of 5 μg or 200 IU daily for infants over 6 months of age, children, and adolescents and for adults age 19 to 50 years, including women who are pregnant or lactating [15]. This amount of the vitamin is thought to be obtainable by exposure to sunlight. In the continental United States, about 1.5 IU vitamin D/cm^2/hour during the winter and about 6 IU/cm^2/hour during the summer can be synthesized in the skin [16]. Alternately, it takes about 10 minutes of summer sun on the face and hands to produce 10 μg (400 IU) of cholecalciferol [17]. In addition to season of the year, latitude and time of day—and, in older individuals, organ function—influence vitamin D production. The AIs for vitamin D for those age 51 to 70 years or >70 years are 10 μg (400 IU) and 15 μg (600 IU), respectively [15]. A vitamin D supplement providing 400 to 800 IU may be necessary for most elderly, particularly those who drink little milk and are partially or totally housebound.

Deficiency: Rickets and Osteomalacia

In infants and children, vitamin D deficiency results in **rickets,** which is characterized by failure of bone to mineralize. In vitamin D–deficient infants, epiphyseal cartilage continues to grow and enlarge without replacement by bone matrix and minerals. These effects are especially visible at the wrists, ankles, and knees, all of which enlarge. In addition, long bones of the legs bow and knees knock as weight-bearing activity such as walking begins. The spine becomes curved, and pelvic and thoracic deformities—such as rachitic rosary, characterized by costochondral beading at the juncture of the ribs and cartilages—occur.

In adults, deprivation of vitamin D leads to mineralization defects referred to as **osteomalacia.** The defect results from changes in calcium and phosphorus absorption and excretion. For example, with vitamin D deficiency, less calcium is absorbed. Declining serum calcium concentrations trigger increased secretion of PTH. With continued poor calcium absorption due to vitamin D deficiency, PTH remains elevated in the blood for prolonged periods. PTH promotes bone resorption and increased urinary phosphorus excretion, among other changes. Indicators of bone resorption include increased urinary excretion of bone collagen by-products such as hydroxyproline, N-telopeptide, pyridonoline, and deoxypyridonoline. Alkaline phosphatase activity increases, while serum concentrations of calcium and vitamin D diminish. Without sufficient serum calcium and phosphorus, the mineralization of bones under the direction of calcitonin cannot occur. Thus, in vitamin D–deficient adults, as bone turnover occurs, the bone matrix is preserved but remineralization is impaired. The bone matrix becomes progressively demineralized, producing radiographic changes and resulting in bone pain and osteomalacia (soft bone).

Natural exposure to sunlight maintains adequate vitamin D nutrition for most of the world's population; however, people with insufficient sun exposure may be at risk for vitamin D deficiency [3]. In addition to inadequate sun exposure, certain diseases, conditions, and populations may be risk factors for vitamin D deficiency. The elderly represent one population group that typically has insufficient vitamin D intake and low sunlight exposure [18]. In addition, aging reduces synthesis of cholecalciferol in the skin and reduces the activity of renal 1-hydroxylase in response to PTH [18]. Impaired vitamin D absorption may occur in disorders characterized by fat malabsorption, such as tropical sprue and Crohn's disease. Disorders affecting the parathyroid, liver, and/or kidney will impair synthesis of the active form of the vitamin. People on anticonvulsant drug therapy may develop an impaired response to vitamin D and exhibit problems with calcium metabolism. Infants may be at risk for deficiency because human milk is low in vitamin D and infants' exposure to sunlight typically is minimal [19].

Vitamin D supplements are widely prescribed for individuals with renal disease because these individuals' kidneys are typically unable to synthesize calcitriol. Rocaltrol (Hoffman-LaRoche) is a commonly used oral calcitriol supplement, while Calcijex (Abbott Laboratories) is given intravenously to individuals with renal disease in the United States. Other preparations, such as Calderol (Organon-USA), which provides 25-OH D_3, also are available for use by individuals with organ malfunction.

Toxicity

Although excessive exposure to sunlight may be the primary risk factor in development of skin cancer, it poses no risk of toxicity through overproduction of endogenous cholecalciferol. Extensive whole-body irradiation with ultraviolet light will generally raise the level of circulating 25-OH D_3 to 40 to 80 ng/mL; levels >~160 ng/mL are associated with possible toxicity [7,15]. Photochemistry regulates the cutaneous production of vitamin D_3, thereby protecting people excessively exposed to sunlight from vitamin D intoxication [3].

Exogenous dietary ingestion of large amounts of vitamin D is the most likely of all vitamins to cause overt toxic reactions. With excessive dietary ingestion of vitamin D, the vitamin is absorbed and incorporated into chylomicrons, the remnants of which deliver the vitamin to the liver. There the vitamin is hydroxylated in position 25 and released to the blood. Although the efficiency of 25-hydroxylase is decreased when the vitamin is present in abundance, the enzyme 25-hydroxylase is not well regulated, and thus an excessive amount of the metabolite can be produced with oversupplementation. Calcidiol in high concentrations may stimulate some of the same actions as calcitriol.

In the 1950s, an epidemic of "idiopathic hypercalcemia" among English infants was traced to an intake of vitamin D between 2,000 and 3,000 IU per day. Symptoms of toxicity in the infants included anorexia, nausea, vomiting, hypertension, renal insufficiency, and failure to thrive. Eight individuals experienced hypervitaminosis from consuming milk ($\frac{1}{2}$–3 cups daily) from a local dairy that contained up to 232,565 IU of vitamin D_3 per quart; the individuals displayed hypercalcemia and hypercalcidiolemia [20]. Dosages of 10,000 IU per day for several months have resulted in hypercalcemia and associated calcification of soft tissues (calcinosis) such as the kidney, heart, lungs, and blood vessels, as well as hyperphosphatemia, hypertension, anorexia, nausea, weakness, renal dysfunction (characterized by polyuria, polydypsia, azotemia, nephrolithiasis, and renal failure), and, in some cases, death [15,21]. The tolerable upper intake level is set at 50 μg (2,000 IU) per day [15].

Assessment of Nutriture

The plasma concentration of 25-OH D_3 (calcidiol) is often used as an index of vitamin D status. Concentrations <15 ng/mL are associated with subclinical deficiency, while concentrations <11 ng/mL suggest vitamin D deficiency; toxicity is considered when 25-OH D_3 concentrations typically exceed ~160 ng/mL [6,7,15]. Elevations in plasma alkaline phosphatase also have been used to detect preclinical rickets.

References Cited for Vitamin D

1. Norman A, Ishizuka S, Okamura W. Ligands for the vitamin D endocrine system: different shapes function as agonists and antagonists for genomic and rapid response receptors or as a ligand for the plasma vitamin D binding protein. J Steroid Biochem Molec Biol 2001;76:49–59.

2. Norman A, Bishop J, Bula C, Olivera C, Mizwicki M, Zanello L, Ishida H, Okamura W. Molecular tools for study of genomic and rapid signal transduction responses initiated by 1α,25$(OH)_2$–vitamin D_3. Steroids 2002;67:457–66.

3. Webb A, Holick M. The role of sunlight in cutaneous production of vitamin D_3. Ann Rev Nutr 1988;8:375–99.

4. Omdahl J, Morris H, May B. Hydroxylase enzymes of the vitamin D pathway: expression, function, and regulation. Ann Rev Nutr 2002;22:139–66.

5. Dawson-Huges B, Harris S, Dallal G. Plasma calcidiol, season and serum parathyroid hormone concentrations in healthy elderly men and women. Am J Clin Nutr 1997;65:67–71.

6. Kinyamu H, Gallagher J, Balhorn K, Petranick K, Rafferty K. Serum vitamin D metabolites and calcium absorption in normal young and elderly free-living women and in women living in nursing homes. Am J Clin Nutr 1997;65:790–97.

7. Holick M. The use and interpretation of assays for vitamin D and its metabolites. J Nutr 1990;120:1464–69.

8. Reichel H, Koeffler H, Norman A. The role of the vitamin D endocrine system in health and disease. N Engl J Med 1989; 320: 980–91.

9. MacDonald P, Baudina T, Tokumaru H, Dowd D, Zhang C. Vitamin D receptor and nuclear receptor coactivators. Steroids 2001; 66:171–76.

10. DeBoland A, Norman A. Evidence for involvement of protein kinase C and cyclic adenosine 3′5′ monophosphate-dependent protein kinase in the 1,25-dihydroxyvitamin D_3–mediated rapid stimulation of intestinal calcium transport (transcaltachia). Endocrinology 1990;127:39–45.

11. Jurutka P, Whitfield G, Hsieh J, Thompson P, Haussler C, Haussler M. Molecular nature of the vitamin D receptor and its role in regulation of gene expression. Rev Endo Metab Dis 2001; 2:203–16.

12. Van Leeuwen J, van Driel M, van den Bemd G, Pols H. Vitamin D control of osteoblast function and bone extracellular matrix mineralization. Crit Rev Euk Gene Expression 2001;11:199–226.

13. Bikle D. Vitamin D: new actions, new analogs, new therapeutic potential. Endocrin Rev 1992;13:765–84.

14. Heldenberg D, Tenenbaum G, Weisman Y. Effect of iron on serum 25-hydroxyvitamin D and 24,25-dihydroxy–vitamin D concentrations. Am J Clin Nutr 1992;56:533–36.

15. Food and Nutrition Board, Institute of Medicine. Dietary Reference Intakes. Washington, DC: National Academy Press, 1997, pp. 250–87.

16. Collins E, Norman A. Vitamin D. In: Rucker RB, Suttie JW, McCormick DB, Machlin LJ, eds. Handbook of Vitamins, 3rd ed. New York: Marcel Dekker, Inc., 2001, pp. 51–114.

17. DeLuca H. Vitamin D: 1993. Nutrition Today 1993;28 (Nov–Dec):6–11.

18. MacLaughlin J, Holick M. Aging decreases the capacity of human skin to produce vitamin D_3. J Clin Invest 1985;76:1536–38.

19. Zeghoud F, Vervel C, Guillozo H, Walrant-Debray O, Boutignon H, Garabedian M. Subclinical vitamin D deficiency in neonates: definition and response to vitamin D supplements. Am J Clin Nutr 1997;65:771–78.

20. Jacobus C, Holick M, Shao Q, Chen T, Holm I, Kolodny J, Fuleihan G, Seely E. Hypervitaminosis D associated with drinking milk. N Engl J Med 1992;326:1173–77.

21. Allen S, Shah J. Calcinosis and metastatic calcification due to vitamin D intoxication: a case report and review. Horm Res 1992;37:68–77.

VITAMIN E

Vitamin E typically has encompassed eight compounds (vitamers). Each of these eight compounds contains a phenolic functional group on a chromanol/chromane ring (sometimes referred to as the head of the molecule) and an attached phytyl side chain (sometimes called the **phytyl tail** of the

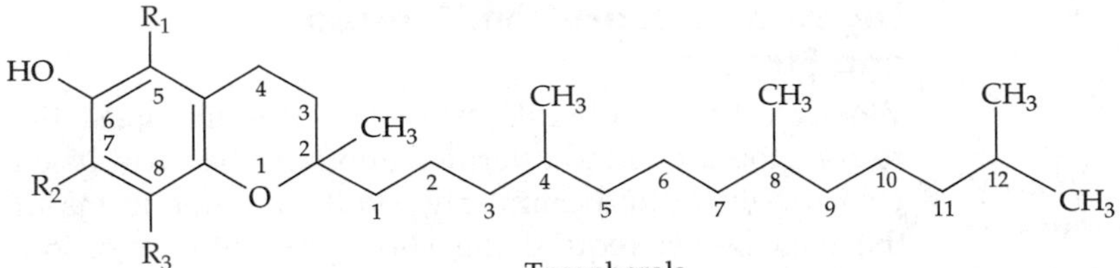

Tocopherols

	R_1	R_2	R_3
α-tocopherol	CH_3	CH_3	CH_3
β-tocopherol	CH_3	H	CH_3
γ-tocopherol	H	CH_3	CH_3
δ-tocopherol	H	H	CH_3

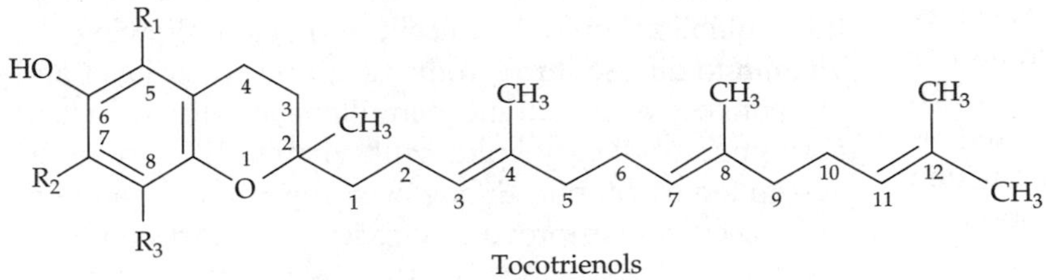

Tocotrienols

	R_1	R_2	R_3
α-tocotrienol	CH_3	CH_3	CH_3
β-tocotrienol	CH_3	H	CH_3
γ-tocotrienol	H	CH_3	CH_3
δ-tocotrienol	H	H	CH_3

Figure 10.17 The structures of the various forms of the tocopherols and tocotrienols.

molecule). The eight compounds (Fig. 10.17) are usually divided into two classes:

- the tocopherols, which have saturated side chains with 16 carbons, and
- the tocotrienols (also called trienols), which have unsaturated side chains with 16 carbons.

Each class is composed of four vitamers that differ in the number and location of methyl groups on the chromanol ring. Vitamers in both classes are designated as α, β, γ, or δ. Only α-tocopherol has biologic activity. All tocopherols and tocotrienols found naturally in foods have an RRR stereochemistry. R and S are used to designate stereoisomers of asymmetrical molecules such as vitamin E.

Synthetic ester forms of α-tocopherol include all-racemic (all-rac) α-tocopheryl acetate and all-rac α-tocopheryl succinate, which are used in vitamin supplements and fortified foods. These synthetic forms of the vitamin often contain a mixture of eight stereoisomers and thus are not as active as the naturally occurring form, RRR α-tocopherol. Of the eight stereoisomers, four are in the 2R-stereoisomeric form (RRR, RSR, RRS, and RSS) and four are in the 2S-stereoisomeric form (SRR, SSR, SRS, and SSS) [1]. The form of the vsitamin should be listed on the food or supplement label.

In the report on vitamin E for the establishment of recommended intakes by the Food and Nutrition Board, vitamin E activity is limited to naturally occurring RRR α-tocopherol and to three synthetic stereoisomeric forms (RSR, RRS, and RSS) of α-tocopherol [1]. In the establishment of a tolerable upper intake level, all supplemental forms of the vitamin are considered [1].

Sources

Vitamin E, in its various forms, is found in both plant and animal foods. Plant foods, especially oils from plants, are considered the richest and main sources of vitamin E. Oils high in α-tocopherol include canola, olive, sunflower, safflower, and cottonseed. Soybean and corn oils contain some α-tocopherol but considerably higher amounts of γ-tocopherol [2,3]. Foods (especially full-fat varieties) made from vegetable oils, such as salad dressings, mayonnaise, and margarine, and foods made from nuts, such as peanut butter, represent good sources of vitamin E [2,3]. Unfortunately, individuals limiting fat intake also limit foods that are high in vitamin E and thus may compromise their ability to meet dietary intake recommendations for the vitamin. Other plant sources of vitamin E include whole-grain cereals, legumes, and some fruits and vegetables. The leaves and other green (chloroplast) portions of plants contain mostly α-tocopherol with small amounts of γ-tocopherol. The main sources of γ-, δ-, and β-tocopherols are nonchloroplast regions of plants. Tocotrienols are found in legumes and cereal grains such as wheat, barley, rice, and oats [2,3]. The bran and germ sections of cereals are especially rich in tocotrienols. Thus, wheat germ oil and wheat bran represent significant sources of tocotrienols.

In foods of animal origin, vitamin E, primarily α-tocopherol, is found concentrated in fatty tissues of the animal. Thus, higher-fat meats can provide some vitamin E. However, compared to plants, animal products represent an inferior source of vitamin E.

Table 10.3 lists the approximate α-tocopherol equivalents found in commonly consumed foods. The contributions of the four tocopherols and the four tocotrienols are included in α-tocopherol equivalents, with adjustments for bioavailability. Prior to the 2000 Dietary Reference Intakes publication with recommendations for vitamin E [1], the vitamin E content of foods and recommendations for the vitamin were expressed as α-tocopherol equivalents. While most food composition tables report the vitamin E content of foods as α-tocopherol equivalents, composition tables providing the actual α-tocopherol content of foods are being developed. While calculations for the direct conversion from α-tocopherol equivalents to α-tocopherol for food are not possible, an analysis of the dietary intake data from the National Health and Nutrition Examination Survey III revealed that about 80% of total dietary vitamin E was in the form of α-tocopherol [1].

Vitamin E, like other fat-soluble vitamins, is susceptible to destruction during food preparation, processing, and/or storage. Tocopherols can be oxidized with lengthy exposure to air. In addition, exposure of the vitamin to light, heat, or metals also can lead to increased destruction.

Table 10.3 Approximate Vitamin E Content of Foods as α-Tocopherol Equivalents

Food	mg/100 g
Oils:	
Wheat germ	192
Corn	21
Cottonseed	38
Peanut	13
Safflower	43
Soybean	18
Sunflower	51
Margarine	15
Nuts	0.69–9
Breads	0.4
Vegetables	0.1–2.0
Fruits	0.1–1.1
Meat, fish	1
Eggs	1

Source: www.nal.usda.gov/fnic/foodcomp

Digestion, Absorption, Transport, and Storage

Whereas the tocopherols are found free in foods, the tocotrienols are found esterified and must be hydrolyzed prior to absorption. Similarly, synthetic ester forms of the tocopherols require digestion prior to absorption. Pancreatic esterase and/or duodenal mucosal esterase are thought to function in the lumen or at the brush border of the intestine to hydrolyze tocotrienols and synthetic ester α-tocopherols for absorption [4].

Absorption of vitamin E as free alcohols occurs primarily in the jejunum by nonsaturable, passive (requiring no carrier) diffusion. Bile salts are required for emulsification, solubilization, and micelle formation allowing the vitamin to diffuse through the unstirred water layer and the enterocyte membrane. Simultaneous digestion and absorption of dietary lipids with vitamin E improve the absorption of vitamin E; however, the optimum amount of fat needed to improve absorption has not been identified [1]. In addition, the extent of absorption of vitamin E is unclear, with results of studies ranging from 20% up to about 80% [5–7]. Similar efficiency of absorption has been demonstrated among RRR and SRR α-tocopherols and RRR and all-rac α-tocopherols [8–12].

In the enterocyte, absorbed tocopherol is incorporated into chylomicrons for transport through the lymph into circulation. During tocopherol transport in the chylomicrons, tocopherol equilibrates or is transferred among the plasma lipoproteins, including HDLs and LDLs, which contain the highest concentrations of the vitamin [13,14]. The half-life for RRR α-tocopherol in humans is about 48 hours, while the stereoisomer SRR α-tocopherol has a half-life of about 13 hours [15].

Chylomicron remnants deliver vitamin E (absorbed tocopherols and tocotrienols) to the liver. Only RRR α-tocopherol appears to be incorporated into very low density lipoproteins (VLDLs) for resecretion back into the blood and transport to other tissues. A specific protein, called α-tocopherol transfer protein (αTTP), which is made in the liver, appears to be necessary for the transfer of tocopherol into VLDLs, which enable distribution of the vitamin to tissues [10,16,17]. A deficiency or absence of αTTP due to gene defects leads to a vitamin E deficiency syndrome. Because of the specificity of the transfer protein, other forms of the vitamin are poorly recognized by the protein and are not resecreted into the circulation via VLDLs [10,16,17].

Tocopherol uptake into cells occurs as lipoproteins are taken up by body tissues. Thus, uptake of the vitamin can occur

- as receptor-mediated uptake of LDLs occurs,
- through lipoprotein lipase-mediated hydrolysis of chylomicrons and VLDLs,

- through HDL-mediated nutrient delivery, or
- possibly by other mechanisms [6,18].

A phospholipid transfer protein also is thought to facilitate vitamin E transfer from lipoproteins to membranes [19].

Within the cell cytoplasm as well as other parts of the cell, including the nucleus, vitamin E appears to bind to specific proteins (tocopherol-binding proteins) for transport. Vitamin E is found within the cell primarily in cell membranes such as the plasma, mitochondrial, and microsomal membranes. Vitamin E's chromanol group likely is directed toward the membrane surface (near the phosphate region of the phospholipid), while its phytyl tail is directed near the hydrocarbon region [20].

There is no single storage organ for vitamin E. The largest amount of the vitamin is concentrated in an unesterified form in the adipose tissue, with smaller amounts in liver, lung, heart, muscle, adrenal glands, spleen, and brain. The concentration of vitamin E in adipose tissues increases linearly with dosage of vitamin E, whereas vitamin E concentration in the other tissues remains constant or increases only at a very slow rate [13]. Release of vitamin E from adipose tissues, however, is slow even during periods of low vitamin E intake. The liver and plasma concentrations of the vitamin provide a readily available source. Vitamin E from other storage sites, such as the heart and muscle, can be utilized at intermediate rates [20].

Functions and Mechanisms of Action

The principal function of vitamin E is the maintenance of membrane integrity, including possible physical stability, in body cells. The mechanism by which vitamin E functions to protect the membranes from destruction is through its ability to prevent the oxidation (peroxidation) of unsaturated fatty acids contained in the phospholipids of the membranes. The phospholipids of the mitochondrial membrane and endoplasmic reticulum contain more unsaturated fatty acids than the cell's plasma membrane and thus are at greater risk of oxidation. However, cell membranes are still vulnerable to oxidation. Tissues with cell membranes especially susceptible to oxidation include the lungs, brain, and erythrocytes. Erythrocyte membranes, for example, are high in polyunsaturated fatty acids and are exposed to high concentrations of oxygen. Because it prevents oxidation, vitamin E is referred to as an antioxidant. A discussion of vitamin E's role as an antioxidant follows, with a brief description of the generation of carbon-centered and peroxyl radicals. More information on how free radicals are generated and how they can damage cell membranes may be found in this chapter's perspective, "The Antioxidant Nutrients, Reactive Species, and Disease."

Antioxidant Role

As an antioxidant, vitamin E can stop reactions involving free radicals (free radical termination) and can destroy singlet molecular oxygen. We will address each of these aspects of vitamin E function.

Free Radical Termination. The structure of vitamin E, specifically its phenolic ring, allows for the donation of hydrogen ions to free radicals. Of the different forms of the vitamin, α-tocopherol is more effective than β-, γ-, or δ-tocopherol in its ability to donate hydrogen atoms. The hydrogen ions from α-tocopherol effectively and quickly react with and terminate a variety of free radicals before the free radicals can destroy cell membranes and other cell components.

Free radicals are generated in the course of many body processes involving enzymatic reactions or with exposure to trace metals or ultraviolet light, among other events. Free radicals can start a series of reactions that can be terminated by vitamin E. The reactions occur in three phases: initiation, **propagation** (ongoing generation), and termination, with the last involving vitamin E. A description of the three phases, including the reactions occuring in each, is presented next.

Initiation typically begins with an initiator such as a free radical. For example, hydroxyl radicals ($^{\bullet}OH$) are very highly reactive, rapidly taking electrons from the surroundings. Often the electron taken by the reactive free hydroxyl radical is from nearby organic molecules. If the organic molecule is a polyunsaturated fatty acid (PUFA) present in the phospholipid portion of the cell membrane, damage to the membrane occurs. Membrane lipid peroxidation is thought to represent a primary event in oxidative cellular damage [21]. Specifically, hydrogen atoms from the methylene groups ($—CH_2—$) found between double bonds in polyunsaturated fatty acids ($—CH{=}CHCH_2CH{=}CH—$) are primary targets for proton abstraction by radicals.

- The reaction between lipid cosmpounds (LH) such as PUFA and free hydroxyl radicals ($^{\bullet}OH$) leads to the formation of a lipid carbon-centered radical ($L^{\bullet}$) and water, as shown here and in Figure 10.18:

$$LH + {}^{\bullet}OH \longrightarrow L^{\bullet} + H_2O$$

- Alternately, lipid compounds (LH) can react with molecular oxygen (O_2) to generate lipid carbon-centered radicals and the **hydroperoxyl radical** $HO_2^{\bullet}$, as follows:

$$LH + O_2 \longrightarrow L^{\bullet} + HO_2^{\bullet}$$

Once lipid carbon-centered radicals are formed, they may react to form additional radicals in propagation

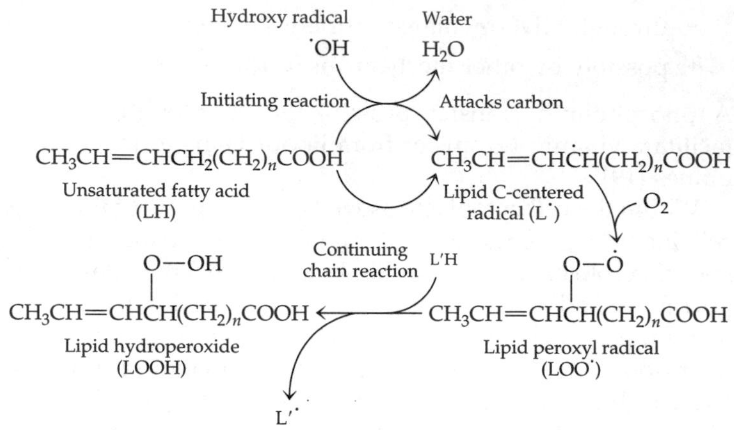

Figure 10.18 Initiating and chain reactions caused by hydroxy free radical attack on an unsaturated fatty acid.

reactions. Propagation is the second step in the process of lipid peroxidation.

• Lipid carbon-centered radicals can react with molecular oxygen in a propagation reaction to form peroxyl radicals, LOO˙, and promote peroxidation, as shown here and in Figure 10.18:

$$L^{\cdot} + O_2 \longrightarrow LOO^{\cdot} \text{(also written } LO_2^{\cdot}\text{)}$$

Peroxyl radicals (LOO˙), once formed, can abstract a hydrogen atom from other organic compounds including more polyunsaturated fatty acids (L′H) in membranes or in lipoproteins to generate lipid peroxides (LOOH) and a chain reaction with the L˙, as shown here and in Figure 10.18:

$$LOO^{\cdot} + L'H \longrightarrow L'^{\cdot} + LOOH$$

Chain reactions involving L˙ must be terminated to minimize cellular damage. Prevention of damage from oxygen radicals depends on a complex protective system of which vitamin E is a part.

Vitamin E located in or near membrane surfaces can react with peroxyl radicals (LOO˙) before they interact with fatty acids in cell membranes or other cell components. Thus, vitamin E terminates chain-propagation reactions. Vitamin E is less effective, however, in terminating peroxidation that generates free hydroxyl radicals (˙OH) or alkoxyl radicals (RO˙).

Vitamin E (EH, reduced state), because of the reactivity of the phenolic hydrogen on its carbon 6 hydroxyl group and the ability of the chromanol ring system to stabilize an unpaired electron [5], can provide a hydrogen for the reduction of peroxyl radicals, as shown:

$$LOO^{\cdot} + EH \longrightarrow LOOH + E^{\cdot}$$

It also provides a hydrogen for the reduction of lipid carbon-centered radicals, as shown:

$$L^{\cdot} + EH \longrightarrow LH + E^{\cdot}$$

E˙ represents oxidized vitamin E. The process is sometimes referred to as "free-radical scavenging." Termination is achieved when two free radicals combine to form a molecule that is not a free radical and cannot continue the reaction.

Note that vitamin E becomes oxidized (E˙) in the termination and must be regenerated to be reused. Regeneration (Fig. 10.19) requires reducing agents, which include vitamin C (ascorbic acid), reduced glutathione (GSH), NADPH, ubiquinol, and dihydrolipoic acid, among others [22,23].

Vitamin E is only one line of defense against oxidative tissue damage. Other parts of the protective system

Figure 10.19 The regeneration of vitamin E (α-tocopherol).

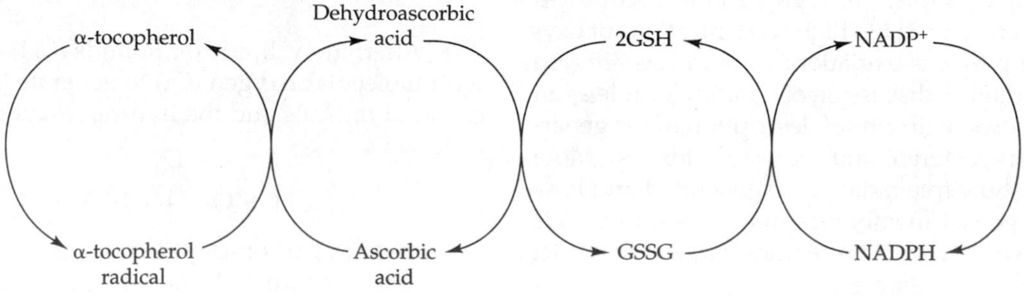

include vitamin C, glutathione, carotenoids, and enzymes that require a variety of trace or microminerals (iron, selenium, zinc, copper, and manganese) for their activation. Therefore, an interrelationship exists among vitamins E and C, carotenoids, and these minerals involved in antioxidant activities. Vitamins C and E appear to work synergistically in inhibiting oxidation [22]. The relationship between vitamin E and other nutrients with antioxidant functions is reviewed in the perspective at the end of this chapter.

Clinical trials with vitamin E alone as well as with other antioxidants suggest that the vitamin may decrease the susceptibility of LDL to oxidation by free radicals [24–29]. High vitamin E intakes have been associated with a lower risk of coronary heart disease in large cohort studies involving men [27] and women [26]. Supplementation with 800 IU of vitamin E, 1 g of vitamin C, and 24 mg of β-carotene significantly reduced the susceptibility of LDL to oxidation in patients with cardiovascular disease [28]. Supplementation with α-tocopherol (800 IU) alone was found to be as effective as a combination of ascorbate (1 g), β-carotene (30 mg), and α-tocopherol (800 IU) in decreasing LDL oxidation [29]. Supplementation with 400 or 800 IU (268 or 567 mg) α-tocopherol in another group of patients with confirmed heart disease reduced the rate of both nonfatal and total heart attacks [30]. These findings have implications for prevention of atherosclerosis. Briefly, atherosclerosis is thought to begin with an accumulation of lipid-laden foam cells in the arterial intima. Radical-induced oxidation of apoprotein B100, for example, in LDL is thought to be involved in promoting scavenger receptor-mediated uptake of the LDL by macrophages. Macrophages, which develop into foam cells, are thought to take up oxidized LDL more readily than nonoxidized LDL. With continued accumulation, fatty streaks develop and represent the initial steps in atherosclerosis. Oxidized LDL may also reduce macrophage motility in the arterial intima, increase monocyte accumulation in endothelial cells, and increase cytotoxicity of endothelial cells to contribute to atherogenicity [26,27]. Thus, vitamin E's ability to prevent or decrease LDL oxidation thwarts the development of atherosclerotic lesions. However, other clinical trials providing vitamin E (400 IU or 300 mg) to individuals who had either a heart attack or diagnosed heart disease showed no beneficial effects in decreasing risk of death [31,32].

Vitamin E has been suggested for the treatment or prevention of other disorders. Cataracts result in part from oxidative damage to proteins that then aggregate and precipitate in the lens to cause lens opacities or cloudiness. Oxygen and oxyradicals are thought to contribute to the development of cataracts. Poor antioxidant status or intake, especially of vitamins E and C, has been shown in many but not all studies to be associated with development of cataracts [33–41].

Vitamin E has also been suggested for individuals with conditions characterized by increased lipid peroxidation. For example, iron toxicity typically leads to increased lipid peroxidation through production of free radicals and causes excessive damage to organs, especially the liver [42]. Individuals with diabetes mellitus also experience increased peroxidation. Vitamin E supplementation (600–900 mg α-tocopherol) by individuals with non-insulin-dependent diabetes mellitus decreased oxidative damage and improved metabolic control [43–45]. Vitamin E was thought to perhaps improve plasma membrane structure and its related activities required for glucose transport and/or metabolism (and thus metabolic control) [43–45]. By diminishing lipid peroxidation and increasing GSH availability, vitamin E could help maintain cell membrane fluidity, which in turn may improve glucose transporter function and thus insulin-dependent cellular glucose uptake [46].

Singlet Molecular Oxygen Destruction. Singlet molecular oxygen, $^1O_2$, generated from lipid peroxidation of membranes, transfer of energy from light (photochemical reactions), or the respiratory burst occurring in neutrophils (enzymatic reactions), for example, is another very reactive and destructive compound that may be formed in the body. Singlet molecular oxygen readily reacts with organic molecules such as protein, lipids, and DNA and thus can damage cellular components unless removed. Quenching is a process by which electronically excited molecules, such as singlet molecular oxygen, are inactivated. Specifically, physical quenching occurs when the singlet excited oxygen is deactivated without light emission and generally involves electron energy transfer [47]. This process was discussed earlier in this chapter in the section on the antioxidant functions of carotenoids (p. 336). However, carotenoids are not alone in their ability to quench singlet oxygen. Vitamin E also has oxygen-quenching abilities. The ability of vitamin E to physically quench singlet oxygen is related to the free hydroxyl group in position 6 of vitamin E's chromane ring (Fig. 10.17). Yet all tocopherols are not equal in their quenching abilities: α-tocopherol was found to be as or more effective in the quenching of singlet molecular oxygen than β-tocopherol, followed in descending order by γ-tocopherol and then δ-tocopherol [47]. Moreover, the $^1O_2$-quenching ability of the carotenoids lycopene and β-carotene is about two orders of magnitude greater than that of vitamin E; however, given the lower plasma concentrations of the carotenoids, vitamin E's role in quenching singlet oxygen is of physiological significance [47].

Other Roles

Other, nonantioxidant roles of vitamin E have been demonstrated. Tocotrienols, for example, appear to affect cholesterol metabolism. Suppression of the activity of the rate-limiting enzyme 3-hydroxy-3-methylglutaryl (HMG) CoA reductase in cholesterol synthesis by tocotrienol has been shown in vitro [48]. These findings are consistent with observations that tocotrienols reduce plasma cholesterol concentrations in animals and in humans [49].

Suppression of tumor growth and cell proliferation also has been attributed to tocotrienols, although in general diets high in vitamin E have not been associated with lower risk of cancers [50–53]. Protein kinase C, important for signal transduction and cell growth and differentiation, may be inhibited by α-tocopherol [53].

Interactions with Other Nutrients

Because the antioxidant functions of vitamin E in the body are closely tied to those of selenium-dependent glutathione peroxidase (an enzyme that converts lipid peroxides into lipid alcohols), an interrelationship exists between vitamin E and selenium. The actions of both nutrients are complementary, and higher concentrations of one nutrient can reduce the effects of lower concentrations of the other nutrient. Similarly, some of vitamin C's functions also complement vitamin E, and vitamin C can regenerate vitamin E following its oxidation.

To a lesser extent, interrelationships exist between vitamin E and sulfur-containing amino acids (S-aa). Cysteine, an S-aa generated from another S-aa, methionine, is necessary for synthesis of glutathione, which serves as the reducing agent in the glutathione peroxidase reaction and has been shown to regenerate (reduce) vitamin E if it has undergone oxidation.

The relationship between vitamin E and dietary polyunsaturated fatty acids has been suggested because the requirement for the vitamin increases or decreases as the degree of unsaturation of fatty acids in body tissues rises or falls; body tissue lipids, in turn, are influenced by dietary lipid intakes [1]. However, foods high in polyunsaturated fatty acids also tend to be relatively good sources of vitamin E.

High intakes of vitamin E can interfere with several aspects of the other fat-soluble vitamins. Vitamin E inhibits β-carotene absorption and/or its conversion to retinol in the intestine [54,55]. Vitamin E may also impair vitamin K absorption [13,20,55–57]. In the vitamin K cycle, vitamin E or α-tocopheryl quinone may block regeneration of the reduced form of vitamin K [13,20,55–57]. Vitamin E also has caused vitamin D–dependent bone mineralization problems in animals [5].

Metabolism and Excretion

Initial oxidation of α-tocopherol generates a tocopheroxyl chromanoxy radical, which may be reduced by vitamin C or glutathione, among other compounds, back to α-tocopherol or may be further oxidized to tocopheryl quinone. In the liver, the tocopheryl quinone may be reduced by α-tocopheryl quinone reductase, using NADPH, to tocopherol hydroquinone. The side chain of the latter may be oxidized to form α-tocopheronic acid. Tocopheronic acid typically is conjugated with glucuronic acid and excreted in the urine. Another urinary metabolite, α-tocopheronolactone, also has been identified.

Oxidation of the phytyl side chain of unoxidized α-tocopherol generates 2,5,7,8-tetramethyl 2-(2′-carboxyethyl) 6-hydroxychroman (abbreviated α-CEHC), which may be conjugated with glucuronic acid and excreted in the urine. Similarly, oxidation of the phytyl side chain of γ-tocopherol produces 2,7,8-trimethyl 2-(2′-carboxyethyl) 6-hydroxychroman (abbreviated γ-CEHC), which also is excreted in the urine.

The major route of excretion for absorbed α-tocopherol is through the bile into the feces. In addition, fecal concentrations of the vitamin and/or its metabolites are relatively higher than urinary concentrations because relatively little vitamin E is absorbed and many of the vitamin forms (such as γ-, δ-, and β-tocopherols and tocotrienols) that are absorbed are not utilized. For example, γ-tocopherol is preferentially metabolized by the liver and excreted. Most of the vitamin E secreted into the bile for elimination is usually conjugated with glucuronic acid prior to excretion.

Recommended Dietary Allowances

The latest (2000) recommendations for the intake of vitamin E differ from those published in 1989 not only in the amount recommended but also in the form of the vitamin [1]. Previous recommendations for vitamin E included the eight naturally occurring forms of the vitamin, while the newest recommendations are only for α-tocopherol. The rationale for this change is the inability of the body to interconvert the different forms of the vitamin and the preferential hepatic secretion of only α-tocopherol. The units of intake for the vitamin have changed from mg α-tocopherol equivalents to mg α-tocopherol. The former units accounted for all eight naturally occurring forms of vitamin E with adjustments for bioavailability.

The RDA for vitamin E for adult men and women (including during pregnancy for women) is 15 mg α-tocopherol [1]. During lactation, women require slightly higher vitamin E intakes, with an RDA of 19 mg [1]. The RDA for vitamin E for adults is based on the vitamin E requirement plus twice the coefficient of variation, rounded to the nearest mg [1]. Recommendations for children age 9 to 13 and 14 to 18 years are 11 and 15 mg, respectively; those for children age 1 to 3 and 4 to 8 years are 6 and 7 mg, respectively [1]. Only an adequate intake (AI) for vitamin E was established for infants. The AI, RDA, and requirement for vitamin E are based on intake of the natural form (RRR) of α-tocopherol and the synthetic all-rac 2R-stereoisomeric forms (RSR, RRS, and RSS) of α-tocopherol used in fortified foods and vitamin supplements [1].

Deficiency

A deficiency of vitamin E in humans is quite rare. Only a few population groups are at risk for deficiency, including those with fat malabsorption disorders such as cystic fibrosis (characterized by pancreatic lipase deficiency) and hepatobiliary system disorders, particularly chronic cholestasis (characterized by decreased bile production). A second group at risk are those with genetic defects in either lipoproteins or the vitamin E transfer protein [11,17,58]. For example, abetalipoproteinemia is a rare genetic disease that may result in vitamin E deficiency due to lack of microsomal transfer protein needed for the assembly or secretion of lipoproteins containing apolipoprotein B [17].

Some symptoms of vitamin E deficiency are skeletal muscle pain (myopathy) and weakness, ceroid pigment accumulation, hemolytic anemia, and degenerative neurological problems, including cerebellar ataxia, loss of vibratory sense, and loss of coordination of limbs [6,53]. Plasma concentrations of total tocopherol relative to total lipids in adults decrease to <5 μg/mL or <0.8 mg/g with vitamin E deficiency [59,60].

Toxicity

Vitamin E appears to be one of the least toxic of the vitamins [61]. Nonetheless, because of an increased tendency for bleeding, a tolerable upper intake level of 1,000 mg supplemental α-tocopherol for adults has been established by the Food and Nutrition Board [1]. This recommendation for an upper level of intake includes any form of supplemental α-tocopherol [1]. In addition to increased bleeding, higher intakes of the vitamin also have been associated with gastrointestinal distress, including nausea, diarrhea, and flatulence; impaired blood coagulation; and occasional reports of muscle weakness, fatigue, and double vision [13,56,61]. Clinical trials with doses of the vitamin in excess of current recommendations are being conducted to examine vitamin E's effectiveness in the prevention and/or treatment of various diseases. Positive findings may ultimately lead to higher recommended intakes of the vitamin for specific populations with or at risk for a particular condition [1].

Assessment of Nutriture

Accurate evaluation of vitamin E status in humans remains difficult with current techniques. Normal serum vitamin E concentrations range from about 5 to 20 μg/mL in adults, with values <5 μg/mL indicative of deficiency. In vitamin E deficiency, plasma α-tocopherol concentrations correlate with vitamin E intake [62]. Thus, plasma concentrations are responsive to dietary intake under limited conditions. In contrast, concentrations of the vitamin plateau with daily intake of at least 200 mg RRR or all-rac α-tocopherol [12].

A crude estimation of vitamin E status can be obtained from an erythrocyte hemolysis test that compares the amount of hemoglobin released by red cells during dilute hydrogen peroxide versus distilled water incubations. The result is expressed as a percentage, with >20% indicating deficiency [20]. Concentrations of α-tocopherol of 6 μg/mL are usually sufficient to prevent hemolysis; however, variables other than vitamin E status influence in vitro hemolysis [63].

References Cited for Vitamin E

1. Food and Nutrition Board, Institute of Medicine. Dietary Reference Intakes. Washington, DC: National Academy Press, 2000, pp. 186–283.

2. Eitenmiller R. Vitamin E content of fats and oils—nutritional implications. Food Tech 1997;51:78–81.

3. Murphy S, Subar A, Block G. Vitamin E intakes and sources in the United States. Am J Clin Nutr 1990;52:361–67.

4. Cheeseman K, Holley A, Kelly F, Wasil M, Hughes L, Burton G. Biokinetics in humans of RRR-alpha-tocopherol: the free phenol, acetate ester, and succinate ester forms of vitamin E. Free Radic Biol Med 1995;19:591–98.

5. Combs G. The Vitamins. New York: Academic Press, 1992, pp. 179–203.

6. Sokol R. Vitamin E deficiency and neurologic disease. Ann Rev Nutr 1988;8:351–73.

7. Bieri J. Vitamin E. In: Brown ML, ed. Present Knowledge in Nutrition. Washington, DC: International Life Sciences Institute Nutrition Foundation, 1990, pp. 117–21.

8. Kiyose C, Muramatsu R, Kameyama Y, Ueda T, Igarashi O. Biodiscrimination of alpha tocopherol stereoisomers in humans after oral administration. Am J Clin Nutr 1997;65:785–89.

9. Traber M, Burton G, Ingold K, Kayden H. RRR- and SRR-alpha-tocopherols are secreted without discrimination in human chylomicrons, but RRR-alpha-tocopherol is preferentially secreted in very low density lipoproteins. J Lipid Res 1990;31:675–85.

10. Traber M, Burton G, Hughes L, Ingold K, Hidaka H, Malloy M, Kane J, Hyams J, Kayden H. Discrimination between forms of vitamin E by humans with and without genetic abnormalities of lipoprotein metabolism. J Lipid Res 1992;33:1171–82.

11. Traber M, Rader D, Acuff R, Brewer H, Kayden H. Discrimination between RRR- and all racemic alpha tocopherols labeled with deuterium by patients with abetalipoproteinemia. Atherosclerosis 1994;108:27–37.

12. Chopra R, Bhagavan H. Relative bioavailabilities of natural and synthetic vitamin E formulations containing mixed tocopherols in human subjects. Int J Vitam Nutr Res 1999;69:92–95.

13. Bieri J, Corash L, Hubbard V. Medical uses of vitamin E. N Engl J Med 1983;308:1063–71.

14. Kagan V, Serbinova E, Forte T, Scita G, Packer L. Recycling of vitamin E in human low density lipoproteins. J Lipid Res 1992;33:385–97.

15. Traber M, Ramakrishnan R, Kayden H. Human plasma vitamin E kinetics demonstrate rapid recycling of plasma RRR-alpha-tocopherol. Proc Natl Acad Sci USA 1994;91:10005–8.

16. Traber M, Kayden H. Preferential incorporation of alpha-tocopherol vs. gamma-tocopherol in human lipoproteins. Am J Clin Nutr 1989;49:517–26.

17. Rader D, Brewer H. Abetalipoproteinemia. New insights into lipoprotein assembly and vitamin E metabolism from a rare genetic disease. JAMA 1993;270:865–69.

18. Traber M, Kayden H. Vitamin E is delivered to cells via the high-affinity receptor for low-density lipoprotein. Am J Clin Nutr 1984;40:747–51.

19. Kostner G, Oettl K, Jauhiainen M, Ehnholm C, Esterbauer H, Dieplinger H. Human plasma phospholipid transfer protein accelerated exchange/transfer of alpha tocopherol between lipoproteins and cells. Biochem J 1995;305:659–67.

20. Machlin L. Vitamin E. In: Machlin LJ. Handbook of Vitamins, 2nd ed. New York: Dekker, 1991, pp. 99–144.

21. Niki E, Yamamota Y, Komuro E, Sato K. Membrane damage due to lipid oxidation. Am J Clin Nutr 1991;53:201S–5S.

22. Niki E, Noguchi N, Tsuchihashi H, Gotoh N. Interaction among vitamin C, vitamin E, and β-carotene. Am J Clin Nutr 1995; 62(suppl):1322S–26S.

23. Stoyanovsky D, Osipov A, Quinn P, Kagan V. Ubiquinone-dependent recycling of vitamin E radicals by superoxide. Arch Biochem Biophys 1995;323:343–51.

24. Jialal I, Grundy S. Effect of dietary supplementation with alpha tocopherol on the oxidative modification of low density lipoprotein. J Lipid Res 1992;33:899–906.

25. Esterbauer H, Dieber-Rotheneder M, Striegl G, Waeg G. Role of vitamin E in preventing the oxidation of low-density lipoprotein. Am J Clin Nutr 1991;53:314S–21S.

26. Stampfer M, Hennekens C, Manson J, Colditz G, Rosner B, Willett W. Vitamin E consumption and the risk of coronary disease in women. N Eng J Med 1993;328:1444–49.

27. Rimm E, Stampfer M, Ascherio A, Giovannucci E, Colditz G, Willett W. Vitamin E consumption and the risk of coronary heart disease in men. N Eng J Med 1993;328:1450–56.

28. Mosca L, Rubenfire M, Mandel C, Rock C, Tarshis T, Tsai A, Pearson T. Antioxidant nutrient supplementation reduces the susceptibility of low density lipoprotein to oxidation in patients with coronary artery disease. J Am Coll Cardiol 1997;30:392–99.

29. Jialal I, Grundy S. Effect of combined supplementation with α-tocopherol, ascorbate, and beta-carotene on low-density lipoprotein oxidation. Circulation 1993;88:2780–86.

30. Stephens N, Parsons A, Schofield P, Kelly F, Cheeseman K, Mitchinson M, Brown M. Randomized controlled trial of vitamin E in patients with coronary disease: Cambridge Heart Antioxidant Study (CHAOS). Lancet 1996;347:781–86.

31. GISSI-Prevenzione Investigators. Dietary supplementation with n-3 polyunsaturated fatty acids and vitamin E after myocardial infarction: results of the GISSI-Prevenzione Trial. Lancet 1999;354:447–55.

32. HOPE Study Investigators. Vitamin E supplementation and cardiovascular events in high risk patients. N Engl J Med 2000; 342:154–60.

33. Taylor A, Jacques P, Epstein E. Relations among aging, antioxidant status, and cataract. Am J Clin Nutr 1995;62(suppl):1439S–47S.

34. Bendich A, Langseth L. The health effects of vitamin C supplementation: a review. J Am Coll Nutr 1995;14:124–36.

35. Jacques P, Taylor A, Hankinson S. Long-term vitamin C supplement use and prevalence of early age-related lens opacities. Am J Clin Nutr 1997;66:911–16.

36. Varma S. Scientific basis for medical therapy of cataracts by antioxidants. Am J Clin Nutr 1991;53:335S–45S.

37. Robertson J, Donner A, Trevithick J. A possible role for vitamins C and E in cataract prevention. Am J Clin Nutr 1991;53:346S–51S.

38. Vitale S, West S, Hallfrisch J, Alston C, Wang F, Moorman C, Muller D, Singh V, Taylor H. Plasma antioxidants and risk of cortical and nuclear cataract. Epidemiology 1993;4:195–203.

39. Knekt P, Heliovaara M, Rissanen A, Aromaa A, Aaran R. Serum antioxidant vitamins and risk of cataract. Br Med J 1992;305:1392–94.

40. Leske M, Chylack L, Wu S. The Lens Opacities Case-Control Study. Risk factors for cataract. Arch Ophthalmol 1991;109:244–51.

41. Jacques P, Chylack L. Epidemiologic evidence of a role for the antioxidant vitamins and carotenoids in cataract prevention. Am J Clin Nutr 1991;53:352S–55S.

42. Omara F, Blakley B. Vitamin E is protective against iron toxicity and iron-induced hepatic vitamin E depletion in mice. J Nutr 1993;123:1649–55.

43. Reaven P. Dietary and pharmacologic regimens to reduce lipid peroxidation in non-insulin dependent diabetes mellitus. Am J Clin Nutr 1995;62(suppl):1483S–89S.

44. Paolisso G, D'Amore A, Giugliano D, Ceriello A, Varricchio M, D'Onofrio F. Pharmacologic doses of vitamin E improve insulin action in healthy subjects and non insulin dependent diabetic patients. Am J Clin Nutr 1993;57:650–56.

45. Davi G, Ciabattoni G, Consoli A, Mezzetti A, Falco A, Santarone S, Pennese E, Vitacolonna E, Bucciarelli T, Costantini F, Capani F, Patrono C. In vivo formation of 8-isoprostaglandin F2α and platelet activation in diabetes mellitus. Effects of improved metabolic control and vitamin E supplementation. Circulation 1999;99:224–29.

46. Whiteshell R, Reyen D, Beth A, Pelletier D, Abumrad N. Activation energy of slowest step in the glucose carrier cycle: correlation with membrane lipid fluidity. Biochem 1989;28:5618–25.

47. Kaiser S, Mascio P, Murphy M, Sies H. Physical and chemical scavenging of singlet molecular oxygen by tocopherols. Arch Biochem Biophys 1990;277:101–8.

48. Parker R, Pearces B, Clark R, Gordon D, Wright J. Tocotrienols regulate cholesterol production in mammalian cells by post-transcriptional suppression of 3-hydroxy-3-methylglutaryl-coenzyme A reductase. J Biol Chem 1993;268:11230–38.

49. Qureshi A, Qureshi N, Wright J, Shen S, Kramer G, Gabor A, Chong Y, DeWitt G, Ong A, Peterson D, Bradlow B. Lowering of serum cholesterol in hypercholesterolemic humans by tocotrienols (palmvitee). Am J Clin Nutr 1991;53:1021S–26S.

50. Gould M, Haag J, Kennan W, Tanner M, Elson C. A comparison of tocopherol and tocotrienol for the chemo-prevention of chemically induced rat mammary tumors. Am J Clin Nutr 1991;53:1068S–70S.

51. Byers T, Guerrero N. Epidemiologic evidence for vitamin C and vitamin E in cancer prevention. Am J Clin Nutr 1995;62(suppl): 1385S–92S.

52. Azzi A, Boscoboinik D, Marilley D, Ozer N, Stauble B, Tasinato A. Vitamin E: a sensor of the cell oxidation state. Am J Clin Nutr 1995;62(suppl):1337S–46S.

53. Traber M, Packer L. Vitamin E: beyond antioxidant function. Am J Clin Nutr 1995;62(suppl):1501S–9S.

54. Food and Nutrition Board, Institute of Medicine. Dietary Reference Intakes. Washington, DC: National Academy Press, 2001, pp. 82–161.

55. Willett W, Stampfer M, Underwood B, Taylor J, Hennekins C. Vitamins A, E and carotene: effects of supplementation on their plasma levels. Am J Clin Nutr 1983;38:559–66.

56. Bendich A, Machlin L. Safety of oral intake of vitamin E. Am J Clin Nutr 1988;48:612–19.

57. Alexander G, Suttie J. The effects of vitamin E on vitamin K activity. FASEB J 1999;13:A535.

58. Sokol R. Vitamin E deficiency and neurologic disorders. In: Packer I, Fuchs J, eds. Vitamin E in Health and Disease. New York: Marcel Dekker, 1993, pp. 815–49.

59. Horwitt M, Harvey C, Dahm C, Searcy L. Relationship between tocopherol and serum lipid levels for determination of nutritional adequacy. Ann NY Acad Sci 1972;203:223–36.

60. Farrell P, Levine S, Murphy D, Adams A. Plasma tocopherol levels and tocopherol-lipid relationship in a normal population of children as compared to healthy adults. Am J Clin Nutr 1978;31:1720–26.

61. Kappus H, Diplock A. Tolerance and safety of vitamin E: a toxicological position report. Free Radic Biol Med 1992;13:55–74.

62. Horwitt M. Vitamin E and lipid metabolism in man. Am J Clin Nutr 1960;8:451–61.

63. Boda V, Finckh B, Durken M, Commentz J, Hellwege H, Kohlschutter A. Monitoring erythrocyte free radical resistance in neonatal blood microsamples using a peroxyl radical–mediated haemolysis test. Scand J Clin Lab Invest 1998;58:317–22.

VITAMIN K

Compounds with vitamin K activity all have a 2-methyl 1,4-naphthoquinone ring. The naturally occurring forms of vitamin K are phylloquinone (2-methyl 3-phytyl 1,4-naphthoquinone), isolated from green plants, and menaquinones, which generally are synthesized by bacteria. Most of the menaquinones (abbreviated MK) contain about 6 to 13 **isoprenoid** units (MK-6–13) in a side chain attached at the number 3 carbon. Phylloquinone and menquinone formerly were designated K_1 and K_2, respectively. While most menaquinones are generated by bacteria, one is made from menadione. Menadione, 2-methyl 1,4-naphthoquinone (formerly called K_3), is not found naturally but rather is a synthetic form of vitamin K that must be alkylated by tissue enzymes for activity. Alkylation of menadione can generate MK-4. Figure 10.20 depicts menadione, phylloquinone, and one of the menaquinones, specifically menaquinone-7 (MK-7), which has seven isoprenoic units.

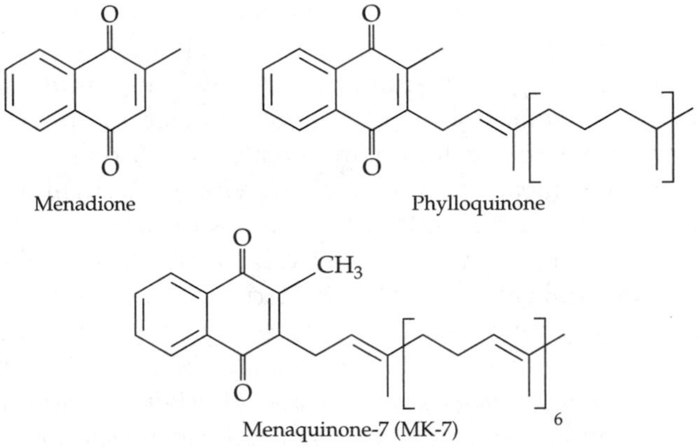

Figure 10.20 Biologically active forms of vitamin K.

Sources

Dietary vitamin K is provided mostly as phylloquinone in plant foods and as a mixture of menaquinones in animal products. Bacteria in the gastrointestinal tract, especially the colon, provide a source of menaquinones for humans. Phylloquinone is thought to provide the majority of the vitamin in the U.S. diet [1]. The average adult consumes about 70 to 80 μg phylloquinone per day [1]. The approximate vitamin K content of various foods is given in Table 10.4.

It is evident from Table 10.4 that dietary vitamin K is provided by plant foods, especially leafy green vegetables, and certain legumes [2–4]. The richest vegetable sources and the main dietary sources of vitamin K include collards, spinach, some salad greens, and broccoli. Oils and margarine represent the second major source of the vitamin [1]. Rapeseed and soybean oils are particularly rich (142–200 μg/100 g) in phylloquinone

Table 10.4 Vitamin K Content of Selected Foods

Phylloquinone μg/100 g			
<10	10–50	>100	>200
Milk	Asparagus	Cabbage	Broccoli
Butter	Celery	Lettuce	Kale
Eggs	Green beans	Brussels sprouts	Swiss chard
Cheese	Avocado	Mustard greens	Turnip
Meats	Kiwi		Watercress greens
Fish	Pumpkin (canned)		Collards
Corn	Peas		Spinach
Cauliflower	Peanut butter		Salad greens
Grains	Lentils		
Fruits (most)	Kidney beans		
Tea (brewed)	Pinto beans		
	Soybeans		
	Coffee (brewed)		

Source: Adapted from Booth et al. Vitamin K1 (phylloquinone) content of foods. J Food Comp and Anal 1993;6:109–20.

[3]. Olive oil contains 55 μg phylloquinone/100 g oil. Sunflower, safflower, walnut, and sesame oils provide only 6 to 15 μg phylloquinone/100 g, while peanut and corn oils contain <3 μg/100 g [3]. Smaller amounts of phylloquinone are found in cereals, fruits, dairy products, and meats. Exposure of the vitamin to light and heat can result in significant vitamin K destruction [3].

Menaquinones are synthesized by a variety of facultative and obligate anaerobic bacteria that reside in the lower digestive tract. Examples of menaquinone-producing obligate anaerobes include *Bacteroides fragilis, Eubacterium, Propionibacterium,* and *Arachnia. Escherichia coli,* a facultative anaerobe, also produces menaquinone [5]. Bacterial synthesis of vitamin K is not sufficient to meet the needs of healthy children or adults [1].

Although rarely needed, vitamin K supplements as phylloquinone (such as Mephyton and Konakion) are available. Water-soluble forms of the vitamin (AquaMephyton, Synkayvite, and Kappadione) are also manufactured for individuals with fat malabsorptive disorders.

Absorption, Transport, and Storage

Phylloquinone is absorbed from the small intestine, particularly from the jejunum. Absorption of vitamin K occurs as part of micelles and thus is enhanced by the presence of dietary fats, bile salts, and pancreatic juice.

Menaquinones that are synthesized by some bacteria in the lower digestive tract are absorbed by passive diffusion from the ileum and colon; however, the ability to absorb and utilize the bacterially produced vitamin varies considerably from human to human and has been difficult to determine accurately [1,6].

Within the intestinal cell, phylloquinones are incorporated into the chylomicron that enters the lymphatic and then the circulatory system for transport to tissues. Chylomicrons transport the majority of phylloquinone [7,8]. Chylomicron remnants deliver vitamin K to the liver. Absorbed menadiones are alkylated in the liver and then, along with phylloquinone and menaquinone, incorporated into very low density lipoproteins, and ultimately carried to extrahepatic tissues in low-density and high-density lipoproteins [8,9].

Phylloquinones are found in higher concentrations in the liver, with lesser amounts in the heart, among other tissues [10,11]. Hepatic concentrations of phylloquinone range from about 2 to 20 ng per liver and are about 10 times lower than those of the menaquinones [5,12]. Menaquinone-4 (MK-4) synthesis from menadione has been demonstrated with MK-4 found in a variety of tissues, including the pancreas, salivary glands, brain, and sternum [10,11]. Circulating plasma concentrations of phylloquinones range from about 0.15 to 1.15 ng/mL [13]. The body pool size of vitamin K, estimated at 50 to 100 μg, is quite low for a fat-soluble vitamin and smaller than that of vitamin B_{12} [9]. Turnover of vitamin K is rapid, approximately once every 2.5 hours [9].

Functions and Mechanisms of Action

Vitamin K is necessary for the posttranslational carboxylation of specific glutamic acid (glutamyl) residues in proteins to form γ-carboxyglutamate residues, which enable the protein to bind to calcium and interact with other compounds such as phospholipids. These interactions are necessary for blood clotting and bone mineralization, among other processes. The role of vitamin K in blood clotting and vitamin K's possible roles in bone and nonosteous tissues are reviewed here.

Vitamin K and Blood Clotting

The vitamin K–dependent posttranslational carboxylation of glutamyl residues forms γ-carboxyglutamate on 4 of 13 proteins required for the coagulation of blood. The four vitamin K–dependent blood-clotting proteins, referred to as factors, are factors II (prothrombin), VII, IX, and X. Proteins C and S, and possibly Z, also require vitamin K for carboxylation, but these proteins function to inhibit the coagulation process.

Overview of Blood Clotting. For blood to clot, fibrinogen, a soluble protein, must be converted to fibrin, an insoluble fiber network, as shown at the bottom of Figure 10.21. Thrombin catalyzes the proteolysis of fibrinogen to yield fibrin. Fibrin molecules aggregate to form a polymer, which then undergoes cross-linking by fibrin-stabilizing factor (activated by thrombin or factor XIII) to form an insoluble clot and stop bleeding (hemorrhage).

Thrombin, however, circulates in the blood as prothrombin, an inactive enzyme (zymogen). Two pathways, extrinsic and intrinsic, can be used to generate prothrombin and thus thrombin for blood clotting. The reactions needed to produce thrombin occur in a cascade as shown in Figure 10.21 and described below. In the intrinsic pathway, the coagulation process is initiated by adsorption of factor XII or XI (both of which circulate in the blood) onto a substance such as collagen. Upon contact, factor XII or XI becomes activated, as indicated by the letter *a* next to the factor. The cascade proceeds in a stepwise process:

- XIa, now an active protease, associates with a protein cofactor and its substrate, factor IX, a vitamin K–dependent carboxylated protein in contact with calcium. Factor IX is converted to IXa by factor XIa.
- Factor IXa continues the cascade of reactions by associating with factor VIIIa and its substrate, factor X. Factor VIIIa is synthesized from factor VIII by thrombin (IIa). Factor X is converted to Xa by active protease factor IXa.
- Factor Xa is another vitamin K–dependent carboxylated protein that interacts with calcium and

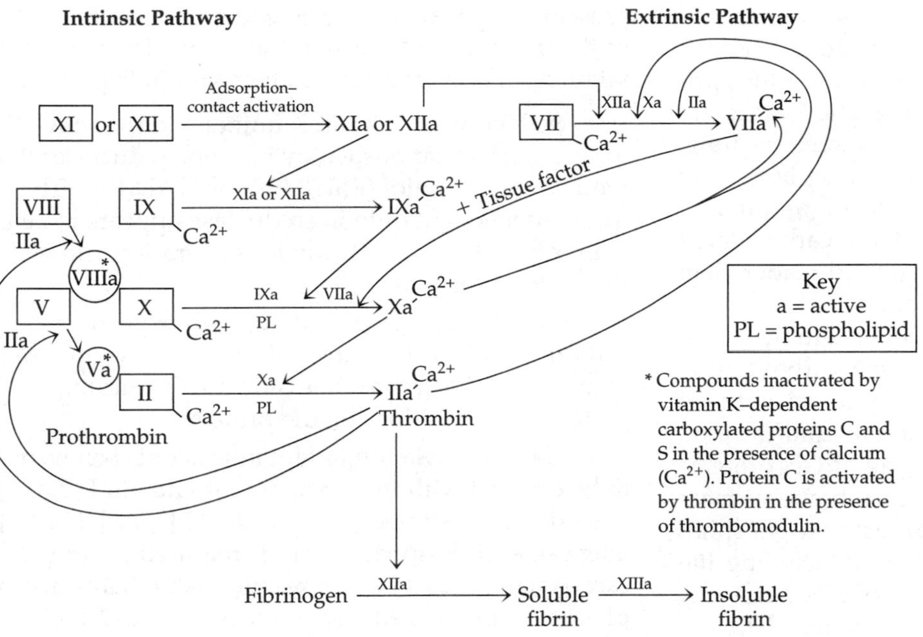

Figure 10.21 The roles of vitamin K–dependent clotting factors in the coagulation of blood.

phospholipids. It also associates with factor Va and its substrate prothrombin (factor II), another vitamin K–dependent carboxylated protein. Factor Va is generated from factor V by thrombin (IIa). Factor Xa hydrolyzes prothrombin (factor II) to produce thrombin (IIa).

- Thrombin catalyzes the conversion of fibrinogen to fibrin for clot formation.

Other proteins, designated C, S, and Z, also have been identified as vitamin K–dependent carboxylated proteins. While the function of protein Z is unknown, proteins C and S appear to inhibit the blood-clotting process and thus exhibit anticoagulant functions. Protein C associates with thrombomodulin and calcium, and in the presence of thrombin it can be converted to protein Ca. This active protease, in association with calcium and protein S, inactivates factors VIIIa and Va to disrupt the clotting process. Protein S has been found not only in the blood but also in bone and thus may have other functions [14].

In the extrinsic pathway, blood-clotting proteins interact with tissue factors in a second cascade of reactions that intercepts with the intrinsic pathway as shown in Figure 10.21 and briefly described here. In the extrinsic pathway, factor VII is converted to VIIa by a variety of blood-clotting proteases, including thrombin and factors Xa and XIIa. Factor VIIa, a carboxylated vitamin K–dependent protein, in association with calcium and a tissue factor, can convert factor IX (a vitamin K–dependent protein associated with calcium) to IXa and can convert factor X (vitamin K–dependent protein associated with calcium and phospholipids) to Xa. As in the intrinsic pathway, factor Xa synthesizes thrombin from prothrombin, and thrombin converts fibrinogen to fibrin for clot formation.

The Role of Vitamin K in Carboxylation of Glutamic Acid Residues. We will use prothrombin as a model to describe the carboxylation process. Remember that blood-clotting factors VII, IX, and X, as well as other proteins such as C, S, and Z and those discussed under bone and nonosteous roles of vitamin K, depend on vitamin K for carboxylation. Prothrombin requires a vitamin K–dependent enzyme for the carboxylation of 10 to 12 glutamic acid residues residing in its N-terminal. Once carboxylated, this glutamic acid portion forms γ-carboxyglutamic acid (Gla), as shown in Figure 10.22. The carboxylation is required for the protein to become functional. The enzyme responsible

Figure 10.22 Production of γ-carboxylglutamic acid (Gla) via vitamin K–dependent carboxylation.

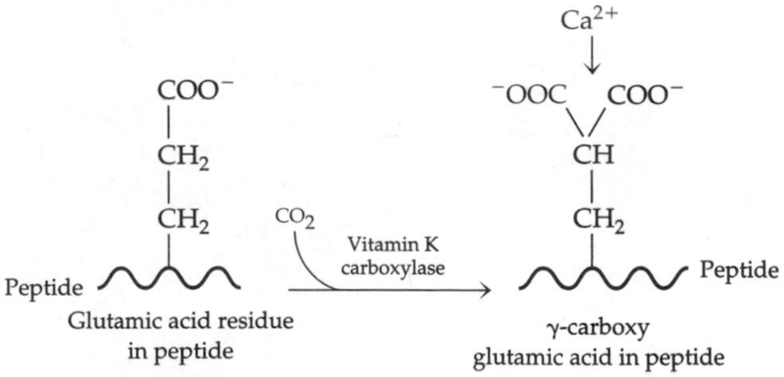

for the γ-carboxylation, referred to as vitamin K–dependent γ-glutamyl carboxylase, is found associated with the rough endoplasmic reticulum (RER), primarily in the liver, where the hemostatic factors are synthesized, but also in other tissues such as lung, spleen, kidney, thyroid, pancreas, cartilage, bone, and skin [9]. The widespread occurrence of γ-glutamyl carboxylase suggests that the need for carboxylated proteins that can bind calcium is much broader than just the regulation of blood coagulation.

The synthesis of Gla residues occurs posttranslationally; however, the directionality of the carboxylation and the multisite specificity of the enzyme are not well understood [15]. Gla residues function to bind calcium. The calcium then mediates the binding of Gla proteins to negatively charged phospholipid membrane surfaces [16]. This adsorption of specific proteins on phospholipid surfaces is essential in hemostasis, including the initiation, progression, and regulation of blood clotting.

The participation of vitamin K in the carboxylation of proteins is a cyclic process (Fig. 10.23) often referred to as the vitamin K cycle. The γ-glutamyl carboxylase enzyme requires dihydrovitamin KH_2, also known as reduced, dihydroxy, or hydroquinone vitamin K. Thus, for carboxylation to occur, vitamin K is needed in the reduced form, vitamin KH_2. However, vitamin K is generally present in the body in its oxidized quinone form because of the presence of oxygen in the blood. The steps of the vitamin K cycle are reviewed here and in Figure 10.23.

- Reduction of vitamin K quinone to the active KH_2 form can be accomplished by quinone reductases that require either dithiol (RSH-HSR) or NAD(P)H. The dithiol-dependent quinone reductase appears to be the main physiological pathway for generating vitamin KH_2 from the quinone.
- Once KH_2 is present, along with oxygen and carbon dioxide as the carboxyl precursor, γ-glutamyl carboxylase can carboxylate (add a CO_2 onto) the glutamic acid residues on the protein.
- The carboxylation of glutamic acid is believed to be coupled with the formation of vitamin K 2,3-epoxide, as illustrated in Figure 10.23 [17,18]. No adenosine triphosphate (ATP) is required for the carboxylation reaction; the reaction is probably accomplished by the free energy produced through the oxidation of vitamin KH_2 to 2,3-epoxide, whereby vitamin K provides reducing equivalents.
- As the cycle continues, vitamin K 2,3-epoxide is converted to vitamin K quinone by an epoxide reductase.
- The quinone is then converted back to the dihydroxy (hydroquinone) vitamin K (KH_2) by one of the

Figure 10.23 The vitamin K cycle.

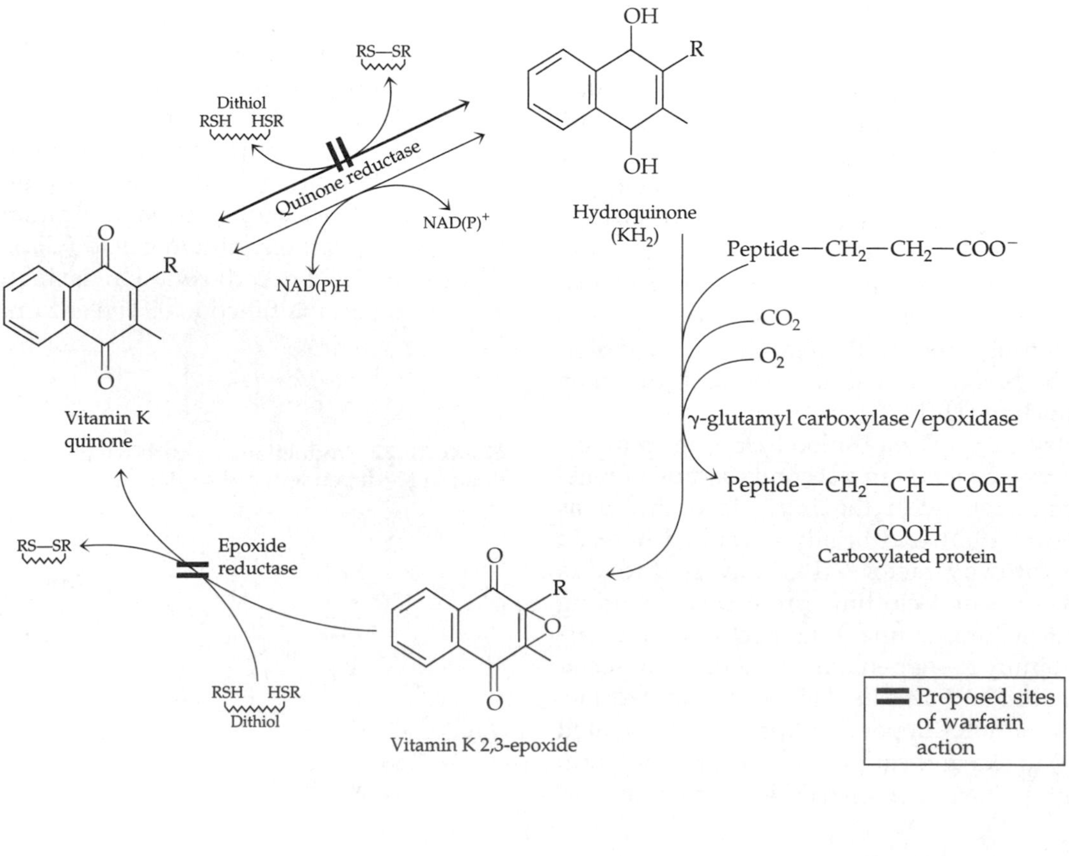

two quinone reductases, requiring either NAD(P)H or 2 RSH (Fig. 10.23) as previously described.

Anticoagulants. Coumadin (warfarin) is an anticoagulant that may be prescribed to individuals at risk for a thrombotic event (such as a heart attack). The anticoagulant antagonizes the synthesis of vitamin K. Warfarin, for example, interferes with the dithiol-catalyzed quinone reductase necessary for reducing oxidized vitamin K to the KH_2 form (Fig. 10.23). Warfarin also may act on the epoxide reductase, again preventing KH_2 regeneration [9]. Ingestion of diets high in vitamin K, as obtained from about a pound of broccoli daily, can lead to warfarin resistance [19]. Thus, individuals who are taking anticoagulant medications are instructed not to consume large quantities of foods rich in vitamin K.

Vitamin K and Bone and Nonosteous Tissue Proteins

Two vitamin K–dependent proteins have been identified in bone and dentine: osteocalcin, also called bone Gla protein (BGP); and matrix Gla protein (MGP). The synthesis of both osteocalcin and MGP appears to be stimulated by 1,25-$(OH)_2$ D_3 and by retinoic acid [20–22]. Osteocalcin is secreted by osteoblasts during bone matrix formation, about at the onset of hydroxyapatite deposition [20,21]. Osteocalcin comprises about 15% to 20% of noncollagen protein in bone. With vitamin K–dependent carboxylation, the three Gla residues facilitate the binding of calcium ions [23]. Although its physiological role remains unclear, osteocalcin appears to be involved in bone remodeling and/or calcium mobilization [20,21]. Lack of osteocalcin in knockout mice has been associated with increased bone formation [24]. Coumadin (warfarin) has been shown to impair osteocalcin's ability to adsorb to hydroxyapatite due to undercarboxylation [14].

MGP is found in bone, dentine, and cartilage and is associated with the organic matrix and mobilization of bone calcium. As with osteocalcin, the physiological role of MGP is uncertain. However, messenger RNA for MGP has been found in a variety of tissues, including brain, heart, kidney, liver, lung, and spleen, suggesting a broad role for the protein. Lack of MGP in knockout mice has been associated with extensive arterial calcification [25].

A third vitamin K–dependent protein, kidney Gla protein (KGP), has been identified in the cortex of the kidney [21]. Further research is needed to delineate the roles of not only KGP but also MGP and osteocalcin.

Interactions with Other Nutrients

The fat-soluble vitamins A and E are known to antagonize vitamin K. Excess vitamin A appears to interfere with vitamin K absorption. Vitamin E's antagonistic effects on vitamin K include possible inhibition vitamin K absorption, function, and/or metabolism [9,26]. Vitamin E or its quinone (α-tocopheryl quinone), for example, is thought to block the regeneration of the reduced form of vitamin K and/or to affect prothrombin formation by another manner [27,28].

A possible interrelationship among vitamins K, D, and A is suggested based on their relationship to the mineral calcium. Vitamin D functions impact calcium metabolism, and vitamin K–dependent proteins bind calcium. Two sites of action of 1,25-$(OH)_2$ D_3 are bone and kidney, and in both these tissues vitamin K–dependent calcium-binding proteins have been identified. Retinoic A as well as 1,25-$(OH)_2$ D_3 has been shown to regulate, in part, production of BGP, MGP, and/or KGP [20–22]. Further research is needed to better characterize the interrelationships.

Metabolism and Excretion

Phylloquinone, degraded much more slowly than menaquinone, is almost completely metabolized to a variety of metabolites (many uncharacterized) prior to its excretion. The metabolism usually involves oxidation of the phytyl side chain at position 3 with subsequent conjugation. Most of the metabolites of phylloquinone are conjugated with glucuronides for excretion primarily in the feces via the bile, with some metabolite excretion via the urine.

Relatively little is known about the metabolism and excretion of menaquinone. Studies suggest that menadione is rapidly metabolized to menadiol, which then reacts with phosphate, sulfate, or glucuronide. Menadiol phosphate and menadiol sulfate are excreted in the bile (and thus ultimately in the feces) and in the urine; menadiol glucuronides are excreted mostly in the feces via the bile.

Adequate Intakes

Lack of data has hampered the Food and Nutrition Board in its efforts to estimate requirements for vitamin K [1]. Adequate intake (AI) recommendations of 120 and 90 μg for adult males and females (including those who are pregnant or lactating), respectively, have been set based on the highest dietary intakes of vitamin K by healthy individuals obtained from the National Health and Nutrition Examination Survey (NHANES) III [1]. Values of vitamin K intake were rounded up to the nearest 5 μg for setting the AIs [1]. Recommended AIs for children age 1 to 3 and 4 to 8 years are 30 and 55 μg, respectively, while those for children age 9 to 13 and 14 to 18 years are 60 and 75 μg, respectively [1]. Recommendations for children also are based on the highest median intake for each age group found in the NHANES III [1].

The 2001 recommendations for vitamin K intake are higher than those established for the first time by the board in 1989. The 1989 recommended dietary allowances for vitamin K for adult males and females were 80 and 65 μg per day, respectively [29]. In the past, a range of intakes has been suggested based on the assumption that a substantial amount of vitamin K could be supplied by intestinal bacteria. However, it is now recognized that bacterial-generated menaquinones are generally not sufficiently produced and/or utilized to maintain adequate vitamin K status [1].

Deficiency

A deficiency of vitamin K is unlikely in healthy adults. The population groups that appear to be most at risk for a vitamin K deficiency are newborn infants and people with severe gastrointestinal malabsorptive disorders or people being treated chronically with antibiotics. Newborns are particularly at risk because their food is limited to milk, which is low in vitamin K; their stores of the vitamin are low due to poor placental transfer; and their intestinal tract is not yet populated by vitamin K–synthesizing bacteria. Supplementation with vitamin K is considered advisable for all newborns; currently it is recommended that 0.5 to 1 mg phylloquinone be injected intramuscularly into infants shortly after birth [1].

People consuming vitamin K–poor diets and on prolonged sulfa and antibiotic drug therapy are at risk for vitamin K deficiency owing to the coupled effects of low dietary intake and antibiotic-induced destruction of gastrointestinal bacteria that manufacture the vitamin and contribute a source of vitamin K. Other conditions and populations associated with increased need for vitamin K intake include those with fat malabsorptive disorders: biliary fistula, obstructive jaundice, steatorrhea or chronic diarrhea, intestinal bypass surgery, chronic pancreatitis, and liver disease. Because vitamin K is fat soluble, it is absorbed best with dietary fat. Consequently, individuals who malabsorb fat also malabsorb fat-soluble vitamins.

Subclinical vitamin K deficiency has been induced in healthy adults fed a diet providing only about 10 μg phylloquinone per day [30]. The 13-day low–vitamin K diet resulted in a significant reduction in plasma vitamin K concentrations. Urinary γ-carboxyglutamate excretion significantly decreased in younger subjects but remained unchanged in older adults. Prothrombin time did not change; however, descarboxyprothrombin (undercarboxylated prothrombin) concentrations increased significantly in subjects [30]. Severe vitamin K deficiency is associated with bleeding episodes (hemorrhage) due to prolonged prothrombin time. The undercarboxylated blood-clotting factors cannot effectively bind calcium and interact with cell membrane phospholipids exposed on tissue injury, an interaction necessary for thrombin generation and clot formation.

A relationship between vitamin K and osteoporosis has been suggested. Subclinical vitamin K deficiency may be associated with alterations in bone mineral density and increased fracture rates, although the results of studies are not consistent.

Toxicity

Ingestion of large amounts of phylloquinone and menaquinone has caused no symptoms of toxicity, and no tolerable upper intake level for vitamin K has been established by the Food and Nutrition Board [1,31]. The synthetic product menadione, however, can cause liver damage when ingested in relatively large amounts. Toxic effects reported in infants supplemented with menadione include hemolytic anemia, hyperbilirubinemia, and severe jaundice [28,31]. Menadione is thought to combine with sulfhydryl groups such as those in glutathione, resulting in glutathione oxidation and excretion and ultimately membrane damage induced by phospholipid oxidation [16].

Assessment of Nutriture

Plasma or serum concentrations of phylloquinone have been shown to reflect recent (within about 24 hours) intakes of the vitamin [32]. Measurement of whole blood clotting times as well as of prothrombin (or other blood-clotting proteins) time is routinely used to identify potential deficiency of vitamin K. Prothrombin time measures the time required for a fibrin clot to form following the addition of calcium and other substances to citrated plasma. A normal prothrombin time is considered to be between about 11 and 14 seconds, while times greater than 25 seconds are associated with major bleeding and may indicate possible vitamin K deficiency. This test, however, is considered relatively insensitive, because plasma prothrombin concentrations typically must decrease considerably (sometimes 50% or more) prior to any effects on prothrombin time [33].

Another means of assessment of vitamin K status that has been used is measurement of undercarboxylated vitamin K–dependent proteins such as prothrombin and osteocalcin or the ratio of under- to fully carboxylated proteins [32]. Vitamin K deficiency results in the secretion of under- or partially carboxylated proteins into the blood. These undercarboxylated proteins, which have been referred to as protein-induced vitamin K absence or antagonism (PIVKA), have been shown to respond to dietary changes in vitamin K [1]. More accurate and valid methods are needed to better assess vitamin K status in humans.

References Cited for Vitamin K

1. Food and Nutrition Board, Institute of Medicine. Dietary Reference Intakes. Washington, DC: National Academy Press, 2001, pp. 162–96.

2. Booth S, Sadowski J, Weihrauch J, Ferland G. Vitamin K1 (phylloquinone) content of foods: a provisional table. J Food Comp Anal 1993;6:109–20.

3. Ferland G, Sadowski J. Vitamin K1 (phylloquinone) content of edible oils: effects of heating and light exposure. J Agric Food Chem 1992;40:1869–73.

4. Booth S, Suttie J. Dietary intake and adequacy of vitamin K. J Nutr 1998;128:785–88.

5. Suttie J. The importance of menaquinones in human nutrition. Ann Rev Nutr 1995;15:399–417.

6. Ichihashi T, Takagishi Y, Uchida K, Yamada H. Colonic absorption of menaquinone-4 and menaquinone-9 in rats. J Nutr 1992;122:506–12.

7. Kohlmeier M, Salomon A, Saupe J, Shearer M. Transport of vitamin K to bone in humans. J Nutr 1996;126:1192S–96S.

8. Lamon-Fava S, Sadowski J, Davidson K, O'Brien M, McNamara J, Schaefer E. Plasma lipoproteins as carriers of phylloquinone (vitamin K1) in humans. Am J Clin Nutr 1998;67:1226–31.

9. Olson R. The function and metabolism of vitamin K. Ann Rev Nutr 1984;4:281–337.

10. Davidson R, Goley A, Engelke J, Suttie J. Conversion of dietary phylloquinone to tissue menaquinone-4 in rats not dependent on gut bacteria. J Nutr 1998;128:220–23.

11. Thijssen H, Drittij-Reijnders M. Vitamin K status in human tissues: tissue specific accumulation of phylloquinone and menaquinone-4. Br J Nutr 1996;75:121–27.

12. Usui Y, Tanimura H, Nishimura N, Kobayashi N, Okanoue T, Ozawa K. Vitamin K concentrations in the plasma and liver of surgical patients. Am J Clin Nutr 1990;51:846–52.

13. Sadowski J, Hood S, Dallal G, Garry P. Phylloquinone in plasma from elderly and young adults: factors influencing its concentration. Am J Clin Nutr 1989;50:100–108.

14. Binkley N, Suttie J. Vitamin K nutrition and osteoporosis. J Nutr 1995;125;1812–21.

15. Benton M, Price P, Suttie J. Multi-site-specificity of the vitamin K–dependent carboxylase: in vitro carboxylation of des-γ-carboxylated bone Gla protein and des-γ-carboxylated pro bone Gla protein. Biochemistry 1995;34:9541–51.

16. Esmon C. Cell mediated events that control blood coagulation and vascular injury. Ann Rev Cell Biol 1993;9:1–26.

17. Kuliopulos A, Hubbard B, Lam Z, Koski I, Furie B, Furie B, Walsh C. Dioxygen transfer during vitamin K dependent carboxylase catalysis. J Am Chem Soc 1992;31:7722–28.

18. Dowd P, Ham S, Hershline R. Role of oxygen in the vitamin K–dependent carboxylation reaction: incorporation of a second atom of ^{18}O from molecular oxygen-$^{18}O_2$ into vitamin K oxide during carboxylase activity. JACS 1992;114:7613–17.

19. Kempin S. Warfarin resistance caused by broccoli. N Eng J Med 1983;308:1229–30.

20. Price P. Role of vitamin K–dependent proteins in bone metabolism. Ann Rev Nutr 1988;8:565–83.

21. The function of the vitamin K–dependent proteins, bone Gla protein (BGP) and kidney Gla protein (KGP). Nutr Rev 1984;42:230–33.

22. Cancela M, Price P. Retinoic acid induces matrix Gla protein gene expression in human cells. Endocrinology 1992;130:102–8.

23. Saupe J, Shearer M, Kohlmeier M. Phylloquinone transport and its influence on gamma-carboxyglutamate residues of osteocalcin in patients on maintenance hemodialysis. Am J Clin Nutr 1993; 58:204–8.

24. Ducy P, Desbois C, Boyce B, Pinero G, Story B, Dunstan C, Smith E, Bonadio J, Goldstein S, Gundberg C, Bradley A, Karsenty G. Increased bone formation in osteocalcin-deficient mice. Nature 1996;382:448–52.

25. Luo G, Ducy P, McKee M, Pinero G, Loyer E, Behringer R, Karsenty G. Spontaneous calcification of arteries and cartilage in mice lacking matrix Gla protein. Nature 1997;386:78–81.

26. Alexander G, Suttie J. The effects of vitamin E on vitamin K activity. FASEB J 1999;13:A535.

27. Bieri J, Corash L, Hubbard V. Medical uses of vitamin E. N Engl J Med 1983;308:1063–71.

28. Bendich A, Machlin L. Safety of oral intake of vitamin E. Am J Clin Nutr 1988;48:612–19.

29. Food and Nutrition Board. Recommended Dietary Allowances, 10th ed. Washington, DC: National Academy Press, 1989, pp. 107–14.

30. Ferland G, Sadowski J, O'Brien M. Dietary induced subclinical vitamin K deficiency in normal human subjects. J Clin Invest 1993;91:1761–68.

31. Council on Scientific Affairs, American Medical Association. Vitamin preparations as dietary supplements and as therapeutic agents. JAMA 1987;257:1929–36.

32. Sokoll L, Booth S, O'Brien M, Davidson K, Tsaioun K, Sadowski J. Changes in serum osteocalcin, plasma phylloquinone, and urinary gamma carboxyglutamic acid in response to altered intakes of dietary phylloquinone in human subjects. Am J Clin Nutr 1997;65:779–84.

33. Suttie JW. Vitamin K and human nutrition. J Am Diet Assoc 1992;92:585–90.

The Antioxidant Nutrients, Reactive Species, and Disease

While different sections in several chapters of this book have addressed the roles of selected nutrients as they relate to antioxidant function, nowhere is this information brought together to provide a comprehensive review of how these individual nutrients function together to protect the body from destructive radicals and destructive nonradical species. That is the purpose of this perspective, which first reviews free radical chemistry. The perspective next addresses how free radicals and selected nonradicals are generated in the body, the damage caused by reactive oxygen species, and finally how the antioxidant nutrients function together to eliminate destructive radical and nonradical oxygen species.

Table 1 Some Reactive Oxygen and Nitrogen Species

Reactive Oxygen Species		Reactive Nitrogen Species	
Oxygen-containing Radicals	**Oxygen-containing Nonradicals**	**Nitrogen-containing Radicals**	**Nitrogen-containing Nonradicals**
Superoxide O_2^{-}	Ozone O_3	Nitric oxide $NO^{\cdot}$	Nitrous acid HNO_2
Hydroxyl $^{\cdot}OH$	Singlet oxygen $^1O_2$	Nitrogen dioxide $NO_2^{\cdot}$	Peroxynitrite ONO_2^{-}
Hydroperoxyl $HO_2^{\cdot}$	Hypochlorous acid HOCL		Alkyl peroxynitrite $LOONO^{\cdot}$
Alkoxyl $LO^{\cdot}$ or $RO^{\cdot}$	Hydrogen peroxide H_2O_2		
Peroxyl $LO_2^{\cdot}$ or $RO_2^{\cdot}$			

Free Radical Chemistry

Back in probably one of your first chemistry courses, you learned about atoms. It is here that a brief review of free radical chemistry begins. Atoms contain protons and neutrons that are found in the nucleus. You may remember that the atomic weight of an element is a function of its number of protons and neutrons, while the atomic number represents solely the number of protons. Atoms also have electrons, which revolve in orbitals (also called shells) around the nucleus. An atomic orbital holds a maximum of two electrons. These electrons are generally found in pairs in the orbitals. The term free radical refers to an atom or molecule that has one or more unpaired electrons. The unpaired electron is found alone in the outer orbital and is usually denoted by a superscript dot next to the element. The **superoxide radical** is denoted by a superscript dot ($O_2^{\cdot}$) or a superscript dash (O_2^{-}) or both ($O_2^{\cdot -}$). The imbalance in electrons in the orbitals results in most cases in the high reactivity of the free radicals. Free radicals that contain oxygen may be referred to as reactive oxygen species (ROS), while free radicals containing nitrogen are called reactive nitrogen species (RNS). The term *reactive* is most appropriately used when comparing different radicals, because reactivity with other compounds is relative. The terms *reactive oxygen species* and *reactive nitrogen species,* however, include not only free radicals containing oxygen and nitrogen, respectively, but also nonradicals, as shown in Table 1.

The radicals listed in Table 1 are not inclusive of all free radical or reactive species. Oxygen itself is a biradical because it has two unpaired electrons, residing in separate orbitals, that cannot form a pair. An example of a reactive sulfur species radical is thiyl ($RS^{\cdot}$), generated from amino acids and thiols. Trichloromethyl ($CCl_3^{\cdot}$), formed during metabolism of carbon tetrachloride (CCl_4) by cytochrome P_{450} enzymes in the liver, is a chloride-based carbon-centered radical, meaning that the unpaired electron resides on the carbon atom.

Generation of Reactive Species

A variety of different reactive species are generated daily from multiple sites in the body. In general, the reactive oxygen species are formed on exposure to substances such as smog, ozone, chemicals, drugs, radiation, and high oxygen, among others, and during normal physiological processes, especially in the defense against microbes and other foreign substances. Radicals also breed more radicals, as seen in several of the reactions shown in this perspective. Production of the superoxide radical; hydrogen peroxide; the hydroxyl radical; the peroxyl, hydroperoxyl, and carbon-centered (alkyl) radicals; and lipid peroxides is reviewed in this section and shown in Figure 1.

The Superoxide Radical

The superoxide radical (designated hereafter as O_2^{-}) is an oxygen-centered radical; that is, the unpaired electron resides on the oxygen. Remember that molecular oxygen has two unpaired electrons in different orbitals. The addition of an electron to molecular oxygen leaves only one unpaired electron:

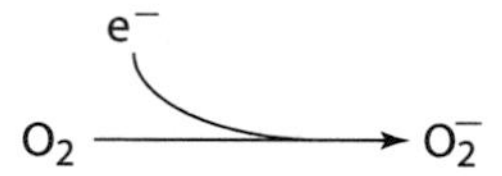

Superoxide radicals can be made when oxygen molecules (O_2) react with different compounds, such as with the catecholamines epinephrine and dopamine or with the vitamin folate, as tetrahydrofolate. The electron transport chain also accidentally produces superoxide radicals due to autooxidation reactions and leaking of electrons from the electron transport chain onto oxygen—that is, a one-electron reduction of oxygen to generate the superoxide radical. This leaking of electrons onto oxygen occurs during the passage of electrons from $CoQH^{\cdot}$ (coenzyme Q) as part of the electron transport chain. In the electron transport chain, electrons ultimately are transferred to oxygen (O_2) for ATP production; however, upon interaction between $CoQH^{\cdot}$ and O_2, shown here, the superoxide radical is formed:

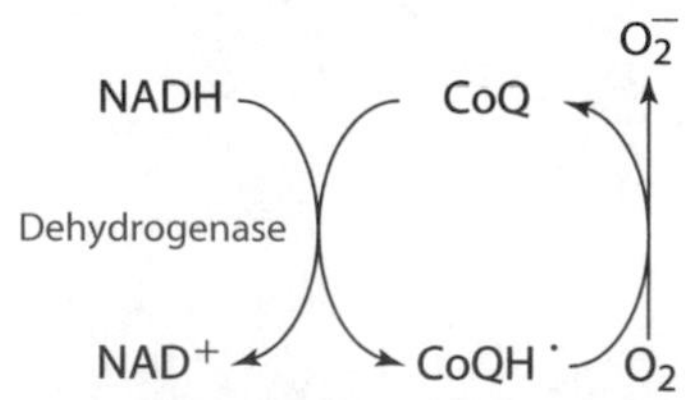

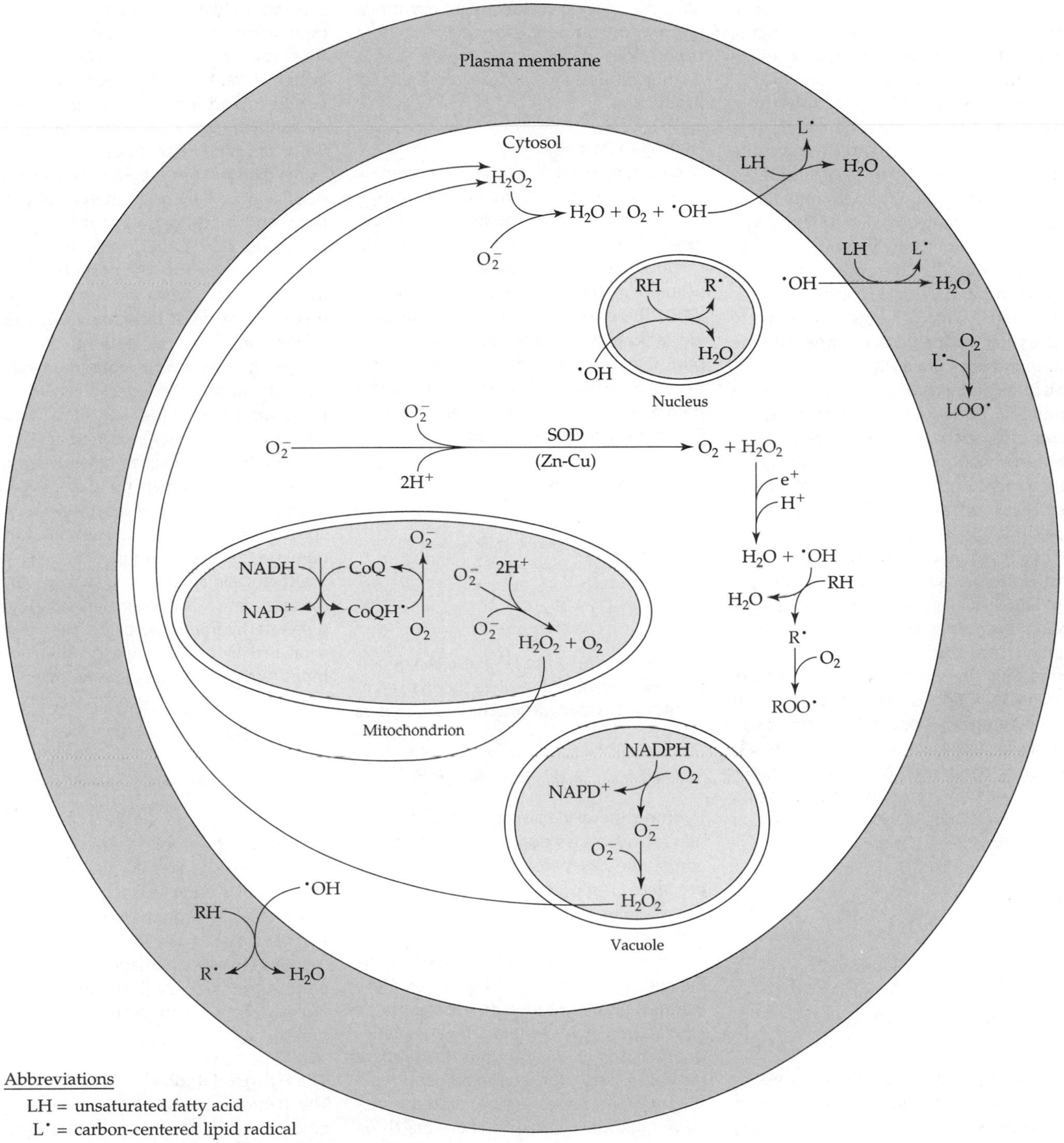

Abbreviations

LH = unsaturated fatty acid
$L^{\bullet}$ = carbon-centered lipid radical
RH = organic compound (e.g., amino acid, nucleic acid)
O_2^- = superoxide radical
${}^{\bullet}OH$ = hydroxy radical
$R^{\bullet}$ = carbon-centered nonlipid radical
H_2O_2 = hydrogen peroxide
$ROO^{\bullet}$ = nonlipid peroxy radical
$LOO^{\bullet}$ = peroxy radical

Figure 1 Generation of reactive species.

Cytochrome P_{450} enzymes also can generate superoxide radicals. These heme enzymes found in the endoplasmic reticulum membrane consist of a cytochrome P_{450} reductase that transfers electrons from NADPH and a second cytochrome P_{450} that binds molecular oxygen and the substrate being hydroxylated. A variety of substrates, including fatty acids, steroids, and therapeutic drugs, are hydroxylated by this system. The reactions catalyzed by some of the cytochrome P_{450} enzymes function to convert nonpolar compounds to polar compounds. This change in polarity enables elimination (fecal or urinary) of the compound from the body.

Superoxide radicals also are produced in significant quantities in activated white blood cells, such as macrophages, monocytes, and neutrophils conducting phagocytosis, to assist in the destruction of foreign substances such as bacteria and viruses. The superoxide radicals in these cells are needed for the subsequent production of other toxic reactive oxygen species, such as hydrogen peroxide (H_2O_2), to further help destroy foreign bacteria and other organisms. In addition, superoxide radicals generated by neutrophils heighten the inflammatory response by acting as a chemoattractant for other neutrophils. Production of superoxide radicals in activated white blood cells is thought to begin with the action of NADPH oxidase as a foreign substance is being engulfed by a white blood cell. This reaction is shown here:

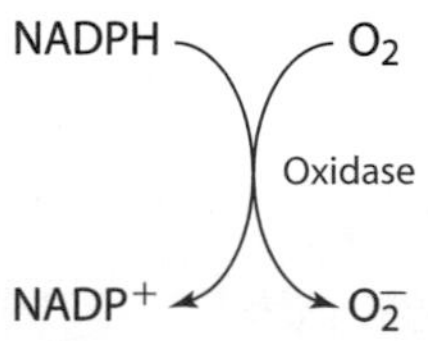

The extensive oxygen-requiring process by which white blood cells destroy organisms is sometimes referred to as the respiratory burst.

Although superoxide radicals assist in the destruction of bacteria, viruses, fungi, and the like in white blood cells, these same radicals can do harm. They are a potent initiator of chain reactions and can lead to the production of other reactive oxygen species, such as hydrogen peroxide and the hydroperoxyl radical. The superoxide radical also can react with nitric oxide to generate several reactive nitrogen species, including peroxynitrite, nitroxyl, and nitrogen dioxide. Fortunately, superoxides are not lipid-soluble and thus do not diffuse too far from their site of production.

Hydrogen Peroxide

Hydrogen peroxide is not a radical because it has no unpaired electrons, but it is considered a reactive oxygen species and easily diffuses throughout cells, causing damage. Hydrogen peroxide is generated through the action of the enzyme superoxide dismutase (SOD). This enzyme, which removes superoxide radicals, is found extracellularly and in both the cell cytoplasm and mitochondria. Extracellular SOD and cytosolic SOD require both zinc and copper, while mitochondrial SOD is manganese dependent.

$$O_2^- + O_2^- + 2H^+ \xrightarrow{\text{Superoxide dismutase}} H_2O_2 + O_2$$

Ascorbate (AH_2), like SOD, also can generate hydrogen peroxide while trying to eliminate superoxide radicals. The reaction is as follows:

$$AH_2 + O_2^- + H^+ \longrightarrow AH^- + H_2O_2$$

Hydrogen peroxide also is produced in significant quantities during the oxidation of compounds in peroxisomes, cytoplasmic organelles responsible for the degradation of molecules such as very long chain (20+ carbons) fatty acids, among others.

Other reactions in the body also generate hydrogen peroxide. In trauma or injury situations such as intestinal ischemia or cardiac ischemia (ischemia means inadequate blood flow and thus inadequate oxygen supply), for example, many reactive oxygen species are generated, especially hydrogen peroxide. There are three possible reasons for the free radical and nonradical production observed in ischemic tissue. First, activation of neutrophils by compounds released by the damaged tissues results in the generation of hydrogen peroxide and superoxide radicals [1–3]. Second, injury may result in disruption of the respiratory chain, with more electrons leaked to oxygen for superoxide radical formation [1–4]. Third, for tissues such as the intestine and possibly endothelial cells of blood vessels, the generation of xanthine oxidase results in free radical formation [1–4]. During ischemia, xanthine dehydrogenase is converted to xanthine oxidase via oxidation of sulfhydryl groups and/or proteolysis. Both xanthine dehydrogenase and xanthine oxidase require molybdenum and riboflavin as FAD and catalyze hypoxanthine and xanthine degradation. In hypoxic tissue, ADP is degraded (because of lack of oxygen for ATP generation), producing lots of hypoxanthine. During the medical treatment of ischemia, oxygen is administered to the patient. While the oxygen helps prevent organ damage, the large quantities of oxygen given with this **reperfusion** provide xanthine oxidase with the oxygen (O_2) needed to oxidize hypoxanthine and xanthine and also generate H_2O_2, as shown on page 479. The production of these reactive oxygen species by xanthine oxidase can further damage the already injured tissue [1–3].

Other cellular oxidases, such as amine oxidase (which is copper dependent), also generate hydrogen peroxide. The reaction catalyzed by amine oxidase, found in the blood and body tissues, is as follows:

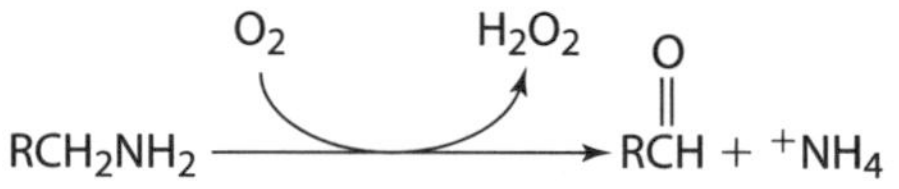

Concentrations of hydrogen peroxide, like superoxide radicals, need to be controlled in the body cells to prevent cellular destruction. Hydrogen peroxide easily diffuses in water and in lipids within cells and to tissues to cause damage. It also can react with superoxide radicals to produce a highly reactive and destructive hydroxyl radical.

The Hydroxyl Radical

The hydroxyl radical ($^{\cdot}OH$) is an oxygen-centered radical. It can be produced when the body is exposed to γ-rays, low-wavelength electromagnetic radiation. These rays split water in the body to form the hydroxyl radical: $H_2O \longrightarrow H^{\cdot} + {}^{\cdot}OH$.

Hydroxyl radicals also are produced from reactions between hydrogen peroxide and superoxide radicals (known as the Haber-Weiss reaction), as shown here,

$$H_2O_2 + O_2^- \longrightarrow O_2 + OH^- + {}^{\cdot}OH$$

or from other electrons and protons, as shown here:

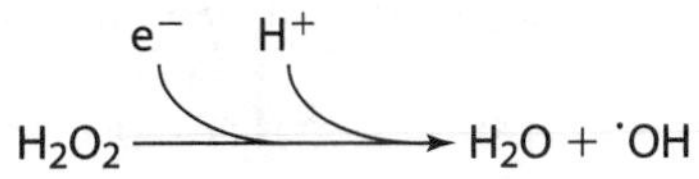

Hydrogen peroxide in contact with free ferrous iron can result in the formation of hydroxyl radicals. However, iron normally is bound to proteins and is not found free in cells. Should the iron be freed (protein-bound—$Fe^{3+} + O_2^- \longrightarrow$ free $Fe^{3+} + O_2^- \longrightarrow O_2 + Fe^{2+}$), the following reaction, known as the Fenton reaction, may generate the hydroxyl radical:

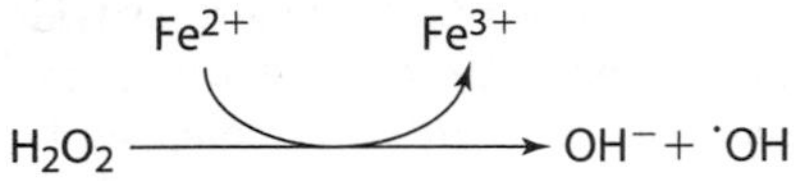

In this reaction, the hydrogen peroxide is functioning as an iron-oxidizing agent. Free copper also is able to react with hydrogen peroxide, but copper, like iron, is found bound to proteins in vivo.

According to Diplock [5], ·OH is a severe threat to living systems. The hydroxyl radical is thought to be one of the most potent of reactive radicals and to attack all molecules in the body [6]. Free hydroxy radicals rapidly take electrons from the surroundings. The hydroxyl radical is thought to be a major initiator of lipid peroxidation. Thus, removal of free hydroxyl radicals is important to prevent the destruction of cell components.

Carbon-Centered, Peroxyl, and Hydroperoxyl Radicals and Lipid Peroxides

Peroxyl (O_2^{2-}) and hydroperoxyl (HO^{2-}) radicals (oxygen centered) can be formed in the body from superoxide radicals reacting with additional electrons and hydrogen, as shown here:

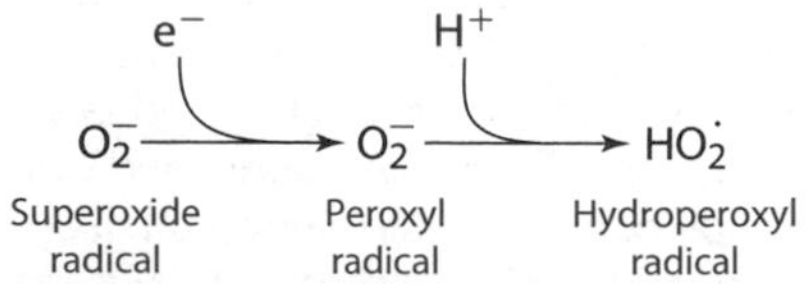

The peroxyl radical, as well as the hydroxyl and alkoxyl radicals, is more reactive than the superoxide radical [6].

Lipid carbon-centered radicals ($L^{\cdot}$) are produced in the body when radicals such as hydroxyl radicals ($^{\cdot}OH$) attack polyunsaturated fatty acids (LH) in the phospholipids of membranes or attack other organic compounds. The initiation reaction in the attack of a polyunsaturated fatty acid may be written as follows:

$$LH + {}^{\cdot}OH \longrightarrow L^{\cdot} + H_2O \text{ (initiation)}$$

Alternately, the reaction may be viewed showing part of the polyunsaturated fatty acid as shown here:

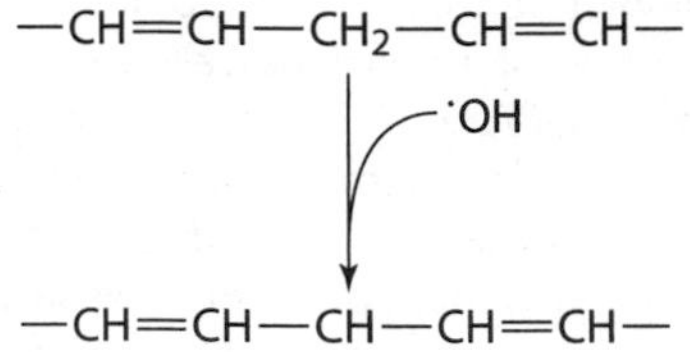

Propagation follows the initiation step, with products formed in one reaction being used as reactants in another reaction. Oxygen, for example, can react with the lipid carbon-centered radical to generate a peroxyl radical as follows:

$$L^{\cdot} + O_2 \longrightarrow LOO^{\cdot}$$

Alternately, this reaction may be expressed as follows:

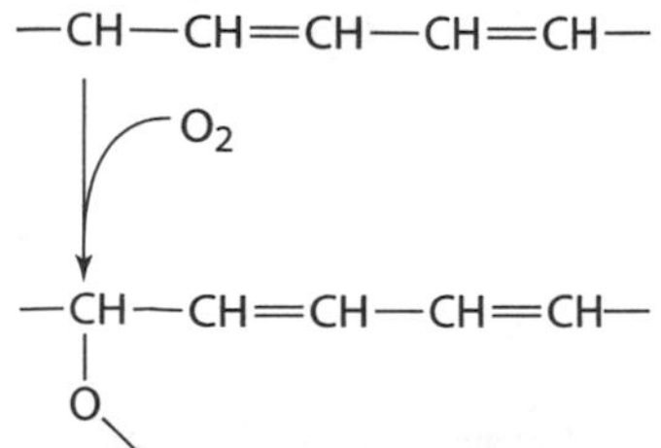

Oxygen also can react with polyunsaturated fatty acids (LH) to form carbon-centered radicals and hydroperoxyl radicals:

$$LH + O_2 \longrightarrow L^{\cdot} + HO_2^{\cdot}$$

In additional propagation reactions, peroxyl radicals ($LOO^{\cdot}$) may attack (abstract a hydrogen atom or proton from) other polyunsaturated fatty acids (L′H) in cell membranes to generate lipid peroxides (LOOH) and another carbon-centered radical.

$$LOO^{\cdot} + L'H \longrightarrow LOOH + L'^{\cdot}$$

This reaction may also be depicted as follows:

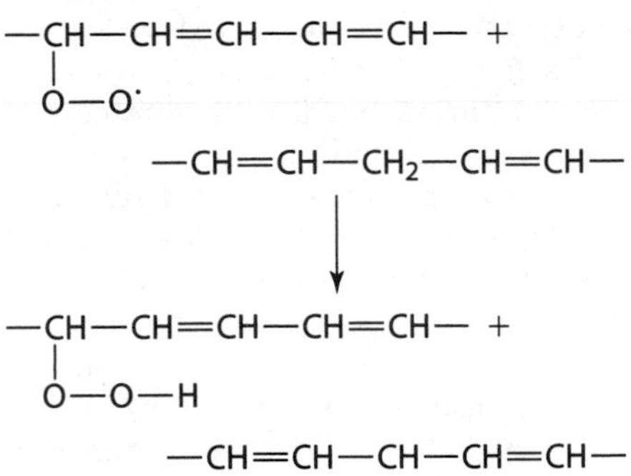

Should lipid peroxides (LOOH), also known as peroxidized fatty acids, come in contact with free iron, for example, alkoxyl ($LO^{\cdot}$) and peroxyl ($LOO^{\cdot}$) radicals also can be generated, as shown in these two reactions:

$$LOOH + Fe^{2+} \longrightarrow LO^{\cdot} + OH^- + Fe^{3+}$$

$$LOOH + Fe^{3+} \longrightarrow LOO^{\cdot} + H^+ + Fe^{2+}$$

Like peroxyl radicals, the alkoxyl radical can in turn initiate chain reactions with other polyunsaturated fatty acids in membranes, as follows:

$$LO^{\cdot} + L'H \longrightarrow LOH + L'^{\cdot}$$

However, again it is important to note that in vivo little or no free iron appears to be available to initiate such reactions.

Singlet Molecular Oxygen

Singlet molecular oxygen ($^1O_2$) possesses higher energy and is more reactive than ground-state oxygen. Specifically, in singlet oxygen the peripheral electron in the oxygen structure is excited to an orbital above the one it normally occupies [5]. This excited form of oxygen can be generated from lipid peroxidation of membranes, by enzymatic reactions such as occur with the respiratory burst in white blood cells, or via photochemical reactions, as shown:

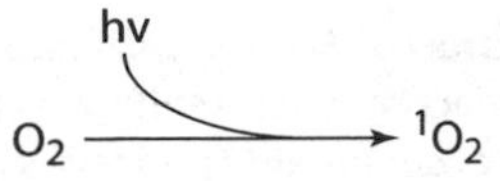

Singlet oxygen, being a reactive oxygen species, can, like free radicals, damage cells and tissues unless it is removed from the body.

Damage Due to Reactive Species

Once formed, free radicals attack, taking electrons from cell constituents (including nucleic acid in DNA in the cell nucleus) as well as from proteins (especially amino acids such as proline, histidine, or arginine and those with sulfhydryl groups such as cysteine) and polyunsaturated fatty acids (PUFAs) found in cell membranes or in the membranes of intracellular organelles such as those of the nucleus, mitochondria, or endoplasmic reticulum. Hydroxyl radical–induced changes in purine and pyrimidine bases in DNA may lead to mutations or breakages, which if not repaired may result, for example, in cancer [4]. Attack on amino acids in proteins by reactive oxygen species may break the peptide bonds in the protein backbone or disrupt the protein structure. Oxidative damage to proteins may cause cross-linking between amino acids or aggregation resulting in changes in the secondary or tertiary structures. Such events may even lead to premature degradation of the protein. Free radical attack on polyunsaturated fatty acids present in the phospholipid portion of the cell membranes can lead to degradation of the lipid. Extensive damage in a red blood cell, for example, may cause hemolysis of the membrane and thus the cell [7–9]. Aqueous peroxyl and peroxy nitrite radicals may induce oxidation of LDLs. Furthermore, radicals give rise to more radicals and thus more damage.

Antioxidant Nutrient Functions

Overproduction of reactive oxygen and nitrogen species and their attack on DNA, proteins, and polyunsaturated fatty acids have been implicated as a cause of or contributor to a variety of conditions and diseases such as cancer, heart disease, cataracts, and complications of diabetes mellitus, among others. Vitamins, along with several other antioxidant compounds, function to help control or eliminate free radicals. The destruction of reactive species by some of the antioxidant nutrients and compounds is reviewed in this section and shown in Figure 2.

Elimination of Superoxide Radicals

The primary mechanism by which the body gets rid of superoxide radicals is conversion of the superoxide radicals to other compounds. Several antioxidant nutrients function to dispose of superoxide radicals. These nutrients include vitamin C as well as three minerals (zinc, copper, and manganese) that function as cofactors for enzymes involved in oxidant defense.

Vitamin C (ascorbate), being water-soluble and hydrophilic, is found in the aqueous parts of the body such as the blood or within the cytoplasm of the cells. Ascorbate (AH_2) can provide electrons to reduce the superoxide radical to form hydrogen peroxide and dehydroascorbate (DHAA).

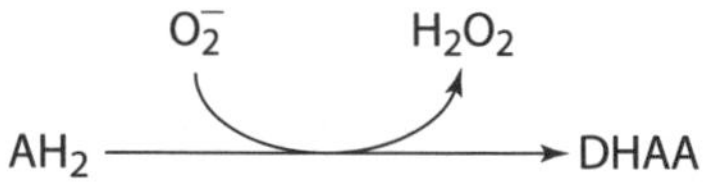

The conversion of superoxide radicals to hydrogen peroxide also is accomplished by the action of an enzyme called superoxide dismutase (SOD). In fact, superoxide dismutase works considerably faster than vitamin C in the inactivation of superoxide radicals. As previously mentioned, superoxide dismutase is found extracellularly as well as intracellularly. The extracellular form is found in exceptionally high concentrations in arterial blood vessels. Both the extracellular and the cytosolic forms of the enzyme are dependent on the presence of two minerals, zinc and copper. SOD in the mitochondria is dependent on manganese for activity. Thus, zinc, copper, and manganese are important minerals involved in the body's oxidant defense system. Superoxide dismutase eliminates superoxide radicals and forms hydrogen peroxide, as shown here:

$$O_2^- + O_2^- + 2H^+ \xrightarrow{\text{Superoxide dismutase}} H_2O_2 + O_2$$

Uric acid may help preserve the activity of superoxide dismutase [10,11].

Elimination of Hydrogen Peroxide

Hydrogen peroxide may be disposed of by several mechanisms in cells and tissues. Vitamin C readily reacts with hydrogen peroxide, as do some enzymes. Two enzymes that function in hydrogen peroxide disposal are glutathione peroxidase and catalase. A third enzyme, myeloperoxidase, utilizes the hydrogen peroxide for the generation of other radicals needed to help fight bacteria and viruses invading body cells. The role of vitamin C as well as that of each of the enzymes and their antioxidant nutrient cofactors will be presented here.

Vitamin C effectively scavenges hydrogen peroxide. Ascorbate (AH_2) reacts with hydrogen peroxide to produce water and dehydroascorbate (DHAA), as shown:

$$AH_2 + H_2O_2 \longrightarrow 2\,H_2O + DHAA$$

Glutathione peroxidase, found in the plasma as well as in the cytoplasm and mitochondria of cells, is an important enzyme necessary not only for removal of hydrogen peroxide but also for reduction of other peroxides. The enzyme requires the mineral selenium (four atoms) as a cofactor, and activity is impaired if selenium or iron status is poor. Because of selenium's role in glutathione peroxidase, the mineral is considered an antioxidant nutrient. The reaction catalyzed by glutathione peroxidase for hydrogen peroxide removal requires the tripeptide glutathione (composed of glycine, cysteine, and glutamic acid) in its reduced form (GSH), as shown:

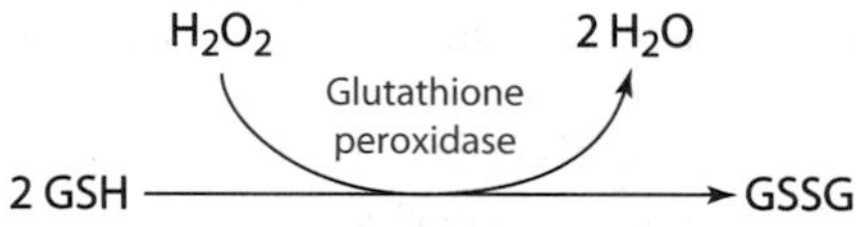

Glutathione is one of many thiols found in both aqueous and lipophilic parts of the body. Thiols are characterized by the presence of sulfhydryl residues (R-SH) and include glutathione, thioredoxin, and lipoic acid, among others. Glutathione (GSH) serves as a reducing agent and during reactions becomes oxidized. In the reaction for hydrogen peroxide removal, each of the two glutathione molecules gives up a hydrogen from its sulfhydryl group (SH). A radical center is formed on the sulfur atom (GS·) until two glutathiyl radicals join to form a disulfide bond (GSSG).

Catalase is another key enzyme involved in the removal of hydrogen peroxide. This enzyme is heme iron–dependent and found mostly in cell peroxisomes (cytoplasmic organelles where lots of hydrogen peroxide is produced during oxidation of very long chain fatty acids among other molecules). Smaller amounts of the enzyme also are found in the cytosol, mitochondria, and microsomes of cells. Neutrophils and other white blood cells contain fairly high quantities of catalase to dispose of hydrogen peroxide no longer needed in the respiratory burst required for phagocytosis of foreign bacteria, viruses, and fungi. Higher concentrations of hydrogen peroxide are

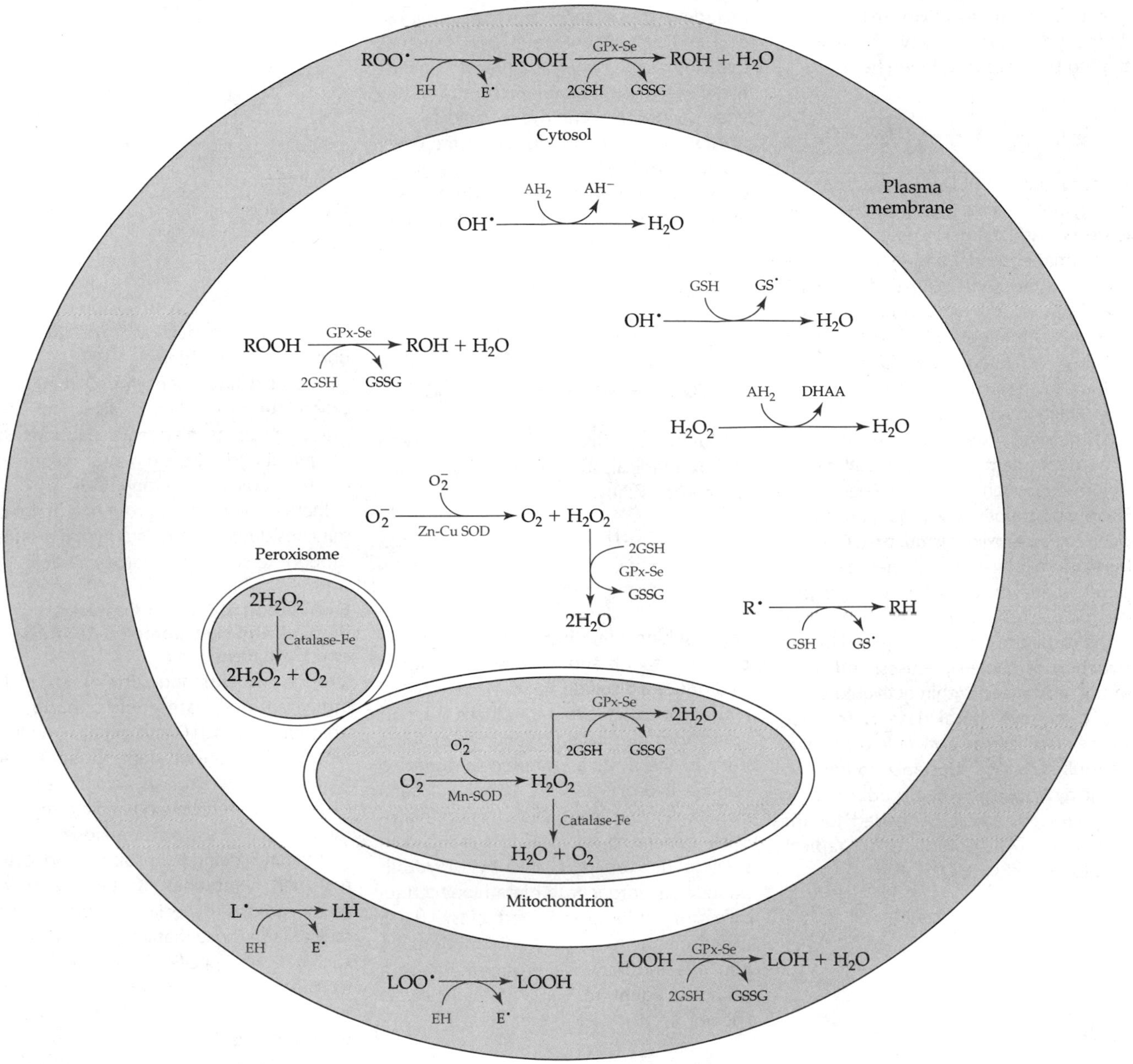

Abbreviations

EH = vitamin E
AH_2 = vitamin C
SOD = superoxide dismutase
GSH = reduced glutathione
GSSG = oxidized glutathione
O_2^- = superoxide radical
$LOO^\bullet$ = peroxy radical
LH = unsaturated fatty acid
$L^\bullet$ = carbon-centered lipid radical
RH = organic nonlipid compound
$R^\bullet$ = carbon-centered nonlipid radical
H_2O_2 = hydrogen peroxide
$ROO^\bullet$ = nonlipid peroxy radical
ROOH = nonlipid peroxides
LOOH = lipid peroxides

Figure 2 The interactions among selected antioxidant nutrients to prevent cell damage.

required for catalase activity than for glutathione peroxidase activity. The reaction catalyzed by catalase is shown here:

$$2\,H_2O_2 \xrightarrow{\text{Catalase}} 2\,H_2O + O_2$$

Thus, accumulation of H_2O_2 is prevented by two enzymes, catalase and glutathione peroxidase. Glutathione peroxidase, because of its dual (mitochondrial and cytosolic) locations in the cell and because of its higher activity with lower hydrogen peroxide concentrations, is thought to be more active in the removal of hydrogen peroxide from body cells than catalase. Figure 2 shows the complex interaction among components of the oxidant defense system, including the roles of iron-dependent catalase (catalase-Fe), selenium-dependent glutathione peroxidase (GPx-Se), and copper-, zinc-, and manganese-dependent superoxide dismutase (SOD).

Myeloperoxidase is a heme iron–dependent enzyme that uses hydrogen peroxide for the respiratory burst. Remember that the respiratory burst is required for the destruction of bacteria, viruses, and other harmful substances. Within activated white blood cells, myeloperoxidase is released from the granules into a vacuole containing the engulfed foreign substance. In this vacuole, the hydrogen peroxide, produced from the superoxide radical, is needed for the production of a potent toxic radical, hypochlorous acid (HOCl).

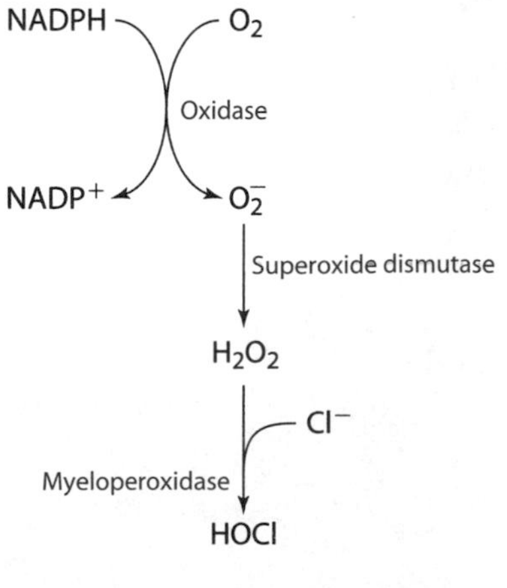

Hypochlorous acid, along with other potent compounds, assists in the destruction of the foreign bacteria's cell membranes to promote death (lysis) of the foreign substance.

Elimination of Hydroxyl Radicals

Vitamin C and other water-soluble compounds such as uric acid, various thiols including glutathione and dihydrolipoic acid, and possibly other substances such as metallothionein serve as defenses against hydroxyl radicals. Vitamin E, in contrast, is less effective in eliminating hydroxyl radicals.

Vitamin C can rapidly and effectively react, in aqueous solutions such as blood, with reactive oxygen species prior to their initiation of oxidative damage [12]. Vitamin C (AH_2) reacts with the hydroxyl radical to produce water and the fairly nonreactive semidehydroascorbate radical (AH^-).

$$^{\cdot}OH \xrightarrow{AH_2 \;\to\; AH^-} H_2O$$

Glutathione may react directly with hydroxyl radicals in aqueous or lipid environments, as shown:

$$^{\cdot}OH \xrightarrow{GSH \;\to\; GS^{\cdot}} H_2O$$

The resulting glutathiyl radical ($GS^{\cdot}$) typically reacts with another glutathiyl radical to produce a disulfide, GSSG.

Dihydrolipoic acid, the reduced form of lipoic acid (also called thioctic acid), functions in the body as a reducing agent to remove hydroxyl radicals (among others) from the environment. Dietary or endogenously generated lipoic acid is reduced in cells to dihydrolipoic acid by dihydrolipamide dehydrogenase, glutathione reductase, or thioredoxin reductase [13]. Dihydrolipoic acid in turn functions in aqueous and lipophilic environments as a reducing agent to eliminate radicals, as shown:

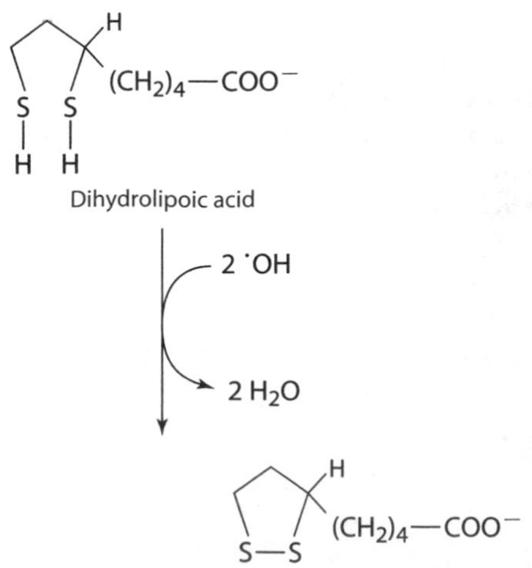

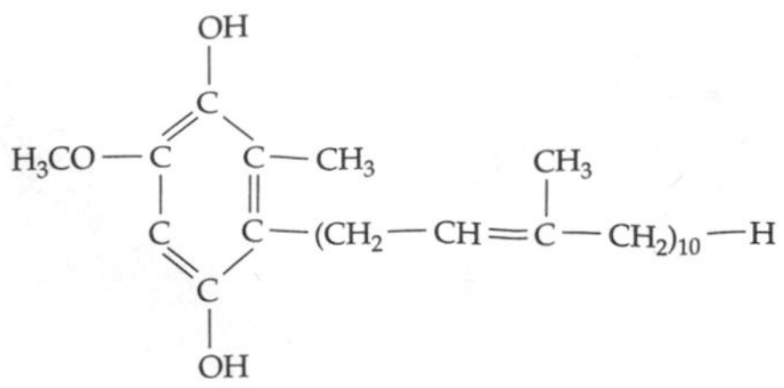

Figure 3 Coenzyme Q or Q_{10} in its reduced form ($CoQH_2$), also called ubiquinol.

Supplementation with α-lipoic acid has been shown to decrease oxidative stress under some conditions [14,15].

Uric acid and coenzyme Q or Q_{10}, also called **ubiquinol** (Fig. 3), also may act as reducing agents in aqueous solutions. Both ubiquinol and uric acid may scavenge various free radicals, including $^{\cdot}OH$.

Metallothionein, a protein rich in cysteine residues and thus sulfhydryl groups, is thought to scavenge hydroxyl radicals [16].

Elimination of Carbon-Centered, Peroxyl, and Hydroperoxyl Radicals and Lipid Peroxides

Several nutrients and compounds, including vitamin E, carotenoids, manganese, ubiquinol, vitamin C, and glutathione, along with the selenium-dependent enzyme glutathione peroxidase, actively eliminate carbon-centered, peroxyl, and hydroperoxyl radicals as well as lipid peroxides.

Vitamin E, being lipid-soluble and located near or in membranes, effectively reacts with many radicals, especially carbon-centered radicals and those that initiate peroxidation, such as $LOO^{\cdot}$. Specifically, vitamin E donates its phenolic hydrogen on the carbon 6 hydroxyl group. Vitamin E's chromanol ring then stabilizes the unpaired electron.

- Vitamin E (EH) terminates carbon-centered radicals (as shown below) before they abstract further hydrogens from other polyunsaturated fatty acids:

$$L^{\cdot} + EH \longrightarrow LH + E^{\cdot}$$

- Vitamin E (EH) prevents peroxidation of polyunsaturated fatty acids by reacting with peroxyl radicals ($LOO^{\cdot}$), as illustrated in this reaction:

$$LOO^{\cdot} + EH \longrightarrow LOOH + E^{\cdot}$$

Thus, vitamin E terminates chain-propagation reactions.

Carotenoids such as β-carotene also have the ability to react directly with peroxyl radicals involved in lipid peroxidation [17].

β-carotene is thought to carry out this role to a lesser extent than vitamin E and perhaps to function more in the interior of the cell while vitamin E functions on or at the surface.

Some transition metals, such as manganese, may be able to scavenge peroxyl radicals as shown here [18]:

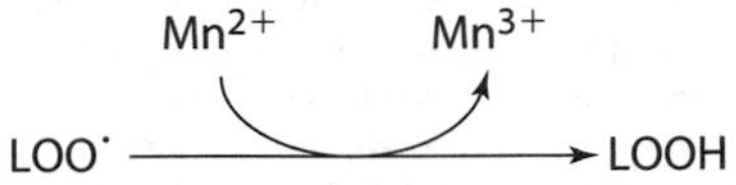

In addition to vitamin E, carotenoids, and manganese, ubiquinol (Fig. 3) has been shown to provide hydrogens to terminate peroxyl radicals and thus appears to be a potent antioxidant [19,20]. Ubiquinol (also called coenzyme Q_{10} or CoQ_{10} as $CoQH_2$), the reduced form of coenzyme Q_{10}, is a small fat-soluble molecule that functions in transporting electrons and ultimately generating ATP in the electron transport chain in the mitochondria. Ubiquinol has been found in small quantities in lipoproteins, where it is thought to be utilized before vitamin E in the termination of peroxyl radicals [20].

$$CoQH_2 + LOO^{\cdot} \longrightarrow CoQH^{\cdot} + LOOH$$

$CoQH^{\cdot}$ may be regenerated into $CoQH_2$ through the electron transport chain in the mitochondria. Supplementation of humans with 100 or 200 mg of ubiquinone-10 (CoQ), the oxidized form of ubiquinol, increased plasma and LDL ubiquinol concentrations and also increased LDL resistance to lipid peroxidation [19].

Vitamin C effectively scavenges alkoxyl and peroxyl radicals, as shown next.

$$AH_2 + LO^{\cdot} \longrightarrow AH^- + LOH$$

Both ascorbate (AH_2) and the ascorbate radical (AH^-) react with peroxyl radicals to produce a lipid peroxide and the ascorbate radical or dehydroascorbate (DHAA), respectively, as shown here:

$$AH_2 + LOO^{\cdot} \longrightarrow AH^- + LOOH$$

$$LOO^{\cdot} + AH^- \longrightarrow LOOH + DHAA$$

While the elimination of $LOO^{\cdot}$ is helpful, the often simultaneous generation of lipid peroxides/peroxidized fatty acids (LOOH) can cause problems if the peroxidized fatty acids are within hydrophobic regions of cell membranes. The problems occur because peroxidized fatty acids are polar compounds and the polarized peroxidized fatty acids, once liberated from the phospholipid in the membrane by the actions of phospholipase A_2, will migrate and destroy the normal architecture of the cell in migrating from the nonpolar region of generation.

Glutathione and the selenium-dependent enzyme glutathione peroxidase function in the elimination of lipid peroxides. Thiols like glutathione act in both aqueous and lipid environments as antioxidants by providing reducing equivalents (hydrogen ions). Glutathione peroxidase utilizes glutathione in its reduced form (GSH) and catalyzes the conversion of the peroxides (LOOH) to hydroxy acids (LOH) as follows:

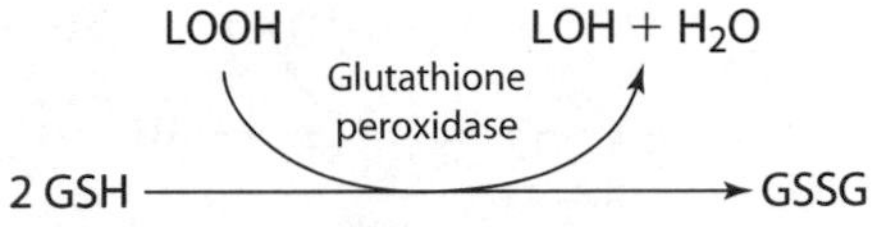

Thioredoxin, which is discussed more on page 376, also can reduce lipid peroxides [21].

Elimination of Singlet Molecular Oxygen

Carotenoids, as well as vitamin C and thiols (especially lipoic acid), may quench singlet molecular oxygen. Carotenoids such as β-carotene and lycopene have the ability to directly quench hundreds of singlet oxygen molecules either in solution or in membrane systems. Quenching is a process by which electronically excited molecules, such as singlet molecular oxygen, are inactivated [22]. The ability of carotenoids to quench singlet oxygen is attributed to the conjugated double-bond systems within the carotenoid structure. The carotenoids can absorb energy from the singlet oxygen without chemical change to return the "excited" $^1O_2$ to its ground state [5]. Carotenoids then release the energy in the form of heat and thus do not need to be regenerated.

$$^1O_2 + \beta\text{-carotene} \longrightarrow {}^3O_2 + \text{excited } \beta\text{-carotene} \longrightarrow \beta\text{-carotene} + \text{heat}$$

Lycopene has been shown to be more effective than β-carotene in quenching singlet oxygen [23,24].

Regeneration of Antioxidants

The provision of reducing equivalents by antioxidants results in oxidation of the antioxidants. Regeneration of the antioxidants is important for further defense against free radicals. It has been estimated that there are fewer than nine vitamin E molecules for every one to two thousand unsaturated fatty acids in cell membrane phospholipids or lipoprotein molecules. Thus, the regeneration or recycling of vitamins is critical for the vitamin to regain its antioxidant function. This section provides discussion of some of the compounds that function in the body to recycle antioxidants.

Vitamin E Regeneration

The regeneration of vitamin E is thought to initially require the migration of the vitamin to the membrane surface. At the cell surface, several compounds have been shown to regenerate vitamin E.

Ascorbate (AH_2) can regenerate α-tocopherol from its radical form ($E^{\cdot}$) and in the process becomes a radical itself, AH^-, which needs to be regenerated.

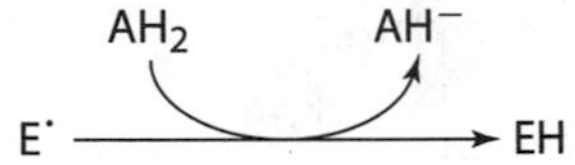

Ubiquinol ($CoQH_2$) also functions to recycle vitamin E, as shown:

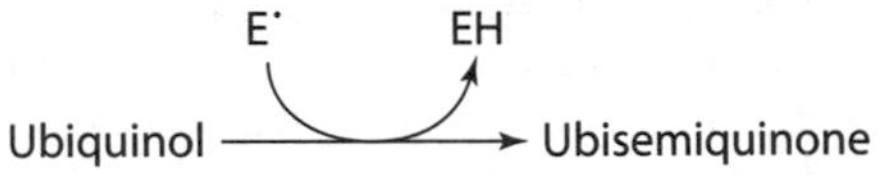

Glutathione in its reduced form (GSH) may donate its hydrogen atom to re-form vitamin E as follows:

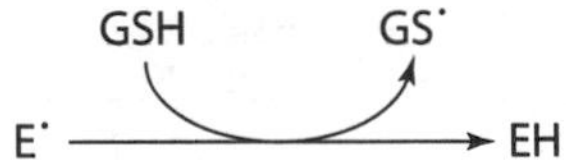

Ubiquinol (Coenzyme QH_2) and Thioredoxin Regeneration

Regeneration of vitamin E by ubiquinol ($CoQH_2$) results in the formation of ubisemiquinone ($CoQH^{\cdot}$). Ubisemiquinone can be converted back to ubiquinol by dihydrolipoic acid (DHLA), as shown here,

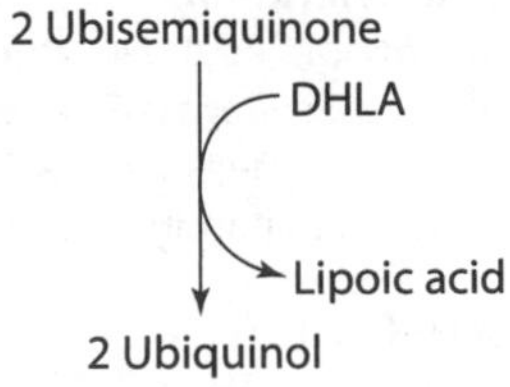

or by the thioredoxin–thioredoxin reductase system. This system, ubiquitous in the body, includes thioredoxin (Trx), a small protein with a dithiol (two sulfhydryl groups, $-(SH)_2$), and the selenium-dependent flavoenzyme (FAD) thioredoxin reductase with a selenocysteine residue at its active site [25,26]. The recycling of ubiquinol is shown here:

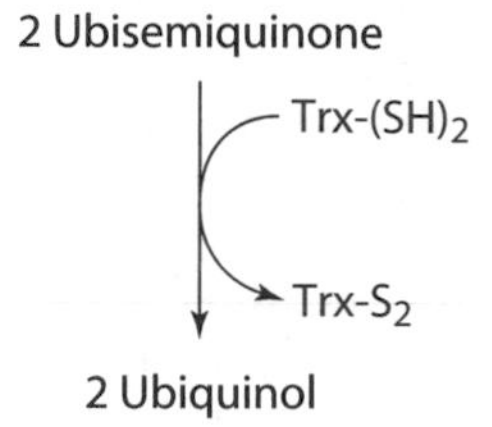

Thioredoxin reductase (TrxR) functions to maintain thioredoxin in its reduced form utilizing reducing equivalents from NADPH, as shown here:

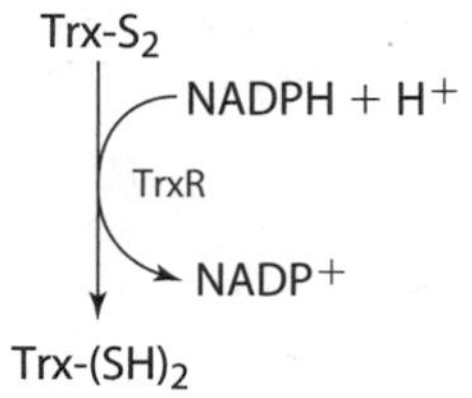

Glutathione Regeneration

Glutathione reductase, a flavoprotein requiring FAD as a cofactor, functions to regenerate oxidized glutathione (GSSG), with niacin as NADPH providing the reducing equivalents, as shown:

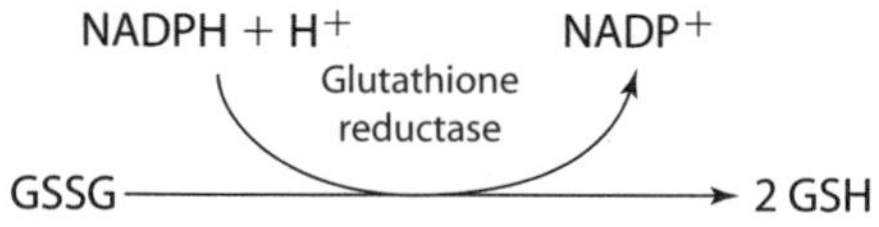

Dihydrolipoic acid (DHLA) also is thought to be able to regenerate glutathione, as shown here:

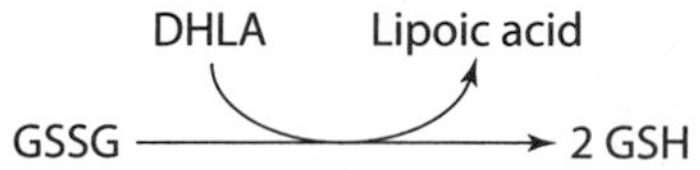

Vitamin C Regeneration

Niacin, dihydrolipoic acid, glutathione, and thioredoxin assist in vitamin C regeneration. Niacin in its coenzyme form NADH allows the regeneration of vitamin C as follows:

$$2\,AH^- + NADH + H^+ \longrightarrow 2\,AH_2 + NAD^+$$

Dihydrolipoic acid provides hydrogens to the dehydro form of vitamin C to recycle ascorbate.

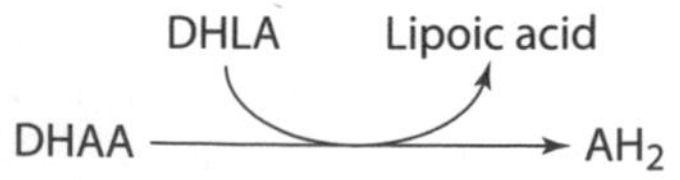

The reaction shown below depicts glutathione (GSH) donating hydrogen atoms to help recycle vitamin C from its radical (AH^-) and dehydroascorbate (DHAA) forms [27]:

$$2\,GSH + 2\,AH^- \longrightarrow GSSG + 2\,AH_2$$
$$DHAA + 2\,GSH \longrightarrow AH_2 + GSSG$$

Not all vitamin C, however, is typically regenerated. Dehydroascorbate is fairly stable in cells but is present in fairly low concentrations.

Thioredoxin also provides reducing equivalents to dehydroascorbate, as shown here:

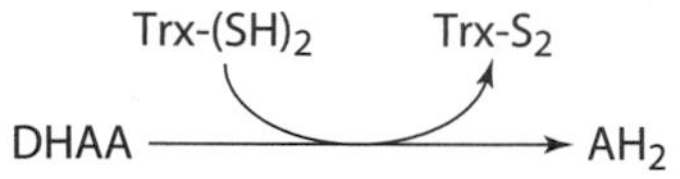

Interactions between the vitamin C radicals also permit ascorbate regeneration. Two vitamin C radicals may interact to produce ascorbate (AH_2) and dehydroascorbate (DHAA) as follows:

$$2\,AH^- \longrightarrow AH_2 + DHAA$$

Antioxidants and Disease

Overproduction of reactive species is thought to contribute to aging and the development of several diseases or conditions, including some cancers, heart disease, cataracts, diabetes mellitus complications, and ischemia-reperfusion injury. In vitro, nutrients often demonstrate specific functions or abilities, such as inhibition of lipoprotein cholesterol oxidation or inhibition of cell proliferation or transformation, that are thought to be able to prevent the development of disease [28–39]. Despite the promising results of many in vitro studies, however, the results of supplementation trials in vivo for disease prevention or treatment are inconsistent [40–47]. Similarly, while many studies have shown that individuals who either consume diets rich in foods (especially fruits and vegetables) containing antioxidant nutrients or have good plasma antioxidant nutrient concentrations have a lower risk of many diseases or conditions, other studies do not support such associations [48–78]. New supplementation trials as well as in vitro and in vivo studies are being conducted to better elucidate the roles and effects of antioxidants. As these studies continue to clarify the roles of the antioxidant nutrients, scientists and other health professionals will continue to reevaluate current recommendations. New guidelines defining optimal levels of nutrients to prevent diseases may be developed.

References Cited

1. Halliwell B, Gutteridge H. Free Radicals in Biology and Medicine. Oxford: Clarendon Press, 1989.
2. McCord J. Free radicals and myocardial ischemia: overview and outlook. Free Radical Biol Med 1988;4:9–14.
3. Baker G, Corry R, Autor A. Oxygen free radical induced damage in kidneys subjected to warm ischemia and reperfusion. Ann Surgery 1985;202:628–41.
4. Halliwell B, Evans P, Kaur H, Aruoma O. Free radicals, tissue injury, and human disease: a potential for therapeutic use of antioxidants? In: Kinney JM, Tuck HN, eds. Organ Metabolism and Nutrition: Ideas for Future Critical Care. New York: Raven Press, 1994, pp. 425–45.
5. Diplock A. Antioxidant nutrients and disease prevention: an overview. Am J Clin Nutr 1991;53:189S–93S.
6. Buettner G. The pecking order of free radicals and antioxidants: lipid peroxidation, α-tocopherol, and ascorbate. Arch Biochem Biophys 1993;300:535–43.
7. Niki E. Action of ascorbic acid as a scavenger of active and stable oxygen radicals. Am J Clin Nutr 1991; 54:1119S–24S.
8. Frei B. Ascorbic acid protects lipids in human plasma and low density lipoprotein against oxidative damage. Am J Clin Nutr 1991;54:1113S–18S.
9. Niki E, Yamamota Y, Komuro E, Sato K. Membrane damage due to lipid oxidation. Am J Clin Nutr 1991;53:201S–5S.
10. Hink H, Santanam N, Sikalov S, McCann L, Nguyen A, Parthasarathy S, Harrison D, Fukai T. Peroxidase properties of extracellular superoxide dismutase: role of uric acid in modulating in vivo activity. Atherosclerosis, Thrombosis, and Vascular Biology 2002;22:1402–8.
11. Landmesser U, Drexler H. Toward understanding of extracellular superoxide dismutase regulation in atherosclerosis: a novel role of uric acid. Atherosclerosis, Thrombosis, and Vascular Biology 2002;22:1367–68.
12. Frei B, England L, Ames B. Ascorbate is an outstanding antioxidant in human blood plasma. Proc Natl Acad Sci USA 1989;86:6377–81.
13. Moini H, Packer L, Saris N. Antioxidant and prooxidant activities of α-lipoic acid and dihydrolipoic acid. Tox Appl Pharm 2002;182:84–90.
14. Marangon K, Devaraj S, Tirosh O, Packer L, Jialal I. Comparison of the effect of alpha lipoic acid and alpha tocopherol supplementation on measures of oxidative stress. Free Rad Biol Med 1999;27:1114–21.
15. Khanna S, Atalay M, Laaksonen D, Gul M, Roy S, Sen C. Alpha lipoic acid supplementation: tissue glutathione homeostasis at rest and after exercise. J Appl Physiol 1999;86:1191–96.
16. Sato M, Bremner I. Oxygen free radicals and metallothionein. Free Rad Biol Med 1993;14:325–37.
17. Burton G, Ingold K. β-carotene: an unusual type of lipid antioxidant. Science 1984;224:569–73.
18. Coassin M, Ursini F, Bindoli A. Antioxidant effect of manganese. Arch Biochem Biophys 1992;299:330–33.
19. Thomas S, Neuzil J, Mohr D, Stocker R. Coantioxidants make α-tocopherol an efficient antioxidant for low density lipoprotein. Am J Clin Nutr 1995; 62 (suppl):1357S–64S.
20. Mohr D, Bowry V, Stocker R. Dietary supplementation with coenzyme Q_{10} results in increased levels of ubiquinol-10 within circulating lipoproteins and increased resistance of human low density lipoprotein to the initiation of lipid peroxidation. Biochim Biophys Acta 1992;1126:247–54.

21. Miranda-Vizuete A, Damdimopoulos A, Spyrou G. The mitochondrial thioredoxin system. Antioxidants and Redox Signaling 2000;2:801–10.

22. Mascio P, Murphy M, Sies H. Antioxidant defense systems: the role of carotenoids, tocopherols, and thiols. Am J Clin Nutr 1991;53:194S–200S.

23. Bohm F, Haley J, Truscott T, Schalch W. Cellular bound β-carotene quenches singlet oxygen in man. J Photochem Photobiol B Biol 1993;21:219–21.

24. Conn P, Schalch W, Truscott T. The singlet oxygen and carotenoid interaction. J Photochem Photobiol B 1991;11:41–47.

25. Nordberg J, Arner E. Reactive oxygen species, antioxidants, and the mammalian thioredoxin system. Free Rad Biol Med 2001;31:1287–312.

26. Deneke S. Thiol-based antioxidants. Curr Top Cell Reg 2000;36:151–80.

27. Martensson J, Han J, Griffith O, Meister A. Glutathione esters delay the onset of scurvy in ascorbate-deficient guinea pigs. Proc Natl Acad Sci USA 1993;90:317–21.

28. Abbey M, Nestel P, Baghurst P. Antioxidant vitamins and low-density-lipoprotein oxidation. Am J Clin Nutr 1993;58:525–32.

29. Esterbauer H, Dieber-Rotheneder M, Striegl G, Waeg G. Role of vitamin E in preventing the oxidation of low-density lipoprotein. Am J Clin Nutr 1991;53:314S–21S.

30. Niki E, Noguchi N, Tsuchihashi H, Gotoh N. Interaction among vitamin C, vitamin E, and β-carotene. Am J Clin Nutr 1995;62(suppl):1322S–26S.

31. Jialal I, Grundy S. Effect of dietary supplementation with alpha tocopherol on the oxidative modification of low density lipoprotein. J Lipid Res 1992;33:899–906.

32. Mosca L, Rubenfire M, Mandel C, Rock C, Tarshis T, Tsai A, Pearson T. Antioxidant nutrient supplementation reduces the susceptibility of low density lipoprotein to oxidation in patients with coronary artery disease. J Am Coll Cardiol 1997;30:392–99.

33. Jialal I, Grundy S. Effect of combined supplementation with α-tocopherol, ascorbate, and beta-carotene on low-density lipoprotein oxidation. Circulation 1993; 88:2780–86.

34. Allard J, Royall D, Kurian R, Muggli R, Jeejeebhoy K. Effects of β-carotene supplementation on lipid peroxidation in humans. Am J Clin Nutr 1994;59:884–90.

35. Bertram J, Bortkiewicz H. Dietary carotenoids inhibit neoplastic transformation and modulate gene expression in mouse and human cells. Am J Clin Nutr 1995;62(suppl):1327S–36S.

36. Bertram J, Pung A, Churley M, Kappock T, Wilkins L, Cooney R. Diverse carotenoids protect against chemically induced neoplastic transformation. Carcinogenesis 1991;12:671–78.

37. Davis M, Austin J, Partridge D. Vitamin C: Its Chemistry and Biochemistry. Cambridge, England: Royal Society of Chemistry, 1991.

38. Tannenbaum S, Wishnok J, Leaf C. Inhibition of nitrosamine formation by ascorbic acid. Am J Clin Nutr 1991;53:247S–50S.

39. Schorah C, Sobala G, Sanderson M, Collis N, Primrose J. Gastric juice ascorbic acid: effects of disease and implications for gastric carcinogenesis. Am J Clin Nutr 1991;53:287S–93S.

40. Harward T, Coe D, Souba W, Kingman N, Seeger J. Glutamine preserves gut glutathione levels during intestinal ischemia/reperfusion. J Surg Res 1994;56:351–55.

41. Stephens N, Parsons A, Schofield P, Kelly F, Cheeseman K, Mitchinson M, Brown M. Randomised controlled trial of vitamin E in patients with coronary disease: Cambridge Heart Antioxidant Study (CHAOS). Lancet 1996;347:781–86.

42. Stampfer M, Hennekens C, Manson J, Colditz G, Rosner B, Willett W. Vitamin E consumption and the risk of coronary disease in women. N Eng J Med 1993; 328:1444–9.

43. Rimm E, Stampfer M, Ascherio A, Giovannucci E, Colditz G, Willett W. Vitamin E consumption and the risk of coronary heart disease in men. N Engl J Med 1993;328:1450–56.

44. GISSI-Prevenzione Investigators. Dietary supplementation with n-3 polyunsaturated fatty acids and vitamin E after myocardial infarction: results of the GISSI-Prevenzione Trial. Lancet 1999;354:447–55.

45. HOPE Study Investigators. Vitamin E supplementation and cardiovascular events in high risk patients. N Engl J Med 2000;342:154–60.

46. Alpha-tocopherol, beta-carotene (ATBC) cancer prevention study group. The effect of vitamin E and beta carotene on the incidence of lung cancer and other cancers in male smokers. N Engl J Med 1994;330:1029–35.

47. Omenn G, Goodman G, Thomquist M, Balmes J, Cullen M, Glass A, Keogh J, Meyskens F, Valanis B, Williams J, Barnhart S, Hammar S. Effects of a combination of beta carotene and vitamin A on lung cancer and cardiovascular disease. N Engl J Med 1996;334:1150–55.

48. Block G. Vitamin C and cancer: epidemiologic evidence of reduced risk. Ann NY Acad Sci 1992;669:280–90.

49. Block G. Vitamin C and cancer prevention: the epidemiologic evidence. Am J Clin Nutr 1991;53:270S–82S.

50. Block G, Patterson B, Subar A. Fruit, vegetables, and cancer prevention: a review of the epidemiological evidence. Nutr Cancer 1992;18:1–29.

51. Block G. The data support a role for antioxidants in reducing cancer risk. Nutr Rev 1992;50:207–13.

52. Byers T, Guerrero N. Epidemiologic evidence for vitamin C and vitamin E in cancer prevention. Am J Clin Nutr 1995;62(suppl):1385S–92S.

53. Ziegler R. Vegetables, fruits and carotenoids and risk of cancer. Am J Clin Nutr 1991;53(suppl):251S–59S.

54. Gaziano J, Hennekens C. The role of beta carotene in the prevention of cardiovascular disease. Ann NY Acad Sci 1993;69:148–54.

55. Morris D, Kritchevsky S, Davis C. Serum carotenoids and coronary heart disease. JAMA 1994;272:1439–41.

56. Poppel G, Goldbolm R. Epidemiologic evidence for β-carotene and cancer prevention. Am J Clin Invest 1995;62(suppl):1393S–1402S.

57. Gey K, Moser U, Jordan P, Sahelin H, Eichholzer M, Ludin E. Increased risk of cardiovascular disease at suboptimal plasma concentrations of essential antioxidants: an epidemiological update with special attention to carotene and vitamin C. Am J Clin Nutr 1993;57(suppl):787S–97S.

58. Weisburger J. Nutritional approach to cancer prevention with emphasis on vitamins, antioxidants, and carotenoids. Am J Clin Nutr 1991;53:226S–37S.

59. Noroozi M, Angerson W, Lean M. Effects of flavonoids and vitamin C on oxidative DNA damage to human lymphocytes. Am J Clin Nutr 1998;67:1210–18.

60. Taylor A, Jacques P, Epstein E. Relations among aging, antioxidant status, and cataract. Am J Clin Nutr 1995;62(suppl):1439S–47S.

61. Bendich A, Langseth L. The health effects of vitamin C supplementation: a review. J Am Coll Nutr 1995;14:124–36.

62. Jacques P, Taylor A, Hankinson S. Long term vitamin C supplement use and prevalence of early age-related lens opacities. Am J Clin Nutr 1997;66:911–16.

63. Varma S. Scientific basis for medical therapy of cataracts by antioxidants. Am J Clin Nutr 1991; 53:335S–45S.

64. Robertson J, Donner A, Trevithick J. A possible role for vitamins C and E in cataract prevention. Am J Clin Nutr 1991;53:346S–51S.

65. Taylor A, Jacques P, Epstein E. Relations among aging, antioxidant status, and cataract. Am J Clin Nutr 1995;62(suppl):1439S–47S.

66. Bendich A, Langseth L. The health effects of vitamin C supplementation: a review. J Am Coll Nutr 1995; 14:124–36.

67. Varma S. Scientific basis for medical therapy of cataracts by antioxidants. Am J Clin Nutr 1991; 53:335S–45S.

68. Robertson J, Donner A, Trevithick J. A possible role for vitamins C and E in cataract prevention. Am J Clin Nutr 1991;53:346S–51S.

69. Vitale S, West S, Hallfrisch J, Alston C, Wang F, Moorman C, Muller D, Singh V, Taylor H. Plasma antioxidants and risk of cortical and nuclear cataract. Epidemiology 1993;4:195–203.

70. Knekt P, Heliovaara M, Rissanen A, Aromaa A, Aaran R. Serum antioxidant vitamins and risk of cataract. Br Med J 1992;305:1392–94.

71. Leske M, Chylack L, Wu S. The Lens Opacities Case-Control Study. Risk factors for cataract. Arch Ophthalmol 1991;109:244–51.

72. Jacques P, Chylack L. Epidemiologic evidence of a role for the antioxidant vitamins and carotenoids in cataract prevention. Am J Clin Nutr 1991;53:352S–55S.

73. Gale C, Martyn C, Winter P, Cooper C. Vitamin C and risk of death from stroke and coronary heart disease in cohort of elderly people. Br Med J 1995;310:1563–66.

74. Singh R, Ghosh S, Niaz M, Singh R, Beegum R, Chibo H, Shoumin Z, Postiglione A. Dietary intake, plasma levels of antioxidant vitamins and oxidative stress in relation to coronary artery disease in elderly subjects. Am J Cardiol 1995;76:1233–38.

75. Simon J, Hudes E, Browner W. Serum ascorbic acid and cardiovascular disease prevalence in U.S. adults. Epidemiology 1998;9:316–21.

76. Knekt P, Peunanen A, Jarvinen R, Seppanen R, Heliovaara M, Aromaa A. Antioxidant vitamin intake and coronary mortality in a longitudinal population study. Am J Epidemiol 1994;139:1180–89.

77. Pandey D, Shekelle R, Selwyn B, Tangney C, Stamler J. Dietary vitamin C and beta-carotene and risk of death in middle-aged men. The Western Electric Study. Am J Epidemiol 1995;142:1269–78.

78. Losonczy K, Harris T, Havlik R. Vitamin E and vitamin C supplementation use and risk of all-cause and coronary heart disease mortality in older persons. The Established Populations for Epidemiologic Studies of the Elderly. Am J Clin Nutr 1996;64:190–96.

Web Sites

cancernet.nci.nih.gov
www.amhrt.org
www.cancer.org
www.preventcancer.org
www.dcpc.nci.nih.gov/5aday
www.nhlbi.nih.gov/nhlbi/cardio/cardio/htm

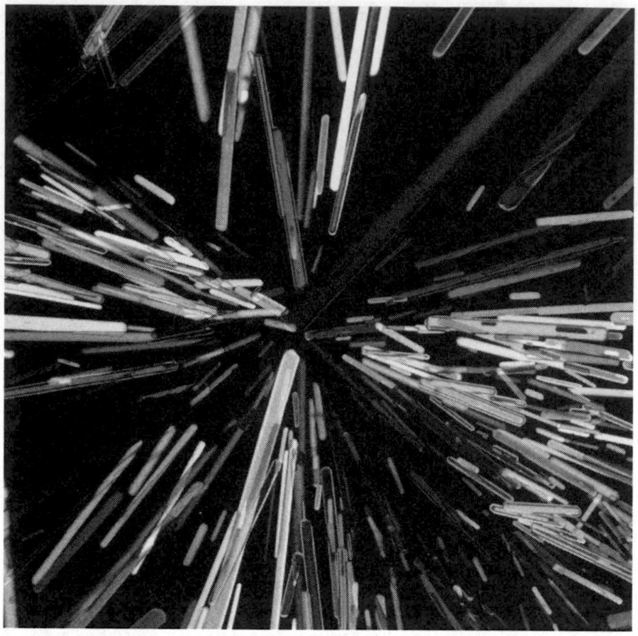

Polarized light micrograph of magnesium sulphate

chapter 11 Macrominerals

THE IMPORTANCE OF MINERALS IN NORMAL NUTRITION and metabolism cannot be overstated, despite the fact that they constitute only about 4% of total body weight. Their functions are many and varied. They provide the medium essential for normal cellular activity, determine the osmotic properties of body fluids, impart hardness to bones and teeth, and function as obligatory cofactors in metalloenzyme activity.

Historically, the awareness that minerals are required in normal nutrition evolved from knowledge of the mineral composition of body tissues and fluids. This knowledge has expanded greatly as a result of accumulating improvements in analytical techniques for quantification of minerals.

Macrominerals, also referred to as major minerals or macronutrient elements, are distinguished from the microminerals (Chaps. 12 and 13) by their occurrence in the body. Using this criterion, various definitions of a macromineral have been expressed, such as the requirement that it constitute at least 0.01% of total body weight or that it occur in a minimum quantity of 5 g in a 60-kg human body. Unfortunately, however, these values clearly are not equivalent. This discrepancy in itself indicates the

Table 11.1 Macrominerals: Functions, Body Content, Deficiency Symptoms, and Recommended Dietary Allowances (RDAs) or Adequate Intakes (AIs)

Mineral	Selected Physiological Functions	Approximate Body Content	Selected Enzyme Cofactors	Deficiency Symptoms	Selected Food Sources	RDA/AI
Calcium	Structural component of bones and teeth; role in cellular processes, muscle contraction, blood clotting, enzyme activation	1,400 g	Adenylate, cyclase, kinases, protein kinase, Ca^{2+}-Mg^{2+} ATPase (others, see Table 11.3)	Rickets, osteomalacia, osteoporosis, tetany	Milk, milk products, sardines, clams, oysters, turnip and mustard greens, broccoli, legumes, dried fruits	1,000 mg*, 19–50 years
Chloride	Primary anion; maintains pH balance, enzyme activation, component of gastric hydrochloric acid	105 g		In infants: loss of appetite, failure to thrive, weakness, lethargy, severe hypokalemia, metabolic acidosis	Table salt, seafood, milk, meat, eggs	
Magnesium	Component of bones; role in nerve impulse transmission, protein synthesis; enzyme cofactor	35 g	Hydrolysis and transfer of phosphate groups by phosphokinase; important in numerous ATP-dependant enzyme reactions	Neuromuscular hyperexcitability, muscle weakness, tetany	Nuts, legumes, whole-grain cereals, leafy green vegetables	400 mg males; 310 mg, females; 19–30 years
Phosphorus	Structural component of bone, teeth, cell membranes, phospholipids, nucleic acids, nucleotide coenzymes, ATP-ADP phosphate transferring system in cells, pH regulation	850 g	Activates many enzymes in phosphorylation and dephosphorylation	Neuromuscular, skeletal, hematologic, and cardiac manifestations; rickets, osteomalacia	Meat, poultry, fish, eggs, milk, milk products, nuts, legumes, grains, cereals	700 mg, 19+ years
Potassium	Water, electrolyte, and pH balances; cell membrane transfer	245 g	Pyruvate kinase, Na^+/K^+-ATPase	Muscular weakness, mental apathy, cardiac arrhythmias, paralysis, bone fragility	Avocado, banana, dried fruits, orange, peach, potatoes, dried beans, tomato, wheat bran, dairy products, eggs	Not established
Sodium	Water, pH, and electrolyte regulation; nerve transmission, muscle contraction	105 g	Na^+/K^+-ATPase	Anorexia, nausea, muscle atrophy, poor growth, weight loss	Table salt, meat, seafood, cheese, milk, bread, vegetables (abundant in most foods except fruits)	Not established
Sulfur	Component of sulfur-containing amino acids, lipoic acid, and 2 vitamins (thiamin, biotin)	175 g		Unknown	Protein foods—meat, poultry, fish, eggs, milk, cheese, legumes, nuts	Not established

Note: Abbreviations: ATP, adenosine triphosphate; ADP, adenosine diphosphate.

* Adequate intake.

desirability of a less ambiguous, standard definition, such as required in amounts >100 mg/day.

The major minerals of the human body traditionally include calcium, phosphorus, magnesium, sodium, potassium, and chloride. Because of their importance in the maintenance of electrolyte balance in body fluids, the macrominerals sodium, chloride, and potassium also are discussed in Chapter 14. Although sulfur is found in the body and is considered a macromineral, the mineral is not discussed as a subsection of this chapter because the body does not use sulfur alone as a nutrient. Sulfur is found in the body associated structurally with vitamins such as thiamin and biotin, and as part of the sulfur-containing amino acids methionine, cysteine, and taurine. Thus, sulfur is commonly found within proteins, especially those found in skin, hair, and nails.

Table 11.1 provides an overview of the macrominerals, including information on general functions, approximate body content, deficiency signs, foods sources, and recommended intakes. A similar overview of the trace minerals may be found in Chapter 12, Table 12.1. Noteworthy is the difference in body content between the macro- and microminerals, with the macromineral content of the body ranging from ~35 to 1,400 g and the micromineral content ranging from <1 mg to ~4 g. In your consideration of the body's mineral content, keep in mind that a pound is equal to 454 g and an ounce is the same as about 28.4 g.

CALCIUM

Calcium is the most abundant divalent cation of the human body, representing about 1.5% to 2% of total body weight, or between ~1,000 and 1,400 g in a 70-kg human. Bones and teeth contain about 99% of the body's calcium. The other 1% is distributed in intra- and extracellular fluids.

Sources

The best food sources of calcium include milk and dairy products, especially cheese and yogurt; selected seafoods, such as salmon and sardines (with bones), clams, and oysters; selected vegetables, such as turnip and mustard greens, broccoli, cauliflower, and kale; legumes and legume products such as tofu (soybean curd); and dried fruits. Other foods providing excellent amounts of calcium include those fortified with calcium, such as fruit juices (especially orange juice) and breads. Many forms of calcium supplements also are available, including, for example, calcium carbonate, calcium acetate, calcium lactate, calcium gluconate, calcium citrate, calcium citrate-malate, and calcium monophosphate.

Meats, grains, and nuts are relatively poor sources of calcium. Vegetables such as spinach, rhubarb, and swiss chard also are poor sources due to the presence of high amounts of oxalic acid, which binds calcium and prevents its absorption, as discussed under "Factors Influencing Absorption" on page 382.

Digestion, Absorption, and Transport

Digestion

Calcium is present in foods and dietary supplements as relatively insoluble salts. Because calcium is absorbed only in its ionized (Ca^{2+}) form, it must first be released from the salts. Calcium is solubilized from most calcium salts in about 1 hour at an acidic pH (as occurs in the stomach). Solubilization, however, does not necessarily ensure better absorption, because within the more alkaline pH of the small intestine calcium may complex with minerals or other selected dietary constituents [1]. Formation of these complexes in the small intestine may limit calcium bioavailability.

Absorption

Two main transport processes (Fig. 11.1) are responsible for the absorption of calcium, which occurs along the length of the small intestine [2].

- One of the transport processes, operative primarily in the duodenum and proximal jejunum, is saturable, requires energy, involves a calcium-binding protein (CBP; also called calbindin D_{9k}), and is regulated by calcitriol. Calcitriol is also referred to as 1,25-dihydroxycholecalciferol or vitamin D, abbreviated 1,25-$(OH)_2$ D_3. The calcitriol-dependent calcium transport system is stimulated on ingestion of low-calcium diets, especially intakes <400 mg, as well as in conditions of growth, pregnancy, and lactation, in which calcium requirements are increased. Growing children, for example, absorb up to 75% of dietary calcium in contrast to adults, who average about 30% absorption [3]. For calcium to be absorbed by this active process, three sequential steps, all regulated by vitamin D, must occur: first, transport across the brush border membrane; second, intracellular movement; third, extrusion across the basolateral membrane. Calcitriol, which is released in response to an increase in parathyroid hormone (PTH) secretion caused by a reduction in plasma levels of ionized calcium, enhances calcium absorption. Calcitriol-induced absorption of calcium involves changes in membrane lipid composition and topology and stimulation of the synthesis of the calcium-binding protein calbindin. With age, however, the vitamin D–regulated absorption of calcium becomes impaired by decreased efficiency in renal calcitriol production in response to PTH. High plasma phosphorus concentrations also may diminish calcitriol production in the kidney. Estrogen deficiency at menopause also decreases vitamin D–mediated calcium absorption. Following brush border absorption, intracellular calcium movement occurs. Specifically, calcium

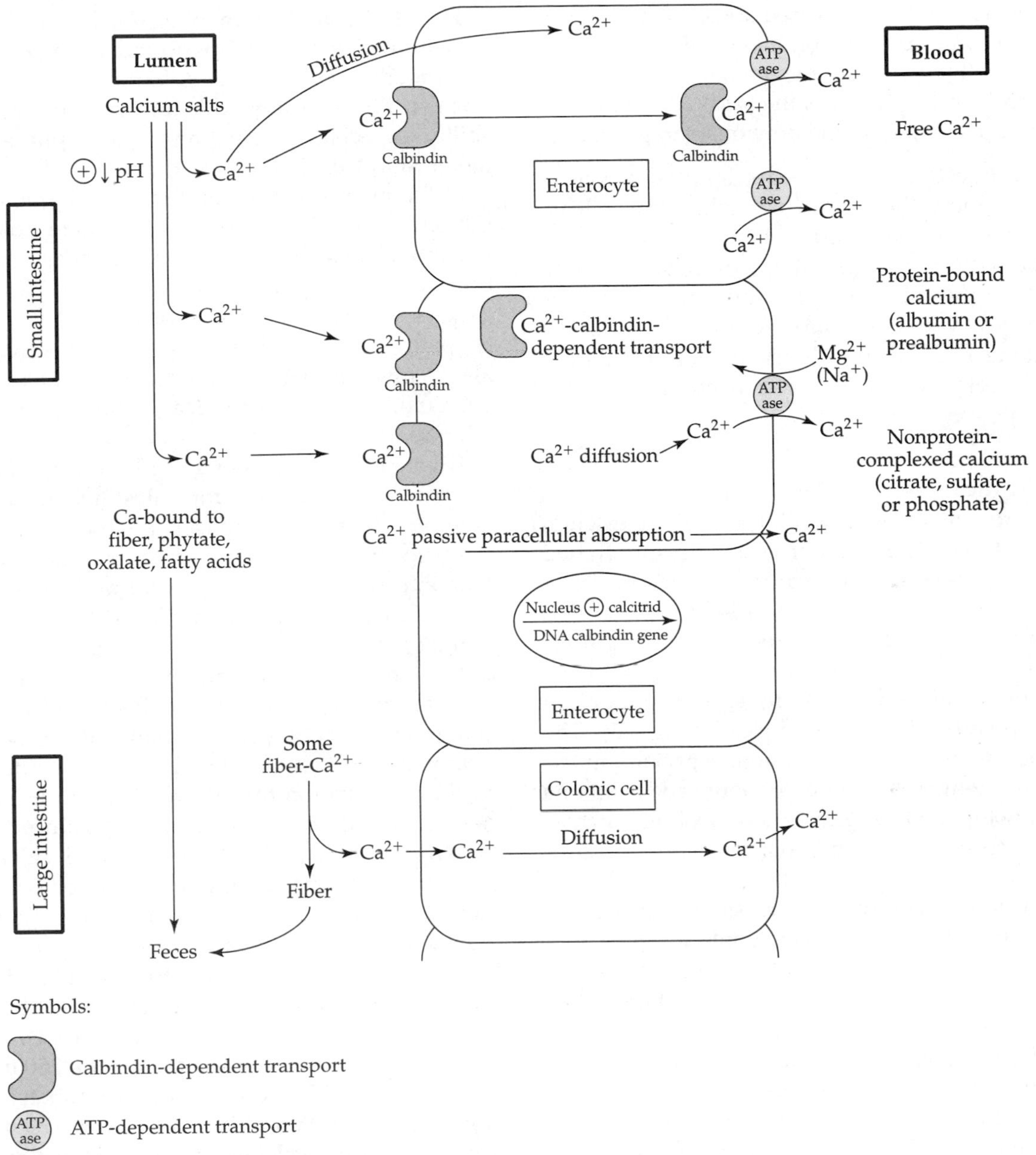

Figure 11.1 Calcium digestion, absorption, and transport.

transport across the intestinal cell may occur via diffusion or via active transport requiring a carrier protein, calbindin D_{9k}. Calbindin D_{9k} not only facilitates brush border absorption but also serves as a transport protein to shuttle the calcium across the cytoplasm of the enterocyte to the basal membrane for extrusion. Other calcium-binding proteins, such as calmodulin, also may facilitate intracellular calcium movement. The extrusion of calcium from the enterocyte into the extracellular fluid requires Ca^{2+}-Mg^{2+} ATPase, an enzyme that hydrolyzes ATP and releases energy for pumping Ca^{2+} out of the cell as Mg^{2+} moves in. The Ca^{2+}-Mg^{2+} pump is ATP dependent and is stimulated by vitamin D. Sodium also may be exchanged for Ca^{2+} in the extrusion process at the intestinal basolateral membrane; however, this system is thought to contribute only to a small extent to calcium extrusion from intestinal cells [4].

- The second of the two processes for calcium absorption occurs throughout the small intestine but mostly in the jejunum and ileum and is nonsaturable and passive. Passive paracellular absorption (i.e., absorption between cells rather than through them) is also thought to occur when calcium concentrations are high. The amount of calcium absorbed via the nonsaturable, paracellular mechanism depends on the supply of calcium in the intestinal lumen, up to a threshold level, such that increased absorption via this mechanism becomes possible on increased intake of the mineral. Intracellular calcium movement through the enterocyte and extrusion across the basal lateral membrane occur as described in the previous paragraph.

The large intestine also appears to play a role in calcium absorption. Bacteria in the colon may release calcium bound to some fermentable fibers such as pectins. About 4% to 10% (or ~8 mg) of dietary calcium is absorbed by the colon per day; this amount may be higher in people who are absorbing less calcium in the small intestine [3]. Calcium-deficient diets have been linked with colon cancer, as discussed later in the section on calcium deficiency.

Factors Influencing Absorption. Several substances are known to enhance or inhibit intestinal calcium absorption (Table 11.2). Vitamin D, as mentioned previously, improves the absorption of calcium. Polymorphisms that exist in the vitamin D receptor (VDR) gene also influence, to a minor extent, calcium absorption [5]. Ingestion of food or lactose along with the calcium source appears to improve overall calcium absorption, possibly by improving solubility [6]. The effects of lactose on calcium diffusion, especially in the ileum, are thought to be more pronounced in infants than in adults [6]. Other sugars, sugar alcohols (such as xylitol), and protein also can enhance calcium absorption [6–8].

Fiber as well as phytate may decrease calcium absorption and retention [9,10]. Nonfermentable fibers such as cellulose or those found in wheat bran can increase the bulk of intestinal contents and decrease transit time, thus decreasing the time available for calcium absorption to occur. Nonfermentable or slowly fermentable fibers such as some of the hemicelluloses stimulate the proliferation of microbes, which in turn bind minerals such as calcium and make them unavailable for absorption. Phytate (also called phytic acid or myoinositol hexaphosphate and shown later in Fig. 11.7) is found in some of the same plant foods in which fiber is found (e.g., legumes, nuts, cereals). Phytates bind calcium and decrease its availability, especially when present in a phytate : calcium molar ratio >0.2 [10].

Calcium absorption in the intestine may also be inhibited by the presence of oxalate (oxalic acid), which chelates the calcium and increases fecal excretion. Oxalate is found in a variety of vegetables (e.g., spinach, rhubarb, swiss chard, beets, celery, eggplant, greens, okra, squash), fruits (e.g., straw-, black-, blue-, and gooseberries, currants), nuts (pecans, peanuts), and beverages (tea, Ovaltine, cocoa), among other foods.

Divalent cations, along with other minerals, can compete with calcium for intestinal absorption. For example, magnesium and calcium, both divalent cations, compete with each other for intestinal absorption whenever an excess of either is present in the gastrointestinal tract. Calcium absorption from low-calcium diets (230 mg) that include supplements of zinc (another divalent cation) also may be impaired [11].

Unabsorbed dietary fatty acids found in significant quantities in the gastrointestinal tract associated with steatorrhea (>7 g of fecal fat per day) can interfere with calcium absorption through the formation of insoluble calcium soaps (calcium–fatty acid complexes) in the lumen of the small intestine. These calcium soaps cannot be absorbed and are excreted in the feces. Steatorrhea is a problem associated with some gastrointestinal tract disorders, such as inflammatory bowel diseases, as well as with disorders affecting the pancreas, such as pancreatitis and cystic fibrosis.

Calcium absorption from calcium supplements varies depending on the calcium salt. Calcium (250 mg) absorption was 39% ± 3% from calcium carbonate, 32% ± 4% from calcium acetate, 32% ± 4% from calcium lactate, 30% ± 3% from calcium citrate, and 27% ± 3% from

Table 11.2 Interactions between Calcium and Selected Nutrients/Substances

Nutrients/Substances Enhancing Calcium Absorption	Nutrients/Substances Inhibiting Calcium Absorption
Vitamin D	Fiber
Sugars and sugar alcohols	Phytate
Protein	Oxalate
	Excessive divalent cations (Zn, Mg)
	Unabsorbed fatty acids
Nutrients Enhancing Urinary Calcium Excretion	**Nutrients Whose Absorption May Be Inhibited by Excessive Calcium**
Sodium	Iron
Protein	Fatty acids
Caffeine	

calcium gluconate [2]. Other studies suggest that calcium absorption from chelated forms of calcium such as calcium citrate, calcium citrate-malate, and calcium gluconate is better than that from calcium carbonate [12,13]. Ingestion of supplements providing 250 mg calcium from calcium citrate-malate resulted in 35% calcium absorption, and from calcium monophosphate 25% calcium absorption. Calcium carbonate, a widely used form of supplemental calcium, is relatively inexpensive and contains about 40% calcium by weight; calcium carbonate from fossilized oyster shell or dolomite, however, may be contaminated with aluminum and lead and should not be used [13]. Bone meal preparations also contain lead and should be avoided [13]. Because the amount of calcium varies among supplements, to obtain 500 mg of calcium an individual would need to ingest 5.49 g calcium gluconate, 3.53 g calcium lactate, 2.37 g calcium citrate, 2.16 g calcium acetate, or 1.26 g calcium carbonate [2].

Overall, calcium absorption in adults averages about 30%, the estimate used in deriving recommendations for intakes for adults [3]. Studies report calcium absorption in the range of 20% to 50% from the diet, with most absorption in the range of 20% to 35% from dairy products [2,3,14–17].

Transport

Calcium is transported in the blood in three forms. Some calcium (~40%) is bound to proteins, mainly albumin and prealbumin. Some calcium (up to ~10%) is complexed with sulfate, phosphate, or citrate. About 50% of calcium is found free (ionized) in the blood.

Regulation of Calcium Concentrations

Calcium concentrations are tightly controlled both intracellularly and extracellularly.

Extracellular Calcium Concentration Regulation. Three main hormones are involved in calcium homeostasis in the blood: PTH, calcitriol, and calcitonin. We will discuss each of these hormones and their actions involving calcium; calcitriol and PTH are discussed together. An overview of calcium regulation is shown in Figure 11.2.

- PTH is secreted from the chief cells of the parathyroid gland. PTH secretion is influenced by plasma concentrations of especially calcium but also magnesium. With low plasma calcium concentrations, PTH secretion is increased and calcitonin secretion from the thyroid gland is diminished. Calcium-sensing receptors on the parathyroid gland and the kidney (tubule) appear to monitor calcium and magnesium concentrations in the blood. Increased concentrations of calcium and magnesium appear to initiate a conformational change in an exterior portion of the receptor that, via IP_3 release (discussed further on p. 386), signals the parathyroid gland to diminish PTH release [18].

- PTH, alone or with calcitriol, acts to increase extracellular fluid (plasma) calcium concentrations through interactions with the kidney, intestine, and bone. In the kidney, PTH increases the synthesis of calcitriol from 25-OH vitamin D via 1-hydroxylase. Calcitriol production results in increased renal tubular reabsorption of calcium via calbindin D_{28k} (another vitamin D–dependent calcium transporter found in the kidneys). Calcitriol performs similar functions in the intestine, where it stimulates the synthesis of calbindin D_{9k}. Specifically, calcitriol is thought to interact with vitamin D receptors in the cytosol of the enterocyte and, following transport to the nucleus, to bind to DNA and induce transcription of genes that code for calbindin D (genomic actions). Calbindin D functions as a calcium-binding protein to promote calcium

Figure 11.2 An overview of blood calcium regulation by parathyroid hormone (PTH) and calcitriol (also called 1,25-$(OH)_2$ vitamin D) in response to low blood calcium concentrations.

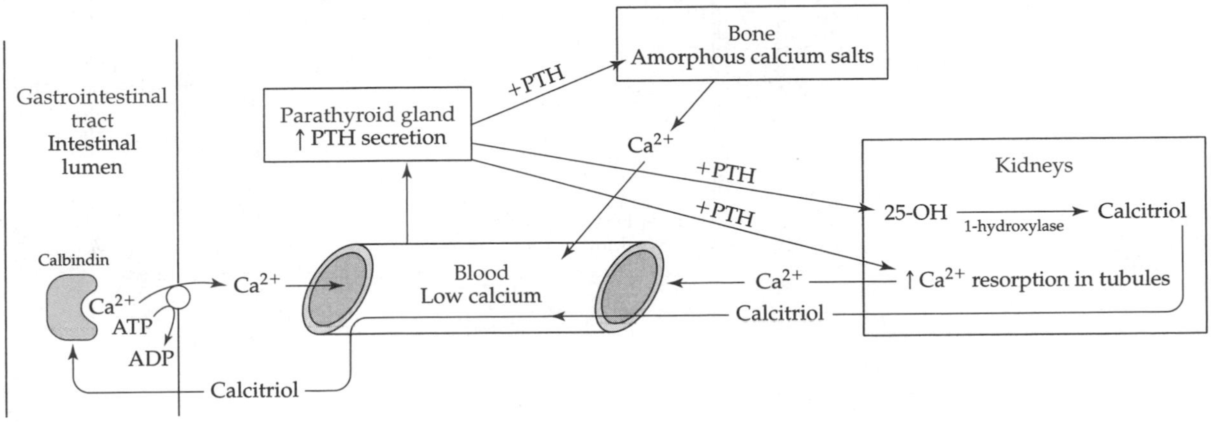

absorption. Calcitriol also is thought to induce changes in the brush border and basal lateral membranes to enhance calcium absorption directly (nongenomic actions). In bone, PTH interacts with receptors on osteoblasts (bone-building cells) that signal osteoclasts (bone-breaking cells). Lysosomal proteases in osteoclasts degrade bone to promote resorption of amorphous calcium salts in bone. Calcium pumps, on activation in the membrane, pump calcium through the membrane and out of bone fluid into the blood. Calcitriol also may be involved in this process.

- Calcitonin is synthesized in the parafollicular cells of the thyroid gland. In contrast to PTH, calcitonin stimulates osteoblasts and serves to lower serum Ca^{2+} by inhibiting the activity of osteoclasts and preventing mobilization of Ca^{2+} from bone. Calcitonin also may inhibit production of active vitamin D and diminish renal calcium reabsorption, thus promoting calcium excretion from the body.

Intracellular Calcium Concentration Regulation. Calcium may enter the cell directly from extracellular sites by transmembrane diffusion or by one of two channels (voltage-dependent slow channels or agonist-dependent channels), which are activated by depolarization, neurotransmitters, or hormones. Second messengers also may increase cytoplasmic calcium levels by stimulating release of calcium from intracellular sites such as the endoplasmic reticulum and the mitochondria. Efflux of organelle-sequestered calcium typically requires a pump such as a Ca^{2+}, Na^+-antiport pump.

Low free Ca^{2+} concentrations (100 nmol/L, or approximately 0.0001 of the concentration in the extracellular fluid) are maintained within cells both through ATP-dependent calcium pumps, which export calcium out of the cell, and through storage of calcium in organelles such as the mitochondria, endoplasmic reticulum, nucleus, and vesicles. Calcium extrusion from cells occurs via ATP-dependent transport systems. These transporters require either sodium or magnesium, and they pump Ca^{2+} out of the cell to help maintain low intracellular concentrations. In addition, to control cytosolic calcium concentrations, Ca^{2+} may be pumped via a Ca^{2+}/Mg^{2+}-ATPase pump and sequestered in the endoplasmic (or sarcoplasmic) reticulum. Another main storage site for calcium within cells is the mitochondria. A Ca^{2+} pump can drive Ca^{2+} out of the cytoplasm into the mitochondrial matrix for storage until needed by the cell. Within the organelles, calcium binds to protein (such as calsequestrin) in the sarcoplasmic reticulum or may complex with phosphate as in the mitochondrion. Figure 11.3 illustrates the mechanisms of cellular control of calcium concentrations.

Raising the concentration of cytosolic Ca^{2+} by the release of calcium from intracellular reservoirs or storage sites in organelles and from extracellular sites allows Ca^{2+} to carry out its cellular functions. Following stimulation and release of Ca^{2+} into the cytoplasm to carry out its functions, concentrations are returned to their normal, low levels by a reversal of the events that raised its concentration. For example, the neurotransmitter may be degraded or the agonist may be released from the cell surface receptor, intracellular second messengers are inactivated, and Ca^{2+} is pumped out of

Figure 11.3 Regulation of intracellular calcium concentrations.

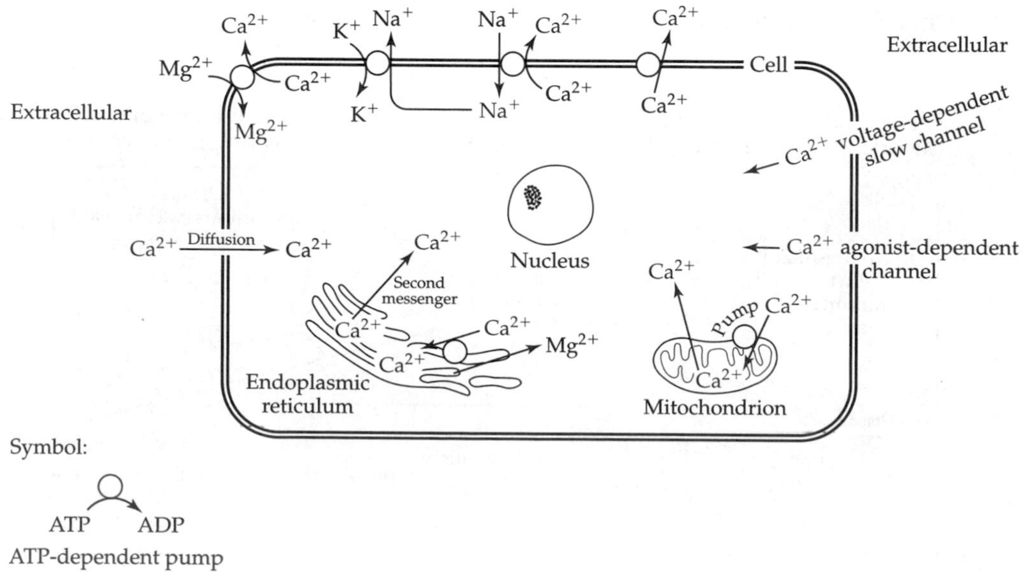

the cell or once again sequestered by intracellular organelles and binders.

Functions and Mechanisms of Action

Calcium functions in the mineralization of bone, of which there are two types: cortical bone and trabecular bone (Fig. 11.4). Most bones possess an outer layer of cortical bone that surrounds trabecular bone. Some bones also contain a cavity for bone marrow. Cortical bone is compact or dense, represents about 75% to 80% of total bone in the body, consists of layers of mineralized collagen, and is found mainly on the surfaces or outer layers of long bones of the limbs. Trabecular bone has a spongy appearance, represents about 20% to 25% of bone in the body, and is found in relatively high concentrations in the axial skeleton (vertebrae and pelvic region). Trabecular bone is more active metabolically, with a high turnover rate, and thus is more rapidly depleted of calcium with poor calcium intake than is cortical bone. Despite the differences between cortical and trabecular bone, all bones require mineralization, which involves mainly calcium, phosphorus, and magnesium but also other minerals.

Figure 11.4 Trabecular bone is the lacy network of calcium-containing crystals that fills the interior. Cortical bone is the dense, ivorylike bone that forms the exterior shell. *Source:* Whitney EN, Rolfes SR. *Understanding Nutrition,* 6th ed. St. Paul: West, 1993, p. 396. Courtesy of Gjon Mill. Used by permission of Wadsworth Publishing Co.

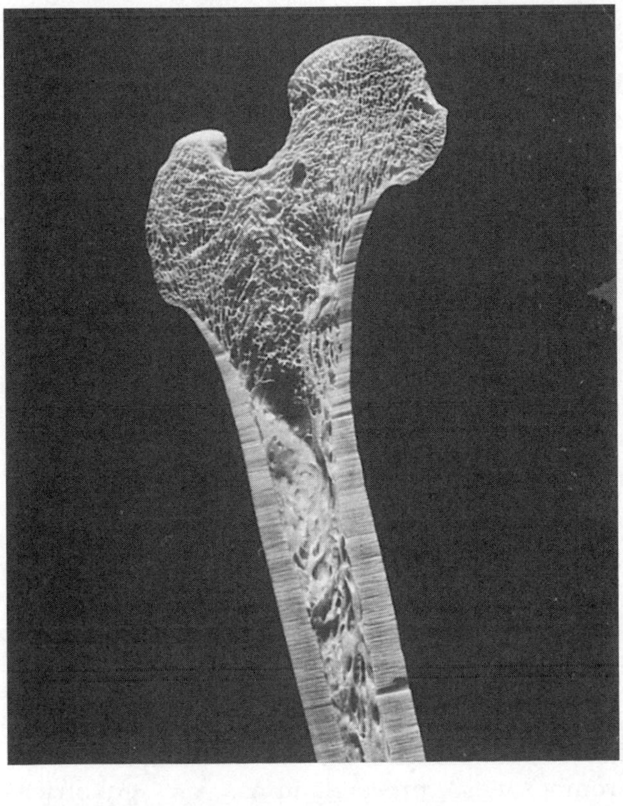

Bone Mineralization

Approximately 99% of total body calcium is found in bones and teeth. About 60% to 66% of the weight of bones is due to minerals, with the remaining 34% to 40% due to water, ground substance, and protein. Minerals, or the mostly inorganic portion of bone, consist largely of calcium and phosphorus but also include fluoride, magnesium, potassium, sodium, strontium, and hydroxyl groups. Hydroxyl groups make up part of **hydroxyapatite,** a crystal lattice–like substance found in bones and teeth. Carbonate is also found in bone, usually associated with calcium, potassium, and sodium. The organic parts of bone contain a range of proteins and ground substance. Proteins in bone include primarily collagen (about 85%–90% of proteins), with smaller amounts of osteonectin, osteopontin, bone sialoprotein, osteocalcin (also called bone Gla protein, abbreviated BGP), and matrix Gla protein (abbreviated MGP). The last two proteins are dependent on vitamin K for carboxylation of their glutamic acid residues and function in calcium binding and matrix modification. Calcium facilitates interactions between proteins or between proteins and phospholipids in cell membranes. Osteonectin is a phosphoprotein that binds both calcium and collagen. Osteopontin binds to both hydroxyapatite and bone cells. Ground substance in bone is made up mostly of glycoproteins and proteoglycans. Glycoproteins consist of proteins covalently bound to typically short chains of carbohydrate. Proteoglycans are similar to glycoproteins but typically are larger, with longer carbohydrate chains; examples include chondroitin 4-sulfate, hyaluronic acid, and keratan sulfate.

Among the three main types of bone cells (osteoblasts, osteocytes, and osteoclasts), osteoblasts are referred to as bone-building cells and originate from the bone marrow. Under the influence of PTH, calcitriol, and estrogen, among other hormones, osteoblasts secrete collagen and other proteins as well as ground substance—that is, the extracellular matrix (also called the bone matrix osteoid) surrounding the bone cells. As the osteoblasts secrete the proteins and ground substance and mineralization occurs, the osteoblasts become embedded in the proteins and the ground substance matrix. With further embedding in the matrix and morphological changes, osteoblasts become osteocytes. Osteocytes—that is, osteoblasts that have been incorporated into bone matrix—are important to maintaining the integrity of the surrounding bone. Osteocytes and other bone cells (osteoblasts and osteoclasts) communicate with one another through long processes that in turn connect to form an osteocytic membrane system. The membrane system, which also contains calcium pumps, separates bone and bone fluid.

During mineralization, calcium, phosphorus, magnesium, and other minerals enter bone fluid from blood and then attach to bone proteins and ground substance. Calcium is first present as Ca^{2+} and/or as amorphous (noncrystal or poorly crystalline) calcium forms, such as $Ca_3(PO_4)_2$. Other amorphous forms of minerals in bone include carbonate bound to calcium, phosphorus, and/or magnesium, and, for example, $Ca_3(PO_4)_2$ (tricalcium phosphate), $Mg_3(PO_4)_2$ (trimagnesium phosphate), and $CaHPO_4 \cdot 2H_2O$ (brushite). These salts ultimately are converted to more crystalline compounds such as $Ca_8H_2(PO_4)_6 \cdot 5H_2O$ (octacalcium phosphate) as well as to hydroxyapatite crystals $Ca_{10}(PO_4)_6(OH)_2$. Osteoblasts are thought to secrete substances onto the bone surface, which enhances the precipitation or deposition of calcium and other minerals. Whether osteoblasts facilitate the movement of calcium and other minerals from the blood to the bone fluid and then to the bone surface is unclear. The process of calcification and mineralization of the bone matrix has yet to be clearly delineated.

Osteoclasts, another type of bone cell, are large, multinucleated (with about two to ten nuclei) cells that function to resorb previously made bone. Osteoclasts contain lysosomes that release acids (such as citrate and lactate), proteases, and hydrolases and other enzymes capable of breaking down the bone protein and matrix and dissolving amorphous mineral complexes. Osteoclasts respond to PTH, calcitriol, and calcitonin. Osteoclasts play an important role in helping maintain normal blood calcium concentrations in times of inadequate calcium intake.

In children and adolescents, skeletal turnover occurs such that formation of bone exceeds resorption of bone. Skeletal turnover continues into adulthood, with peak bone mass occurring in early adulthood. During the fifth decade, bone mass begins to decline. Although the need for calcium in bone modeling is continuous, its greatest benefits in promoting the formation of a sturdy skeletal mass occur during linear bone growth and the years immediately following. The dietary factors involved in osteoporosis, a condition characterized by decreased bone mass, are discussed in the perspective "Osteoporosis and Diet" at the end of this chapter.

Other Roles

The small amount (1%) of remaining body calcium (that is not associated with bone, or nonosseous) is found both intracellularly within organelles such as the mitochondria, endoplasmic reticulum (sarcoplasmic reticulum in muscle), nucleus, and vesicles and extracellularly in the blood, lymph, and body fluids. Of the calcium in the blood plasma, about 50% is ionized (Ca^{2+}). It is this ionized calcium that is active, which means that the numerous regulatory functions of calcium are performed by $<0.5\%$ of the total body calcium. Nonosseous calcium is essential for a number of processes, including, for example, blood clotting (see Fig. 10.21 under vitamin K), nerve conduction, muscle contraction, enzyme regulation, and membrane permeability.

Calcium fluxes across membranes within cells as well as across the plasma membrane mediate the actions of a variety of hormones and neurotransmitters to affect intracellular processes. The consequential rising of cytosolic Ca^{2+} concentration allows Ca^{2+} to carry out these cellular functions. The rise in intracellular free calcium concentrations is achieved either by release of calcium from intracellular reservoirs or storage sites by second messengers or by influx from extracellular sites via transmembrane diffusion or via channels activated by depolarization, neurotransmitters, or hormones.

An example of intracellular calcium release and functions is shown in Figure 11.5 and discussed next. Hormones or neurotransmitters bind to cell membrane receptors, initiating a series of hydrolytic reactions on cell membrane phospholipids. Specifically, the reactions can result in the hydrolysis of cell membrane phospholipids such as phosphatidylinositol by phospholipase C, a membrane protein. From the inner cell membrane, phosphatidylinositol is coverted first to phosphatidyl 4-phosphate and next to phosphatidylinositol 4,5-diphosphate (PIP_2). PIP_2 is then hydrolyzed to generate two compounds, inositol 1,4,5-triphosphate (IP_3) and diacylglycerol (DAG). IP_3 is water-soluble, whereas DAG is lipid-soluble. IP_3 functions as a second messenger; it diffuses to the endoplasmic reticulum, where it triggers the release of calcium into the cytoplasm. DAG also acts as a second messenger, whereby it activates protein kinase C (PKC), which is associated with membrane phospholipids. When associated with phospholipids and DAG, PKC has an increased binding affinity for Ca^{2+} such that the Ca^{2+} requirement of PKC can be met by resting Ca^{2+} concentrations. Without DAG, higher concentrations of Ca^{2+} are needed to activate PKC [19]. The exact role of PKC is unknown, but it is involved in mediating sustained cellular responses [20]. In general, protein kinases catalyze the phosphorylation of amino acids found within proteins, a process that alters the protein's function and thus the cell's function or activity.

Increased free Ca^{2+} concentrations in the cell may affect the cell functions directly or may function through binding to calcium-binding proteins. Increased free Ca^{2+} can trigger neutrophils and activate platelet phospholipase A_2. Phospholipase A_2 acts on carbon 2 of the glycerol backbone of phospholipids (e.g., phosphatidylcholine) to liberate fatty acids (e.g., arachidonic acid from phosphatidylcholine). The arachidonic acid can be metabolized to form thromboxanes, prostaglandins, or leukotrienes.

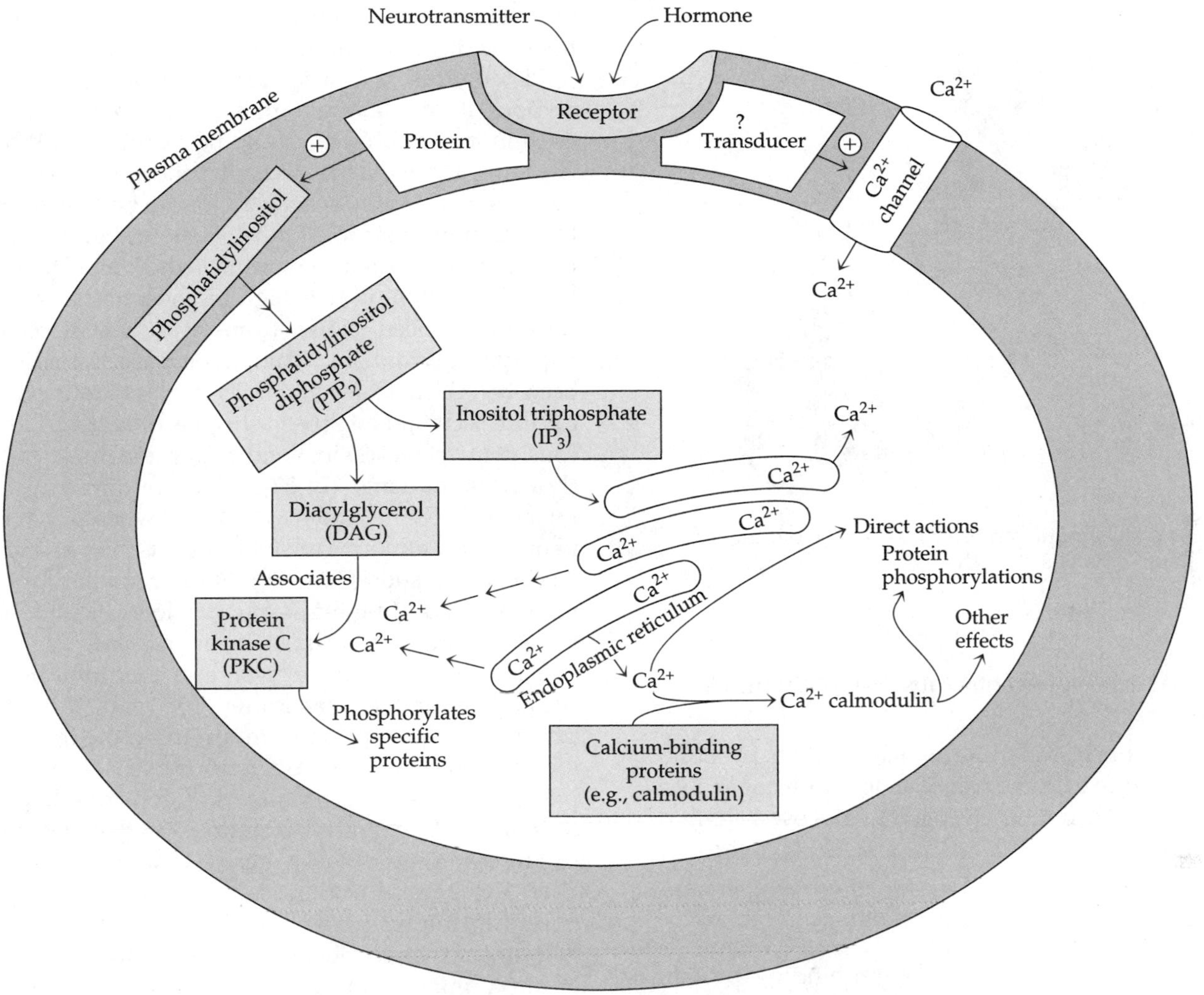

Figure 11.5 Some intracellular actions of calcium.

Phosphodiesterase, which hydrolyzes cyclic AMP (cAMP) to 5′AMP, is also dependent on Ca^{2+}. Cyclic AMP, formed from ATP by adenylate cyclase, activates protein kinases, thereby influencing intermediary metabolism. The actions of cAMP and Ca^{2+} are thought to be mutually dependent. Other enzymes that may be affected either directly by increased free Ca^{2+} or through Ca^{2+} bound to any number of calcium-binding proteins are listed in Table 11.3.

Calcium functions in a variety of processes through interactions with binding proteins. In fact, increased intracellular Ca^{2+} concentrations promote the binding of calcium to any of several calcium-binding proteins. Calmodulin, one example of a calcium-binding protein, appears to be operative in most cells. Calmodulin consists of two similar globular lobes joined by a long helix. Each lobe contains two Ca^{2+}-binding sites, and thus calmodulin in total binds four calcium ions per molecule (Fig. 11.6). Binding of Ca^{2+} activates calmodulin by changing its conformation, thereby allowing it to stimulate or interact with a variety of macromolecular processes or enzymes. Some examples of the calmodulin-dependent enzymes include

- calcineurin, a phosphatase that dephosphorylates and inactivates calcium channels;
- myosin light-chain kinase, which phosphorylates the light chain of myosin and, following

Table 11.3 Selected Enzymes Regulated by Calcium and/or Calmodulin

Adenylate cyclase	Guanylate cyclase
Ca-dependent protein kinase	Myosin kinase
Ca/Mg-ATPase	NAD kinase
Ca/phospholipid-dependent protein kinase	Nitric oxide synthase
Cyclic nucleotide phosphodiesterase	Phospholipase A_2
Glycerol 3-phosphate dehydrogenase	Phosphorylase kinase
Glycogen synthase	Pyruvate carboxylase
	Pyruvate dehydrogenase
	Pyruvate kinase

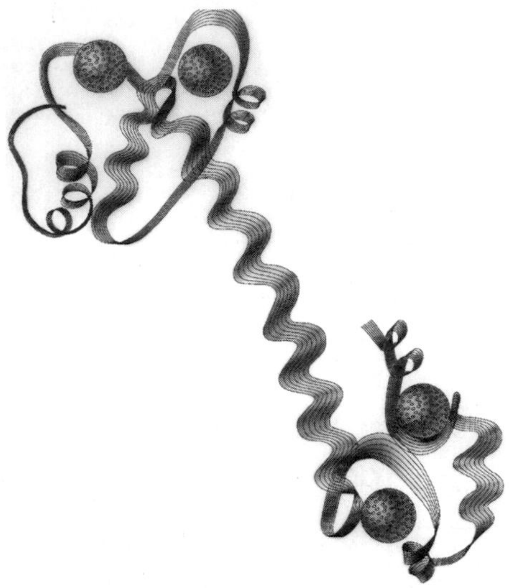

Figure 11.6 Schematic representation of the binding of four calcium ions (Ca^{2+}) by the calcium-binding protein calmodulin.

a sequence of events, causes smooth muscle contraction;

- phosphorylase kinase, which activates phosphorylase (the enzyme responsible for glycogenolysis, that is, degrading glycogen to glucose 1-PO_4); and
- calcium calmodulin kinases, of which there are several with several functions.

A second example of a calcium-binding protein is troponin C, which is found in skeletal muscle. Skeletal muscle stimulated by nerve impulses (acetylcholine as neurotransmitter) triggers increased concentrations of calcium. The calcium can then bind to the troponin C, allowing muscle contraction. The structure of troponin C, with its four binding sites for calcium, closely resembles that of calmodulin. Like calmodulin, the conformational change in troponin C due to Ca^{2+} binding permits an interaction between actin and myosin, resulting in muscle contraction [20]. Once the plasma membrane repolarizes, calcium is pumped back into the sarcoplasmic reticulum, troponin C releases its bound calcium, and myosin and actin no longer interact [20]. Some other calcium- or calmodulin-dependent enzymes are listed in Table 11.3.

Interactions with Other Nutrients

Calcium interacts with several nutrients not only at the absorptive surface of the intestinal cell but also within the body. Some interrelationships between calcium and other nutrients and substances have been discussed in the section on calcium absorption. Additional interactions are discussed here and listed in Table 11.2.

Phosphorus is particularly interesting in that for decades it was thought that certain dietary ratios of calcium to phosphorus should be maintained. While the need for specific ratios is still believed to be true for infants and children, specific ratios are no longer thought to be as important for adults. Diets low in calcium and high in phosphorus are common in the United States. Prolonged ingestion of diets high in phosphorus and low in calcium has been shown to result in a mild secondary hyperparathyroidism. This hyperparathyroidism has been theorized to lead to calcium loss from bone and calcium secretion into the gastrointestinal tract. However, consistent increases in bone resorption have not been shown in humans [21,22]. Also, resorption of bone minerals has been shown to be lower when plasma phosphorus concentrations are high (versus low) at any given PTH concentration [3,21–29]. Further studies investigating the effects of high-phosphorus, low-calcium diets on bone resorption and acquisition are needed.

The use of calcium supplements to inhibit phosphorus absorption has been known for years. Inhibition of phosphorus absorption is important in the treatment of kidney diseases, because with renal failure plasma phosphorus concentrations rise considerably above normal due to impaired excretion. For decades, calcium in large amounts (2–3 g per day or in ratios greater than 3 to 1) was prescribed for patients with kidney failure to inhibit phosphorus absorption and thereby help lower plasma phosphorus concentrations.

Many interactions among calcium and other nutrients or substances (including protein, sodium, caffeine, alcohol, and boron) occur in the kidney and promote loss of calcium from the body. Dietary protein, for example, promotes calcium losses [30–33]. Doubling protein intake without changing the intake of other nutrients, for example, results in up to a 50% increase in urinary calcium. Ingestion of an additional 1 g protein promotes an increased urinary calcium excretion of about 1 to 1.7 mg [33]. Sulfate generated from metabolism of the sulfur-containing amino acids in the protein may bind with the calcium and inhibit its reabsorption and/or increase its urinary excretion [31–33]. However, many protein-containing foods also contain phosphorus, which decreases calcium excretion. Ingestion of foods containing both nutrients tends to minimize negative effects on calcium balance. Additional studies examining indicators of bone turnover and bone accrual with varying intakes of calcium, phosphorus, and protein are needed [34].

Sodium and calcium excretion are linked in the proximal renal tubule. Sodium consumption of 500 mg, for example, can increase urinary calcium excretion by about 10 mg [35,36]. Moreover, urinary sodium excretion is negatively correlated with changes in bone density in the hip of postmenopausal women [36].

Caffeine (300–400 mg) not only increases urinary calcium (0.25 mmol or 10 mg per day) by reducing renal reabsorption but also causes increased secretion of calcium into the gut, thereby leading to increased endogenous fecal losses [27,37–39]. Caffeine and alcohol intake have each been positively associated with risk of fracture in middle-aged women [39,40].

Other minerals also have been shown to promote calcium losses from the body. For example, boron supplements (3 mg) when given with magnesium supplements (200 mg) increased urinary calcium losses [41].

Calcium also interacts with some nutrients to inhibit their absorption into the body. Calcium in the form of dietary supplements (providing up to 600 mg calcium in various forms, such as calcium citrate) or in natural food form significantly decreases nonheme iron absorption in a dose-dependent relationship [42–44]. Calcium is thought to affect iron absorption within the enterocyte and not at the brush border. This relationship has been documented in several studies and occurs primarily when calcium and iron are ingested together with food.

Lead absorption is inversely related to dietary calcium intake [45]. Poor dietary calcium intake also is associated with lead accumulation in blood and organs [46].

Calcium also can diminish the absorption of fatty acids and thus influence serum lipid concentrations and the fatty acid profile of bile. Calcium may work by inhibiting bile acid reabsorption in the ileum, necessitating the use of body cholesterol for the synthesis of additional bile. Calcium also may directly bind the fatty acids in the small intestine to form insoluble "soaps" that are excreted in the feces. Ingestion of calcium carbonate (providing 1,200–3,000 mg calcium) has resulted in significant decreases in total and low-density lipoprotein cholesterol and significant increases in high-density lipoprotein cholesterol [47–51]. Such changes may decrease the risk for heart disease. Calcium supplementation of 2 or 3 g daily decreased chenodeoxycholate concentrations in bile and the lithocholate: deoxycholate ratio in the feces [52]. Such changes are favorable to the colonic environment and may help prevent colon cancer.

Excretion

Calcium is excreted in the urine and feces, although up to about 182 mg (average, 60 mg) may be lost daily from the skin, especially with extreme sweating [53]. Most calcium is filtered and reabsorbed by the kidney such that urinary calcium losses range from about 100 to 240 mg per day, with an average of about 170 mg [53,54]. Urinary calcium excretion may be decreased by PTH secretion as well as in the presence of phosphorus, potassium, magnesium, and boron, and it may be increased in the presence of sodium, protein, boron plus magnesium, and caffeine [31–42,55].

Fecal losses of calcium from endogenous sources range from about 45 to 100 mg per day [53]. Fecal losses may increase with consumption of fiber, phytate, and oxalate, and of magnesium in excess, and in people with fat-malabsorbing disorders.

Adequate Intakes

In 1997, recommendations by the Food and Nutrition Board for adequate intakes of calcium were set at 1,000 mg daily for adult men and women age 19–50 years, including women during pregnancy and lactation [3]. For adults age 51 years and older, the calcium recommendations increase to 1,200 mg per day [3]. Additional calcium was not recommended for women on hormone or estrogen replacement during the postmenopausal period, as it has been shown not to prevent bone (trabecular) loss that occurs within the first 5 years after menopause [56].

A National Institutes of Health (NIH) panel on osteoporosis also has issued recommendations for calcium intake. Echoing the adequate intake recommendations, the NIH panel recommends that adults ingest 1,000 mg per day; however, for postmenopausal women not treated with estrogen, an intake of 1,500 mg/day is suggested [57]. The distinction between women treated and not treated with estrogen is made by the NIH panel because estrogen influences bone mineralization and postmenopausal women experience a rapid loss of bone minerals without estrogen replacement. A level of 1,500 mg is thought to be associated with maximum calcium retention, and intakes >1,500 mg daily are thought to represent the threshold amount whereby additional intake would not be expected to produce further rises in calcium retention [57,58]. Also recommended by the NIH panel is an intake of 1,500 mg for men age 65 years and older versus 1,200 mg for men and women age 51 years and older by the Food and Nutrition Board [3]. The inside covers of the book provide the AIs for calcium for other age groups.

The Food and Drug Administration has approved some health claims related to calcium. One example claim is "Regular exercise and a healthy diet with enough calcium help teen and young adult white and Asian women maintain good bone health and may reduce the risk of osteoporosis later in life" [59]. Another claim added to the aforementioned statement in foods providing 40% or more of the daily value (1,000 mg) states, "Adequate calcium intake is important, but daily intakes above about 2,000 mg are not likely to provide any additional benefit" [59]. Foods citing these claims should not provide more phosphorus than calcium on a weight-for-weight basis [59].

Deficiency

Inadequate calcium intake, poor calcium absorption, and/or excessive calcium losses contribute to calcium deficiency. Poor calcium intakes affect mostly bone and muscle. Rickets occurs in children when the amount of calcium accretion per unit of bone matrix is deficient. Low levels of free ionized Ca^{2+} in the blood (hypocalcemia) may result in **tetany,** a condition characterized by intermittent muscle contractions that fail to relax, especially in muscles of the arms and legs (extremities). Muscle pain, muscle spasms, and paresthesia (numbness or tingling in the hands and feet) also are common signs of tetany. In adults deficient in calcium, osteoporosis—the loss of bone mass (protein matrix and bone minerals)—occurs [60,61]. Two types of osteoporosis have been described:

- type I, which occurs mostly in postmenopausal women between the ages of 50 and 65 years and affects mainly the vertebrae and distal radius, and
- type II, which occurs in men and women over the age of about 70 years and affects the vertebrae, hips, pelvis, humerus, and tibia [39].

Both type I and type II contribute to bone loss (decreased mass), increased bone fragility, and fracture risk in individuals. Osteoporosis and diet are discussed further in a perspective at the end of the chapter.

Much of the U.S. population, particularly females over 12 years of age, fails to consume the recommended amounts of calcium. Inadequate calcium intake during the period of bone mineralization is a concern because of the high incidence of osteoporosis among elderly women and the significant correlation shown to exist between present bone density and past calcium intake [3]. Several studies have reported positive effects from consumption of adequate dietary calcium and/or from calcium supplementation on age-related bone loss [62]. Populations associated with an increased need for calcium include those with high-fiber/high-phytate diets, fat malabsorption, immobilization (which promotes calcium loss from bone), decreased gastrointestinal transit time, and long-term use of thiazide diuretics (which increase calcium excretion in the urine).

In addition to osteoporosis, deficient (long-term) calcium intakes also are associated with the development of hypertension, colon cancer, and obesity or higher body weights. An inverse relationship exists between calcium and blood pressure (as intake of calcium decreases, prevalence of hypertension increases), with a steep slope at calcium intakes <600 mg/day [63,64]. The perspective "Macrominerals and Hypertension" at the end of this chapter addresses this relationship. Calcium also is thought to decrease the risk of colon cancer through its ability to bind bile acids and free fatty acids, which act as promoters of cancer by inducing colon cell hyperproliferation. Colon cancer has been linked with calcium-deficient diets in some but not all studies [3,14,63,65–69]. Adequate intakes of calcium (>800 mg/day) are thought to be protective against colon cancer; however, evidence in humans is considered insufficient to recommend the intake of calcium to prevent colon cancer [3]. Low intakes of calcium and dairy products have also been associated with obesity and higher body weights in humans. The modulation of body weight by calcium is under investigation, but it is thought to be related to alterations in intracellular calcium concentrations and regulation of fatty acid synthesis and lipolysis [70–73].

Toxicity

Intakes of calcium in amounts up to 2,500 mg daily appear to be safe for most individuals [3]. A tolerable upper intake level of 2,500 mg calcium has been recommended for those age 1 year and older [3].

Milk alkali syndrome has been documented in a few dozen individuals consuming excessive quantities of calcium in the form of milk and antacids in the treatment of ulcers. The large intakes of calcium resulted in hypercalcemia and deposition of calcium in soft tissues, along with systemic alkalosis. Soft tissue calcification typically occurs in patients with renal failure when the plasma calcium concentration times the plasma phosphorus concentration is high. Constipation also can occur with ingestion of large amounts of calcium, and for people with idiopathic **hypercalciuria** (urinary calcium levels >4 mg/kg of body weight per day) excessive calcium intakes may increase the risk of developing calcium-containing kidney stones [3,74].

Assessment of Nutriture

No routine biochemical method appears to assess calcium status accurately. Serum calcium (composed of protein-bound calcium, diffusible calcium complexes, and ionized calcium) is so exquisitely regulated that it usually indicates little about calcium status. Serum calcium concentrations normally range from about 8.5 to 10.5 mg/dL for adults, with slightly higher levels in children. Serum ionized calcium, Ca^{2+}, can reflect alterations in calcium metabolism. Assuming the presence of normal albumin concentrations, the ratio between bound calcium and ionized calcium remains constant. When albumin concentrations are depressed, corrections are needed to adjust for the corresponding decrease that occurs in the protein-bound fraction of calcium. For each 1 g/dL decrease in serum albumin, serum calcium will decrease 0.8 mg/dL. The following equations can be used for estimating protein-bound calcium:

$$\text{Protein-bound calcium (mg/dL)} = 0.44 + 0.76 \times \text{albumin (g/dL)} \quad \text{or}$$

$$= 0.8 \times (\text{normal albumin} - \text{actual albumin}) + \text{measured calcium (mg/dL)}$$

Bone densitometry can be assessed through computerized tomography (CT) scans. Though less accurate and precise than dual-energy X-ray absorptiometry (discussed below), CT can measure variances in tissue density (such as in vertebral bone). X rays are taken as the individual is held in a scanner. Radiation pulses are emitted, collected, and processed to reconstruct the image and calculate bone density.

Neutron activation, an in vivo procedure in which gamma rays are counted following administration of ^{48}Ca into the body and exposure of the body to a low neutron flux, allows assessment of total body calcium content. Results of neutron activation correlate with single-photon absorptiometry, which measures total bone mineral content. Single-photon absorptiometry exposes a portion of a limb, usually the radius (forearm) or os calcis (heel) to radiation. The quantity of bone mineral is inversely proportional to the amount of photon energy transmitted from the bone, as measured by a scintillation counter.

Dual-energy X-ray absorptiometry (abbreviated DEXA or DXA) can be used to measure both body fat and bone mineral content (total and selected sites such as the vertebrae or femur). The procedure involves scanning specific sites at two different energy levels using an X-ray tube. Radiation exposure is very low, and the procedure is relatively quick. Dual-energy X-ray absorptiometry may be used to assess changes in mass over time and is thought to represent the best method for assessing bone mineral density [75]. Further, measurement of bone mass is thought to be the best tool for assessing calcium status. Information on the use of bone mineral density to diagnose osteoporosis is provided in the perspective "Osteoporosis and Diet" at the end of this chapter.

References Cited for Calcium

1. Heaney R, Recker R, Weaver C. Absorbability of calcium sources: the limited role of solubility. Calcif Tissue Int 1990;46:300–304.

2. Sheikh MS, Santa Ana CA, Nicar MJ, Schiller LR, Fordtran JS. Gastrointestinal absorption of calcium from milk and calcium salts. N Engl J Med 1987;317:532–36.

3. Food and Nutrition Board, Institute of Medicine. Dietary Reference Intakes. Washington, DC: National Academy Press, 1997, pp. 71–145.

4. Bronner F. Transcellular calcium transport. In: Bronner F, ed. Intracellular Calcium Regulation. New York: Wiley-Liss, 1990, pp. 415–37.

5. Wishart J, Horowitz M, Need A, Scopacasa F, Morris H, Clifton P, Nordin B. Relations between calcium intake, calcitriol, polymorphisms of the vitamin D receptor gene, and calcium absorption in premenopausal women. Am J Clin Nutr 1997;67:798–802.

6. Ziegler EE, Fomon SJ. Lactose enhances mineral absorption in infancy. J Pediatr Gastr Nutr 1983;2:288–94.

7. Schaafsma G. Calcium in extracellular fluid homeostasis. In: Nordin BEC. Calcium in Human Biology. London: Springer-Verlag, 1988, pp. 241–59.

8. Hamalainen M. Bone repair in calcium-deficient rats: comparison of xylitol + calcium carbonate with calcium carbonate, calcium lactate and calcium citrate on the repletion of calcium. J Nutr 1994;124:874–81.

9. Harland BF, Oberleas D. Phytate in foods. Wld Rev Nutr Diet 1987;52:235–59.

10. Greger JL. Mineral bioavailability/new concepts. Nutr Today 1987;22:4–9.

11. Spencer H. Minerals and mineral interactions in human beings. J Am Diet Assoc 1986;86:864–67.

12. Anderson JJB. Nutritional biochemistry of calcium and phosphorus. J Nutr Biochem 1991;2:300–307.

13. Whiting S. Safety of some calcium supplements questioned. Nutr Rev 1994;52:95–97.

14. Weaver C. Assessing calcium status and metabolism. J Nutr 1990;120:1470–73.

15. Recker R, Bammi A, Barger-Lux M, Heaney R. Calcium absorbability from milk products, an imitation milk and calcium carbonate. Am J Clin Nutr 1988;47:93–95.

16. Johnson PE, Lykken GI. Manganese and calcium absorption and balance in young women fed diets with varying amounts of manganese and calcium. J Trace Elem Exp Med 1991;4:19–35.

17. Schwartz R, Apgar BJ, Wien EM. Apparent absorption and retention of Ca, Cu, Mg, Mn, and Zn from a diet containing bran. Am J Clin Nutr 1986;43:444–55.

18. Brown EM. Extracellular Ca^{2+} sensing, regulation of parathyroid cell function, and role of Ca^{2+} and other ions as extracellular (first) messengers. Physiol Rev 1991;71:371–411.

19. Wasserman R. Cellular calcium: action of hormones. In: Bronner F, ed. Intracellular calcium regulation. New York: Wiley-Liss, 1990, pp. 385–419.

20. Rasmussen H. The calcium messenger system (parts 1 and 2). N Engl J Med 1986;314:1094–101, 1164–70.

21. Calvo M, Kumar R, Heath H. Elevated secretion and action of parathyroid hormone in young adults ingesting high phosphorus, low calcium diets assembled for ordinary foods. J Clin Endocrinol Metab 1988;66:823–29.

22. Calvo M, Kumar R, Heath H. Persistently elevated parathyroid hormone secretion and action in young women after four weeks of ingesting high phosphorus, low calcium diets. J Clin Endocrinol Metab 1990;70:1334–40.

23. Calvo MS. Dietary phosphorus, calcium metabolism and bone. J Nutr 1993;123:1627–33.

24. Calvo S, Park Y. Changing phosphorus content of the U.S. diet: potential for adverse effects on bone. J Nutr 1996;126:1168S–80S.

25. Bizik BK, Ding W, Cerklewski FL. Evidence that bone resorption of young men is not increased by high dietary phosphorus obtained from milk and cheese. Nutr Res 1996;16:1143–46.

26. Heaney RP, Recker RR. Calcium supplements: anion effects. Bone Miner 1987;2:433–39.

27. Heaney RP, Recker RR. Effects of nitrogen, phosphorus, and caffeine on calcium balance in women. J Lab Clin Med 1982; 99:46–55.

28. Zemel M, Linkswiler H. Calcium metabolism in the young adult male as affected by level and form of phosphorus intake and level of calcium intake. J Nutr 1981;11:315–24.

29. Karkkainen M, Lamberg-Allardt C. An acute intake of phosphorus increases parathyroid hormone secretion and inhibits bone formation in young women. J Bone Miner Res 1996;11:1905–11.

30. Whiting S, Anderson D, Weeks S. Calciuric effects of protein and potassium bicarbonate but not sodium chloride or phosphate can be detected acutely in women and men. Am J Clin Nutr 1997; 65:1465–67.

31. Heaney R. Protein intake and the calcium economy. J Am Diet Assoc 1993;93:1259–60.

32. Itoh R, Nishiyama N, Suyama Y. Dietary protein intake and urinary excretion of calcium: a cross-sectional study in a healthy Japanese population. Am J Clin Nutr 1998;67:438–44.

33. Mahalko JR, Sandstead HH, Johnson LK, Milne DB. Effect of a moderate increase in dietary protein on the retention and excretion of Ca, Cu, Fe, Mg, P, and Zn by adult males. Am J Clin Nutr 1983; 37:8–14.

34. Delmas PD. Clinical use of biochemical markers of bone remodeling in osteoporosis. Bone 1992;13:S17–S21.

35. Nordin B, Need A, Morris H, Horowitz M. The nature and significance of the relationship between urinary sodium and urinary calcium in women. J Nutr 1993;123:1615–22.

36. Devine A, Criddle R, Dick I, Kerr D, Prince R. A longitudinal study of the effect of sodium and calcium intake on regional bone density in postmenopausal women. Am J Clin Nutr 1995;62:740–45.

37. Massey LK. Dietary factors influencing calcium and bone metabolism: introduction. J Nutr 1993;123:1609–10.

38. Massey L, Whiting S. Caffeine, urinary calcium, calcium metabolism and bone. J Nutr 1993;123:1611–14.

39. Harward M. Nutritive therapies for osteoporosis: the role of calcium. Med Clin N Am 1993;77:889–98.

40. Hernandez-Avila M, Colditz G, Stampfer M, Rosner B, Speizer F, Willett W. Caffeine, moderate alcohol intake, and risk of fractures of the hip and forearm in middle-aged women. Am J Clin Nutr 1991; 54:157–63.

41. Hunt C, Herbel J, Nielsen F. Metabolic responses of postmenopausal women to supplemental dietary boron and aluminum during usual and low magnesium intake: boron, calcium, and magnesium absorption and retention and blood mineral concentrations. Am J Clin Nutr 1997;65:803–13.

42. Cook J, Dassenko S, Whittaker P. Calcium supplementation: effect on iron absorption. Am J Clin Nutr 1991;53:106–11.

43. Hallberg L, Rossander-Hulten L, Brune M, Gleerup A. Calcium and iron absorption: mechanism of action and nutritional importance. Eur J Clin Nutr 1992;46:317–27.

44. Hallberg L, Brune M, Erlandsson M, Sandberg A-S, Rossander-Hulten L. Calcium: effect of different amounts on nonheme- and heme-iron absorption in humans. Am J Clin Nutr 1991;53:112–19.

45. Barton J, Conrad M, Harrison L, Nuby S. Effects of calcium on the absorption and retention of lead. J Lab Clin Med 1978; 91:366–76.

46. Bogden J, Gertner S, Christakos S. Dietary calcium modifies concentrations of lead and other metals and renal calbindin in rats. Can J Nutr 1992;122:1351–60.

47. Fleischman A, Yacowitz H, Hayton T, Bierenbaum M. Long term studies on the hypolipemic effect of dietary calcium in mature male rats fed cocoa butter. J Nutr 1967;91:151–58.

48. Bell L, Halstenton CE, Halstenton CJ, Macres M, Keane W. Cholesterol lowering effects of calcium carbonate in patients with mild to moderate hypercholesterolemia. Arch Intern Med 1992; 152:2441–44.

49. Paydas S, Seyrek N, Sagliker Y. Does oral $CaCO_3$ and calcitriol administration for secondary hyperparathyroidism treatment affect the lipid profile in HD patients? Dialysis and Transplant 1996; 25:344–47, 383.

50. Carlson L, Olsson A, Oro L, Rossner S. Effects of oral calcium upon serum cholesterol and triglycerides in patients with hyperlipidemia. Atherosclerosis 1971;14:391–400.

51. Gardner TA, Yates LA, Soffed O, Gropper SS. Calcium carbonate binder therapy: impact on serum lipids in hemodialysis patients. Dialysis and Transplant 1999;28:641–52.

52. Lupton J, Steinbach G, Chang W, O'Brien C, Wiese S, Stoltzfus C, Glober G. Calcium supplementation modifies the relative amounts of bile acid in bile and affects key aspects of human colon physiology. J Nutr 1996;126:1421–28.

53. Charles P, Eriksen EF, Hasling C, Sondergard K, Mosekilde L. Dermal, intestinal, and renal obligatory losses of calcium: relation to skeletal calcium loss. Am J Clin Nutr 1991;54:266S–73S.

54. Calvo MS, Eastell R, Offord KP, Bergstralh EJ, Burritt MF. Circadian variation ionized calcium and intact parathyroid hormone: evidence of sex differences in calcium homeostasis. J Clin Endocrinol 1991;72:69–76.

55. Lemann J, Pleuss J, Gray R. Potassium causes calcium retention in healthy adults. J Nutr 1993;123:1623–26.

56. Elders PJ, Lips P, Netelenbos JC, van Ginkel FC, Kohe E, van der Vijgh WJ, van der Stelt PF. Long-term effect of calcium supplementation on bone loss in perimenopausal women. J Bone Mineral Res 1994;9:963–70.

57. National Institutes of Health, Consensus Development Panel on Optimal Calcium Intake. Optimal calcium intake. JAMA 1994;272:1942–48.

58. Matkovic V, Heaney R. Calcium balance during human growth: evidence for threshold behavior. Am J Clin Nutr 1992;55:992–96.

59. www.cfsan.fda.gov

60. Sowers M. Epidemiology of calcium and vitamin D in bone loss. J Nutr 1993;123:413–17.

61. Nieves J, Komar L, Cosman F, Lindsay R. Calcium potentiates the effect of estrogen and calcitonin on bone mass: review and analysis. Am J Clin Nutr 1998;67:18–24.

62. Heaney RP. Calcium, dairy products and osteoporosis. J Am Coll Nutr 2000;19:83S–99S.

63. Barger-Lux M, Heaney R. The role of calcium intake in preventing bone fragility, hypertension, and certain cancers. J Nutr 1994; 124:1406S–11S.

64. McCarron D, Morris C, Young E, Roullet C, Drueke T. Dietary calcium and blood pressure: modifying factors in specific populations. Am J Clin Nutr 1991;54:215S–19S.

65. Bostick RM, Potter JD, Fosdick L, Grambsch P, Lampe JW, Wood JR, Louis TA, Ganz R, Grandits G. Calcium and colorectal epithelial cell proliferation: a preliminary randomized, double-blinded, placebo-controlled clinical trial. J Natl Cancer Inst 1993;85:132–41.

66. Kleibeuker JH, Welberg JW, Mulder NH, van der Meer R, Cats A, Limburg AJ, Kreumer WM, Hardonk MJ, deVries EG. Epithelial cell

proliferation in the sigmoid colon of patients with adenomatous polyps increases during oral calcium supplementation. Br J Cancer 1993;67:500–503.

67. Meyer F, White E. Alcohol and nutrients in relation to colon cancer in middle-aged adults. Am J Epidemiol 1993;138:225–36.

68. Slattery ML, Sorenson AW, Ford MH. Dietary calcium intake as a mitigating factor in colon cancer. Am J Epidemiol 1988; 128:504–14.

69. Garland C, Shekelle RB, Barrett-Connor E, Criqui MH, Rossof AH, Paul O. Dietary vitamin D and calcium and risk of colorectal cancer: a 19 year prospective study in men. Lancet 1985;1:307–9.

70. Zemel MB. Calcium modulation of hypertension and obesity: mechanisms and implications. J Am Coll Nutr 2001;20:428S–35S.

71. Heaney RP, Davies KM, Barger-Lux J. Calcium and weight: clinical studies. J Am Coll Nutr 2001;21:152S–55S.

72. Zemel MB. Nutritional and endocrine modulation of intracellular calcium: implications in obesity, insulin resistance and hypertension. Molec Cell Biochem 1998;188:129–36.

73. Carruth BR, Skinner JD. The role of dietary calcium and other nutrients in moderating body fat in preschool children. Int J Obesity 2001;25:559–66.

74. Brown W, Wolfson M. Diet as culprit or therapy. Stone disease, chronic renal failure, and nephrotic syndrome. Med Clin N Am 1993;77:783–94.

75. Heymsfield S, Wang Z. Human body composition. Ann Rev Nutr 1997;17:527–58.

Websites

www.cfsan.fda.gov
www.nhlbi.nih.gov
www.nationaldairycouncil.org
www.calciuminfo.com
www.consensus.nih.gov

PHOSPHORUS

Among the inorganic elements, phosphorus is second only to calcium in abundance in the body. Approximately 560 to 850 g are present in a 70-kg human, representing about 0.8% to 1.2% of body weight. Of total body phosphorus, about 85% is in the skeleton, 1% is in the blood and body fluids, and the remaining 14% is associated with soft tissue such as muscle. In the body, phosphorus typically is found in combination with other inorganic elements or with organic compounds.

Sources

Phosphorus is widely distributed in foods. The best food sources of phosphorus are listed in Table 11.1 and include meat, poultry, fish, eggs, milk, and milk products. Nuts, legumes, cereals, and grains also contain phosphorus; however, animal products are superior sources of available phosphorus compared with most plant foods. Coffee and tea also provide small amounts of phosphorus, as do soft drinks. Cola-type soft drinks contain phosphoric acid and, depending on consumption habits, can contribute substantially to dietary intake. In addition to dietary sources, phosphate-containing supplements are available commercially, including K-Phos and Neutra-Phos K, which also provide potassium. Such supplements can be helpful for individuals whose phosphorus stores have been depleted due to malnutrition.

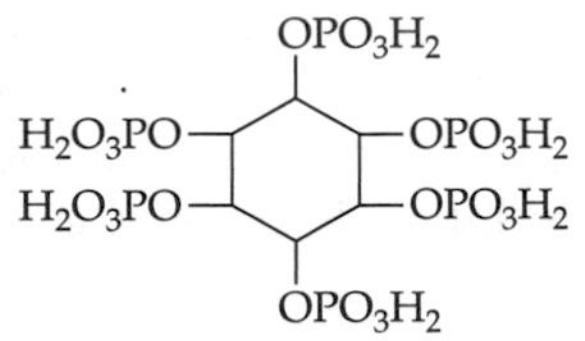

Figure 11.7 Phytic acid (phytate).

Phosphorus is not usually found free in nature. Dietary phosphorus occurs in both an inorganic form and an organic form. In its organic form, phosphorus is bound to a variety of compounds such as proteins, sugars, and lipids. The relative amounts of inorganic and organic phosphorus vary with the type of diet. For example, about one-third of the phosphorus in milk is in the form of inorganic phosphates. Meats contain phosphorus that is largely bound to organic compounds and thus requires hydrolysis for absorption to occur. Over 80% of the phosphorus in grains, such as wheat, rice, and corn, is found as phytate (Fig. 11.7; also called phytic acid or myoinositol hexaphosphate). Phosphorus in the form of phytate is also found in beans, legumes, and nuts. The bioavailability of phosphorus from phytate is limited to about 50%, as discussed in the section "Factors Influencing Absorption."

Digestion, Absorption, Transport, and Storage

Digestion

Regardless of its dietary form, most phosphorus is absorbed in its inorganic form. Organically bound phosphorus is hydrolyzed enzymatically in the lumen of the small intestine and released as inorganic phosphate. Phospholipase C, a zinc-dependent enzyme, for example, hydrolyzes the glycerophosphate bond in phospholipids. Alkaline phosphatase, another zinc-dependent enzyme whose activity is stimulated by calcitriol, functions at the brush border of the enterocyte to free phosphorus from some, but not all, bound forms. For example, it cannot free phytate-bound phosphorus.

Absorption

Phosphorus absorption occurs in its inorganic form throughout the small intestine. However, radiophosphorus perfusion studies suggest that phosphorus absorption occurs primarily in the duodenum and jejunum. About

50% to 70% of dietary phosphorus is absorbed, with absorption from animal products at the upper end of the range and that from phytate-containing foods at the lower end. Variations in intake have not been shown to affect absorption [1].

Phosphorus absorption appears to occur by two processes:

- a saturable, carrier-mediated active transport system dependent on sodium and enhanced by calcitriol and
- a concentration-dependent diffusion process [2].

Factors Influencing Absorption. A number of factors either positively or negatively influence phosphorus absorption, as shown in Table 11.4. One stimulus of phosphorus absorption is vitamin D as calcitriol, which stimulates absorption in both the duodenum and the jejunum [2].

Several substances have been shown to inhibit phosphorus absorption. Phytate (Fig. 11.7) is the major form of phosphate in grains and legumes. The poor bioavailability of phosphorus from phytates is due to the absence of phytase in mammalian digestion. Phytase is a phosphate esterase that liberates phosphate from phytic acid. Yeasts in breads possess phytase that can hydrolyze some of the phytates to yield some phosphorus available for absorption. In addition, bacteria in the gastrointestinal tract can liberate some phosphorus from phytates as long as the phytates are not complexed with cations such as calcium, zinc, and iron [3]. When consumed with cations such as Ca^{2+} or Zn^{2+}, phytate forms cation-phytate complexes and prevents these nutrients from being absorbed (Fig. 12.9 shows a phytate-cation complex).

Several minerals, including magnesium, aluminum, and calcium, also impair phosphorus absorption. Phosphorus absorption may be reduced by dietary magnesium, and, conversely, a deficiency of luminal magnesium enhances the absorption of phosphate. The two minerals are thought to form a complex, $Mg_3(PO_4)_2$, within the gastrointestinal tract to render each other unavailable for absorption. Aluminum hydroxide (3 g) given with a meal has been shown to reduce phosphorus absorption from 70% to 35%. Aluminum, magnesium (as hydroxides), and calcium (as carbonate or acetate) are common components of antacids and for years were given in pharmacological doses to bind dietary phosphate in people with **hyperphosphatemia** (high blood phosphorus concentrations) due to kidney disease.

Table 11.4 Factors Enhancing and Inhibiting Intestinal Phosphorus Absorption

Substances Enhancing Absorption	Substances Inhibiting Absorption
Vitamin D	Phytate
	Excessive intakes of: Magnesium Calcium Aluminum

Transport and Storage

Phosphorus is quickly absorbed from the intestine and into the blood, appearing in the blood within about an hour after ingestion in animal studies. Phosphorus is found in the blood in both organic and inorganic forms. About 70% of phosphorus is present as organic phosphate, such as that found as phospholipids in lipoproteins. Of the remaining 30% of phosphorus, most (approximately 85%) is as HPO_4^{2-} and $H_2PO_4^-$, with trace amounts of PO_4^{3-}. Some inorganic phosphates are associated with other minerals, such as calcium, magnesium, or sodium [4].

Inorganic phosphorus is sometimes referred to as ultrafilterable phosphate. In adults, plasma inorganic phosphate ranges from about 2.5 to 4.5 mg/dL. Dietary phosphate, age and stage of growth, time of day, various hormones, and renal function all contribute to the variability of the serum phosphate concentration. Circulating phosphate is in equilibrium with skeletal and cellular inorganic phosphate as well as with that of organic phosphates formed in intermediary metabolism. Phosphorus is found in all cells of the body, with bone and muscle containing the majority. Figure 11.8 provides an overview of phosphorus digestion, absorption, and transport.

Functions and Mechanisms of Action

Phosphorus has many functions in the body, with involvement in several biologically important compounds. Examples include roles in bone mineralization, energy transfer and storage, nucleic acid formation, cell membrane structure, and acid-base balance. We will briefly discuss each of these roles.

Bone Mineralization

Phosphate is of prime importance in the development of skeletal tissue, which in itself accounts for 85% of body phosphorus. In bone, phosphorus is found in amorphous calcium phosphate forms, including, for example, $Ca_3(PO_4)_2$, $CaHPO_4{\cdot}2H_2O$, $Ca_3(PO_4)_2{\cdot}3H_2O$, and in more crystalline forms such as hydroxyapatite, $Ca_{10}(PO_4)_6(OH)_2$, which is laid down on collagen in the ossification process of bone formation. In amorphous bone, the ratio of calcium to phosphorus is about 1.3 : 1, similar to extracellular fluid; however, in crystalline bone, the ratio is about 1.5 : 1.

Parathyroid hormone (PTH), calcitriol, and calcitonin influence phosphorus metabolism. Calcitonin promotes

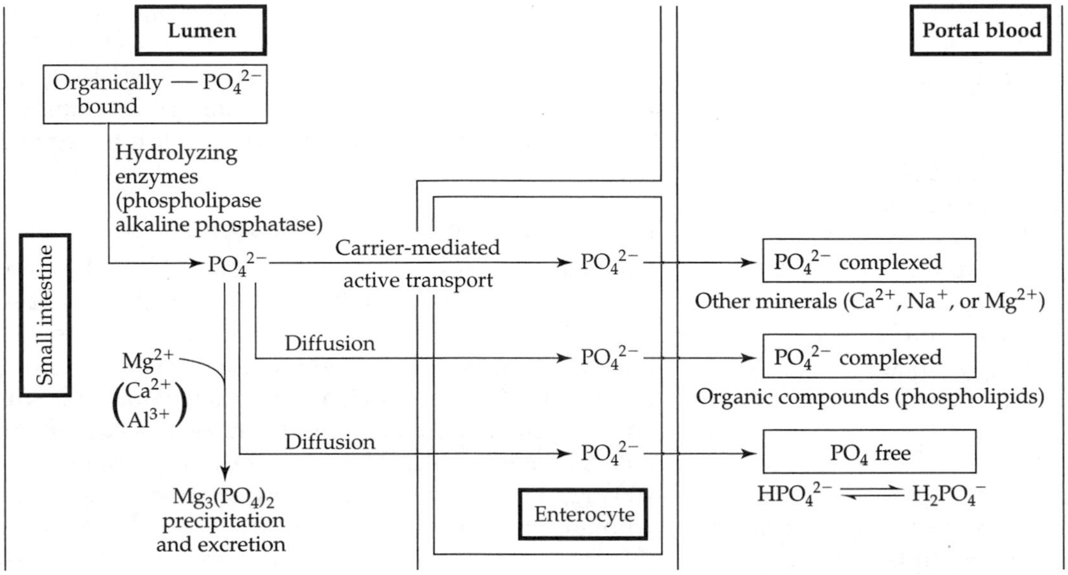

Figure 11.8 Digestion, absorption, and transport of phosphorus.

bone mineralization, while PTH stimulates resorption of phosphate from bone, as it does calcium. However, in contrast to calcium, PTH stimulates excretion of phosphorus in urine. The PTH-induced urinary excretion of phosphorus typically is sufficient to override bone resorption of phosphorus so as to effect a net decrease in plasma phosphate. Calcitriol (1,25-dihydroxy vitamin D), in conjunction with PTH, also enhances phosphate resorption from bone. Calcitriol also stimulates phosphate absorption in the intestine, possibly through enhanced alkaline phosphatase activity. See the calcium section of this chapter for a further discussion of bone mineralization and the roles of calcium and phosphorus (p. 385). Phosphorus that is not part of bone is found either in extracellular fluids such as blood or in soft tissues. Within cells, phosphorus is the major anion and is involved in a host of processes.

Nucleotide/Nucleoside Phosphates

Structural Roles. Phosphate is an important component of the nucleic acids DNA and RNA, alternating with pentose sugars to form the linear backbone of these molecules. DNA and RNA are discussed in more detail in Chapter 1.

Energy Storage and Transfer. Phosphorus is of vital importance in intermediary metabolism of the energy nutrients in the form of high-energy phosphate bonds, such as the nucleoside triphosphate adenosine triphosphate (ATP). More information on ATP can be found on page 59. In addition to its presence in ATP, phosphorus is found in creatine phosphate (also called phosphocreatine). Creatine phosphate is synthesized in muscle from ATP and creatine and can provide energy to muscles as needed (e.g., during exercise) by transferring its PO_4 to ADP via creatine kinase. More information on the functions of creatine phosphate can be found on page 190.

Another nucleoside triphosphate, uridine triphosphate (UTP), functions to activate substances in intermediary metabolism. For example, UTP hydrolysis provides for the coupling of uridine monophosphate (UMP) and glucose 1-phosphate to form uridine diphosphate (UDP)-glucose. UDP-glucose is critical for the synthesis of glycogen, as discussed in the section "Glycogenesis" on page 84.

Intracellular Second Messenger. Phosphorus as part of cyclic adenosine monophosphate (cAMP), which is derived from ATP, functions as a second messenger to affect cellular metabolism. cAMP, which acts within cells by activating certain protein kinases, is generated in response to the binding of certain hormones to cell receptors. Inositol triphosphate (IP_3) also functions as a second messenger to trigger intracellular calcium release. Its actions are mediated by protein kinases. The role of protein kinases as they function in enzyme activation is discussed next.

Phosphoproteins

Phosphorus also is of vital importance in intermediary metabolism of the energy nutrients through the phosphorylation of different substrates in the body. Protein kinases activated by cAMP, a phosphate-containing second messenger, function to phosphorylate specific target proteins within the cell, thereby changing cellular activities. Many enzymatic activities, for example, are controlled by alternating phosphorylation or dephosphorylation. An example of the role of phosphorylation and dephosphorylation of enzymes can be found in the discussion of glycogen degradation (p. 85).

Structural Roles

Cell membranes are made up in part of lipids, including phospholipids, which (as their name implies) contain phosphorus. Phospholipids, with their polar and nonpolar regions, are important to the bilayer structure of cell membranes. Some examples of phospholipids are phosphatidylcholine, phosphatidylinositol, phosphatidylserine, and phosphatidylethanolamine. More information on phospholipids is found on page 133.

Acid-Base Balance

Phosphate also functions in acid-base balance in the body. Within cells, phosphate is the main intracellular buffer. Within the kidney, for example, filtered phosphate reacts with secreted hydrogen ions, releasing sodium ions in the process, as shown here:

$$Na_2HPO_4 + H^+ \longrightarrow NaH_2PO_4 + Na^+$$

This action removes free hydrogen ions and therefore increases pH. The following reaction also effects a rise in pH:

$$HPO_4^{2-} + H^+ \longrightarrow H_2PO_4^-$$

These reactions may be reversed to effect a lowering of pH.

Oxygen Availability

Phosphate is involved indirectly in oxygen delivery. In red blood cells, synthesis of 2,3-diphosphoglycerate, which influences oxygen release from hemoglobin, requires phosphorus. Decreased 2,3-diphosphoglycerate associated with phosphorus deficiency can diminish release of oxygen to tissues.

Excretion

About 67% to 90% of phosphorus is excreted in inorganic form in the urine. The remaining 10% to 33% of phosphorus is excreted in the feces. Unlike calcium, high dietary phosphorus leads to high serum phosphorus, which leads to increased urinary phosphorus excretion. In other words, maintenance of the phosphate balance is achieved largely through renal excretion. The amount of dietary phosphorus and absorbed phosphorus has approximately a linear relationship with urinary phosphorus if the amount of phosphorus filtered is greater than the tubular maximum for phosphorus [1]. The tubular maximum for phosphorus (TmP) is the amount (mmol) of phosphorus reabsorbed per unit time. However, if phosphorus intake and plasma phosphorus concentrations are low, then most filtered phosphorus is reabsorbed. This reabsorption helps maintain the plasma phosphorus concentration. PTH concentrations are inversely related to TmP. Therefore, high levels of PTH decrease TmP and thus increase the amount of phosphorus excreted in the urine. Other hormones that inhibit the tubular reabsorption of phosphorus include estrogen and thyroid hormones.

Recommended Dietary Allowances

An estimated requirement (580 mg/day) for phosphorus was determined based on the relationship between dietary phosphorus intake and plasma phosphorus concentrations as well as a known efficiency of intestinal absorption [5]. A coefficient of variation of 10% was added to the requirement and rounded to establish the recommended intake. The 1997 RDA for phosphorus is 700 mg/day for males and females (including those who are pregnant or lactating) age 19 years and older [5]. These values are slightly lower than the 1989 RDA of 800 mg/day for phosphorus. The inside covers of the book provide the RDAs for phosphorus for other age groups.

Deficiency

Phosphorus deficiency is rare. It is typically confined to people (such as those with renal disease) who are receiving large amounts of antacids containing calcium, magnesium, and/or aluminum (which bind phosphorus in the gastrointestinal tract). In addition, individuals who are malnourished and are being refed enterally through a tube or parenterally (intravenously) without being given additional phosphorus have been known to exhibit phosphate deficiency syndrome. This situation is often referred to as "refeeding syndrome." Deficiency of phosphorus, usually manifested biochemically by low serum phosphorus concentrations (<1.5 mg/dL), is associated with anorexia, hypophosphatemic rickets and bone loss, skeletal muscle and cardiac myopathy, weakness, neurological problems (ataxia and paresthesia), and disturbances in oxygen delivery.

Toxicity

Toxicity from phosphorus is rare. Problems have been reported only in infants when calcium : phosphorus ratios are altered significantly in favor of phosphorus. Phosphorus toxicity is characterized predominantly by hypocalcemia and tetany. A tolerable upper intake level of 4 g phosphorus has been recommended for those age 9 to 70 years; after age 70 years, the tolerable level drops to 3 g phosphorus daily [5]. For pregnant and lactating women, the tolerable upper intake levels are 3.5 and 4 g, respectively [5].

Assessment of Nutriture

The assessment of phosphorus nutriture is not a major consideration because deficiency is so rare. Serum phosphorus concentrations and urinary excretion are most often assessed; however, their specificity and sensitivity are low. Serum phosphate concentrations, for example, can be maintained at the expense of tissues.

References Cited for Phosphorus

1. Lemann J Jr. Calcium and phosphate metabolism: an overview in health and in calcium stone formers. In: Coe FL, Favus MJ, Pak CY, Parks JH, Preminger GM, eds. Kidney Stones: Medical and Surgical Management. Philadelphia, PA: Lippincott-Raven, 1996, pp. 259–88.
2. Chen TC, Castillo L, Korychka-Dahl M, DeLuca HF. Role of vitamin D metabolites in phosphate transport of rat intestine. J Nutr 1974;104:1056–60.
3. Sandberg A, Larsen T, Sandstrom B. High dietary calcium level decreases colonic phytate digestion in pigs fed a rapeseed diet. J Nutr 1993;123:559–66.
4. Lobaugh B. Blood calcium and phosphorus regulation. In: Anderson JJB, Garner SC, eds. Calcium and Phosphorus in Health and Disease. Boca Raton, FL: CRC Press, 1996, pp. 27–43.
5. Food and Nutrition Board, Institute of Medicine. Dietary Reference Intakes. Washington, DC: National Academy Press, 1997, pp. 146–89.

MAGNESIUM

Magnesium as a cation in the human body ranks fourth in overall abundance, but intracellularly it is second only to potassium. A 70-kg human contains about 35 g magnesium (0.05% of body weight), of which approximately 55% to 60% is located in bone, another 20% to 25% in soft tissues, and about 1% in extracellular fluids.

Sources

Magnesium is found in a wide variety of foods and beverages. Beverages rich in magnesium are coffee, tea, and cocoa. Foods (and food components) particularly high in magnesium are nuts, legumes, whole-grain cereals (especially oats and barley), spices, seafoods, and green leafy vegetables. Chlorophyll found in the green leafy vegetables contains the magnesium. Other particularly good food sources of magnesium are chocolate, blackstrap molasses, corn, peas, carrots, brown rice, and parsley. Tap water also may represent a source of magnesium. Water can be high in magnesium (hard water) or high in sodium (soft water).

Magnesium salts—such as magnesium sulfate ($MgSO_4$, or Epsom salts), magnesium oxide (MgO), magnesium chloride ($MgCl_2$), magnesium lactate, magnesium acetate, magnesium gluconate, and magnesium citrate—are commonly available supplemental forms of the mineral. Slow Mag® (magnesium chloride) and Mag-Tab SR® (magnesium lactate) tablets provide ~60 to 84 mg magnesium per tablet. Supplements are sometimes needed for individuals with diseases causing fat malabsorption, such as inflammatory bowel diseases and pancreatic diseases. To maximize absorption, magnesium supplements should not be taken at the same time as other mineral supplements, such as iron.

Food processing and preparation may substantially reduce the magnesium content of some foods. For example, the refining of whole wheat with removal of the germ and outer layers can reduce the magnesium content by 80% [1].

Absorption and Transport

Absorption

Magnesium absorption occurs throughout the small intestine, mainly in the distal jejunum and ileum [2]. Two transport systems are thought to be responsible for magnesium absorption in the intestinal tract:

- a saturable, carrier-mediated active transporter that operates mostly at low magnesium intakes and
- simple diffusion, which is thought to function more with higher intakes [3,4].

The colon also may play a role in the absorption of magnesium, especially if disease has interfered with magnesium absorption in the small intestine [4,5].

About 40% to 60% of magnesium is thought to be absorbed in adults with usual intakes [2,3,6–8]. Absorption declines to about 11% to 35% with intake ranging from about 550 to 850 mg magnesium, and magnesium absorption is more efficient (up to 75% absorption) when magnesium status is poor or marginal and/or when magnesium intake is low [3,5,7,9]. For example, 65% of magnesium is absorbed with an intake of 36 mg versus only 11% absorption with an intake of 973 mg magnesium [3]. Efflux of magnesium out of cells is via a sodium- and energy-dependent carrier and possibly a calcium-dependent carrier [10,11]. Figure 11.9 illustrates magnesium absorption and transport.

Factors Influencing Absorption. Magnesium absorption may be influenced by a variety of other factors, as outlined in Table 11.5. For example, dietary phytate and nonfermentable fiber have been shown to impair magnesium absorption, but only to a small extent [12–15]. Unabsorbed fatty acids present in high quantities, as with steatorrhea, may bind to magnesium to form soaps. These magnesium–fatty acid soaps are excreted in the feces [6]. Other minerals, especially calcium and phosphorus, can inhibit magnesium absorption. The inhibition is most apparent when magnesium consumption is low and intake of the other minerals is high. For example, as stated earlier, magnesium and phosphorus can form a complex, $Mg_3(PO_4)_2$, within the gastrointestinal tract to render each other unavailable for absorption.

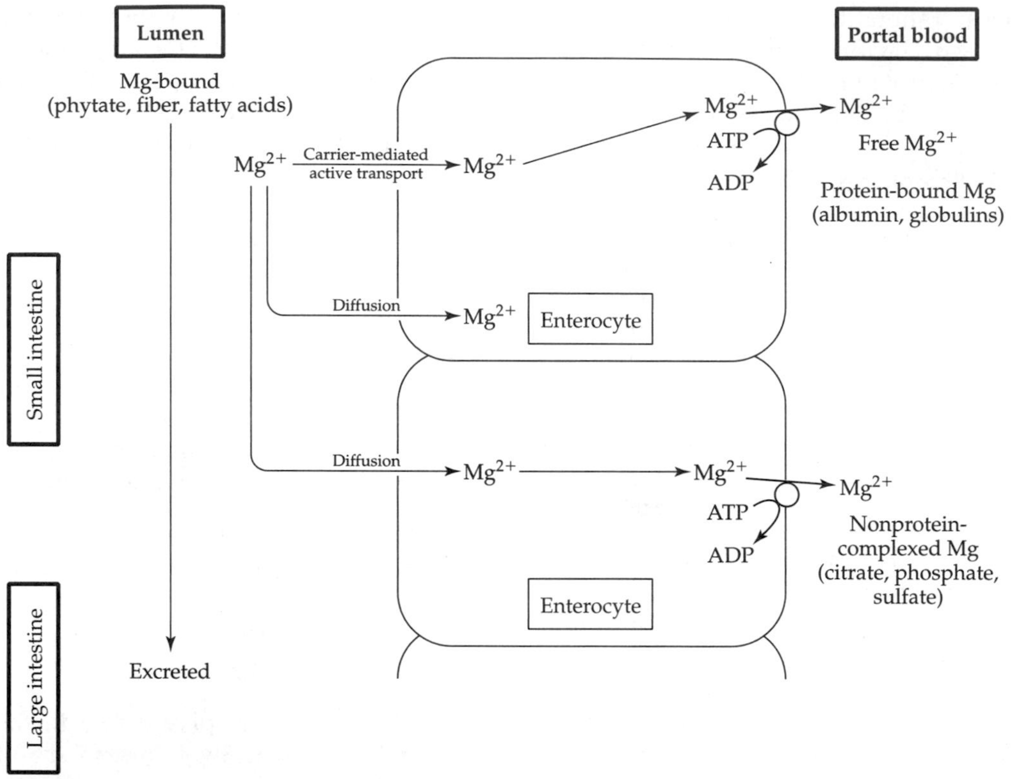

Figure 11.9 Magnesium absorption and transport.

Some factors are thought to improve magnesium absorption. Vitamin D, in pharmacological doses in some but not all studies, has been shown to increase magnesium absorption by active transport [4,6,16,17]. Carbohydrates can increase magnesium absorption. For example, fructose enhances absorption in humans by an unidentified mechanism [18,19]. In addition, lactose consumption by infants or individuals who are lactose intolerant can improve magnesium absorption [14,20]. The role of dietary protein in magnesium absorption is unclear; some but not all studies suggest improved absorption, while some suggest changes in retention [14]. Coatings used on magnesium supplements also affect magnesium absorption. Magnesium absorption from enteric-coated (cellulose acetate phthalate) magnesium supplements (such as Slow-Mag®, containing magnesium chloride) was substantially (67%) less than that from magnesium chloride encapsulated in gelatin [3].

Table 11.5 Substances/Nutrients Affecting Intestinal Absorption or Interacting with Magnesium at an Extraintestinal Site

Substances Enhancing Absorption	Substances Inhibiting Absorption	Nutrient Interactions
Vitamin D	Phytate	Calcium
Carbohydrates:	Fiber	Phosphorus
Lactose	Excessive unabsorbed fatty acids	Potassium
Fructose		Protein

Transport

In the plasma (Fig. 11.9), most magnesium (50%–55%) is found free, about 33% is bound to protein, and 13% is complexed with citrate, phosphate, sulfate, or other ions. Of the 33% of magnesium that is protein bound, most (about 30%) is bound to albumin, with the remaining usually bound to globulins. Concentrations of magnesium in the plasma are maintained between about 1.6 and 2.2 mg/dL; however, the homeostatic mechanism of control is unclear. Maintenance of these constant values appears to depend on gastrointestinal absorption, renal excretion, and transmembranous cation flux rather than on hormonal regulation [1]. Several hormones appear to affect but not regulate magnesium metabolism. Parathyroid hormone, for example, increases intestinal magnesium absorption, diminishes renal magnesium excretion, and enhances bone magnesium resorption, thereby raising plasma magnesium concentrations.

Functions and Mechanisms of Action

About 55% to 60% of magnesium in the body is found associated with bone. Bone magnesium is divided between that found associated with phosphorus and calcium as part of the crystal lattice (~70%) and that found on the surface in an amorphous form (~30%). Bone surface magnesium is thought to represent an exchangeable magnesium pool that is able to maintain serum levels. In contrast, the magnesium in the crystal lattice is probably deposited at the time of bone formation [21]. Magnesium may be present in bone as $Mg(OH)_2$ or $Mg_3(PO_4)_2$, for example.

Magnesium that does not function as part of bone is found in extracellular fluids (1%); in soft tissues, primarily muscle (about 25%); and in organs such as the liver and kidneys [1,6]. Within cells, magnesium is bound to phospholipids as part of cell membranes (plasma, endoplasmic reticulum, and mitochondria), where it may help in membrane stabilization. Magnesium is also associated with nucleic acids and protein (enzymes). Magnesium, with an approximate intracellular concentration of 8 to 10 mmol/L, is important for over 300 different enzyme reactions either as a structural cofactor or as an allosteric activator of enzyme activity [5,6].

Up to about 90% of intracellular magnesium may be associated with ATP or ADP and associated enzymes. Mg-ATP, for example, is utilized by hexokinase and phosphofructokinase. Mg-ADP is required by phosphoglycerate kinase and pyruvate kinase. In ATP, magnesium binds to phosphate groups, forming a complex that assists in the transfer of ATP phosphate. Figure 11.10 depicts magnesium as a ligand for the phosphate groups of ATP. Protein kinases transfer the γ-phosphate of magnesium ATP to a substrate [21].

Listed here are some of magnesium's roles in the body [21,22]:

- Glycolysis: hexokinase and phosphofructokinase (p. 87).
- Krebs cycle: oxidative decarboxylation.
- Hexosemonophosphate shunt: transketolase reaction.
- Creatine phosphate formation: creatine kinase.
- β-oxidation: initiation by thiokinase (acyl CoA synthetase).
- Activities of alkaline phosphatase and pyrophosphatase.
- Nucleic acid synthesis.
- DNA synthesis and degradation, as well as the physical integrity of the DNA helix.
- DNA and RNA transcription.
- Amino acid activation.
- Protein synthesis (e.g., with ribosomal aggregation and binding messenger RNA to ribosome subunits).
- Cardiac and smooth muscle contractability (direct action as well as influence on calcium ion transport and use).
- Vascular reactivity and coagulation (possible role).
- Cyclic adenosine monophosphate (cAMP) formation via adenylate cyclase. Because of its function in the formation of cAMP, magnesium mediates, in part, the effects of numerous hormones, including parathyroid hormone.
- Ion channel regulation, especially potassium channels.

Figure 11.10 Modes by which Mg^{2+} provides stability to ATP.

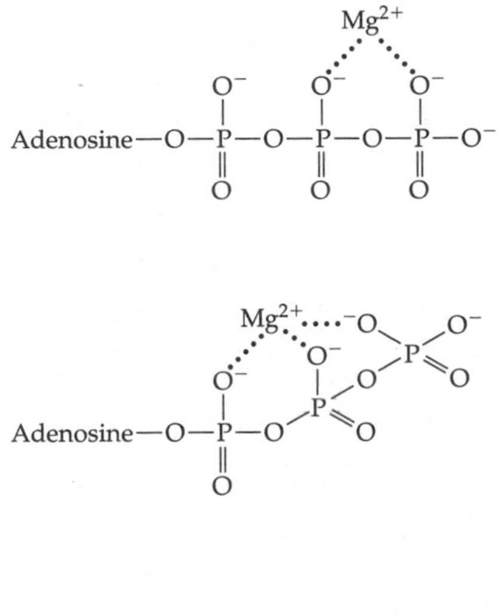

Interactions with Other Nutrients

Magnesium has interrelationships with a number of other nutrients. The first we will discuss here is that with calcium. Magnesium is needed for PTH secretion, which is important in calcium homeostasis. High magnesium concentrations, however, appear to inhibit PTH release, similar to calcium. Magnesium also is needed for PTH effects on the bone, kidney, and gastrointestinal tract. The hydroxylation of vitamin D in the liver requires magnesium. Calcium and magnesium use overlapping transport systems in the kidney and thus compete in part with each other for reabsorption. Magnesium may mimic calcium by binding to calcium-binding sites and eliciting the appropriate physiological response [5,22–24]. Magnesium also may cause an alteration in calcium distribution by changing the flux of calcium across the cell membrane or by displacing calcium on its intracellular binding sites. Magnesium may further inhibit release of calcium from the sarcoplasmic reticulum in response to increased influx from extracellular sites and may activate the Ca^{2+}-ATPase pump to decrease intracellular Ca^{2+} concentrations [24]. The ratio of calcium to magnesium has been shown to affect muscle contraction. Magnesium may compete with calcium for nonspecific binding sites on troponin C and myosin [24]. Additional effects of magnesium are seen in the smooth muscles [22,24]. For example, calcium binding initiates acetylcholine release and smooth muscle contraction, and magnesium bound to the calcium sites prevents calcium binding and inhibits contraction [23]. The magnesium-calcium relationship has implications for people with respiratory disease, because increased intracellular calcium promotes bronchial smooth muscle contraction [23]. Magnesium may also influence the process of blood coagulation. In blood coagulation, the actions of calcium and magnesium are antagonistic, with calcium promoting and magnesium inhibiting the process.

Magnesium inhibits phosphorus absorption. As magnesium intake increases, phosphorus absorption decreases. The two minerals are thought to precipitate as $Mg_3(PO_4)_2$. Magnesium acetate (600 mg), for example, has been shown to reduce phosphorus absorption from about 77% to 34% [3].

A close interrelationship also exists between magnesium and potassium. Magnesium influences the balance between extracellular and intracellular potassium, but its mechanism of action is unclear. Studies have shown that magnesium depletion is associated with increased potassium efflux from cells and subsequent renal excretion but is not associated with changes in the function of Na^+/K^+-ATPase, which requires magnesium as an activator [25]. When magnesium and potassium deficiencies coexist, as may occur with some diuretic drug therapies, magnesium infusions, but not potassium infusions—can normalize muscle potassium [5]. Finally, dietary protein intake impacts magnesium retention. Increasing dietary protein to a marginally adequate level in subjects previously ingesting low-magnesium and very low protein diets improved magnesium retention. However, when protein intake was further increased, magnesium retention was decreased [4,5].

Excretion

Most magnesium not retained by the body is excreted via the kidneys. Of the filtered magnesium, about 65% is reabsorbed in the loop of Henle, and another 20% to 30% is reabsorbed in the proximal tubule [7,26]. Thus, only about 5% of the filtered magnesium is excreted in the urine [5,7]. With changes in dietary intake of magnesium, changes in absorption and excretion of magnesium result to maintain, at least in part, homeostasis [7,22,27]. Diuretic medications, as well as protein, alcohol, and caffeine consumption, increase urinary magnesium excretion [28,29]. In contrast, PTH inhibits magnesium excretion by facilitating its reabsorption in the tubule.

Fecal magnesium concentrations represent unabsorbed magnesium and a small amount of endogenous magnesium. About 25 to 50 mg magnesium from endogenous sources is usually excreted daily in the feces [1]. Magnesium also may be lost in sweat, in amounts estimated to be approximately 15 mg/day [5].

Recommended Dietary Allowances

The RDAs for magnesium published in 1997 suggest 400 mg magnesium for males and 310 mg magnesium for females age 19 to 30 years, and 420 mg magnesium for males and 320 mg magnesium for females age 31 years and older [30]. Pregnant women age 19 to 30 years should ingest 350 mg, and those age 31 to 50 years should consume 360 mg magnesium [30]. During lactation, women age 19 to 30 years should ingest 310 mg, and those age 31 to 50 years should ingest 320 mg [30]. The inside covers of the book provide the RDAs for magnesium for other age groups.

Deficiency

Deficiency of magnesium or disturbances in magnesium homeostasis in humans are usually associated with the presence of other illnesses. Poor magnesium status may be related to cardiovascular disease, renal disease, diabetes mellitus, toxemia of pregnancy, hypertension, or postsurgical complications [5,6,24,31,32]. Other conditions that would increase the likelihood of developing a deficiency include excessive vomiting and/or diarrhea (that is, malabsorptive disorders), protein malnutrition, excessive alcohol use, refeeding syndrome, diuretic use, parathyroid disease, or burns.

Pure magnesium deficiency due to inadequate dietary intake has not been reported, but deficiency has been induced in humans under research protocols. Symptoms associated with deficiency or disturbances in balance include nausea, vomiting, anorexia, muscle weakness, spasms and tremors, personality changes, and hallucinations [26]. Changes in cardiovascular and neuromuscular function (such as neuromuscular hyperexcitability) may lead to cardiac arrhythmia and death. Hypomagnesemia, associated with deficiency, represents a plasma magnesium concentration of less than ~1.5 mg/dL and develops within a relatively short time following a magnesium deficit [27,33]. Other biochemical changes include low blood concentrations of not only magnesium but also calcitriol, potassium, and calcium [32,33]. Effects on PTH concentrations vary, but concentrations are usually low due to diminished parathyroid hormone secretion and typically result in hypocalcemia (low blood calcium) [33,34]. The observed **hypokalemia** (low blood potassium) results from altered cellular transport systems that maintain the potassium gradient [35]. Calcitriol synthesis may be altered due to decreases in PTH secretion and/or renal resistance to PTH [33].

Toxicity

An excessive intake of magnesium is not likely to cause toxicity except in the case of people with impaired renal function. Normal kidneys are able to remove magnesium so rapidly that significant increases in serum level do not occur [5]. Excessive intake of magnesium salts (3–5 g), such as from $MgSO_4$, may, however, have a cathartic effect, leading to diarrhea and possible dehydration [30]. Other signs, including nausea, flushing, double vision, slurred speech, and weakness, usually appear at plasma magnesium concentrations of ~9 to 12 mg/dL. Acute magnesium toxicity from excessive intravenous administration of magnesium has resulted in nausea, depression, and paralysis [30]. Muscular paralysis and cardiac and/or respiratory failure are associated with plasma magnesium concentrations over ~15 mg/dL. A tolerable upper intake level of 350 mg magnesium from nonfood sources has been recommended for individuals age 9 years and older (including during pregnancy and lactation) [30]. The lowest observed adverse-effect level is 360 mg.

Assessment of Nutriture

Assessment of magnesium status is difficult because extracellular magnesium represents only about 1% of total body magnesium and appears to be homeostatically regulated. Despite low sensitivity and specificity (e.g., normal serum levels may persist despite severe intracellular deficits), serum magnesium concentrations are routinely measured to assess magnesium status [5,7]. When serum magnesium is below normal, an inadequate amount of intracellular magnesium is a certainty. Erythrocyte magnesium concentrations decrease more slowly with magnesium deficiency than plasma or serum concentrations and may reflect longer-term magnesium status because of the life span of the red blood cell [7]. Peripheral lymphocyte magnesium concentrations correlate with skeletal and cardiac muscle magnesium content and thus represent a possible indicator of magnesium status [6].

More definitive determination of magnesium status may involve measurement of renal magnesium excretion, which decreases with magnesium deficiency. Renal magnesium excretion should be measured before and after the administration of an intravenous magnesium load. Decreased excretion determined over two 24-hour periods following administration of the magnesium load indicates deficiency [21]. Alternately, an oral magnesium load test may be used [36]. Normal serum and urinary magnesium concentrations are ~1.6 to 2.6 mg/dL and ~36 to 207 mg per 24 hours, respectively.

References Cited for Magnesium

1. National Research Council. Recommended Dietary Allowances, 10th ed. Washington, DC: National Academy Press, 1989, pp. 187–94.
2. Kayne LH, Lee DB. Intestinal magnesium absorption. Min Electrolyte Metab 1993;19:210–17.
3. Fine K, Santa Ana C, Porter J, Fordtran J. Intestinal absorption of magnesium from food and supplements. J Clin Invest 1991; 88:396–402.
4. Hardwick LL, Jones MR, Brautbar N, Lee DB. Magnesium absorption: mechanisms and the influence of vitamin D, calcium, and phosphate. J Nutr 1991;121:13–23.
5. Wester PO. Magnesium. Am J Clin Nutr 1987;45(suppl):1305–12.
6. Rude R. Magnesium metabolism and deficiency. Endocrin Metab Clin N Am 1993;22:377–95.
7. Elin RJ. Assessment of magnesium status. Clin Chem 1987; 33:1965–70.
8. Spencer H, Lesniak M, Gatza CA, Osis D, Lender M. Magnesium absorption and metabolism in patients with chronic renal failure and in patients with normal renal function. Gastroenterology 1980;79:26–34.
9. Schwartz R, Apgar BJ, Wien EM. Apparent absorption and retention of Ca, Cu, Mg, Mn, and Zn from a diet containing bran. Am J Clin Nutr 1986;43:444–55.
10. Romani A, Marfella C, Scarpa A. Cell magnesium transport and homeostasis: role of intracellular compartments. Miner Electrolyte Metab 1993;19:282–89.
11. Gunther T. Mechanisms and regulation of Mg^{2+} efflux and Mg^{2+} influx. Mineral Electrolyte Metab 1993;19:259–65.
12. Siener R, Hesse A. Influence of a mixed and a vegetarian diet on urinary magnesium excretion and concentration. Br J Nutr 1995;73:783–90.
13. Wisker E, Nagel R, Tanudjaja TK, Feldheim W. Calcium, magnesium, zinc, and iron balances in young women: effects of a low-phytate barley fiber concentration. Am J Clin Nutr 1991;54:553–59.
14. Brink EJ, Beynen AC. Nutrition and magnesium absorption: a review. Prog Food Nutr Sci 1992;16:125–62.
15. Coudray C, Demigne C, Rayssiguier Y. Effects of dietary fibers on magnesium absorption in animals and humans. J Nutr 2003;133:1–4.
16. Brickman AS, Hartenbower DL, Norman AW, Coburn JW. Action of 1,25 $(OH)_2$- and 1α (OH)-vitamin D_3 on magnesium metabolism in man. Clin Res 1975;23:315A.
17. Hodgkinson A, Marshall DH, Nordin BEC. Vitamin D and magnesium absorption in man. Clin Sci 1979;57:121–23.
18. Holbrook JT, Smith JC, Reiser S. Dietary fructose or starch; effects on copper, zinc, iron, manganese, calcium and magnesium balance in humans. Am J Clin Nutr 1989;49:1290–94.
19. Milne DB, Nielsen FH. The interaction between dietary fructose and magnesium adversely affects macromineral homeostasis. J Am Coll Nutr 2000;19:31–37.
20. Ziegler EE, Fomon SJ. Lactose enhances mineral absorption in infancy. J Pediatr Gastr Nutr 1983;2:288–94.
21. Shils M. Magnesium. In: Shils ME, Olson JA, Shike M. Modern Nutrition in Health and Disease, 8th ed. Philadelphia, PA: Lea and Febiger, 1994, pp. 164–84.
22. Levine B, Coburn J. Magnesium, the mimic/antagonist of calcium. N Engl J Med 1984;310:1253–55.
23. Landon R, Yound E. Role of magnesium in regulation of lung function. J Am Diet Assoc 1993;93:674–77.

24. Iseri L, French J. Magnesium: nature's physiologic calcium blocker. Am Heart J 1984;108:188–93.

25. Dorup I, Clausen T. Correlation between magnesium and potassium contents in muscle: role of Na^+-K^+ pump. Am J Physiol 1993;264:C457–C463.

26. Rude RK, Singer FR. Magnesium deficiency and excess. Ann Rev Med 1981;32:245–59.

27. Kelepouris E, Agus Z. Hypomagnesemia: renal magnesium handling. Sem Nephrol 1998;18:58–73.

28. Mahalko JR, Sandstead HH, Johnson LK, Milne DB. Effect of a moderate increase in dietary protein on the retention and excretion of Ca, Cu, Fe, Mg, P, and Zn by adult males. Am J Clin Nutr 1983;37:8–14.

29. McCollister RJ, Flink EB, Lewis MD. Urinary excretion of magnesium in man following the ingestion of ethanol. Am J Clin Nutr 1963;12:415–20.

30. Food and Nutrition Board, Institute of Medicine. Dietary Reference Intakes. Washington, DC: National Academy Press, 1997, pp. 190–249.

31. Frakes M, Richardson L. Magnesium sulfate therapy in certain emergency conditions. Am J Emerg Med 1997;15:182–87.

32. Ma J, Folsom AR, Melnick SL, Eckfeldt JH, Sharrett AR, Nabulsi AA, Hutchinson RG, Metcalf PA. Associations of serum and dietary magnesium with cardiovascular disease, hypertension, diabetes, insulin, and carotid arterial wall thickness: the ARIC study. J Clin Epidemiol 1995;48:927–40.

33. Fatemi S, Ryzen E, Flores J, Endres DB, Rude RK. Effect of experimental human magnesium depletion on parathyroid hormone secretion and 1,25-dihydroxyvitamin D metabolism. J Clin Endocrin Metab 1991;73:1067–72.

34. Rude RK, Oldham SB, Singer FR. Functional hypoparathyroidism and parathyroid hormone end organ resistance in human magnesium deficiency. Clin Endocrinol 1976;5:209–24.

35. Hamill-Ruth R, McGory R. Magnesium repletion and its effects on potassium homeostasis in critically ill adults: results of a double-blind randomized, controlled trial. Crit Care Med 1996;24:38–45.

36. Durlach J, Bac P, Durlach V, Guiet-Bara A. Neurotic, neuromuscular and autonomic nervous form of magnesium imbalance. Magnesium Res 1997;10:169–95.

SODIUM

Approximately 30% of the ~105 g of sodium in the body (70-kg human) is located on the surface of bone crystals. From that site, it can be released into the bloodstream should **hyponatremia** (low serum sodium) develop. The remainder of the body's sodium is in the extracellular fluid, primarily plasma, and in nerve and muscle tissue. Sodium constitutes about 93% of the cations in the body, making it by far the most abundant member of this family.

Sources

The major source of sodium in the diet is added salt in the form of sodium chloride. Sodium comprises 40% by weight of sodium chloride. Because salt is so extensively used in food processing and manufacturing, it is estimated that processed foods account for nearly 75% of total sodium consumed. Canned meats and soups, condiments, pickled foods, and traditional snacks (chips, pretzels, crackers, etc.) are particularly high in added salt. Naturally occurring sources of sodium such as milk, meat, eggs, and most vegetables furnish only about 10% of consumed sodium. Salt added during cooking and at the table provides roughly 15% of total sodium, and water supplies <10%. Terms such as free, very low, low, reduced, or light in conjunction with sodium on food labels are associated with specific amounts of sodium per serving. For example, free means <5 mg sodium per serving, very low means ≤35 mg per serving, and low means ≤140 mg sodium per serving. The term reduced or less indicates at least 25% less sodium per serving than the appropriate reference food. The term light may be used if the food is low in calories and fat and the sodium content has been reduced by at least 50%. The Daily Value on food labels for sodium is 2,400 mg. Depending on the method of assessment, estimates of ingested sodium by Americans range from ~1,800 to 5,000 mg/day.

Sodium intake has been linked with high blood pressure (hypertension) in some individuals, as discussed in the perspective "Macrominerals and Hypertension" at the end of this chapter. The Food and Drug Administration has approved health claims stating "Diets low in sodium may reduce the risk of high blood pressure, a disease associated with many factors" as well as "Development of hypertension or high blood pressure depends on many factors. [This product] can be part of a low-sodium and low-salt diet that might reduce the risk of hypertension or high blood pressure" [1].

Absorption, Transport, and Function

About 95% to 100% of ingested sodium is absorbed, with the remaining 0% to 5% excreted in the feces. There are three basic pathways for absorption of sodium across the intestinal mucosa. One of these pathways (the Na^+/glucose cotransport system) functions broadly throughout the small intestine. Another pathway (an electroneutral Na^+ and Cl^- cotransport system) is active in both the small intestine and the proximal portion of the colon, and the third pathway (an electrogenic sodium absorption mechanism) operates principally in the colon.

The Na^+/glucose cotransport system involves a carrier on the brush border (apical) membrane of the small intestine. Na^+ and glucose bind to the carrier, which shuttles them from the outer surface to the inner surface of the cell membrane. There both are released before the carrier returns to the outer surface. Absorbed Na^+ is then pumped out across the basolateral membrane by the Na^+/K^+-ATPase pump, while the glucose diffuses across the membrane by a facilitated transport pathway. The Na^+ gradient created by the Na^+/K^+-ATPase pump provides the energy needed to maintain the absorptive direction of the ion. Cotransport of Na^+ by this mechanism also can occur with solutes other than glucose, including amino acids, di- and tripeptides, and many B vitamins.

The electroneutral Na^+ and Cl^- cotransport mechanism has been proposed because of the observation that a significant portion of sodium uptake requires the presence of chloride, and vice versa [2]. Precisely how this system functions has not yet been established. However, it is believed that the cotransport is composed of Na^+/H^+exchange working in concert with a Cl^-/HCO_3^- mechanism [3]. The mechanism allows the entrance of both Na^+ and Cl^- into the cell, where they are exchanged for H^+ and HCO_3^-. Protons and HCO_3^- are produced within the cell by the action of carbonic anhydrase on CO_2. Absorbed Na^+ is pumped across the basolateral membrane by the Na^+/K^+-ATPase pump, followed by Cl^-, which crosses by diffusion.

The colonic mechanism is called an electrogenic sodium absorption mechanism because the absorbed sodium ion is the only ion moving transcellularly, allowing its transport to be monitored by electrical equipment. It enters the luminal membrane of the colonic mucosal cell through Na^+-conducting pathways called Na^+ channels, diffusing inwardly by the downhill concentration gradient of the ion. The absorbed sodium is accompanied by water and anions, resulting in net water and electrolyte movement from the luminal side to the bloodstream side of the colon epithelium. It is pumped out across the basolateral membrane on the bloodstream side of the cell by the Na^+/K^+-ATPase pump.

All three of these mechanisms are depicted schematically in Figure 11.11. It is important to recognize that the common driving force for sodium absorption in all the processes is the inwardly directed gradient maintained by the basolateral Na^+ pump.

Once absorbed into the body, sodium is transported freely in the blood. Serum sodium concentrations, as well as those of potassium and chloride, are maintained within a fairly narrow range by several hormones, including antidiuretic hormone (ADH) or vasopressin, aldosterone, atrial natriuretic hormone, renin, and angiotensin II.

Within the body, sodium plays important roles in the maintenance of fluid balance, nerve transmission/impulse conduction, and muscle contraction. While proteins play a role in fluid balance, they normally remain either intracellular or extracellular. Sodium, potassium, and chloride therefore display the most movement across cell membranes to maintain osmotic pressure and thus fluid balance. Sodium's roles in nerve transmission and muscle contraction involve sodium as part of the

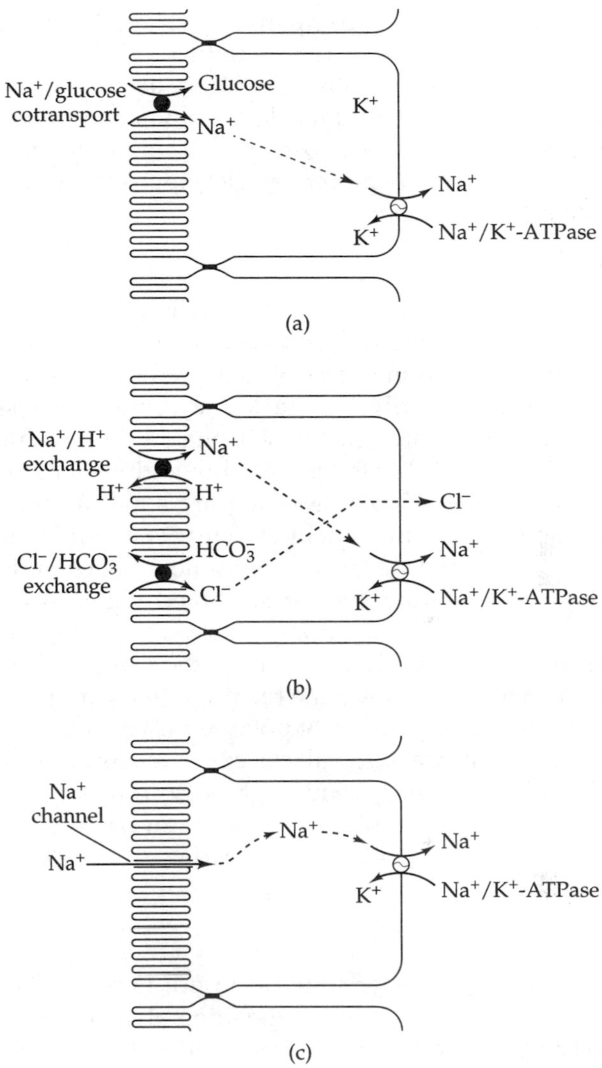

Figure 11.11 Absorption mechanisms for sodium in the intestine. (a) Na^+/glucose cotransport. A carrier on the brush border membrane of the enterocyte cotransports sodium together with a solute such as glucose into the cell. Once in the cell, Na^+ is pumped across the basolateral membrane by Na^+/K^+-ATPase, while glucose exits through the membrane by facilitated diffusion. (b) Electroneutral Na^+ and Cl^- absorption. The Na^+/H^+ exchange works in concert with a Cl^-/HCO_3^- exchange. Sodium is then pumped basolaterally, with Cl^- diffusing passively. (c) Electrogenic Na^+ absorption. Sodium enters the luminal membrane via a Na^+ channel.

Na^+/K^+-ATPase pump found in the plasma membrane of cells. With the exchange of sodium for potassium and the hydrolysis of ATP, an electrochemical potential gradient generates nerve or impulse conduction.

Interactions with Other Nutrients

It has long been recognized (prior to 1940) that dietary sodium intake affects urinary calcium excretion. Studies have shown that accompanying the calciuria are decreases in fecal calcium excretion. Such calcium-elevating effects partially offset the urinary calcium losses [4–6]. The sodium-calcium interaction and its possible association with osteoporosis are presented in more detail in the perspective "Osteoporosis and Diet" at the end of this chapter.

Excretion

Because nearly all the ingested sodium is absorbed, much larger amounts are absorbed than are required by the body. Sodium in excess of that needed by the body is excreted primarily by the kidneys. Sodium losses also take place through the skin via sweating. Under conditions of moderate temperature and level of exercise, sodium losses via sweating are small. However, because the sodium content of sweat is about 50 mEq (milliequivalents)/L, it can be reasoned that conditions of high temperature and/or sustained vigorous exercise can account for significant losses. Renal excretion and retention of sodium are under the control of aldosterone, which promotes the retention (reabsorption) of sodium and the excretion of potassium. The hormone is released from the adrenal cortex in response to low sodium or, more important, high potassium concentrations. The renal regulation of sodium, as well as of potassium and chloride, is presented in greater detail in Chapter 14.

Deficiency

Dietary deficiencies of sodium do not normally occur because of the abundance of the mineral across a broad spectrum of foods. Serum concentrations of sodium normally are regulated within the range of ~135 to 145 mEq/L. However, with excessive sweating involving a loss of more than about 3% of total body weight, deficiencies of sodium have been reported. Symptoms include muscle cramps, nausea, vomiting, dizziness, shock, and coma.

Recommended Intakes and Assessment of Nutriture

The National Research Council (1989), while establishing no RDA, recommends a minimum intake of 500 mg sodium/day, an amount thought to represent the requirement for the mineral and to provide for variations in physical activity and climatic exposure, which account for sodium losses through sweating [7]. An intake of only 115 mg/day of sodium is thought to be sufficient to replace obligatory losses (without active sweating) and provide for growth.

Sodium is measured routinely in clinical laboratories, especially to determine electrolyte balance (see Chap. 14). Sodium in the serum and other biological fluids is usually quantified by the technique of ion-selective electrode **potentiometry.** This method measures Na^+ in the same way a pH meter measures protons. Twenty-four-hour urinary sodium excretion is most often used as a reflection of sodium intake.

POTASSIUM

Potassium is the major intracellular cation. In fact, in contrast to sodium, about 95% to 98% of the body's potassium is found within body cells. Potassium constitutes up to ~0.35% of total body weight, or up to ~245 g in a 70-kg human.

Sources

Potassium is widespread in the diet and is especially abundant in unprocessed foods, such as fruits (especially orange juice, bananas, canteloupe, and watermelon), vegetables (avocados and leafy green vegetables), and fresh meats. Other good sources of potassium are potatoes, whole grains, legumes, and milk. In addition to unprocessed sources, salt substitutes often contain potassium in place of sodium.

Diets high in potassium are associated with lower blood pressure; this topic is discussed further in the perspective "Macrominerals and Hypertension" at the end of this chapter. The Food and Drug Administration has approved the health claim "Diets containing foods that are good sources of potassium and low in sodium may reduce the risk of high blood pressure and stroke" [1]. To use this claim, a food must contain at least 350 mg (10% daily value) potassium; must have ≤140 mg sodium, ≤3 g total fat, ≤1 g saturated fat, and ≤20 mg cholesterol; and must provide ≤15% of energy (kcal) from saturated fat [1]. For food labeling purposes, to be considered a "rich," "excellent," or "high" source of potassium (any nutrient), a food must contain 20% or more of the daily value; to be a "good" source of potassium, the food must contain 10% to 19% of the daily value [1].

Absorption, Transport, and Function

The mechanisms by which potassium is absorbed from the gastrointestinal tract are not as clearly understood as the mechanisms of sodium absorption. Only recently have actual intestinal transport mechanisms for potassium been recognized and investigated. Over 90% of ingested potassium is absorbed, and while the sites along the gastrointestinal tract at which absorption takes place have not been precisely identified, both the small intestine and the colon appear to play a role [8–10].

It is believed that K^+ may be absorbed across the brush border (apical) membrane of the colonic mucosal cell by a K^+/H^+-ATPase pump. This pump exchanges intracellular H^+ for luminal K^+, the mechanism by which H^+, along with Cl^- (secreted via Cl^- channels), is secreted into the stomach as HCl. Alternatively, K^+ may enter the cell via apical membrane channels that also serve as secretory pathways. To enter the blood, the K^+ accumulated in the cell then diffuses across the basolateral membrane via the K^+ channel.

Potassium influences the contractility of smooth, skeletal, and cardiac muscle and profoundly affects the excitability of nerve tissue. It is also important in maintaining electrolyte and pH balance.

Interactions with Other Nutrients

Like sodium, potassium has an effect on the urinary excretion of calcium. However, its effect is opposite to that of sodium in that it decreases calcium excretion while sodium increases it. Replacement of some of the NaCl in the diet with KCl to reduce the amount of NaCl consumed has been shown to reduce the excretory rate of calcium [11].

Excretion

Most potassium is excreted from the body via the kidneys, with only small amounts excreted in the feces. As with sodium, potassium balance is achieved largely through the kidneys, with aldosterone being the major regulatory hormone. Aldosterone acts reciprocally on sodium and potassium. Although it stimulates the reabsorption of sodium in the kidney tubules, it accelerates the excretion of potassium. Renal control of potassium is discussed further in Chapter 14.

Deficiency and Toxicity

Hyperkalemia (abnormally high serum potassium) is toxic, resulting in severe cardiac arrhythmias and even cardiac arrest. It is nearly impossible to produce hyperkalemia by dietary means in an individual with normal circulation and renal function because of potassium's delicate control within a narrow concentration range. Similarly, hypokalemia (abnormally low serum potassium) does not occur by dietary deficiency because of the abundance of potassium in common foods. Hypokalemia is associated with muscular weakness, nervous irritability, and mental disorientation and can result from profound fluid loss, such as that which occurs with severe vomiting and diarrhea or with use of some diuretic medications. Hypokalemia also may occur as part of refeeding syndrome, which occurs when malnourished individuals are being refed (usually intravenously or through a tube) a diet lacking enough supplemental potassium to replace that lost from the cells during the starvation period and needed for the body as it synthesizes new lean body mass.

Recommended Intakes and Assessment of Nutriture

The National Research Council (1989), while not establishing any RDA, suggests a dietary intake of 2,000 mg potassium per day but further states that 3,500 mg per day may be more desirable in view of the increased intake of fruits and vegetables recommended for prevention and control of hypertension [7]. The normal serum concentration of potassium, as K^+, is ~3.6 to 5.0 mEq/L. Serum potassium levels, like those of sodium, are determined primarily by ion-selective electrode potentiometry.

CHLORIDE

Chloride is the most abundant anion in the extracellular fluid, with approximately 88% of chloride found in extracellular fluid and just 12% intracellular. Its negative charge neutralizes the positive charge of the sodium ions with which it is usually associated. In this respect, it is of great importance in the maintenance of electrolyte balance. Total body chloride content is similar to that of sodium, representing about 0.15% of body weight, or about 105 g in a 70-kg human.

Sources

Nearly all the chloride consumed in the diet is associated with sodium in the form of sodium chloride, or salt. Salt, which is about 60% chloride, is abundant in a large number of foods, particularly in snack items and processed foods. Chloride also is found in eggs, fresh meats, and seafood. It is estimated that the average adult consumes between 50 and 200 mEq/day.

Absorption, Transport, and Secretion

Chloride is almost completely absorbed in the small intestine. Its absorption closely follows that of sodium in the establishment and maintenance of electrical neutrality. The absorptive mechanisms, however, generally are different. For example, in the Na^+-glucose cotransport system (described in the section on sodium), chloride follows the actively absorbed Na^+ passively through a so-called paracellular, or tight junction, pathway. The absorbed Na^+ creates an electrical gradient that provides the energy for the accompanying inward diffusion of Cl^-. The electroneutral Na^+/Cl^- cotransport absorption system also contributes to the movement of chloride into the mucosal cells, although the relative contribution of this system to total chloride absorption is not well established. Sodium absorbed by the electrogenic Na^+ absorption mechanism also is accompanied by chloride, which follows the absorbed sodium passively (paracellularly) to maintain electrical neutrality. It is clear, therefore, that regardless of which

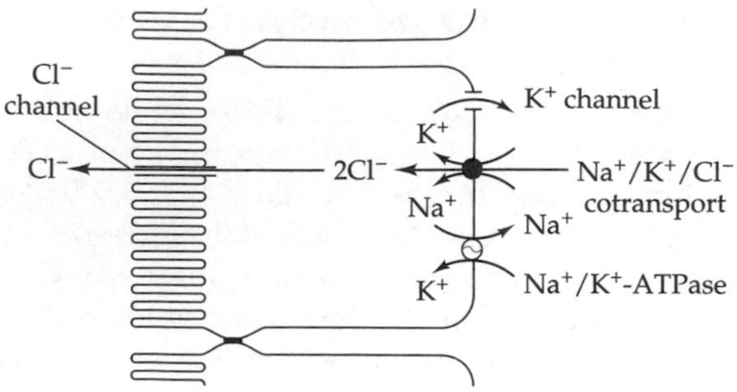

Figure 11.12 Intestinal chloride secretory mechanism. Chloride is cotransported along with Na^+ and K^+ from the circulation across the basolateral membrane and into the mucosal cell. Chloride then exits the cell into the lumen through Cl^- channels in the apical membrane. The driving force is provided by active removal of Na^+ by the Na^+/K^+-ATPase pump and the recycling of potassium through K^+ channels on the basolateral membrane.

absorptive mechanism is functioning, wherever sodium goes, chloride cannot be far behind!

Secretory mechanisms for the electrolytes throughout the gastrointestinal tract center on chloride, which is the major secretory product of the stomach and the rest of the gastrointestinal tract. The well-defined mechanism is an electrogenic Cl^- secretion. Cl^- is the only ion actively secreted by the epithelium, and its movement can be monitored by changes in electrical potentials. Cells take up chloride from the blood across the basolateral membrane via an $Na^+/K^+/Cl^-$ cotransport pathway. An appropriate gradient is set up by the Na^+/K^+-ATPase pump, which maintains a low concentration of intracellular sodium. Potassium channels on the basolateral membrane allow potassium recycling out of the cell. Chloride accumulating in the cell exits through the apical membrane into the lumen via the Cl^- channels. Figure 11.12 illustrates the chloride secretory mechanism. Dysfunction of chloride transport is found in individuals with cystic fibrosis. The genetic disorder results from a mutation in a protein called the cystic fibrosis transmembrane conductance regulator [12]. Defects in the protein result in the production of extremely thick mucus that obstructs many of the body's glands and causes malfunction of many organs, especially the lungs and pancreas.

Functions

Chloride has important functions in addition to its role as a major electrolyte. The formation of gastric hydrochloric acid requires chloride, which is secreted along with protons from the parietal cells of the stomach. Chloride is released by white blood cells during phagocytosis to assist in the destruction of foreign substances. Also, chloride acts as the exchange anion for HCO_3^- in red blood cells. Sometimes referred to as the chloride shift, this latter process requires a protein transporter that moves Cl^- and HCO_3^- in opposite directions across the cell membrane. The purpose is to allow the transport of tissue-derived CO_2 back to the lungs in the form of plasma HCO_3^-. Waste CO_2 from tissues enters the red blood cell, where it is converted to HCO_3^- by carbonic anhydrase. The transporter protein (chloride bicarbonate exchanger) then transports the HCO_3^- out of the cell into the plasma as it simultaneously transports plasma Cl^- into the cell. In the absence of chloride, bicarbonate transport ceases.

Excretion

Chloride excretion occurs through three primary routes: the gastrointestinal tract, the skin, and the kidneys, with losses through each route closely reflecting those of sodium. Excretion of chloride through the gastrointestinal tract normally is very small, ~1 to 2 mEq/day for the average adult, and mostly represents unabsorbed chloride. Losses through the skin are essentially the same as for sodium, that is, normally quite small except in cases of high temperature and vigorous exercise. The major route of chloride excretion is through the kidney, where it is primarily regulated indirectly through sodium regulation.

Deficiency

Dietary deficiency of chloride does not occur under normal conditions. As is the case for the other electrolytes, deficiency arises chiefly through alimentary disturbance such as severe diarrhea and vomiting. Convulsions typically occur with chloride deficiency.

Recommended Intakes and Assessment of Nutriture

The National Research Council (1989) recommends a chloride intake of 750 mg/day to meet requirements; however, no RDA has been established [7]. In view of losses through sweating, however, this value may need to be adjusted upward for people with physically rigorous lifestyles or those chronically exposed to high temperatures.

The serum concentration of chloride is ~101 to 111 mEq/L. Its measurement is generally used to establish the chloride status of the body. However, like all serum solutes, concentration depends on the body water status. It is possible, for example, for total body store of chloride to be diminished and fluid concentrations of chloride to appear normal and even be elevated if body water accompanies the losses. Two widely used methods for determining chloride concentration in serum are ion-selective electrode potentiometry and a **coulometric**

titration (a method of measuring the volume of reagent required for a reaction) with silver ions.

References Cited for Sodium, Potassium, and Chloride

1. www.cfsan.fda.gov
2. Frizzell RA, et al. Sodium-coupled chloride transport by epithelial tissues. Am J Physiol 1979;236:F1–8.
3. Barrett KE, Dharmsathaphorn K. Transport of water and electrolytes in the gastrointestinal tract: physiological mechanisms, regulation, and methods of study. In: Maxwell MH, Kleeman CR. Clinical Disorders of Fluid and Electrolyte Metabolism. Narins RG, ed. New York: McGraw-Hill, 1994, pp. 506–7.
4. Nordin B, Need A, Morris H, Horowitz M. The nature and significance of the relationship between urinary sodium and urinary calcium in women. J Nutr 1993;123:1615–22.
5. Devine A, Criddle R, Dick I, Kerr D, Prince R. A longitudinal study of the effect of sodium and calcium intake on regional bone density in postmenopausal women. Am J Clin Nutr 1995;62:740–45.
6. Shortt C, Flynn A. Sodium-calcium interrelationships with specific reference to osteoporosis. Nutr Res Rev 1990;3:101–15.
7. National Research Council. Recommended Dietary Allowances, 10th ed. Washington, DC: National Academy Press, 1989.
8. Hayslett JP, Binder HJ. Mechanism of potassium adaptation. Am J Physiol 1982;243:F103–12.
9. Kliger AS, et al. Demonstration of active potassium transport in the mammalian colon. J Clin Invest 1981;67:1189–96.
10. Agarwal R, Afzalpurkar R, Fordtran J. Pathophysiology of potassium absorption and secretion by the human intestine. Gastroenterology 1994;107:548–71.
11. Bell RR, Eldrid MM, Watson FR. The influence of NaCl and KCl on urinary calcium excretion in healthy young women. Nutr Res 1992;12:17–26.
12. Riordan JR, et al. Identification of the cystic fibrosis gene: cloning and characterization of complementary DNA. Science 1989;245:1066–75.

Web Sites

www.cfsan.fda.gov

Macrominerals and Hypertension

Dietary factors influence blood pressure just as they do other physiological processes of the body. Although high blood pressure, called hypertension, has primarily and most publicly been linked to sodium intake, other nutrients play a role in blood pressure control.

Hypertension is thought to affect about 25% of Americans. The condition is one in which there is an increase in vascular resistance most often due to a decreased luminal diameter of the arteries and/or arterioles. Systolic and diastolic blood pressure values ≥140 and 90 mm Hg, respectively, are indicative of hypertension. Hypertension is often classified as primary (also called essential) or secondary. Causes of essential hypertension are generally unknown and are thought to be multifactorial, perhaps related to malfunction of sodium excretion or of the renin-angiotensin or kallikrein-kinin systems, hyperactivity of the nervous system, and/or abnormal prostaglandin production, among other factors. Essential hypertension accounts for >90% of hypertension cases. The remaining cases of hypertension occur secondary to other conditions, such as kidney, endocrine, or neurological diseases. Whether hypertension is essential or secondary, the condition increases the risk of stroke and heart disease. Although some risk factors for hypertension are not controllable (e.g., genetic predisposition, race, aging), others can be modified by an individual's commitment to dietary and lifestyle changes.

Unfortunately, hypertension is a heterogeneous disease, having a variety of precipitating factors, and thus dietary modification works for some but not all hypertensive individuals. This perspective discusses some of the nutrients associated with essential hypertension. The nutrients most often associated with blood pressure are the macrominerals sodium, potassium, calcium, and magnesium. Each of these will be discussed, along with sucrose and alcohol, which also have been shown to influence blood pressure.

Sodium

Sodium, as salt, was one of the first nutrients linked to hypertension. Specifically, increased salt intakes directly correlate with increased blood pressure. However, some individuals with hypertension (~40%–60%) and a genetic predisposition appear to be much more sensitive to an excess of salt than others. Thus, in some but not all hypertensive individuals, high dietary salt intakes raise blood pressure, and dietary salt restriction results in blood pressure reduction [1–6]. Hypertensive individuals likely to benefit from sodium reduction include those who are African American, obese, or over 65 years of age or who have low plasma renin activity, as well as those taking antihypertensive medications [1,2,7,8].

No one mechanism is thought to be responsible for salt-induced elevations in blood pressure. In salt-sensitive individuals, salt ingestion is thought to cause sodium and water retention and extracellular volume expansion, with the resulting release of a substance or substances that increase heart and blood vessel contractile activity and affect the renin-angiotensin-aldosterone system [1,9]. Alternatively, sodium may infiltrate or cause abnormal handling of other ions into and out of vascular smooth muscle, causing contraction and elevations in blood pressure [1,10]. Sensitivity to sodium correlates with low plasma renin activity (reflecting volume overload), a decreased capacity of the renin-angiotensin system to respond to physiological stimuli, and insulin resistance [8]. Sodium restriction appears to increase plasma renin activity and sympathetic nervous system activity [8].

Potassium

Potassium is yet another nutrient known to impact blood pressure. Epidemiological studies, as well as national surveys, clearly show an association between higher potassium intakes (alone or relative to sodium intakes) and a lower prevalence of hypertension [1,11–13]. Supplementation trials with potassium have further supported such findings. A meta-analysis of 30 controlled trials found that potassium supplementation was associated with significant reductions in both systolic and diastolic blood pressure [14]. Generally, the blood-pressure-lowering effects of potassium supplementation were more apparent in hypertensive individuals than in normotensive individuals [11–15]. Furthermore, effects of potassium were greater in individuals ingesting higher sodium intakes [14].

The mechanisms by which potassium affects blood pressure are multiple. Potassium promotes urinary sodium excretion **(natriuresis)** and thus diminishes body sodium. Increased potassium intakes also are associated with reduced urinary calcium and magnesium excretion; calcium and magnesium, discussed in the next two sections, influence blood pressure [11]. Potassium may induce vascular smooth muscle relaxation and thus reduce peripheral resistance [13]. It can inhibit platelet aggregation and arterial thrombosis and also inhibit proliferation of smooth vascular muscle cells to decrease vascular resistance [8]. Potassium may interact with the kinin system; for example, potassium is known to increase urinary kallikrein [1]. Potassium also may affect renin to regulate blood pressure [13].

Calcium

A possible relationship between calcium and the development of hypertension was first recognized with the discovery in the early 1970s that communities characterized by hard water (high calcium content) had a lower death rate from cardiovascular disease [16,17]. Since that time, much evidence from epidemiological studies, laboratory studies involving animals and humans, and clinical trials has accumulated to support the relationship between calcium and blood pressure [17]. A meta-analysis of over 30 randomized calcium supplementation (median intake, 1 g calcium) studies found that calcium supplementation significantly resulted in small reductions in systolic, but not diastolic, blood pressure [18,19]. Further, a meta-analysis of studies involving pregnant women concluded that consumption of calcium during pregnancy reduced the risk of pregnancy-induced hypertension [20].

However, a segment of the hypertensive population appears to be more responsive to calcium supplementation than other segments. The difference in response to oral calcium among hypertensives may be due to the heterogeneity of the disease. People who appear to benefit from oral calcium therapy are those who have low calcium intakes (especially <400 mg), low serum ionized-calcium concentrations, or elevated serum PTH and vitamin D (calcitriol) and those who have been classified as having low renin activity and as being "salt sensitive" [21–25].

How dietary calcium can exhibit an anti-hypertensive effect in "calcium-sensitive" hypertensives is uncertain. Calcium has a membrane-stabilizing, vasorelaxing effect on the smooth muscle cells [8,25]. It also affects the central and peripheral sympathetic nervous systems and modifies calcium homeostasis as well as the actions of PTH and calcitriol; calcium may suppress PTH-induced elevation in calcium concentration to in turn reduce vascular tone [22,25]. Increased intracellular calcium concentrations have been shown to directly correlate with increased blood pressure and age. Calcium may also exert its effects through interaction with other nutrients. For example, increased calcium intake causes natriuresis [26]. Calcium may correct sodium-induced decreases of ionized serum calcium as would occur with sodium-induced calciuria [27].

Magnesium

Epidemiological data as well as animal and human studies suggest an inverse relationship between blood pressure and magnesium intake. For example, the Nurses' Health Study found that magnesium intake had an independent and significant inverse association with blood pressure [10,11,28]. Yet the results of studies providing magnesium supplementation to treat hypertension have been contradictory.

How magnesium directly affects blood pressure is not clear. Magnesium is known to promote relaxation of vascular smooth muscle as well as to interact with calcium [25,26]. In fact, low serum magnesium (indicative of low magnesium status) is associated with increased smooth muscle tension, vasospasms, and higher blood pressure [9]. Increased blood pressure also is associated with both calcium and magnesium excretion [29]. Magnesium is a required cofactor for enzymes involved in fatty acid metabolism for the synthesis of prostaglandins, and prostaglandins in turn can influence blood pressure. The blood-pressure-lowering effects of fish oil, rich in eicosapentaenoic acid and docoshexaenoic acid, have been attributed, in part, to enhanced production of PGI_3, a prostaglandin that promotes vasodilation and inhibits platelet aggregation, and to decreased formation of thromboxane A_2, which promotes vasoconstriction and platelet aggregation.

Other Dietary Factors

Sucrose also has been shown to elevate blood pressure. Several animal studies have demonstrated sucrose-induced rises in blood pressure. The effects are thought to be short term and to result from volume expansion and antinatriuretic effects that accompany sucrose ingestion [15].

Alcohol consumption is thought to account for up to ~20% of hypertension, especially in middle-aged men [7,30,31]. Changes in hormones (such as stimulation of the sympathetic, endothelin, or renin-angiotensin-aldosterone system or of insulin or cortisol), changes in vascular tone (e.g., inhibition of vascular relaxing substances such as nitric oxide and/or increased intracellular concentrations of calcium or electrolytes in vascular smooth muscle), as well as changes in baroreflex sensitivity have been suggested as mechanisms by which alcohol may influence blood pressure [10,31,32].

The randomized trial Dietary Approaches to Stop Hypertension (DASH) reported that diets rich in fruits and vegetables and low-fat dairy products but low in fat were effective in reducing blood pressure versus a control diet low in fruits and vegetables and average in fat (~36% of kcal) [33]. The DASH diet provides 3 g sodium, 8 to 10 servings of fruits and vegetables, and 2 to 3 servings of low-fat dairy products; limits red meat, fats, and sugar-sweetened foods and beverages; and emphasizes nuts, seeds, and legumes. The DASH-sodium study, which compared the effects of the DASH diet versus a control diet with three sodium intakes (3.3 g, 2.4 g, and 1.5 g), further showed that additional blood pressure reduction could be achieved through reduction in dietary sodium. Similarly, consumption of diets that meet or exceed the RDAs of calcium, potassium, and magnesium is not associated with hypertension even when the diet is high in sodium chloride [34]. Thus, use of supplements may not be necessary to achieve reductions in blood pressure. Diets that ensure adequate dietary intakes of calcium, potassium, and magnesium are recommended by the Joint National Committee on Prevention, Detection, Evaluation, and Treatment of High Blood Pressure for the treatment of hypertension [35].

References Cited

1. Haddy F, Pamnani M. Role of dietary salt in hypertension. J Am Coll Nutr 1995;14:428–38.
2. Luft F, Weinberger M. Heterogeneous responses to changes in dietary salt intake: the salt-sensitivity paradigm. Am J Clin Nutr 1997;65:612S–17S.
3. Cowley A. Genetic and nongenetic determinants of salt sensitivity and blood pressure. Am J Clin Nutr 1997;65:587S–93S.
4. Weinberger M. Salt sensitivity of blood pressure in humans. Hypertension 1996;27(3 pt 2):481–90.
5. Staessen J, Lijnen P, Thijs L, Fagard R. Salt and blood pressure in community based intervention trials. Am J Clin Nutr 1997;65:661S–70S.
6. Cutler J, Follmann D, Allender P. Randomized trials of sodium reduction: an overview. Am J Clin Nutr 1997;65:643S–51S.
7. Joint National Committee on the Detection, Evaluation, and Treatment of High Blood Pressure. National High Blood Pressure Education Program. Arch Intern Med 1993;153:154–83.
8. Buemi M, Senatore M, Corica F, Aloisi C, Romeo A, Tramontana D, Frisina N. Diet and arterial hypertension: is the sodium ion alone important? Medicinal Res Rev 2002;22:419–28.
9. Das UN. Nutritional factors in the pathobiology of human essential hypertension. Nutrition 2001;17:337–46.
10. Suter PM, Sierro C, Vetter W. Nutritional factors in the control of blood pressure and hypertension. Nutr Clin Care 2002;5:9–19.
11. Reusser M, McCarron D. Micronutrient effects on blood pressure regulation. Nutr Rev 1994;52:367–75.
12. Barri Y, Wingo C. The effects of potassium depletion and supplementation on blood pressure: a clinical review. Am J Med Sci 1997;314:37–40.
13. Stein P, Black H. The role of diet in the genesis and treatment of hypertension. Med Clin N Am 1993; 77:831–47.
14. Whelton P, He J, Culter J, Brancati F, Appel L, Follmann D, Klag M. Effects of oral potassium on blood pressure: meta-analysis of randomized controlled clinical trials. JAMA 1997;277:1624–32.
15. Kotchen T, Kotchen J. Dietary sodium and blood pressure: interactions with other nutrients. Am J Clin Nutr 1997;65:708S–11S.
16. Henry H, McCarron DA, Morris CD, et al. Increasing calcium intake lowers blood pressure: the literature reviewed. J Am Diet Assoc 1985;85:182–85.
17. Cappuccio F, Elliott P, Allender P, Pryer J, Follman D, Cutler J. Epidemiologic association between dietary calcium intake and blood pressure: a meta-analysis of published data. Am J Epidemiol 1995;142:935–45.
18. Bucher H, Cook R, Guyatt G, Lang J, Cook D, Hatala R, Hunt D. Effects of dietary calcium supplementation on blood pressure: a meta-analysis of randomized controlled trials. JAMA 1996;275:1016–22.
19. Allender P, Cutler J, Follmann D, Cappuccio F, Pryer J, Elliott P. Dietary calcium and blood pressure: a meta-analysis of randomized clinical trials. Ann Intern Med 1996;124:825–31.
20. Bucher H, Guyatt G, Cook R, Lang J, Cook D, Hatala R, Hunt D. Effects of calcium supplementation on pregnancy-induced hypertension and pre-eclampsia: a meta-analysis of randomized controlled trials. JAMA 1996;275:1113–17.
21. Aalberts J, Weegels P, van der Heyden L, et al. Calcium supplementation: effect on blood pressure and

urinary mineral excretion in normotensive male lactoovovegetarians and omnivores. Am J Clin Nutr 1988;48:131–38.

22. Witteman J, Willet W, Stampfer M. Dietary calcium and magnesium and hypertension: a prospective study. Circulation 1987;76(suppl IV):35.

23. Sowers J, Zemel M, Zemel P, Standley P. Calcium metabolism and dietary calcium in salt sensitive hypertension. Am J Hyperten 1991;4:557–63.

24. Morris C, Reusser M. Calcium intake and blood pressure: epidemiology revisited. Semin Nephrol 1995;15:490–95.

25. Hatton D, Yue Q, McCarron D. Mechanisms of calcium's effects on blood pressure. Semin Nephrol 1995;15:593–602.

26. Massey LK. Dietary factors influencing calcium and bone metabolism: introduction. J Nutr 1993;123:1609–10.

27. Gruchow H, Sobocinski K, Barboriak J. Calcium intake and the relationship of dietary sodium and potassium to blood pressure. Am J Clin Nutr 1988;48:1463–70.

28. Witteman J, Willet W, Stampfer M. A prospective study of nutritional factors and hypertension among U.S. women. Circulation 1989;80:1320–27.

29. Wu X, Ackermann U, Sonnenberg H. Potassium depletion and salt sensitive hypertension in Dahl rats: effect on calcium, magnesium, and phosphate excretion. Clin Exp Hyperten 1995;17:989–1008.

30. Stamfer J, Stamler R, Neaton J. Blood pressure, systolic and diastolic, and cardiovascular risks: U.S. population data. Arch Intern Med 1993;153:598–615.

31. Cushman WC. Alcohol consumption and hypertension. J Clin Hyperten 2001;3:166–70.

32. Beilin LJ. Alcohol, hypertension and cardiovascular disease. J Hyperten 1995;13:939–42.

33. Appel L, Moore T, Obarzanek E, Vollmer W, Svetkey L, Sacks F, Bray G, Vogt T, Cutler J, Windhauser M, Lin P, Karanja N. A clinical trial of the effects of dietary patterns on blood pressure. N Engl J Med 1997;336:1117–24.

34. McCarron D. Role of adequate dietary calcium intake in the prevention and management of salt-sensitive hypertension. Am J Clin Nutr 1997;65:721S–26S.

35. Joint National Committee on Prevention, Detection, Evaluation, and Treatment of High Blood Pressure. The sixth report. Arch Intern Med 1997;157:2413–46.

Additional References

Colin PR. Dietary modification and changes in blood pressure. Curr Opin Nephrol Hypertens 2001;10: 359–63.

McAlister FA, et al. The 2000 Canadian recommendations for the management of hypertension, part I. Can J Cardiol 2001;17:543–49.

Zamke KB, et al. The 2000 Canadian recommendations for the management of hypertension, part II. Can J Cardiol 2001;17:1249–63.

Web Sites

www.bloodpressure.com
www.americanheart.org
nhlbi.nih.gov/guidelines/hypertension
nlm.nih.gov/medlineplus/highbloodpressure.html
www.cdc.gov/nchs/fastats/hyprtens.htm

Osteoporosis and Diet

One in every 3 women and 1 in every 12 men will suffer a fracture due to osteoporosis sometime during their lives [1]. Treatment of the fracture, however, will not necessarily restore health. About 20% of individuals with hip fractures due to osteoporosis die within 1 year of sustaining the fracture [2]. About 33% of individuals who have had an osteoporosis-induced hip fracture are no longer able to care for themselves and move into nursing homes within the year following the fracture, and another 17% (while not requiring nursing home care) are not able to return to their previous, prefracture lifestyle [3,4]. Osteoporosis affecting the vertebrae is associated with loss in height, vertebral pain, and the rounding of the shoulders or **kyphosis** (hunchback-type curvature of the spine, also called **dowager's hump**). The kyphosis in turn reduces the space in the chest and abdominal cavity, resulting in decreased lung capacity and thus shortness of breath, abdominal pain, reduced appetite, and premature satiety [5]. Many individuals who suffer an osteoporosis-induced vertebral fracture spend their remaining years in severe, chronic pain and with limited mobility. The limited mobility causes excessive bed rest, which further weakens the individual's muscles and bones and predisposes the person to falling and suffering further fractures. The excessive bed rest also increases the person's risk for pressure sores, also called decubitus ulcers.

In the United States, osteoporosis affects approximately 28 to 30 million people, 80% of whom are women. The condition results in about 1.5 million fractures per year. Fractures affecting the spine occur most frequently (over 700,000), followed by fractures of the hip (600,000) and wrist (250,000) [6]. The cost of treating osteoporotic fractures exceeds $14 billion per year. The condition is considered a major health threat [3].

Osteoporosis is a systemic skeletal disease characterized by the deterioration of the microarchitecture of bone tissue and low bone mineral density [3]. The condition results in fragile bones at increased risk for fracture. While bone turnover occurs throughout life, after about age 30 to 35 years bone resorption (breakdown) exceeds bone formation. This bone resorption, including mineral loss, occurs at a rate of up to ~10% per decade in both men and women. However, it is during the first 5 to 8 years after menopause that the rate of loss accelerates considerably in women. The decline in estrogen production that occurs with menopause, coupled with the generally smaller body and bone mass of women, contributes to the higher prevalence of osteoporosis in women than in men.

Osteoporosis affects both cortical and trabecular bone, although trabecular bone has a higher turnover rate and is affected to a greater extent than is cortical bone. Cortical or compact bone is found mostly in the shaft of long bones of the limbs but also on the outer walls of all bones. Trabecular bone is the honeycomb or lattice-type bone found in the vertebrae of the spine, the pelvis, and the ends of long bones. Thus, sites containing trabecular bone—the vertebral bodies (~95% trabecular bone), the femoral neck (~45% trabecular bone), and the radius (~5% trabecular bone)—are the principal sites affected with osteoporosis, especially in women (Fig. 1) [7]. In addition, teeth also may become loose or fall out due to loss of some trabecular bone in the jaw.

Two types of osteoporosis have been described. Type I osteoporosis is characterized by demineralization of mostly trabecular bone and occurs mostly in postmenopausal women about 50 to 65 years of age, or about 10 to 15 years after menopause [8]. Type I osteoporosis, also called postmenopausal osteoporosis, is linked to menopause and reduced estrogen production. Type II osteoporosis is characterized by demineralization of both cortical and trabecular bone. It occurs in both men and women over approximately 70 to 75 years of age [8]. In type II osteoporosis, trabecular and cortical bone are slowly lost due to age-induced decreased bone cell activity, especially osteoblast activity. In addition, decreased synthesis of calcitriol (caused by decreased 1-hydroxylase activity in the kidney) and decreased intestinal calcium absorption occur with aging and contribute to type II osteoporosis. When these events are coupled with low calcium intake and/or high phosphorus intake, parathyroid hormone concentrations increase. However, aging in itself also causes mild above-normal elevations in serum parathyroid hormone concentrations. High blood parathyroid hormone concentrations stimulate bone resorption and promote bone demineralization.

Diagnosis of osteoporosis is based on measurements of bone mineral density, primarily via dual-energy X-ray absorptiometry (DEXA). Bone mineral density represents the average concentration of minerals per unit area, or how tightly the bone mineral tissue is compressed in a given area. Bone density is reported for comparison purposes as a T score or Z score. T scores represent the number of standard deviations (SDs) away from the mean bone density of gender- and race-matched young (25- to 45-year-old) adults. A T score equal to 0 means that the individual's bone mineral density is at the mean for young adults of the same gender and race. The World Health Organization defines osteoporosis as a bone density T score of greater than 2.5 SDs below (i.e., >-2.5) the young adult mean [3]. Osteopenia is defined as a bone density T score of -1 to -2.5. For every 1 SD below the mean, the risk of fracture doubles. Thus, those with osteoporosis are at considerable risk for fracture, and those with osteopenia are at risk for fracture as well as for the development of osteoporosis. Z scores are similar to T scores but represent the number of SDs from the mean bone density of age-matched as well as gender- and race-matched individuals. Thus, for older individuals, T scores will likely be lower than Z scores.

The high prevalence of osteoporosis among women makes this condition a public health problem. Women who are most at risk are those with a family history of the disorder, those who are Caucasian or Asian, and those with a small frame size and/or low body mass (especially BMI <19 kg/m^2). Individuals using medications such as glucocorticoids, thyroid hormones (excess), and antiepileptic drugs also are at increased risk for bone loss and thus osteoporosis. Although the effects of aging and genetic factors (and sometimes drug therapies) cannot be eliminated, other factors contributing to the development of osteoporosis may be modified. Factors interfering with the attainment of peak bone mass as well as factors accelerating the rate of bone loss are influential in the development of osteoporosis. Some of the factors influencing attainment of peak bone mass and/or accelerating the rate of bone loss will be addressed in this perspective. These factors include estrogen, physical activity, and intakes of calcium, vitamin D, and sodium. In addition, some of the effects of phosphorus, protein, vitamins C and K, and fluoride intakes will be reviewed, along with the effects of caffeine and alcohol consumption and smoking.

Estrogen

Estrogen has positive effects on bone formation and mineralization, and its influence is especially evident at puberty. Estrogen deficiency, on the other hand, promotes bone resorption in all age groups, but in adolescence estrogen deficiency also prevents attainment of peak bone mass. While estrogen's effects are thought to be mediated by changes in the activities of osteoblasts (bone-forming cells) and osteoclasts (bone-destroying cells), the exact mechanisms by which estrogen affects bone formation and resorption have not been elucidated.

Estrogen concentrations decrease in women around the time of menopause (perimenopause). Estrogen concentrations also may be low in young women athletes and in young women with eating disorders, especially anorexia nervosa. This estrogen deficit, whether it occurs in older women at menopause, in adolescent girls, or in young women, increases the risk for development of osteoporosis unless estrogen levels can be quickly restored.

Because of the protective effect of estrogen on bone, many physicians believe that estrogen replacement should be recommended on an individual basis, especially for women who are immediately postmenopausal or are going through menopause [9]. Estrogen replacement in the form of oral contraceptive agents also is important for young women who have low estrogen concentrations secondary to an eating disorder and/or considerable physical activity (see the Chap. 15 perspective on eating disorders and the female athlete triad). Moreover, use of oral contraceptive agents in women over the age of 40 years has been shown to decrease subsequent risk of hip fractures after menopause and to improve bone mineral density [10,11]. Estrogen or estrogen replacement therapy (ERT) for peri- or postmenopausal women attenuates bone loss to slow turnover rates and decreases vertebral and nonvertebral fracture rates. It also may increase vertebral and hip bone density [12]. ERT and recovery from amenorrhea, however, have not been associated with normalization of bone density [13]. Moreover, ERT does not protect very well against the spinal dowager's hump, suggesting that bone loss from the spine is likely due to factors other than or in addition to decreased estrogen levels [14].

Use of ERT, however, is not without risk. Major side effects include vaginal bleeding, increased risk of breast cancer as well as of uterine cancer, and increased risk of cardiovascular events [12]. Additional studies are under way to determine whether changing dosage and/or alternating use of progestins with estrogen might minimize some of the side effects.

Figure 1 Major sites affected by osteoporosis.

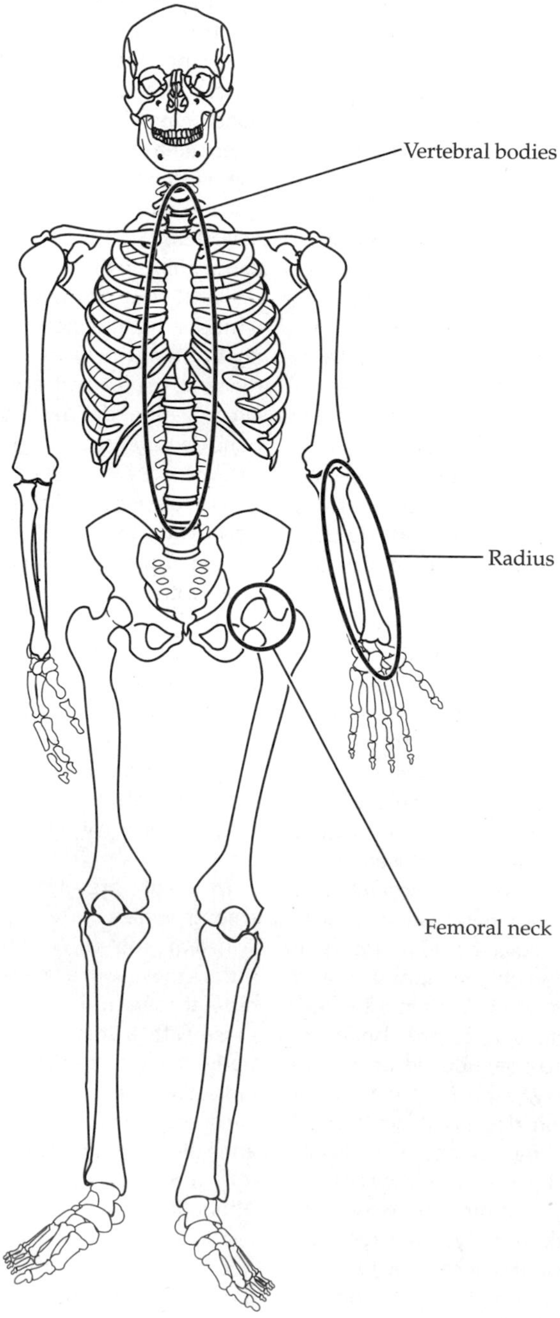

Physical Activity

The effects of the absence of physical activity on bone are apparent in individuals on complete bed rest, due to injury for example. Similarly, the negative influence of weightlessness, as occurs with space travel, on mineral balance has long been recognized. It follows, therefore, that weight bearing by the bone will influence mineral balance positively. This supposition has proved to be true. Weight-bearing exercises, including the carrying of one's own body weight or weight training, on a regular basis have a protective effect on bone, improving bone mineral density or decreasing the age-related demineralization of bone [15,16]. Physical activity in college-age women has been positively correlated with rate of gain in spinal bone density [17]. Beyond the benefits to bone, improvements in muscle strength and balance associated with exercise (even walking 4 hours per week) diminish the likelihood of falling and thus of fracturing bones [12,18]. Extreme physical activity, however, when associated with amenorrhea (lack of menstruation and thus low blood estrogen), is counterproductive to maintaining bone mass.

Calcium

Adequate intake of calcium is important throughout life. Sufficient calcium during childhood, adolescence, and young adulthood is especially critical for attainment of the full genetic expression of peak skeletal mass that occurs sometime in early adulthood. Attainment of dense bones during the early years offers the best protection against weakened, osteoporotic bones in later years.

Adequate calcium intake (whether obtained through dietary sources or through food plus supplements) in children and adolescents has been shown to improve bone mineral density and thus help achieve peak bone mass [19,20]. Calcium intakes of teenagers, for example, have been shown to correlate with adult bone density [21]. Recommended calcium intakes for children and adults are provided on the inside covers of this book; unfortunately, average calcium intakes of females typically are below the recommendations, not only during adolescence but throughout life. The inadequate calcium intake means that less calcium is available to be absorbed and to maintain plasma calcium concentrations. Parathyroid hormone concentrations in turn rise to maintain plasma calcium concentrations, promoting bone resorption and thus bone loss. Thus, to prevent osteoporosis, ingestion of adequate calcium as well as vitamin D is imperative.

While peak bone mass is achieved by early adulthood, calcium is needed throughout life for function in bone as well as in other body tissues, such as blood and muscles. The accelerated loss of bone that occurs in women after menopause and the age-related increases in parathyroid hormone concentrations can be ameliorated in part by adequate intakes of calcium (typically 1,000–1,200 mg or more) and vitamin D (typically 400–800 IU or more) [3,22–25]. Supplementation with calcium and (typically) vitamin D and estrogen has been shown to improve or prevent the loss of bone mineral density, especially in the spine, and/or to decrease vertebral and nonvertebral fractures in postmenopausal women [26,27].

Vitamin D

As you may remember from Chapter 10, calcitriol, 1,25-$(OH)_2$ D_3, accelerates the absorption of calcium from the gastrointestinal tract. Specifically, the vitamin hormone interacts with receptors in the enterocyte and, following transport to the nucleus, increases transcription of genes that code for calbindin. Calbindin functions as a calcium-binding protein and enhances calcium absorption. Calcitriol is also thought to induce changes in the brush border and basolateral membranes to enhance calcium absorption directly. Calcitriol also may be involved in the PTH-mediated calcium reabsorption in the kidney and the PTH-mediated calcium resorption by bone.

While everyone needs to ingest adequate amounts of vitamin D, elderly people appear to benefit from vitamin D supplementation. Poor vitamin D status is common in the elderly because of marginal intake of the vitamin, little exposure to sunlight, and decreased efficiency of transformation of the vitamin into its active metabolite, calcitriol (1,25-dihydroxy cholecalciferol) due to decreased renal 1-hydroxylase activity. Furthermore, the amount of vitamin D_3 produced in aging skin during exposure to the ultraviolet rays of the sun may be decreased to half that produced in young skin [28]. Serum 25-hydroxy vitamin D concentrations are used to assess vitamin D status. When concentrations diminish to <10 ng/mL, vitamin D supplements of 400 to 800 IU effectively improve vitamin D status. In addition, various analogues of vitamin D are being studied for their effectiveness in improving bone formation [29]. Recommended intakes for vitamin D in adults increase from 200 IU (5 μg) for adults through age 50 years to 400 IU (10 μg) for adults age 51 to 70 years and increase further to 600 IU (15 μg) for adults over the age of 70 years [25]. The tolerable upper intake level for vitamin D is 2,000 IU (50 μg) [25]. Optimal effective doses of vitamin D associated with osteoporosis treatment range from about 400 to 1,000 IU [3].

Several studies have shown that supplementation of both vitamin D and calcium improves bone density and diminishes fractures. For example, vitamin D supplements (400 IU) coupled with calcium supplements (377 mg/day as calcium citrate malate) increased bone mineral density in the spine and decreased risk of vertebral fractures in postmenopausal women [30]. In a study supplying 1.2 g calcium as tricalcium phosphate and 800 IU vitamln D, the risk of hip and other nonvertebral fractures significantly decreased and proximal femur bone density increased in elderly women [22].

Sodium

While vitamin D improves the body's calcium status, sodium has been shown to be detrimental to body calcium. Sodium is excreted in the urine with calcium, so a direct relationship exists between sodium and calcium excretion. For example, a sodium load of 100 mmol (2.3 g) per day increased urinary calcium excretion by 1 mmol (40 mg) per day [31,32]. In females age 8 to 13 years, urinary sodium excretion was found to be a major determinant of urinary calcium excretion [33].

This relationship between urinary sodium and calcium excretion is also associated with bone. Urinary sodium excretion has been negatively correlated with changes in bone density (bone loss) in the hip region of postmenopausal women [34]. Other analyses, however, suggest that dietary sodium does not significantly affect biomarkers of bone resorption, especially in young adults, and thus an increased sodium intake is not a major risk factor in the development of osteoporosis [35,36].

Phosphorus

Diets adequate in phosphorus are important for bone health. Definitive answers as to the effects of high dietary phosphorus when consumed with low calcium (common in the United States) on bone turnover in humans cannot be given without further research. What is known is that high plasma phosphorus concentrations, by stimulating parathyroid hormone secretion, increase indirectly the reabsorption of calcium by the renal tubules so that less calcium is lost in the urine. Yet phosphorus also causes loss of calcium by increasing calcium secretion into the gastrointestinal tract, and the increased parathyroid hormone concentrations promote bone resorption, increasing plasma calcium concentrations at the expense of bone.

Prolonged ingestion of diets high in phosphorus and low in calcium results in a mild secondary hyperparathyroidism [37,38]. Again, the high parathyroid hormone concentrations stimulate bone resorption, with possible long-term detrimental effects on bone mineral content [37–39]. Vitamin D synthesis (calcitriol, or 1,25-dihydroxycholecalciferol) in response to the elevated parathyroid hormone concentrations varies. Longer intakes of high-phosphorus/low-calcium diets appear to be associated with no rise in calcitriol synthesis, which is needed to improve calcium absorption [37]. However, high-phosphorus diets, while increasing parathyroid hormone concentrations, have not been shown in humans to consistently enhance concentrations of compounds (biomarkers) that indicate increased bone resorption and/or turnover [37,40–42]. Further research to address the effects of such diets on both bone resorption and bone accretion is needed to clarify the effects of diets high in phosphorus on the development of osteoporosis in humans.

Protein

Adequate protein intake is necessary for bone health, yet concerns have been raised that high protein intakes may be detrimental to bone. Proteins and a variety of the constituent amino acids (especially the sulfur-containing amino acids methionine and cysteine, which may bind calcium) have been shown to increase excretion of calcium in the urine. Dietary protein directly influences calcium; doubling of protein intake without changing intake of other nutrients results in about a 50% increase in urinary calcium [43–45]. Significant positive correlations between protein intake and urinary calcium excretion have been demonstrated in adults age 20 to 79 years [46]. However, in natural foods, proteins are usually combined with substances that counteract their effect on calcium excretion. For example, because many protein-containing foods also contain phosphorus, ingestion of foods containing both nutrients tends to minimize negative effects on urinary calcium excretion [47]. In a group of college-age women, the rate of gain of spinal bone density was positively correlated with the calcium : protein intake ratio [17]. Other studies have also shown positive associations between protein intake and bone mass [48]. Moreover, in recovery from bone fractures, higher intakes of both energy and protein have been shown to improve recovery times and to attenuate the decrease in bone mineral density associated with the fracture [49,50].

Vitamins C and K

Vitamins C and K are important for the synthesis and function of various proteins found in bone. Collagen is one of the main proteins found in bone, and the synthesis of collagen is dependent on vitamin C (see p. 264). Positive correlations between vitamin C intake and bone mineral density have been shown in adolescents and in adult women [48,51].

In addition to collagen, bone also contains many other proteins, including osteocalcin and matrix Gla protein. Osteocalcin and matrix Gla protein require vitamin K to function (see p. 365). With inadequate vitamin K status, these two proteins are not carboxylated as they normally would be and thus have limited ability to bind calcium and aid in bone mineralization. Serum undercarboxylated osteocalcin concentrations (a sign of poor vitamin K status) have been found to be correlated with bone mineral density in the **Ward's triangle** (a region within the hip) and femoral neck in women during the first decade of menopause [52]. Serum undercarboxylated osteocalcin concentrations also have been shown to be predictive of increased risk of hip fractures in elderly women [53]. In addition, low vitamin K intakes have been found to be associated with an increased incidence of hip fractures in elderly men and women [54].

Fluoride

Use of fluoride is not recommended or approved for the prevention or treatment of osteoporosis [4,55]. While fluoride has been shown to reduce the incidence of dental caries, its effectiveness in the prevention and treatment of osteoporosis is inconsistent. Fluoride, usually administered as sodium fluoride (40–80 mg/day), stimulates bone formation (osteoblast activity). In some studies, use of fluoride along with calcium increased mostly trabecular bone mass and to some extent cortical bone and decreased fracture rates in postmenopausal women [7,56–58]. However, supplements of 75 mg fluoride together with 1,500 mg calcium failed to reduce the risk of vertebral fractures and increased the risk of nonvertebral fractures in postmenopausal women [59]. In addition, abnormal bone quality has been found to accompany increases in bone density following use of fluoride. Other research has shown that highly fluoridated water fails to protect against bone loss [60]. While the formulation, dose, delivery mode, and duration of fluoride therapy may account for observed differences among studies, additional studies are thought to be needed before recommendations for fluoride therapy may be issued [7,9,56,57,59].

Smoking

Smoking negatively impacts bone health. Smoking is associated with lower bone density and, in women, with earlier menopause and increased postmenopausal bone loss [61,62]. Smoking decreases circulating estrogen concentrations, thereby contributing to bone loss [61]. Smoking has also been shown to be a significant predictor of bone loss in men [63].

Alcohol

Chronic and excessive ingestion of alcohol damages bone and increases the risk of osteoporosis. The mechanisms by which alcohol exerts its effects are unclear but are thought to be multifactorial [64]. Alcohol consumption has been significantly associated with increased rates of bone loss in men [63]. People consuming excessive alcohol generally have lower bone mass and reduced osteoblast activity and are at increased risk, in a dose-response relationship, of hip and forearm fractures [64,65]. Factors associated with excessive alcohol intake affecting bone loss include insufficient intake of nutrients (especially calcium, protein, and/or vitamin D) coupled with poor absorption of nutrients, as well as elevated parathyroid hormone concentrations [64].

Caffeine

Caffeine minimally impacts calcium balance and therefore may be weakly associated with the development of osteoporosis. Caffeine reduces the renal reabsorption of calcium, which leads to increased urinary calcium losses. However, it has been estimated that one cup of caffeinated coffee promotes the loss of only about 6 mg calcium in the urine [65,66]. Caffeine in amounts of 300 to 400 mg increased urinary calcium by 10 mg/day [67]. However, caffeine may also promote increased secretion of calcium into the gut to enhance calcium loss from the body; whether the secreted calcium is reabsorbed and the extent of the secretion have not been determined [8]. Caffeine intake has been positively associated with risk of hip fracture in middle-aged women [65]. However, no association was reported between current caffeine intake and bone density in postmenopausal women [68].

Summary

Maintenance of desirable skeletal status clearly is multifactorial. While nutrients such as calcium and vitamin D have been shown to play considerable roles in bone health, many other nutrients (some probably still undiscovered) play minor but important roles. Inadequate amounts of dietary boron or magnesium, for example, can promote bone problems. Moreover, diets with added copper, manganese, and zinc, for example, have been shown to be more effective in arresting bone loss in postmenopausal women than diets with no added nutrients or with only added calcium or trace minerals [69]. A person's genetic makeup cannot be changed, nor can the physiological changes accompanying aging be reversed. The individual usually does have the option, however, of choosing a lifestyle in which good nutrition (a variety of foods and recommended intakes of all nutrients) and weight-bearing exercise are practiced regularly. In addition to a good diet and exercise, attention to the hormonal environment is also critical to attenuating bone loss during periods of low estrogen concentration such as may occur with eating disorders or excessive exercise or during the peri- and postmenopausal stages of life for women. With monitoring of bone density and early diagnosis of problems, appropriate interventions may be started to slow or halt the progression of osteoporosis [6].

References Cited

1. Cooper C, Campion G, Melton U. Hip fracture in the elderly: a worldwide projection. Osteoporosis Int 1992;2:285–89.

2. Rotella D. Osteoporosis: challenges and new opportunities for therapy. Curr Opin Drug Disc Devel 2002;5:477–86.

3. NIH Consensus Development Panel on Osteoporosis. Osteoporosis prevention, diagnosis, and therapy. JAMA 2001;285:785–95.

4. Sayegh R, Stubblefield P. Bone metabolism and the perimenopause. Obstet Gynecol Clin N Am 2002; 29:495–510.

5. Pachucki-Hyde L. Assessment of risk factors for osteoporosis and fracture. Nursing Clin N Am 2001; 36:401–8.

6. Hall J, Riley R. Nutritional strategies to reduce the risk of osteoporosis. Med Surg Nurs 1999;8:281–93.

7. Phipps K. Fluoride and bone health. J Publ Health Dent 1995;55:53–56.

8. Harward M. Nutritive therapies for osteoporosis: the role of calcium. Med Clin N Am 1993;77:889–98.

9. Khosla S, Riggs L. Treatment options for osteoporosis. Mayo Clin Proc 1995;70:978–82.

10. Michaelsson K, Baron J, Farahmand B, Persson I, Ljunghall S. Oral contraceptive use and risk of hip fracture: a case control study. Lancet 1999;353:1481–84.

11. Kuohung W, Borgatta L, Stubblefield P. Low dose oral contraceptive and bone mineral density: an evidence-based analysis. Contraception 2000;61:77–82.

12. Nelson H. Postmenopausal osteoporosis and estrogen. Am Fam Physic 2003;68:606–12.

13. Kaufman B, Warren M, Dominguez J, Wang J, Heymsfiedl S, Pierson R. Bone density and amenorrhea in ballet dancers are related to a decreased resting metabolic rate and lower leptin levels. J Clin Endo Metab 2002;87:2777–83.

14. Avioli L. Calcium and osteoporosis. Ann Rev Nutr 1984;4:471–91.

15. Heaney R. Bone mass, nutrition, and other lifestyle factors. Nutr Rev 1996;54:S3–S10.

16. Vuori I. Peak bone mass and physical activity: a short review. Nutr Rev 1996;54:S11–S14.

17. Recker R, Davies K, Hinders S, Heaney R, Stegman M, Kimmel D. Bone gain in young adult women. JAMA 1992;268:2403–8.

18. Feskanich D, Willett W, Colditz G. Walking and leisure-time activity and risk of hip fracture in postmenopausal women. JAMA 2002;288:2300–2306.

19. Johnston C, Miller J, Slemenda C, Reister T, Hui S, Christian J, Peacock M. Calcium supplementation and increases in bone mineral density in children. N Engl J Med 1992;327:82–87.

20. Lloyd T, Andon M, Rollings N, Martel J, Landis J, Demers L, Eggli D, Kleselhorst K, Kulin H. Calcium supplementation and bone mineral density in adolescent girls. JAMA 1993;270:841–44.

21. Nieves J, Golden A, Siris E. Teenage and current calcium intake are related to bone mineral density of the hip and forearm in women aged 30–39 years. Am J Epidemiol 1995;141:342–51.

22. Chapuy M, Arlot M, Duboeuf F, Brun J, Crouzet B, Arnaud S, Delmas P, Meunier P. Vitamin D_3 and calcium to prevent hip fractures in elderly women. N Engl J Med 1992;327:1637–42.

23. Chapuy M, Arlot M, Delmas P, Meunier P. Effect of calcium and cholecalciferol treatment for three years on hip fractures in elderly women. BMJ 1994;308:1081–82.

24. Tuck S, Francis R. Osteoporosis. Postgrad Med J 2002;78:526–32.

25. Food and Nutrition Board. Dietary Reference Intakes for Calcium, Phosphorus, Magnesium, Vitamin D and Fluoride. Washington, DC: National Academy Press, 1997.

26. Reid I, Ames R, Evans M, Gamble G, Sharpe S. Effect of calcium supplementation on bone loss in postmenopausal women. N Engl J Med 1993;328:460–64.

27. Nieves J, Komar L, Cosman F, Lindsay R. Calcium potentiates the effect of estrogen and calcitonin on bone mass: review and analysis. Am J Clin Nutr 1998;67:18–24.

28. MacLauglin J, Holick M. Aging decreases the capacity of human skin to produce vitamin D_3. J Clin Invest 1985;76:1536–38.

29. Nishi Y. Active vitamin D and its analogs as drugs for the treatment of osteoporosis: advantages and problems. J Bone Miner Metab 2002;20:57–65.

30. Dawson-Hughes B, Dallah G, Krall E, Harris S, Sokoll L, Falconer G. Effect of vitamin D supplementation on wintertime and overall bone loss in healthy postmenopausal women. Ann Intern Med 1991;115:505–12.

31. Massey L. Dietary factors influencing calcium and bone metabolism: introduction. J Nutr 1993;123:1609–10.

32. Nordin B, Need A, Morris H, Horowitz M. The nature and significance of the relationship between urinary sodium and urinary calcium in women. J Nutr 1993;123:1615–22.

33. Matkovic V, Illich J, Andon M, Hsieh L, Tzagournis M, Lagger B, Goel P. Urinary calcium, sodium, and bone mass of young females. Am J Clin Nutr 1995;62:417–25.

34. Devine A, Criddle R, Dick I, Kerr D, Prince R. A longitudinal study of the effect of sodium and calcium intakes on regional bone density in postmenopausal women. Am J Clin Nutr 1995;62:740–45.

35. Cohen A, Roe F. Review of risk factors for osteoporosis with particular reference to a possible aetiological role of dietary salt. Food Chem Toxicology 2000;38:237–53.

36. Lin P-H, Ginty F, Appel L, Aickin M, Bohannon A, Garnero P, Barclay D, Svetkey L. The DASH diet and sodium reduction improve markers of bone turnover and calcium metabolism in adults. J Nutr 2003; 133:3130–36.

37. Calvo M, Kumar R, Heath H. Persistently elevated parathyroid hormone secretion and action in young women after four weeks of ingesting high phosphorus, low calcium diets. J Clin Endocrinol Metab 1990;70: 1334–40.

38. Anderson J. The role of nutrition in the functioning of skeletal tissue. Nutr Rev 1992;50:388–94.

39. Calvo M. Dietary phosphorus, calcium metabolism and bone. J Nutr 1993;123:1627–33.

40. Zemel M, Linkswiler H. Calcium metabolism in the young adult male as affected by level and form of phosphorus intake and level of calcium intake. J Nutr 1981;11:315–24.

41. Bizik B, Ding W, Cerklewski F. Evidence that bone resorption of young men is not increased by high dietary phosphorus obtained from milk and cheese. Nutr Res 1996;16:1143–46.

42. Karkkainen M, Lamberg-Allardt C. An acute intake of phosphorus increases parathyroid hormone secretion and inhibits bone formation in young women. J Bone Miner Res 1996;11:1905–11.

43. Teegarden D, Lyle R, McCabe G, McCabe L, Proulx W, Michon K, Knight A, Johnston C, Weaver C. Dietary calcium, protein, and phosphorus are related to bone mineral density and content in young women. Am J Clin Nutr 1998;68:749–54.

44. Massey L. Dietary factors influencing calcium and bone metabolism: introduction. J Nutr 1993;123: 1609–10.

45. Whiting S, Anderson D, Weeks S. Calciuric effects of protein and potassium bicarbonate but not sodium chloride or phosphate can be detected acutely in women and men. Am J Clin Nutr 1997;65:1465–67.

46. Itoh R, Nishiyama N, Suyama Y. Dietary protein intake and urinary excretion of calcium: a cross-sectional study in a healthy Japanese population. Am J Clin Nutr 1998;67:438–44.

47. Wardlaw G. Putting osteoporosis in perspective. J Am Diet Assoc 1993;93:1000–1006.

48. Freudenheim J, Johnson N, Smith E. Relationships between usual nutrient intake and bone-mineral content of women 35–65 years of age: longitudinal and cross-sectional analysis. Am J Clin Nutr 1986; 44:863–76.

49. Schurch M, Rizzoli R, Slosman D, Vadas L, Vergnaud P, Bonjour J. Protein supplements increase serum insulin-like growth factor 1 levels and attenuate proximal femur bone loss in patients with recent hip fracture: a randomized, double-blind, placebo-controlled trial. Ann Intern Med 1998;128:801–9.

50. Jallut D, Tappy L, Kohut M, Bloesch D, Munger R, Schutz Y, Chiolero R, Felber J, Livio J, Jequier E. Energy balance in elderly patients after surgery for a femoral neck fracture. JPEN 1990;14:563–68.

51. Gunnes M, Lehmann E. Dietary calcium, saturated fat, fiber, and vitamin C as predictors of forearm cortical and trabecular bone mineral density in healthy children and adolescents. Acta Paediatr 1995;84:388–92.

52. Knapen M, Kruseman A, Wouters R, Vermeer C. Correlation of serum osteocalcin fractions with bone mineral density in women during the first 10 years after menopause. Calcif Tiss Int 1998; 63:375–79.

53. Szulc P, Arlot M, Chapuy M, Duboeuf F, Meunier P, Delmas P. Serum undercarboxylated osteocalcin correlates with hip bone mineral density in elderly women. J Bone Miner Res 1994;9:1591–95.

54. Booth S, Tucker K, Chen H, Hannan M, Gagnon D, Cupples L, Wilson P, Ordovas J, Schaefer E, Dawson-Hughes B, Kiel D. Dietary vitamin K intakes are associated with hip fracture but not with bone mineral density in elderly men and women. Am J Clin Nutr 2000; 71:1201–8.

55. Crandall C. Parathyroid hormone for treatment of osteoporosis. Ann Intern Med 2002;162:2297–2309.

56. Pak C, Sakhaee K, Piziak V, Peterson R, Breslau N, Boyd P, Poindexter J, Herzog J, Sakhaee A, Haynes S, Huet B, Reisch J. Slow release sodium fluoride in the management of postmenopausal osteoporosis: a randomized controlled trial. Ann Intern Med 1994;120:625–32.

57. Kleerekoper M, Mendlovic D. Sodium fluoride therapy of postmenopausal osteoporosis. Endocrin Rev 1993;14:312–23.

58. Eisinger J, Clairet D. Effects of silicon, fluoride, etidronate and magnesium on bone mineral density: a retrospective study. Magnesium Res 1993;6:247–49.

59. Riggs B, Hodgson S, O'Fallon W, Chao E, Wahner H, Muhs J, Cedel S, Melton L. Effect of fluoride treatment on the fracture rate in postmenopausal women with osteoporosis. N Engl J Med 1990;322:802–9.

60. Sowers M, Wallace R, Lemke J. The relationship of bone mass and fracture history to fluoride and calcium intake: a study of three communities. Am J Clin Nutr 1986;44:889–98.

61. Jensen J, Christiansen C, Rodbro P. Cigarette smoking, serum estrogens, and bone loss during hormone-replacement therapy early after menopause. N Engl J Med 1985;313:973–77.

62. Krall E, Dawson-Hughes B. Smoking and bone loss among postmenopausal women. J Bone Min Res 1991;4:331–38.

63. Slemenda C, Christian J, Read T, Reister T, Williams C, Johnston C. Long-term bone loss in men: effects of genetic and environmental factors. Ann Intern Med 1992;117:286–91.

64. Laitinen K, Valimaki M. Alcohol and bone. Calcif Tissue Int 1991;49(suppl):S70–73.

65. Hernandez-Avila M, Colditz G, Stampfer M, Rosner B. Caffeine, moderate alcohol intake, and risk of fractures of the hip and forearm in middle-aged women. Am J Clin Nutr 1991;54:157–63.

66. Heaney R, Recker R. Effects of nitrogen, phosphorus and caffeine on calcium balance in women. J Lab Clin Med 1982;99:46–55.

67. Massey LK, Whiting SJ. Caffeine, urinary calcium, calcium metabolism and bone. J Nutr 1993;123:1611–14.

68. Lloyd T, Rollings N, Eggli D, Kieselhorst K, Chinchilli V. DIetary caffeine intake and bone status of postmenopausal women. Am J Clin Nutr 1997; 65:1826–30.

69. Strause L, Saltman P, Smith K, Bracker M, Andon M. Spinal bone loss in postmenopausal women supplemented with calcium and trace minerals. J Nutr 1994;124:1060–64.

Iron
Zinc
Copper
Selenium
Chromium
Iodine
Manganese
Molybdenum
Fluoride

For each of the microminerals listed, the following subtopics (if known and when applicable) are discussed:

Sources
Digestion, Absorption, Transport, Uptake, and Storage
Functions and Mechanisms of Action
Interactions with Other Nutrients
Excretion
Recommended Dietary Allowances or Adequate Intakes
Deficiency
Supplements
Toxicity
Assessment of Nutriture

perspective
Nutrient–Drug Interactions

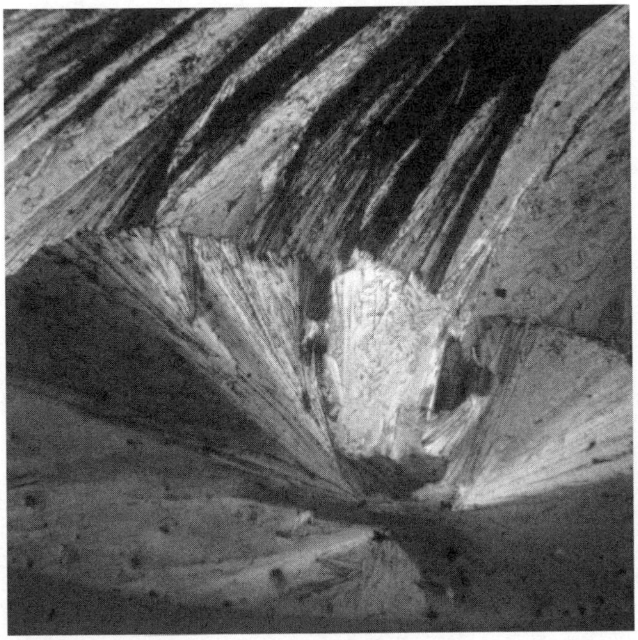

Polarized light micrograph of manganese sulfate

chapter 12 Microminerals

A PRECISE DEFINITION FOR THE essential microminerals (or trace minerals or trace elements) has not been established. These minerals initially gained the description "trace" because their concentrations in tissue were not easily quantified by early analytical methods. Today, however, trace minerals can be analyzed by a variety of techniques [1]. The term *trace* when applied to minerals or elements is still used and can be defined as minerals that comprise <0.01% of total body weight [2]. Others define trace elements as nutrients the body needs in concentrations of one part per million or less [2]. Iron appears to be the mineral that divides the macrominerals from the microminerals; consequently, some define an essential trace mineral as a mineral needed by the body in a concentration equal to or lower than that of iron [3]. Alternately, *trace* may be applied to minerals needed by the body in amounts <100 mg per day.

The term *essential* as applied to trace elements also was specified in the 1980s. An element is considered essential if a dietary deficiency of that element consistently results in a suboptimal biological function that is preventable or reversible by physiological amounts of the element [4].

Table 12.1 The Microminerals: Approximate Body Content, Selected Function, Deficiency Symptoms, Food Sources, and Recommended Intake Dietary Allowance (RDA) or Adequate Intake (AI)

Mineral	Approximate Body Content	Selected Physiological Roles	Selected Enzyme Cofactor Roles	Selected Deficiency Symptoms	Food Sources	RDA or AI (Adults)
Chromium	4–6 mg	Normal use of blood glucose and function of insulin		Glucose intolerance, glucose and lipid metabolism abnormalities	Mushrooms, prunes, asparagus, organ meats, whole-grain breads and cereals	35 μg*, male; 25 μg*, female
Copper	50–150 mg	Utilization of iron stores, lipids, collagen, pigment, neurotransmitter synthesis	Oxidases, monooxygenases, superoxide dismutase	Anemia, neutropenia, bone abnormalities	Liver, shellfish, whole grains, legumes, eggs, meat, fish	900 μg
Fluorine	Unknown	Maintenance of teeth and bone structure		Dental caries, bone problems	Fish, meat, legumes, grains, drinking water (variable)	4 mg*, male; 3 mg*, female
Iodine	15–20 mg	Thyroid hormones synthesis		Enlarged thyroid gland, myxedema, cretinism, increase in blood lipids, gluconeogenesis, and extracellular retention of NaCl and H_2O	Iodized salt, salt-water seafood, sunflower seeds, mushrooms, liver, eggs	150 μg
Iron	2–4 g	Component of hemoglobin and myoglobin for O_2 transport and cellular use	Heme enzymes, catalase, cytochromes, myeloperoxidase, nonheme enzymes carnitine and collagen synthesis	Listlessness, fatigue, anemia, palpitations, sore tongue, angular stomatitis, dysphagia, decreased resistance to infection	Organ meats (liver), meat, molasses, clams, oysters, nuts, legumes, seeds, green leafy vegetables, dried fruits, enriched/whole-grain breads/cereals	8 mg, male; 18 mg, female
Manganese	10–20 mg	Brain function, collagen, bone, growth, urea, synthesis, glucose and lipid metabolism, CNS function	Arginase, pyruvate carboxylase, PEP, carboxykinase, superoxide dismutase	In animals, possibly humans: impaired growth, skeletal abnormalities, impaired CNS function	Wheat bran, legumes, nuts, lettuce, beet tops, blueberries, pineapple, seafood, poultry, meat	2.3 mg*, male; 1.8 mg*, female
Molybdenum	Unknown	Metabolism of purines, pyrimidines, pteridines, aldehydes, and oxidation	Xanthine dehydrogenase/oxidase, aldehyde oxidase, sulfite oxidase	Hypermethioninemia, ↑ urinary xanthine, sulfite excretion, ↓ urinary sulfate and urate excretion	Soybeans, lentils, buckwheat, oats, rice, bread	45 μg
Selenium	15 mg	Protects cells against destruction by hydrogen peroxide and free radicals	Glutathione peroxidase, 5′-deiodinase	Myalgia, cardiac myopathy, ↑ cell fragility, pancreatic degeneration	Grains, meat, poultry, fish, dairy products	55 μg
Zinc	1.5–2.5 g	Energy metabolism, metabolism, protein synthesis, collagen formation, alcohol detoxification, carbon dioxide elimination, sexual maturation, taste and smell functions	DNA-RNA polymerase, carbonic anhydrase, carboxypeptidase, alkaline phosphatase, deoxythymidine kinase	Poor wound healing, subnormal growth, anorexia, abnormal taste/smell; changes in hair, skin, nails; retarded reproductive system development	Oysters, wheat germ, beef, liver, poultry, whole grains	11 mg, male; 8 mg, female

*Indicates adequate intake.

More stringent criteria [5] proposed to establish essentiality of a mineral include the following:

- It is present in all healthy tissue of living things.
- Its concentration from one animal to the next is fairly constant.
- Its withdrawal from the body induces reproducibly the same physiological and structural abnormalities, regardless of species studied.
- Its addition either reduces or prevents these abnormalities.
- The abnormalities induced by deficiencies are always accompanied by specific biochemical changes.
- These biochemical changes can be prevented or cured when the deficiency is prevented or cured.

Elements established as essential may not necessarily comply with all the criteria listed, in part because of limitations imposed by the degree of sophistication of the analytical methodology available. Essentiality, therefore, is technically easier to ascertain for elements that occur in relatively high concentration than for those ultratrace elements occurring at very low concentrations and having a low requirement.

For six essential trace minerals (iron, zinc, copper, iodine, selenium, and molybdenum), recommended dietary allowances (RDAs) have been established for humans. Adequate intakes have been estimated for another three essential trace minerals (fluoride, manganese, and chromium). The inside covers of this book provide the recommended intakes for the microminerals. Very little is known about the need of humans for ultratrace elements, including nickel, silicon, vanadium, arsenic, and boron; therefore, no recommendations for intake exist.

Each essential trace mineral is necessary for one or more functions in the body, and its function or functions, like those of other essential nutrients, are optimal when mineral intake and body concentrations of the nutrient fall within a specific range. Whenever the intake or body concentration is too low or too high, function is impaired and death can result.

This chapter discusses the sources, digestion, absorption, transport, functions, interactions with other nutrients, excretion, recommended intakes, deficiency, toxicity, and assessment of nutriture for the microminerals. Chapter 13 addresses these topics for several ultratrace elements. Table 12.1 provides an overview of the trace elements, including information on selected functions, approximate body content, sources, deficiency symptoms, and recommended intakes. As pointed out at the beginning of Chapter 11, the differences in body content between the macro- and microminerals is quite large. The body's content of the macrominerals ranges from ~35 to 1,400 g, while that of the trace elements ranges from <1 mg to ~4 g (remember that an ounce weighs about 28.4 g).

References Cited

1. Mertz W. The essential trace elements. Science 1981;213:1332–38.

2. Taylor A. Detection and monitoring of disorders of essential trace elements. Ann Clin Biochem 1996;33:486–510.

3. Tracing the facts about trace minerals. Tufts Univ Diet and Nutr Letter, March 1987;5:3–6.

4. Nielsen FH. Ultratrace elements in nutrition. Ann Rev Nutr 1984;4:21–41.

5. Underwood EJ, Mertz W. Trace Elements in Human and Animal Nutrition. San Diego: Academic Press, 1987, vol. 2, pp. 1–19.

IRON

The human body contains ~2 to 4 g iron, or ~38 mg iron/kg body weight for women and ~50 mg iron/kg body weight for men. Over 65% of body iron is found in hemoglobin, up to about 10% is found as myoglobin, about 1% to 5% is found as part of enzymes, and the remaining body iron is found in the blood or in storage. Table 12.2 gives an approximate distribution of iron per kilogram of body weight in adult males and females [1–3]. The total amount of iron found in a person not only is related to body weight but also is influenced by other physiological conditions, including age, gender, pregnancy, and state of growth.

Iron, a metal, exists in several oxidation states varying from Fe^{6+} to Fe^{2-}, depending on its chemical environment. The only states that are stable in the aqueous environment of the human body and in food are the ferric (Fe^{3+}) and the ferrous (Fe^{2+}) forms.

Table 12.2 Approximate Distribution of Iron in Adult Males and Females (mg/kg body weight)

	Males	Females
Functional iron		
Hemoglobin	31	28
Myoglobin	5	4
Heme enzymes	1	1
Nonheme enzymes	1	1
Transport iron		
Transferrin	0.05	0.05
Storage iron		
Ferritin and Hemosiderin	12	4
Total iron:	50.05	38.05

Sources

Although iron is widely distributed in food, its content in an average Western diet is estimated at no more than 5 to 7 mg iron per 1,000 kcal. Dietary iron is found in one of two forms in foods, heme and nonheme. Heme iron is derived mainly from hemoglobin and myoglobin and thus is found in animal products, especially meat, fish, and poultry. About 50% to 60% of the iron in meat, fish, and poultry is heme iron; the rest is nonheme iron. Nonheme iron is found primarily in plant foods (nuts, fruits, vegetables, grains, tofu) and dairy products (milk, cheese, eggs), although dairy products have very little iron and represent a very poor iron source. Nonheme iron is usually bound to components of foods and must be hydrolyzed, digested, or solubilized in the gastrointestinal tract prior to absorption into the intestinal cells.

Foods particularly high in iron, such as liver and organ meats, are not popular items in most Western diets. More popular foods that are relatively good sources of iron include red meats, oysters and clams, beans (lima, navy), dark green leafy vegetables, and dried fruits. Other good sources of iron are listed in Table 12.1.

In addition to amounts of iron found naturally in foods, foods such as breads, rolls, pasta, cereals, grits, and flour are fortified with iron. Fortified flour, for example, contains 20 mg iron per lb, while corn grits, corn meal, and rice contain from 13 to 26 mg per lb. Pasta has 13 to 16.5 mg per lb, and bread, rolls, and buns contain 12.5 mg iron per lb. Elemental iron, ferrous ascorbate, ferrous carbonate, ferrous citrate, ferrous fumarate, ferrous gluconate, ferrous lactate, ferric ammonium citrate, ferric chloride, ferric citrate, ferric pyrophosphate, and ferric sulfate are approved and used for food fortification.

Digestion, Absorption, Transport, Storage, and Uptake

Heme Iron Digestion and Absorption

Heme iron must be hydrolyzed from the globin portion of hemoglobin or myoglobin prior to absorption. This digestion is accomplished by the proteases in both the stomach and the small intestine and results in the release of heme iron. Heme, containing the iron bound to the porphyrin ring (referred to as a metalloporphyrin; Fig. 12.1), remains soluble, especially in the presence of the degradation products (amino acids and peptides) of globin, and is readily absorbed intact into the mucosal cell (enterocyte) of the small intestine. Characterization of the heme transporter in the intestinal cells has not been completed.

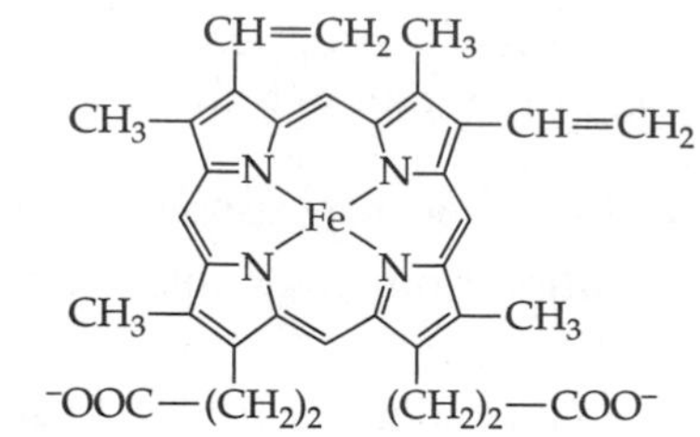

Figure 12.1 Heme iron, a metalloporphyrin.

Iron absorption can occur throughout the small intestine, but it is most efficient in the proximal portion, particularly the duodenum. Within the mucosal cell, the absorbed heme porphyrin ring is hydrolyzed by heme oxygenase into inorganic ferrous iron and protoporphyrin (Fig. 12.2). The released iron may associate with proteins that make up the paraferritin complex (see p. 424 for a discussion of the paraferritin complex) and can be used by the intestinal mucosal cell, excreted with the sloughing of the enterocytes, or, following transport out of the enterocyte, used by other body tissues.

Nonheme Iron Digestion and Absorption

Nonheme iron bound to components of foods must be enzymatically freed in the gastrointestinal tract for absorption to occur (Fig. 12.2). Gastric secretions, including hydrochloric acid and the protease pepsin in the stomach and proteases in the small intestine, aid in the release of nonheme iron from food components.

Once released from food components, most nonheme iron is present as ferric (Fe^{3+}) iron in the stomach. Ferric iron remains fairly soluble as long as the pH of the environment is acidic. Some of the ferric iron may even be reduced to the ferrous state (Fe^{2+}). Once it passes from the stomach into the distal duodenum and jejunum, ferric iron mixes with alkaline juices secreted into the intestine from the pancreas. In this more alkaline environment, ferric iron may complex to produce ferric hydroxide ($Fe(OH)_3$), a relatively insoluble compound that tends to aggregate and precipitate, making the iron less available for absorption. While ferrous iron remains fairly soluble at pH 8, some ferrous iron may be oxidized to the ferric form in the alkaline pH of the intestine. Ferrireductases, including duodenal cytochrome b (Dcytb), have been identified on the brush border membrane of enterocytes and function in the duodenum to reduce ferric iron to the ferrous state.

Thus, following digestion (release from food components), nonheme iron may be present in either the ferric

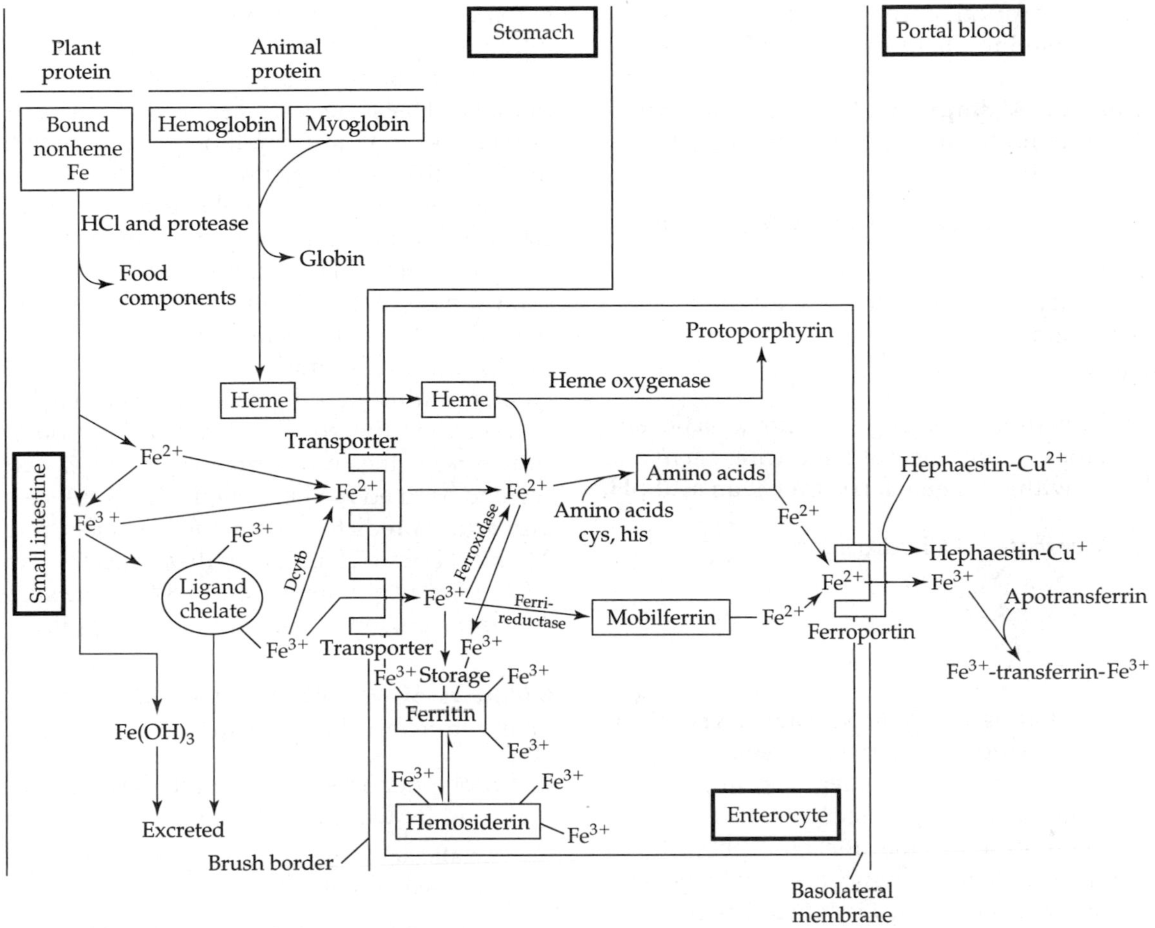

Figure 12.2 Overview of iron digestion, absorption, and transport.

or the ferrous state in the small intestine. Ferrous iron may be absorbed across the brush border and into the intestinal mucosal cell by binding to any of several transporters located in the intestinal cell brush border membrane. Examples of these protein carrier transporters include natural resistance associated macrophage protein 2 (abbreviated nramp 2) and divalent cation or mineral transporter 1 (abbreviated DCT or DMT), which may be an isoform of nramp 2. In the gastrointestinal tract, these transporters are found primarily in the duodenum and transport not only iron but also, to a lesser extent, other divalent cations such as zinc, manganese, copper, nickel, and lead. Synthesis of both transport proteins appears to be affected by iron status, with increased transporter synthesis associated with low iron stores or status.

The mechanisms of absorption of ferric iron are not clearly delineated. It is known that absorption is best from an acidic environment and is facilitated by chelation of the iron with ligands or **chelators** that help solubilize the ferric iron. A membrane protein known as integrin is thought to facilitate iron (as well as zinc) absorption through the microvillous brush border membrane of the enterocyte. Integrin is thought to exist as part of a complex called the paraferritin complex, which includes mobilferrin and a flavin-dependent ferrireductase. The roles of mobilferrin and this ferrireductase in the transport and reduction of iron in the cytosol are discussed on page 424. The role of ligands and chelators in the absorption of iron is discussed next.

Factors Influencing Iron Absorption

Several compounds (known as chelators or ligands) may bind with nonheme iron to either inhibit or enhance its absorption. Chelators are small organic compounds that form a complex with a metal ion. Ligands are compounds that also bind or complex with minerals. Whether chelated iron or iron attached to a ligand is absorbed or excreted depends in part on the nature of the iron-chelate/ligand complex. If the iron-chelate/ligand complex maintains solubility and the iron is loosely bonded, the iron can be released at the mucosal cell and absorption enhanced. However, if the iron chelate/ligand is strongly bonded and insoluble, the absorption of iron will not occur and the iron will be excreted in the feces as part of the chelate.

Enhancers of Iron Absorption. Some dietary factors that have been found to enhance nonheme iron absorption include

- acids, such as ascorbic, citric, lactic, and tartaric;
- sugars;
- meat, poultry, and fish or their digestion products; and
- mucin.

Ascorbic acid (vitamin C), along with citric, lactic, and tartaric acids, for example, acts as a reducing agent and forms a chelate with nonheme ferric iron at an acid pH.

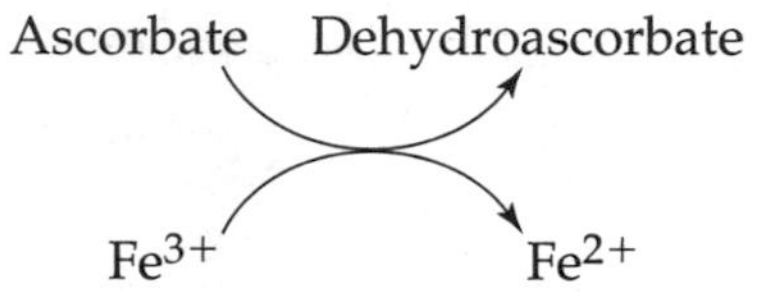

This chelate (a ferrous ascorbate chelate if vitamin C served as the reducing agent) remains soluble in the small intestine and thus can improve intestinal absorption of nonheme iron. Sugars such as fructose and sorbitol also promote nonheme iron absorption. Meat, poultry, and fish factors that enhance nonheme iron absorption have not been clearly identified. The enhancement is not a general property of animal proteins but is due to the digestion products from animal tissues high in the contractile proteins actin and myosin [4]. Both of these proteins are digested into peptides that contain relatively large amounts of the amino acid cysteine. The cysteine-containing peptides are thought to be responsible for the increased absorption of iron [4–6]. It is further suspected that meat is not just a source of solubilizing ligands (e.g., the cysteine-containing peptides that bind iron) but may also improve iron absorption through stimulation of enhancing intestinal secretions [4]. Amino acids, including histidine and cysteine among others, also may form chelates with iron and enhance iron absorption. These amino acid–iron chelates are thought to be absorbed intact using amino acid carrier proteins. EDTA (ethylene diaminetetraacetate), although generally shown to inhibit iron absorption, may improve iron absorption from, for example, meals with low iron bioavailability [7].

Mucin, an endogenously synthesized chelator, is a small protein made in both gastric and intestinal cells. Gastric mucin (sometimes called gastroferrin) is released into the gastrointestinal tract, while some mucin is also found on the surface of the mucosal cell in the intestine. Chelation of iron by mucin facilitates iron absorption. However, mucin also chelates with lower-affinity chromium and zinc, among other minerals. Mucin binds multiple ferric iron molecules at an acid pH and maintains ferric iron solubility in the alkaline pH of the small intestine. Histidine, ascorbic acid, and fructose, other chelators of iron, also are thought to donate the iron to mucin in the small intestine.

The amount of iron available for absorption can be estimated from the quantity of vitamin C and/or meat, fish, or poultry that is ingested with the nonheme iron source, assuming ~500 mg body iron stores. Seventy-five units of ascorbic acid and/or meat, fish, or poultry (MFP) factor (one unit = 1.3 g raw or 1 g cooked meat, fish, or poultry or 1 mg ascorbic acid) has been shown to maximize the effect on iron absorption when consumed with the iron source [8]. Units in excess of 75 seem to have no further benefit. The absence of enhancing factors predicts a nonheme iron absorption of only 2% to 3%, but 75 units of these factors can increase absorption of nonheme iron to 8% (some suggest up to 20% if the person is also iron deficient) [5].

Inhibitors of Iron Absorption. Many dietary factors inhibit iron absorption, including

- polyphenols such as tannin derivatives of gallic acid (in tea and coffee);
- oxalic acid (in spinach, chard, berries, chocolate, and tea, among others);
- phytates, also called phytic acid, inositol hexaphosphate, or polyphosphate (in maize, whole grains, legumes);
- EDTA (a preservative);
- phosvitin, a protein containing phosphorylated serine residues found in egg yolks; and
- nutrients such as calcium, calcium phosphate salts, zinc, manganese, and nickel.

Polyphenols are found in fairly high concentrations in both tea and coffee. These phenolic compounds when consumed with a source of iron have been shown to reduce iron absorption over 60%. Coffee consumption, with or just after a meal, may reduce iron absorption by 40% [9].

Phytates and oxalates bind, via oxygen, many minerals, including not only iron but also zinc, copper, and calcium. The phytate mineral and oxalate mineral complexes are insoluble and poorly absorbed. Fermentation of bread has been shown to reduce the phytate content and improve the absorption of some minerals, but in general mineral absorption is better without the presence of phytates or oxalates. (Fig. 12.9, in the section on zinc, shows the structures of both phytate and oxalate.)

Several nutrients, when ingested in large amounts, have been shown to reduce nonheme iron absorption.

Calcium and phosphorus are thought to interact with iron and inhibit its absorption through Fe:Ca:PO_4 chelate formation at the intestinal mucosa. Alternately, the inhibitory effect of calcium on iron absorption may be within the intestinal mucosal cells at a step in iron transport that is common for both heme and nonheme iron transport [10]. Several studies [10–13] have demonstrated that ingestion of calcium in amounts of 300 to 600 mg and in the forms of calcium phosphate, calcium citrate, calcium carbonate, and calcium chloride, when given with up to 18 mg iron as ferrous sulfate or when incorporated into food, substantially decreases iron absorption by up to 70%. Similar reductions in iron absorption have been shown with milk ingestion [12]. Thus, to maximize iron absorption from a supplement, the iron supplement should not be taken with a source of calcium.

Zinc and iron also interact and may negatively impact each other's absorption. The two minerals are thought to compete for the same common absorptive pathway, such as DCT 1, as well as to interact at another, more distal, site. Inhibition of iron absorption has been demonstrated with the coingestion of zinc, usually as zinc sulfate, in amounts greater than iron as ferrous sulfate. For example, ingestion of 15 mg and 45 mg zinc as zinc sulfate given in a water solution with 3 mg iron as ferrous sulfate significantly reduced iron absorption [14]. Zinc in a 1 : 1 and a 2.5 : 1 (27 mg zinc and 68.5 mg zinc doses) molar ratio with iron in solution inhibited nonheme iron absorption by 66% and 80%, respectively [15]. A review of studies assessing iron and zinc interactions suggests that the interactions result primarily when the two minerals are given in solution and do not occur when they are given in a meal [16]; however, a study in which flour was cofortified with equal amounts of iron and zinc as zinc sulfate significantly reduced iron absorption in children [17].

Manganese and iron also appear to interact. Manganese (as manganese chloride) when ingested in water or with a meal in a 2.5 : 1 or 5 : 1 ratio with iron (as ferrous sulfate) reduced iron absorption by 22% to 40% [14].

Nickel has been shown to interact synergistically with iron as ferric sulfate only, but not as a mixture of ferric and ferrous sulfates, to affect hematopoiesis. Nickel appears to facilitate the use of ferric iron but somehow to antagonize ferrous iron absorption, particularly in severe iron deficiency. DCT 1 transports both Fe^{2+} and Ni^{2+}. Increased nickel transport likely would result when intake of other divalent cations, especially ferrous iron, is diminished. The enhancement of Fe^{3+} absorption by nickel is not understood. There is speculation that nickel may function as a cofactor in enhancing the complexing of the Fe^{3+} with a ligand.

Other intraluminal factors inhibitory to iron absorption include rapid transit time, malabsorption syndromes, achylia (absence of digestive juices), and excess alkalinization as may occur with excessive use of antacids or with decreased gastric acidity. Overall absorption of iron from the U.S. diet is estimated at about 10% to 18%, but a person's iron status also affects iron absorption.

The regulation of absorption is closely tied to the level of the body's iron stores and may range from 10% (for a person with normal iron status) up to 35% (for persons who are iron deficient) [18]. In other words, iron absorption can rise to 3 to 6 mg daily when the body is depleted of iron and can fall to 0.5 mg or less daily when iron stores are high. Sites of iron storage and blood-forming tissues such as the liver and bone marrow are thought to release compounds that in turn affect the intestinal cells, to either increase or decrease iron absorption as needed. One proposed regulator of iron absorption is the protein hepcidin, which is thought to be released from the liver when iron stores are high. Upon release, hepcidin is thought to interact with other proteins, including HFE, β_2-microglobulin, and transferrin receptors, found on the surface of crypt cells in the small intestine. The interaction of hepcidin with these proteins, coupled with cellular uptake of iron into the crypt cells, results in absorptive brush border membrane enterocytes that express fewer brush border membrane transport proteins (DCT 1 and nramp 2) and fewer other proteins (Dcytb, ferroportin, and hepaestin, discussed later) that normally facilitate iron absorption. Thus, in times of high iron stores, iron absorption in the near future will be diminished. Conversely, when iron stores are low, the absence or low levels of hepcidin coupled with low cellular iron uptake would cause crypt cells to evolve within the next 24 to 48 hours into brush border enterocytes that express higher concentrations of transport proteins and enzymes to enhance iron absorption.

Intestinal Cell Iron Use

The preceding sections have reviewed digestion and absorption, including factors inhibiting and enhancing iron absorption into the enterocyte. Following absorption across the brush border membrane into the enterocyte, iron must be either

- transported through the enterocyte and into the blood for use by the body tissues,
- stored in the intestinal cell for future use or elimination, or
- used by the intestinal cell in a functional capacity.

We will discuss transport across the enterocyte first.

Because of the potential for free iron to initiate oxidative damage, little iron is thought to freely diffuse through or across the mucosal cell. Proteins and/or amino acids are thought to transport or ferry the iron throughout the cell. Cysteine and histidine are two examples of amino acids thought to be able to transport iron across the mucosal cell. In addition, ferric iron may be bound to another cytosolic protein, mobilferrin, which is found in two forms: monomeric mobilferrin and mobilferrin that is part of a paraferritin complex. Mobilferrin (both forms) appears to interact with integrin, located in the enterocyte membrane, and binds minerals, especially iron but also calcium, zinc, and copper. Specifically, mobilferrin is capable of binding one iron molecule, which it then shuttles across the cytosol of the mucosal cell. Also present with mobilferrin in the paraferritin complex is an intracellular flavin, NADPH-dependent ferrireductase, that reduces ferric iron to its ferrous state (this ferrireductase is called paraferritin in some literature). Other flavins ($FAD/FADH_2$ or NAD/NADH), along with vitamin C, also may be able to reduce the ferric iron within the cytosol.

Iron not being transported across the cell for release into the blood may be incorporated into apoferritin in the intestinal cell for short-term storage. Apoferritin is a protein that acts as a shell for iron storage. This protein's shell further serves as a ferroxidase, using oxygen to convert the ferrous iron to the ferric state for deposition and storage. The stored ferric iron can be reduced back to the ferrous state and released from the ferritin molecule should iron be needed later by the mucosal or other nonintestinal cells. If not needed, the iron remains as ferritin and is excreted when the short-lived (2–3 days) mucosal cells are sloughed off into the lumen of the gastrointestinal tract. Ferritin synthesis in the intestine is directly affected by iron, with increased synthesis associated with high iron stores and decreased synthesis associated with low iron stores. Ferritin is discussed in further detail in the section on iron storage.

Iron moving through the mucosal cell may be used by the cell for a variety of functions, especially as a cofactor for enzymes (see p. 429). Iron that is not needed within the enterocyte may be released into the blood following transport across the basolateral membrane.

Iron transport across the intestinal-cell basolateral membrane is thought to involve binding to another membrane transport protein called ferroportin (Fp), also known as Ireg 1 or MTP 1. Transport of ferrous iron across the basolateral membrane is coupled with its oxidation to Fe^{3+} by a copper-containing protein called hephaestin. The oxidation of iron to the ferric state is essential for the transport of iron in the blood.

$$Fe^{2+} \longrightarrow Fe^{3+} \text{ (which can now bind to transferrin)}$$
$$\text{Hephaestin-}Cu^{2+} \curvearrowright \text{Hephaestin-}Cu^{1+}$$

Transport

Iron in its oxidized ferric state is transported in the blood attached to the protein transferrin. We will review iron oxidation, transferrin's role in iron transport, and the importance of protein in iron binding in the body.

As mentioned in the previous section, iron must first be oxidized before it can bind to transferrin for transport in the blood. Hephaestin found in the intestinal cells and ceruloplasmin found throughout the body are both copper-containing proteins with ferroxidase activity. These proteins catalyze the oxidation of ferrous iron to its ferric form so it can bind tightly to transferrin in the plasma. The role of copper as part of hephaestin and ceruloplasmin is crucial to iron metabolism. Copper deficiency results in accumulation of iron in sites such as the intestine and liver and a reduction in iron transport to tissues. The role of ceruloplasmin in the oxidation of iron may be depicted as follows:

$$Fe^{2+} \longrightarrow Fe^{3+} \text{ (which can now bind to transferrin)}$$
$$\text{Ceruloplasmin-}Cu^{2+} \curvearrowright \text{Ceruloplasmin-}Cu^{1+}$$

Transferrin, a glycoprotein made primarily in the liver, has two binding sites for minerals. The binding site near the C-terminal end of transferrin has a high affinity for ferric iron. The binding site near the N-terminal end also has a high affinity for ferric iron but will also bind other minerals, such as chromium, followed in descending order by copper > manganese > cadmium > zinc and nickel. Tight binding of ferric iron to transferrin also requires the presence of an anion, usually bicarbonate, at each binding site. Transferrin in the plasma is typically about one-third saturated with ferric iron. If all binding sites of the transferrin were occupied, then the transferrin would be fully (100%) saturated.

The role of proteins in the transport as well as storage of iron is important because of iron's redox activity. The binding of iron by proteins serves as a defense mechanism. Left unbound, the iron's redox activity can lead to the generation of harmful free radicals. Free ferrous iron (Fe^{2+}), for example, readily reacts with hydrogen peroxide (H_2O_2) in a reaction known as the Fenton reaction:

$$Fe^{2+} + H_2O_2 \longrightarrow Fe^{3+} + OH^- + {}^{\bullet}OH$$

This reaction generates a hydroxyl anion and a free hydroxyl radical (${}^{\bullet}OH$), which is extremely reactive and damaging to cells (see the perspective in Chap. 10). In addition, the binding of iron by protein is important to ensure that bacteria that may be present in the body, as with an infection, are unable to utilize the iron for their own (bacterial) growth. Free iron—but not protein-bound iron—is readily used by bacteria for proliferation and growth. Multiplication of bacteria requires acquisition of nutrients such as iron from the host. Thus, keeping iron attached to proteins in the body prevents bacterial acquisition of the iron. Transferrin not only binds and transports newly absorbed dietary iron that has been transported across the basolateral membrane of the mucosal cell but also transports iron that has been released following the degradation of iron-containing compounds in the body. In fact, most of the iron entering the plasma for distribution by transferrin is contributed from hemoglobin destruction and release from storage. Thus, transferrin ferries iron throughout the body, delivering both new and recycled iron to tissues either for use or for storage. Transferrin has a half-life of about 7 to 10 days.

Storage

Iron not needed in a functional capacity is stored in three principal sites: the liver, bone marrow, and spleen. Transferrin delivers iron to these sites, especially the liver parenchyma, which is thought to store about 60% of iron. The remaining 40% is found in reticuloendothelial (RE) cells within the liver, spleen, and bone marrow (and possibly between muscle fibers). Most of the iron stored in reticuloendothelial cells is derived from phagocytosis of red blood cells and subsequent degradation of the erythrocyte hemoglobin.

Ferritin is the primary storage form of iron in cells. Ferritin is synthesized in a variety of tissues, especially within the liver, spleen, bone marrow, and intestine, and consists of apoferritin in which iron molecules have been deposited. Apoferritin, which is shaped like a hollow sphere, is composed of 24 protein subunits. Ferritin's subunits are classified based on molecular mass as H or L, and the proportions of H and L subunits within ferritin vary between tissues. The L form, for example, predominates in the liver and spleen. Iron enters apoferritin through channels or pores. The pores serve as the site of the oxidation of ferrous iron into ferric oxyhydroxide crystals ($4\ Fe^{2+} + O_2 + 6\ H_2O \longrightarrow 4\ FeOOH + 8\ H^+$) or ferrihydrite ($5\ Fe_2O_3 \cdot 9\ H_2O$), and molecular oxygen functions as the electron acceptor. Ferric oxyhydroxide or ferrihydrite is deposited in the interior of the protein shell (Fig. 12.3). As many as 4,500 iron atoms can be stored in ferritin.

Ferritin is not a stable compound but rather is constantly being degraded and resynthesized, providing an

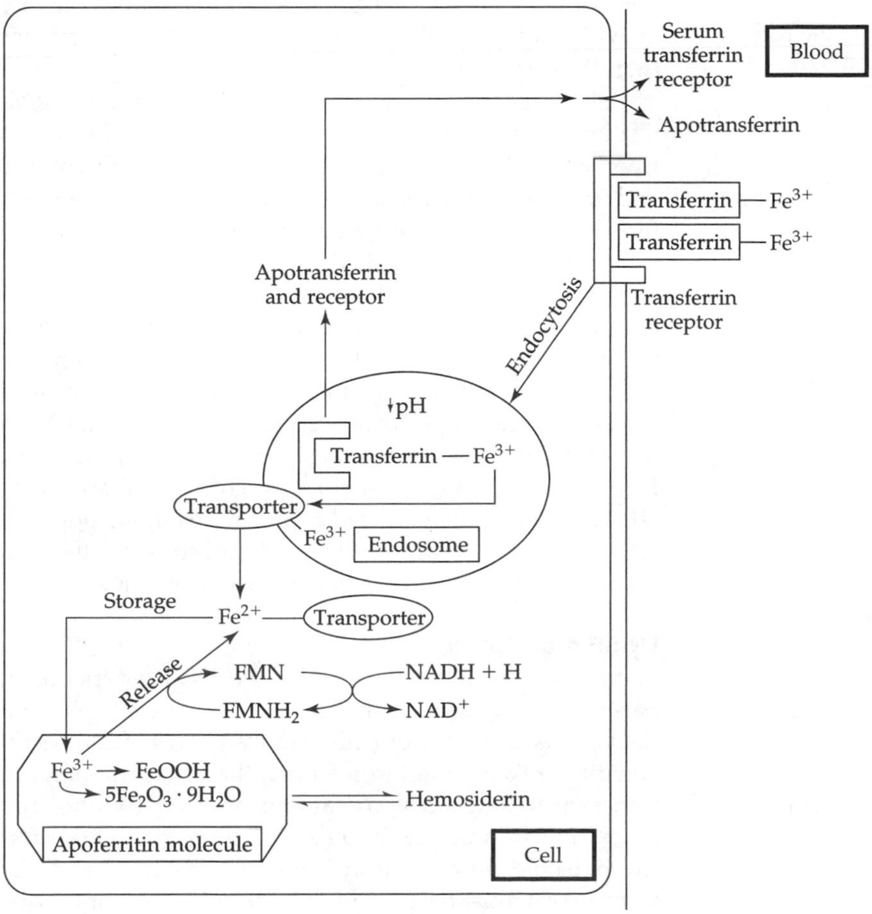

Figure 12.3 Overview of iron uptake, metabolism and storage.

available intracellular iron pool. Cellular iron is thought to influence in part the synthesis of apoferritin at the translation level (Fig. 12.4). Specifically, an iron regulatory/response element binding protein (IRE-BP) responds to the cell's iron status. This IRE-BP's ability to respond depends on the cell's iron status. With lots of iron, the IRE-BP exists as a 4Fe-4S cluster and exhibits aconitase activity. In contrast, with less iron, the IRE-BP exists as a 3Fe-4S cluster and functions as a binding protein. As a binding protein, the IRE-BP binds to iron response elements (IREs) located in the 5′ untranslated region of ferritin mRNA. IREs are stem loop structures of about 30 nucleotides found in the mRNA. In low-iron situations, the IRE-BP acts as a binding protein and binds to the IRE in ferritin mRNA, and this binding of IRE-BP to the ferritin mRNA acts as a repressor to inhibit the translation of the ferritin protein. Thus, less ferritin protein is made in cells when cellular iron content is low. From a physiological standpoint this makes sense, because ferritin functions to store iron and not much ferritin would be needed if the cell's iron content was low. Under the opposite conditions, in which the cell has a relatively high iron content, the IRE-BP (containing a 4Fe-4S cluster) exhibits aconitase activity. Without the binding of the IRE-BP (4Fe-4S), the ferritin mRNA undergoes translation. Thus, more ferritin protein is made in cells when cellular iron concentrations are high.

Figure 12.4 The influence of intracellular iron on the translation of ferritin mRNA and transferrin receptor mRNA.

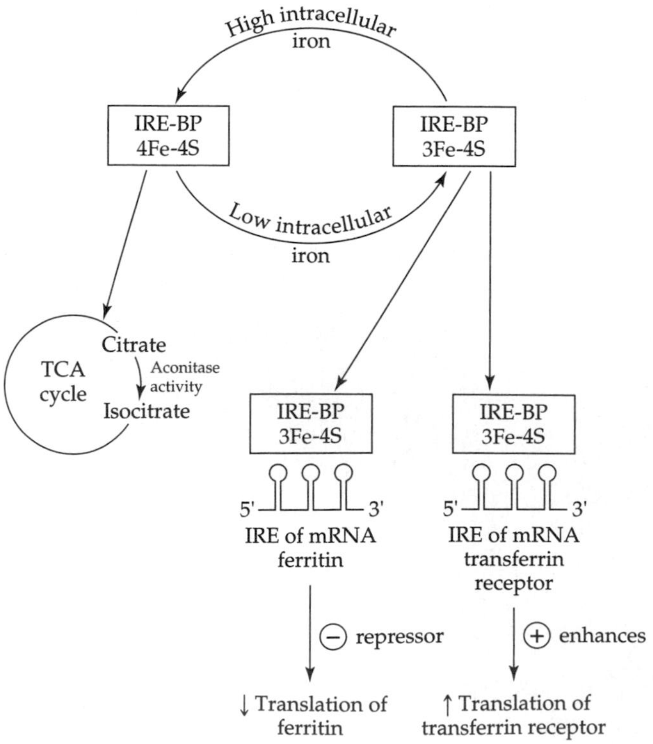

Abbreviations:
IRE = iron response element
IRE-BP = IRE binding proteins

Equilibration occurs between tissue ferritin and serum ferritin. Thus, serum ferritin is used as an index of body iron stores: 1 ng ferritin/mL serum equals ~10 mg body iron stores. Normal serum ferritin concentrations (for adults) exceed ~12 ng/mL; however, because ferritin acts as an acute phase reactant protein, it is not a reliable indicator of iron stores during and possibly for several weeks following inflammation or illness. In other words, serum ferritin concentrations may be elevated or within the normal range in the blood despite an individual's having little to no iron. Assessment of iron status is discussed further on page 434.

Hemosiderin is another iron storage protein. Hemosiderin is thought to be a degradation product of ferritin, representing, for example, aggregated ferritin or a deposit of degraded apoferritin and coalesced iron atoms. The content of iron in hemosiderin may be as high as 50%. The ratio of ferritin to hemosiderin in the liver varies according to the level of iron stored in the organ, with ferritin predominating at lower iron concentrations and hemosiderin predominating at higher concentrations (iron overload) [19]. Although iron in hemosiderin can be labilized to supply free iron, the rate at which iron is released from hemosiderin is slower than that from ferritin.

Release of iron from stores (Fig. 12.3) requires mobilization of Fe^{3+} and the use of reducing substances such as riboflavin ($FMNH_2$), niacin (NADH), and/or vitamin C and/or possibly a chelator to enable diffusion through ferritin pores. However, following the reduction of iron to release it from storage, Fe^{2+} is transported to the cell surface, where it must be reoxidized to allow transport out of the cell. This reoxidation of iron to enable binding to transferrin for transport to tissues requires ceruloplasmin, as previously described in the section on iron transport. The superoxide radical ($O_2^{\cdot}$) also has been found to initiate iron release from ferritin in vitro. However, only one or two iron molecules from ferritin are released even with extended exposure to superoxide radicals. The size and age of ferritin's iron core, not the iron content of ferritin's protein shell, affect iron release [20].

Uptake by Tissues

The amount of iron taken up by the tissues depends in part on the transferrin saturation level. For example, iron delivery is greater from diferric transferrin (transferrin containing two bound iron atoms) than from monoferric transferrin (transferrin containing only one bound iron atom). For iron uptake into tissues to occur, the transferrin molecule bound to iron (either diferric or monoferric transferrin) must first bind to transferrin receptors (TfRs) on cells (Fig. 12.3). Liver cells and crypt cells in the intestine appear to contain an isoform of the transferrin receptor, referred to as TfR2, which binds diferric transferrin. Transferrin receptors are found on almost all cell surfaces and consist of two subunits that each bind one transferrin molecule. Once the transferrin molecule is bound to the receptor, the complex is thought to be internalized by endocytosis and to form a vesicle (also called an endosome) in the cytoplasm of the cell. Next, in an ATP-dependent process, protons are pumped into the endosome and reduce the pH to about 5.5. In the presence of the acidic pH and possibly other factors, iron molecules are released from the transferrin molecule. The apotransferrin is then thought to return to the cell surface and plasma. Use of the released iron requires its transport across the endosomal membrane. DCT 1 or nramp 2 (transporters that are also found on the brush border membrane of the intestinal cells), along with a protein called stimulator of iron transport (SFT), is thought to transport the iron across the endosomal membrane.

The number of transferrin receptors on cells increases or decreases depending on intracellular iron concentrations. In other words, intracellular iron affects the genetic expression of transferrin receptors on the cell, as shown in Figure 12.4. As with ferritin mRNA, mRNA for the transferrin receptor contains (five) IREs in the 3′ untranslated region. Remember that IREs are stem loop structures of about 30 nucleotides found in the mRNA. Within the cytoplasm, again as with ferritin, IRE binding proteins (IRE-BPs), with multiple iron-sulfur clusters, respond to the cell's iron status. In a low-cellular-iron situation, the IRE-BP contains a 3Fe-4S cluster and readily binds to the IRE, thereby stabilizing the transferrin receptor mRNA. The stabilized transferrin receptor mRNA exhibits a longer half-life, and consequently more transferrin receptor mRNA is translated into transferrin receptor proteins. Once made, these transferrin receptor proteins become embedded in the cell's plasma membrane to promote cellular iron uptake. Thus, in conditions of low cellular iron, transferrin receptor synthesis is increased.

In the situation of relatively high intracellular iron, fewer transferrin receptors will be translated due to the following sequence of events. With adequate or high cellular iron, the IRE-BP exists as a 4Fe-4S cluster and exhibits aconitase activity and thus does not act as a binding protein for the IRE of the transferrin receptor mRNA. Without the IRE-BP bound to the IRE of transferrin receptor mRNA, the mRNA is not as stable and is more quickly degraded. This decreased stability and increased degradation in turn diminish the translation of the mRNA and result in the production of fewer transferrin receptor proteins. The synthesis of fewer transferrin receptor proteins means that fewer receptors will be available on the cell surface and less iron will be brought into the cell. Thus, the level of transferrin receptor expression is indicative of the cell's need for iron uptake.

Functions and Mechanisms of Action

Iron functions in the body as part of several proteins. In many body proteins, iron is present as part of heme. In other proteins, iron is found in a cluster with sulfur (2Fe-2S, 4Fe-4S, or 3Fe-4S), by itself as a single atom, or as part of a bridge with oxygen (Fe—O—Fe). Heme proteins represent the largest group and include hemoglobin, myoglobin, cytochromes involved in electron transport, and enzymes such as monooxygenases, dioxygenases, and oxidases. Iron sulfur proteins also include several enzymes involved in electron transport, as well as a few nonredox enzymes such as aconitase and ferrochelatase. Proteins that contain single iron atoms are mostly mono- and dioxygenase enzymes, and the one iron oxygen bridge protein also is an enzyme, ribonucleotide reductase.

Hemoglobin and Myoglobin

The essentiality of iron is due in part to its presence in heme, which functions as a prosthetic group for some proteins. The atom of iron in the center of the heme molecule allows the transport of oxygen to tissues (hemoglobin); the transitional storage of oxygen in tissues, particularly muscle (myoglobin); and the transport of electrons through the respiratory chain (cytochromes).

Hemoglobin is synthesized in red blood cells and carries about 98.5% of the total oxygen found in the blood. Hemoglobin consists of a globin portion, which is made up of four polypeptides, and four heme groups. Each polypeptide chain is associated with one of the heme molecules. Heme is an iron-containing derivative of porphyrin. Porphyrins, in turn, are cyclic compounds made up of four pyrrole rings joined together by methenyl bridges (—CH—). Nitrogen atoms in each of the four pyrrole rings bind to the iron atom (Fig. 12.5), and these bonds hold the iron atom in the plane of the porphyrin ring. The iron atom in the center of the heme has two remaining coordinate bonds available for binding. One is with an amino acid (often the nitrogen atom of histidine) of the protein to which the heme is attached. For example, in hemoglobin, the iron in the heme binds to the nitrogen of an amino acid in the protein globin; heme is found in a hydrophobic pocket of the protein. The sixth and last coordinate bond in heme proteins that bind oxygen—namely, hemoglobin and myoglobin—exists between the iron and oxygen. The oxygen is held quite loosely so that transfer to tissues can be rapid. In heme proteins that do not bind oxygen, the sixth coordinate bond is with atoms of

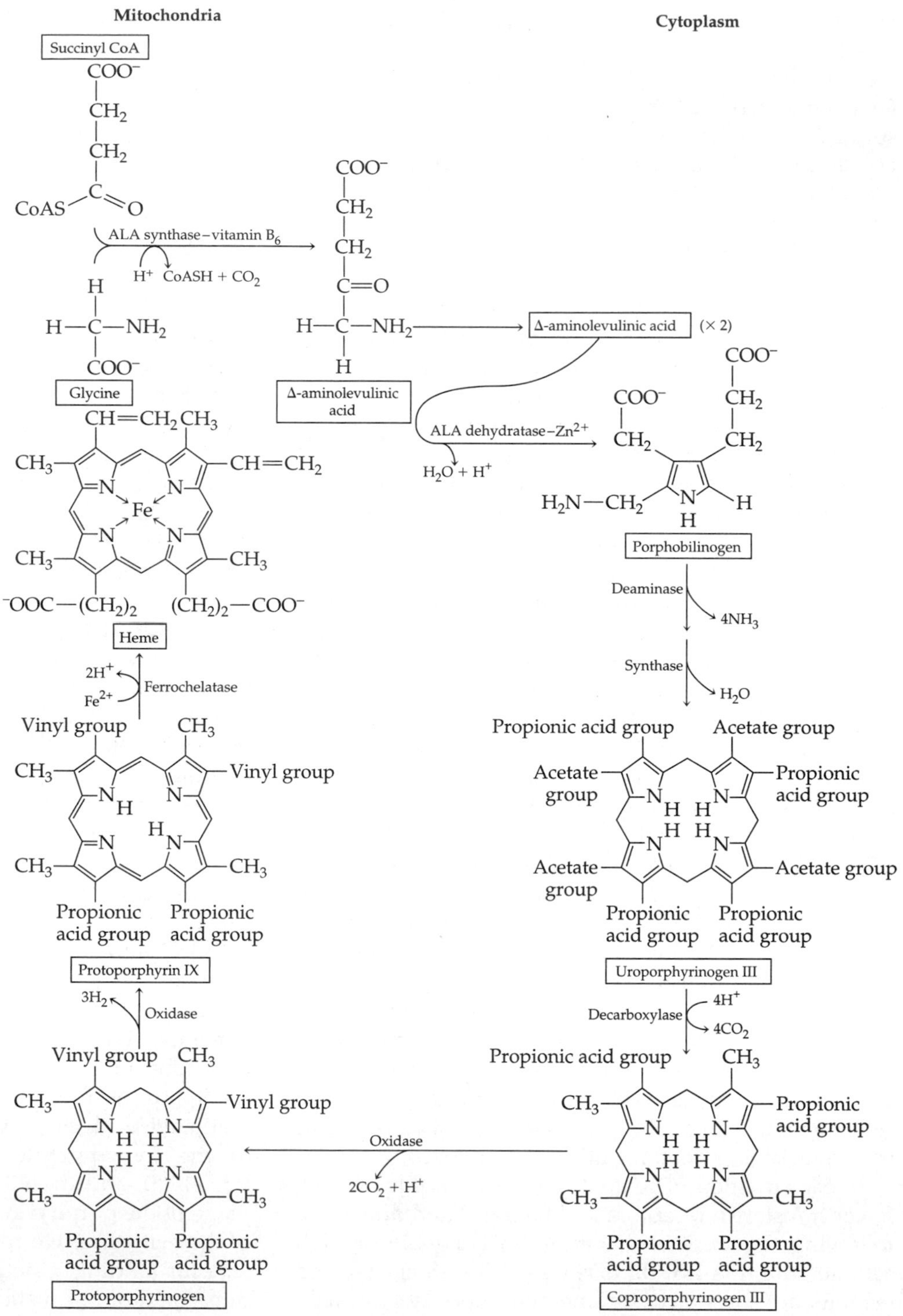

Figure 12.5 Heme biosynthesis. Vinyl group: $CH{=}CH_2$; propionic acid group: $(CH_2)_2COO^-$; acetate group: CH_2COO^-.

amino acid groups in the protein (such as an enzyme) with which the heme group is associated.

Heme synthesis and the attachment of globin occur primarily in the red blood cells of bone marrow. Heme synthesis accounts for the largest utilization of functional iron in the body. In fact, each red blood cell is thought to contain millions of hemoglobin molecules, and all the red blood cells in the body together contain about two-thirds of total body iron. Erythropoietic cells in bone marrow possess transferrin receptors on their cell surface. Transferrin delivers the iron for heme synthesis to the erythropoietic cells in the bone marrow. The synthesis of heme (Fig. 12.5) occurs as follows:

- Heme synthesis begins in the mitochondria, where glycine and succinyl CoA combine to form Δ-aminolevulinic acid (ALA). The reaction is catalyzed by Δ-aminolevulinic acid synthase, a vitamin B_6–dependent enzyme that is inhibited by the final end product (heme) and whose synthesis is also thought to be regulated by iron.
- Next, ALA enters the cytoplasm, where a zinc-dependent dehydratase catalyzes the condensation of two ALA molecules to form porphobilinogen. This enzyme is sensitive to lead, which binds to its sulfhydryl groups to inactivate the enzyme.
- Next, in a series of cytosolic reactions involving a deaminase, a synthase, and a decarboxylase, four porphobilinogens condense to form a tetrapyrrole that cyclizes. Side chains are modified, and coproporphyrinogen III is formed and enters the mitochondria.
- Coproporphyrinogen is converted in the mitochondria to protoporphyrinogen.
- Protoporphyrinogen is oxidized to form protoporphyrin IX.
- Last, an iron (Fe^{2+}) atom is inserted into protoporphyrin IX to yield heme. The insertion of iron into the heme is catalyzed by ferrochelatase, a 2Fe-2S cluster protein. The transcription of the ferrochelatase enzyme appears to be regulated by iron.

Unlike hemoglobin, which is a tetrameric protein, myoglobin consists of a single hemoprotein chain. Myoglobin, which is found in the cytoplasm of the muscle cells, facilitates the diffusion rate of dioxygen from capillary red blood cells to the cytoplasm and mitochondria of muscle cells.

Cytochromes and Other Enzymes Involved in Electron Transport

Heme-containing cytochromes in the electron transport chain (Fig. 3.16), such as cytochromes b and c, pass along single electrons. The transfer of electrons along the chain is made possible by the change in the oxidation state of iron. In the reduced cytochromes, the iron atom is in the ferrous state. The iron atom of the reduced cytochrome becomes oxidized to the ferric state when a single electron is transferred to the next cytochrome. The iron atom of the cytochrome receiving the electron then becomes reduced. Other heme iron-containing cytochromes include cytochrome b_5 (involved in lipid metabolism) and the cytochrome P_{450} family (heme enzymes found in the endoplasmic reticulum membrane and involved in drug metabolism and steroid hormone synthesis).

Nonheme iron sulfur enzymes involved in electron transport include NADH dehydrogenase, succinate dehydrogenase, and ubiquinone–cytochrome c reductase. Whether iron is carrying oxygen or transporting electrons, its essentiality in energy transformation is without question.

Monooxygenases and Dioxygenases

Body enzymes involved in a variety of processes besides the respiratory chain also require iron. Many monooxygenases, for example, contain iron. Monooxygenases function to insert one of two oxygen molecules into a substrate. Examples of single iron–containing monooxygenases include

- phenylalanine monooxygenase,
- tyrosine monooxygenase, and
- tryptophan monooxygenase.

These enzymes insert an oxygen molecule into the aromatic amino acids phenylalanine, tyrosine, and tryptophan, respectively. Monooxygenases may be further classified based on the cosubstrate that participates in the reaction. The cosubstrate functions to furnish the hydrogen atoms that reduce the second oxygen molecule to water. Phenylalanine monooxygenase, tyrosine monooxygenase, and tryptophan monooxygenase all use tetrahydrobiopterin as a cosubstrate, and during the reactions tetrahydrobiopterin is oxidized to dihydrobiopterin. The reaction catalyzed by phenylalanine monooxygenase (also called phenylalanine hydroxylase because the main substrate, phenylalanine, becomes hydroxylated) is shown in Figure 9.6 (p. 267). This enzyme converts phenylalanine to tyrosine; vitamin C is also involved in this reaction to reduce iron.

Many dioxygenases also contain iron. Dioxygenases catalyze the insertion of two oxygen atoms into a substrate. There are many important iron-requiring dioxygenases in the body, including

- tryptophan dioxygenase (amino acid metabolism),
- homogentisate dioxygenase (amino acid metabolism),
- trimethyl lysine dioxygenase and 4-butyrobetaine dioxygenase (carnitine synthesis),
- lysine dioxygenase and proline dioxygenase (procollagen synthesis),
- nitric oxide synthase, and
- β-carotene dioxygenase (vitamin A synthesis).

Some of these reactions are discussed hereafter. For example, tryptophan dioxygenase (a heme-containing enzyme, also called a pyrrolase) converts the amino acid tryptophan to N-formylkynurenine (Fig. 9.18, p. 287), representing the first step of tryptophan metabolism. Iron deficiency has been shown to reduce the efficacy of tryptophan as a precursor of niacin [21]. In humans, 60 mg tryptophan can be converted to 1 mg niacin. Homogentisate dioxygenase is also involved in amino acid metabolism, specifically that of tyrosine. During tyrosine metabolism, tyrosine is transaminated to produce hydroxyphenylpyruvate, which is then converted to homogentisate. Homogentisate in turn is converted to 4-maleylacetoacetate by homogentisate dioxygenase, a single iron–dependent enzyme (Fig. 9.6).

Two of the four steps required for carnitine synthesis involve iron-dependent dioxygenases. Recall that carnitine is an important nitrogen-containing compound necessary for the transport of long-chain fatty acids into the mitochondria for oxidation. The first step in carnitine synthesis (Fig. 9.5), in which trimethyl lysine is converted to 3-OH trimethyl lysine, requires a single iron–containing trimethyl lysine dioxygenase, and the final step, in which 4-butyrobetaine is converted to carnitine, requires 4-butyrobetaine dioxygenase, another single iron–containing enzyme. α-ketoglutarate is a required cosubstrate in both of these reactions, and during the reactions the keto acid becomes oxidatively decarboxylated to succinate. Vitamin C also participates in the reactions as a reducing agent.

Hydroxylation rections for procollagen synthesis are shown in Figure 9.4. Both lysine and proline dioxygenases contain single iron atoms. As described in the steps for carnitine synthesis, α-ketoglutarate is a required cosubstrate, and vitamin C serves as a reducing agent.

Two isoforms of nitric oxide synthase, a dioxygenase needed for the synthesis of nitric oxide (a potent biological effector molecule), require heme iron.

Peroxidases

Other important reactions required to protect the body also use iron-containing enzymes, such as catalase and myeloperoxidase.

- Catalase, with four heme groups, converts hydrogen peroxide to water and molecular oxygen: $2H_2O_2 \longrightarrow 2H_2O + O_2$. Catalase helps prevent cellular damage induced by hydrogen peroxide (see the perspective in Chap. 10).

- Myeloperoxidase (also called chloroperoxidase), another heme-containing enzyme, is found in the plasma as well as in granules within neutrophils (white blood cells). During phagocytosis of bacteria, myeloperoxidase is released into the phagocytic vesicle within the neutrophil. The phagocytic vesicle contains a variety of compounds, including hydrogen peroxide (H_2O_2), free hydroxyl radicals ($^{\cdot}OH$), and other ions such as chloride (Cl^-). Myeloperoxidase catalyzes the following reaction:

$$H_2O_2 + Cl^- \longrightarrow H_2O + {}^-OCl$$

The ^-OCl (hypochlorite) formed in the reaction is a strong cytotoxic oxidant that is important for the destruction of foreign substances such as bacteria. Activity of myeloperoxidase may be impaired with iron deficiency, resulting in increased susceptibility to or severity of infection.

Peroxidases also are important in the production of thyroid hormones.

- Thyroperoxidase, a heme-dependent enzyme, is necessary for organification of iodide (the addition of $2I^-$ to thyroglobulin-tyrosine) and conjugation of iodinated tyrosine residues on thyroglobulin (see p. 469). These reactions are necessary for the synthesis of the thyroid hormones T_3 and T_4.

Oxidoreductases

Some oxidoreductases that are iron-dependent include

- aldehyde oxidase, which uses oxygen to convert aldehydes (RCOH) to alcohols (RCOOH);
- sulfite oxidase, an iron sulfur-containing enzyme that converts sulfite (SO_3) to sulfate (SO_4); and
- xanthine oxidase and dehydrogenase, both iron-sulfur cluster and molybdenum-containing enzymes that convert hypoxanthine generated from purine catabolism to xanthine and then convert xanthine to uric acid for excretion (see Fig. 12.25). Remember that purine bases are found in DNA.

Other Iron-Containing Proteins

Another iron-dependent enzyme involved in DNA synthesis and thus cell replication is ribonucleotide reductase, which converts adenosine diphosphate (ADP) into deoxy ADP (dADP). This enzyme contains iron as part of a bridge with oxygen ($Fe^{3+}—O^{2-}—Fe^{3+}$).

In glycolysis, glycerol phosphate dehydrogenase, a flavoprotein, has a nonheme iron component. Phosphoenolpyruvate carboxykinase, important in gluconeogenesis, also requires iron for its functioning. In the Krebs cycle, aconitase, which converts citrate to isocitrate in the mitochondria of the cell, contains a 4Fe-4S cluster. Aconitase also functions in the cytosol of the cell as an iron regulatory protein to affect translation of iron transport and storage proteins; as an iron regulatory protein, aconitase contains a 3Fe-4S cluster. The role of iron regulatory proteins in the translation of ferritin and transferrin receptors is discussed on pages 426 and 427.

Iron as a Pro-oxidant

As a pro-oxidant, free ferrous iron may catalyze the nonenzymatic Fenton reaction

$$Fe^{2+} + H_2O_2 \longrightarrow Fe^{3+} + OH^- + {}^{\cdot}OH$$

In this reaction, ferrous iron reacts with hydrogen peroxide to generate ferric iron and free radicals. In a reaction known as the Haber Weiss reaction, the superoxide radical, O_2^-, may react with another hydrogen peroxide molecule to generate molecular oxygen and free hydroxyl radicals such as $^{\cdot}OH$, a dangerous membrane oxidant.

$$O_2^- + H_2O_2 \longrightarrow O_2 + {}^{\cdot}OH + OH^-$$

Interactions with Other Nutrients

The interactions of iron with ascorbic acid in enhancing iron absorption and maintaining iron in the appropriate valence state for enzyme function have been discussed previously (pp. 422 and 429). The potential also may exist for vitamin C–induced release of ferric iron from ferritin, with subsequent reduction of iron to the ferrous form [22]. Whether such reactions result in Fenton reactions and occur in vivo is unclear.

An interrelationship also exists between iron and copper because of the role of the copper-containing ceruloplasmin as a ferroxidase. In the 1920s, studies revealed that iron therapy was unable to cure anemia in rats; however, ashed foodstuffs containing copper replenished blood hemoglobin concentrations [23]. Without the copper-dependent ferroxidase activity, iron cannot be mobilized from ferritin stores.

Another nutrient with which iron appears to interact is zinc. Ingestion of both nutrients as a 25 : 1 molar ratio of nonheme iron (ferrous sulfate) to zinc diminished the absorption of zinc from water to 34% in humans; however, when the same ratio of iron to zinc was given with a meal, no inhibitory effects were demonstrated [24]. Ratios of nonheme iron to zinc of 2 : 1 and 3 : 1 also have been shown to inhibit zinc absorption, while similar ratios of heme iron to zinc had no effect on zinc absorption [25]. Thus, excessive intake of nonheme iron, as may occur with supplements, may have a detrimental effect on zinc absorption.

Another association is that between vitamin A and iron. Reduced vitamin A status alters iron distribution among tissues. Low plasma retinol concentrations are associated with decreased plasma iron and blood hemoglobin and hematocrit as well as increased hepatic iron accumulation in rats [26].

Iron and lead also interact. Lead inhibits the activity of Δ-aminolevulinic acid dehydratase, a zinc-dependent enzyme required in heme synthesis. Lead also inhibits the activity of ferrochelatase, the enzyme that incorporates iron into heme. In addition, increased absorption of lead occurs with iron deficiency in animals and could be problematic for children, who are often iron-deficient and may have increased exposure to lead [27]. The mechanism by which iron deficiency improves lead absorption is unknown, but it may involve uptake through common divalent metal/cation transporters.

Iron deficiency is associated with decreased selenium concentrations as well as with glutathione peroxidase synthesis and activity [28–30]. Glutathione peroxidase, a selenium-requiring enzyme, catalyzes the reduction of hydrogen peroxide with the use of glutathione (GSH) as follows:

$$2\,GSH + H_2O_2 \xrightarrow{\text{Glutathione peroxidase}} GSSG + 2\,H_2O$$

(See also p. 458.) In addition, the enzyme converts organic peroxides (ROOH) to their hydroxy (or alcohol) form.

$$2\,GSH + ROOH \xrightarrow{\text{Glutathione peroxidase}} GSSG + ROH + H_2O$$

The mechanism behind the interaction between iron and selenium is not known. Iron is thought to be involved in the pretranslational regulation of the glutathione peroxidase synthesis. Alternately, iron deficiency may affect selenium absorption or increase selenium use in the body.

Turnover

While dietary iron is important in maintaining the long-term adequacy of body iron, the amount of iron absorbed (about 0.06% of the total body iron content) cannot meet the daily iron needs of the body. Rather, the avid conservation and constant recycling of body iron ensure its adequacy.

Most of the iron entering the plasma for distribution or redistribution by transferrin is contributed by sites of hemoglobin destruction and sites of ferritin and hemosiderin degradation (Fig. 12.6). Hemoglobin is degraded primarily by phagocytes of the reticuloendothelial system (found in the liver, spleen, and bone marrow). Stored iron as ferritin and hemosiderin is degraded primarily in the liver, spleen, and bone marrow. We will briefly review hemoglobin degradation. Ferritin degradation was discussed under the earlier section on iron storage.

Most old (senescent) red blood cells, which live for about 120 days, are taken up by macrophages in the spleen and degraded (phagocytosed); however, reticuloendothelial cell macrophages in bone marrow and Kupffer cells in the liver also may degrade the red blood cells. During red blood cell degradation, the heme portion of the hemoglobin molecule in the red blood cell is catabolized by heme oxygenase to biliverdin and subsequently to bilirubin, which is then secreted into the bile for excretion from the body. With the degradation of heme, ~20 to 25 mg iron per day is released from hemoglobin catabolism. This iron may be reused, for example, for erythropoiesis or for incorporation into iron-dependent enzymes, or the iron may be deposited for storage.

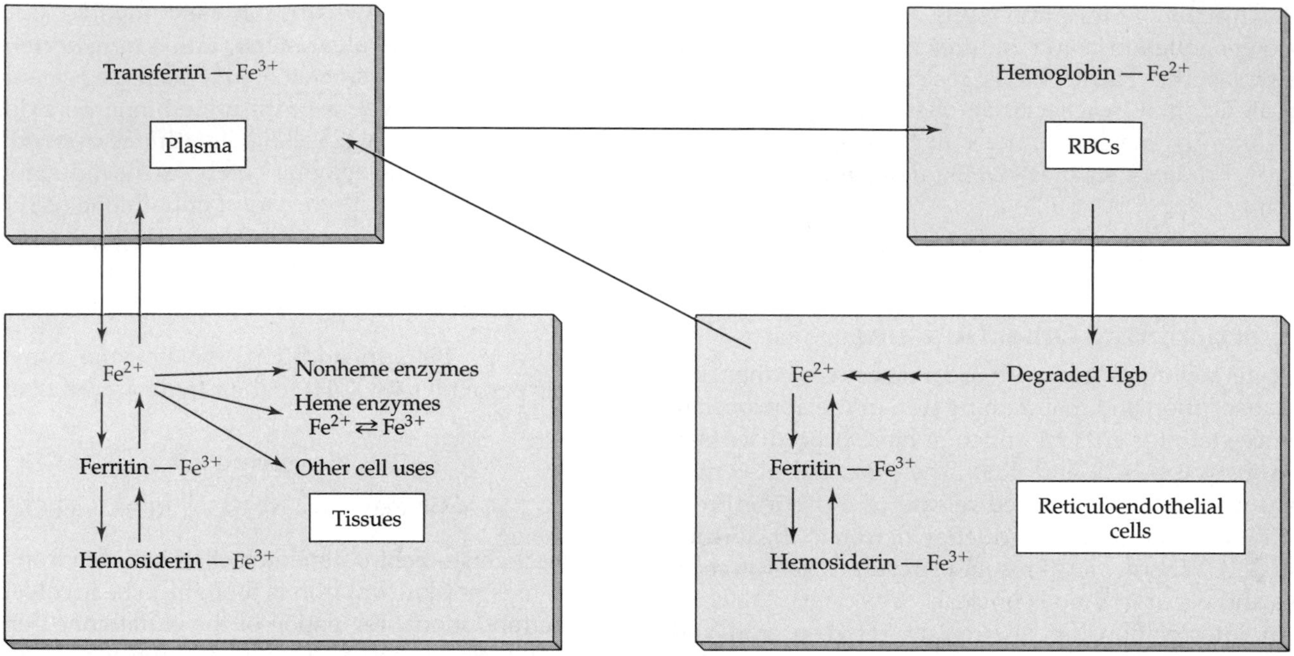

Figure 12.6 Internal iron exchange.

Although the majority of red blood cells are degraded in the reticuloendothelial system, some (up to ~10%) red blood cell lysis occurs within the blood. Two proteins, haptoglobin and hemopexin, function to remove the released hemoglobin and any free heme, respectively, from the blood. Haptoglobin, synthesized by the liver, forms complexes with free hemoglobin, while hemopexin, also synthesized in the liver, forms a complex with free heme in the blood. The proteins then deliver the iron-containing compounds to the liver, where further degradation occurs to enable reuse of the iron. With significant hemolysis, the quantity of iron passing through the plasma can expand to six to eight times normal. In contrast, should erythropoiesis decline dramatically, as occurs on descent from high altitudes, the quantity of iron in the plasma pool may decrease to as little as one-third of normal. Figure 12.6 represents schematically the internal iron exchange in the body.

Excretion

Daily iron losses by an adult male are ~0.9 to 1.0 mg/day (12–14 mg/kg/day), while basal iron losses for women (postmenopausal) are a bit lower, ~0.7 to 0.9 mg/day, because of women's smaller surface area. Losses of iron occur from three main sites:

- the gastrointestinal tract,
- skin, and
- the kidney.

Of these sites, most (0.6 mg) iron losses are via the gastrointestinal tract. Of the 0.6 mg, about 0.45 mg is due to minute (~1 mL) blood loss (which occurs even in healthy people), and another 0.15 mg is due to losses in bile and desquamated mucosal cells. The skin losses of ~0.2 to 0.3 mg iron are due to desquamation of surface cells from the skin. Finally, a very small amount, about 0.08 mg, is lost in the urine. Losses of iron, however, may increase in people with gastrointestinal ulcers or intestinal parasites, or with hemorrhage induced by surgery or due to injury.

Total iron losses of premenopausal women are estimated to be ~1.3 to 1.4 mg/day because of iron loss in menses. The average loss of blood during a menstrual cycle is ~35 mL, with an upper limit of ~80 mL. The iron content of blood is ~0.5 mg/100 mL of blood, which translates into a loss of nearly 17.5 mg iron per period. Averaged out over a month, iron loss in menses is ~0.5 mg/day; in some women, however, iron loss due to menses alone may exceed 1.4 mg/day. Balancing iron losses from the body with iron absorption is very important to health. Iron deficiency remains one of the most common nutritional deficiencies worldwide.

Recommended Dietary Allowances

The requirement and RDA for iron for adult men age 19 to over 70 years are 6 mg/day and 8 mg/day, respectively; for postmenopausal women, the requirement and RDA for iron are 5 mg/day and 8 mg/day, respectively [31]. Due to higher losses associated with menses, premenopausal women require 8.1 mg iron/day, and recommended intakes are 18 mg/day [31]. During pregnancy, though no menstrual losses occur, iron needs for the fetus and for expansion of blood volume and/or for tissue and storage are considered to be such that the RDA for iron is 27 mg/day; the RDA is 9 mg/day during lactation [31]. The inside cover of the book provides additional RDAs for iron for other age groups.

Deficiency: Iron Deficiency with and without Anemia

Iron intake is frequently inadequate in four population groups:

- infants and young children (6 months to about 4 years), because of the low iron content of milk and other preferred foods, rapid growth rate, and insufficient body reserves of iron to meet needs beyond about 6 months;
- adolescents in their early growth spurt, because of rapid growth and the needs of expanding red blood cell mass;
- females during childbearing years, because of menstrual iron losses; and
- pregnant women, because of their expanding blood volume, the demands of fetus and placenta, and blood losses to be incurred in childbirth.

In addition, many nonpregnant females during childbearing years fall short of the RDA for iron because of restricted caloric intakes and because only 5 to 7 mg iron can be expected per 1,000 kcal from the average Western diet.

Other conditions and populations have an increased need for iron intake due to increased iron losses or impaired iron absorption. Conditions associated with increased iron losses include hemorrhage, renal disease, renal replacement therapy, decreased gastrointestinal transit time, steatorrhea, and parasites. Impaired iron absorption may occur with protein calorie malnutrition, renal disease, achlorhydria (the absence of hydrochloric acid in gastric juice), prolonged use of alkaline-based drugs such as antacids, and parasites.

Figure 12.7 depicts the gradual depletion of iron content in the body and demonstrates the fact that anemia does not occur until iron depletion is severe. Iron deficiency without anemia, however, can occur. Symptoms of iron deficiency, mostly demonstrated in children, include pallor, listlessness, behavioral disturbances, impaired performance in some cognitive tasks, some irreversible impairment of learning ability, and short

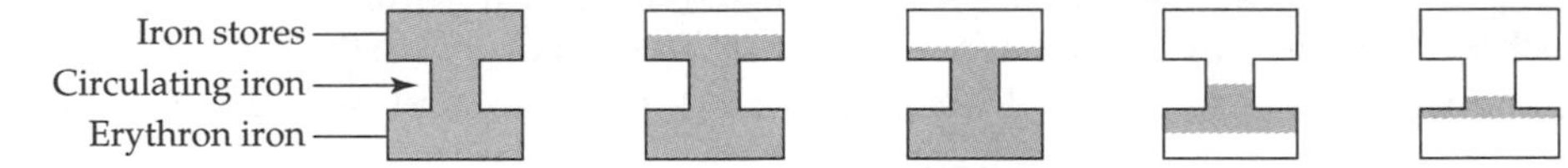

	Normal	Early Negative Iron Balance	Iron Depletion	Iron-Deficient Erythropoiesis	Iron Deficiency Anemia
Reticuloendothelial marrow iron	2–3+	1+	0–1+	0	0
Transferrin iron-binding capacity (μg/dL)	330±30	330–360	360	390	410
Plasma ferritin (μg/L)	100±60	<25	20	10	<10
Iron absorption (%)	5–10	10–15	10–15	10–20	10–20
Plasma iron (μg/dL)	115±50	<120	115	<60	<40
Transferrin saturation (%)	35±15	30	30	<15	<15
Sideroblasts (%)	40–60	40–60	40–60	<10	<10
Erythrocyte protoporphyrin (μg/dL)	30	30	30	100	200
Erythrocytes	Normal	Normal	Normal	Normal	Microcytic Hypochromic
Serum transferrin receptors	Normal	Normal–high	High	Very high	Very high
Ferritin iron	Normal	Normal–low	Low	Very low	Very low

Figure 12.7 Sequential changes in iron status associated with iron depletion. *Source:* Adapted from Victor Herbert, Recommended dietary intakes (RDI) of iron in humans, Am J Clin Nutr 1987;45:679–86 (© Am J Clin Nutr, American Society for Clinical Nutrition), and Victor Herbert, J Nut 1996;126: 1213S–20S. Used with permission.

attention span [32]. In adults, work performance and productivity are most commonly impaired with iron deficiency [33,34]. Iron deficiency may impair the degradation of γ-aminobutyric acid (GABA), an inhibitory neurotransmitter in the brain, or may inhibit dopamine-producing neurons [32]. Possible impairment of the immune system, decreased resistance to infection, and impaired capacity to maintain body temperature have also been shown [32].

Further discussion of iron deficiency with and without anemia as it relates to changes that occur in indices of iron status are discussed in the section "Assessment of Nutriture."

Supplements

Oral supplements of ferrous iron are available in complexes with sulfate, succinate, citrate, lactate, tartarate, fumarate, and gluconate. Intravenous administration of iron dextrans also can be given. Oral iron supplements provide nonheme iron, and thus absorption of the iron is enhanced when ingested with a source of vitamin C or other enhancing factors. Amino-acid iron chelates, such as iron glycine, are also marketed; however, in humans, absorption of iron administered as a chelate has not been shown to be superior to iron given as ferrous sulfate or ferrous ascorbate [35–37]. Initial effects of oral iron supplements on red blood cell counts and hemoglobin concentrations take about 2 weeks. Iron therapy to build up body stores of iron may be needed for 6 months to 1 year.

Toxicity: Hemochromatosis

Accidental iron overload (toxicity) has been observed in young children following excessive ingestion of iron pills or vitamin and mineral pills. Other people susceptible to iron overload have a genetic disorder known as **hemochromatosis.** It is estimated that about 50 per 10,000 persons in the United States are homozygous for the disorder. Hemochromatosis is most often seen in adult Caucasian males and begins to occur around 20 years of age. The condition is characterized by increased (at least two times normal) iron absorption. Mutations in the HFE gene have been shown to be responsible for the condition and result in the inability of the body, primarily the intestinal cells, to accurately sense iron stores and down-regulate intestinal iron absorption. Thus, in individuals with hemochromatosis, iron absorption continues despite high iron stores. The absorbed iron is progressively deposited within tissues, especially the liver, heart, and pancreas, among others, causing extensive organ damage and ultimately organ failure. Iron deposition in the liver, for example, leads to cirrhosis usually by about 50 years of age. Heterozygotes for the condition do not develop severe organ dysfunction but do have abnormal iron status. Treatment of the condition usually involves frequent phlebotomy (removal of blood) and may require administration of deferroxamine, which can chelate iron and increase urinary iron excretion.

Other people at particularly high risk for iron overload are those with iron-loading anemias, thalassemia, and sideroblastic anemia. The elevated erythropoiesis in people so affected causes increased iron absorption. However, while previous studies once linked high body iron (serum ferritin >200 μg/L) to heart disease, a larger group of studies has shown no such association.

Assessment of Nutriture

Numerous measurements are used for the assessment of iron nutriture. The most common indices are hemoglobin (amount of iron-containing protein found in red blood cells per unit, usually deciliter or liter, of blood) and hematocrit (that proportion of the total blood volume that is red blood cells). However, while these indices indicate the presence of anemia, they are among the last to change as iron deficiency develops.

In the first stages of iron deficiency, iron stores in the liver, spleen, and bone marrow are diminished. While iron stores may be aspirated and measured from bone marrow, the routine test involves measurement of plasma ferritin. Decreases in plasma ferritin concentration are thought to parallel the decrease in the amount of iron found in stores. Plasma ferritin concentrations $<\sim 12$ μg/L are associated with iron deficiency. However, if inflammation or infection is present, serum ferritin concentration rises, an occurrence unrelated to iron stores. Thus, serum ferritin may appear within normal range or high when the actual amount of iron in the protein is quite low. Measurement of the iron content of serum ferritin or of percentage saturation of serum ferritin with iron is thought to be a better indicator than measurement of serum ferritin itself in people with inflammation or infection.

As iron deficiency progresses into the second stage, iron stores typically remain low and transport iron decreases. Thus, plasma ferritin concentrations continue to be diminished, and circulating iron begins to decrease. Iron circulates in the blood bound to transferrin. With deficiency, transferrin saturation decreases to $<16\%$. (Remember that transferrin is normally about one-third saturated.) Transferrin saturation can be calculated by multiplying the serum iron concentration by 100 and then dividing by the total iron-binding capacity (TIBC). TIBC represents the amount of iron that plasma transferrin can bind and normally ranges from ~250 to 400 μg/dL. Levels >400 are suggestive of iron deficiency. Serum iron concentrations, which represent the amount of iron bound to transferrin, also are affected with iron deficiency, decreasing to $<\sim 50$ μg/dL (normal values range from ~50–165 μg/dL).

As circulating iron diminishes, functional or cellular iron also becomes limiting. With diminished iron, free protoporphyrin concentrations in erythrocytes rise. Protoporphyrin is a precursor of heme (for hemoglobin) and accumulates within red blood cells when iron is not available. Erythrocyte protoporphyrin levels >70 μg/dL red blood cells are associated with iron deficiency. In iron deficiency, the number of transferrin receptors on the cell surface, especially of immature red cells, also increases. The increased receptor number represents an up-regulation to enable cells to better compete for transferrin-bound iron. With iron deficiency, concentrations of serum transferrin receptors (sTfR), truncated forms of the membrane receptor protein, increase to >8.5 mg/L and are thought to be directly proportional to the functional tissue iron deficit after depletion of iron stores.

In the final stages of iron deficiency, anemia occurs, as indicated by low blood hemoglobin concentrations. Blood hemoglobin concentrations of <12 g/dL and <13 g/dL for females and males, respectively, are suggestive of iron deficiency anemia. Hematocrit concentrations of <37% and <40% for women and men, respectively, also are typical of iron deficiency anemia. Characterization of red blood cells with respect to size (mean corpuscular volume, or MCV) and amount of hemoglobin in them (mean corpuscular hemoglobin, or MCH, and mean corpuscular hemoglobin concentration, or MCHC) may be assessed and typically are lower than normal in the final stages of iron deficiency anemia. Descriptions of these assessments follow.

- MCV (fl) represents the size of the red blood cell. It is calculated by dividing hematocrit by red blood cells and then multiplying by 10.
- MCH (pg/rbc) represents the average hemoglobin content of each individual red blood cell. It is calculated by dividing hemoglobin by red blood cells and then multiplying by 10.
- MCHC represents the amount of hemoglobin in grams per deciliter (%) of red blood cells. It is calculated by dividing hemoglobin by hematocrit and then multiplying by 100.

In summary, red blood cells are pale (hypochromic) and small (microcytosis) with iron deficiency anemia. Figure 12.7 illustrates the changes that occur in the various measurements.

References Cited for Iron

1. Finch CA, Huebers H. Perspectives in iron metabolism. N Engl J Med 1982;306:1520–28.

2. Leibel RL. Behavioral and biochemical correlates of iron deficiency. J Am Diet Assoc 1977;77:378–404.

3. Hallberg L. Iron absorption and iron deficiency. Hum Nutr Clin Nutr 1982;36C:259–78.

4. Hurrell R, Lynch S, Trinidad T, Dassenko S, Cook J. Iron absorption in humans: bovine serum albumin compared with beef muscle and egg white. Am J Clin Nutr 1988;47:102–7.

5. Monsen, E. Iron nutrition and absorption: dietary factors which impact iron bioavailability. J Am Diet Assoc 1988;88:786–90.

6. Taylor P, Martinez-Torres C, Romano E, Layrisse M. The effect of cysteine-containing peptides released during meat digestion on iron absorption in humans. Am J Clin Nutr 1986;43:68–71.

7. MacPhail A, Ratel R, Bothwell T, Lamparelli R. EDTA and the absorption of iron from food. Am J Clin Nutr 1994;59:644–48.

8. Monsen E, Balintfy J. Calculating dietary iron bioavailability: refinement and computerization. J Am Diet Assoc 1982;80:307–11.

9. Morck T, Lynch S, Cook J. Inhibition of food iron absorption by coffee. Am J Clin Nutr 1983;37:416–20.

10. Hallberg L, Rossander-Hulten L, Brune M, Gleerup A. Calcium and iron absorption: mechanism of action and nutritional importance. Eur J Clin Nutr 1992;46:317–27.

11. Cook J, Dassenko S, Whittaker P. Calcium supplementation: effect on iron absorption. Am J Clin Nutr 1991;53:106–11.

12. Hallberg L, Brune M, Erlandsson M, Sandberg A-S, Rossander-Hulten L. Calcium: effect of different amounts on nonheme- and heme-iron absorption in humans. Am J Clin Nutr 1991; 53:112–19.

13. Snedeker S, Smith S, Greger J. Effect of dietary calcium and phosphorus levels on the utilization of iron, copper, and zinc by adult males. J Nutr 1982;112:136–43.

14. Rossander-Hulten L, Brune M, Sandstrom B, Lonnerdal B, Hallberg L. Competitive inhibition of iron absorption by manganese and zinc. Am J Clin Nutr 1991;54:152–56.

15. Crofton R, Gvozdanovic D, Gvozdanovic S, Khin C, Brunt P, Mowat N, Agget P. Inorganic zinc and the intestinal absorption of ferrous iron. Am J Clin Nutr 1989;50:141–44.

16. Whittaker P. Iron and zinc interactions in humans. Am J Clin Nutr 1998;68:442S–46S.

17. Herman S, Griffin IJ, Suwarti S, Ernawati F, Permaesih D, Pambudi D, Abrams SA. Cofortification of iron-fortified flour with zinc sulfate, but not zinc oxide, decreases iron absorption in Indonesian children. Am J Clin Nutr 2002;76:813–17.

18. Hallberg L, Hulten L, Gramatkovski E. Iron absorption from the whole diet in men: how effective is the regulation of iron absorption? Am J Clin Nutr 1997;66:347–56.

19. Finch C, Huebers H. Perspectives in iron metabolism. N Engl J Med 1982;306:1520–28.

20. Bolann B, Ulvik R. On the limited ability of superoxide to release iron from ferritin. Eur J Biochem 1990;193:899–904.

21. Oduho G, Han Y, Baker D. Iron deficiency reduces the efficacy of tryptophan as a niacin precursor. J Nutr 1994;124:444–50.

22. Herbert V, Shaw S, Jayatilleke E. Vitamin C–driven free radical generation from iron. J Nutr 1996;126:1213S–20S.

23. Waddell J, Steenbock H, Elvehjem C, Hart E. Iron salts and iron-containing ash extracts in the correction of anemia. J Biol Chem 1927;77:777–95.

24. Sandstrom B, Davidsson L, Cederblad A, Lonnerdal B. Oral iron, dietary ligands and zinc absorption. J Nutr 1985;115:411–14.

25. Solomons N, Jacob R. Studies on the bioavailability of zinc in humans: effects of heme and nonheme iron on the absorption of zinc. Am J Clin Nutr 1981;34:475–82.

26. Houwelingen FV, Van Den Berg GJ, Lemmens AG, Sijtsma KW, Beynen AC. Iron and zinc status in rats with diet-induced marginal deficiency of vitamin A and/or copper. Biol Trace Elem Res 1993;38:83–95.

27. Goyer R. Nutrition and metal toxicity. Am J Clin Nutr 1995; 61(suppl):646S–50S.

28. Moriarty P, Picciano M, Beard J, Reddy C. Classical selenium-dependent glutathione peroxidase expression is decreased secondary to iron deficiency in rats. J Nutr 1995;125:293–301.

29. Yetgin S, Huncal F, Basaran G, Ciliv G. Serum selenium status in children with iron deficiency anemia. Acta Hematol 1992; 88:185–88.

30. Lee Y, Layman D, Bell R. Glutathione peroxidase activity in iron-deficient rats. J Nutr 1981;111:194–200.

31. Food and Nutrition Board, Institute of Medicine. Dietary Reference Intakes. Washington, DC: National Academy Press, 2001, pp. 290–393.

32. Scrimshaw NS. Iron deficiency. Scientific Am 1991;265:46–52.

33. Prasad A, Prasad C. Iron deficiency: non-hematological manifestations. Prog Food Nutr Sci 1991;15:255–83.

34. Johnson M, Fischer J, Bowman B, Gunter E. Iron nutriture in elderly individuals. FASEB J 1994;8:609–21.

35. Fox T, Eagles J, Fairweather-Tait S. Bioavailability of iron glycine as a fortificant in infant foods. Am J Clin Nutr 1998;67:664–68.

36. Pineda O, Ashmead D, Perez J, Lemus C. Effectiveness of iron amino acid chelate on the treatment of iron deficiency anemia in adolescents. J Appl Nutr 1994;46:2–13.

37. Olivares M, Pizarro F, Pineda O, Name J, Hertrampf E, Walter T. Milk inhibits and ascorbic acid favors ferrous bis-glycine chelate bioavailability in humans. J Nutr 1997;127:1407–11.

Suggested Readings

Beard J, Dawson B, Pinero D. Iron metabolism. Nutr Rev 1996;54:295–317.

Clarke S, Abraham S. Gene expression: nutrient control of pre- and posttranscriptional events. FASEB J 1992;6:3146–52.

Conrad ME, Umbreit JN. Iron absorption. Am J Hemat 1993; 42:67–73.

Klausner R, Rouault T, Harford J. Regulating the fate of mRNA: the control of cellular iron metabolism. Cell 1993;72:19–28.

Lash A, Saleem A. Iron metabolism and its regulation. Ann Clin Lab Sci 1995;25:20–30.

Leibold E, Guo B. Iron-dependent regulation of ferritin and transferrin receptor expression by the iron-responsive element binding protein. Ann Rev Nutr 1992;12:345–68.

Pietrangelo A. Physiology of iron transport and the hemochromatosis gene. Am J Physiol Liver Physiol 2002;282:G403–14.

Powell JJ, Jugdaohsingh R, Thompson RPH. The regulation of mineral absorption in the gastrointestinal tract. Proc Nutr Soc 1999; 58:147–53.

Umbreit JN, Conrad ME, Moore EG, Latour LF. Iron absorption and cellular transport: the mobilferrin/paraferritin paradigm. Sem in Hematology 1998;35:13–34.

Uzel C, Conrad ME. Absorption of heme iron. Sem Hematology 1998;35:27–34.

Worwood M. The laboratory assessment of iron status—an update. Clin Chim Acta 1997;259:3–23.

Web Site

www.cfsan.fda.gov

ZINC

The human body contains ~1.5 to 2.5 g of zinc. Zinc is found in all organs and tissues (primarily intracellularly) and in body fluids. Most of the zinc in humans is found in bone, liver, kidney, muscle, and skin. Zinc, a metal, can exist in several different valence states, but it is almost universally found as the divalent ion (Zn^{2+}).

Sources

Zinc is typically associated with the protein fraction and/or the nucleic acid fraction of foods. Specifically, zinc is found in food complexed with amino acids that are part of peptides and proteins and with nucleic acids. The zinc content of foods varies widely (Table 12.3). Very good sources of zinc are red meats (especially organ meats) and seafood (especially oysters and mollusks). Animal products are thought to provide between 40% and 70% of zinc consumed by most people in the United States. Other good animal sources of zinc include poultry, pork, and dairy products. Whole grains (especially bran and germ) and vegetables (leafy and root) represent good plant sources of zinc. Fruits and refined cereals are poor zinc sources. Zinc from plant sources not only is lower in content but also is absorbed to a lesser extent than zinc from meat [1].

Table 12.3 Zinc Content of Selected Foods

Food/Food Group	Zinc (mg/100 g)
Seafood	
Oysters	17–91
Crabmeat	3.8–4.3
Shrimp	1.1
Tuna	0.5–0.8
Meat and poultry	
Liver	3.1–3.9
Chicken	1.0–2.0
Beef, ground	3.9–4.1
Veal	3.1–3.2
Pork	1.6–2.1
Eggs and dairy products	
Eggs	1.1
Milk	0.4
Cheeses	2.8–3.2
Legumes (cooked)	0.6–1.0
Grains and cereals	
Rice and pasta (cooked)	0.3–0.6
Bread (wheat)	1.0
Bread (white)	0.6–0.8
Vegetables	0.1–0.7
Fruits	<0.1

Source: www.nal.usda.gov/fnic/foodcomp.

Processing of certain foods may affect the zinc available for absorption. Heat treatment can cause food zinc to form complexes that are resistant to hydrolysis, thereby making zinc unavailable for absorption. Maillard reaction products—that is, amino acid–carbohydrate complexes resulting from browning, for example—are particularly notable for inhibiting zinc's availability for absorption.

In addition to dietary food sources, endogenous sources for zinc are also available. Specifically, zinc is found in pancreatic and biliary secretions that are released into the gastrointestinal tract. Carboxypeptidase, for example, is a zinc metalloenzyme. Following carboxypeptidase activity, the enzyme itself is hydrolyzed and zinc is released. The released zinc is then available for absorption and reuse in the body.

Digestion, Absorption, Transport, Uptake, and Storage

Digestion

Zinc, like iron, needs to be hydrolyzed from most amino acids and nucleic acids prior to absorption. Zinc is believed to be liberated from food during the digestive process, most likely by proteases and nucleases in the stomach and small intestine. Hydrochloric acid also appears to play an important role in zinc digestion and/or absorption. The ingestion of antacids, H_2 receptor blockers (such as Zantac®, Tagamet®, or Pepcid®), or proton pump blockers (such as Prevacid® or Prilosec®) increases gastric pH, resulting in decreased zinc absorption [2]. The role of gastric acid in zinc digestion and/or absorption has not been elucidated but may be related to impaired hydrolysis of zinc from nucleic or amino acids, changes in zinc's ionic state, or alterations in the enterocyte membrane to affect permeability and thus zinc absorption.

Absorption

The main site of zinc absorption in the gastrointestinal tract is the proximal small intestine, most likely the jejunum. However, the relative contribution of each segment of the small intestine (duodenum, jejunum, and ileum) toward overall zinc absorption has not been demonstrated. Zinc is absorbed into the enterocyte by a carrier-mediated process, with low zinc intakes absorbed more efficiently than higher intakes. Nramp 2 (natural resistance associated macrophage protein 2) and DC/MT 1 (divalent cation or mineral transporter 1, a possible isoform of nramp 2) are thought to transport zinc, among other divalent cations (especially Fe^{2+}), into the intestinal cell. The need for energy (ATP) in zinc's absorptive process is unclear. In addition to carrier-mediated transport, passive diffusion (nonsaturable) and/or paracellular zinc absorption also are thought to occur with high zinc intake (Fig. 12.8). Studies have shown that zinc absorption varies from approximately 10% to 59%.

The form in which zinc is absorbed into the enterocyte is uncertain. Zinc may move across the brush border as an ion or as part of a chelated complex. Most evidence supports the absorption of zinc as a complex with ligands derived from both exogenous and endogenous sources.

Factors Influencing Zinc Absorption

As is the case with iron, chelators or ligands may bind to zinc. Whether these substances are enhancers or inhibitors depends on the digestibility and absorbability of the zinc chelates formed.

Enhancers of Zinc Absorption. Several endogenous substances are thought to serve as ligands with zinc, especially in the presence of inhibitors. Possible endogenous ligands include citric acid and picolinic acid, the latter of which is a metabolite of the tryptophan-to-niacin pathway (p. 287), as well as prostaglandins. Amino acid ligands include histidine, cysteine, and possibly other amino acids (lysine and glycine). Pancreatic secretions are thought to contain an unidentified constituent that enhances zinc absorption. In addition, glutathione (a tripeptide composed of cysteine, glutamate, and glycine) or products of protein digestion, such as tripeptides, are purported to serve as ligands. In these ligands, zinc typically binds to sulfur (e.g., cysteine alone, or as part of glutathione) or nitrogen (e.g., histidine).

Absorption of zinc also appears to be enhanced by low zinc status. Specifically, absorption of zinc by carrier-mediated mechanisms is enhanced with low zinc status, suggesting that the total amount of zinc absorbed is homeostatically regulated. However, how zinc status regulates absorption of the mineral is unclear.

Inhibitors of Zinc Absorption. Many compounds in food may complex with zinc and inhibit its absorption. Inhibitors include

- phytate,
- oxalate,
- polyphenols,
- fibers, and
- nutrients (including vitamins and divalent cations).

Phytate, also called phytic acid, inositol hexaphosphate, or inositol polyphosphate, is found in plant foods particularly cereals such as maize and bran and

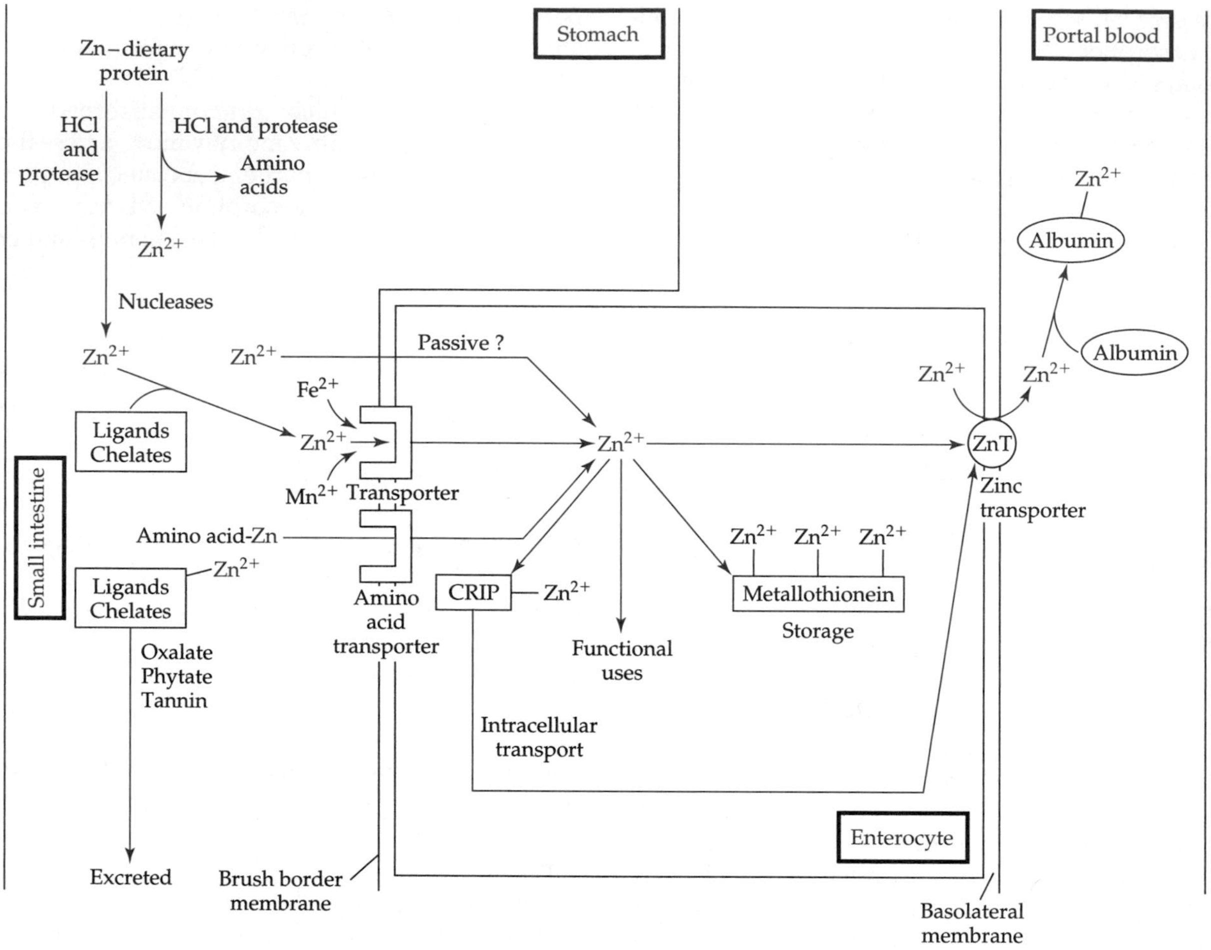

Figure 12.8 Digestion, absorption, enterocyte use, and transport of zinc. Abbreviation: CRIP, cysteine-rich intestinal proteins.

legumes. It binds to zinc (as well as other minerals) via oxygen. The zinc-phytate complex is large, insoluble, and poorly absorbed [3]. However, fermentation of bread has been shown to reduce the phytate content and improve zinc absorption. Figure 12.9 depicts the binding of zinc by phytate.

Oxalate or oxalic acid, another inhibitor of zinc absorption, is found in a variety of foods, most notably spinach, chard, berries, chocolate, and tea. The binding of zinc by oxalate is also via oxygen, as shown in Figure 12.9. Polyphenols such as tannins in tea and certain fibers found in whole grains, fruits, and vegetables also bind zinc and inhibit its absorption.

Interactions between zinc and nutrients such as the vitamin folic acid and a variety of divalent cations (Fe^{2+}, Ca^{2+}, Cu^{2+}) may occur and inhibit zinc absorption. Folic acid (350 μg) ingestion for 2 weeks has been shown to decrease zinc (50 mg) absorption by 21% [4]. However, another study that provided 800 μg folic acid and either 3.5 mg or 14.5 mg zinc for two 25-day periods found no adverse effects on zinc status [5]. Given the use of folate supplements to prevent neural tube defects in women during childbearing years, additional studies are warranted.

Figure 12.9 The binding of zinc by oxalate and phytate.

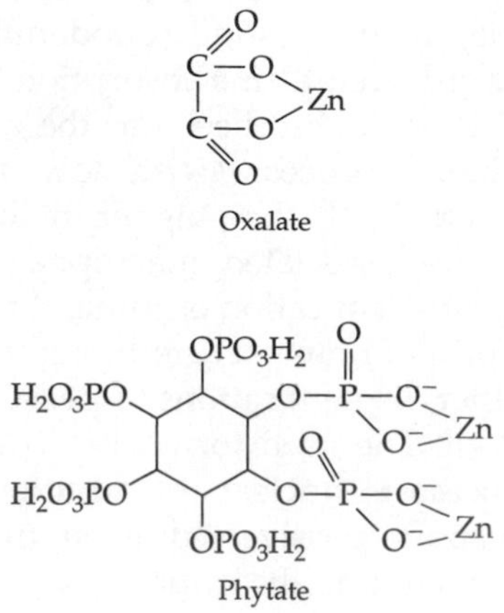

The interaction between zinc and other divalent cations is probably related to the fact that these cations compete with one another for binding ligands in the intestinal lumen or within the cell as well as for receptor sites on the brush border of the enterocytes. Iron and zinc interact primarily when coingested in solution; the effects are not always apparent when given with a meal [6]. Inhibition of zinc absorption is most common when the amount of the nonheme iron exceeds that of zinc. For example, ferrous sulfate and zinc sulfate ingested together in a ratio of 2 : 1 (50 mg : 25 mg) and 3 : 1 (75 mg : 25 mg) decreased zinc absorption in humans [7]. Heme iron does not have the same effects on zinc, nor does ingestion of nonheme iron with zinc from food [7]. These studies suggest that to maximize zinc absorption the zinc supplement should not be consumed with nonheme iron supplements.

The effects of calcium on zinc absorption and balance appear to vary. Some studies in humans have shown that ingestion of from 500 mg to ~2 g of calcium as calcium carbonate, hydroxyapatite, or calcium citrate malate has no effect on zinc absorption, while other studies providing similar amounts of calcium as milk, calcium phosphate, and calcium carbonate found a reduction in net zinc absorption and zinc balance in postmenopausal women [8–11].

Although copper has the potential to interfere with zinc absorption, this has not been reported. In fact, the opposite appears to occur; that is, zinc supplements inhibit copper absorption and can lead to copper deficiency (see the section "Interactions with Other Nutrients," p. 443).

Intestinal Cell Zinc Use

Movement of zinc through the enterocyte is not a well-delineated process. As indicated in Figure 12.8, zinc entering the enterocyte has several possible fates. The zinc may be either

- used functionally within the enterocyte,
- stored bound to the proteins in the enterocyte, or
- transported through the cell and across the basolateral membrane into the plasma for use by other tissues.

The use of zinc within the enterocyte is similar to its use in other body cells and is discussed further in the section "Functions and Mechanisms of Action." Cysteine-rich intestinal proteins (CRIPs) and metallothionein in the enterocyte serve as intracellular binding ligands for zinc as well as for other minerals, primarily copper in the case of metallothionein. Initially, zinc appears to accumulate on CRIP; however, with increased zinc concentrations, metallothionein concentrations rise. Thionein protein has an unusually high content of cysteine (30% cysteine residues), which functions in metal binding. The zinc captured and held bound to metallothionein in the enterocytes is typically lost into the lumen with the sloughing of these cells. Reduced zinc absorption is directly correlated with metallothionein formation from orally administered zinc and newly synthesized thionein polypeptides [12]. In fact, gene expression of thionein is induced by diets high in zinc [13]. Metallothionein is discussed in further detail in the section on storage.

Zinc not bound to metallothionein or used within the enterocyte is transported across the basolateral membrane of the enterocyte. Several zinc transporters (ZnTs) have been identified. ZnT-1 is found in many tissues throughout the body, including the enterocyte basolateral membrane. ZnT-1 preferentially transports zinc out of the duodenal and jejunal intestinal cells and does not require sodium or ATP [14]. Other zinc transporters, such as ZnT-2, ZnT-3, and ZnT-4, have been isolated in the intestine, kidney, testes, mammary glands, and brain, for example [14]. These transporters may be involved in intracellular zinc movement.

Transport

Zinc passing into portal blood from the intestinal cell is mainly transported loosely bound to albumin (Fig. 12.8). From the enterocyte, most zinc is taken to the liver, where the mineral is initially concentrated. Upon departing from the liver, albumin as well as other compounds, such as transferrin, α-2 macroglobulin, and immunoglobulin (Ig) G, binds and transports zinc in the blood. Albumin is thought to transport up to ~60% of zinc. Transferrin, α-2 macroglobulin, and immunoglobulin (Ig) G are thought to transport ~15% to 40% of the zinc in the blood (Fig. 12.10). Two amino acids, histidine and cysteine, loosely bind ~2% to 8% of the zinc for transport; these amino acids form a ternary (histidine-zinc-cysteine) complex in the blood.

Zinc is complexed and released from its plasma carriers on a continual basis. Some of this released zinc can pass back into the enterocyte and perhaps even through the cell into the intestinal lumen. The albumin-bound zinc appears to be the most readily taken up by tissues, and it is this fraction of plasma zinc that is thought to be important in the regulation of zinc absorption [13].

Uptake by Tissues

The mechanism of zinc uptake by tissues is unknown. Multiple transport systems (ZnT) and amino acid carrier systems for uptake of amino acid–bound zinc have been identified. Some zinc carriers are not thought to be highly selective, while others are tissue-specific.

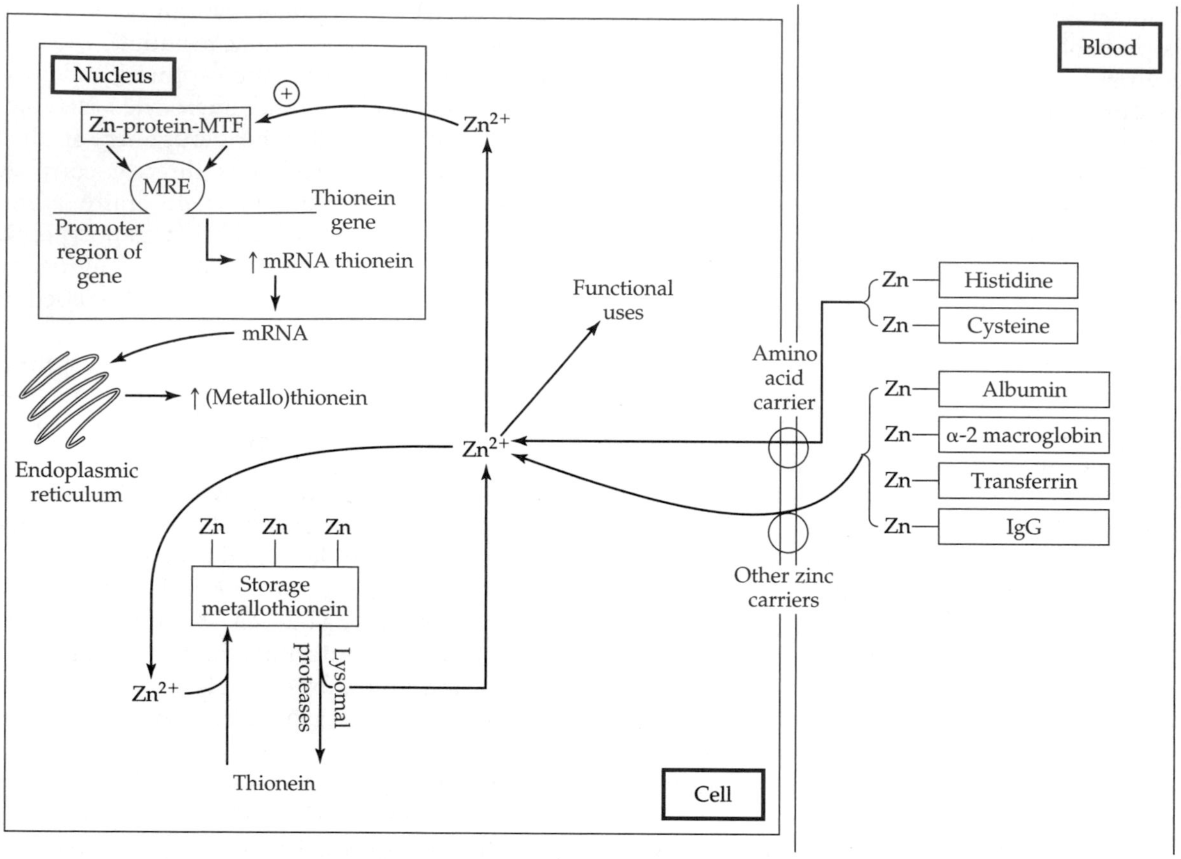

Figure 12.10 Uptake, storage and use of zinc in cells. Abbreviations: MRE, metal regulatory elements; MTF, metal transcription factor.

An increase in amino acid use by tissues leads to increased uptake of zinc, and vice versa. Given that numerous metalloenzymes within the cell require zinc as a component, it is reasonable to assume that enzyme synthesis and zinc uptake are correlated.

Distribution and Storage

Zinc is found in all body organs, most notably the liver, kidney, muscle, skin, and bones. However, the zinc content of most soft tissues (including muscle, brain, lung, and heart) is relatively stable. This soft-tissue zinc does not respond to or equilibrate with other zinc pools to release zinc should dietary zinc intake be low. Furthermore, while zinc is found in bones as part of apatite, bones release the mineral very slowly and cannot be depended on as a supplier of zinc during dietary deprivation. Instead, when dietary zinc intake is insufficient to meet the body's needs, plasma zinc–containing enzymes and metallothionein provide zinc. Catabolism of selected "less essential" zinc-containing metalloproteins (enzymes) as well as liver metallothionein occurs so that zinc can be redistributed to meet particularly crucial needs for the mineral.

Zinc is thought to be stored in most tissues as part of the protein thionein, which when mineral bound is known as metallothionein. Metallothionein is found in most tissues of the body, including the liver, pancreas, kidney, intestine, and red blood cell. Various forms of the protein appear to exist. These forms are designated by number as metallothionein (MT)-1 through MT-4. MT-1 and MT-2 appear to be the most common tissue forms. As discussed in the section "Intestinal Cell Use," metallothionein contains a high proportion of cysteine residues (20 of 61 amino acids), each of which binds metals. In addition to binding zinc (7 g atoms/mol), metallothionein binds copper, cadmium, and mercury.

Liver and red blood cell metallothionein-bound zinc diminishes as dietary zinc intake decreases and thus is thought to reflect zinc status or stores. Zinc, and possibly other minerals, appears to affect the gene expression of thionein. Specifically, metal regulatory elements (MREs) made of specific nucleotide sequences are found in the promoter region of the thionein gene [15,16]. Zinc may interact with the MREs alone or through a transcription factor (sometimes called a metal transcription factor, abbreviated MTF) to induce thionein synthesis [15,16]. Thionein gene expression is also influenced by glucagon and the monokine interleukin 1. Interleukin 1, synthesized and secreted by monocytes and activated macrophages, is thought to induce thionein gene transcription during infection [16]. During infection, plasma zinc concentrations typically decrease and hepatic zinc concentrations rise; the sequestering of zinc by liver metallothionein in turn prevents bacterial use of zinc for replication.

Release of zinc from metallothionein involves lysosomal proteases (Fig. 12.10). At an acid pH, these proteases degrade metallothionein to release the apoprotein thionein and zinc, which is then available for use by cells or other tissues.

Functions and Mechanisms of Actions

Zinc has many seemingly divergent functions, probably due to the numerous metalloenzymes of which it is a component. As a component of metalloenzymes, zinc provides structural integrity to the enzyme by binding directly to amino acid residues and/or participates in the reaction at the catalytic site. Zinc appears to be part of more enzyme systems than the rest of the trace minerals combined. Zinc affects many fundamental life processes (Table 12.4). Enzymes (at least 70 and perhaps over 200) from every enzyme class have been shown to require zinc. We will discuss a few of these zinc-dependent enzymes next.

Zinc-Dependent Enzymes

- *Carbonic anhydrase*, found primarily in the erythrocytes and in the renal tubule, is essential for respiration. It catalyzes the following reaction, thereby allowing rapid disposal of carbon dioxide:

$$CO_2 + H_2O \xrightarrow{\text{Carbonic anhydrase}} H_2CO_3 \xrightarrow[\text{Dissociation}]{} H^+ + HCO_3^-$$

The H^+ dissociated from carbonic acid reduces oxyhemoglobin as oxygen is released to the tissues; the bicarbonate passes into the plasma to participate in buffering reactions. The amount of zinc associated with carbonic anhydrase and carried by the erythrocytes is approximately eight to nine times as much as that distributed to tissues in plasma [13]. Carbonic anhydrase has a very high affinity for the mineral zinc, which plays a catalytic role. Catabolism of this enzyme apparently does not occur even with zinc deprivation.

- *Alkaline phosphatase* contains four zinc ions per enzyme molecule. Two of the four ions are required for enzyme activity. The other two are needed for structural purposes. The enzyme, found mainly in bone and in the liver (with small amounts in the plasma), lacks substrate specificity, hydrolyzing monoesters of phosphates from various compounds. Enzyme activity decreases with zinc deficiency.

Table 12.4 Selected Functions of Zinc

Metalloenzyme component
Oxidoreductase
Hydrolase
Lyase
Isomerase
Transferase
Ligase
Gene expression
Cell replication
Membrane and cytoskeletal stabilization
Structural role in hormones

- *Alcohol dehydrogenase* also contains four zinc ions per enzyme molecule, with two of the four required for catalytic activity and two required for structural purposes (protein conformation). This enzyme is important in the conversion of alcohols to aldehydes (e.g., retinol to retinal, which is needed for the visual cycle and night vision). NADH also participates in the reaction.

- *Carboxypeptidase A* (Fig. 12.11), an exopeptidase secreted by the pancreas into the duodenum, is necessary for the digestion of protein. Zinc is bound tightly to carboxypeptidase A and is essential for enzymatic activity. Carboxypeptidase A activity decreases with zinc deficiency.

- *Aminopeptidase* is also involved in protein digestion. Aminopeptidases have been shown to contain one zinc atom needed for catalytic activity. The enzyme cleaves amino acids from the amino terminal end of the protein or polypeptide that is being digested in the intestinal tract.

- *Δ-aminolevulinic acid dehydratase,* involved in heme synthesis, is also zinc-dependent. This thiol (SH)-containing enzyme is made up of eight subunits, each of which binds one zinc atom. Zinc is essential for the maintenance of free thiols in the enzyme. The enzyme catalyzes the condensation of two Δ-aminolevulinic acids to form porpho bilinogen (Fig. 12.5). Lead, if present in the body in high concentrations (as occurs with lead poisoning), has been shown to replace zinc in the dehydratase.

- *Superoxide dismutase (SOD)* found in the cell cytoplasm requires two atoms each of zinc and copper for function; zinc appears to have a structural role in the enzyme. An extracellular form of the

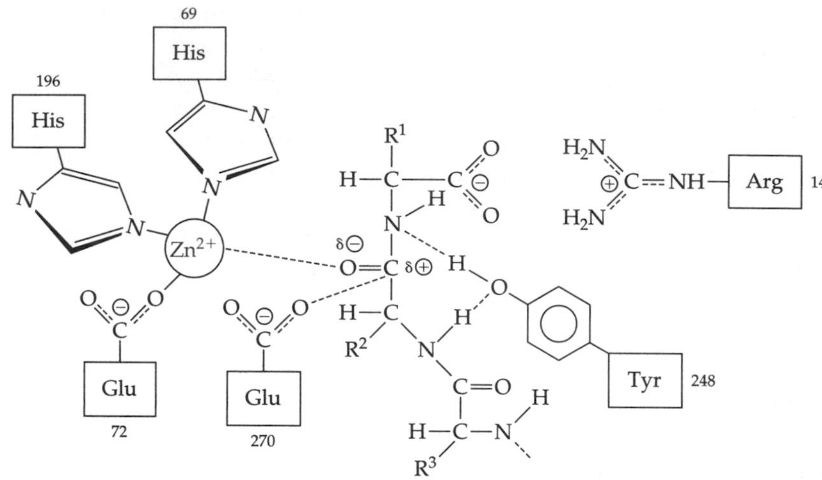

Figure 12.11 Partial structure of carboxypeptidase A.

enzyme that is also zinc- and copper-dependent has been characterized and appears to be more sensitive to zinc than is the cytosolic form of the enzyme. The cytosolic and extracellular forms of SOD both serve important antioxidant defense roles in the body by catalyzing the removal of superoxide radicals, O_2^-:

$$2O_2^- + 2H^+ \xrightarrow{\text{Superoxide dismutase}} H_2O_2 + O_2$$

Further information on SOD is found in the section on copper (p. 451), and in the Chapter 10 perspective.

• *Collagenases* function in the digestion of collagen in the gastrointestinal tract. Zinc plays a catalytic role in the enzyme's function.

• *Phospholipase C* requires three zinc atoms for catalytic activity. This enzyme hydrolyzes the glycerophosphate bond in phospholipids.

• *Polyglutamate hydrolase,* also called γ-glutamylhydrolase, is a zinc-dependent enzyme necessary for the digestion of folate in the gastrointestinal tract. Folate is found in foods bound to several (poly)glutamate residues. In order for folate to be absorbed, most of the glutamate residues need to be removed. Polyglutamate hydrolase catalyzes the hydrolysis of the glutamate residues from folate to yield monoglutamate folate, which is then actively transported into the intestinal cells. Thus, poor zinc intake or status can diminish folate absorption.

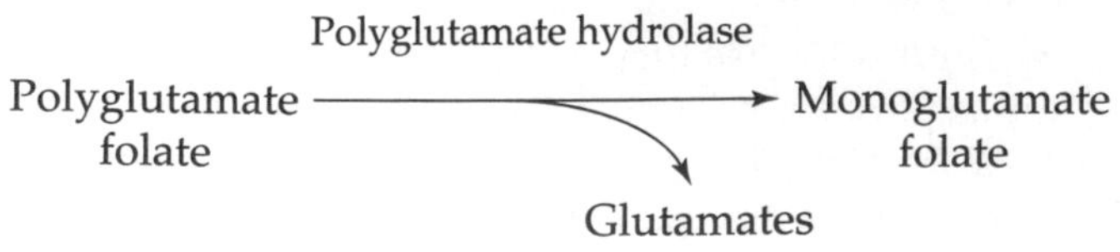

• *Polymerases, kinases, nucleases, transferases, phosphorylases,* and *transcriptases* all require zinc. Paramount in nucleic acid synthesis are the zinc metalloenzymes DNA and RNA polymerase and deoxythymidine kinase. Deoxythymidine kinase is necessary for the conservation or salvaging of thymine, the pyrimidine unique to DNA. Catabolism of RNA appears to be regulated by zinc because of zinc's influence on ribonuclease activity. Enzymes such as deoxynucleotidyl transferase, nucleoside phosphorylase, and reverse transcriptase also depend on zinc. Chapter 1 provides additional information on the roles of some of these zinc-dependent enzymes in transcription and translation.

Other Roles

Physiological functions of zinc include tissue or cell growth, cell replication, bone formation, skin integrity, cell-mediated immunity, and generalized host defense. The role of zinc in tissue growth is related primarily to its function in the regulation of protein synthesis, which includes its influence on polysome conformation as well as the synthesis and catabolism of the nucleic acids.

With respect to transcription, zinc appears to interact with nuclear proteins that bind to promoter sequences of specific genes (Fig. 12.10). Thus, zinc helps regulate transcription. Specifically, zinc serves as a necessary structural component of DNA-binding proteins (also called transcription factors) that contain zinc fingers. *Zinc fingers* is a term used to indicate the shape (configuration) of the proteins, which look like fingers, and the presence of the mineral zinc bound to the protein. The fingerlike configuration results from the twisting and coiling of the cysteine and histidine residues to which zinc binds in that segment of the protein. DNA-binding proteins that contain zinc fingers also bind other substances, such as retinoic acid, thyroxine, 1,25-$(OH)_2$ vitamin D, and other steroid hormones such as estrogen and androgens. Thus, hormones such as retinoic acid or 1,25-$(OH)_2$ vitamin D would enter the cell nucleus (see the section on vitamins A and D in Chap. 10) and bind to specific protein-containing zinc fingers. In the presence of zinc, which is required for the binding of the protein to the DNA, the protein (with the hormone attached to it) binds to the DNA to affect gene expression.

The effect of zinc on cell membranes may be through direct effects on the membrane proteins' conformation and/or on protein-to-protein interactions [17]. Zinc may affect the activity of several enzymes attached to plasma membranes, including alkaline phosphatase, carbonic anhydrase, and superoxide dismutase, among others [17]. These particular enzymes that control the structures and functions of the membranes to which they are attached are in turn controlled by zinc [12]. Zinc itself also is believed to stabilize membrane structure by stabilizing phospholipids and thiol (SH) groups that need to be maintained in a reduced state [18] and to guard the membrane against peroxidative damage by occupying sites on the membrane that might instead be occupied by pro-oxidant metals such as iron or by quenching free radicals through association with metallothionein [19]. Zinc may also stabilize membranes by promoting associations between membrane skeletal and cytoskeletal proteins [17]. Zinc in cells is found bound to tubulin, a protein that makes up the microtubules. Microtubules are thought to act as a framework for structural support of the cell as well as being needed for movement.

Zinc influences carbohydrate metabolism. Specifically, zinc is associated with insulin within stored granules in pancreatic beta cells. Zinc deficiency decreases insulin response, resulting in impaired glucose tolerance. Zinc also appears to influence the basal metabolic rate (BMR); a decrease in thyroid hormones and BMR has been observed in subjects receiving a zinc-restricted diet [20]. Zinc is also important for taste; it is a component of gustin, a protein involved in taste acuity.

Although many functions of zinc are known, many of its roles are not known. The effects of zinc deficiency on the body fail to explain fully the manifestations of zinc deprivation. It is "the small fraction of total body zinc that exchanges relatively rapidly with plasma zinc that is responsible for many of the known physiological functions of zinc" [21].

Interactions with Other Nutrients

Some of the interactions that result in the inhibition of the absorption of zinc have been addressed in the section on absorption. Interactions between zinc and nutrients that do not affect zinc absorption will be briefly discussed here.

Zinc and vitamin A interact in several ways. From the discussion on zinc functions, you may remember that zinc is required for alcohol dehydrogenase. Retinol (vitamin A) serves as a substrate for this enzyme, which converts retinol to retinal (retinaldehyde). In addition, zinc is necessary for the hepatic synthesis of retinol-binding protein, which transports vitamin A in the blood [22]. Zinc deficiency is associated with decreased mobilization of retinol from the liver as well as decreased concentrations of several transport proteins found in the blood, including albumin, transferrin, and prealbumin [22,23].

The detrimental effect of excessive zinc intake on copper absorption is thought to be due to zinc's stimulation of thionein synthesis. Thionein polypeptides have a higher affinity for copper than for zinc. Thus, when zinc intake causes increased synthesis of thionein, dietary copper easily becomes trapped as part of metallothionein within the enterocyte [24–28]. The formation of copper metallothionein traps the copper in the enterocyte, preventing its passage into the plasma. The danger of copper deficiency precipitated by zinc supplementation has led to the recommendation of a tolerable upper intake level of elemental zinc of 40 mg daily [29].

Diminished calcium absorption has occurred with ingestion of zinc supplements when calcium intake is low (230 mg calcium) [8]. However, absorption appears to be unaffected when calcium intakes are at adequate (recommended) levels [30].

Cadmium appears to bind to sites to which zinc would normally bind and to disrupt normal zinc functions. For example, cadmium can replace zinc in zinc fingers, causing the fingers to no longer function as they would with zinc present.

Excretion

The three primary routes of zinc loss from the body are via the

- gastrointestinal tract,
- kidney, and
- skin (integument and sweat).

The majority of zinc is lost from the body through the gastrointestinal tract in the feces. Endogenous zinc in the form of enzyme metalloproteins is secreted by the salivary glands, intestinal mucosa, pancreas (main source), and liver into the gastrointestinal tract. Although some of this zinc is reabsorbed, some also is excreted in the feces. Zinc is also contributed to the gastrointestinal lumen by sloughed intestinal cells and possibly by enterocytes that may permit a bidirectional flow of the mineral.

In contrast to intestinal zinc losses, renal and dermal losses of zinc, as well as zinc losses in semen and menses, are relatively constant. The majority of zinc filtered by the kidneys is reabsorbed by the tubules. Thus, only a small amount of zinc (~0.3–0.7 mg/day) is excreted in the urine. The zinc appearing in the urine is believed to be derived from the small percentage of plasma zinc that is complexed with histidine and cysteine. Zinc losses of ~0.4 to 0.6 mg/day occur with exfoliation of skin and with sweating. Other minor routes of zinc loss include (for men) semen (0.1 mg/day) and (for women) menses (0.1 mg/day). Hair contains ~0.1 to 0.2 mg zinc/g hair.

Recommended Dietary Allowances

An allowance for zinc appeared for the first time in the 1974 RDAs. The subcommittees on the 1989 and 2001 editions of the RDAs based zinc recommendations on the intake needed to maintain balance as well as on estimates of zinc absorption and body losses. Total zinc losses for adult men and women were calculated at 3.84 mg and 3.3 mg, respectively [29]. Zinc losses for men consisted of 0.63 mg urinary zinc, 0.54 mg integumental and sweat zinc, 0.1 mg semen zinc, and 2.57 mg endogenous intestinal zinc; for women, urinary zinc losses were 0.44 mg, integumental and sweat zinc losses were 0.46 mg, menses zinc losses were 0.1 mg, and endogenous intestinal zinc losses were 2.3 mg [29]. To account for absorption, the daily requirements for zinc for adult men and women were set at 9.4 mg and 6.8 mg, respectively, and the RDAs were set at 11 mg and 8 mg, respectively. These recommendations are lower than those set in 1989, which were 15 mg/day for adult men and 12 mg/day for adult women [31]. The 2001 RDA for zinc during pregnancy is 11 mg/day to cover the calculated need for growth of the fetus and placenta [29]. The zinc recommendation for lactating women is 12 mg/day [29]. The inside cover of the book provides additional RDAs for zinc for other age groups.

Deficiency

Few tissues contain large stores of zinc. Thus, should intake be inadequate and increased absorption fail to provide enough zinc, body reserves of zinc used for release and redistribution are quickly exhausted. Consequently, a deficient intake of zinc results in the catabolism of some of the zinc metalloenzymes. Normally, zinc is removed from those metalloenzymes that hold it less securely. The activities of three metalloenzymes—alkaline phosphatase in bone, carboxypeptidase A in pancreas, and deoxythymidine kinase in subcutaneous connective tissue—decrease with zinc deprivation. The zinc released by these is redistributed throughout the body to satisfy the more crucial cellular needs. Certain metalloenzymes with very high affinity for zinc, such as carbonic anhydrase, may be little influenced by a general zinc deprivation. The extent to which the metalloenzyme loses zinc during a deficiency depends on the geometry of the nitrogen, oxygen, and/or sulfur atoms that comprise the binding site [13].

Some population groups, especially the elderly and vegetarians, have been found to consume less than adequate amounts of zinc [32]. Conditions associated with an increased need for intake include alcoholism, chronic illness, stress, trauma, surgery, and malabsorption.

Signs and symptoms of zinc deficiency include growth retardation (an early response to zinc deficiency in children due to inadequate cell division needed for growth) [33], skeletal abnormalities due to impaired development of epiphyseal cartilage, defective collagen synthesis and/or cross-linking, poor wound healing, dermatitis (especially around body orifices), delayed sexual maturation in children, hypogeusia (blunting of sense of taste), night blindness, alopecia (hair loss), impaired immune function, and impaired protein synthesis, among others [22,34,35].

Supplements

Zinc is found in many forms in supplements (oral tablets, lozenges, and sprays), including zinc oxide, zinc sulfate, zinc acetate, zinc chloride, and zinc gluconate. Each of the forms differs in the amount of zinc provided and in absorption. Zinc gluconate, for example, is approximately 14.3% zinc, whereas zinc sulfate is 23% zinc and zinc chloride is 48% zinc. Zinc chloride and zinc sulfate are very soluble, as is zinc acetate. In contrast, zinc carbonate and zinc oxide are fairly insoluble. A comparison of zinc preparations suggested that zinc acetate was one of the best-tolerated zinc preparations when compared with zinc sulfate, zinc aminoate, zinc methionine, and zinc oxide; zinc oxide was least absorbed [36]. Zinc supplements are directed to be consumed on an empty stomach and without simultaneous ingestion of other mineral supplements. Gastric irritation is a common side effect.

Zinc lozenges are purported to assist in the treatment of colds. A meta-analysis of zinc salt lozenges and colds found no statistically significant benefit associated with the use of zinc lozenges for the treatment of colds [37]. However, several limitations were associated with the studies, and the use of zinc in the treatment of colds appears to require further study [37].

Toxicity

Excessive intakes of zinc can cause toxicity. An acute toxicity with 1 to 2 g zinc sulfate (225–450 mg zinc) can produce a metallic taste, nausea, vomiting, epigastric pain, abdominal cramps, and bloody diarrhea [26,31]. Chronic ingestion of zinc in amounts of about 40 mg (lower for some individuals) results in a copper deficiency [24–26,29,31]. The tolerable upper intake level for zinc has been set at 40 mg daily based on this interaction with copper [29].

Assessment of Nutriture

Evaluation of zinc nutriture is difficult owing to homeostatic control of body zinc. A variety of static indices have been used to assess zinc status, including measurements of zinc in red blood cells, leukocytes, neutrophils, and plasma or serum. The most common basis for assessment is serum or plasma zinc, with fasting concentrations <70 μg/dL suggesting deficiency [33]. Zinc (fasting) in the plasma decreases only when the dietary intake is so low that homeostasis cannot be established without use of zinc from the exchangeable pool that includes plasma zinc [33]. Low fasting plasma zinc thus indicates that little zinc is present in the exchangeable zinc pool and reflects a loss of zinc from bone and liver [34]. Interpretation of plasma zinc must be made with caution, because concentrations are influenced by many factors unrelated to zinc depletion, including meals, time of day (diurnal variation), stress, infection, hypoalbuminemia, steroid therapy, and oral contraceptive administration [38,39]. Postprandial zinc concentrations have been found to be more sensitive to low dietary zinc intakes than fasting plasma zinc concentrations [40].

Metallothionein also has been used to assess zinc status. Red blood cell (erythrocyte) concentrations of metallothionein appear to respond to changes in dietary zinc; however, the use of metallothionein as an indicator of zinc status requires additional study [41].

Urinary zinc and hair zinc have also been used to assess zinc status, but they are not valid indicators. Urinary zinc excretion remains fairly constant over a range of intakes and diminishes only with severe zinc deficiency. Low hair zinc may be associated with chronic intake of dietary zinc in suboptimal amounts; however, the concentration of zinc in hair depends not only on delivery of zinc to the root but also on the rate of hair growth, which is affected by other conditions (including protein status). Additional research and the development of standardized procedures (to eliminate contamination from, for example, shampoo and confounding variables such as variations due to hair color, sampling sites, etc.) are required before hair zinc may be useful for assessing zinc status.

Measurement of the activity of zinc-dependent enzymes also has been employed as an index of zinc status. Unfortunately, no enzyme is considered at present to be a valid and reliable indicator of zinc status. Studies using enzymes as indicators typically have measured carbonic anhydrase or alkaline phosphatase. Ideally, measurements of activity should be taken before and after zinc supplementation. An oral zinc tolerance test has been used to assess zinc absorption from different meals or supplements. This test typically involves ingestion of 25 or 50 mg zinc as zinc acetate with a test meal or supplement. Changes in plasma zinc concentration are assessed and compared in the same subjects following consumption of different test meals or supplements on different occasions under standardized conditions [42].

References Cited for Zinc

1. Hunt J, Matthys L, Johnson L. Zinc absorption, mineral balance, and blood lipids in women consuming controlled lacto-ovovegetarian and omnivorous diets for 8 wk. Am J Clin Nutr 1998;67:421–30.

2. Sturniolo GC, Montino MC, Rossetto L, Martin A, D'Inca R, D'Odorico A, Naccarato R. Inhibition of gastric acid secretion reduces zinc absorption in man. J Am Coll Nutr 1991;10:372–75.

3. Ellis R, Kelsay J, Reynolds R, Morris E, Moser P, Frazier C. Phytate: zinc and phytate × calcium: zinc millimolar ratios in self-selected diets of Americans, Asian Indians and Nepalese. J Am Diet Assoc 1987; 87:1043–47.

4. Simmer K, Iles CA, James C, Thompson R. Are iron folate supplements harmful? Am J Clin Nutr 1987;45:122–25.

5. Kauwell G, Bailey L, Gregory J, Bowling D, Cousins R. Zinc status is not adversely affected by folic acid supplementation and zinc intake does not impair folate utilization in human subjects. J Nutr 1995; 125:66–72.

6. Whittaker P. Iron and zinc interactions in humans. Am J Clin Nutr 1998;68:442S–46S.

7. Solomons N, Jacob R. Studies on the bioavailability of zinc in humans: effects of heme and nonheme iron on the absorption of zinc. Am J Clin Nutr 1981;34:475–82.

8. Spencer H. Minerals and mineral interactions in human beings. J Am Diet Assoc 1986;86:864–67.

9. Dawson-Hughes B, Seligson FH, Hughes VA. Effects of calcium carbonate and hydroxyapatite on zinc and iron retention in postmenopausal women. Am J Clin Nutr 1986;44:83–88.

10. McKenna A, Ilich J, Andon M, Wang C, Matkovic V. Zinc balance in adolescent females consuming a low- or high-calcium diet. Am J Clin Nutr 1997;65:1460–64.

11. Wood R, Zheng J. High dietary calcium intakes reduce zinc absorption and balance in humans. Am J Clin Nutr 1997;65:1803–9.

12. Prasad A. Clinical, biochemical and nutritional spectrum of zinc deficiency in human subjects: an update. Nutr Rev 1983;41:197–208.

13. DiSilvestro R, Cousins R. Physiological ligands for copper and zinc. Ann Rev Nutr 1983;3:261–88.

14. McMahon R, Cousins R. Mammalian zinc transporters. J Nutr 1998;128:667–70.

15. Cousins R, Lee-Ambrose L. Nuclear zinc uptake and interactions and metallothionein gene expression are influenced by dietary zinc in rats. J Nutr 1992;122:56–64.

16. Bremner I, Beattie J. Metallothionein and the trace minerals. Ann Rev Nutr 1990;10:63–83.

17. Bettger W, O'Dell B. Physiological roles of zinc in the plasma membrane of mammalian cells. J Nutr Biochem 1993;4:194–207.

18. Role of zinc in enzyme regulation and protection of essential thiol groups. Nutr Rev 1986;44:309–11.

19. Sato M, Bremner I. Oxygen free radicals and metallothionein. Medicine 1993;14:325–37.

20. Wada L, King J. Effect of low zinc intakes on basal metabolic rate, thyroid hormones and protein utilization in adult men. J Nutr 1986; 116:1045–53.

21. Miller L, Hambidge M, Naake V, Hong Z, Westcott J, Fennessey P. Size of the zinc pools that exchange rapidly with plasma zinc in humans: alternative techniques for measuring and relation to dietary zinc intake. J Nutr 1994;124:268–76.

22. Christian P, West K. Interactions between zinc and vitamin A: an update. Am J Clin Nutr 1998;68:435S–41S.

23. Bates J, McClain C. The effect of severe zinc deficiency on serum levels of albumin, transferrin, and prealbumin in man. Am J Clin Nutr 1981;34:1655–60.

24. Festa M, Anderson H, Dowdy R, Ellersieck M. Effect of zinc intake on copper excretion and retention in men. Am J Clin Nutr 1985; 41:285–92.

25. Fischer P, Giroux A, L'Abbe M. Effect of zinc supplementation on copper status in adult man. Am J Clin Nutr 1984;40:743–46.

26. Fosmire G. Zinc toxicity. Am J Clin Nutr 1990;51:225–27.

27. Hoffman H, Phyliky R, Fleming C. Zinc-induced copper deficiency. Gastroenterology 1988;94:508–12.

28. Sandstead H. Requirements and toxicity of essential trace elements, illustrated by zinc and copper. Am J Clin Nutr 1995; 61(suppl):621S–24S.

29. Food and Nutrition Board, Institute of Medicine. Dietary Reference Intakes. Washington, DC: National Academy Press, 2001, pp. 442–501.

30. Solomons N. Mineral interactions in the diet. J Dent Child 1982; 49:445–48.

31. National Research Council. Recommended Dietary Allowances, 10th ed. Washington, DC: National Academy Press, 1989, pp. 205–13.

32. Pennington J, Young B. Total diet study nutritional elements, 1982–1989. J Am Diet Assoc 1991;91:179–83.

33. King J. Assessment of zinc status. J Nutr 1990;120:1474–79.

34. Ploysangam A, Falciglia G, Brehm B. Effect of marginal zinc deficiency on human growth and development. J Trop Pediatr 1997; 43:192–98.

35. Baer M, King J, Tamura T, Margen S, Bradfield R, Weston W, Daugherty N. Nitrogen utilization, enzyme activity, glucose intolerance and leukocyte chemotaxis in human experimental zinc depletion. Am J Clin Nutr 1985;41:1220–35.

36. Prasad A, Beck F, Nowak J. Comparison of absorption of five zinc preparations in humans using oral zinc tolerance test. J Trace Elem Exp Med 1993;6:109–15.

37. Jackson J, Peterson C, Lesho E. A meta-analysis of zinc salt lozenges and the common cold. Arch Intern Med 1997;157:2372–76.

38. Wallock L, King J, Hambidge K, English-Westcott J, Pritts J. Meal-induced changes in plasma, erythrocyte, and urinary zinc concentrations in adult women. Am J Clin Nutr 1993;58:695–701.

39. King J, Hambidge K, Westcott J, Kern D, Marshall G. Daily variation in plasma zinc concentrations in women fed meals at six-hour intervals. J Nutr 1994;124:508–16.

40. Mellman D, Hambidge K, Westcott J. Effect of dietary zinc restriction on postprandial changes in plasma zinc. Am J Clin Nutr 1993; 58:702–4.

41. Thomas E, Bailey L, Kauwell G, Lee D, Cousins R. Erythrocyte metallothionein response to dietary zinc in humans. J Nutr 1992; 122:2408–14.

42. Henderson L, Brewer G, Dressman J, Swidan S, DuRoss D, Adair C, Barnett J, Berardi R. Use of zinc tolerance test and 24-hour urinary zinc content to assess oral zinc absorption. J Am Coll Nutr 1996; 15:79–83.

COPPER

The copper content of the human adult body is on the order of 50 to 150 mg. Copper is found in the body in either of two valence states, cuprous state (Cu^{1+}) or cupric state (Cu^{2+}).

Sources

The copper content of food varies widely, reflecting the origin of the food and the conditions under which the food was produced, handled, and prepared for use. The richest sources of copper are organ meats and shellfish, as shown in Table 12.5. Plant food sources rich in copper include nuts, seeds, legumes, and dried fruits. Potatoes and whole grains also are good sources of copper. In the United States, the median intake of copper from foods by adults is calculated to be 1,000 to 1,600 μg/day [1].

Endogenous sources of copper also may be found in the gastrointestinal tract. Copper is secreted daily into the gastrointestinal tract in digestive juices in relatively large amounts. For example, the copper contents of saliva and gastric juice are ~400 μg and 1,000 μg, respectively; pancreatic and duodenal juices may contain up to 1,300 μg and 2,200 μg, respectively [2].

Table 12.5 Copper Content of Selected Foods

Food/Food Group	Copper (mg/100 g)	Food/Food Group	Copper (mg/100 g)
Seafood		Meat and poultry	
Oysters	4.40	Liver	4.48
Crabmeat	0.64	Chicken	0.06
Shrimp	0.30	Beef, sirloin	0.15
Lobster	1.94	Pork	0.09
Eggs and dairy products		Legumes (cooked)	0.25
Eggs	0.02	Nuts and seeds	1.10–2.22
Milk	0.009	Fruits	
Cheeses	0.03	Fresh	0.04–1.11
Grains and cereals		Dried	0.19–0.34
Rice and pasta (cooked)	0.07–0.10	Vegetables	0.02–0.13
		Potatoes	0.20
Bread white/wheat	0.13/0.29		

Source: www.nal.usda.gov/fnic/foodcomp

Digestion, Absorption, Transport, Uptake, and Storage

Digestion

Most copper, primarily as Cu^{2+} but some as Cu^{1+}, in foods is bound to organic components, especially amino acids that make up food proteins. Thus, digestion is needed to free the bound copper before absorption can occur. Gastric hydrochloric acid and pepsin facilitate the release of bound copper in the stomach. Additional proteolytic enzymes in the small intestine may hydrolyze proteins to further release copper. Copper digestion is shown in Figure 12.12.

Absorption

Although copper is absorbed throughout the small intestine, especially the duodenum, the stomach also appears to possess some absorptive capacity. This may be attributable to the solubilizing effect of the acidic environment on copper, which facilitates its transport across the gastric mucosa. However, compared to intestinal copper absorption, gastric copper absorption contributes relatively little to overall absorption.

The mechanisms for the absorption of copper across the brush border of the small intestine are not completely understood. It is possible that luminal copper

Figure 12.12 Overview of copper digestion, absorption, enterocyte metabolism, and transport.

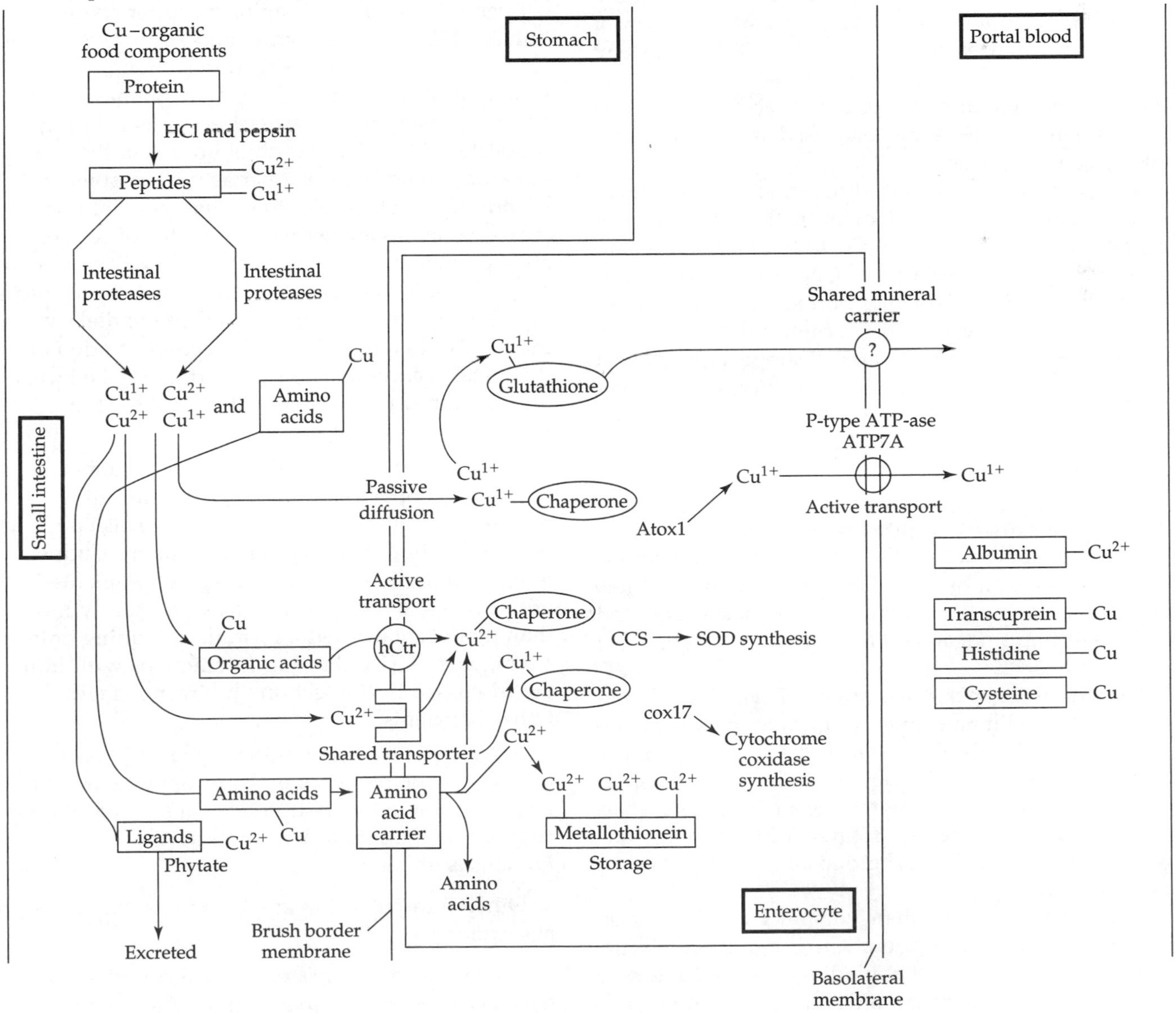

must be bound to more absorbable ligands for effective transport. Even if copper is transported in the free ionic form, the presence of such ligands may be needed in order to present the metal to brush border receptors in a way that increases uptake.

Copper appears to be absorbed both by active carrier-mediated transporters and by a nonsaturable, passive diffusion process (Fig. 12.12). As is true for other transport systems, low concentrations of dietary copper are transported primarily via the active carrier-mediated pathway, whereas the diffusion process accommodates higher concentrations. Examples of copper transporters include hCtr1, 2, and 3. The hCtr1 transporter has been demonstrated in several body tissues, with the highest expression in the liver, heart, and pancreas and intermediate expression in the intestine [3–6]. Natural resistance associated macrophage protein (nramp 2) and divalent cation/mineral transporter 1 (DC/MT), a possible isoform of nramp, also may transport Cu^{2+} to a limited extent; however, Fe^{2+}, Zn^{2+}, and Mn^{2+} are favored over copper. Copper may also utilize amino acid active transport systems, such as the one used by histidine, for absorption.

Typically, the gastrointestinal tract absorbs over 50% of ingested copper. However, the percentage of copper absorbed is influenced by copper status and dietary copper availability. Copper absorption is significantly higher during periods of low dietary copper than during periods of higher dietary copper. Absorption, for example, may average only 20% at copper intakes of >5 mg/day but increases to over 50% at intakes of <1 mg/day [2,7–9]. Copper absorption was calculated at 75% based on intakes of ~350 μg [1,9].

Factors Influencing Copper Absorption

Copper transport across the brush border membrane may be influenced by a variety of dietary components, with some having a positive effect on absorption and others exerting a negative influence.

Enhancers of Copper Absorption. Examples of substances that facilitate copper absorption include amino acids, especially histidine, which may bind to copper and allow absorption through an amino acid transport system, as well as sulfur-containing amino acids such as methionine and cysteine. Copper also forms ligands with amino acid sulfhydryl groups in compounds such as glutathione.

Organic acids, other than vitamin C, in foods also improve copper absorption. Citric, gluconic, lactic, acetic, and malic acids act as binding ligands to improve solubilization of copper and thus absorption [10]. Citrate has been shown to form a stable complex with copper to improve its absorption.

Inhibitors of Copper Absorption. Many substances diminish copper absorption, including some substances in food.

- *Phytate* (inositol hexaphosphate or inositol polyphosphate; see Fig. 12.9), found mainly in plant foods (cereals, legumes), is a known inhibitor of copper (among other minerals, including iron, zinc, and calcium).

In addition to substances in foods, several trace minerals typically ingested in supplement forms are known to impede copper absorption.

- *Zinc* in amounts as low as 18.5 mg but typically in amounts over 40 mg has been shown to impair copper absorption and diminish copper status in humans [11–15]. The detrimental effect of excessive zinc intake on copper absorption is thought to result from zinc's stimulation of thionein synthesis. Thionein, a protein that possesses an unusually high proportion (25%–30%) of thiol groups in the form of cysteine, avidly binds copper as well as other metals to form metallothionein. Intestinal metallothionein may function as a negative modulator of copper absorption and, in this respect, act as a "detoxifying agent," binding copper and reducing its transmucosal flux (passage into the plasma) when the dietary intake and therefore the luminal concentration of the metal is excessive [16]. At normal intake levels of copper, however, the regulatory role of the protein remains unclear.
- *Iron* ingested in relatively large amounts decreases copper absorption in both rats and humans [17–20]. Excessive iron intake also appears to impede copper absorption in humans. Copper absorption in infants fed formula supplemented with iron (10.8 mg iron/L) was significantly lower than that of infants fed a formula providing only 1.8 mg iron/L [18]. Further interactions with iron are discussed in the section "Interactions with Other Nutrients."
- *Molybdenum* as tetrathiomolybdate $(MoS_4)^{2-}$ forms an insoluble complex with copper to inhibit its absorption in the gastrointestinal tract of rats and ruminants. The significance of these findings for humans is unknown.

Other nutrients also are known to impair copper absorption.

- *Calcium* and *phosphorus*, two major minerals, have been shown to impair copper absorption.

Calcium (2,382 mg as calcium gluconate) and phosphorus (2,442 mg as glycerol phosphate) were shown to increase fecal copper excretion compared with diets containing only moderate amounts of calcium (780 mg as calcium gluconate) with either high phosphorus (2,442 mg as glycerol phosphate) or moderate phosphorus (843 mg as glycerol phosphate) [19]. Urinary copper losses were also significantly greater on the high-calcium, high-phosphorus diet than on the moderate-calcium, moderate-phosphorus diet [19].

- Vitamin C may interact with copper to decrease its absorption. Presumably, vitamin C reduces copper from a cupric state (Cu^{2+}) to a less absorbable cuprous state (Cu^{1+}) [20,21]. Vitamin C has also been suggested to decrease copper retention.
- Excessive antacid ingestion may diminish copper absorption and induce deficiency. Copper at a neutral pH will bind to hydroxides (OH), forming insoluble compounds that are not readily absorbable.

Other factors also appear to influence copper absorption, including the body's copper status. The efficiency of absorption of copper changes to regulate in part whole-body copper status. Changes in fecal excretion also mediate the process. Thus, with high copper intake, less copper is absorbed. As body copper stores increase, copper excretion via the bile increases. Moderately low copper intakes result in the reverse (increased absorption, decreased excretion) to some extent. With copper intakes of ~0.38 mg/day, regulation does not sufficiently compensate to prevent depletion of body copper [7].

Intestinal Cell Use

Once within the intestinal cell, copper may be stored, used by the cell, or transported through the cell for subsequent transport across the basolateral membrane. Storage of copper occurs as part of metallothionein (see p. 440 for a description of metallothionein). Unless released from storage, this copper will be lost with intestinal cell turnover, approximately every 2 to 3 days. In addition to intestinal cell use and storage, some copper will be transported across the enterocyte's cytosol for export across the basolateral membrane into the plasma.

Intracellular copper transport is not well characterized. Like iron, however, free copper ions may damage cells through nonenzymatic Fenton and Haber Weiss reactions (see p. 430). Consequently, copper is found in the body typically bound to proteins. Amino acids and glutathione (a tripeptide composed of glycine, cysteine, and glutamate) are proposed copper (Cu^{1+}) carriers. In addition, **chaperones** (soluble intracellular proteins) function to bind intracellular copper and deliver it to various locations. Several chaperones have been identified, including cox17, atox1 (also referred to as hAtx or Hah1), and CCS (copper chaperone for superoxide dismutase). Cox17 is thought to transport Cu^{1+} for cytochrome c oxidase synthesis, while CCS delivers copper for the synthesis of superoxide dismutase (SOD) [3–6]. Atox1 ferries Cu^{1+} to cytosolic P (phosphorylation)-type ATPases necessary for cellular export of copper.

Copper transport across the intestinal cell's basolateral membrane into the plasma is thought to occur primarily by active transport via a P-type ATPase referred to as ATP7A [22–24]. Generally, ATPase transporters carry metals in their reduced state; however, whether this is true for copper transport is unclear. Mutations in the ATP7A gene are thought to result in Menkes' disease, a disorder characterized by defective copper transport, especially in the intestine and brain where the ATP7A typically functions. Individuals with Menkes' disease have increased intestinal cell copper concentrations and impaired delivery of copper to peripheral tissues. The condition is also characterized by vascular and neurological problems that are only partially alleviated by intravenous administration of copper.

Transport and Uptake

From the intestinal cell, copper is transported in portal blood to the liver bound loosely to albumin. Specifically, the N-terminus of albumin has a high affinity for copper (Cu^{2+}). Copper also may be transported bound to transcuprein (Tc) and to amino acids such as histidine and cysteine [23] (Figs. 12.12 and 12.13).

The observations that the uptake of copper by hepatocytes is a saturable, temperature-dependent process and that no competition with other metal ions occurs suggest a specific, facilitated diffusion mechanism. Transport across the cell membrane may involve the formation of certain amino acid–copper complexes and may also involve albumin [24].

Once within cells, more than half of the accumulated copper is found in the supernatant fraction and one-fourth within the nuclei. Copper first appears to bind to metallothionein and then is slowly transferred to the copper enzymes, especially apoceruloplasmin. Six copper ions (in the form of Cu^{1+} and Cu^{2+}) are attached posttranslationally to apoceruloplasmin to form ceruloplasmin (Fig. 12.13) [25,26]. Three of the six copper atoms are involved in electron transfer, while the other three function at the catalytic site and give the protein a blue color. Although copper does not appear to influence apoceruloplasmin synthesis,

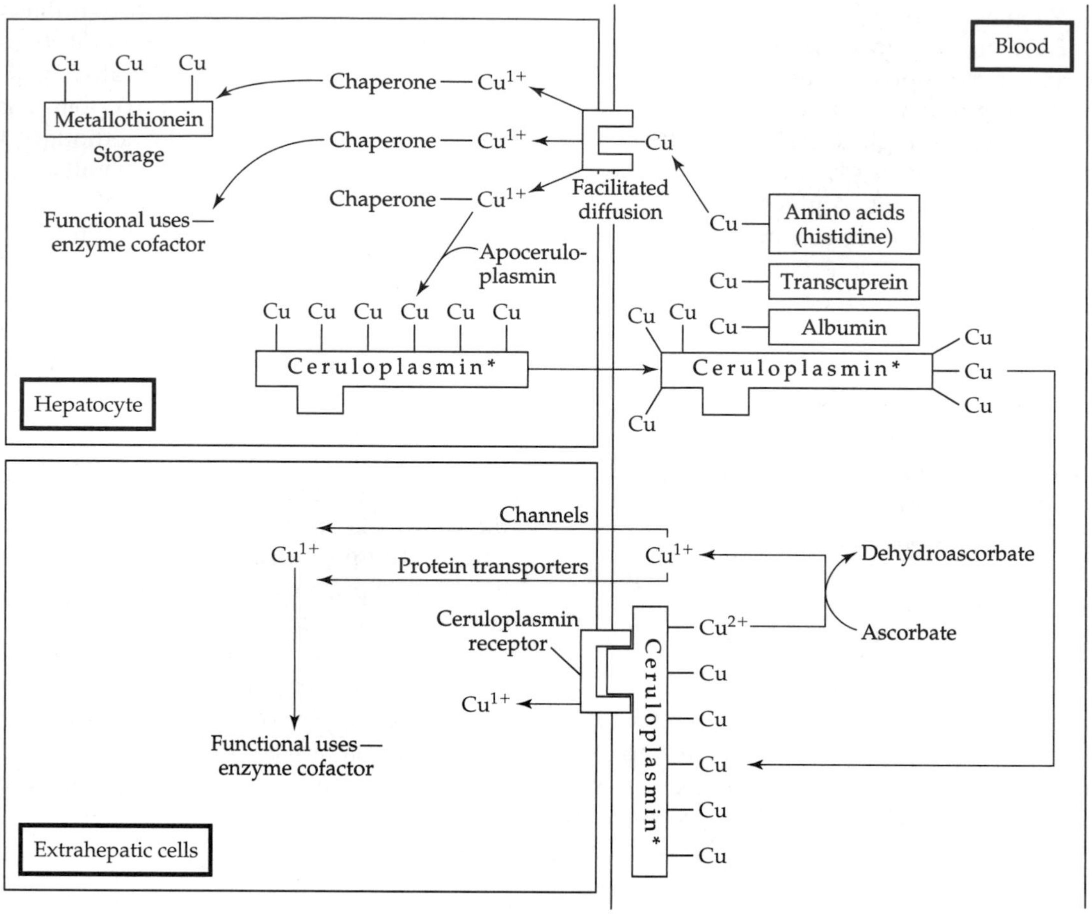

*Ceruloplasmin contains six sites for copper in either the Cu^{1+} or Cu^{2+} oxidation state.

Figure 12.13 Transport, uptake, and metabolism of copper in hepatocytes and extrahepatic cells.

ceruloplasmin activity is diminished or absent without sufficient copper, and ceruloplasmin's half-life is shortened.

Ceruloplasmin is released into the blood from the liver and constitutes about 60% (or perhaps up to 95%) of circulating copper in the blood after meals [10, 26–28]. The remaining copper in the blood circulates loosely bound to albumin, transcuprein, and histidine [25,29]. The basic aspects of mammalian copper metabolism are summarized in Figure 12.13.

Ceruloplasmin delivers copper to tissues. Uptake of ceruloplasmin copper by extrahepatic cells involves binding of ceruloplasmin to specific receptors [28]. The copper ions that are not at ceruloplasmin's active oxidase site are released [26]. Release is thought to involve the reduction of copper from Cu^{2+} to Cu^{1+}. Following dissociation from the ceruloplasmin, copper enters the cell either directly through channels or after binding protein transporters such as hCtrl, 2, or 3. Ascorbic acid enhances copper transfer and is probably involved in the reduction of the copper (Fig. 12.13) [28].

Storage

Compared to other trace minerals, little copper (<~150 mg) is found in the body. What copper is found in the body is found within a variety of cells and tissues. Following intake, both the liver and the kidney rapidly extract copper from the blood. Other copper-containing tissues include the brain, heart, bone, muscle, skin, intestine, spleen, hair, and nails.

Within cells and tissues, copper is bound to amino acids or proteins. The liver appears to be the main storage site for copper, which is thought to be bound to metallothionein. Copper positively influences hepatic and renal, but not intestinal, thionein synthesis. Metallothionein, in addition to storing up to about 12 copper atoms (as well as zinc atoms), protects cells by scavenging damaging superoxide and hydroxyl radicals. The amount of copper available to extrahepatic tissues is thought to be regulated by the liver through the synthesis of ceruloplasmin, through copper incorporation into metallothionein, and through excretion of copper into the bile.

Functions and Mechanisms of Action

The essentiality of copper is due, in part, to its participation as an enzyme cofactor and as an allosteric component of enzymes. Several copper-requiring metalloenzymes and the reactions they catalyze are described next. In many enzymes, copper functions as an intermediate in electron transfer.

Ceruloplasmin

Ceruloplasmin, an α-2 glycoprotein, is not simply a transporter of copper in the blood. It is also a multifaceted oxidative enzyme (oxidase) and antioxidant that may be found in the blood but also may be found bound to cell surface receptors on the plasma membranes of cells. Ceruloplasmin, also known as ferroxidase I, is responsible for the oxidation of minerals, most notably ferrous (Fe^{2+}) iron but also manganese (Mn^{2+}). The oxidation of Fe^{2+} to Fe^{3+} is needed in order for iron to bind to transferrin for transport to tissues such as the bone marrow.

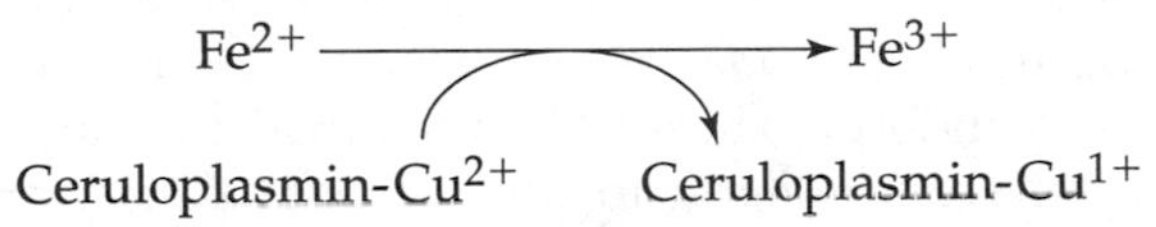

Another proposed function of ceruloplasmin is as a modulator of the inflammatory process and a scavenger of oxygen radicals to protect cells. As a modulator of the inflammatory process, many proteins, including ceruloplasmin, serve as acute-phase proteins. Acute-phase proteins rise in the blood with, for example, infection or other inflammatory events (injury). This rise in the blood is important, because during infections phagocytosis of invading organisms by white blood cells generates superoxide radicals, among other damaging compounds. These compounds are normally generated, but they are generated in larger amounts with inflammation and must be eliminated (by ceruloplasmin, superoxide dismutase, or other enzymes) to prevent further damage to body cells.

Superoxide Dismutase

Superoxide dismutase (SOD), found both in the cytosol of cells and extracellularly, is copper- and zinc-dependent (another form in the mitochondria is manganese-dependent). In the enzyme, copper is thought to be linked with zinc through an imidiazole group, and both minerals are linked to the enzyme protein via histidine and aspartate residues. Copper (Cu^{2+}) is found at the enzyme's active site, where the superoxide substrate binds to the enzyme. Removal of copper, but not zinc, results in reduced cytosolic SOD activity but has no effect on the enzyme's synthesis [29]. Specifically, superoxide dismutase catalyzes the removal (dismutation) of the superoxide radicals (O_2^-). During the reaction, copper is reduced along with the oxygen radical to initially generate molecular oxygen (O_2) and then, by reoxidation, hydrogen peroxide (H_2O_2) [29].

$$2O_2^- + 2H^+ \xrightarrow{\text{Superoxide dismutase}} O_2 + H_2O_2$$

Superoxide radicals can cause peroxidative damage of phospholipid components of cell membranes. In other words, without SOD, superoxide radicals can form more destructive hydroxyl radicals that damage both unsaturated double bonds in cell membranes, fatty acids, and other molecules in cells (see the perspective in Chap. 10). SOD therefore assumes a very important protective function. SOD is found in the cytosol of most cells of the body. Extracellular SOD is secreted and bound to heparan sulfate on the surface of cells and is found in relatively large concentrations in the arterial wall, where it may serve an important role in antioxidant defense (among other possible functions). Increased peroxidation of cell membranes is found with copper deficiency.

Cytochrome c Oxidase

Cytochrome c oxidase contains three copper atoms per molecule. One subunit of the enzyme contains two copper atoms and functions in electron transfer. The second subunit contains another copper atom involved in reducing molecular oxygen. Cytochrome c oxidase functions in the terminal oxidative step in mitochondrial electron transport (p. 66). Specifically, the enzyme transfers an electron such that molecular oxygen (O_2) is reduced to form water molecules and enough free energy is generated to permit ATP production. Severe copper deficiency ultimately impairs the activity of this enzyme.

Amine Oxidases

Amine oxidases are also copper-dependent. Copper appears to function as an allosteric structural component of these enzymes, and TOPA quinone (6-hydroxydopa) serves as an organic cofactor [30]. Histidine residues in the enzyme serve as ligands for the copper. Amine oxidases, found both in the blood and in body tissues, catalyze the oxidation of biogenic amines such as tyramine, histamine, and dopamine to form aldehydes and ammonium ions (NH_4 is generated from the cleaved amine group).

In the reaction, oxygen (O_2) is reduced to form hydrogen peroxide (H_2O_2). Other amino substrates include serotonin (5-hydroxytryptamine), norepinephrine, and polyamines.

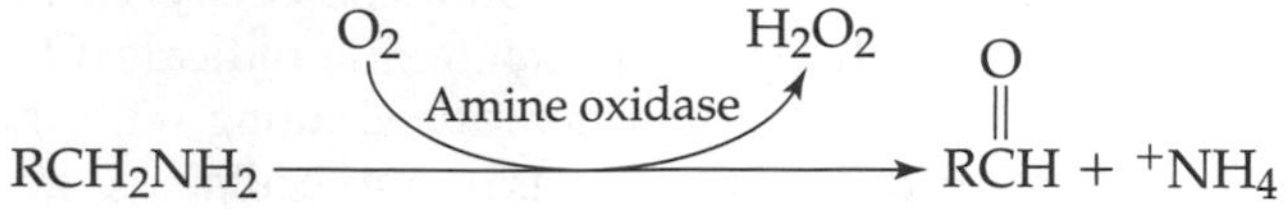

Tyrosine Metabolism—Dopamine Monooxygenase and p-hydroxyphenylpyruvate Hydroxylase

In tyrosine metabolism (Fig. 9.6, p. 267), norepinephrine and homogentisate production are both copper-dependent. Norepinephrine synthesis begins with tyrosine, which is converted in an iron-dependent reaction to 3,4-dihydroxyphenylalanine (also called L-dopa). The L-dopa is further metabolized to dopamine. It is from dopamine that norepinephrine is made via dopamine monooxygenase. This enzyme contains up to eight copper atoms per molecule and requires molecular oxygen and vitamin C for its function, as shown.

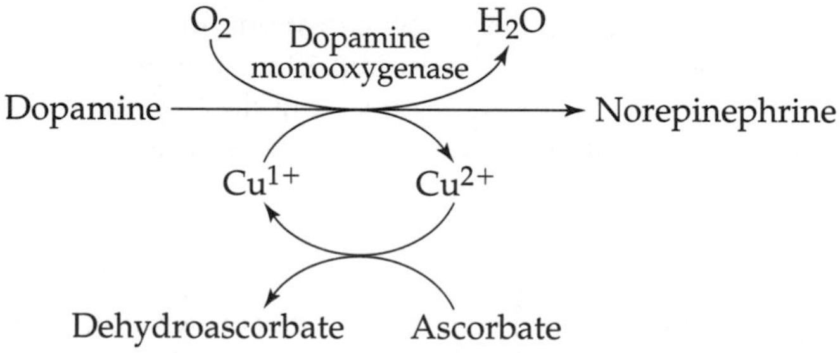

In tyrosine catabolism (Fig. 9.6, p. 267), the conversion of p-hydroxyphenylpyruvate to homogentisate also requires a copper-dependent hydroxylase and vitamin C, as shown.

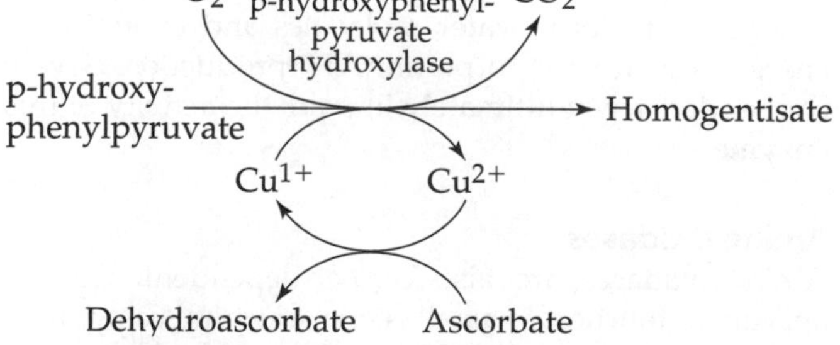

Lysyl Oxidase

Lysyl oxidase is secreted by connective tissue cells (bone, blood vessels, etc.) and serves to generate cross-linking between connective tissue proteins, including collagen and elastin. Specifically, lysyl oxidase catalyzes the removal of the epsilon amino group (oxidative deamination) of lysyl and hydroxylysyl residues of a collagen or elastin polypeptide and the oxidation of the terminal carbon atom of an aldehyde to form cross-links. The cross-linking is needed to stabilize the extracellular matrix. Lysyl oxidase activity decreases with inadequate copper intake, negatively impacting connective tissues [31].

Peptidylglycine α-amidating Monooxygenase

Amidation of peptide hormones, such as bombesin, calcitonin, gastrin, and cholecystokinin, is necessary for hormone function. The amidation requires a copper-dependent enzyme known as peptidylglycine α-amidating monooxygenase, which is found mostly in the brain. This enzyme cleaves a carboxy terminal glycine residue off peptides that have a C-terminal glycine. The amino group of glycine is retained by the peptide as a terminal amide. The oxidized residue is released as glyoxylate. Peptidylglycine α-amidating monooxygenase also requires vitamin C to reduce Cu^{2+} back to Cu^{1+}. This reaction is shown in Figure 9.8.

Other Roles

Copper plays a variety of other roles in the body that are not well understood; these roles may or may not involve enzymes. Some of these other roles include angiogenesis, immune system function, nerve myelination, and endorphin action. As a pro-oxidant, copper (if free) behaves similarly to iron. Copper (Cu^{2+}) reacts with superoxide radicals and catalyzes the formation of hydroxyl radicals through the Fenton reaction:

$$O_2^- + Cu^{2+} \longrightarrow O_2 + Cu^{1+}$$

$$Cu^{1+} + H_2O_2 \longrightarrow Cu^{2+} + OH^- + {}^{\cdot}OH$$

Associated with the generation of reactive oxygen species is increased oxidative damage to DNA (base oxidation and strand breaks), proteins, and lipids (peroxidation), especially membrane lipids.

Copper influences gene expression through binding to specific transcription factors, also called binding proteins. In some cases, copper has been shown to influence transcription by binding to transcription factors that in turn bind to promoter sequences on DNA. Once the Cu-bound transcription factors are bound to DNA, transcription may be enhanced or suppressed.

Interactions with Other Nutrients

Copper is known to interact with a number of inorganic and organic dietary constituents. Those that affect copper absorption have been discussed previously (p. 448). Additional interactions will be mentioned in this section.

Among organic dietary substances, ascorbic acid (1.5 g for 64 days) resulted in decreased serum ceruloplasmin activity; however, concentrations remained within the normal range [20]. Intakes of 605 mg vitamin C for 3 weeks also resulted in a 21% decrease in serum ceruloplasmin oxidase activity [21]. The effects of vitamin C may be mediated through the reduction of the cupric ion to its cuprous form by the ascorbate or through the formation of a poorly absorbable complex, or both.

It is well established that a strong, mutual antagonism exists between copper and zinc, most likely caused by the induction of intestinal metallothionein by zinc. This results in excessive intracellular binding of the copper, reducing its luminal-to-serosal (e.g., from the lumen of the gastrointestinal tract across the basolateral membrane) flux, and entry into the blood. Zinc intakes ranging from 18.5 to 300 mg daily have resulted in a copper deficiency [11–15]. Furthermore, copper deficiency induced by intakes of zinc (110–165 mg) for 10 months did not respond to cessation of zinc and 2 months of oral copper supplementation. Cupric chloride given intravenously for 5 days (total dose, 10 mg) was needed to correct the deficiency, suggesting that elimination of excess zinc by the body is a slow process and continues to inhibit copper absorption until it is eliminated [14].

Another interaction of copper of practical importance involves iron. The importance of copper in normal iron metabolism is evidenced by the anemia that results from prolonged copper deficiency. It is known that the anemia is caused by an impaired mobilization and use of iron due to the reduced ferroxidase activity of ceruloplasmin, which is responsible for oxidation of iron to its trivalent (Fe^{3+}) state. Only as Fe^{3+} can iron be bound to its transport protein, transferrin. High iron intakes appear to interfere with copper mobilization from stores, copper use in the body, and copper absorption in infants and children [17,18,32,33].

As discussed in brief regarding factors inhibiting copper absorption, in animals (ruminants and rats) dietary copper forms insoluble complexes with molybdenum and sulfur in the form of tetrathiomolybdate $(MoS_4)^{2-}$. While such findings have not been reported in humans, urinary copper excretion in humans has been shown to rise from 24 to 77 μg/day as molybdenum intake increased from 160 to 1,540 μg/day [8]. No changes in fecal copper excretion were noted, suggesting that molybdenum may have increased copper mobilization from tissues and promoted excretion [8].

Copper and selenium also appear to interact. Copper deficiency has been shown to decrease the activity of the selenium-dependent enzymes glutathione peroxidase and 5′-deiodinase [34,35]. Antagonistic interactions of copper with cadmium, silver, and mercury have been reported but have more theoretical than practical importance.

Excretion

Most absorbed copper is secreted by the liver into the bile for excretion in the feces. Dietary copper intake directly influences biliary copper excretion such that low dietary copper intake results in low fecal copper excretion [7]. In other words, biliary copper excretion is regulated to maintain copper balance. Wilson's disease, an inherited disorder of copper metabolism, is characterized by defective biliary copper excretion. Consequently, copper accumulates mainly in the liver but also in other organs, including the brain, kidney, eye (cornea), and spleen. With typical copper intakes, endogenous fecal copper excretion is $<\sim 300$ μg/day [1].

Only a small amount of copper (<20 μg) is excreted through the kidneys via the urine. Furthermore, urinary copper excretion does not change significantly with changes in copper intake except under extreme conditions [36].

Similarly, only small amounts (<50 μg) of copper are lost in sweat and with desquamation of skin cells, and dermal excretion does not significantly change with changes in intake. Women experience trace losses of copper via normal menstrual flow; however, a woman's copper status, unlike her iron status, is not compromised by menstruation. Trace amounts of copper also are lost with loss of hair and nails and, in males, in semen. Together, losses from menses or semen, along with losses from hair and nails, are not thought to exceed surface losses [1].

Recommended Dietary Allowances

A recommendation for an estimated safe and adequate daily dietary intake (ESADDI) for copper was first made in the 1980 RDAs. The 1989 estimated safe and adequate range for copper intake for adults was 1.5 to 3 mg/day [37]. Over the past decade, results of depletion and repletion studies, along with other studies permitting factorial analysis of obligatory losses over a range of intake, have enabled an estimate of copper requirements to be made. The requirement for copper for adult men and women was determined to be 700 μg [1]. The RDA for copper for adult men and women was set at 900 μg/day, based on a 30% coefficient of variation of the requirement and rounding to the nearest 100 μg [1]. Recommendations during pregnancy and lactation are 1,000 μg and 1,300 μg, respectively [1]. RDAs for copper for other age groups are found on the inside cover of the book.

Deficiency

Various clinical manifestations are associated with human copper deficiency. Recognized manifestations include hypochromic anemia, leukopenia (specifically, neutropenia, a lower-than-normal number of neutrophils), hypopigmentation or depigmentation of skin and hair, impaired immune function, bone abnormalities (especially demineralization), and cardiovascular and pulmonary dysfunction [38,39]. Changes in cholesterol concentrations have been reported in some but not all studies [40–42].

The likelihood of copper deficiency increases in persons consuming excessive amounts of zinc (40 mg/day) or antacids as well as in persons with conditions that promote increased loss of copper from the body, as occurs with nephrosis or gastrointestinal malabsorptive disorders such as celiac disease, tropical sprue, and inflammatory bowel diseases.

Toxicity

Copper toxicity (toxicosis) is fairly rare in the United States, although acute poisonings have occurred because of water contamination or accidental ingestion. Copper intakes of 64 mg (250 mg copper sulfate) have resulted in nausea, vomiting, and diarrhea. Other symptoms of toxicity include hematuria (blood in urine), jaundice, oliguria (little urine production), or anuria (no urine production) [43]. Copper is lethal in amounts about 1,000 times normal dietary intake [44].

Wilson's disease, a genetic disorder characterized by copper toxicity, results from mutation(s) in the gene coding for ATP7B in hepatocytes [22]. The absence or dysfunction of ATP7B disrupts copper movement through the Golgi network into bile and into the secretory pathway for incorporation into selected proteins. In Wilson's disease, copper accumulates in organs, resulting in disturbed function of organs, especially the liver, kidney, and brain. Kayser-Fleischer (greenish gold) rings due to copper deposition also are visible in the cornea. At present, treatment of Wilson's disease involves avoidance of high-copper foods along with D-penicillamine therapy to bind body copper and increase its excretion [45]. Zinc supplements (>40 mg daily) along with tetrathiomolybdate also may be recommended to decrease copper absorption.

Supplements

The main form of copper used in mineral-fortified food products is copper sulfate; however, cupric oxide is still found in many vitamin-mineral supplements for humans [46]. The use of cupric oxide as a source of copper is discouraged because the copper has been shown to be unavailable for absorption from the gastrointestinal tract of animals; in fact, it is no longer used as a copper supplement in animal nutrition [46]. In addition to copper sulfate (~25% copper), other bioavailable and water-soluble forms of copper include cupric chloride (~47% copper), cupric acetate (~35% copper), and copper carbonate (~57% copper) [46].

Assessment of Nutriture

Assessment of copper status is best made using multiple indicators. Serum, plasma, or red blood cell copper is frequently used, but these indicators are likely inadequate to assess short-term changes in copper status. The lower end of the normal range for serum copper concentrations is reported to be 10 μmol/L. The change in plasma or serum copper concentration that occurs when subjects consume inadequate copper is quite variable between individuals and is further affected by several factors unrelated to diet. Extremely low copper intake (~0.38 mg/day), however, appears to be sufficient to significantly decrease not only plasma copper but also ceruloplasmin concentration and activity as well as urinary copper excretion [47]. Many other studies also have shown decreases in serum ceruloplasmin concentrations and activity with copper deficiency. The lower end of the normal range for serum ceruloplasmin is 180 mg/L, although levels <20 mg/L have been reported with copper deficiency [48,49]. The ratio of ceruloplasmin enzyme activity to protein concentration is thought to be better than either measurement alone [50,51].

Response of serum ceruloplasmin to copper supplements also may be used to assess copper status. Typically, supplemental copper results in normalization of serum copper and neutrophil count followed by serum ceruloplasmin [38]. Ceruloplasmin increases following supplementation only in copper-deficient subjects. Another useful indicator of copper status is measurement of the activity of copper-dependent enzymes such as superoxide dismutase (SOD) (normal 0.47–0.067 mg/g) in the red blood cell. SOD activity is sensitive to longer-term copper deficiency [48]. Platelet copper concentrations, along with platelet or leukocyte cytochrome c oxidase or skin lysyl oxidase activity, also have shown response to changes in copper status.

Hair copper concentrations have not been shown to correlate with either serum or organ copper, yet they are reduced with a prolonged period of copper deficiency. Hair copper concentrations are not thought to be useful indicators of copper status, nor is urinary copper excretion, which normally is very low and is responsive to change only when intake is so low that other indicators have already declined [48].

References Cited for Copper

1. Food and Nutrition Board, Institute of Medicine. Dietary Reference Intakes. Washington, DC: National Academy Press, 2001, pp. 224–57.

2. Linder M, Hazegh-Azam M. Copper biochemistry and molecular biology. Am J Clin Nutr 1996;63:797S–811S.

3. Huffman DL, O'Halloran TVO. Function, structure, and mechanism of intracellular copper trafficking proteins. Annu Rev Biochem 2001;70:677–701.

4. Harrison MD, Jones CE, Dameron CT. Copper chaperones: function, structure and copper-binding properties. JBIC 1999;4:145–53.

5. Cullotta VC, Lin SJ, Schmidt P, Lomp LW, Casareno RL, Gitlin J. Intracellular pathways of copper trafficking in yeast and humans. Adv Exp Med Biol 1999;448:247–54.

6. Rosenzweig AC. Copper delivery by metallochaperone proteins. Acc Chem Res 2001;34:119–28.

7. Turnlund J, Keyes W, Peiffer G, Scott K. Copper absorption, excretion, and retention by young men consuming low dietary copper determined using stable isotope ^{65}Cu. Am J Clin Nutr 1998; 67:1219–25.

8. Turnlund J. Copper nutriture, bioavailability, and the influence of dietary factors. J Am Diet Assoc 1988;88:303–8.

9. Johnson P, Milne D, Lykken G. Effects of age and sex on copper absorption, biological half-life, and status in humans. Am J Clin Nutr 1992;56:917–25.

10. DiSilvestro R, Cousins R. Physiological ligands for copper and zinc. Ann Rev Nutr 1983;3:261–88.

11. Festa M, Anderson H, Dowdy R, Ellersieck M. Effect of zinc intake on copper excretion and retention in men. Am J Clin Nutr 1985; 41:285–92.

12. Fischer P, Giroux A, L'Abbe M. Effect of zinc supplementation on copper status in adult man. Am J Clin Nutr 1984;40:743–46.

13. Fosmire G. Zinc toxicity. Am J Clin Nutr 1990;51:225–27.

14. Hoffman H, Phyliky R, Fleming C. Zinc-induced copper deficiency. Gastroenterology 1988;94:508–12.

15. Sandstead H. Requirements and toxicity of essential trace elements, illustrated by zinc and copper. Am J Clin Nutr 1995; 61(suppl):621S–24S.

16. Cousins R. Absorption, transport and hepatic metabolism of copper and zinc: special reference to metallothionein and ceruloplasmin. Physiol Rev 1985;65:238–44.

17. Yu S, West C, Beynen A. Increasing intakes of iron reduce status, absorption and biliary excretion of copper in rats. Brit J Nutr 1994; 71:887–95.

18. Haschke F, Ziegler E, Edwards B, Fomon S. Effect of iron fortification of infant formula on trace minerals absorption. J Pediatr Gastroenterol Nutr 1986;5:768–73.

19. Snedeker S, Smith S, Greger J. Effect of dietary calcium and phosphorus levels on the utilization of iron, copper, and zinc by adult males. J Nutr 1982;112:136–43.

20. Finley E, Cerklewski F. Influence of ascorbic acid supplementation on copper status in young adult men. Am J Clin Nutr 1983; 37:553–56.

21. Jacob R, Skala J, Omaye S, Turnlund J. Effect of varying ascorbic acid intakes on copper absorption and ceruloplasmin levels of young men. J Nutr 1987;117:2109–15.

22. Bingham M, Ong T, Summer K, Middleton R, McArdle H. Physiologic function of the Wilson disease gene product, ATP7B. Am J Clin Nutr 1998;67(suppl):982S–87S.

23. Linder MC, Wooten L, Cerveza P, Cotton S, Shulze R, Lomeli N. Copper transport. Am J Clin Nutr 1998;67(suppl):965S–71S.

24. Harris E. The transport of copper. In: Prasad AS, ed. Essential and Toxic Trace Elements in Human Health and Disease: An Update. New York: Wiley-Liss, 1993, pp. 163–79.

25. Hellman NE, Gitlin JD. Ceruloplasmin metabolism and function. Ann Rev Nutr 2002;22:439–58.

26. Zaitseva I, Zaitsev V, Card G, Moshkov K, Bax B, Ralph A, Lindley P. The X-ray nature of human serum ceruloplasmin at 3.1 A: nature of the copper centres. J Biol Inorg Chem 1996;1:15–23.

27. Scott K, Turnlund J. Compartmental model of copper metabolism in adult men. J Nutr Biochem 1994;5:342–50.

28. Percival S, Harris E. Copper transport from ceruloplasmin: characterization of the cellular uptake mechanisms. Am J Physiol 1990; 258:C140–46.

29. Harris E. Copper as a cofactor and regulator of copper, zinc, superoxide dismutase. J Nutr 1992;123:636–40.

30. Mu D, Medzihradszky K, Adams G, Mayer P, Hines W, Burlingame A, Smith A, Cai D, Klinman J. Primary structures for a mammalian cellular and serum copper amine oxidase. J Biol Chem 1994;269:9926–32.

31. Werman M, Bhathena S, Turnlund J. Dietary copper intake influences skin lysyl oxidase in young men. J Nutr Biochem 1997;8:201–4.

32. Barclay S, Aggett P, Lloyd D, Duffty P. Reduced erythrocyte superoxide dismutase activity in low birth weight infants given iron supplements. Pediatr Res 1991;29:297–301.

33. Morais MB, Fisberg M, Suzuki HV, Amancio OMS, Machado NL. Effects of oral iron therapy on serum copper and serum ceruloplasmin in children. J Trop Pediatr 1994;40:51–52.

34. Olin K, Walter R, Keen C. Copper deficiency affects selenoglutathione peroxidase and selenodeiodinase activities and antioxidant defense in weanling rats. Am J Clin Nutr 1994;59:654–58.

35. Jenkinson S, Lawrence R, Burk R, Williams D. Effects of copper deficiency on the activity of the selenoenzyme glutathione peroxidase and on excretion and tissue retention of $^{75}SeO_3^{2-}$. J Nutr 1982;112:197–204.

36. Turnlund J, Keen C, Smith R. Copper status and urinary and salivary copper in young men at three levels of dietary copper. Am J Clin Nutr 1990;51:658–64.

37. National Research Council. Recommended Dietary Allowances, 10th ed. Washington, DC: National Academy Press, 1989, pp. 224–30.

38. Tamura H, Hirose S, Watanabe O, Arai K, Murakawa M, Matsumura O, Isoda K. Anemia and neutropenia due to copper deficiency in enteral nutrition. JPEN 1994;18:185–89.

39. Cordano A. Clinical manifestations of nutritional copper deficiency in infants and children. Am J Clin Nutr 1998; 67(suppl):1012S–16S.

40. Lei K. Dietary copper: cholesterol and lipoprotein metabolism. Ann Rev Nutr 1991;11:265–83.

41. Copper deficiency and hypercholesterolemia. Nutr Rev 1987; 45:116–17.

42. Reiser S, Powell A, Yang C, Canary J. Effect of copper intake on blood cholesterol and its lipoprotein distribution in men. Nutr Rep Internl 1987;36:641–49.

43. Chuttani H, Gupta P, Gulati S, Gupta D. Acute copper sulfate poisoning. Am J Med 1965;39:849–54.

44. Bremner I. Manifestations of copper excess. Am J Clin Nutr 1998;67(suppl):1069S–73S.

45. Smithgall J. The copper-controlled diet: current aspects of dietary copper restriction in management of copper metabolism disorders. J Am Diet Assoc 1985;85:609–11.

46. Baker DH. Cupric oxide should not be used as a copper supplement for either animals or humans. J Nutr 1999;129:2278–79.

47. Turnlund J. Human whole-body copper metabolism. Am J Clin Nutr 1998;67(suppl):960S–64S.

48. Turnlund J, Scott K, Peiffer G, Jang A, Keyes W, Keen C, Sakanashi T. Copper status of young men consuming a low-copper diet. Am J Clin Nutr 1997;65:72–78.

49. Danks DM. Copper deficiency in humans. Ann Rev Nutr 1988; 8:235–57.

50. Milne D. Assessment of copper status. Clin Chem 1994;40:1479–84.

51. Milne D. Copper intake and assessment of copper status. Am J Clin Nutr 1998;67(suppl):1041S–45S.

Additional Reading

Genetic and environmental determinants of copper metabolism. Am J Clin Nutr 1998;67(May suppl).

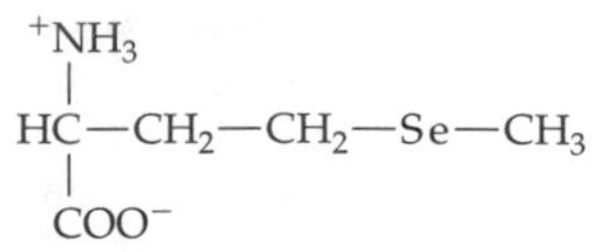

Selenomethionine

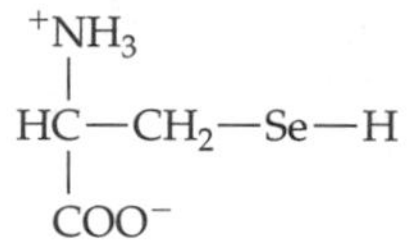

Selenocysteine

Figure 12.14 Selenomethionine and selenocysteine.

SELENIUM

Selenium, a nonmetal, exists in several oxidation states, including Se^{2-}, Se^{4+}, and Se^{6+}. The chemistry of selenium is similar to that of sulfur; consequently, selenium can substitute for sulfur in amino acids such as methionine, cysteine, and cystine. The total body selenium content is ~15 mg.

Sources

Perhaps more than any other essential trace element, selenium varies greatly in its soil concentration throughout the regions of the world. Soil concentration is directly related to selenium's concentration in food plants. Actually, this heterogeneous distribution has benefited science by providing a clear correlation between selenium-poor regions of the world (such as parts of China) and the incidence of disease associated with selenium deficiency. Because of the wide disparity in soil selenium concentrations, tables listing the mineral's content in assorted foods are only generally appropriate. Animal products (especially organ meats) are thought to contain more selenium (~0.4–1.5 μg/g) than plant sources. Seafood is also thought to represent one of the better sources of selenium, although the bioavailability of selenium from fish (especially fish containing mercury) may be low due to the formation of unabsorbable mercury-selenium complexes [1,2]. Muscle meats typically provide between 0.1 and 0.4 μg selenium/g. As mentioned, selenium in plants is extremely variable. Cereals and grains may contain from less than 0.1 μg/g to over 0.8 μg/g. Dairy products contain less than ~0.3 μg/g.

Absorption, Transport, Uptake, Storage, and Metabolism

Selenium occurs naturally in foods almost exclusively in the form of organic compounds, primarily

- selenomethionine (Fig. 12.14),
- selenocystine, and
- selenocysteine (Fig. 12.14).

These organic forms are thought to represent selenium analogues of sulfur-containing amino acids. The element substitution is made possible by the chemical similarity between selenium and sulfur. These selenium analogues become incorporated into plant proteins.

Inorganic forms of selenium include selenite (H_2SeO_3) and selenate (H_2SeO_4). These inorganic forms may be found in some vegetables. In addition, in parts of the world where selenium levels in natural foodstuffs are low, animal feeds generally are supplemented with sodium selenite.

Absorption

The organic and inorganic forms of selenium are all efficiently absorbed, although to different extents, from the gastrointestinal tract. Selenium absorption is shown in Figure 12.15. The duodenum appears to be the primary absorptive site, with some absorption occurring in the jejunum and ileum but virtually none in the stomach.

Balance and stable isotopic tracer studies have generally shown selenium, as selenomethionine, to be more effectively absorbed than selenite [3]. Selenoamino acid absorption, which occurs through amino acid transport systems, is estimated to be over 80%. Selenomethionine, however, is thought to be better absorbed than selenocysteine. Selenite absorption has been shown to exceed 85% in some studies [4]. Selenates are thought to be better absorbed than selenites [5].

Factors Influencing Selenium Absorption. Factors enhancing selenium absorption include vitamins C, A, and E, as well as the presence of reduced glutathione in the intestinal lumen. Heavy metals (such as mercury [2,6]) and phytates are thought to inhibit selenium absorption through chelation and precipitation.

Transport

Following absorption from the intestine, selenium is bound to transport proteins for travel through the blood to the liver and other tissues. In human blood, selenium

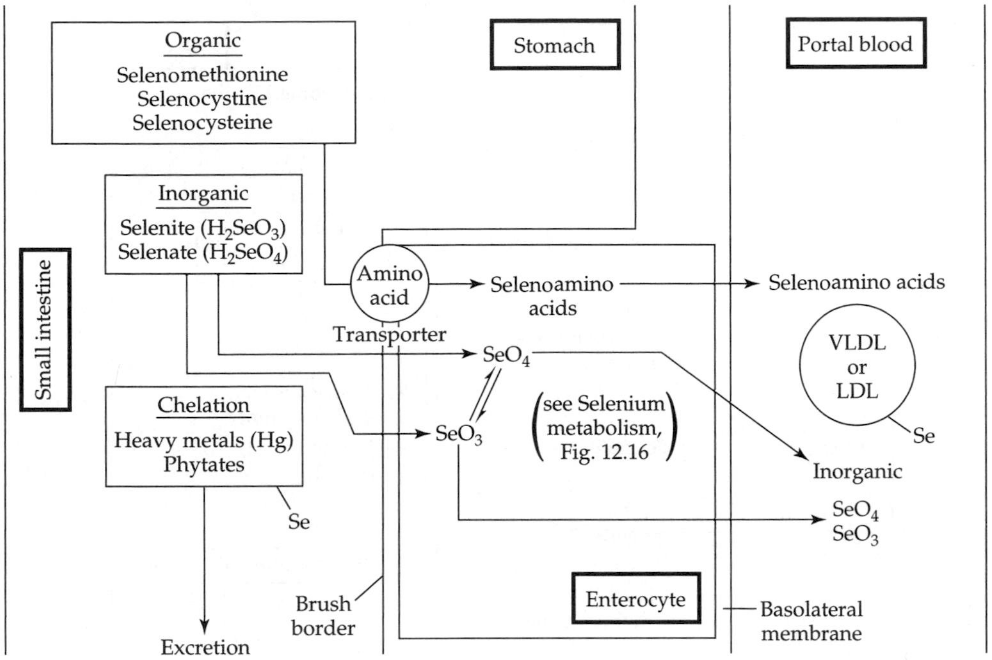

Figure 12.15 Overview of selenium digestion, absorption, and transport. Abbreviations: VLDL, very low density lipoprotein; LDL, low-density lipoprotein.

binds to sulfhydryl groups in α- and β-globulins such as very low density lipoproteins and low-density lipoproteins, respectively. The selenocysteine-containing plasma protein, selenoprotein P, also appears to function as a selenium transport protein, carrying the majority (>50%) of selenium in the plasma [7–9]. Selenoprotein P contains up to ten selenocysteine residues but may be synthesized with fewer should selenium be limited. This glycoprotein is synthesized mostly in the liver and to lesser degrees in the kidney, heart, and lungs. It circulates in the blood and also is found associated with capillary endothelial cells.

Uptake and Storage

The mechanism by which selenium is freed from plasma transport proteins is not known. Tissues containing relatively high selenium concentrations include the kidney, liver, heart, pancreas, and muscle. The lungs, brain, bone, and red blood cells also contain selenium. Uptake of selenium into the red blood cell is thought to occur by diffusion; selenite uptake exceeds that of selenate, which in turn exceeds selenomethionine uptake [10]. Mechanisms by which other forms of selenium are taken up by tissues are unclear. Whether the methods of uptake vary among tissues also is not known.

Higher tissue concentrations of selenium have resulted when selenium was administered as selenomethionine as opposed to selenite. The reverse is true with respect to the uptake of selenium by its major metalloenzyme, glutathione peroxidase. That is, dietary selenium in inorganic forms such as selenite leads to greater incorporation of the mineral into glutathione peroxidase than when selenomethionine, the organic form, is the dietary form [11].

Metabolism

Within tissues such as the liver, selenoamino acids and inorganic forms of selenium undergo metabolism. Selenomethionine, which is derived from the diet, may be either stored as selenomethionine in an amino acid pool, used for protein synthesis just as the amino acid methionine is used, or catabolized to ultimately yield other selenoamino acids, selenocysteine and selenocystine. Selenomethionine metabolism is similar to methionine metabolism (Fig. 7.27, p. 203). Selenium metabolism is shown in Figure 12.16.

Selenocysteine, which is derived either from selenomethionine metabolism or from the diet, may be degraded by selenocysteine β-lyase to yield free elemental selenium. Free selenium is typically converted in the body to selenide, with hydrogens provided by glutathione or other thiols. Selenide, in turn, can be methylated and excreted in the urine or can be converted to selenophosphate, an important intermediate in the synthesis of the body's selenium-dependent enzymes.

Inorganic selenium also undergoes metabolism (Fig. 12.16). Selenate from the diet may be converted in the body to selenite, which is further metabolized to selenodiglutathione and subsequently to selenide. Selenide is metabolized as described above to generate methylated forms for excretion or to form selenophosphate for further

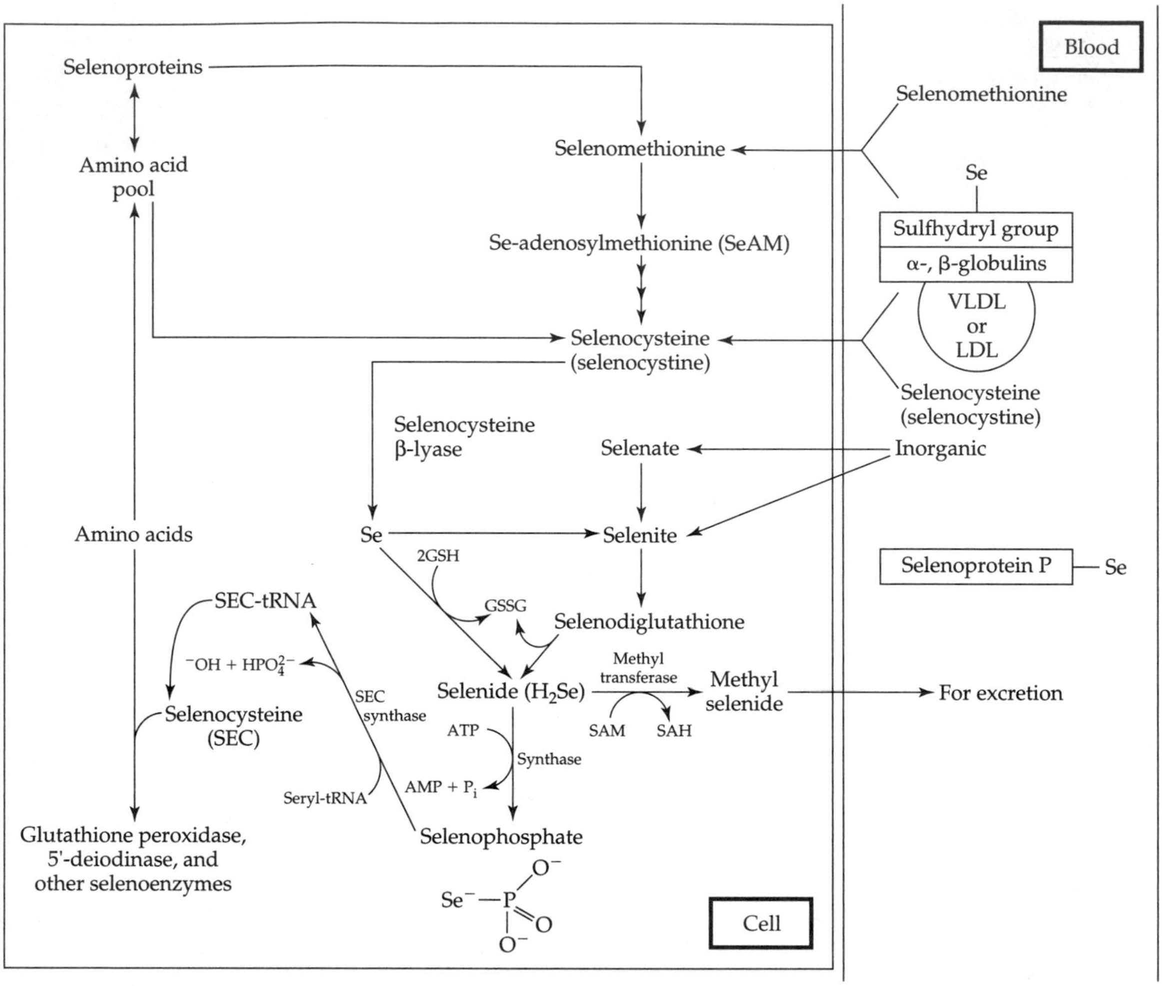

Figure 12.16 Selenium metabolism.

use in the synthesis of selenoenzymes such as 5′-deiodinase or glutathione peroxidase.

Functions and Mechanisms of Action

Various incompletely understood roles for selenium in mammalian metabolism have been postulated. Some of the less defined roles are its involvement in the maintenance or induction of the cytochrome P_{450} system, in pancreatic function, in DNA repair and enzyme activation, in immune system function, and in detoxification of heavy metals. The better-characterized roles of selenium are related to its functions as integral parts of specific enzymes in the body, although only a few selenium-dependent enzymes are well studied. We will discuss some of the known selenium-dependent enzymes in humans.

Glutathione peroxidase (GPX)

Perhaps one of the most clearly established functions of selenium is as an essential cofactor for the enzyme glutathione peroxidase. Five glutathione peroxidase enzymes (designated GPX1, 2, 3, 4, and 5) have been characterized, and each catalyzes the same basic reaction but in different tissues. GPXs 1–4 are selenium dependent, containing four selenocysteine residues. GPX1 and GPX4, for example, are found in most body tissues but most notably the liver, kidney, and red blood cell. GPX2 is found predominantly in the gastrointestinal tract and liver. GPX3 is found in the plasma (extracellular) as well as in the kidney, heart, and lung, among other tissues [12]. Within tissues, glutathione peroxidase is found mainly (~70%) in the cytosol of cells and to a lesser extent (~30%) in the mitochondrial matrix. GPX3 and selenoprotein P together are thought to account for over 90% of the selenium in the plasma.

Glutathione peroxidase catalyzes the removal from tissues of hydrogen peroxides (H_2O_2) and other organic hydroperoxides (designated LOOH for a lipid hydroperoxide or ROOH for a general organic hydroperoxide). Glutathione, a tripeptide of glycine, cysteine, and glutamate found in most cells of the body, is needed in its reduced form for the reaction and furnishes the reducing equivalents for the following reaction.

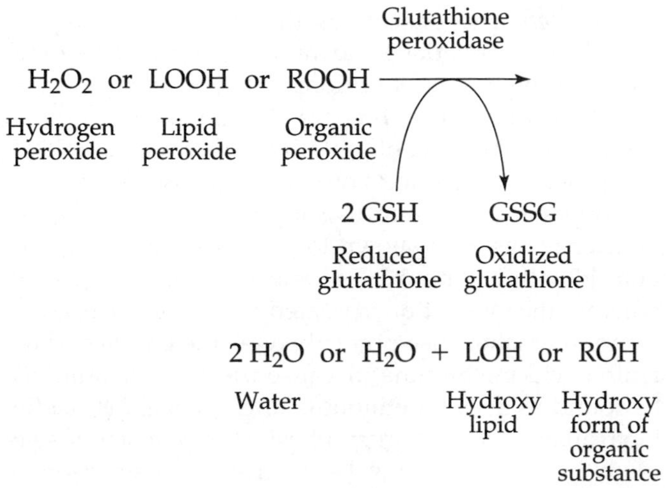

Organic peroxides are derived from nucleic acids and other molecules, including unsaturated fatty acids, in which case the peroxide is referred to as a lipid (versus organic) peroxide. Hydrogen peroxides are generated in many cells throughout the body as part of normal metabolism and may be generated in large amounts by activated white blood cells as they phagocytize foreign substances. The reaction, catalyzed by glutathione peroxidase, neutralizes or eliminates hydrogen peroxide and organic (including lipid) peroxides. In fact, glutathione peroxidase is more active than catalase (see p. 430) in reducing organic peroxides and hydrogen peroxides. If not removed, these peroxides could damage cellular membranes and other cell components.

Selenium availability has been shown to affect mRNA concentrations of glutathione peroxidase (GPX1) in the liver. With selenium deficiency, less mRNA is made for hepatic glutathione peroxidase and enzyme activity is diminished [6,13,14]. Available selenium is shifted to other, more critical selenoproteins such as selenoprotein P. With selenium supplementation, there is a rapid increase in mRNA to control levels; the increase in enzyme activity is gradual. The generation of hydrogen peroxides and lipid and organic peroxides and the coordinated roles of selenium (as part of glutathione peroxidase), vitamin E, iron (as catalase and myeloperoxidase), and zinc and copper (as superoxide dismutase), which also function as antioxidants to prevent free radical–induced cell damage, are discussed in the perspective at the end of Chapter 10.

The regeneration of reduced glutathione (GSH) from its oxidized state (GSSG) is imperative in order for cells to be able to maintain appropriate redox states. Glutathione reductase, aflavoenzyme, catalyzes the reduction in a reaction dependent on NADPH + H^+, derived from the hexosemonophosphate shunt. The regeneration of reduced glutathione is shown here:

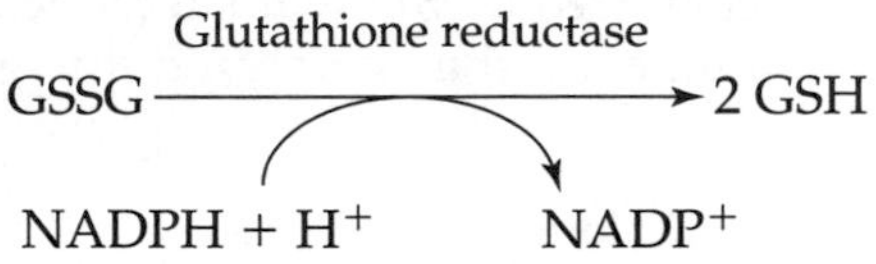

Iodothyronine Deiodinases (IDI or DI)

Selenium is also necessary for iodine metabolism. Iodothyronine deiodinases have been shown to be selenocysteine-containing proteins with selenocysteines present at the active site [6,15–17]. Three types of deiodinases have been characterized. Type I is found in the endoplasmic reticulum of the liver, kidney, and muscle. Types II and III are found in tissues such as the skin, pituitary, adipose, and brain [6,15–17].

Deiodinases catalyze the deiodination (removal of iodine) of thyroid hormones and some of their metabolites. For example, 5′-deiodinase (5′-DI) converts the thyroid hormone thyroxine (T_4), which is secreted from the thyroid gland, to its 3,5,3′-triiodothyronine (T_3) form. This reaction, which is catalyzed mainly in the liver, is especially important because the T_3 form of the hormone is the main active form in the body. T_3 is the body's primary hormonal regulator of metabolism as well as of normal growth and development.

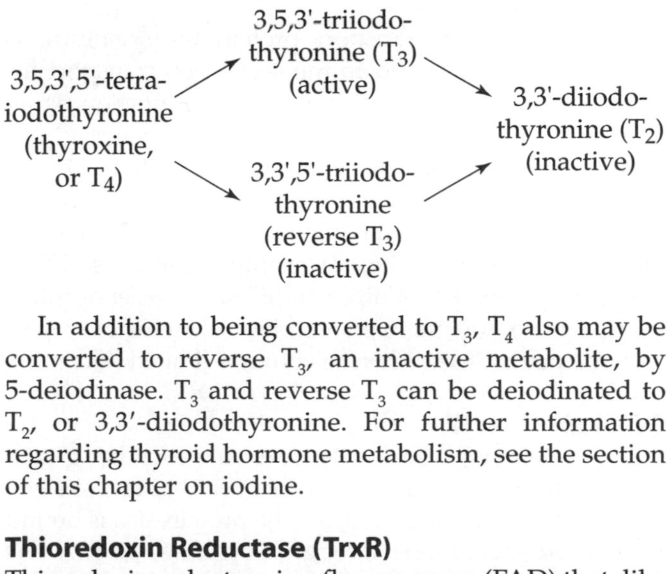

In addition to being converted to T_3, T_4 also may be converted to reverse T_3, an inactive metabolite, by 5-deiodinase. T_3 and reverse T_3 can be deiodinated to T_2, or 3,3′-diiodothyronine. For further information regarding thyroid hormone metabolism, see the section of this chapter on iodine.

Thioredoxin Reductase (TrxR)

Thioredoxin reductase is a flavoenzyme (FAD) that, like GPX and 5′-DI, contains selenocysteine at its active site. The enzyme is found in the blood as well as within cells and tissues such as the skin and liver and helps maintain the redox state [18]. Specifically, thioredoxin reductase transfers reducing equivalents from NADPH through its bound FAD to reduce disulfide bonds within (intramolecular) the oxidized form of its substrate thioredoxin. In its reduced state, thioredoxin, a thiol like glutathione, is able to provide oxidized compounds with hydrogens (i.e., reducing equivalents). The reaction catalyzed by thioredoxin reductase, shown below, is similar to that catalyzed by glutathione reductase.

$$\underset{\text{Oxidized thioredoxin}}{TrxS_2} \xrightarrow[\text{NADPH + H}^+ \;\rightarrow\; \text{NADP}^+]{\text{Thioredoxin reductase}} \underset{\text{Reduced thioredoxin}}{Trx(SH)_2}$$

Selenophosphate Synthetase

At least two forms of selenophosphate synthetase have been identified in the body. One isoform has been shown to contain selenocysteine and catalyzes the synthesis of selenophosphate from selenide, as shown here:

$$\underset{\text{Selenide}}{H_2Se} \xrightarrow[\text{ATP} \;\rightarrow\; \text{AMP} + P_i]{\text{Selenophosphate synthetase}} \underset{\text{Selenophosphate}}{HSePO_3^{2-}}$$

Selenophosphate is a key compound needed in the body to synthesize other selenocysteine-containing enzymes such as glutathione peroxidase, 5′-deiodinase, and thioredoxin reductase (Fig. 12.16).

Selenoprotein P

Selenoprotein P, a transport protein for selenium, is described both here and in the section on transport for selenium. Selenoprotein P is thought to function as an antioxidant through the removal of damaging radicals such as peroxynitrite ($ONOO^-$). Peroxynitrite is synthesized by activated white blood cells from superoxide radicals ($O_2^{\cdot}$) and nitrogen monooxide ($NO^{\cdot}$) [7–9]. If not inactivated, peroxynitrite, for example, can cause DNA single strand breaks and lipid peroxidation. Selenoprotein P appears to preferentially receive selenium over glutathione peroxidases when selenium is limited [9].

Selenoprotein W

Selenoprotein W, also a selenocysteine-containing protein, is found mostly in the cytosol of cardiac and skeletal muscle as well as other tissues. The protein also is bound to reduced glutathione through a cysteine residue. The function of this protein is unclear at present, but it is speculated to have antioxidant roles in the body [19–21].

Interactions with Other Nutrients

The interrelationship between selenium and the other antioxidant nutrients is discussed in the perspective at the end of Chapter 10.

The presence of significant amounts of lead in the body appears to significantly lower tissue selenium concentrations. Although this mechanism is unclear, the fact that both elements bind to sulfhydryl groups provides reason for speculation [22].

Iron deficiency decreases the synthesis of hepatic glutathione peroxidase and reduces hepatic and other tissue selenium concentrations [23]. The mechanism(s) of action are unclear but are thought to result from decreased translation of glutathione peroxidase mRNA and possibly from effects on selenium absorption.

Copper and selenium also appear to interact. Copper deficiency has been shown to decrease the activities of both glutathione peroxidase and 5′-deiodinase [24,25]; whether the interaction is related to iron is unclear.

An interaction also occurs between selenium and the amino acid methionine. Because dietary selenium can be found as selenomethionine and, as such, is readily bioavailable for protein synthesis, the potency of selenium in this form may be reduced if a situation of methionine deficiency exists [2]. The explanation for this observation is that if methionine is deficient, selenomethionine substitutes for it in the synthesis of body proteins [2,26]. Selenium then becomes available only as these proteins subsequently become degraded in the course of normal turnover.

Excretion

Selenium is excreted from the body almost equally in the urine and feces. Excretion is thought to be the means by which selenium homeostasis is maintained. Major urinary metabolites of selenium include methylselenol [$(CH_3)_2Se$], dimethylselenide [$(CH_3)_2Se$], and trimethylselenium [$(CH_3)_3Se^+$], among others [27]. Selenium losses via the lungs and skin also contribute to daily selenium excretion. Pulmonary elimination of selenium, usually associated with ingestion of large amounts of the mineral, is via exhalation of dimethylselenide, which is quite volatile and has a garlicky odor.

Recommended Dietary Allowances

Recommendations in the form of an estimated safe and adequate daily dietary intake (ESADDI) were developed for selenium in 1980. These recommendations were based primarily on calculations of selenium requirements for animals and were set at 50 to 200 μg/day [28]. In 1989, RDAs for selenium were established (70 μg for men and 55 μg for women), [29]. The RDAs have subsequently been modified as additional studies have been conducted over the last decade. In 2000, the Food and Nutrition Board set an RDA for selenium for adult men and women of 55 μg/day [30]. Based mostly on balance studies as well as on repletion studies of men with selenium deficiency in regions of China, the requirement for selenium for adults was determined to be 45 μg. The requirement was based on calculation of the amount of selenium necessary for plateau concentrations of selenoproteins in the plasma. To set the RDA, a 20% coefficient of variation was added and the final number was rounded to the nearest five. RDAs for selenium for pregnancy and lactation were set at 60 μg and 70 μg, respectively [30]. The additional selenium is needed for fetal deposition during pregnancy and for inclusion in milk during lactation [30]. The inside cover of the book provides RDAs for selenium for other age groups.

Deficiency

Selenium deficiency has been linked to a number of livestock animal diseases and also to regional human diseases such as Keshan disease and Kashin-Beck's disease in China [31]. Keshan disease is characterized by cardiomyopathy involving cardiogenic shock and/or congestive heart failure, along with multifocal necrosis of heart tissue, which becomes replaced with fibrous tissue [31]. Kashin-Beck's disease is characterized by osteoarthropathy involving degeneration and necrosis of the joints and of epiphyseal-plate cartilages of the legs and arms [31]. Several factors, including selenium deficiency, are thought to contribute to the development of Kashin-Beck's disease.

Selenium deficiency also has been observed in people receiving total parenteral nutrition [32–34]. Major symptoms of deficiency included poor growth, muscle pain and weakness, loss of pigmentation of hair and skin, and whitening of nail beds. Poor growth may be associated with the role of selenium in thyroid hormone metabolism.

Toxicity

Selenium toxicity, also called selenosis, has been observed both in miners and in individuals consuming excess selenium intake from supplements. Physical manifestations as well as biochemical abnormalities may occur depending on ingested amounts. Signs and symptoms of toxicity include nausea, vomiting, fatigue, diarrhea, hair and nail brittleness and loss, paresthesia, interference in sulfur metabolism (primarily oxidation of sulfhydryl groups), and inhibition of protein synthesis [35]. Acute poisoning from gram amounts of selenium is lethal, with damage occurring to most organ systems [35]. A tolerable upper intake level of 400 μg/day has been set by the Food and Nutrition Board [30]. The lowest observed adverse effect level (LOAEL) for selenium is 910 μg [29].

Assessment of Nutriture

The concentrations of selenoproteins in the blood are a reflection or function of dietary intake within a specific range. For plasma selenium concentrations, a value of 7 μg/dL (0.8 μmol/L) appears to be the cutoff [30,36,37]. If a person's plasma selenium concentration is $<$7 μg/dL, then dietary selenium will impact the plasma selenium concentration. When plasma concentrations exceed this value, factors other than diet also affect plasma concentrations [30].

The activities and concentrations of selenoproteins also have been used to assess selenium status. The most commonly used enzymes are selenoprotein P and glutathione peroxidase in tissues (GPX1) and in the plasma (GPX3). GPX3 has been thought to be more accurate and more reflective of tissue levels than other forms [30]. Glutathione peroxidase in platelets has a relatively rapid turnover and a high selenium content, and enzyme activity responds rapidly to changes in selenium intake [1]. Like serum or plasma selenium, enzyme activity plateaus as intake increases, thus serving as an index of selenium status in populations with low intake [29,30].

Toenail clippings have been suggested as being reflective of selenium status for up to 1 year prior to sampling; however, nails and hair have been shown to be influenced by the forms of selenium ingested and, in the case of hair, by its color and contamination from shampoos and other products [30,38–40]. Urinary selenium concentration may reflect status, but it can be affected by diet. It has also been shown to identify selenium toxicity but may be proportional to status [30,36,39,40].

References Cited for Selenium

1. Levander O. Considerations in the design of selenium bioavailability studies. Fed Proc 1983;42:1721–25.

2. Forbes R, Erdman J. Bioavailability of trace mineral elements. Ann Rev Nutr 1983;3:213–31.

3. McAdam P, Lewis S. Absorption of selenite and L-selenomethionine in healthy young men using a ^{74}Se tracer. Fed Proc 1985;44:1671.

4. Sandstrom B, Davidsson L, Eriksson R, Alpsten M, Bogentoft C. Retention of selenium (^{75}Se), zinc (^{65}Zn) and manganese (^{54}Mn) in humans after intake of a labelled vitamin and mineral supplement. J Trace Elem Electrolytes Health Dis 1987;1:33–38.

5. Thomson C, Robinson M. Urinary and fecal excretions and absorption of a large supplement of selenium: superiority of selenate over selenite. Am J Clin Nutr 1986;44:659–63.

6. Burk R, Hill K. Regulation of selenoproteins. Ann Rev Nutr 1993;13:65–81.

7. Arteel GE, Klotz L, Buchczyk DP, Sies H. Selenoprotein P. Meth Enzymol 2002;347:121–25.

8. Moschos MP. Selenoprotein P. Cell Molec Life Sci 2000;57:1836–45.

9. Mostert V. Selenoprotein P: properties, functions, and regulation. Arch Biochem Biophys 2000;376:433–38.

10. Combs G, Combs S. The Role of Selenium in Nutrition. Orlando: Academic Press, 1986.

11. Whanger P, Butler J. Effects of various dietary levels of selenium as selenite or selenomethionine on tissue selenium levels and glutathione peroxidase activity in rats. J Nutr 1988;118:846–52.

12. Avissar N, Ornt D, Yagil Y, Horowitz S, Watkins R, Kerl E, Takahashi K, Palmer I, Cohen H. Glutathione peroxidase activity in human plasma originates mainly from kidney proximal tubular cells. FASEB J 1993;7:A277.

13. Kato T, Read R, Rozga J, Burk R. Evidence for intestinal release of absorbed selenium in a form with high hepatic extraction. Am J Physiol 1992;262:G854–58.

14. Evenson J, Sunde R. Selenium incorporation into seleno proteins in the selenium-adequate and selenium-deficient rat. Proc Soc Exp Biol Med 1988;187:169–80.

15. Berry M, Larsen P. The role of selenium in thyroid hormone action. Endocrine Rev 1992;13:207–19.

16. Bianco AC, Salvatore D, Gereben B, Berry MJ, Larsen PR. Biochemistry, cellular and molecular biology, and physiological roles of the iodothyronine selenodeiodinases. Endocrine Rev 2002; 23:38–89.

17. Arthur JR, ed. Interrelationships between selenium deficiency, iodine deficiency, and thyroid hormones. Am J Clin Nutr 1993; 57:235S–318S.

18. Soderberg A, Sahaf B, Rosen A. Thioredoxin reductase, a redox-active selenoprotein, is secreted by normal and neoplastic cells: presence in human plasma. Cancer Res 2000;60:2281–89.

19. Whanger PD. Selenoprotein W: a review. Cell Molec Life Sci 2000; 57:1846–52.

20. Whanger PD. Selenoprotein W. Meth Enzymol 2002;347:179–87.

21. Jeong D, Kim TS, Chung YW, Lee BJ, Kim IY. Selenoprotein W is a glutathione-dependent antioxidant in vivo. FEBS Letters 2002; 517:225–28.

22. Neatherly M, Miller W, Gentry R, et al. Influence of high dietary lead on selenium metabolism in dairy calves. J Dairy Sci 1987; 70:645–52.

23. Moriarty P, Picciano M, Beard J, Reddy C. Iron deficiency decreases Se-GPX mRNA level in the liver and impairs selenium utilization in other tissues. FASEB J 1993;7:A277.

24. Olin K, Walter R, Keen C. Copper deficiency affects selenoglutathione peroxidase and selenodeiodinase activities and antioxidant defense in weanling rats. Am J Clin Nutr 1994;59:654–58.

25. Jenkinson S, Lawrence R, Burk R, Williams D. Effects of copper deficiency on the activity of the selenoenzyme glutathione peroxidase and on excretion and tissue retention of $^{75}SeO_3^{2-}$. J Nutr 1982; 112:197–204.

26. Waschulewski I, Sunde R. Effect of dietary methionine on utilization of tissue selenium from dietary selenomethionine for glutathione peroxidase in the rat. J Nutr 1988;119:367–74.

27. Robinson J, Robinson M, Levander O, Thomson C. Urinary excretion of selenium by New Zealand and North American human subjects on different intakes. Am J Clin Nutr 1985;41:1023–31.

28. National Research Council. Recommended Dietary Allowances, 9th ed. Washington, DC: National Academy Press, 1980, pp. 162–64.

29. National Research Council. Recommended Dietary Allowances, 10th ed. Washington, DC: National Academy Press, 1989, pp. 217–24.

30. Food and Nutrition Board, Institute of Medicine. Dietary Reference Intakes. Washington, DC: National Academy Press, 2000, pp. 284–324.

31. Ge K, Yang G. The epidemiology of selenium deficiency in the etiological study of endemic diseases in China. Am J Clin Nutr 1993;57:259S–63S.

32. Abrams C, Siram S, Galsim C, Johnson-Hamilton H, Munford F, Mezghebe H. Selenium deficiency in long-term total parenteral nutrition. Nutr Clin Prac 1992;7:175–78.

33. Van Rij A, Thomson C, McKenzie J, Robinson M. Selenium deficiency in total parenteral nutrition. Am J Clin Nutr 1979;32:2076–85.

34. Vinton N, Dahlstrom K, Strobel C, Ament M. Macrocytosis and pseudoalbinism: manifestations of selenium deficiency. J Pediatr 1987;111:711–17.

35. Clark RF, Strukle E, Williams SR, Manoguerra AS. Selenium poisoning from a nutritional supplement. JAMA 1996;275:1087–88.

36. Diplock A. Indexes of selenium status in human populations. Am J Clin Nutr 1993;57:256S–58S.

37. Neve J, Vertongen F, Capel P. Selenium supplementation in healthy Belgian adults: response in platelet glutathione peroxidase activity and other blood indices. Am J Clin Nutr 1988;48:139–43.

38. Garland M, Morris J, Stampfer M, Colditz G, Spate V, Baskett C, Rosner B, Speizer F, Willett W, Hunter D. Prospective study of toenail selenium levels and cancer among women. J Natl Cancer Inst 1995;87:497–505.

39. Ovaskainen M, Virtamo J, Alfthan G, Haukka J, Pietinen P, Taylor P, Huttunen J. Toenail selenium as an indicator of selenium intake among middle-aged men in an area with low soil selenium. Am J Clin Nutr 1993;57:662–65.

40. Longnecker M, Stampfer M, Morris J. A 1 year trial of the effect of high selenium bread on selenium concentrations in blood and toenails. Am J Clin Nutr 1993;57:408–13.

CHROMIUM

Chromium, a metal, exists in several oxidation states, from Cr^{2-} to Cr^{6+}. The metal has ubiquitous presence. It is found in air, water, and soil. Trivalent chromium, or Cr^{3+}, is the stablest of the oxidation states and often binds to ligands containing nitrogen, oxygen, or sulfur to form hexacoordinate or octahedral complexes. The trivalent form of chromium is thought to be the most important form in humans. The chromium content of humans is estimated to be ~4 to 6 mg.

Sources

Numerous analytic difficulties and biological uncertainties have been associated with the determination of chromium in food. However, with advances in methodology and contamination control, chromium in foods now may be measured with accuracy.

In foods, chromium exists in the trivalent form (Cr^{3+}). Good sources of dietary chromium include meats and poultry (especially organ meats) and grains (especially whole grains) [1,2]. Other foods provide variable amounts of chromium. Examples of foods relatively high in chromium include cheese, mushrooms, various condiments and spices, as well as tea, beer, and wine [1,2]. Brewer's yeast is notable because of its suspected high content of the biologically active organically complexed form of chromium known as **glucose tolerance factor (GTF).**

Food processing and refining can affect the chromium content of foods. Refining of sugar, for example, diminishes chromium. Thus, molasses and brown sugar are higher in chromium than white sugar. In contrast, chromium is easily solubilized from stainless steel cookware or cans into acidic foods. Thus, use of stainless steel cookware may increase the amount of chromium in food [3].

Absorption, Transport, and Storage

Absorption

In acidic solutions, as would be found in the stomach, Cr^{3+} is soluble and may form complexes with ligands. Chromium is thought to be absorbed throughout the small intestine, especially in the jejunum [4]. While the mode of absorption is still not known, chromium is suspected to be absorbed either by diffusion or by a carrier-mediated transporter. About 0.4% to 2.5% of chromium intake is absorbed into intestinal cells for use by the body [5–8].

Factors Influencing Chromium Absorption

Like other trace minerals, chromium absorption may be influenced by dietary factors.

Enhancers of Chromium Absorption. Within the stomach, amino acids or other ligands may chelate inorganic chromium. Amino acids such as methionine and histidine, for example, act as ligands to improve chromium absorption [9]. Such chelations typically help chromium remain soluble and prevent olation (see next paragraph) once it reaches the alkaline pH of the small intestine. Solubility improves chromium absorption. For example, picolinate as a ligand helps maintain solubility, is relatively stable, and is lipophilic, which enhances absorption through the lipid membranes of cells. Vitamin C may enhance chromium absorption. Consumption of 1 mg chromium as chromium chloride along with 100 mg ascorbate was associated with increased plasma chromium concentrations versus chromium ingestion in the absence of ascorbate [10–12].

Inhibitors of Chromium Absorption. Inorganic chromium in a neutral or alkaline environment reacts with hydroxyl ions (OH^-), which readily polymerize to form high-molecular-weight compounds in a process called olation. This results in precipitation of chromium and thus reduced absorption. Ingestion of antacids significantly reduces blood and tissue chromium concentrations through decreased absorption [10]. Phytates found mostly in grains and legumes also diminish chromium absorption.

Transport

In the blood, inorganic Cr^{3+} binds competitively with transferrin and is transported along with iron bound to transferrin. If transferrin sites are unavailable for chromium, albumin is thought to transport chromium. Globulins and possibly lipoproteins also are thought to transport the mineral if present in very high concentrations. Some chromium also may circulate unbound in the blood. How organically complexed chromium is transported in the blood remains uncertain.

Storage

The human body contains ~4 to 6 mg chromium [13]. Tissues especially high in chromium include the kidney, liver, muscle, spleen, heart, pancreas, and bone. Tissue chromium concentrations have been shown to decline with age [14]. Chromium is thought to be stored in tissues with ferric iron because of its transport by transferrin.

Functions and Mechanisms of Action

Chromium is known to potentiate the action of insulin; however, the mechanism by which this occurs is still under investigation. For decades, the biological action of chromium has been believed to be due to its complexing with nicotinic acid and amino acids to form the organic compound glucose tolerance factor (GTF) [15,16]. While GTF was first identified in brewer's yeast, this factor has never been purified nor its exact structure characterized. Nevertheless, the belief remains that the biologically active molecule is a dinicotinato chromium complex coordinated with amino acids that stabilize the complex. Mertz [15,16] proposed that the initial product of in vivo synthesis was a tetra-aquo dinicotinato chromium complex, as shown in Figure 12.17. Because this complex is unstable in the alkaline pH of the organism, Mertz proposed that the coordinated water molecules are replaced by amino acid ligands, thereby stabilizing the complex and preventing its precipitation. The amino acids acting as ligands are believed to be those making up glutathione (glutamate, cysteine, and glycine). GTF, following stimulation by the release of insulin, is thought to potentiate the actions of insulin by initiating the disulfide bridging between insulin and the insulin receptor (Fig. 12.18). Although the insulin receptor has been purified and characterized, however, no evidence has been uncovered indicating that chromium is a component of the receptor's subunits or is part of an accessory protein for insulin binding [13,17,18].

More recent studies have shown that chromium may be involved in pancreatic insulin secretion or insulin receptor production, expression, and/or activity to potentiate or enhance insulin's effectiveness [17–19]. The effectiveness of insulin is greater in the presence of

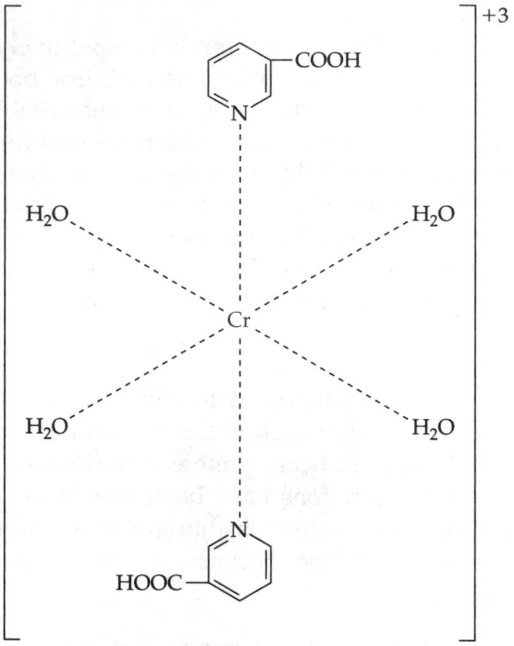

Figure 12.17 Tetra-aquo dinicotinato chromium complex. Water molecules are believed to be replaced by amino acids (glutamic acid, cysteine, and glycine) to stabilize the complex. *Source:* From Nutrition Reviews 33(1975):129–35. © International Life Sciences Institute—Nutrition Foundation. Used with permission.

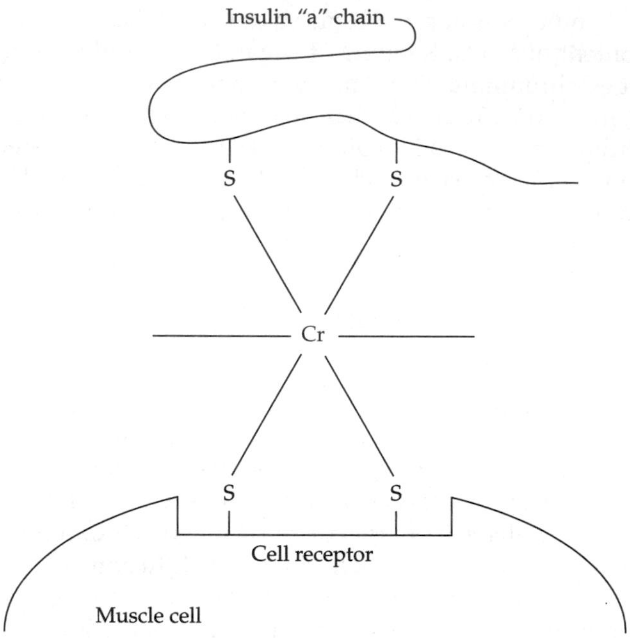

Figure 12.18 Proposed interaction of Cr as part of GTF and insulin and cell's insulin receptor. *Source:* Modified from Mertz W, Toepfer EW, Roginski EE, Polansky MM. Present knowledge of the role of chromium. Fed Proc 1974;33:2276.

chromium than in its absence [19]. The role of chromium in stimulating insulin activity is thought to occur as described next and shown in Figure 12.19. With increased plasma insulin, chromium uptake bound to transferrin increases via transferrin receptors. Within cells, four chromium atoms bind to apochromodulin, a low-molecular-weight chromium (LMWCr) binding substance, to form holochromodulin (Cr_4-chromodulin), also called chromodulin. Chromodulin is an oligopeptide composed of glycine, cysteine, aspartate, and glutamate. Chromodulin, but not apochromodulin, has been shown to bind to the cytosolic beta subunit of the insulin receptor and to stimulate the kinase activity of the insulin receptor [20–23]. The kinase activity of the insulin receptor is involved in multiple phosphorylation reactions that impact not only insulin activity but also the activities of enzymes involved in nutrient metabolism.

Roles in glucose and lipid metabolism have been suggested for chromium, likely via its effects on insulin. For example, chromium may improve glucose intolerance if impaired and if the individual has suboptimal chromium status. Chromium also may affect lipoprotein lipase activity and/or, in some unknown way, affect cholesterol metabolism. Several studies have reported improvements in blood lipid profiles of people following chromium supplementation. Significant increases in blood HDL cholesterol, along with decreases in total and LDL cholesterol concentrations, have been demonstrated with chromium supplementation [6,15,17,18,24,25]. Chromium as a supplement has been purported to effect changes in body composition and strength performance. However, most well-controlled studies providing chromium supplementation have shown no significant effects on strength gains, muscle accretion, or fat loss [26–30].

Another proposed role for chromium is in nucleic acid metabolism. It is postulated that Cr^{3+} is involved in maintaining the structural integrity of nuclear strands and in the regulation of gene expression [31]. RNA synthesis in vitro, as directed by DNA, is enhanced by chromium binding to the template [32].

Interactions with Other Nutrients

Because chromium is transported in the blood bound to transferrin, the primary iron-binding protein, one might surmise the potential for chromium, if given in large amounts, to displace iron from the transferrin. Indeed, ingestion of chromium (~200 μg) as chromium chloride and chromium picolinate was associated with a

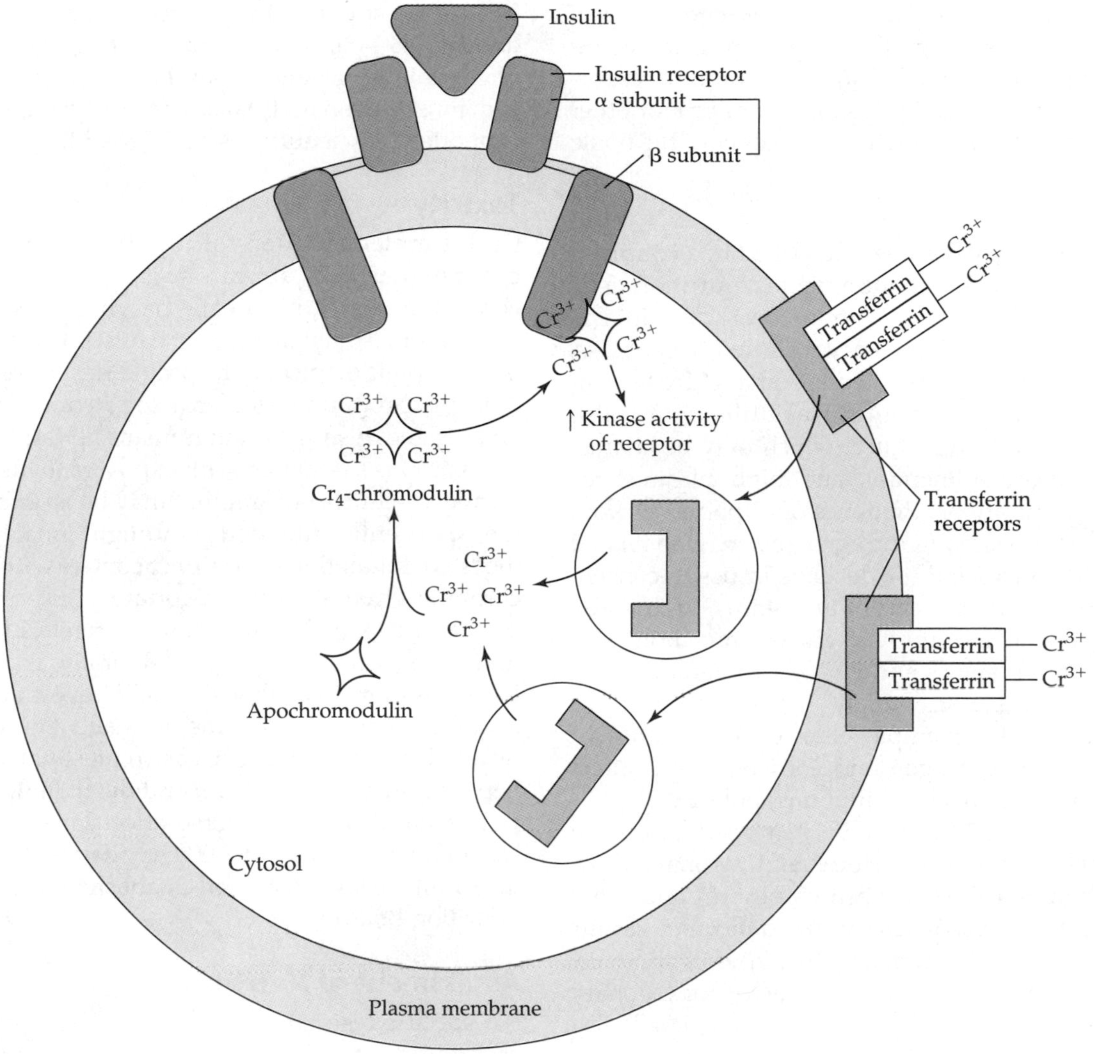

Figure 12.19 Proposed role of chromium (Cr^{3+}) as part of chromodulin in potentiating insulin's actions.

significant decrease in serum ferritin, total iron-binding capacity, and transferrin saturation in 36 men [28]. Other studies, however, report that chromium picolinate ingestion (924 μg) had no effects on hematologic indexes in men [30].

Excretion

Most absorbed chromium is excreted from the body in the urine. In fact, urinary chromium represents about 95% of chromium excretion and mainly reflects recent intake (not status). In absolute terms, urinary chromium is ~0.2 to 0.4 μg/day, and 0.5% to 2% of intake is excreted with intakes of 40 μg and 10 μg, respectively [6,8,33–35]. Consumption of diets high in simple sugars (35% simple sugars, 15% complex carbohydrates) has been shown to raise urinary chromium in some subjects by 300% in contrast to consumption of diets high in complex (starch) carbohydrates (35% complex carbohydrates, 15% simple sugars) [36]. In addition to urinary losses, small amounts of chromium are lost with desquamation of skin cells. Fecal chromium represents mostly unabsorbed dietary chromium, not endogenous chromium excreted via the bile into the feces.

Adequate Intakes

An estimated safe and adequate daily dietary intake (ESADDI) for chromium was first reported in the 1980 RDAs. In 1989, an ESADDI for chromium of 50 to 200 μg/day was recommended for adults [37]. The latest recommendation for chromium is in the form of an adequate intake (AI) and was set based on estimated mean chromium intakes in the United States. The AIs for chromium for adult men and women through age 50 years are 35 μg and 25 μg, respectively; these values drop to 30 μg and 20 μg for men and women, respectively, over 50 years of age [7]. During pregnancy and lactation, intakes of 30 μg and 45 μg chromium, respectively, are recommended [7]. AIs for chromium for other age groups are provided on the inside cover of the book.

Deficiency

Chromium deficiency has been described in a couple of individuals who received intravenous nutrition feed (total parenteral nutrition) without oral food intake. Signs and symptoms of deficiency included weight loss, peripheral neuropathy, elevated plasma glucose concentrations or impaired glucose utilization (also referred to as insulin resistance, which may be characterized by hyperinsulinemia), and high plasma free fatty acid concentrations. Evidence of impaired glucose tolerance increases among the aged and may be related to inadequate intake and/or declines in tissue concentrations [38]. Improved chromium status, if initially suboptimal, results in improved glucose metabolism in individuals with diabetes and glucose intolerance.

Severe trauma and stress may increase the need for chromium. Stress, for example, elevates the secretion of hormones such as glucagon and cortisol, which alters glucose and ultimately chromium metabolism.

Chromium needs also may be increased in certain diseases, such as diabetes mellitus and coronary heart disease, although a link between chromium and these diseases is not conclusive. Chromium deficiency results in insulin resistance characterized by hyperinsulinemia, which has been implicated as a risk factor for coronary heart disease [39–41]. Mild chromium deficiency also has been shown to be a risk factor for a group of symptoms (except hypertension) similar to Syndrome X [40]. Syndrome X, a constellation of abnormalities that increase the risk of coronary heart disease, includes hyperinsulinemia, resistance to insulin-stimulated glucose uptake, glucose intolerance, hypertriglyceridemia (high concentrations of triglycerides in the blood), decreased blood HDL concentrations, and hypertension [41].

Supplements

Chromium is available in supplement form as inorganic salts, such as with chloride, or as an organic complex, such as with acetate, nicotinic acid alone or with amino acids, or picolinic acid. Although all forms appear to be absorbed and utilized, the form of the supplement appears to affect tissue concentrations in rats. While chromium picolinate, because of its increased solubility (lipophilic), has been touted as superior to other forms of chromium, chromosomal damage has been demonstrated in hamster cells with use of chromium picolinate [42]; other studies have indicated potential for organ damage [43–48]. Advertisements suggesting that the use of chromium picolinate may help a person lose fat and gain muscle (lean body) mass do not appear to be entirely supported by scientific research [26–30].

Toxicity

Oral supplementation of up to about 1,000 μg of chromium as Cr^{3+} appears to be safe [7,46]. However, chromium (Cr^{3+}) picolinate has been shown to produce chromosomal damage in hamster cells [42]. In addition, chromium picolinate providing between 600 and 2,400 μg chromium has been associated with renal failure and hepatic dysfunction in humans [43,44].

Toxicity is associated with exposure to the hexavalent form (Cr^{6+}) of chromium that may be absorbed through the skin, enter the body through inhalation, or be ingested. Inhalation of or direct contact with hexavalent chromium may result in respiratory disease or in dermatitis and skin ulcerations, respectively. Liver damage may also occur. Cr^{6+} ingested orally is about 10 to 100 times more toxic than Cr^{3+} [47]. Ingestion of chromic acid (CrO_3), which contains hexavalent chromium, has resulted in severe acidosis, gastrointestinal hemorrhage, hepatic injury, renal failure, and death [45].

The no observed adverse effect level (NOAEL) for chromium Cr^{3+} is set at 1,000 μg/day [48]. No tolerable upper intake level has been established by the Food and Nutrition Board to date.

Assessment of Nutriture

No specific tests are currently available to determine chromium status prior to supplementation [15]. Although a plasma chromium level of ~0.5 ng/mL is considered normal, the chromium content of physiological fluids is not indicative of status [33]. Fasting plasma chromium is not in equilibrium with tissue chromium. Responses of plasma chromium to an oral glucose load are inconsistent. Urinary chromium appears to reflect only recent intake, not status [33]. Hair chromium concentrations may indicate the status of a large population but not of individuals [15]. Relative chromium status has been evaluated retrospectively through following the effects of chromium supplementation on various parameters such as blood glucose and lipids, but this assessment is not valid in determining absolute nutriture.

References Cited for Chromium

1. Khan A, Bryden N, Polansky M, Anderson R. Insulin potentiating factor and chromium content of selected foods and spices. Biol Trace Elem Res 1990;24:183–88.

2. Kumpulainen J. Chromium content of foods and diets. Biol Trace Elem Res 1992;32:9–18.

3. Kuligowski J, Halperin K. Stainless steel cookware as a significant source of nickel, chromium, and iron. Arch Environ Contam Toxicol 1992;23:211–215.

4. Anderson R. Chromium. In: Mertz W, ed. Trace Elements in Human and Animal Nutrition, 5th ed. San Diego: Academic Press, 1987;1:225–44.

5. Offenbacher E, Spencer H, Dowling H, Pi-Sunyer F. Metabolic chromium balances in men. Am J Clin Nutr 1986;44:77–82.

6. Anderson R, Polasky M, Bryden N, Canary J. Supplemental chromium effects on glucose, insulin, glucagon, and urinary chromium losses in subjects consuming controlled low chromium diets. Am J Clin Nutr 1991;54:909–16.

7. Food and Nutrition Board, Institute of Medicine. Dietary Reference Intakes. Washington, DC: National Academy Press, 2001, pp. 197–223.

8. Anderson R, Kozlovsky A. Chromium intake, absorption, and excretion of subjects consuming self selected diets. Am J Clin Nutr 1985;41:1177–83.

9. Dowling H, Offenbacher E, Pi-Sunyer X. Effects of amino acids on the absorption of trivalent chromium and its retention by regions of the rat small intestine. Nutr Res 1990;10:1261–71.

10. Seaborn C, Stoecker B. Effects of antacid or ascorbic acid on tissue accumulation and urinary excretion of ^{51}chromium. Nutr Res 1990; 10:1401–7.

11. Offenbacher E. Promotion of chromium absorption by ascorbic acid. Trace Elem Electrolytes 1994;11:178–81.

12. Davis ML, Seaborn CD, Stoecker BJ. Effects of over-the-counter drugs on ^{51}chromium retention and urinary excretion in rats. Nutr Res 1995;15:201–10.

13. Is chromium essential for humans? Nutr Rev 1988;46:17–20.

14. Mertz W. Chromium levels in serum, hair, and sweat decline with age. Nutr Rev 1997;55:373–75.

15. Mertz W. Chromium in human nutrition: a review. J Nutr 1993; 123:626–33.

16. Mertz W. Effects and metabolism of glucose tolerance factor. Nutr Rev 1975;33:129–35.

17. Evans G. The effect of chromium picolinate on insulin controlled parameters in humans. Int J Biosocial Med Res 1989; 11:163–80.

18. Evans G, Bowman T. Chromium picolinate increases membrane fluidity and rate of insulin internalization. J Inorgan Biochem 1992; 46:243–50.

19. Striffler J, Polansky M, Anderson R. Dietary chromium enhances insulin secretion in perfused rat pancreas. J Trace Elem Exper Med 1993;6:75–81.

20. Saad M. Molecular mechanisms of insulin resistance. Brazilian J Med Biol Res 1994;27:941–57.

21. Vincent JB. Elucidating a biological role for chromium at a molecular level. Acct Chem Res 2000;33:503–10.

22. Davis C, Vincent J. Chromium oligopeptide activates insulin receptor kinase activity. Biochemistry 1997;36:4382–85.

23. Roth R, Lui F, Chin J. Biochemical mechanisms of insulin resistance. Hormone Res 1994;41(suppl2):51–55.

24. Anderson R. Nutritional factors influencing the glucose/insulin system: chromium. J Am Coll Nutr 1997;16:404–10.

25. Thomas V, Gropper S. Effect of chromium nicotinic acid supplementation on selected cardiovascular disease risk factors. Biol Trace Elem Res 1996;55:297–305.

26. Clarkson P. Effects of exercise on chromium levels: is supplementation required? Sports Med 1997;23:341–49.

27. Hasten D, Rome E, Franks D, Hegsted M. Effects of chromium picolinate on beginning weight training students. Int J Sports Nutr 1992;2:343–50.

28. Lukaski H, Bolonchuk W, Siders W, Milner D. Chromium supplementation and resistance training: effects on body composition, strength and trace element status of men. Am J Clin Nutr 1996;63:954–65.

29. Clancy S, Clarkson P, DeCheke M, Nosaka K, Freedson P, Cunningham J, Valentine B. Effects of chromium picolinate supplementation on body composition, strength, and urinary chromium loss in football players. Int J Sports Nutr 1994;4:142–53.

30. Campbell W, Beard J, Joseph L, Davey S, Evans W. Chromium picolinate supplementation and resistive training by older men: effects on iron-status and hematologic indexes. Am J Clin Nutr 1997;66:944–49.

31. Stoecker B. Chromium. In: Brown ML, ed. Present Knowledge in Nutrition. Washington, DC: International Life Sciences Institute Nutrition Foundation, 1990, pp. 287–93.

32. Nielsen F. Chromium. In: Shils M, Olson J, Shike M, eds. Modern Nutrition in Health and Disease. Philadelphia: Lea and Febiger, 1994, pp. 264–68.

33. Anderson R, Polansky M, Bryden N, Patterson K, Veillon C, Glinsmann W. Effects of chromium supplementation on urinary chromium excretion of human subjects and correlation of chromium excretion with selected clinical parameters. J Nutr 1983;113:276–81.

34. Anderson RA, Polansky MM, Bryden NA, Roginski EE, Patterson KY, Reamer DC. Effect of exercise (running) on serum glucose, insulin, glucagon and chromium excretion. Diabetes 1982;31:212–16.

35. Paschal DC, Ting BG, Morrow JC, Pirkle JL, Jackson RJ, Sampson EJ, Miller DT, Caldwell KL. Trace metals in urine of United States residents: reference range concentrations. Environmental Res 1998;76:53–59.

36. Kozlovsky A, Moser P, Reiser S, et al. Effects of diets high in simple sugars on urinary chromium losses. Metabolism 1986;35:515–18.

37. National Research Council. Recommended Dietary Allowances, 10th ed. Washington, DC: National Academy Press, 1989, pp. 241–43.

38. Bunker V, Lawson M, Delves H, et al. The uptake and excretion of chromium by the elderly. Am J Clin Nutr 1984;39:797–802.

39. Zavaroni I, Bonora E, Pagliara M, Dall'aglio E, Luchetti L, Buonanno G, Bonati PA, Bergonzani M, Gnudi L, Passeri M, Reaven G. Risk factors for coronary artery disease in healthy persons with hyperinsulinemia and normal glucose tolerance. N Engl J Med 1989;320:702–6.

40. Reaven G. The role of insulin resistance and hyperinsulinemia in coronary heart disease. Metabolism 1992;41:16–19.

41. Reaven GM. The role of insulin resistance in human disease. Diabetes 1988;37:1595–1607.

42. Stearns D, Wise J, Patierno S, Wetterhahn K. Chromium (III) picolinate produces chromosome damage in Chinese hamster ovary cells. FASEB J 1995;9:1643–48.

43. Wasser WG, Feldman NS, D'Agati VD. Chronic renal failure after ingestion of over-the-counter chromium picolinate. Ann Intern Med 1997;126:410–11.

44. Cerulli J, Grabe DW, Gauthier I, Malone M, McGoldrick MD. Chromium picolinate toxicity. Ann Pharmacotherapy 1998;32:428–31.

45. Loubieres Y, de Lassence A, Bernier M, Vieillard-Baron A, Schmitt JM, Page B, Jardin F. Acute, fatal, oral chromic acid poisoning. Clin Toxicol 1999;37:333–36.

46. Anderson R. Chromium as an essential nutrient for humans. Regulatory Toxicol and Pharmacol 1997;26:S35–S41.

47. Katz S, Salem H. The toxicology of chromium with respect to its chemical speciation. J Appl Toxicol 1993;13:217–24.

48. Hathcock J. Vitamins and minerals: efficacy and safety. Am J Clin Nutr 1997;66:427–37.

IODINE

Iodine, a nonmetal, typically is found and functions in its ionic form, iodide (I^-). Hence, the term *iodide* is used throughout this discussion of the trace element. About 15 to 20 mg iodide is found in the human body.

Sources

The iodide concentration in human foods is extremely variable because, as is so often the case, it reflects the regionally variable soil concentrations of the element and the amount and nature of fertilizer used in plant cultivation. Thus, the iodide content of grains, vegetables, and fruits varies with the iodide content of the soil, and the iodide content of meats depends on the iodide of the soil and plants that the animals ate. The amount of iodide in drinking water is an indication of the iodide content of the rocks and soils of a region and closely parallels the incidence of iodine deficiency among the inhabitants of that region. Numerous investigations spanning decades have demonstrated unequivocally the relationship of low levels of iodide in drinking water to the incidence of goiter (see the section on iodine deficiency). For example, the iodide content of water from goitrous areas in India, Nepal, and Ceylon ranged from 0.1 to 1.2 mg/L, compared to 9.0 mg/L found in nongoitrous Delhi [1].

Iodide is found in seafoods as well as in water; however, large differences in iodide content exist between seawater fish and freshwater fish. Edible sea fish contain ~300 to 3,000 μg/kg, in contrast to only 20 to 40 μg/kg of freshwater fish.

An additional source of iodide is breads and grain products made from bread dough. Dough oxidizers or conditioners contain iodates (IO^{3-}) as food additives to improve cross-linking of the gluten. Such iodates provide about 500 mg iodide per 100 g bread [2].

Digestion, Absorption, Transport, and Storage

Dietary iodine (I) is either bound to amino acids or found free, primarily in the form of iodate (IO^{3-}) or iodide (I^-) (Fig. 12.20). During digestion, iodate, for example from breads, is reduced to iodide by glutathione [3].

Iodide is absorbed rapidly and completely throughout the gastrointestinal tract, including the stomach. Very little iodide appears in the feces. The small quantities of iodinated amino acids and other organic forms of iodide are absorbed, but not as efficiently as the iodide ion. The thyroid hormones thyroxine (T_4) and triiodothyronine

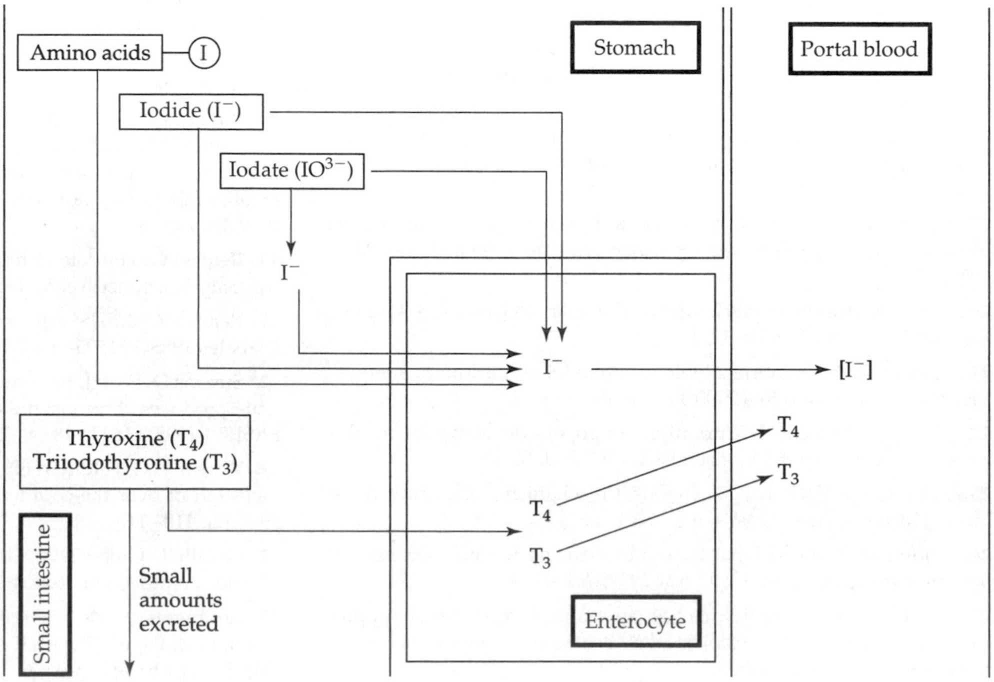

Figure 12.20 Digestion and absorption of iodine.

(T_3) also are absorbed unchanged, with a bioavailability of about 75%, allowing T_4 medication to be administered orally [4].

Following absorption, free iodide appears in the blood (Fig. 12.20). Iodide is distributed throughout the extracellular fluid, from which it is capable of permeating all tissues. The element selectively concentrates, however, in the thyroid glands. Lesser amounts of iodide are found in ovaries, placenta, skin, and salivary, gastric, and mammary glands. The kidneys also take up excess iodide for excretion. It is the thyroid gland that traps iodide most aggressively, doing so by way of a sodium-dependent, active transport system against an iodide gradient that is often 40 to 50 times the plasma concentration. The thyroid gland contains 70% to 80% of the total body iodide and takes up about 120 μg of iodide per day.

Because the thyroid gland and its synthesis of the thyroid hormones are the focal points of iodide metabolism, information on the transport of iodide into nonthyroidal tissue is sparse. It is likely, however, that salivary gland uptake proceeds by an active transport mechanism similar to that of the thyroid [5].

Functions and Mechanisms of Action

The main function of iodide is for the synthesis of the thyroid hormones thyroxine (T_4) and triiodothyronine (T_3) by the thyroid gland. The thyroid gland is made of multiple acini, also called follicles. The follicles are spherical in shape and are surrounded by a single layer of thyroid cells. The follicles are filled with colloid, a proteinaceous material. Both amino acids and iodide are needed to synthesize thyroid hormones. The events in thyroid hormone synthesis are shown in Figure 12.21 and described here:

- The thyroid cells actively collect iodide. In fact, the thyroid gland must trap about 60 mg of iodide daily against a steep gradient of the element to ensure an adequate supply of hormones [6]. The trapping mechanism operates through an Na^+/K^+-ATPase pump (Fig. 12.21) [7].
- Once within the cell, iodide (I^-) is oxidized to iodine (I), which is then bound to the number 3 position of tyrosyl residues of the glycoprotein thyroglobulin (a process called organification of the iodine). The binding of iodine to the tyrosyl residues of thyroglobulin (Thg)

Figure 12.21 Overview of iodine intrathyroidal metabolism and hormonogenesis, and thyroid transport and cellular uptake. Abbreviations: T_4, 3,5,3′,5′-tetraiodothyronine; T_3, 3,5,3′-triiodothyronine; rT_3, reverse T_3; Thg, thyroglobulin; MIT, 3-monoiodotyrosine; DIT, 3,5-diiodotyrosine.

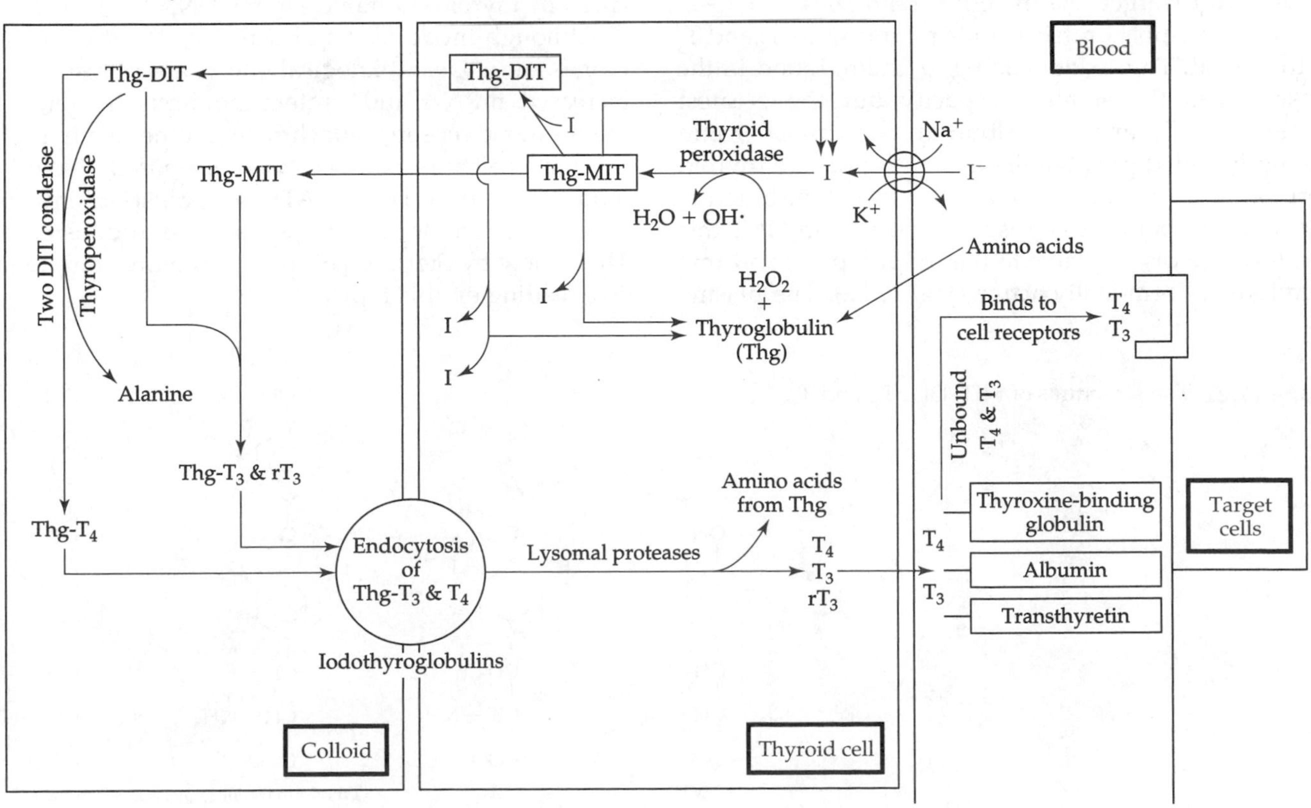

is catalyzed by thyroperoxidase and generates thyroglobulin-3-monoiodotyrosine (Thg-MIT) (Fig. 12.21). Hydrogen peroxide acts as the electron acceptor.

- Next, MIT is iodinated in the number 5 position to form thyroglobulin-3,5-diiodotyrosine (Thg-DIT). In the colloid, two DITs condense or couple to form Thg-3,5,3′,5′-tetraiodothyronine (Thg-T_4) with the elimination of an alanine side chain. Thyroperoxidase catalyzes this coupling reaction.
- DIT also condenses or couples with MIT to form 3,5,3′-triiodothyronine (T_3) and reverse T_3(rT_3).
- DIT and MIT not used for thyroid hormone synthesis in the thyroid cells are deiodinated, and the iodine is made available for recycling in the formation of new iodothyroglobulin. The structures of MIT, DIT, thyroxine (T_4) and 3,5,3′-triiodothyronine (T_3) are shown in Figure 12.22.

Transport of Thyroid Hormones in the Blood

To release the thyroid hormones into the blood, iodothyroglobulin must be resorbed in the form of colloid droplets by endocytosis back into the thyroid cell (Fig. 12.21). Within the thyroid cell, the iodothyroglobulin (Thg-T_4 and Thg-T_3) is hydrolyzed by lysosomal proteases, and T_4 and T_3 are released into the blood. In the blood, T_4 and T_3 associate with transport proteins and are distributed to target cells in peripheral tissues.

Three transport proteins bind and transport T_4 and T_3 in the blood. Thyroxine-binding globulin, found in the plasma, has the smallest capacity but the greatest affinity for T_4 and T_3. Albumin and transthyretin (formerly called prealbumin) also transport the thyroid hormones. A very small fraction (<0.1%) of the blood T_4 and T_3 is not bound to transport proteins, and it is this free form that is available to the cell receptors and that therefore is hormonally active (Fig. 12.22). The plasma concentration of T_4 is nearly 50 times that of T_3, but T_3 is many times more potent on an equal molar basis. For a more in-depth discussion of thyroid hormone synthesis, see the review by Taurog [8].

Several tissues—the liver, kidney, brain, pituitary, and brown adipose tissue, to name a few—can deiodinate T_4 to generate T_3 and rT_3. Most T_3 in the blood has been synthesized in the liver from T_4. A selenium-dependent 5′-deiodinase generates T_3, and a 5-deiodinase generates rT_3. Conversion of T_4 to T_3 is impaired with selenium deficiency [9].

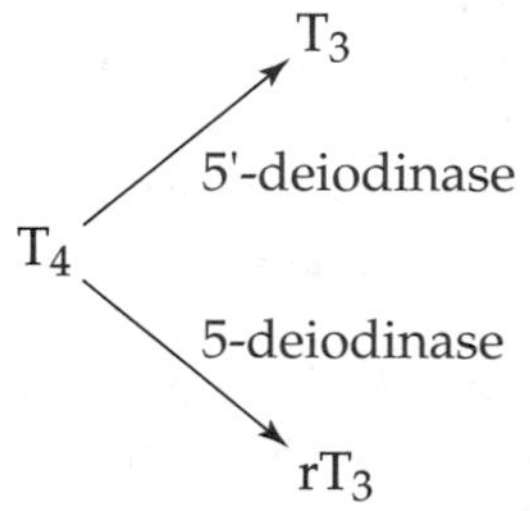

The multiple effects of the thyroid hormones result from the hormones' occupancy of nuclear receptors, with subsequent effects on gene expression. The receptors appear to be the same in all tissues, binding T_3 more avidly than T_4 and requiring fivefold to sevenfold higher concentrations of T_4 to achieve comparable physiological effects. Zinc may play a role in the binding of the zinc fingers of the receptor protein (which in turn is influenced by thyroid hormones) to the DNA.

Although mechanisms of action of the thyroid hormones are unclear, biological effects are in response to increased mRNA and protein synthesis triggered by the hormone receptor attachment. Numerous hypotheses for mechanisms have been proposed, including modulation of (Na^+/K^+-ATPase) transport systems, adrenergic receptor sensitivity, and neurotransmitters. The review by Sterling [10] provides more comprehensive reading on this topic.

Figure 12.22 The structures of MIT, DIT, T_3, and T_4.

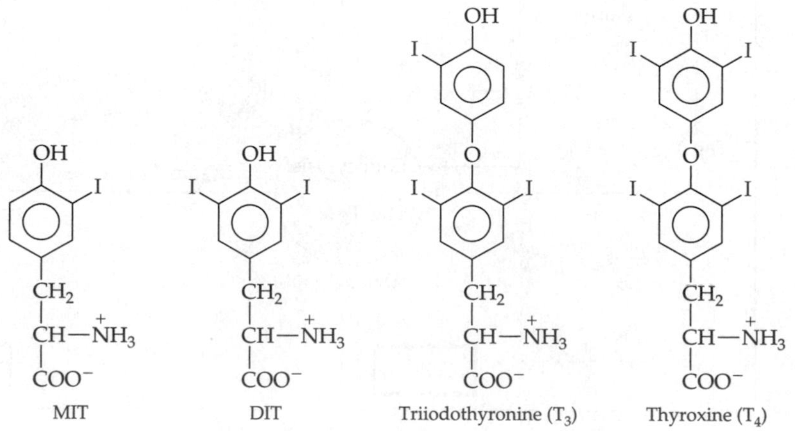

The effects of thyroid hormones on metabolism are many and varied. Thyroid hormones stimulate the basal rate of metabolism, oxygen (O_2) consumption, and heat production and are necessary for normal nervous system development and linear growth. Directly or indirectly, most organ systems are under the influence of these hormones.

Interactions with Other Nutrients

Arsenic appears to be goitrogenic in mice. In studies with mice, arsenic is believed to antagonize the mechanism of iodine uptake by the thyroid gland, causing compensatory goiter.

A more established interaction is that between iodide and goitrogens. Substances that interfere with iodide metabolism in any way that inhibits thyroid hormonogenesis are called goitrogens because their effect is to secondarily augment TSH release and consequently thyroid gland enlargement. Goitrogens may affect iodide uptake by the gland, organification of the iodide, or hormone release from the thyroid cells.

Most goitrogenic compounds act by competing with iodide in its active transport into the thyroid cells. Halide ions such as bromide (Br^-) and astatide (At^-) function in this way, as do thiocyanate (SCN^-), perrhenate (ReO_4^-), and pertechnetate (TcO_4). Perchlorate (ClO_4^-), along with perrhenate and pertechnetate, interferes with organification as well as uptake. Lithium (Li^-), used to treat some psychiatric disorders, inhibits hormone release from the gland. Other classes of goitrogens include polycyclic hydrocarbons, phenol compounds derived from coal, among other substances. These substances also interfere with iodide metabolism.

That some natural foods are goitrogenic was evidenced many years ago when it was discovered that rabbits fed a fresh cabbage diet developed goiters that could be reversed by iodine supplementation. It was later shown that vegetables of the cabbage family contained, along with small quantities of thiocyanates, a potent goitrogen that later became known as goitrin (Fig. 12.23). Numerous edible plants contain goitrin, including cabbage, kale, cauliflower, broccoli, rutabaga, turnips, brussels sprouts, and mustard greens. It is doubtful, however, that these foods are consumed in sufficient quantity to implicate them in the etiology of endemic goiter. Perhaps the only food to be identified directly with goiter etiology is cassava, which is consumed in large quantities in Third World countries [11]. Cassava contains cyanogen glucosides, of which thiocyanates are a major metabolite. Thiocyanates prevent the uptake of iodine by the thyroid gland.

Figure 12.23 Goitrin.

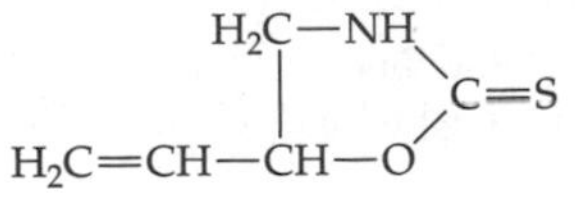

Excretion

The kidneys have no mechanism to conserve iodide, and they therefore provide the major route (~80%–90%) for iodide excretion [12,13]. The urinary output of iodide correlates closely with both the plasma iodide concentration and diet such that daily urinary iodine can be used to calculate iodine intake using the following formula: Daily iodine intake = Urinary iodine × 0.0235 × body weight, with urinary iodine measured in μg/L and weight measured in kg [14].

Fecal excretion of iodide (up to 20% of the total excreted) in humans is relatively low, ranging from 6.7 to 42.1 μg/day [12]. Some iodide is also lost in sweat, a loss that can be of consequence in hot, tropical regions where iodide intake is marginally adequate.

Recommended Dietary Allowances

Because of its important link to thyroid function, iodide nutriture has been investigated thoroughly for over half a century. Dating as far back as the 1930s, intake requirements have been published based on results of balance studies and on calculations of average daily urinary losses. Adult daily requirements established by those early studies ranged from 100 to 200 μg. The minimum amount (requirement) of iodide to prevent goiter is estimated to be between 50 and 75 μg/day or ~1 μg/kg of body weight.

The intake estimates have not changed significantly over the years. Both the 1989 and 2001 RDA for iodine is 150 μg/day for adults of both sexes and provides a margin of safety to allow for unquantified levels of goitrogens in the diet [2,14]. Although the recommendations apply equally to both sexes, iodide needs are higher during pregnancy and lactation: 220 μg and 290 μg, respectively [14]. The inside cover of the book provides additional RDAs for iodine for other age groups.

Deficiency

Thyroid Hormone Release as Related to Iodide Deficiency

The release of thyroid hormones by the thyroid gland is controlled. Thyrotropin-releasing hormone released from the hypothalamus acts on the pituitary gland to stimulate thyroid-stimulating hormone (TSH). TSH, in response to thyrotropin-releasing hormone, is secreted from the anterior pituitary and increases the activity of the thyroid gland to generate T_4. TSH output is regulated by T_4 through negative feedback to the pituitary.

A decline in the blood level of T_4 triggers release of pituitary TSH, resulting in hyperplasia of the thyroid. Elevated T_4 inhibits release of TSH and thyrotropin-releasing hormone.

Iodine Deficiency and Iodine Deficiency Disorders

Iodine deficiency prevails in many areas of the world and is associated most often with dietary insufficiency of iodine. Iodine deficiency is the main cause of goiter (although other factors such as ingestion of goitrogens may cause the disorder). Simple goiter is associated most often with insufficient dietary iodine and is characterized by enlargement of the thyroid gland. The enlargement is caused by overstimulation by TSH. Iodide deficiency causes depletion of thyroid iodine stores and therefore reduced output of T_4 and T_3. As stated above, the decline in the blood level of T_4 triggers release of pituitary TSH, resulting in hyperplasia of the thyroid gland. The growth of the gland is self-restricting, however, because in its enlarged state it traps and processes available iodide more efficiently. The gland returns to normal size as dietary iodide is increased to adequate amounts. When the prevalence of goiter in any population exceeds 10%, it is called endemic goiter [15].

Because of the effects of iodide deficiency on growth, development, and other health factors, the term iodide deficiency disorders (IDDs) has been implemented. Iodine deficiency in a fetus results from iodide deficiency of the mother, and cretinism, of which there are two types, results. Neurological cretinism in the infant is characterized by mental deficiency, hearing loss or deaf mutism, and motor disorders such as spasticity and muscular rigidity [6,15]. Hypothyroid cretinism results in thyroid failure. Early treatment of cretinism with iodine can often correct the condition.

The addition of iodide to table salt and the administration of iodized oil or potassium iodide has done much to alleviate the problem of endemic goiter in some goitrous regions of the world [16]. Yet iodide deficiency continues to be a major health problem in many underdeveloped countries, and in China it may be coupled with selenium deficiency [17].

Toxicity

The lowest observed adverse effect level (LOAEL) occurs at iodide intakes of ~1,700 μg/day. A tolerable upper intake level for iodine has been set at 1,100 μg/day in response to changes in serum thyrotropin concentrations from varying iodine intakes.

Assessment of Nutriture

Iodide nutritional status assessment is generally directed at populations living in areas suspected of being iodide-deficient. The assessment is based on both the physical examination and the chemical testing of individuals. The data collected for assessment studies are extensive and include at least the following:

- total population count, including the number of children under 15 years of age;
- the incidence of goiter as established by physical examination and cretinism in the population;
- the quantification of urinary iodide excretion;
- the quantification of iodide in the drinking water; and
- determination of serum T_4 levels in various age groups.

The chemistry of tests measuring urinary iodide excretion is based on the ability of iodide ion to reduce cerric ion (Ce^{4+}), which is yellow, to its colorless, cerrous state (Ce^{3+}), as shown here:

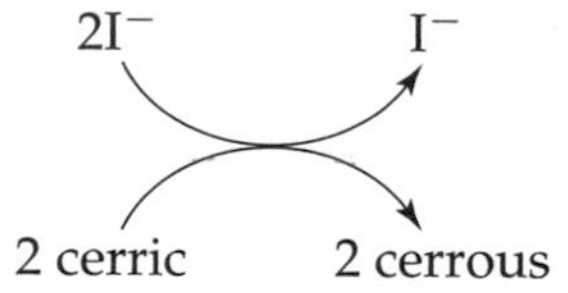

The extent of the color change, which is directly proportional to the iodide concentration in the specimen, is monitored spectrophotometrically. All iodine in the specimen, therefore, must first be reduced to iodide. Urinary iodine concentrations of <50 μg/g creatinine are considered to indicate risk [18]. However, use of the iodine : creatinine ratio in casual urine samples has been shown to be unsuitable as an indicator for evaluating iodine status in some populations [19]. Radioactive iodide (^{131}I) uptake may also be measured to assess thyroid function. The greater the overall uptake and the quicker the uptake of the radioactive iodide by the thyroid gland, the greater the likelihood of iodide deficiency [18].

References Cited for Iodine

1. Karmarkar M, Deo M, Kochupillai N, Ramalingaswami V. Pathophysiology of Himalayan endemic goiter. Am J Clin Nutr 1974; 27:96–103.

2. National Research Council. Recommended Dietary Allowances, 10th ed. Washington, DC: National Academy Press, 1989, pp. 213–17.

3. Taurog A, Howells E, Nachimson H. Conversion of iodate to iodide in vitro and in vivo. J Biol Chem 1966;241:4686–93.

4. Hays MT. Localization of human thyroxine absorption. Thyroid 1991;1:241–48.

5. Harden RMcG, Alexander W, Shimmins J, Kostalas H, Mason D. Quantitative aspects of the inhibitory effect of the iodide ion on parotid salivary iodide and pertechnetate secretion in man. J Lab Clin Med 1968;71:92–100.

6. Clugston G, Hetzel B. Iodine. In: Shils ME, Olson JA, Shike M, eds. Modern nutrition in health and disease. Philadelphia: Lea and Febiger, 1994, pp. 252–63.

7. O'Neill B, Magnolato D, Semenza G. The electrogenic, Na^+-dependent I^- transport system in plasma membrane vesicles from thyroid glands. Biochim Biophys Acta 1987;896:263–74.

8. Taurog A. Hormone synthesis: thyroid iodine metabolism. In: Ingbar SH, Braverman LE, eds. Werner's the Thyroid. Philadelphia: Lippincott 1986, pp. 53–97.

9. Arthur J, ed. Interrelationships between selenium deficiency, iodine deficiency, and thyroid hormones. Am J Clin Nutr 1993;57: 235S–318S.

10. Sterling K. Thyroid hormone action at the cellular level. In: Ingbar SH, Braverman LE, eds. Werner's the Thyroid. Philadelphia: Lippincott, 1986, pp. 219–33.

11. Maberly G, Waite K, Eastman C, et al. In: Ui N, Torizuka K, Nagataki A, et al., eds. Current Problems in Thyroid Research. Amsterdam: Excerpta Medica 1983, p. 341.

12. Vought R, London W, Lutwak L, Dublin T. Reliability of estimates of serum inorganic iodine and daily fecal and urinary iodine excretion from single casual specimens. J Clin Endocr Metab 1963;23:1218–28.

13. Nath SK, Moinier B, Thuillier F, Rongier M, Desjeux JR. Urinary excretion of iodide and fluoride from supplemented food grade salt. Interntl J Vit Nutr Res 1992;62:66–72.

14. Food and Nutrition Board, Institute of Medicine. Dietary Reference Intakes. Washington, DC: National Academy Press, 2001, pp. 258–89.

15. Lamberg B. Iodine deficiency disorders and endemic goitre. Eur J Clin Nutr 1993;47:1–8.

16. Todd C, Dunn J. Intermittent oral administration of potassium iodide solution for the correction of iodine deficiency. Am J Clin Nutr 1998;67:1279–83.

17. Ma T, Guo J, Wang F. The epidemiology of iodine-deficiency diseases in China. Am J Clin Nutr 1993;57:264S–66S.

18. Gibson R. Principles of Nutritional Assessment. New York: Oxford University Press, 1990, pp. 527–32.

19. Furnee C, Haar F, West C, Hautvast J. A critical appraisal of goiter assessment and the ratio of urinary iodine to creatinine for evaluating iodine status. Am J Clin Nutr 1994;59:1415–17.

MANGANESE

Although widely distributed in nature, manganese occurs in only trace amounts in animal tissues. The body of a healthy 70-kg man is estimated to contain a total of 10 to 20 mg of the metal. In the body, manganese typically exists in either of two states, Mn^{2+} or Mn^{3+}.

Sources

Whole-grain cereals, dried fruits, nuts, and leafy vegetables are among the common manganese-rich foods. Tea also contains large amounts of manganese, but manganese in tea is not well absorbed. The wide content range of the mineral in cereal grains is due partly to plant species differences and partly to the efficiency with which the milling process separates the manganese-rich and manganese-poor parts of the grain. White flour, for example, has a much lower manganese concentration than the wheat grain from which it was produced. Table 12.6 lists the manganese content of selected foods.

Table 12.6 Manganese Content of Selected Foods and Beverages

Foods/Food Group	Manganese Content (mg/100 g)
Bread, whole grains	0.50–2.05
Flour, whole grain	3.80
Bread, white	0.05
Flour, white	0.79
Legumes	0.24–0.58
Nuts	0.83–4.71
Root vegetables	0.05–0.62
Other vegetables	0.15–1.94
Fruits	0.04–1.60
Fruits (dried)	0.09–0.39
Milk and cheeses	< 0.01
Beer	0.01
Wine	
White	0.46
Red	0.60
Coffee (brewed)	0.02–0.03
Tea (brewed)	0.18–0.22

Source: www.nal.usda.gov/fnic/foodcomp.

Absorption, Transport, and Storage

Absorption

Little information is available on the mechanism of manganese absorption, although it has been established that the process occurs equally well throughout the length of the small intestine [1]. Dietary manganese absorption varies considerably, with values of 1% to 14% reported, but absorption is often <5% [2–7]. Gender differences also have been reported, with women absorbing more manganese than men [2]. Manganese absorption from $MnCl_2$ (manganese chloride) has been shown to be greater than that from plant foods such as lettuce, spinach, and sunflower seeds [3].

The absorption process itself appears to be quickly saturable and probably involves a low-capacity, high-affinity, active transport mechanism as demonstrated in rats. With excessive high manganese intake, absorption decreases to protect against toxicity; excretion also increases, as discussed in the section on manganese excretion. Manganese is thought to be absorbed in the Mn^{2+} state. Within the duodenum, ingested manganese as Mn^{2+} may be converted to Mn^{3+}.

Factors Influencing Absorption. Relative to many of the other trace minerals, little information is available on factors influencing manganese absorption. There is evidence for enhancement of absorption by low-molecular-weight ligands such as histidine and citrate [8].

Studies in animals and humans suggest that fiber, phytate, and oxalate may precipitate manganese in the gastrointestinal tract, making the manganese unavailable for absorption [8–10]. Several minerals also inhibit manganese absorption. Iron, for example, competes with manganese for absorption. High dietary nonheme iron can depress both manganese absorption and status in animals and humans, and iron deficiency can enhance manganese absorption and retention [11–14]. The two minerals are thought to compete for common binding sites; however, negative correlations between serum ferritin and manganese absorption and retention also have been shown [5]. Copper also has been shown to decrease manganese absorption and retention, while ascorbic acid diminished Mn-dependent superoxide dismutase activity in rats [14].

Transport and Storage

Manganese entering into the portal circulation from the gastrointestinal tract may either remain free or become bound as Mn^{2+} to α-2 macroglobulin before traversing the liver, where it is almost totally removed. From the liver, some manganese may remain free (Mn^{2+}), or as Mn^{2+} it may be bound to albumin or α-2 macroglobulin, or Mn^{2+} may be oxidized by ceruloplasmin to Mn^{3+} and may complex with transferrin [15,16]. Mn^{3+} bound to transferrin is taken up by transferrin receptors into extrahepatic tissues, including the brain.

Manganese is cleared rapidly from the blood and accumulates preferentially in the mitochondria of tissues, a process that may be mediated by a Ca^{2+} carrier [17]. Within the mitochondria, manganese is present as hydrate Mn^{2+} or Mn^{3+} and as $Mn^{3+}(PO_4)_2$, a matrix precipitate [18]. Manganese is found in most organs and tissues and does not tend to concentrate significantly in any particular one, although its concentration is highest in bone, liver, pancreas, and kidney. In bone, manganese is found as part of the apatite. Hair also can accumulate manganese.

Functions and Mechanisms of Action

At the molecular level, manganese, like other trace elements, can function both as an enzyme activator and as a constituent of metalloenzymes, but the relationship of these functions to the gross physiological changes observed in manganese deficiency is not well correlated. Reviews pertaining to this topic have been published [19].

In the activation of enzyme-catalyzed reactions, manganese may bind to the substrate (such as ATP) or to the enzyme directly, with induction of conformational changes. Enzymes from about every class can be activated by manganese in this manner and are numerous and diverse in function. They include enzymes from these enzyme classes: transferases including kinases, hydrolases, oxido-reductases, ligases, and lyases. The activity of most of these enzymes, however, is not affected by a manganese deficiency, largely because the activation is not manganese specific. The metal can be replaced by other divalent cations, primarily magnesium. One exception to this apparent lack of specificity is the manganese-specific activation of the glycosyl transferases. Examples of some manganese-dependent enzymes from each enzyme class are described next.

Transferases

Many transferases require manganese. Two examples are xylosyl transferases and glycosyl transferases. Glycosyl transferases catalyze the transfer of a sugar moiety such as galactose from uridine diphosphate (UDP) to an acceptor molecule, as shown by the general reaction:

$$\begin{matrix}\text{UDP-sugar} \\ + \\ \text{acceptor}\end{matrix} \xrightarrow{\text{Glycosyl transferase}} \begin{matrix}\text{UDP} \\ + \\ \text{acceptor-sugar}\end{matrix}$$

Several sugars participate in these reactions. Galactose is a more common participate and when bound to UDP may be transferred to an acceptor molecule by the glycosyl transferase. Glycosyl transferases are necessary for proteoglycan, including mucopolysaccharide, synthesis. Remember that mucopolysaccharides, among other proteoglycans, are important components of bone and connective tissue such as collagen.

Hydrolases

Manganese also activates prolidase, a dipeptidase with specificity for dipeptides. Prolidase is found in dermal fibroblasts and catalyzes the final step in collagen degradation. Arginase, which contains four manganese atoms per molecule, is a cytosolic enzyme responsible for urea formation (p. 197) and found in high concentrations in the liver. The Mn^{2+} may allosterically activate arginase through a pH-mediated role [20]. Low-manganese diets in animals have been shown to decrease arginase activity [21].

Lyases

Phosphoenolpyruvate carboxykinase (PEPCK), also activated by manganese, converts oxaloacetate to phosphoenolpyruvate and carbon dioxide. This reaction is important in gluconeogenesis (p. 96). The activity of phosphoenolpyruvate carboxykinase decreases in animals with manganese deficiency.

Oxido-Reductases

Superoxide dismutase, a manganese-dependent (Mn^{3+}-SOD) metalloenzyme (not manganese activated), functions in a manner similar to copper- and zinc-dependent SOD (p. 451) to prevent lipid peroxidation by superoxide radicals. Manganese SOD, however, is found in the mitochondria, whereas copper-zinc SOD is found both extracellularly and in the cytoplasm. Thus, SOD in the mitochondria likely serves to eliminate superoxides before they damage mitochondrial function. The activity of the electron transport/respiratory chain generates large amounts of superoxide radicals, necessitating substantial Mn-SOD activity. It is likely that the cell ultrastructural abnormalities associated with manganese deficiency are due to unchecked lipid peroxidation in the cellular membranes because of reduced Mn-SOD activity or simply because of reduced availability of manganese to directly scavenge free radicals. Manganese (Mn^{2+}), one of several minerals able to scavenge free radicals, quenches peroxyl radicals as shown in this equation [22]:

$$Mn^{2+} + ROO\cdot \longrightarrow Mn^{3+} + ROOH$$

Low-manganese diets in animals have been shown to decrease Mn-SOD activity.

Ligases/Synthetases

Pyruvate carboxylase, which contains four manganese atoms, converts pyruvate to oxaloacetate (p. 96), a tricarboxylic acid–cycle intermediate. Because magnesium can replace manganese in pyruvate carboxylase, minimal changes in pyruvate carboxylase activity occur [21]. Glutamine synthetase (Fig. 7.32) may be a manganese metalloenzyme or may be activated by manganese or magnesium.

Other Roles

Manganese also may act as a modulator of second messenger pathways in tissues. For example, manganese increases cAMP accumulation through binding to ATP and ADP. Manganese can activate guanylate cyclase, and manganese may affect cytoplasmic calcium levels and thus regulate calcium-dependent processes (see Fig. 11.5) [18].

Interactions with Other Nutrients

Only a few interactions between manganese and other trace elements are thought to be of significance nutritionally. One relationship of nutritional significance—that between manganese and iron—was discussed earlier in the section on absorption. Some degree of interaction may occur between manganese and calcium and between manganese and zinc in such a way as to affect the bioavailability of manganese [23]. However, because of the paucity of information and the divergent results of some relevant studies, the nature of such interactions remains inconclusive.

Excretion

Manganese is excreted primarily via the bile in the feces. Excess absorbed manganese from the diet is quickly excreted by the liver into the bile to maintain homeostasis [2]. Very little manganese is excreted in the urine. Moreover, urinary manganese does not correlate with intake and does not increase even when dietary intake of the mineral is excessive [24–26]. However, excretion of manganese through sweat and skin desquamation has been shown to contribute to manganese losses [27].

Adequate Intakes

In 1980, the Food and Nutrition Board first recommended an estimated safe and adequate daily dietary intake for manganese of 2.5 to 5 mg for adults, and in 1989 this range was modified to 2 to 5 mg [28]. This recommendation was thought to represent a dietary intake level achieved by most individuals who exhibit no signs of deficiency or toxicity [28]. The 2001 recommendation, like previous recommendations, is based on median intakes due to insufficient data to calculate the requirement for manganese. The latest recommended intakes are 2.3 mg for adult men and 1.8 mg for adult women [29]. With pregnancy and lactation, recommendations increase to 2 mg and 2.6 mg, respectively [29]. The inside cover of the book gives additional recommendations for manganese for other age groups.

Deficiency

Studies on a wide variety of species have demonstrated that manganese deficiency is associated with striking and diverse physiological malfunctions. Manganese deficiency generally does not develop in humans unless the mineral is deliberately eliminated from the diet. Human studies in which men received either 0.11 mg manganese per day for 39 days (the diet was also devoid of vitamin K, making it difficult to separate the effects of the manganese and vitamin K deficiencies) or 0.35 mg manganese per day resulted in negative manganese balance [24,27,28]. Symptoms and signs of deficiency included nausea; vomiting; dermatitis; decreased serum manganese; decreased fecal manganese excretion; increased serum calcium, phosphorus, and alkaline phosphatase (thought to be associated with skeletal bone changes); decreased growth of hair and nails; changes in hair and beard color; and low blood cholesterol concentrations [27–29]. Other effects reported included the occurrence of neonatal ataxia and loss of equilibrium, cell ultrastructure abnormalities, compromised reproductive function, abnormal glucose tolerance, and impaired lipid metabolism [27–29]. In rats, dietary manganese deficiency also altered plasma ammonia and urea concentrations in association with decreased arginase activity [19].

Toxicity

Manganese toxicity can occur in individuals with liver failure, because it is through bile excretion that manganese homeostasis is maintained. Manganese toxicity secondary to liver failure is characterized by manganese accumulation within the liver and other organs such as the brain; the latter results in neurologic abnormalities [30,31]. Miners who have inhaled dust fumes high in manganese (about 5 mg/m^3 or more) experience Parkinsonism-like symptoms. Manganese toxicity in individuals chronically exposed to airborne manganese in concentrations as low as 1 mg/m^3 also have been reported to experience problems, including prolonged reaction time, tremors, and diminished memory capacity [32]. The lowest observable adverse effect level is 15 mg, while the no observable adverse effect level and the tolerable upper intake level for manganese have been set at 11 mg/day [29].

Assessment of Nutriture

Assessment of manganese status typically is based on concentrations of manganese in mononuclear blood cells as well as in plasma, serum, and blood [7,33]. Serum concentrations have been found to be somewhat sensitive to large variations in intake but do not necessarily correlate with intake [26]. It has been suggested that mononuclear blood cell concentrations of manganese may be a better indicator than blood or serum concentrations [33]. Enzyme activity also has been used to assess status. In animals, mitochondrial Mn-SOD in some tissues and blood arginase activities have been shown to be diminished with low manganese intake or deficiency [12,14,34]. In humans, manganese supplementation significantly increased lymphocyte Mn-SOD activity and serum manganese concentrations from baseline without changes in manganese excretion [25]. Additional laboratory tests to assess body manganese status are still under investigation.

References Cited for Manganese

1. Thomson A, Olatunbosun D, Valberg L. Interrelation of intestinal transport system for manganese and iron. J Lab Clin Med 1971; 78:642–55.

2. Finley J, Johnson P, Johnson L. Sex affects manganese absorption and retention by humans from a diet adequate in manganese. Am J Clin Nutr 1994;60:949–55.

3. Johnson P, Lykken G, Korynta E. Absorption and biological half-life in humans of intrinsic and extrinsic ^{54}Mn tracers from foods of plant origin. J Nutr 1991;121:711–17.

4. Hunt JR, Matthys LA, Johnson LK. Zinc absorption, mineral balance, and blood lipids in women consuming controlled lacto-ovovegetarian and omnivorous diets for 8 weeks. Am J Clin Nutr 1998;67:421–30.

5. Finley JW. Manganese absorption and retention by young women is associated with serum ferritin concentration. Am J Clin Nutr 1999;70:37–43.

6. Johnson PE, Lykken GI. Manganese and calcium absorption and balance in young women fed diets with varying amounts of manganese and calcium. J Trace Elem Exp Med 1991;4:19–35.

7. Freeland-Graves JH. Manganese: an essential nutrient for humans. Nutrition Today 1988;23:13–19.

8. Garcia-Aranda J, Wapnir R, Lifshitz F. In vivo intestinal absorption of manganese in the rat. J Nutr 1983;113:2601–7.

9. Davidsson L, Almegren A, Juillerat M, Hurrell R. Manganese absorption in humans: the effect of phytic acid and ascorbic acid in soy formula. Am J Clin Nutr 1995;62:984–87.

10. Schwartz R, Apgar BJ, Wien EM. Apparent absorption and retention of Ca, Cu, Mg, Mn, and Zn from a diet containing bran. Am J Clin Nutr 1986;43:444–45.

11. Keen C, Frannson G, Lonnerdal B. Supplementation of milk with iron bound to lactoferrin using weanling mice: effects on tissue manganese, zinc, and copper. J Pediatr Gastroenterol Nutr 1984;3:256–61.

12. Davis CD, Ney DM, Greger JL. Manganese, iron, and lipid interactions in rats. J Nutr 1990;120:507–13.

13. Davis CD, Malecki EA, Greger JL. Interactions among dietary manganese, heme iron, and nonheme iron in women. Am J Clin Nutr 1992;56:926–32.

14. Johnson PE, Korynta ED. Effects of copper, iron, and ascorbic acid on manganese availability to rats. Proc Soc Exp Biol Med 1992;199:470–80.

15. Critchfield J, Keen C. Manganese^{+2} exhibits dynamic binding to multiple ligands in human plasma. Metabolism 1992;41:1087–92.

16. Rabin O, Hegedus L, Bourre JM, Smith QR. Rapid brain uptake of manganese (II) across the blood-brain barrier. J Neurochem 1993;61:509–17.

17. Jeng A, Shamoo A. Isolation of a Ca^{2+} carrier from calf heart inner mitochondrial membrane. J Biol Chem 1980;255:6897–903.

18. Korc M. Manganese as a modulator of signal transduction pathways. In: Prasad AS, ed. Essential and Toxic Trace Elements in Human Health and Disease: An Update. New York: Wiley-Liss, 1993, pp. 235–55.

19. Keen C, Lonnerdal B, Hurley L. Manganese. In: Frieden E, ed. Biochemistry of the Essential Trace Elements. Norfolk, VA: Plenum, 1984, pp. 89–132.

20. Kuhn N, Ward S, Piponski M, Young T. Purification of human hepatic arginase and its manganese (II) dependent and pH-dependent interconversion between active and inactive forms: a possible pH sensing function of the enzyme on the ornithine cycle. Arch Biochem Biophys 1995;320:24–34.

21. Brock A, Chapman S, Ulman E, Wu G. Dietary manganese deficiency decreases rate of hepatic arginase activity. J Nutr 1994;124:340–44.

22. Coassin M, Ursini F, Bindoli A. Antioxidant effect of manganese. Arch Biochem Biophys 1992;299:330–33.

23. Forbes R, Erdman J. Bioavailability of trace mineral elements. Ann Rev Nutr 1983;3:213–31.

24. Freeland-Graves J, Behmardi F, Bales C, Bougherty V, Lin P-H, Crosby J, Trickett P. Metabolic balance of manganese in young men consuming diets containing five levels of dietary manganese. J Nutr 1988;118:764–73.

25. Davis C, Greger J. Longitudinal changes of manganese dependent superoxide dismutase and other indexes of manganese and iron status in women. Am J Clin Nutr 1992;55:747–52.

26. Greger JL, Davis CD, Suttie JW, Lyle BJ. Intake, serum concentrations, and urinary excretion of manganese by adult males. Am J Clin Nutr 1990;51:457–61.

27. Friedman B, Freeland-Graves J, Bales C, Behmardi F, Shorey-Kutschke R, Willis R, Crosby J, Trickett P, Houston S. Manganese balance and clinical observations in young men fed a manganese-deficient diet. J Nutr 1987;117:133–43.

28. National Research Council. Recommended Dietary Allowances, 10th ed. Washington, DC: National Academy Press, 1989, pp. 230–35.

29. Food and Nutrition Board, Institute of Medicine. Dietary Reference Intakes. Washington, DC: National Academy Press, 2001, pp. 394–419.

30. Hauser R, Zesiewicz T, Rosemurgy A, Martinez C, Olanow C. Manganese intoxication and chronic liver failure. Ann Neurol 1994; 36:871–75.

31. Reynolds A, Kiely E, Meadows N. Manganese in long term paediatric parenteral nutrition. Arch Dis Child 1994;71:527–31.

32. Wennberg A, Iregren A, Struwe G, Cizinsky G, Hagman M, Johansson L. Manganese exposure in steel smelters a health hazard to the human worker. Scand J Work Environ Health 1991;17:255–62.

33. Matsuda A, Kimura M, Takeda T, Kataoka M, Sato M, Itokawa Y. Changes in manganese content of mononuclear blood cells in patients receiving total parenteral nutrition. Clin Chem 1994;40:829–32.

34. Thompson K, Lee M. Effects of manganese and vitamin E deficiencies on antioxidant enzymes in streptozotocin-diabetic rats. J Nutr Biochem 1993;4:476–81.

Additional Readings

Freeland-Graves J, Turnlund JR. Deliberations and evaluations of the approaches, endpoints, and paradigms for manganese and molybdenum dietary recommendations. J Nutr 1996;126:2435S–40S.

Greger J. Dietary standards for manganese: overlap between nutritional and toxicological studies. J Nutr 1998;128:368S–71S.

Greger JL. Nutrition versus toxicology of manganese in humans: evaluation of potential biomarkers. Neurotoxicology 1999;20:205–12.

Sandstrom B, Davidsson L, Cederblad A, Eriksson R, Lonnerdal B. Manganese absorption and metabolism in man. Acta Pharmacol Toxicol 1996;59:60–62.

MOLYBDENUM

The need for molybdenum was established in humans through the observation that a genetic deficiency of specific enzymes that require molybdenum as a cofactor resulted in severe pathology in human patients. In the body, molybdenum, a metal, is found primarily in either of two valence states, Mo^{4+} or Mo^{6+}. In biological systems, molybdenum generally is bound to either sulfur or oxygen.

Sources

Molybdenum is widespread among foods, but like many other minerals the molybdenum content of a given plant food may vary greatly depending on the concentration of molybdenum in the soil. It follows that the metal's content in meats in turn reflects its concentration in the regional forage. Better sources of molybdenum in the diet are legumes, which can provide up to 184 μg/100 g; meat, fish, and poultry, which contain up to ~129 μg/100 g; and grains and grain products, which provide up to ~117 μg/100 g [1,2]. Nuts and vegetables usually contain <50 μg/100 g, while fruits and dairy products are especially low in molybdenum, providing <12 μg/100 g [1,2].

Absorption, Transport, and Storage

Little is known about the sites from which absorption of molybdenum occurs in humans. The mechanism of absorption is thought to be passive, although some animal studies suggest the possible involvement of carriers. Absorption in humans ranges from ~50% to over 90% [3–5]. Transport of molybdenum in the blood is thought to occur as molybdate (MoO_4^{2-}). The mineral may be bound to albumin and/or α-2 macroglobulin.

The molybdenum content of human tissues is quite low under normal dietary conditions, averaging 0.1 to 1.0 μg/g of wet weight. Molybdenum is found in tissues as molybdate, free molybdopterin, or molybdopterin that is bound to enzymes. The liver, kidney, and bone contain the most molybdenum in terms of both absolute amount and concentration [6]. Other tissues, such as the small intestine, lungs, spleen, brain, thyroid and adrenal glands, and muscle, also contain molybdenum.

Functions and Mechanisms of Action

The biochemical role of molybdenum centers around the redox function of the element and its necessity as a cofactor for three metalloenzymes (sulfite oxidase, aldehyde oxidase, and xanthine dehydrogenase/oxidase), all of which catalyze oxidation-reduction reactions [7].

One of the more exciting revelations in molybdenum biochemistry has been the identification and characterization of molybdopterin, the molybdenum-containing cofactor. Molybdopterin is an alkylphosphate-substituted pterin to which molybdenum is coordinated through two sulfur atoms [8–10]. It is through molybdopterin that the molybdenum is anchored to the apoenzyme at its catalytic site. The molybdenum is further bonded either to two oxygen molecules (referred to as dioxomolybdopterin) or to one oxygen and one sulfur (referred to as oxosulfidomolybdopterin), as shown in Figure 12.24.

Sulfite Oxidase

Sulfite oxidase, a mitochondrial intermembrane enzyme found in many body tissues, especially the liver, heart, and kidney, has iron-sulfur clusters and two molybdopterin (dioxo cofactor form) and two cytochrome residues. The enzyme catalyzes the

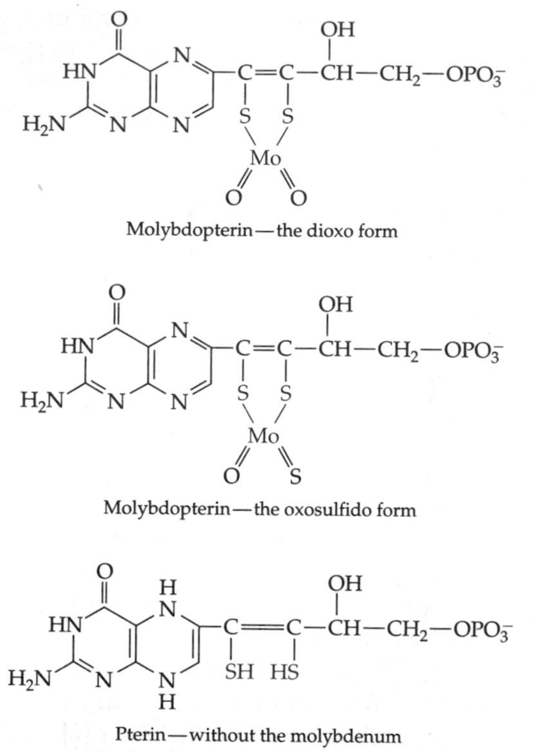

Figure 12.24 Molybdopterin structures.

terminal step in the metabolism of sulfur-containing amino acids (methionine and cysteine), in which sulfite (SO_3^{2-}) is converted to sulfate (SO_4^{2-}), as shown here:

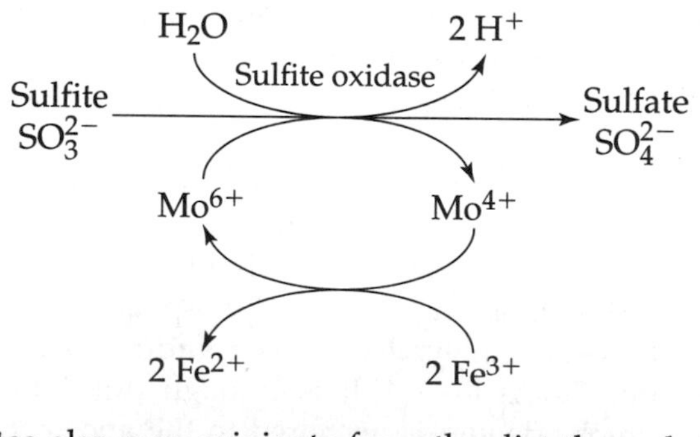

Sulfites also may originate from the diet through their addition to some foods as an antimicrobial agent. Cytochrome c is the physiological electron acceptor for the reaction. Sulfate generated from this reaction typically is excreted in the urine or reused for the synthesis of sulfoproteins, sulfolipids, and mucopolysaccharides (a component of mucus).

Aldehyde Oxidase

Aldehyde oxidase is a molybdoenzyme (using the oxosulfido form) that is very similar to xanthine oxidase (see next) in size, cofactor composition, and substrate specificity. It presumably functions primarily in the liver as a true oxidase, using molecular oxygen as its physiological electron acceptor. The enzyme's primary substrates are thought to include a variety of aldehydes, including drugs [11]. Other enzymes, however, such as an NADH-dependent aldehyde dehydrogenase also found in the liver, are thought to catalyze reactions similar to those catalyzed by this aldehyde oxidase.

Xanthine Dehydrogenase and Xanthine Oxidase

Xanthine dehydrogenase and xanthine oxidase (referred to as oxidoreductases) are iron-dependent, (iron-sulfur centers nonheme-containing) enzymes that also require FAD and molybdopterin in the oxosulfido cofactor form. Xanthine dehydrogenase is found in a variety of tissues, including the liver, lungs, kidneys, and intestine. Xanthine oxidase is found in the intestine, thyroid cells, and possibly other tissues. Healthy tissues may contain about 10% of their total xanthine enzymes in the oxidase form [12]. Conversion of xanthine dehydrogenase to xanthine oxidase may occur following oxidation of essential sulfhydryl groups or by proteolysis of the dehydrogenase form. Xanthine oxidase has been implicated as a cause of damage in postischemic reperfused tissue.

The xanthine dehydrogenase and oxidase enzymes are capable of hydroxylating various purines, pteridines, pyrimidines, and other heterocyclic nitrogen-containing compounds. Hypoxanthine, derived from purine catabolism, is oxidized in most tissues by xanthine dehydrogenase to generate xanthine and then uric acid (see Fig. 12.25). Xanthine dehydrogenase transfers electrons from the substrate onto NAD^+ to form NADH + H^+. Oxidation of hypoxanthine and xanthine by xanthine oxidase also results in uric acid, but in these reactions O_2 accepts the electrons from $FADH_2$ and hydrogen peroxide (H_2O_2) or a superoxide radical is formed.

Although low-molybdenum diets or inclusion in the diet of tungstate, a molybdenum antagonist, predictably reduces the level of xanthine oxidase activity in rat intestine and liver, it is interesting to note that no apparent clinical effects result from the perturbation. Furthermore, the human inheritable disorder xanthinuria, in which large amounts of xanthine are excreted in the urine, provides additional evidence of the body's ability to tolerate low xanthine dehydrogenase or oxidase activity. The condition is essentially free of clinical manifestations, except for the possible development of kidney calculi (stones) caused by the high urinary xanthine concentration. Therefore, whether any of the reactions catalyzed by xanthine dehydrogenase or

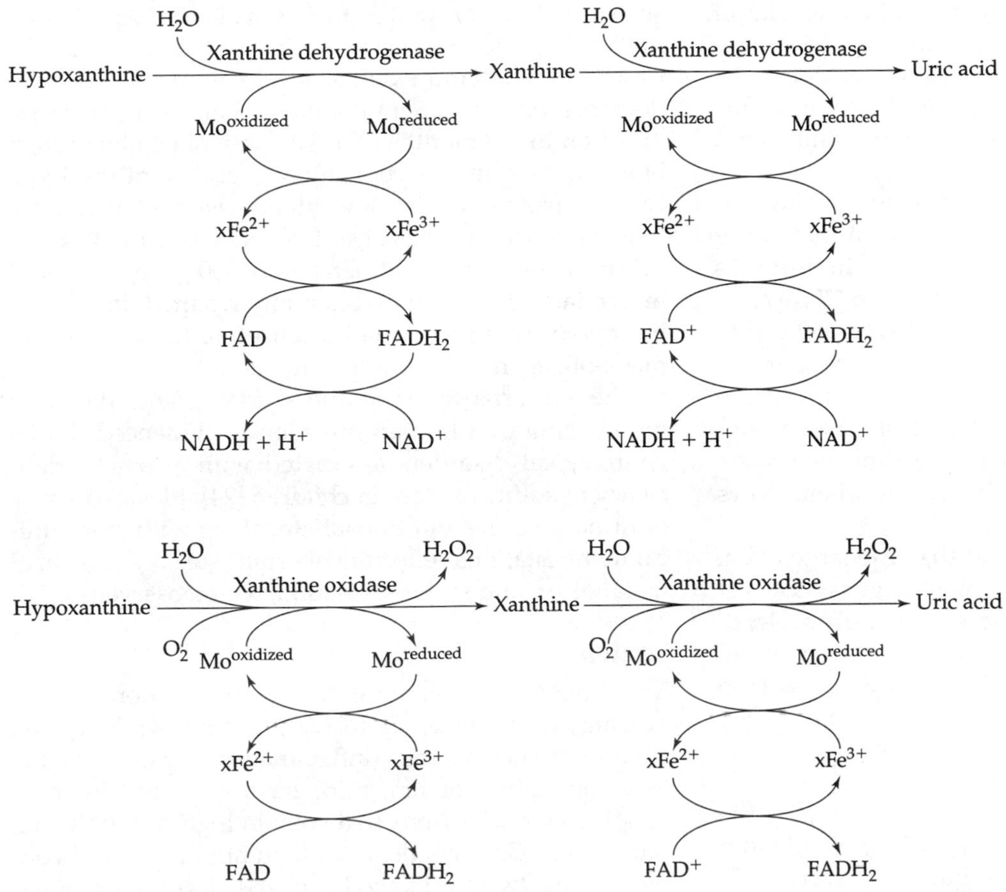

Figure 12.25 The actions of xanthine dehydrogenase and xanthine oxidase on the substrate hypoxanthine.

oxidase are necessary for human health is not firmly established [13].

The effects of xanthine oxidase activity, however, have been shown to be quite damaging in people being treated for ischemia (local or temporary deficiency of blood supply and thus relative oxygen deprivation), for example. Degradation of ATP in hypoxic tissue yields hypoxanthine. Reperfusion of the intestine with oxygen (as occurs with medical treatment of, e.g., intestinal ischemia) helps prevent total destruction of the tissue due to lack of oxygen and nutrients, but it also provides xanthine oxidase with the oxygen needed to oxidize the relatively large concentrations of hypoxanthine. Oxidation of hypoxanthine generates large amounts of hydrogen peroxide, which further induces tissue damage (referred to as reperfusion injury; see the perspective in Chap. 10). However, the injury also is thought to be mediated in part by neutrophil accumulation and activation, and the reactive oxygen species formed may be involved in signal transduction pathways [14].

Another role for molybdenum, in addition to its biochemical role, may involve modulation (likely inhibition through direct interaction) of the glucocorticoid receptor complex [15].

Interactions with Other Nutrients

Tungsten has long been recognized as a potent antagonist of molybdenum [16], and in fact its administration into test animals has become the major means for artificially creating a state of molybdenum deficiency.

Another interaction involves molybdenum, sulfur, and copper. It has been shown, particularly in ruminants, that a high dietary intake of sulfate or molybdenum depressed the tissue uptake of copper and, conversely, that sulfate and copper decreased molybdenum retention [17]. The proposed explanation for this is that sulfide and hydrosulfide ions are generated in the rumen by reduction of ingested sulfate. The reactive sulfide then displaces oxygen from molybdate ions, yielding oxythiomolybdates and tetrathiomolybdates. Molybdenum is not readily absorbed in the form of thiomolybdates, and, furthermore, thiomolybdates bind copper avidly, rendering that metal less physiologically available [18]. It is important to recognize, however, that in humans and other nonruminants such an interaction is not as important because of the low yield of sulfides and hydrosulfides resulting from sulfate reduction during digestion. However, the feeding of tetrathiomolybdates to nonruminant test animals does result in a compromised uptake of copper. Therefore, the antagonistic effect of molybdenum or sulfate on copper availability appears to be due to the tendency of molybdenum to sequester reactive sulfide groups. These groups subsequently bind copper ions, which then become less available.

A relationship between molybdenum intake and copper excretion has been documented in one study in humans. Urinary copper excretion in humans has been shown to rise from 24 μg/day to 77 μg/day as molybdenum intake increased from 160 μg to 1,540 μg/day [19]. No changes in fecal copper excretion were noted, suggesting perhaps that molybdenum increased copper mobilization from tissues and promoted excretion [19]. These effects, however, were not confirmed in a later study by Turnlund and Keys [20].

Other nutrients and substances that appear to affect molybdenum availability, by mechanisms not yet understood, include manganese, zinc, iron, lead, ascorbic acid, methionine, cysteine, and protein. A possible relationship with silicon is discussed on page 496.

Excretion

Most molybdenum is excreted from the body in the urine. Furthermore, urinary excretion of molybdenum increases as dietary molybdenum intake increases [4,5]. In other words, retention of molybdenum in the body is low when dietary intake is high, and the kidney is thought to play a role in molybdenum homeostasis [4,5]. Small amounts of molybdenum are excreted from the body in the feces by way of the bile [4]; small amounts also can be lost in sweat (20 μg) and in hair (0.01 μg/g hair).

Recommended Dietary Allowances

In 1980, an estimated safe and adequate daily dietary intake range for molybdenum for adults of 150 to 500 μg was recommended. In 1989, this range was adjusted to 75 to 250 μg [21]. In the last decade, balance as well as depletion and repletion studies have suggested a minimum requirement of 25 μg molybdenum per day [4,5]. Based on 75% absorption, an estimated average requirement for adults was set at 34 μg [22]. The 2001 RDA for molybdenum for adults (men and women) is 45 μg (130% of the requirement), with 50 μg suggested during pregnancy and lactation [22]. The inside cover of the book provides additional RDAs for molybdenum for other age groups.

Deficiency

Molybdenum deficiency is rarely encountered unless the diet is particularly rich in antagonistic substances such as sulfate, copper, or tungstate. Low molybdenum intakes have been associated with esophageal cancer in China. Molybdemun deficiency in humans has been documented in a patient maintained on total parenteral nutrition for 18 months [23]. The patient exhibited high blood methionine, hypoxanthine, and xanthine concentrations, as well as low blood levels of uric acid. Urinary concentrations of sulfate were low, and those of sulfite were high. Treatment with 300 μg ammonium molybdate (163 μg molybdenum) resulted in clinical improvement and normalization of sulfur amino acid metabolism and uric acid production.

The importance of sulfite oxidase, and therefore molybdenum, in human nutrition is evidenced by the neurological disorders associated with a genetic deficiency of sulfite oxidase in children [24]. Elevated levels of urinary sulfite and thiosulfate, along with biochemical manifestations reflecting aberrant sulfur amino acid metabolism and sulfite oxidation, were observed.

Toxicity

Molybdenum appears to be relatively nontoxic to humans, with intakes up to 1,500 μg/day [4]. However, symptoms such as gout (inflammation of the joints due to accumulation of uric acid) have appeared in some people living in regions that contain high soil molybdenum levels. Gout results from high blood uric acid concentrations (which likely have arisen from increased xanthine dehydrogenase activity) that have accumulated in and around joints. A tolerable upper intake level for molybdenum has been set at 2 mg [22].

Assessment of Nutriture

Molybdenum appears to distribute itself fairly equally between the plasma and red blood cells. Although a few studies have reported the molybdenum concentrations of human plasma and blood, the use of these as indicators of molybdenum status has not been validated.

References Cited for Molybdenum

1. Pennington J, Jones J. Molybdenum, nickel, cobalt, vanadium, and strontium in total diets. J Am Diet Assoc 1987;87:1646–50.

2. Tsongas TA, Meglen RR, Walravens PA, Chappell WR. Molybdenum in the diet: an estimate of the average daily intake in the United States. Am J Clin Nutr 1980;33:1103–7.

3. Turnlund JR, Weaver CM, Kim SK, Keyes WR, Gizaw Y, Thompson KH, Peiffer GL. Molybdenum absorption and utilization in humans from soy and kale intrinsically labeled with stable isotopes of molybdenum. Am J Clin Nutr 1999;69:1217–23.

4. Turnlund JR, Keyes WR, Peiffer GL. Molybdenum absorption, excretion, and retention studied with stable isotopes in young men at five intakes of dietary molybdenum. Am J Clin Nutr 1995;62:790–96.

5. Turnlund J, Keyes W, Peiffer G, Chiang G. Molybdenum absorption, excretion, and retention studied with stable isotopes in young men during depletion and repletion. Am J Clin Nutr 1995;61:1102–9.

6. Scott K, Turnlund J. Compartmental model of molybdenum metabolism in adult men fed five levels of molybdenum. FASEB J 1993;7:A288.

7. Moriwaki Y, Yamamota T, Higashino K. Distribution and pathophysiologic role of molybdenum-containing enzymes. Histol Histopathol 1997;12:513–24.

8. Kramer S, Johnson J, Ribeiro A, Millington D, Rajagopalan K. The structure of the molybdenum cofactor. J Biol Chem 1987; 262:16357–63.

9. Rajagopalan K. Molybdenum: an essential trace element in human nutrition. Ann Rev Nutr 1988;8:401–27.

10. Mize C, Johnson J, Rajagopalan K. Defective molybdopterin biosynthesis: clinical heterogeneity associated with molybdenum cofactor deficiency. J Inher Metab Dis 1995;18:283–90.

11. Beedham C. Molybdenum hydroxylases as drug-metabolizing enzymes. Drug Metab Rev 1985;16:119–56.

12. McCord J. Free radicals and myocardial ischemia: overview and outlook. Free Radicals & Medicine 1988;4:9–14.

13. Coughlan M. The role of molybdenum in human biology. J Inher Metab Dis 1983;6(suppl1):70–77.

14. Meneshian A, Bulkley G. The physiology of endothelial xanthine oxidase: from urate catabolism to reperfusion injury to inflammatory signal transduction. Microcirc 2002;9:161–73.

15. Bodine P, Litwack G. Evidence that the modulator of the glucocorticoid-receptor complex is the endogenous molybdate factor. Proc Natl Acad Sci USA 1988;85:1462–66.

16. Johnson J, Rajogopalan K. Molecular basis of the biological function of molybdenum. J Biol Chem 1974;249:859–66.

17. Suttle N. The interactions between copper, molybdenum, and sulphur in ruminant nutrition. Ann Rev Nutr 1991;11:121–40.

18. Mills C, Davis G. Molybdenum. In: Mertz W, et al. Trace Elements in Human and Animal Nutrition. San Diego: Academic Press, 1987, vol. 1, pp. 449–54.

19. Turnlund J. Copper nutriture, bioavailability, and the influence of dietary factors. J Am Diet Assoc 1988;88:303–8.

20. Turnlund JR, Keyes WR. Dietary molybdenum: effect on copper absorption, excretion, and status in young men. In: Roussel AM, Anderson RA, Favier A, eds. Trace Elements in Man and Animals, 10th ed. New York: Kluwer Academic, 2000.

21. National Research Council. Recommended Dietary Allowances, 10th ed. Washington, DC: National Academy Press, 1989, pp. 243–46.

22. Food and Nutrition Board, Institute of Medicine. Dietary Reference Intakes. Washington, DC: National Academy Press, 2001, pp. 420–41.

23. Abumrad N, Schneider A, Steel D, Rogers L. Amino acid intolerance during prolonged total parenteral nutrition reversed by molybdate therapy. Am J Clin Nutr 1981;34:2551–59.

24. Johnson J, Wuebbens M, Mandell R, Shih V. Molybdenum cofactor deficiency in a patient previously characterized as deficient in sulfite oxidase. Biochem Med Metab Biol 1988;40:86–93.

FLUORIDE

Whereas fluorine (F) is a gaseous chemical element, fluoride (F^-) exists and is composed of fluorine bound to a metal, nonmetal, or organic compound. Fluoride predominates in nature and exerts physiological effects in the human body, where it is present in only trace amounts. The term *fluoride* will be used throughout this section. Analogous to this terminology is the use of the terms *iodide* and *chloride*.

Sources

Community drinking water fluoridation has been practiced for nearly 50 years in the United States following the discovery in 1942 of the inverse relationship between fluoride intake and the incidence of dental caries [1]. This discovery has in turn affected the distribution of fluoride in foods and beverages intended for human consumption. Several beverages, including ready-to-use infant formulas, are made with fluoridated water. Other beverages vary greatly in their fluoride content depending on the use or nonuse of fluoridated water in their processing.

The fluoride content in most food groups is low, usually <~0.05 mg/100 g [2]. However, a few foods contain higher amounts of fluoride, including some grains and cereal products, some marine fish (if consumed with the bones), and tea. Marine fish can contain from ~0.01 to 0.17 mg/100 g [2]. Tea, both caffeinated and decaffeinated, is rich in F^- because tea leaves accumulate the element in fairly high amounts. Brewed tea contains from 1 to 6 mg/L, with decaffeinated forms higher in fluoride than caffeinated [3,4]. Table 12.7 provides the fluoride content of various food groups.

Digestion, Absorption, Transport, and Storage

Absorption of fluoride is nearly 100% when it is consumed as sodium fluorosilicate in fluoridated water or as sodium fluoride or monofluorophosphate in toothpaste. Absorption of fluoride diminishes to ~50% to 80% when it is consumed with solid foods or with

Table 12.7 Fluoride Content of Various Food Groups

Food Group	Fluoride Content Range (mg/100 g)
Dairy products	0.002–0.082
Meat, poultry	0.004–0.092
Grain, cereal products	0.008–0.201
Potatoes	0.008–0.084
Green leafy vegetables	0.008–0.070
Legumes	0.015–0.057
Root vegetables	0.009–0.048
Other vegetables, vegetable products	0.006–0.017
Fruits	0.002–0.013
Fats, oils	0.002–0.044
Sugar adjuncts	0.002–0.078

Sources: Taves DR. Dietary intake of fluoride ashed (total fluoride) vs unashed (inorganic fluoride) analysis of individual foods. Br J Nutr 1983;49:295–301.

Rao G. Dietary intake and bioavailability of fluoride. Ann Rev Nutr 1984;4:115–136.

Food and Nutrition Board, Institute of Medicine. *Dietary Reference Intakes.* Washington, DC: National Academy Press, 1997, p. 294.

calcium-containing beverages. Calcium, along with other minerals (both di- and trivalent), is thought to form insoluble complexes with fluoride to decrease its absorption. In foods, fluoride also may be found bound to proteins. Protein-bound fluoride requires hydrolysis by gastric pepsin or other intestinal proteases prior to absorption, and its absorption is less than that found in water or toothpaste. Fluoride is relatively poorly absorbed (37%–54%) from foods such as bone meal [5].

Humans, given small amounts of soluble fluoride, achieve maximum blood fluoride levels within ~30 to 45 minutes [6]. This rapidity of absorption is accounted for by the fact that it occurs to a great extent in the stomach, a rather unique characteristic among the elements. Fluoride is also absorbed throughout the small intestine, but at a reduced rate.

Fluoride absorption is believed to occur by passive diffusion. Fluoride's rapid gastric absorption can be explained by the fact that it exists primarily as hydrogen fluoride, also called hydrofluoric acid (HF), at the low pH of the gastric contents rather than as ionic fluoride. The rate of diffusion across membranes, in general, correlates directly with the lipid solubility of the diffusing substance. Gastric diffusion is also inversely related to pH. The pH dependence of gastric absorption is consistent with the hypothesis that HF is being absorbed [6]. Hydrogen fluoride is a weak acid with a pKa (the negative logarithm of an acid dissociation constant, Ka) of 3.4, dissociating according to the equation $HF \longrightarrow H^+ + F^-$. Assuming a gastric pH of ~1.5, the ratio of HF to F^-, readily calculable from the Henderson-Hasselbalch equation (p. 512), would be nearly 200 : 1. The gastric luminal form of fluoride is therefore largely diffusible. Fluoride absorption does not appear to be influenced by its plasma levels except at a very high, perhaps toxic, concentration [7].

Some fluoride is transported in the blood as ionic fluoride or hydrofluoric acid, not bound to plasma proteins. Some fluoride is strongly bound and is referred to as nonionic or the organic form. Organically bound fluoride occurs in variable concentrations that are independent of total fluoride intake and plasma ionic fluoride levels. What is not known is the extent to which environmental contamination by industrially generated fluorocarbons may contribute to the variability. Ionic fluoride concentration, in contrast, correlates directly with dietary intake even up to very large oral doses, indicating that plasma ionic fluoride is not precisely controlled by homeostatic mechanisms.

Absorbed fluoride leaves the blood very quickly and is distributed rapidly throughout the body. Most fluoride is found in bones and teeth. Fluoride associated with bone is found in both an amorphous state (rapidly exchangeable pool) and a crystalline state (slowly exchangeable pool). In its more crystalline state, fluoride is sequestered in bones by apatite, a basic calcium phosphate with the theoretic formula $Ca_{10}(PO_4)_6(OH)_2$. Mineralized tissues account for nearly 99% of total body fluoride, with bone being by far the major depot. As the amount of absorbed fluoride increases, so does the quantity taken up by hard tissue. However, the percentage retained at high absorption rates becomes lower because of accelerated urinary excretion [7]. Skeletal growth rate influences fluoride balance, exemplified by the fact that young, growing people incorporate more fluoride into the skeleton than adults and excrete less in the urine.

Functions and Mechanisms of Action

The major functions of fluoride are related to its effects on the mineralization of teeth and bones. Specifically, it promotes mineral precipitation from amorphous solutions of calcium and phosphate, leading to the formation of apatite, a crystalline structure. The apatite is deposited as crystallites within an organic (protein) matrix.

Fluoride can be incorporated into the apatite structure by replacement of hydroxide ions. This can occur during initial crystal formation or by displacement from previously deposited mineral, according to the following equation:

$$Ca_{10}(PO_4)_6(OH)_2 + xF^- \longrightarrow Ca_{10}(PO_4)_6(OH)_2 - xF_x^-$$

With the deposition of fluoride in the hydroxyapatite in the enamel, fluorohydroxyapatite is formed. This compound has been shown to be less acid-soluble than hydroxyapatite and thus more resistant to cavity formation [8,9]. The extent of fluoride incorporation varies with animal species, age, fluoride exposure, and rate of tissue turnover. In bone and dental enamel of humans and other higher mammals, the ratio of substitution of F^- for OH^- is from ~1 : 20 to 1 : 40.

Mineral deposition and stimulation of new bone formation also have been attributed to fluoride [10,11]. Enamel's matrix protein has a high affinity for fluoride, which has led to the speculation that fluoride's major role in mineralization may be its participation in the nucleation of crystal formation rather than its association with the mineral phase [12]. In addition to its role in mineralization, fluoride appears to decrease acid production by oral plaque–producing bacteria [11].

Fluoride therapy, typically as sodium fluoride (40–80 mg/day), in conjunction with calcium supplements appears to stimulate osteoblasts. Osteoblasts function in the formation of new bone. Increases in trabecular bone formation and, to a lesser extent, cortical bone formation have been observed in postmenopausal women receiving fluoride and calcium supplements [10,13–15]. Sustained-release fluoride supplements have been shown to work better than other, more quickly absorbed forms; however, not all studies involving fluoride have shown beneficial effects [16,17].

Interactions with Other Nutrients

It has been reported that aluminum, calcium, magnesium, and chloride reduce fluoride uptake and use, whereas phosphate and sulfate increase its uptake [18]. Sodium chloride, for example, decreases the skeletal uptake of fluoride [19]. This point is of interest because kitchen or table salt has been used as a vehicle for fluoride supplementation in some countries. The mechanisms of the interactions are not established.

Aluminum-containing antacid use also sharply reduces the absorption of fluoride as well as phosphorus. It is speculated that aluminum forms insoluble complexes with fluoride in the intestine [20]. The contribution of the pH effect of the antacid on fluoride availability requires further investigation.

Excretion

Excretion of fluoride takes place rapidly via the urine, which accounts for approximately 90% of total excretion. Some renal tubular reabsorption occurs by passive diffusion of undissociated HF. Because the amount of HF is increased relative to the amount of F^- as acidity is increased, tubular reabsorption and urinary pH are inversely related [6]. That is, the extent of reabsorption is inversely related to the pH of the fluids in the tubules. Fecal elimination accounts for most of the remaining losses, with only minor losses occurring in sweat.

Adequate Intakes

The 1997 Dietary Reference Intakes reported adequate intakes of 4 and 3 mg fluoride/day for adult males and females, respectively [21]. No increases are recommended for women during pregnancy or lactation. Fluoridation of water at 1 to 2 ppm (i.e., 1 or 2 parts fluoride per 1 million parts water) continues to be recommended by the Council on Dental Therapeutics of the American Dental Association to optimize dental health [22,23]. The inside cover of the book provides additional AIs for fluoride for other age groups.

Deficiency

Fluoride deficiency in test animals has been reported to result in curtailed growth, infertility, and anemia. However, these findings are not well documented and clearly cannot be extrapolated to predict similar effects on humans. In humans, what is unequivocal is that an optimal level of fluoride is necessary to reduce the incidence of dental caries and perhaps also to maintain the integrity of skeletal tissue. It is on this basis that the element is considered essential.

Toxicity

Chronic toxicity of fluoride, referred to as fluorosis, is characterized by changes in bone, kidney, and possibly nerve and muscle function [6,23]. Dental fluorosis or mottling of teeth has been observed in children receiving 2 to 8 mg fluoride/kg body weight. Acute toxicity manifests as nausea, vomiting, diarrhea, acidosis, and cardiac arrhythmias. Death has been reported following ingestion of between 5 and 10 g sodium fluoride or ~32 to 64 mg fluoride/kg body weight, although it may occur with intakes as low as 5 mg fluoride/kg body weight [6,23]. The tolerable upper intake levels for fluoride range from 1.3 mg/day for children age 1 to 3 years to 10 mg/day for children older than 8 years and adults [21].

Assessment of Nutriture

Normal ranges for ionic fluoride have been established at 0.01 to 0.2 μg F^-/mL plasma and 0.2 to 1.1 mg F^-/mL urine. The element is most commonly determined in its ionic form by fluoride ion–specific electrode potentiometry, a technique analogous to the hydrogen ion–specific electrode potentiometry of the common pH meter.

References Cited for Fluoride

1. National Research Council. Recommended Dietary Allowances, 10th ed. Washington, DC: National Academy Press, 1989, pp. 235–40.

2. Taves DR. Dietary intake of fluoride ashed (total fluoride) vs unashed (inorganic fluoride) analysis of individual foods. Br J Nutr 1983;49:295–301.

3. Wei SH, Hattab FN, Mellberg JR. Concentration of fluoride and selected other elements in teas. Nutrition 1989;5:237–40.

4. Chan JT, Koh SH. Fluoride content in caffeinated, decaffeinated and herbal teas. Caries Res 1996;30:88–92.

5. Krishnamachari K. Fluoride. In: Mertz W, ed. Trace Elements in Human and Animal Nutrition. San Diego: Academic Press, 1987, vol. 1, pp. 365–415.

6. Whitford G. The physiological and toxicological characteristics of fluoride. J Dent Res 1990;69:539–49.

7. Whitford G, Williams J. Fluoride absorption: independence from plasma fluoride levels. Proc Soc Exp Biol Med 1986;181:550–54.

8. Chow LC. Tooth-bound fluoride and dental caries. J Dent Res 1990;69(spec iss):595–600.

9. Marquis RE. Antimicrobial actions of fluoride for oral bacteria. Can J Microbiol 1995;41:955–64.

10. Kleerekoper M, Mendlovic D. Sodium fluoride therapy of postmenopausal osteoporosis. Endocrin Rev 1993;14:312–23.

11. Bowden GH. Effects of fluoride on the microbial ecology of dental plaque. J Dent Res 1990;69(spec iss):653–59.

12. Crenshaw M, Bawden J. Fluoride binding by organic matrix from early and late developing bovine fetal enamel determined by flow rate dialysis. Arch Oral Biol 1981;26:473–76.

13. Fluoride and bone health. J Publ Health Dent 1995;55:53–56.

14. Pak C, Sakhaee K, Piziak V, Peterson R, Breslau N, Boyd P, Poindexter J, Herzog J, Sakhaee A, Haynes S, Huet B, Reisch J. Slow

release sodium fluoride in the management of postmenopausal osteoporosis: a randomized controlled trial. Ann Intern Med 1994; 120:625–32.

15. Eisinger J, Clairet D. Effects of silicon, fluoride, etidronate and magnesium on bone mineral density: a retrospective study. Magnesium Res 1993;6:247–49.

16. Pak C. Sustained release sodium fluoride in the management of established menopausal osteoporosis. Am J Med 1997;313:23–32.

17. Riggs B, Hodgson S, O'Fallon W, Chao E, Wahner H, Muhs J, Cedel S, Melton L. Effect of fluoride treatment on the fracture rate in postmenopausal women with osteoporosis. N Engl J Med 1990;322:802–9.

18. Rao G. Dietary intake and bioavailability of fluoride. Ann Rev Nutr 1984;4:115–36.

19. Ericsson Y. Influence of sodium chloride and certain other food components on fluoride absorption in the rat. J Nutr 1968;96:60–68.

20. Spencer H, Kramer L. Osteoporosis: calcium, fluoride, and aluminum interactions. J Am Coll Nutr 1985;4:121–28.

21. Food and Nutrition Board, Institute of Medicine. Dietary Reference Intakes. Washington, DC: National Academy Press, 1997, pp. 288–313.

22. American Dental Association. Accepted Dental Therapeutics, 39th ed. Chicago: American Dental Association, 1982.

23. Heifetz S, Horowitz H. The amounts of fluoride in current fluoride therapies: safety considerations for children. J Dent Child 1984;51:257–69.

perspective

Nutrient–Drug Interactions

Nutrient–drug interactions represent nutrient-induced changes in the kinetics of a drug or drug-induced changes in nutrient metabolism or nutritional status. Such interactions can be extremely detrimental. Some nutrient interactions can lead to failure of the drug to perform its desired actions or can lead to drug toxicity. Alternately, some drug interactions can promote nutrient deficiencies or toxicities. In addition to direct interactions, drugs also may influence nutrition status through multiple other mechanisms such as diminishing appetite, altering taste, or promoting nausea, vomiting, and/or diarrhea. This perspective reviews some examples of foods or nutrients that affect the absorption, distribution, metabolism, actions (functions), or excretion of drugs, as well as some examples of drugs that affect the absorption, metabolism, or excretion of nutrients.

Effects of Foods/Nutrients on Drug Absorption

Foods or nutrients in foods can alter drug absorption by their presence as a physical barrier or through effects on transit time (i.e., motility of the gastrointestinal tract), secretions, drug dissolution, chelation, or carrier uptake, among other effects. Many drugs should be taken without food or beverage to prevent interference with drug absorption. For example, the absorption of Fosamax (alendronate), used to treat osteoporosis, is greatly diminished with concurrent ingestion of food or beverages (other than water). Similarly, the antibiotics Erythromycin and Penicillin (ampicillin), along with the antihypertensive drugs Capoten (captopril) and Univasc or Uniretic (moexipril), should be ingested only with water; food should not be consumed for at least 1 hour. Alternately, the absorption of many other drugs is enhanced with coingestion of food or even specific dietary nutrients such as a high-fat meal.

Foods or antacids, which contain relatively high amounts of magnesium, calcium, and aluminum, need to be avoided or should be ingested separately (by several hours) from antibiotics such as Tetracycline, Achromycin, and Sumycin (tetracycline); Cipro (ciprofloxacin); Maxaquin (lomefloxacin); and Levaquin (levofloxacin), as well as from other groups of antibiotics, antimicrobials, or antifungals such as Rifadin (rifampin) and Nizoral (ketoconaxole). The divalent minerals in the antacids or from the foods chelate (bind to) the antibiotics and decrease absorption of the drugs.

The maintenance of an appropriate gastrointestinal tract pH is important for the dissolution and/or absorption of some drugs. Thus, ingestion of foods or antacids that can promote gastrointestinal secretions and/or alter pH may be detrimental. The antifungal agent Nizoral (ketoconazole), for example, needs an acidic pH in order to dissolve. Other drugs are damaged in an acidic pH and thus need to be ingested without food or beverage (except water).

Effects of Foods on Drug Metabolism

Many drugs that undergo substantial first-pass metabolism in the gastrointestinal tract have been shown to be affected by coingestion of grapefruit juice, including the immunosuppressant Neoral (cyclosporine); some HMG CoA reductase inhibitors (used to treat high blood cholesterol) such as Zocor (simvastatin), Mevacor (lovastatin), and Lipitor (atorvastatin); and Pletal (cilostazol), which is used to treat intermittent claudication/peripheral vascular disease. References with more comprehensive lists of drugs known to interact with grapefruit juice are listed at the end of this perspective. The exact compound(s) in grapefruit juice thought to be responsible for the interaction are not clear. Grapefruit juice is rich in many phytochemicals, especially flavonoids such as the flavanone naringenin and its glycoside naringin and the flavonol kaempferol. Ingestion of grapefruit juice is thought to decrease (down-regulate) the isozyme of cytochrome P_{450} known as CYP 3A4, which is found in the intestine. This enzyme normally begins intestinal cell metabolism of many drugs. Consequently, the down-regulation of this enzyme by ingestion of grapefruit juice causes the drugs to be absorbed without any metabolism and causes blood concentrations of the drugs to be much higher than desired. The high blood drug concentrations, in turn, can result in undesirable side effects, including toxicity.

In addition to alterations in drug distribution caused by grapefruit juice, a high protein intake (two to three times recommendations) has been shown to alter the distribution of the anti-Parkinson drugs Dopar and Larodopa (levodopa). The effects are thought to result from competition for carriers at the blood-brain barrier between the drug and large neutral amino acids (such as phenylalanine, tyrosine, and tryptophan). These large neutral amino acids appear in the blood following consumption of large amounts of protein. Vitamin B_6 also can increase the metabolism of levodopa by enhancing its conversion to dopamine before the drug crosses the blood-brain barrier. Vitamin B_6 is found in liver and other protein-rich foods such as meats and legumes as well as seeds and whole grains. Thus, ingestion of levodopa with large amounts of protein or vitamin B_6 or overall consumption of a diet high in protein or vitamin B_6 is contraindicated.

Effects of Foods/Nutrients on the Actions of Drugs

Some foods or nutrients can enhance or oppose the actions of drugs. Foods containing amines, especially tyramine, dopamine, or histamine, are known to interact with a group of drugs known as monoamine oxidase inhibitors (MAOI), used mostly to treat some forms of depression. MAOIs such as Parnate (tranylcypromine sulfate) and Nardil (phenelzine sulfate) prevent the enzyme monoamine oxidase from catabolizing amines in diet as well as amines made endogenously. Amines consist of vasoactive or pressor amines (e.g., tyramine, serotonin, and histamine) and neurotransmitters or psychoactive amines (e.g., dopamine and norepinephrine). The antituberculosis drug INH (isoniazid) exhibits MAOI-like activity. The problem arises when people on MAOI or INH eat foods high in amines, especially tyramine or histamine, which may be found in fairly large quantities in some foods. Consumption of these foods ordinarily presents no problem to individuals because the amines can quickly be inactivated by monoamine oxidase (MAO). However, in individuals taking MAOIs or INH, these reactions do not occur. Consequently, high dietary amines coupled with high endogenous norepinephrine may result in excessive vasoconstriction, manifested as severe headache, acute hypertension or a hypertensive crisis, and cardiac dysrhythmia. Individuals on MAOIs are counseled against ingesting foods high in amines, such as aged cheeses (cheddar, Camembert, Stilton, boursalt), yeast extracts (e.g., marmite), and brewer's yeast. Smoked, salted, or pickled fish such as herring or cod, as well as sausage, salami, pepperoni, corned beef, and bologna, also are high in tyramine. Foods moderately high to high in tyramine include meat extracts; tenderizers; red wines, including Chianti, vermouth, sherry, and burgundy; and cheeses such as blue, natural brick, Brie, Gruyère, mozzarella, Parmesan, Romano, and Roquefort. Broad beans (fava, Chinese pea pods), chocolate, large amounts of caffeine, liver (chicken or beef), and selected fruits may also contain high amounts of tyramine. Histamine is not typically found in large quantities in foods, with the exception of improperly stored or spoiled fish. Dopamine is found in fava and broad beans and snowpeas.

A nutrient known to antagonize the action of the anticoagulant Coumadin (warfarin) is vitamin K. Coumadin works by inhibiting reactions in the vitamin-K cycle that generate the active form of vitamin K needed for blood clotting (see p. 365). By inhibiting production of active vitamin K, the drug prolongs the clotting time of blood. Large intakes of vitamin K oppose the actions of the drug, promoting blood clotting and leading to drug resistance. Ingestion of large quantities of foods rich in vitamin K, including green vegetables as well as some legumes (soybeans, garbanzo beans) and liver, should be avoided.

Caffeine, a component of coffee, tea, many soft drinks, and chocolate, counters the actions of tranquilizers and may exacerbate some adverse effects of the bronchodilators Theobid, Theo-Dur, Theolair, Slo-Phyllin, Uniphyl, and Exiolphyllin (theophylline). Specifically, high intakes of caffeine coupled with use of theophylline promote increased nervousness, insomnia, and tremors.

Effects of Foods/Nutrients on Drug Excretion

Sodium and the mineral lithium in the antimanic drugs Eskalith, Lithobid, or Lithotabs (lithium carbonate) are known to interact in the kidney. Specifically, the sodium and lithium compete with each other for reabsorption into the tubules of the kidney. Thus, high intakes of sodium promote excretion of lithium and thereby diminish the effects of the drug, while low intakes of sodium promote reabsorption of lithium and thereby enhance the likelihood of drug toxicity.

Effects of Drugs on Nutrient Absorption

Drugs may alter the absorption of nutrients through several mechanisms. For example, drugs may alter the transit time of nutrients through the gastrointestinal tract to speed up or slow down the passage of contents. Typically, when contents move quickly through the gastrointestinal tract, fewer nutrients are absorbed. Alternately, when contents move slowly through the gastrointestinal tract, more nutrients are absorbed. Changes in the pH of the gastrointestinal tract also may alter nutrient absorption. For example, H_2 receptor blockers such as Tagamet (cimetidine) and Zantac (ranitidine) and proton-pump inhibitors such as Prilosec (omeprazole) and Prevacid (lansoprazole), which decrease hydrochloric acid secretion into the stomach and thus increase gastric pH, diminish the absorption of several nutrients, especially vitamin B_{12} and iron. H_2 receptor blockers and proton pump inhibitors are used to treat ulcers and gastroesophageal reflux disease (GERD). The ability of some drugs to chelate or adsorb nutrients or gastrointestinal secretions also diminishes nutrient absorption. For example, bile acid sequestrants such as Questran (cholestyramine) adsorb bile and thus decrease the absorption of carotenoids and the fat-soluble vitamins A, D, E, and K. In addition, the drug chelates other nutrients (including folate) and some divalent minerals (including iron, magnesium, calcium, and zinc). Bile acid sequestrant drugs are used to treat high blood cholesterol concentrations, a risk factor for heart disease.

Effects of Drugs on Nutrient Metabolism

In addition to altering nutrient absorption, drugs may alter the metabolism of nutrients in body tissues. INH (isoniazid), used in the treatment of tuberculosis, for example, diminishes the conversion of pyridoxine (vitamin B_6) to its functional coenzyme form in the liver and thus can cause a vitamin B_6 deficiency. Another group of drugs known to alter vitamin metabolism includes the anticonvulsants Phenobarbital (phenobarbital) and Dilantin (phenytoin). These drugs alter the metabolism of vitamin D, leading to (in severe cases) the deficiency conditions rickets and/or osteomalacia if vitamin supplements (as 25-OH cholecalciferol) are not given. Specifically, the anticonvulsants are thought to diminish the hepatic conversion of vitamin D as cholecalciferol to 25-OH cholecalciferol. Interestingly, these anticonvulsants also affect the vitamin folate by diminishing its absorption in the intestine.

Effects of Drugs on Nutrient Excretion

Drugs may increase or decrease the excretion of nutrients from the body. Diuretics such as Lasix (furosemide), Bumex (bumetanide), and other loop diuretics used to treat high blood pressure promote the urinary excretion of sodium and water (important in lowering blood pressure); however, the drugs also increase losses of potassium, chloride, and magnesium from the ascending portion of the loop of Henle. Dietary replacement of the minerals, especially potassium, is important to prevent low blood potassium concentrations.

Summary

Nutrient–drug interactions can severely affect both the nutritional status and the effectiveness of pharmacological treatment of individuals. While accredited healthcare facilities are mandated to educate patients about interactions between foods and drugs, many individuals remain unaware of such interactions and their consequences.

References

Ameer B, Weintraub R. Drug interactions with grapefruit juice. Clin Pharm 1997;33:103–21.

Brown R, Dickerson R. Drug–nutrient interactions. Am J Managed Care 1999;5:345–52.

Chan L. Drug–nutrient interaction in clinical nutrition. Curr Opin Clin Nutr Metab Care 2002;5:327–32.

Fuhr U. Drug interactions with grapefruit juice. Drug Safety 1998;18:251–72.

Greenblatt D, Patiki K, van Moltke L, Shader R. Drug interactions with grapefruit juice: an update. J Clin Psychopharm 2001;21:357–59.

Harris J. Interaction of dietary factors with oral anticoagulants: review and applications. J Am Diet Assoc 1995;95:580–84.

Kane G, Lipsky J. Drug–grapefruit juice interactions. Mayo Clin Proc 2000;75:933–42.

Kirk J. Significant drug–nutrient interactions. Am Fam Physic 1995;51:1175–82.

Maka D, Murphy L. Drug–nutrient interactions: a review. AACN Clinical Issues 2000;11:580–89.

McCabe B. Dietary tyramine and other pressor amines in MAOI regimens: a review. J Am Diet Assoc 1986; 86:1059–64.

Miyagawa C. Drug–nutrient interactions in critically ill patients. Crit Care Nurs 1993;69–90.

Schmidt L, Dalhoff K. Food–drug interactions. Drugs 2002;62:1481–502.

Segal S, Kaminski S. Drug–nutrient interactions. Am Druggist 1996;213:42–49.

Tschanz C, Stargel W, Thomas J. Interactions between drugs and nutrients. Adv Pharmacol 1996;35:1–26.

Web Sites

www.nlm.nih.gov/medlineplus/druginformation.html

www.fda.gov

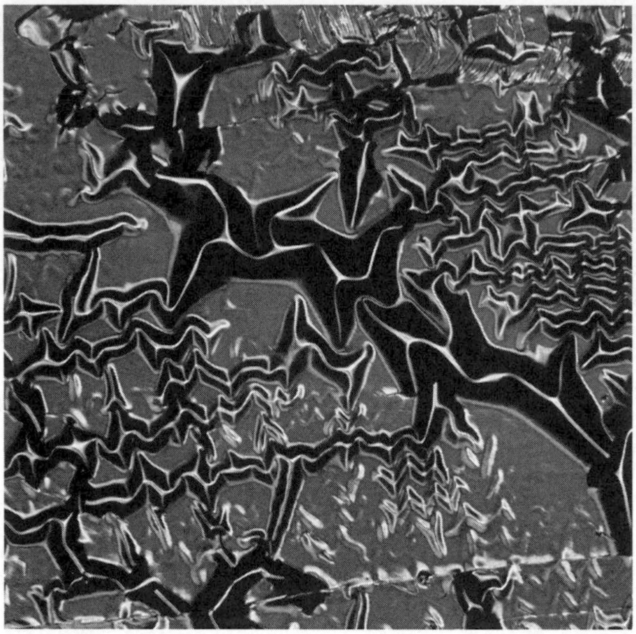

Polarized light micrograph of a thin layer of nickel(II) oxide, reflected

chapter 13 Ultratrace Elements

ULTRATRACE ELEMENTS MAY BE DEFINED AS those elements with estimated, established, or suspected requirements <1 mg/day [1]. Based on this definition, as many as 19 elements may be classified as ultratrace elements: aluminum, arsenic, boron, bromine, cadmium, chromium, copper, fluoride, germanium, iodine, lead, lithium, molybdenum, nickel, rubidium, selenium, silicon, tin, and vanadium [2]. For the purposes of this text, this chapter focuses only on those elements for which there is fairly strong evidence of essentiality but for which the Food and Nutrition Board has established neither an adequate intake (AI) nor a recommended dietary allowance (RDA) [1–4]. Chromium, fluoride, iodine, molybdenum, and selenium, while considered ultratrace elements by the above definition, have been included in Chapter 12, "Microminerals," based on their well-established essentiality and the establishment of either an AI, an estimated safe and adequate daily dietary intake, or an RDA by the Food and Nutrition Board [3,4].

This chapter discusses the sources, absorption, transport, functions, interactions with other nutrients, excretion, recommended intake, deficiency, toxicity, and assessment of nutriture for five ultratrace elements—arsenic,

Table 13.1 Ultratrace Elements: Selected Functions, Deficiency Symptoms, and Food Sources

Mineral	Selected Possible Physiological Roles	Selected Deficiency Symptoms in Animals	Food Sources
Arsenic	Methyl group use, normal growth	Curtailed growth	Seafoods
Boron	Bone development, cell membrane, embryogenesis, metabolic regulator, inflammation	Altered bone mineral metabolism, depressed growth	Fruits, vegetables legumes, nuts
Nickel	Possibly involved in hormonal membrane or enzyme activity	Depressed growth, impaired hematopoiesis	Nuts, legumes, grains, cacoa products
Silicon	Connective tissue and bone formation, prolylhydroxylase activity	Decreased collagen, long bone and skull abnormalities	Beer, unrefined grains, root vegetables
Vanadium	Mimics insulin action, inhibition of Na^+/K^+-ATPase	Reduced growth, hematologic changes, metabolism changes	Shellfish, spinach, parsley, mushrooms, whole grains

boron, nickel, silicon, and vanadium—for which available information provides multiple lines of evidence of essentiality. A brief discussion also is provided for the element cobalt, which, though considered essential, is needed in the body only as part of vitamin B_{12} (cobalamin). Table 13.1 provides an overview of selected functions, food sources, and deficiency symptoms for these nutrients.

References Cited

1. Nielsen F. Ultratrace elements in nutrition: current knowledge and speculation. J Trace Elem Exp Med 1998;11:251–74.

2. Nielsen F. Ultratrace minerals. In: Shils M, Olson J, Shike M, Ross A, eds. Modern Nutrition in Health and Disease, 9th ed. Baltimore, MD: Williams and Wilkins, 1999, pp. 283–303.

3. Food and Nutrition Board. Recommended Dietary Allowances. Washington, DC: National Academy Press, 1989, pp. 213–46.

4. Food and Nutrition Board. Dietary Reference Intakes for Vitamin A, Vitamin K, Arsenic, Boron, Chromium, Copper, Iodine, Iron, Manganese, Molybdenum, Nickel, Silicon, Vanadium, and Zinc. Washington, DC: National Academy Press, 2001, pp. 502–53.

ARSENIC

More than any other trace mineral, arsenic, which is colorless and odorless, conjures an image of toxicity as a poison rather than of nutritional essentiality. The malevolent aspect of arsenic continues to attract attention because a great deal more of the arsenic literature addresses its toxicological rather than its nutritional properties. Nevertheless, there is accumulating evidence that arsenic is an essential element.

Sources

Arsenic is present throughout the earth's continental crust at an estimated concentration of 1.5 to 2.0 μg/g. It is present in water, rocks, and soils, although its concentration varies considerably from region to region based on the geological history of a particular soil as well as on pollution from unnatural sources. Fallout sources such as pesticides, smelters, and coal-fired power plants can, through aerosols and floating dust, enrich a particular area with arsenic, which then affects humans and animals through its incorporation into foods and foodstuffs. Foods of marine origin are rich in arsenic, with fish containing up to 80 μg/g and oysters up to 10 μg/g [1,2]. Arsenic is also present in meats (0.005–0.1 μg/g) and cereal and grain products (0.05–0.4 μg/g) as well as dairy (milk, 0.01–0.05 μg/g; eggs, 0.01–0.1 μg/g) [2]. Dietary intakes of arsenic usually total <30 μg/day [1,2].

Arsenic is found in foods in both organic and inorganic forms, and it exists in nature in both the trivalent As(III) and pentavalent As(V) ionic states. The major arsenicals found in water and foods are pentavalent arsenate (AsO_4) and trivalent arsenite (AsO_2). Foods also contain arsenic in methylated forms. The arsenicals in foods include methylarsonic acid, dimethylarsinic acid, trimethylarsine [$As(CH_3)_3$], arsenobetaine, arsenocholine, trimethylarsonium lactate, and O-phosphatidyltrimethylarsonium lactate (Fig. 13.1). Of the arsenicals, inorganic arsenite and trivalent organoarsenicals are the most toxic, while the pentavalent, methylated arsenic compounds are less toxic.

Absorption, Transport, and Metabolism

Absorption, as well as retention and excretion, of arsenicals varies with their chemical form and solubility, the quantity administered, and the animal species involved in the study. Most inorganic arsenic is absorbed as arsenate and arsenite, with the former being less toxic [3].

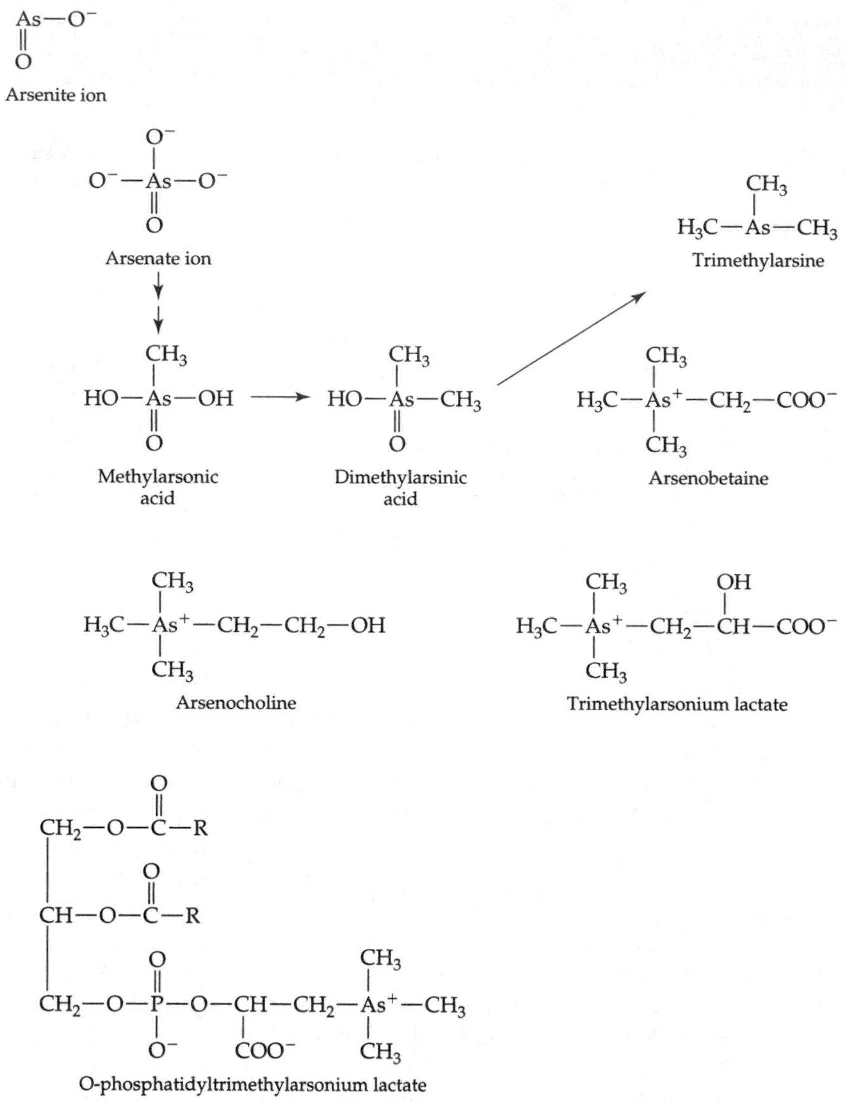

Figure 13.1 Forms of arsenic of biological importance.

For example, >90% of inorganic arsenate and arsenite is absorbed from water, and between 60% and 75% of these inorganic forms of the element is absorbed with food in humans [3]. Similarly, of the organic arsenicals shown in Figure 13.1, >90% of arsenobetaine and between 70% and 80% of arsenocholine are absorbed.

Absorption of organic and inorganic arsenicals is thought to occur by simple diffusion across the intestinal mucosa. Typically, the greater the lipid solubility of the arsenical, the greater the likelihood of its absorption by simple diffusion.

From the intestine, arsenic is transported in the blood to the liver, which takes up both inorganic and organic forms of the element following absorption. In the liver, arsenate-As(V) is reduced to the more toxic trivalent arsenite, which is then methylated to become a relatively less toxic monomethylarsonic acid (Fig. 13.1). The reaction is catalyzed by arsenite methyltransferase. In addition, another methyl group may be added to monomethylarsonic acid by monomethylarsenic acid methyltransferase to form dimethylarsinic acid. Methyl groups are provided by glutathione, choline, and S-adenosylmethionine (SAM) [4]. Thomas and coworkers provide a review of arsenic methylation for the interested reader [5]. In systemic blood, arsenic is found in two forms, methylated and protein-bound.

Organic arsenic, such as arsenobetaine or arsenocholine, that is absorbed is thought to undergo little or no metabolism, as indicated by the fact that the urinary arsenic excreted following the ingestion of arsenic-rich seafoods remained in the original, organically bound form [6].

Tissues that contain the most arsenic include skin, hair, and nails. Within tissues, inorganic arsenic, especially as As(III), is found bound primarily to thiol/sulfhydryl (SH) groups of proteins, such as the zinc storage protein metallothionein [7–9]. Methylated forms of the element do not bind to tissues as much as unmethylated inorganic forms. The organic form arsenocholine may be used like choline in the synthesis of phospholipids.

Functions and Deficiency

Arsenic appears to be needed for the formation and utilization of methyl groups, generated in methionine metabolism to S-adenosylmethionine (SAM). SAM is a major methyl donor in the body and functions in the synthesis of a variety of compounds (see p. 202). Arsenic, however, has not been shown to be an activator or inhibitor of a specific enzyme in methionine metabolism. Arsenic deficiency impairs metabolism of methionine, resulting in decreased SAM concentrations and decreased S-adenosylmethionine decarboxylase activity [10]. Similarly, taurine production from methionine is depressed in arsenic-deficient rats and hamsters [11]. Arsenic-deficient rats fed guanidoacetate experienced growth deficits versus arsenic-supplemented rats [12]. Decreased methylation of guanidoacetate to form creatine and decreased methylation of histones and DNA also are reported with arsenic deprivation [12,13]. Synthesis of polyamines, which for example are derived from SAM (see Fig. 7.27), is impaired with arsenic deficiency. Synthesis of heat shock proteins, via effects on methylation of histones, has been attributed to roles of arsenic in gene expression [13,14]. Other reported effects of arsenic deprivation in animals include curtailed growth, reduced conception rate, and increased neonatal mortality.

Interactions with Other Nutrients

Arsenic seems to interact antagonistically with selenium and iodine. Because selenate and arsenate are both oxyanions with similar chemical properties, each may competitively inhibit the uptake and tissue retention of the other. The interaction of arsenic with iodine is exemplified by the observation that it is goitrogenic in mice. Arsenic is believed to antagonize the mechanism of iodine uptake by the thyroid, causing compensatory goiter.

Excretion

Ingested arsenic is excreted rapidly via the kidneys, representing the major route of excretion. The main urinary metabolites of arsenic include methylarsinic acid, dimethylarsinic acid, and trimethylated arsenic [7,15]. With consumption of organic forms of the element, arsenobetaine and arsenocholine, along with arsenosugars, are excreted in the urine [8]. Concentrations of the metabolites in the urine, however, vary depending on the dietary form of arsenic ingested [15]. Typically, <50 μg arsenic/day is excreted in the urine of healthy adults.

Recommended Intake, Toxicity, and Assessment of Nutriture

There are insufficient data to estimate a human dietary requirement for arsenic, although a requirement of 12 to 25 μg has been suggested [11,12,16]. No tolerable upper intake level for arsenic has been established by the Food and Nutrition Board [17].

Inorganic forms of arsenic are more toxic than organic forms of the element and appear to be carcinogenic [18,19]. Acute toxicity results in gastrointestinal distress (leading to dehydration and electrolyte imbalance), encephalopathy, anemia, and hepatotoxicity. Arsenic appears to be fatal at intakes of 70 to 300 mg [20]. Chronic toxicity is associated with skin hyperpigmentation, hyperkeratosis, muscle weakness, peripheral neuropathy, excessive sweating, liver damage, delirium, encephalopathy, vascular changes, and cancers of the oral cavity, skin, lungs, colon, bladder, and kidney [21–23]. In Taiwan, ingestion of arsenic-containing drinking water has been associated with the development of Blackfoot disease, a peripheral vascular condition [21,22].

Reported levels of arsenic in body fluids include 2 to 62 ng/mL whole blood and 1 to 20 ng/mL plasma or serum. Hair arsenic levels range from ~0.1 to 1.1 μg/g. Chronic or acute exposure to the metal elevates these values. Hair analysis has been particularly useful in this respect because hair arsenic content, unlike that of the fluids, represents an average content over an extended period and does not fluctuate in parallel with intermittent exposure to the element.

The current method of choice for the determination of arsenic in biological fluids is atomic absorption spectrometry, although mass spectrometry, neutron activation analysis, and emission spectroscopy have been used successfully.

References Cited for Arsenic

1. Nielsen F. Ultratrace minerals. In: Shils M, Olson J, Shike M, Ross A, eds. Modern Nutrition in Health and Disease, 9th ed. Baltimore, MD: Williams and Wilkins, 1999, pp. 283–303.

2. Anke M. Arsenic. In: Mertz W, ed. Trace Elements in Human and Animal Nutrition. Orlando, FL: Academic Press, 1986, vol. 2, p. 360.

3. Hopenhayn C, Smith A, Goeden H. Human studies do not support the methylation threshold hypothesis for the toxicity of inorganic arsenic. Environ Res 1993;60:161–77.

4. Thompson D. A chemical hypothesis for arsenic methylation in mammals. Chem Biol Interactions 1993;88:89–114.

5. Thomas D, Styblo M, Lin S. The cellular metabolism and systemic toxicity of arsenic. Toxic Appl Pharmacol 2001;176:127–44.

6. Tam G, Charbonneau S, Bryce F, Sandi E. Excretion of a single oral dose of fish-arsenic in man. Bull Environ Contam Toxicol 1982; 28:669–73.

7. Vahter M, Marafante E. Intracellular interaction and metabolic fate of arsenite and arsenate in mice and rabbits. Chem Biol Interact 1983;47:29–44.

8. Vahter M, Concha G, Nermell B. Factors influencing arsenic methylation in humans. J Trace Elem Exp Med 2000;13:173–84.

9. Toyama M, Yamashita M, Hirayama N, Murooka Y. Interactions of arsenic with human metallothionein-2. J Biochem 2002;132:217–21.

10. Nielsen F. Ultratrace elements of possible importance for human health: an update. In: Prasad AS, ed. Essential and Toxic Trace Elements in Human Health. New York: Wiley-Liss, 1993, pp. 355–76.

11. Uthus E, Nielsen F. Determination of the possible requirement and reference dose level for arsenic in humans. Scand J Work Environ Health 1993;19(suppl1):137–38.

12. Uthus E. Evidence for arsenic essentiality. Environ Geochem Health 1992;14:55–58.

13. Desrosiers R, Tanguay R. Further characterization of the post-translational modifications of core histones in response to heat and arsenite stress in *Drosophila*. Biochem Cell Biol 1986;64:750–57.

14. Bernstam L, Nriagu J. Molecular aspects of arsenic stress. J Toxic Environ Hlth 2000;3:293–322.

15. Yamato N. Concentrations and chemical species of arsenic in human urine and hair. Bull Environ Contam Toxicol 1988;40:633–40.

16. Nielsen F. Boron, manganese, molybdenum, and other trace elements. In: Bowman B, Russell R, eds. Present Knowledge in Nutrition, 8th ed. Washington, DC: International Life Sciences Institute Nutrition Foundation, 2001, pp. 384–99.

17. Food and Nutrition Board. Dietary Reference Intakes for Vitamin A, Vitamin K, Arsenic, Boron, Chromium, Copper, Iodine, Iron, Manganese, Molybdenum, Nickel, Silicon, Vanadium, and Zinc. Washington, DC: National Academy Press, 2001, pp. 502–53.

18. Goldman M, Dacre J. Inorganic arsenic compounds: are they carcinogenic, mutagenic, teratogenic? Environ Geochem Hlth 1991;13:179–91.

19. Meng Z. Effects of arsenic on DNA synthesis in human lymphocytes stimulated by phytohemagglutinin. Biol Trace Elem Res 1993;39:73–80.

20. Abernathy CO, Ohanian EV. Noncarcinogenic effects of inorganic arsenic. Environ Geochem Health 1992;14:35–41.

21. Hall A. Chronic arsenic poisoning. Toxicol Letters 2002;128:69–72.

22. Weir E. Arsenic and drinking water. Can Med Assoc J 2002;166:69–72.

23. Abernathy C, Thomas D, Calderon R. Health effects and risk assessment of arsenic. J Nutr 2003;133:1536S–38S.

BORON

Boron, as boric acid and sodium borate (called borax), was used to preserve foods such as fish, meat, cream, butter, and margarine for over 50 years—that is, until about the 1920s, when it was considered dangerous for humans but deemed essential for plants. Not until the 1980s did evidence for the essentiality of boron in animals start mounting again.

Sources

Foods of plant origin such as fruits, vegetables, nuts, and legumes are particularly rich in boron [1–3]. In addition, wine, cider, and beer contribute to dietary intake. Specific foods particularly rich in boron include avocado, peanuts, peanut butter, pecans, raisins, grapes, and wine [4,5]. Generally, raisins, legumes, nuts, and avocados provide ~1.0 to 4.5 mg boron/100 g, and fruits and vegetables contain 0.1 to 0.6 mg boron/100 g [4,6,7]. Meat, fish, and dairy products are poor sources of the element, usually providing <~0.6 mg boron/100 g [1–3,7]. Drinking water and water-based beverages vary considerably in boron content based on geographic location [3]. Boron also is a contaminant or a major ingredient in some antibiotics, gastric antacids, lipsticks, lotions, creams, and soaps, for example [3]. Boron appears in foods as sodium borate; boric acid, which exists mainly as $B(OH)_2$, $B(OH)_3$, and $B(OH)_4^-$, or as organic borate esters [5,8]. Intake of boron is estimated to be 0.8 to 1.5 mg/day [4,8].

Absorption, Transport, Storage, and Excretion

Greater than 85% of ingested boron is thought to be rapidly absorbed via passive diffusion from the gastrointestinal tract; however, most boron, which is absorbed as $B(OH)_3$, is excreted in the urine as $B(OH)_3$ [8,9]. Boron is found in the blood as boric acid $B(OH)_2$, orthoboric acid $B(OH)_3$, and the borate anion $B(OH)_4^-$. Boron is found mainly in bone, teeth, nails, and hair. Total body boron content ranges from ~3 to 20 mg, with little found in soft tissues. It is excreted primarily (>70%) via the urine, with <13% usually lost via the feces and small amounts lost in sweat [8]. Urinary boron is thought to be a relatively sensitive indicator of intake within an intake range of 0.35 to 10 mg boron [8].

Functions and Deficiency

Boron is thought to have several functions in the body, including roles in embryogenesis, bone development, cell membrane function and stability, metabolic regulation, and mediation of the inflammatory response. For example, with respect to embryogenesis, in some but not all animals (e.g., not in rodents) boron depletion has resulted in embryonic defects, suggesting a possible role in reproduction and/or development. Depressed growth is also frequently observed in boron-depleted animals [2,10]. The composition, structure, and strength of bones also appear to involve boron, possibly via modulation of extracellular matrix turnover. For example, boron enhanced collagenase and cathepsin D activity in fibroblasts to modulate the turnover of the extracellular matrix [11]. Boron also enhanced the actions of estridiol on trabecular bone and promoted absorption and retention of minerals in bone in ovariectomized rats [12]. With respect to bone mineral content, responses to boron have been most marked in animals that also have had either calcium, vitamin D, or magnesium deprivation [13].

In addition to effects on embryogenesis and bone, boron may play a role in cell membrane stability and/or function [14,15]. Boron's effects on the cell membrane may be via modulating calcium uptake into the cell and/or modulating the ability of hormones (including vitamin D, calcitonin, insulin, and estrogen) to exert their actions [10,14]. Boron also may affect cell membrane function or stability through effects on trans-membrane signaling [10,14,15].

As a metabolic regulator, boron decreases serum glucose and increases serum triglyceride concentrations. Boron may directly interact with nutrient substrates, enzymes, or coenzymes or exert its effects through other mechanisms [16,17]. Boron-deficient chicks, for example, exhibit increased insulin secretion, possibly mediated through effects of boron on ion transport [14,17].

Finally, boron is thought to regulate the body's inflammatory response. As a mediator of the inflammatory process, boron may suppress (through reversible formation of analogues and competition with coenzymes) the activities of several serine proteases (e.g., elastase, chymase, and cathepsin) released by inflammation-activated white blood cells [17]. Alternately, boron may decrease leukotriene synthesis and/or decrease the generation or removal of reactive oxygen species produced by neutrophils as part of the respiratory burst [17]. Other studies suggest that boron acts via suppression of T-cell activity and alterations in antibody concentrations [17]. In addition to actions on serine proteases involved with the inflammatory response, boron is thought to affect other serine proteases, such as those involved in blood coagulation [17]. Because of its anti-inflammatory effects, boron is purported to reduce the severity of rheumatoid arthritis (among other inflammatory conditions).

Recommended Intake, Toxicity, and Assessment of Nutriture

A recommended intake of boron has not been established. Dietary intakes of <1 mg have been reported, but the amount needed to meet requirements is unknown [4,8].

Acute toxicity of boron in humans results in nausea, vomiting, diarrhea, dermatitis, and lethargy [18]. Increased urinary excretion of riboflavin also has been reported with boron toxicity [19]. Chronic boron toxicity is associated with nausea; poor appetite and subsequent weight loss; anemia; patchy, dry erythema; and seizures [20]. A tolerable upper intake level of 20 mg boron per day has been established based on animal studies [21].

Inductively coupled plasma emission spectrometry has been used to determine plasma and other body fluid concentrations of boron; however, whether these tissue concentrations are indicative of nutritional status is unknown. Plasma boron concentrations usually range from ~20 to 75 ng/mL [22].

References Cited for Boron

1. Anderson D, Cunningham W, Lindstrom T. Concentrations and intakes of H, B, S, K, Na, Cl, and NaCl in foods. J Food Comp Anal 1994;7:59–82.

2. Nielsen F. The saga of boron in food: from a banished food preservative to a beneficial nutrient for humans. Curr Topics Plant Biochem Physiol 1991;10:274–86.

3. Hunt C, Shuler T, Mullen L. Concentration of boron and other elements in human foods and personal-care products. J Am Diet Assoc 1991;91:558–68.

4. Meacham S, Hunt C. Dietary boron intakes of selected populations in the United States. Biol Trace Elem Res 1998;66:65–78.

5. Rainey C, Nyquist L, Christensen R, Strong P, Culver D, Coughlin J. Daily boron intake from the American diet. J Am Diet Assoc 1999;99:335–40.

6. Naghii M. The significance of dietary boron with particular reference to athletes. Nutr Health 1999;13:31–37.

7. Devirian T, Volpe S. The physiological effects of dietary boron. Crit Rev Food Sci Nutr 2003;43:219–31.

8. Sutherland B, Woodhouse L, Strong P, King J. Boron balance in humans. J Trace Elem Exp Med 1999;12:271–84.

9. Nielsen F, Penland J. Boron supplementation of peri-menopausal women affects boron metabolism and indices associated with macromineral metabolism, hormonal status, and immune function. J Trace Elem Exp Med 1999;12:251–61.

10. Nielsen F. Biochemical and physiologic consequences of boron deprivation in humans. Environ Hlth Perspectives 1994;102:59–63.

11. Nzietchueng R, Dousset B, Franck P, Benderdour M, Nabet P, Hess K. Mechanisms implicated in the effects of boron on wound healing. J Trace Elem Med Biol 2002;16:239–44.

12. Sheng M, Taper L, Veit H, Qian H, Ritchey S, Lau K. Dietary boron supplementation enhanced the action of estrogen, but not that of parathyroid hormone, to improve trabecular bone quality in ovariectomized rats. Biol Trace Elem Res 2001;82:109–23.

13. Hunt C, Herbel J, Nielsen F. Metabolic responses of postmenopausal women to supplemental dietary boron and aluminum during usual and low magnesium intake: boron, calcium and magnesium absorption and retention and blood mineral concentrations. Am J Clin Nutr 1997;65:803–13.

14. Nielsen F. The emergence of boron as nutritionally important throughout the life cycle. Nutrition 2000;16:512–14.

15. Nielsen F. Boron in human and animal nutrition. Plant Soil 1997;193:199–208.

16. Hunt C. The biochemical effects of physiologic amounts of dietary boron in animal nutrition models. Environ Health Perspect 1994;102(suppl7):35–43.

17. Hunt C. Regulation of enzymatic activity. One possible role of dietary boron in higher animals and humans. Biol Trace Elem Res 1998;66:205–25.

18. Linden C, Hall A, Kulig K, Rumack B. Acute ingestions of boric acid. Clin Toxicol 1986;24:269–79.

19. Pinto J, Huang Y, McConnell R, Rivlin R. Increased urinary riboflavin excretion resulting from boric acid ingestion. J Lab Clin Med 1978;92:126–34.

20. Gordon A, Prichard J, Freedman M. Seizure disorders and anaemia associated with chronic borax intoxication. Can Med Assoc J 1973;108:719–21.

21. Food and Nutrition Board. Dietary Reference Intakes for Vitamin A, Vitamin K, Arsenic, Boron, Chromium, Copper, Iodine, Iron, Manganese, Molybdenum, Nickel, Silicon, Vanadium, and Zinc. Washington, DC: National Academy Press, 2001, pp. 502–53.

22. Nielsen F. Dietary supplementation of physiological amounts of boron increases plasma and urinary boron of perimenopausal women. Proc ND Acad Sci 1996;50:52.

NICKEL

Nickel is used industrially in various capacities, such as production of stainless steel and nickel-cadmium batteries. Nickel is released into the environment with combustion of nickel-containing products. With respect to its use in humans, nickel's essentiality was first suggested in the 1930s; however, not until the mid-1970s did studies focus on its possible roles.

Sources

Foods of plant origin have a significantly higher nickel content than foods of animal origin. Nuts, legumes, grains and grain products, and chocolate (and items made from chocolate) are particularly rich in the metal, providing up to ~228 μg/100 g [1]. Fruits and vegetables are generally of intermediate nickel content, providing up to ~48 μg/100 g [1]. Nickel content of foods of animal origin, such as fish, milk, and eggs, generally is low [1,2]. Intake of nickel by adults is typically <100 μg/day [1,2].

The chemical form of nickel in foods is unknown, but in plants it is probably largely inorganic and is dependent on the nickel content of the soil. Dietary nickel derived from contamination of processed foods is likely inorganic as well.

Absorption, Transport, and Storage

Nickel absorption from foods is thought to be <10%. Absorption of nickel is higher (up to 50%) from water than from beverages (such as coffee, tea, cow's milk, and orange juice) to which nickel has been added [2–4]. With ingestion of high doses of nickel (up to 50 μg/kg body weight), nickel absorption was 27 ± 17% following an overnight fast and 0.7 ± 0.4% with a meal [3].

The absorption of ingested nickel across the intestinal brush border is via energy-dependent mechanisms or by passive diffusion [5,6]. Nickel ions appear to compete with iron for a common transport system in the proximal small intestine [6,7]. Transport across the basolateral membrane is thought to occur by diffusion or as part of a complex with an amino acid or binding ligand.

On entering the blood, nickel becomes bound mainly to albumin and to a lesser extent to amino acids, including histidine, cysteine, and aspartic acid [8]. Other serum proteins, such as α-2 macroglobulin, also may transport nickel in the blood.

Although nickel is widely distributed among human tissues, its concentration throughout the body is extremely low, occurring at nanogram/gram levels. The highest concentrations of nickel are found in the thyroid and adrenal glands as well as in hair, bone, and soft tissues such as the lungs, heart, kidneys, and liver.

Functions and Deficiency

A specific role of nickel in human and animal nutrition has not yet been defined, although roles for nickel in plants and microorganisms have been documented [9]. In plants, for example, nickel serves as a cofactor for urease, which catalyzes the hydrolysis of urea into carbon dioxide and ammonia. In bacteria, several hydrogenases appear to be nickel dependent. In the several enzyme systems, however, the role of nickel can be substituted for other minerals, such as magnesium. An example of such a replacement is the formation of the C3 convertase enzyme (C3b,Bb and C4b,2b) of the human complement system, which classically requires Mg^{2+} for activity. The substitution of nickel for magnesium in this complex enhanced both the stability and the activity of the enzyme [10], raising a question as to nickel's possible physiological role in the complement system. It has also been demonstrated that nickel can substitute for zinc in the carboxypeptidases and in horse liver alcohol dehydrogenase [9]. Nickel may be involved with folate and vitamin B_{12} in the metabolism of methionine either in the initial stages involving conversion to homocysteine and/or with vitamin B_{12} in the later stages in which propionyl CoA is converted to succinyl CoA [11,12].

Signs of nickel deprivation continue to be described for some animal species. Among the more consistent signs are depressed growth, altered distribution of some minerals, changes in blood glucose, and impaired hematopoiesis, which probably is due to altered iron metabolism.

Interactions with Other Nutrients

Because nickel shares with other metals the property of being readily chelated by and complexed with a wide variety of ligands, it follows that nickel can compete with those ions for ligand sites. Nickel interacts with many ions in this manner, including as many as 13 essential minerals. The interactions of particular nutritional interest are those involving iron, copper, and zinc. As discussed in the section on absorption, nickel antagonizes ferrous iron absorption [6,7]. Nickel is thought to replace copper at functional sites and thus exacerbates copper deficiency [13]. With respect to zinc, nickel appears to affect zinc metabolism, possibly by causing redistribution of zinc in the body [13].

Excretion

Most absorbed nickel is excreted in the urine. Within the renal cells, nickel is first complexed with low-molecular-weight compounds such as uronic acid and neutral sugar oligosaccharides. Small amounts of absorbed nickel also are excreted through the bile (1.5–3.3 μg/day) [14]. Sweat nickel concentrations, however, can be fairly high (69.9 μg/L) with active secretion of the element by sweat glands, even in acclimatized individuals [15].

Recommended Intake, Toxicity, and Assessment of Nutriture

Extrapolation from animal studies suggests that humans probably need <100 μg nickel/day [16]. A tolerable upper intake level for adults for nickel is 1.0 mg/day in the form of soluble nickel salts (such as nickel sulfate, which may contaminate water) [17].

Signs of toxicity in humans include nausea, vomiting, and shortness of breath; in animals, signs include lethargy, ataxia, irregular breathing, and hypothermia, among others, including possible death [17]. Nickel is also a known carcinogen with demonstrated effects on DNA, including hypermethylation of DNA, inhibition of acetylation of histones, condensation of chromatin, and gene silencing [18].

As for most of the ultratrace metals, the preferred technique for nickel determination is flameless atomic absorption spectrophotometry. This technique offers the degree of sensitivity necessary for determination in the nanogram range. The reference range for nickel in the serum or plasma of healthy adults is 1 to 23 ng/mL; however, valid methods to assess the nickel status of humans are unavailable.

References Cited for Nickel

1. Pennington J, Jones J. Molybdenum, nickel, cobalt, vanadium, and strontium in total diets. J Am Diet Assoc 1987;87:1644–50.

2. Solomons N, Viteri F, Shuler T, Nielsen F. Bioavailability of nickel in man: effects of foods and chemically defined dietary constituents on the absorption of dietary nickel. J Nutr 1982;112:39–50.

3. Sunderman F, Hopfer S, Sweeney K, Marcus A, Most B, Creason J. Nickel absorption and kinetics in human volunteers. Proc Soc Exp Biol Med 1989;191:5–11.

4. Patriarca M, Lyon T, Fell G. Nickel metabolism in humans investigated with an oral stable isotope. Am J Clin Nutr 1997;66:616–21.

5. Tallkvist J, Tjalve H. Transport of nickel across monolayers of human intestinal Caco-2 cells. Toxicol Appl Pharmacol 1998; 151:117–22.

6. Tallkvist J, Wing A, Tjalve H. Enhanced intestinal nickel absorption in iron-deficient rats. Pharmacol Toxicol 1994:75:244–49.

7. Nielsen F. Studies on the interaction between nickel and iron during intestinal absorption. In: Anke M, Bauman W, Braunlich H, et al., eds. Spurenelement-Symposium. Leipzig, East Germany: Karl-Marx-Universität, 1983, pp. 11–98.

8. Tabata M, Sarkar B. Specific nickel (II)-transfer process between the native sequence peptide representing the nickel (II)-transport site of human serum albumin and L-histidine. J Inorgan Biochem 1992; 45:93–104.

9. Walsh C, Orme-Johnson W. Nickel enzymes. Biochem 1987; 26:4901–6.

10. Fishelson Z, Muller-Eberhard H. C3 convertase of human complement: enhanced formation and stability of the enzyme generated with nickel instead of magnesium. J Immunol 1982;129:2603–7.

11. Nielsen F. Nutritional requirements for boron, silicon, vanadium, nickel, and arsenic: current knowledge and speculation. FASEB J 1991;5:2661–67.

12. Uthus E, Poellot R. Dietary folate affects the response of rats to nickel deprivation. Biol Trace Elem Res 1996;52:23–35.

13. Nielsen F. Nickel. In: Frieden E, ed. Biochemistry of the Essential Ultratrace Elements. New York: Plenum Press, 1984, pp. 301–4.

14. Rezuke W, Knight J, Sunderman F. Reference values for nickel concentrations in human tissue and bile. Am J Ind Med 1987; 11:419–26.

15. Omokhodion F, Howard J. Trace elements in the sweat of acclimatized persons. Clin Chim Acta 1994;231:23–28.

16. Food and Nutrition Board. Dietary Reference Intakes for Vitamin A, Vitamin K, Arsenic, Boron, Chromium, Copper, Iodine, Iron, Manganese, Molybdenum, Nickel, Silicon, Vanadium, and Zinc. Washington, DC: National Academy Press, 2001, pp. 502–53.

17. Nielsen F. Ultratrace elements in nutrition: current knowledge and speculation. J Trace Elem Exp Med 1998;1:251–74.

18. Cangul H, Broday L, Salnickow K, Sutherland J, Peng W, Zhang Q, Poltaratsky V, Yee H, Zoroddu M, Costa M. Molecular mechanisms of nickel carcinogenesis. Toxicol Letters 2002;127:69–75.

SILICON

Silicon occupies a unique position among the essential trace elements in that it is second only to oxygen in earth-wide abundance. Quartz, which is crystallized silica, is the most abundant mineral in the earth's crust. The element occurs naturally as dioxide silica, SiO_2, and as water-soluble silicic acid, $Si(OH)_4$, formed by hydration of the oxide. In plants, silicon is deposited as the solid, hydrated oxide $SiO_2 \cdot nH_2O$, known as silica gel, following polymerization of silicic acid.

Whereas early investigations concentrated on silicon's toxicity, such as silicon-related urolithiasis (stones in the urinary tract) and particularly silicosis (a respiratory condition caused by the inhalation of dust), since about the mid-1970s research has focused on the possible roles or functions of silicon in animals and humans.

Sources

Data on the distribution of silicon in human foods and diets are sparse. It is known, however, that foods of plant origin normally are much richer in silicon than those of animal origin. Whole cereal grains and root vegetables appear to be especially rich sources of the element [1,2]. Beverages, including water, coffee, and beer, also contribute to silicon intake [1]. Silicon intakes by adults are estimated to be 14 to 62 mg/day [1,3,4].

Absorption, Transport, Storage, and Excretion

The mechanism of absorption of silicon is not well understood, and future studies will likely be complicated by the fact that its dietary forms are so diverse. Silica, monosilicic acid, phytolithic silica, and silicon found in organic combination (e.g., with pectin and mucopolysaccharides) are a few of its ingestible forms. In fluids, silicon may be present as orthosilicic acid, $Si(OH)_4$. The most soluble form of silicon is metasilicate, which as sodium metasilicate has commonly been used in supplementation studies.

Estimates of the absorption of silicon range from 1% to >70% depending on the form of silicon ingested, the production of a soluble form in the gastrointestinal tract, and the presence of fiber [5,6]. For example, nearly 97% of dietary silicon contained in a high-fiber diet remained unabsorbed and was lost in the feces, compared to a fecal excretion of only 60% when a low-fiber diet was consumed [2]. In studies on rats, changes in absorption were also shown to relate to age, sex, and various hormones [7].

Silicon in the body is found bound as well as in free forms such as silicic acid, $Si(OH)_4$ [8]. Once silicic acid is absorbed into the blood, it is almost entirely free (i.e., not bound to proteins), thus accounting for its rapid decrease in plasma concentration, its diffusion into tissue fluids, and its rapid urinary excretion [9]. After intravenous administration of ^{31}Si silicic acid, the label was most rapidly taken up by liver, lung, skin, and bone, with slower entry occurring in heart, muscle, spleen, and testes. Negligible uptake into the brain was reported, indicating active exclusion by the blood-brain barrier. Generally, silicon concentrates in the body's connective tissues, such as bone, skin, and tendons.

The kidney is the major excretory organ of absorbed silicon; 77% of labeled silicic acid was excreted in the urine of rats within 4 hours [9]. Urinary silicon excretion is significantly correlated with silicon intake [4].

Functions and Deficiency

The physiological role of silicon is focused on the normal formation, growth, and development of bone, connective tissue, and cartilage, functioning in both a metabolic and a structural capacity. The effect of silicon on bone is to hasten formation and mineralization, as well as to promote turnover and growth. In test animals, high-silicon diets were associated with increased calcium content of the bone and accelerated bone maturity. Silicon deficiency resulted in smaller, less flexible long bones and in deformation of the skull. In studies on chicks, the skull deformation was subsequently found to be due to a significantly reduced collagen content in the connective tissue matrix [10]. In rats, silicon affected bone mineral content, formation, and turnover [11]. Decreases in femoral and vertebral calcium, copper, potassium, and zinc concentrations and increased plasma alkaline phosphatase activity have been reported with silicon deprivation in rats [12].

The detrimental effect of silicon deficiency on collagen formation is linked to the mineral's requirement in the synthesis of proline and hydroxyproline, the residues of which are of particular importance in collagen's primary structure. Proline is incorporated as such into the procollagen peptide but becomes hydroxylated posttranslationally by prolyl hydroxylase. The reaction (Fig. 13.2) also requires iron and vitamin C. Silicon is required for maximal prolyl hydroxylase activity, although the mechanism is not yet understood [13,14]. Silicon also appears to be needed for ornithine aminotransferase, an enzyme required for collagen formation and whose activity is diminished with silicon deficiency [15].

In addition to its positive influence on collagen synthesis, silicon also is needed for the formation of glycosaminoglycans such as hyaluronic acid, chondroitin sulfate, and keratin sulfate. Glycosaminoglycans are linked covalently to proteins as components of the extracellular ground substance or organic matrix that surrounds the collagen, elastic fibers, and cells. A structural role for silicon in glycosaminoglycan formation has also been proposed, because silicon has been found to be chemically linked within the glycosaminoglycan framework [8].

Interactions with Other Nutrients

The only mineral element in a normal diet that may be of any consequence with respect to the availability of silicon is molybdenum. The interaction was first discovered when silicon supplementation of a diet high in liver failed to significantly elevate the plasma silicon concentration and both plasma and tissue silicon levels subsequently were shown to be markedly and inversely affected by molybdenum intake [16]. The reverse is also true: silicon supplementation reduces the plasma concentration and cellular uptake of dietary molybdenum. Until the mechanism of

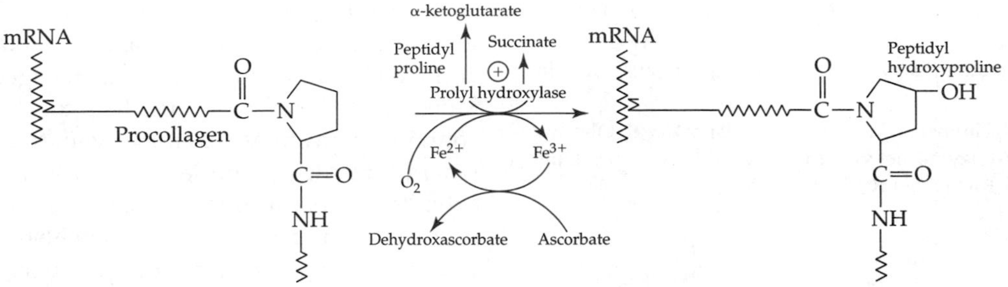

Figure 13.2 The posttranslational hydroxylation of peptidyl proline in a growing procollagen chain. In addition to prolyl hydroxylase, the reaction also requires ascorbate, α-ketoglutarate, ferrous iron, and oxygen. The symbol ⊕ designates the sites at which silicon positively affects collagen synthesis.

intestinal absorption of the two elements is better understood, the manner in which they interact remains unknown.

Recommended Intake, Toxicity, and Assessment of Nutriture

The minimum silicon requirement compatible with human health is largely unknown, as are the dietary forms that render the mineral most available. Requirements for silicon have been largely confined to assessing the relationship of dietary silicon intake, expressed as mg/g of dry diet, to observed growth and skeletal development in test animals. Such studies indicate that the dietary silicon requirement may be relatively high compared to that of other trace elements. For humans, estimates of the requirement for silicon based on animal studies range from 2 to 5 mg/day, while recommendations for intake range from ~5 to 35 mg/day [4,5].

No tolerable upper intake level has been established for silicon. The major potential adverse effect reported is kidney stones; however, it is frequent, chronic (years) use of large amounts of silicon-containing antacids (e.g., magnesium trisilicate, which can provide 6.5 mg elemental silicon per tablet) that appears to be related to a few cases of kidney stones [3,17]. Toxicity of silicon has also been associated with diminished activities of several enzymes that prevent free radical damage, including glutathione peroxidase, superoxide dismutase, and catalase [18].

As in the case of most of the trace elements, levels of silicon in biological fluids of healthy adults have been reported but may not accurately represent nutriture. Chemical assessment generally is performed on serum or plasma, which contains ~0.4 to 10.0 mg silicon/L. Mass spectrometry, emission spectroscopy, and atomic absorption spectrophotometry are a few of the techniques for determining silicon concentration in biological specimens. Of these, atomic absorption spectrophotometry has been the method of choice for most laboratories.

References Cited for Silicon

1. Pennington J. Silicon in foods and diet. Food Additives Contaminants 1991;8:97–118.
2. Kelsay J, Behall K, Prather E. Effect of fiber from fruits and vegetables on metabolic responses of human subjects II: calcium, magnesium, iron, and silicon balances. Am J Clin Nutr 1979;32:1876–80.
3. Food and Nutrition Board. Dietary Reference Intakes for Vitamin A, Vitamin K, Arsenic, Boron, Chromium, Copper, Iodine, Iron, Manganese, Molybdenum, Nickel, Silicon, Vanadium, and Zinc. Washington, DC: National Academy Press, 2001, pp. 502–53.
4. Jugdaohsingh R, Anderson S, Tucker K, Elliott H, Kiel D, Thompson R, Powell J. Dietary silicon intake and absorption. Am J Clin Nutr 2002;75:887–93.
5. Nielsen F. Ultratrace minerals. In: Shils M, Olson J, Shike M, Ross A, eds. Modern Nutrition in Health and Disease, 9th ed. Baltimore, MD: Williams and Wilkins, 1999, pp. 283–303.
6. Benke G, Osborn T. Urinary silicon excretion by rats following oral administration of silicon compounds. Food Cosmet Toxicol 1978;17:123–27.
7. Charnot Y, Peres G. Silicon, endocrine balance and mineral metabolism. In: Bendz G, Lindquist I, eds. Biochemistry of Silicon and Related Problems. New York: Plenum Press, 1978, pp. 269–80.
8. Seaborn C, Nielsen F. Silicon: a nutritional beneficence for bones, brains, and blood vessels. Nutr Today 1993; 28:13–18.
9. Adler A, Etzion Z, Berlyne G. Uptake, distribution, and excretion of ^{31}silicon in normal rats. Am J Physiol 1986;251:E670–73.
10. Carlisle E. A silicon requirement for normal skull formation in chicks. J Nutr 1980;110:352–59.
11. Seaborn C, Nielsen F. Dietary silicon affects acid and alkaline phosphatase and ^{45}calcium uptake in bone of rats. J Trace Elem Exper Med 1994;7:11–18.
12. Seaborn C, Nielsen F. Dietary silicon and arginine affect mineral element composition of rat femur and vertebra. Biol Trace Elem Res 2002;89:239–50.
13. Carlisle E. Silicon: a requirement in bone formation independent of vitamin D. Calc Tissue Intern 1981;33:27–34.
14. Carlisle E, Alpenfels W. The role of silicon in proline synthesis. Fed Proc 1984;43:680.
15. Seaborn C, Nielsen F. Silicon deprivation decreases collagen formation in wounds and bone, and ornithine transaminase enzyme activity in liver. Biol Trace Elem Res 2002;89:251–61.

16. Carlisle E. A silicon-molybdenum interrelationship in vivo. Fed Proc 1979;38:553.

17. Haddad F, Kouyoumdjian A. Silica stones in humans. Urol Int 1986;41:70–76.

18. Najda J, Goss M, Gminski J, Weglarz L, Siemianowicz K, Olszowy Z. The antioxidant enzyme activity in the conditions of systemic hypersilicemia. Biol Trace Elem Res 1994;42:63–70.

VANADIUM

Vanadium was first discovered in the early 1800s and named for a Swedish goddess, Vanadis [1]. The element exists in several oxidation states, from V^{2+} to V^{5+}. In solution, vanadium produces a range of colors, which accounts for its being named after the goddess. In its pentavalent state it is yellowish orange, whereas in its divalent state it is blue [1]. V^{3+} has been shown to form complexes with amino acids such as alanine and aspartate [2]. In biological systems, vanadium is found primarily in the pentavalent state, V^{5+}, known as vanadate or monovanadate (VO_3^-, VO^{3-}, or $H_2VO_4^-$) or in the tetravalent state, V^{4+}, vanadyl ion (VO^{2+}).

Sources

The content of vanadium in foods is very low, and consequently so is the average dietary intake. Most fats and oils contain particularly low levels of the mineral, <0.3 μg/100 g [3]. A few items, including black pepper, parsley, dill seed, canned apple juice, fish sticks, and mushrooms, contain relatively high concentrations, and shellfish such as oysters are particularly rich in the element, with up to ~12 μg/100 g [3,4]. Cereals and grain products contribute fairly substantial amounts of vanadium (up to 15 μg/100 g) to the diet, as do sweeteners (up to 4.7 μg/100 g) [4]. Beer and wine also provide a source of vanadium [3,4]. Vanadium intake in the U.S. diet is thought to range from 10 to 60 μg/day, with many diets containing <15 μg [1,3,4]. Supplements providing vanadium as vanadyl sulfate and sodium metavanadate are available.

Absorption, Transport, and Storage

Absorption of vanadium varies with its oxidation states. For example, vanadate is thought to be reduced to vanadyl (VO^{2+}) in the stomach before absorption. Compared to vanadyl, vanadate is 3 to 5 times more efficiently absorbed, likely due to its transport via the transport system for phosphate, which it mimics chemically [5]. Overall, vanadium absorption is generally <5% [5]. However, studies on vanadium absorption in rats have documented absorption ranging from 10% to as high as 40% [6]. These rat studies suggest caution in assuming that vanadium will always be poorly absorbed.

In blood cells and in plasma and other body fluids, vanadate is converted to vanadyl. Glutathione, NADH, and ascorbic acid can act as reducing agents for vanadate. Vanadyl in the plasma and hepatocytes binds to iron-containing proteins to form vanadyl-transferrin and vanadyl-ferritin complexes. Studies show that V^{3+} exhibits greater binding to the N-terminal end of transferrin than V^{4+} and V^{5+}; however, whether significant quantities of V^{3+} are present in biological systems is unclear [7].

Vanadium is thought to enter cells as vanadate through transport systems for phosphate and possibly other anions. Similar to reactions in the plasma, intracellular vanadate is reduced primarily by glutathione to vanadyl, which is then almost exclusively bound to a variety of ligands, many of which are phosphates and iron-containing proteins; <1% remains unbound [8]. Vanadyl may be converted back to vanadate by NADPH oxidation pathways [9].

Little vanadium is found in the body; the total body pool of vanadium is only ~100 μg [3]. Most tissues contain <10 ng V/g tissue [10,11]. Distribution studies indicate that while kidney cells retain most of the absorbed mineral soon after its administration, accumulation later shifts principally to bone, with somewhat lesser amounts in the spleen and liver. This is understandable in view of the high content in bone of inorganic phosphate, to which vanadyl binds tenaciously [8].

Functions

Vanadium is very active pharmacologically, exerting a broad assortment of effects that are well documented. However, the reader is cautioned not to confuse essentiality with pharmacological activity, because the latter is generally manifested only above a concentration threshold that is considerably greater than that required to fulfill the need for essentiality.

No specific biochemical function has been identified for vanadium. Many of vanadium's effects in vivo are predictable from a consideration of its aqueous chemistry. First, as vanadate it will compete with phosphate at the active sites of phosphate transport proteins, phosphohydrolases, and phosphotransferases. Second, as vanadyl it will compete with other transition metal ions for binding sites on metalloproteins and for small ligands such as adenosine triphosphate (ATP). Third, it will participate in redox reactions within the cell, particularly with substances that can reduce vanadate nonenzymatically, such as glutathione.

A few of the more thoroughly investigated pharmacological effects of vanadium are briefly discussed next. Vanadium inhibits Na^+/K^+-ATPase, an enzyme involved in the phosphorylation by ATP of the carrier protein for sodium ions by permitting the transport of the ions against a concentration gradient. Vanadate is known to inhibit the enzyme by binding to its ATP hydrolysis site. Vanadate has been shown to form ternary complexes with myosin and ADP to inhibit interactions with actin [12].

Vanadium, as vanadate, is believed to stimulate adenylate cyclase by promoting an association of an otherwise inactive guanine nucleotide regulatory protein (G protein) with the catalytic unit of the enzyme [13]. Adenylate cyclase catalyzes the formation of cyclic 3′,5′-adenosine monophosphate (cAMP) from ATP. Cyclic AMP then stimulates protein kinases, which catalyze the phosphorylation of various enzymes and other cellular proteins in cytoplasm, membranes, mitochondria, ribosomes, and the nucleus. The phosphorylation is nearly always stimulatory, and it results secondarily from the hormone-induced stimulation of adenylate cyclase. This is the basis for cAMP's putative role as a second messenger of hormone action.

The effect of vanadate on the transport of amino acids across the intestinal mucosa exemplifies both its inhibitory effect on Na^+/K^+-ATPase and its stimulation of adenylate cyclase. At higher concentrations, vanadate inhibits the mucosal-to-serosal flux of alanine, commensurate with a decrease in Na^+/K^+-ATPase function. However, at a lower concentration (too low to affect Na^+/K^+-ATPase), it is stimulatory to alanine transport; this is attributable to an increase in adenylate cyclase activity and cAMP formation [14].

Vanadium, as vanadate and vanadyl, mimics the action of insulin. Vanadium stimulates glucose uptake into cells, enhances glucose metabolism, and inhibits catecholamine-induced lipolysis [15]. Insulin works by binding to insulin receptors, which span the lipid membranes of cells. Insulin binding to cell membrane receptors results in tyrosine-specific protein kinase–stimulated phosphorylation of tyrosine residues on the receptor. Serine and threonine phosphorylation of the receptor also may occur. The phosphorylation leads to multiple cascades of reactions whereby glucose is taken up into insulin-dependent cells such as the muscle, among other reactions. Vanadium is thought to mimic insulin function; however, vanadate phosphorylates tyrosyl residues not in the insulin receptor, but in cytosolic protein kinases and in non–insulin receptor protein kinases in the plasma membrane [9]. Activation of the cytosolic protein tyrosine kinases affects glucose and lipid metabolism, while activation of the plasma membrane protein tyrosine kinases triggers phosphatidylinositol 3-kinase, inhibits lipolysis, and stimulates glucose uptake [9]. Vanadate also has been shown to inhibit phosphotyrosine phosphatase, thereby prolonging the activity of phosphorylated enzymes [16]. There is also evidence that sodium vanadate exerts an insulinotropic effect by stimulating the release of insulin from rat islet cells [17].

Although vanadate's chemical similarity to phosphate accounts in large part for its biochemical action, vanadium (as the vanadyl cation) has also been shown to be physiologically active, particularly in its substitution for other metals such as zinc, copper, and iron in metalloenzyme activity. Studies examining vanadium deficiency have suggested that the element is associated with iodine metabolism and/or thyroid gland function [18]. Controlled depletion of vanadium has been reported to adversely affect growth rate, perinatal survival, physical appearance, hematocrit, and other manifestations in various animal species [19].

Excretion

Renal excretion is the major route for the elimination of absorbed vanadium. Amounts of vanadium in the urine are generally <0.8 μg/L urine. Urinary metabolites include vanadium diascorbate and vanadyl transferrin complex [20]. In addition to losses in the urine, small amounts (~1.0 ng/g) of vanadium are excreted via the bile.

Recommended Intake, Toxicity, and Assessment of Nutriture

The human requirement for vanadium is not established, although 10 μg/day has been suggested as meeting the requirement [21]. A tolerable upper intake level of 1.8 mg elemental vanadium per day has been established [22]. Toxicity has been shown in humans with intakes above ~10 mg. Toxic manifestations include green tongue (due to deposition of green-colored vanadium in the tongue), diarrhea, gastrointestinal cramps, disturbances in mental function, hypertension, and renal toxicity [1,11,22]. However, doses of 100 mg and 125 mg vanadyl sulfate and sodium metavanadate, respectively, are being tried in clinical trials with individuals with diabetes [23,24].

The techniques most commonly used for assessment are neutron activation analysis and flameless atomic absorption spectrophotometry, with the latter the practical choice of most analytic laboratories. Plasma or serum vanadium concentrations in healthy adults are quite low, with concentrations <0.4 mg/L and often <0.001 mg/L [3].

References Cited for Vanadium

1. Harland B, Harden-Williams B. Is vanadium of human nutritional importance yet? J Am Diet Assoc 1994;94:891–94.

2. Bukietynska K, Podsiadly H, Karwecka Z. Complexes of vanadium (III) with L-alanine and L-aspartic acid. J Inorg Biochem 2003; 94:317–25.

3. Byrne A, Kosta L. Vanadium in foods and in human body fluids and tissues. Sci Total Environ 1978;10:17–30.

4. Pennington J, Jones J. Molybdenum, nickel, cobalt, vanadium, and strontium in total diets. J Am Diet Assoc 1987;87:1644–50.

5. Nielsen F. Boron, manganese, molybdenum, and other trace elements. In: Bowman B, Russell R, eds. Present Knowledge in Nutrition, 8th ed. Washington, DC: International Life Sciences Institute Nutrition Foundation, 2001, pp. 384–99.

6. Bogden J, Higashino H, Lavenhar M, Bauman J, Kemp F, Aviv A. Balance and tissue distribution of vanadium after short-term ingestion of vanadate. J Nutr 1982;112:2279–85.

7. Nagaoka M, Yamazaki T, Maitani T. Binding patterns of vanadium ions with different valance states to human serum transferrin studied by HPLC/high resolution ICP-MS. Biochem Biophys Res Comm 2002;296:1207–14.

8. Nechay B, Nanninga L, Nechay P, Post R, Grantham J, Macara I, Kubena L, Phillips T, Nielsen F. Role of vanadium in biology. Fed Proc 1986;45:123–32.

9. Goldwaser I, Gefel D, Gershonov E, Fridkin M, Shechter Y. Insulin-like effects of vanadium: basic and clinical implications. J Inorg Biochem 2000;80:21–25.

10. Nielsen F. Vanadium in mammalian physiology and nutrition. In: Sigel H, Sigel A, eds. Metal Ions in Biological Systems. Physiology and Biochemistry. Dordrecht: Kluwer, 1990, pp. 51–62.

11. Nielsen F. Ultratrace minerals. In: Shils M, Olson J, Shike M, Ross A, eds. Modern Nutrition in Health and Disease, 9th ed. Baltimore, MD: Williams and Wilkins, 1999, pp. 283–303.

12. Aureliano M. Vanadate oligomer interactions with myosin. J Inorg Biochem 2000;80:141–43.

13. Krawietz W, Downs R, Spiegel A, Aurbach G. Vanadate stimulates adenylate cyclase via the guanine nucleotide regulatory protein by a mechanism differing from that of fluoride. Biochem Pharmacol 1982;31:843–48.

14. Hajjar J, Fucci J, Rowe W, Tomicic T. Effect of vanadate on amino acid transport in rat jejunum. Proc Soc Exp Biol Med 1987;184:403–9.

15. Heyliger C, Tahiliani A, McNeill J. Effect of vanadate on elevated blood glucose and depressed cardiac performance of diabetic rats. Science 1985;227:1474–77.

16. Stankiewicz P, Gresser M. Inhibition of phosphatase and sulfatase by transition-state analogues. Biochem 1988;27:206–12.

17. Fagin J, Ikejiri K, Levin S. Insulinotropic effects of vanadate. Diabetes 1987;36:1448–52.

18. Nielsen F. Ultratrace elements of possible importance for human health: an update. In: Prasad AS, ed. Essential and Toxic Trace Elements in Human Health. New York: Wiley-Liss, 1993, pp. 355–76.

19. Nielsen F. Vanadium. In: Mertz W, ed. Trace Elements in Human and Animal Nutrition. San Diego: Academic Press 1987;1:275–300.

20. Kramer H, Krampitz G, Backer A, Meyer-Lehnert H. Ouabain-like factors in human urine: identification of a Na-K-ATPase inhibitor as vanadium-diascorbate adduct. Clin Exp Hyperten 1998;20:557–71.

21. Nielsen F. Ultratrace elements in nutrition: current knowledge and speculation. J Trace Elem Exp Med 1998;11:251–74.

22. Food and Nutrition Board. Dietary Reference Intakes for Vitamin A, Vitamin K, Arsenic, Boron, Chromium, Copper, Iodine, Iron, Manganese, Molybdenum, Nickel, Silicon, Vanadium, and Zinc. Washington, DC: National Academy Press, 2001, pp. 502–53.

23. Boden G, Chen X, Ruiz J, van Rossum G, Turco S. Effects of vanadyl sulfate on carbohydrate and lipid metabolism in patients with non-insulin dependent diabetes mellitus. Metabolism 1996;45:1130–35.

24. Goldfine A, Simonson D, Folli F, Patti M, Kahn C. In vivo and in vitro studies of vanadate in human and rodent diabetes mellitus. Molec Cell Biochem 1995;153:217–31.

COBALT

There is little evidence that cobalt plays a role in human nutrition other than its being a part of vitamin B_{12} (cobalamin). Although ionic cobalt can substitute for other metals in metalloenzyme activity in vitro, a fact that we will review briefly, no evidence exists for its acting in that capacity in vivo. In this respect, the metal is unique among the essential trace elements in that the requirement in the human is not for an ionic form of the metal but for a preformed metallovitamin that cannot be synthesized from dietary metal. Therefore, it is the vitamin B_{12} content of foods and diet that is of importance in human nutrition rather than ionic cobalt status.

There have been reports regarding the dependency of certain enzymes on cobalt as an activator or on the metal's ability to substitute for other metal ion activators. Cobalt, in the form of CoC^{2+}, for example, appears to regulate the activity of certain phosphoprotein phosphatases, such as casein and phosvitin phosphatases [1,2]. In another study on phosphoprotein phosphatases, only Co^{2+} and Mn^{2+} could reactivate enzymes inactivated by ATP, ADP, and PP_i, with cobalt being significantly the more potent reactivator [3]. Cobalt, along with Mn^{2+} and Ni^{2+}, can also substitute for Zn^{2+} in the metalloenzymes, angiotensin-converting enzyme [4], carboxypeptidase [5], and carbonic anhydrase [6].

The reader is cautioned against interpreting such findings as implying the possible essentiality of ionic cobalt. There is no evidence from deprivation studies on animals that the metal is a requirement for these enzymes in vivo.

References Cited for Cobalt

1. Japundzic I, Levi E, Japundzic M. Cobalt-dependent protein phosphatases from human cord blood erythrocytes. I. Submolecular structure and regulation of activity of E3 casein phosphatase. Enzyme 1988;39:134–43.

2. Japundzic I, Levi E, Japundzic M. Cobalt-dependent protein phosphatases from human cord blood erythrocytes. II. Further characterization of E2 casein phosphatase. Enzyme 1988;39:144–50.

3. Khandelwal R, Kamani S. Studies on inactivation and reactivation of homogeneous rabbit liver phosphoprotein phosphatases by inorganic pyrophosphate and divalent cations. Biochim Biophys Acta 1980;613:95–105.

4. Bicknell R, Holmquist B, Lee F, Martin M, Riordan J. Electronic spectroscopy of cobalt angiotensin converting enzyme and its inhibitor complexes. Biochem 1987;26:7291–97.

5. Auld D, Holmquist B. Carboxypeptidase A. Differences in the mechanisms of ester and peptide hydrolysis. Biochem 1974;13:4355.

6. Lindskog S. Carbonic anhydrase. In: Spiro TG, ed. Zinc Enzymes. New York: Wiley, 1983, pp. 86–97.

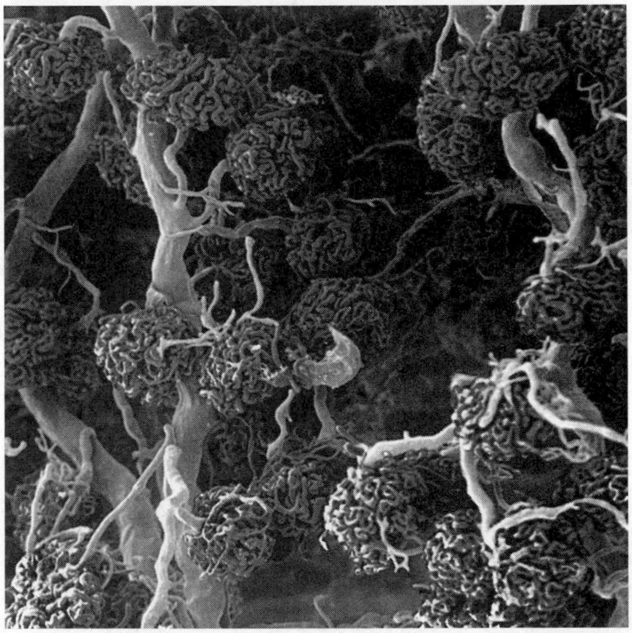

Scanning electron micrograph of human kidney glomeruli and blood vessels

chapter 14 Body Fluid and Electrolyte Balance

CHAPTER 1, IN PARTICULAR, and the subsequent chapters dealing with nutrient metabolism have emphasized the specialized nature of cells comprising the organ systems of the body. Despite the great diversity of specialized cellular functions, the composition of the body fluids (the internal environment) enveloping the cells remains relatively constant under normal conditions. This constant composition, or **homeostasis,** of the internal environment is necessary for optimal activity of the cells. It is maintained by homeostatic mechanisms involving most of the body's organ systems, the most important of which are the circulatory, respiratory, and renal excretory systems as well as the central nervous system (CNS) and the endocrine regulation system. Many minor disturbances inevitably occur in water distribution, electrolyte balance, and pH of the body fluids during metabolism. As disturbances arise, compensatory mechanisms of the regulatory organs make appropriate corrections to maintain homeostasis.

WATER DISTRIBUTION IN THE BODY

Water accounts for ~60% of the total body weight in a normal adult, making it the most abundant constituent of the human body. In terms of volume, the total body water in a man of average weight (70 kg) is roughly 42 L. Water provides the medium for the solubilization and passage of a multitude of nutrients, both organic and inorganic, from the blood to the cells and for the return of metabolic products to the blood. It also serves as the medium in which the vast number of intracellular metabolic reactions take place.

Total body water can theoretically be compartmentalized into two major reservoirs, the intracellular compartment, which includes all water enclosed within cell membranes, and the extracellular compartment, which includes all water external to cell membranes. Of the 42 L of total body water, the intracellular and extracellular compartments account for about 28 L and 14 L, respectively. The anatomic extracellular water is functionally subdivided into the plasma (the cell-free, intravascular water compartment) and the interstitial fluid (ISF). The ISF directly bathes the extravascular cells and provides the medium for the passage of nutrients and metabolic products back and forth between the blood and cells. In addition, potential spaces in the body (i.e., pericardial, pleural, peritoneal, and synovial) that are normally empty except for a small volume of viscous lubricating fluid need to be considered part of the ISF compartment. The body water compartment volumes are summarized in Table 14.1 for a 70-kg man.

The fraction of total body weight that is water and the percentage of total body water that is extracellular or intracellular do not remain constant during growth. Expressed as a percentage of body weight, total body water decreases during gestation and early childhood, reaching adult values by about 3 years of age. During this time, the extracellular water (as percentage of body weight) decreases while the intracellular water (as percentage of body weight) increases (Table 15.8).

Table 14.1 Fluid Compartment Values

	Percentage of Body Weight	Percentage of Total Body Water	Volume (L) in 70-kg Man
Total body water	60	—	42
Extracellular water	20	33	14
Plasma	5	8	3.5
Interstitial fluid	15	25	10.5
Intracellular water	40	67	28

MAINTENANCE OF FLUID BALANCE

Most of the daily available water enters by the oral route as beverages and as liquids contained in foods. A relatively small amount of water is formed within the body as a product of metabolic reactions. These two sources together account for a daily intake of ~2,500 mL fluid, of which the oral route contributes ~2,300 mL, or >90%.

The routes by which water is lost from the body can vary according to environmental and physiological conditions such as ambient temperature and extent of physical exercise. At an ambient temperature of 68°F, ~1,400 mL of the 2,300 mL taken in is normally lost in the urine, 100 mL in the sweat, and 200 mL in the feces. The remaining 600 mL leaves the body as insensible water loss, so called because the subject is not aware of the water loss as it is occurring. Evaporation from the respiratory tract and diffusion through the skin are examples of insensible water loss.

Osmotic Pressure

One of the more important factors determining the distribution of water among the water compartments of the body is **osmotic pressure.** When a membrane permeable to water but impermeable to solute particles separates two fluid compartments of unequal solute concentrations, there is a net movement of water through the membrane from the solution with higher water (lower solute) concentration toward the solution with lower water (higher solute) concentration. The movement of water across a semipermeable membrane is called **osmosis.** Osmosis can be blocked by applying an external pressure across the membrane in the opposite direction to the water flow. The amount of pressure required to exactly oppose osmosis into a solution across a semipermeable membrane separating the solution from pure water is the osmotic pressure of the solution.

The theoretic osmotic pressure of a solution is proportional to the number of solute particles per unit volume of solution. This concentration is expressed in terms of the osmolarity, or osmoles per liter (osm/L), of solute particles. One mole of a nonionic solute, such as glucose or urea, is the same as 1 osm, but 1 mol of a solute that dissociates into two or more ions is equivalent to 2 osm or more. For example, 1.0 mol of sodium chloride equals 2.0 osm because of its dissociation into sodium and chloride ions. The theoretic osmotic pressure presupposes that the solute particles are unable to pass freely through the membrane. When the membrane is permeable to a solute, it does not contribute to the actual, or *effective,* osmotic pressure. The higher the permeability of a membrane to a solute, the lower the effective osmotic pressure of a solution of that solute at a given osmolarity. As an example, cell membranes are much more permeable to a nonionic substance such as urea than to sodium and chloride. Therefore, the effective osmotic pressure of a solution of urea across the cell membrane would be much less than that of a solution of sodium chloride of the same osmolarity.

The term *osmolality* is sometimes encountered in the expression of osmotic pressure. Like osmolarity, it denotes the concentration of solute particles. However, rather than being a weight-per-volume expression of concentration, osmolality refers to solute concentration on a weight-per-weight basis (weight of solute to weight of solvent). Specifically, it is the moles of solute particles per kilogram of solvent. Although osmolality is less convenient than osmolarity as a unit of concentration, it has the advantage of being unaffected by temperature, which can cause expansion or contraction of solvent volume.

The effective osmotic pressure of plasma and interstitial fluid across the capillary endothelium that separates them is due mainly to large molecules, such as proteins, that cannot permeate the endothelium. Protein concentration is much higher in the plasma than in the interstitial fluid, conferring on the plasma a relatively high osmotic pressure, or water-attracting property. Proteins and other macromolecules too large to traverse the capillary endothelium are sometimes called **colloids,** and the osmotic pressure attributed to them is appropriately termed the colloid osmotic pressure.

Filtration Forces

Water distribution across the capillary endothelial surface is controlled by the balance of forces that tend to move water from the plasma to the interstitial fluid (filtration forces) and forces that move water from the interstitial fluid into the plasma (reabsorption forces). The major filtration force in the capillaries is hydrostatic pressure (P_{pl}) caused by the pumping of the heart. A much weaker filtration force is the ISF colloid osmotic pressure (Π_{isf}); this force is weak because of the negligible concentration of protein in the ISF. Another weak filtration force is a small, negative ISF hydrostatic pressure (P_{isf}). The major reabsorption force countering the filtration forces is the plasma osmotic pressure (Π_{pl}), which is approximately 28 mm Hg.

At the arteriolar end of the capillaries, the average values of these forces are P_{pl} (hydrostatic pressure), 25 mm Hg; Π_{isf} (colloid osmotic pressure), 5 mm Hg; P_{isf} (interstitial hydrostatic pressure), −6 mm Hg; Π_{pl} (plasma osmotic pressure), 28 mm Hg. The net result of these four forces can be described by Starling's equation:

$$\text{Filtration pressure} = (P_{pl} + \Pi_{isf}) - (\Pi_{pl} + P_{isf})$$

Substituting the average values, we have

$$\begin{aligned}\text{Filtration pressure} &= (25 + 5) - (28 + (-6)) \\ &= (25 + 5) - (28 - 6) \\ &= 30 - 28 + 6 \\ &= 8 \text{ mm Hg}\end{aligned}$$

This positive filtration pressure indicates that a net filtration of water from the plasma to the ISF occurs at the arteriolar end of the capillaries. When filtration pressure is negative, a net reabsorption of water from the ISF to the plasma will occur. This describes the situation at the venule end of the capillaries, where P_{pl} is significantly reduced while the concentration of plasma protein, and therefore Π_{pl}, correspondingly increases. The net effect of these forces on the water distribution between plasma and ISF along the course of the capillary is shown in Figure 14.1.

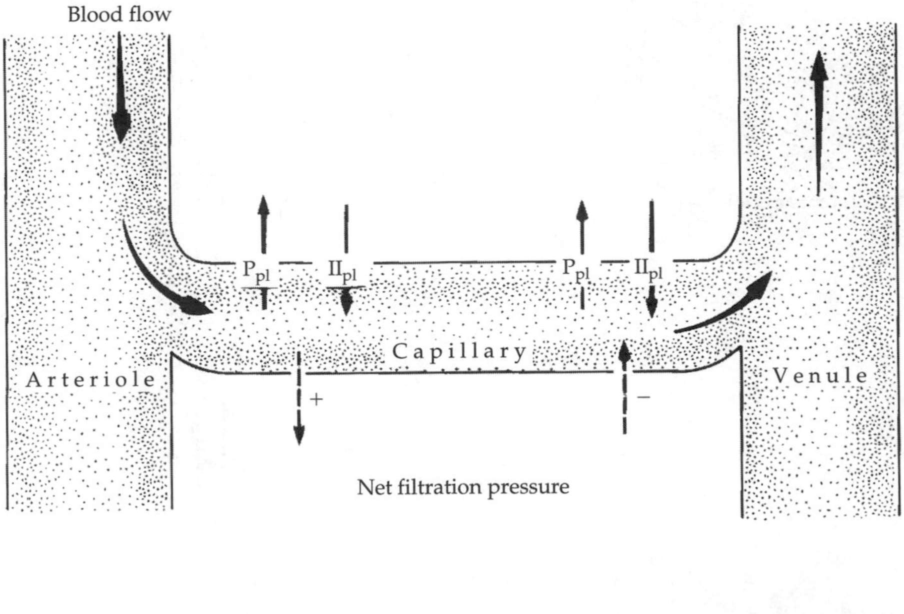

Figure 14.1 Starling's hypothesis of water distribution between plasma and interstitial fluid compartments. The relative magnitudes of the pressures, P_{pl} (plasma hydrostatic pressure) and Π_{pl} (plasma osmotic pressure), are represented by the thickness of their respective arrows. There is a positive net filtration pressure at the arteriolar end of the capillary and a negative net filtration pressure at the venule end.
Source: Kleinman LI, Lorenz JM. Physiology and pathophysiology of body water and electrolytes. In: Kaplan LA, Pesce AJ. *Clinical Chemistry: Theory, Analysis, and Correlation,* 2nd ed. St. Louis: Mosby, 1989, p. 373.

From what we have discussed to this point, it is important to understand that osmotic pressure, together with proper intake of fluids and their output by body mechanisms, is a very important factor in the maintenance of fluid balance and compartmentalization. The body's extracellular water volume, for example, is determined mainly by its osmolarity. The osmolarity, in turn, acts as the signal to the regulatory factors responsible for maintaining fluid homeostasis. The regulation of extracellular water osmolarity and volume is largely the responsibility of the hypothalamus, the renin-angiotensin-aldosterone system, and the kidney.

THE KIDNEY'S ROLE

The functional unit of the kidney is the nephron. Each kidney contains ~1 to 1.5 million nephrons. The five components of the nephron are the Bowman's capsule, proximal convoluted tubule, loop of Henle, distal convoluted tubule, and collecting duct. The excretion process starts in the Bowman's capsule, the blind, dilated end of the renal tubule, which encapsulates a tuft of ~50 capillaries linking the afferent (flowing into the capsule) and efferent (flowing from the capsule) arterioles that surround the tubule segments after they leave the capsule. The capillary network in the Bowman's capsule is called the glomerulus, and it accounts for the particularly rich blood supply that the kidney enjoys. It is estimated that 25% of the volume of blood pumped by the heart into the systemic circulation is circulated through the kidneys, a particularly significant situation in view of the fact that the kidneys constitute only ~0.5% of total body weight. The major components of the nephron are shown schematically in Figure 14.2.

The glomerular capillary network acts as a filter in removing water and other substances, including electrolytes, glucose, amino acids, and metabolic waste products, from plasma. The filtered substances make up what is known as the glomerular filtrate. In the absence of disease, no blood cells (or proteins that exceed a molecular weight of ~50,000 daltons) normally enter the glomerular filtrate because their larger size prevents their passage through the pores of the capillary endothelium.

Each segment of the tubules is functionally distinct in its permeability to water and the solutes of the glomerular filtrate. The tubular segments are surrounded by a network of capillaries into which glomerular filtrate materials can be selectively reabsorbed into the bloodstream as a salvage mechanism. These peritubular capillaries may also secrete certain substances from the

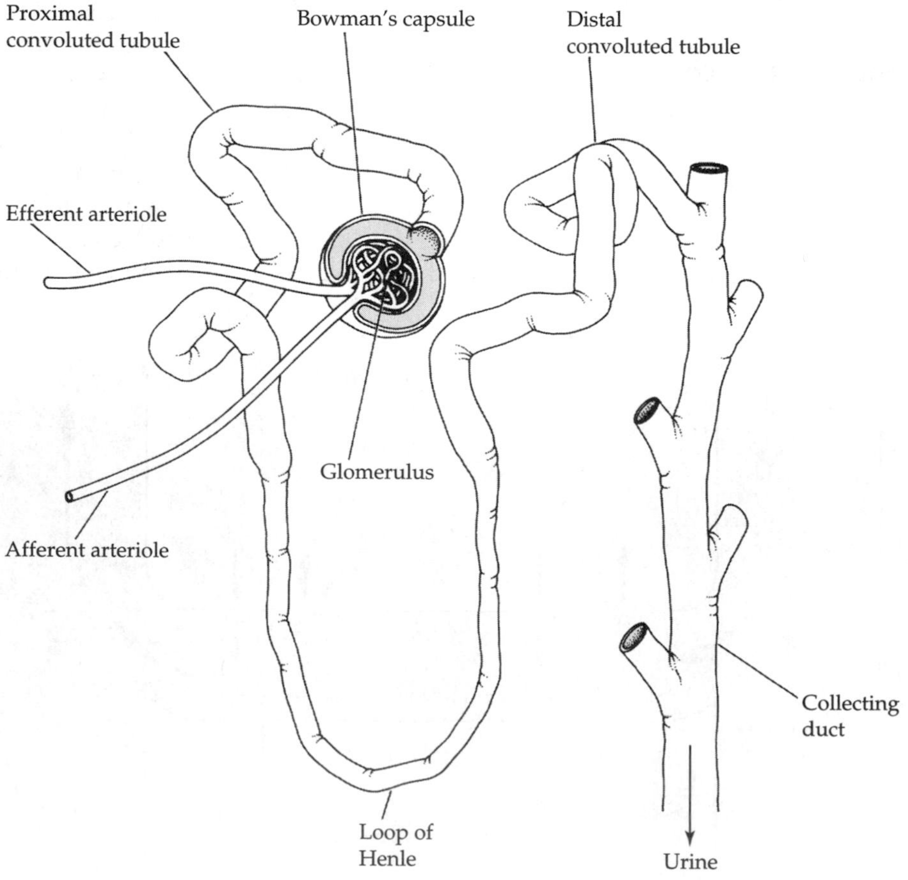

Figure 14.2 A schematic representation of the major components of the nephron.

blood into the renal tubule. The removal of potentially toxic waste products, a major function of the kidneys, is accomplished through the formation of urine. The basic processes involved in urine formation are

- *filtration,* through which the glomerular filtrate is formed;
- *reabsorption* of selected filtrate substances into the bloodstream; and
- *secretion* of materials into the tubules from the surrounding capillaries.

It is through these same processes that the kidneys are able to regulate fluid and electrolyte homeostasis for the proper functioning of cells throughout the body. In healthy individuals, the kidneys are highly sensitive to fluctuations in diet and in fluid and electrolyte intake, and they compensate by varying the volume and consistency of the urine. The glomerular capillaries differ from other capillaries in the body in that the hydrostatic pressure within them is approximately three times greater than in other capillaries. As a result of this high pressure, substances are filtered through the semipermeable membrane into the Bowman's capsule at a rate of ~130 mL/minute. This amounts to over 187,000 mL of filtrate formed per day, yet only ~1,400 mL of urine is produced during this time. This means that $<1\%$ of the filtrate is excreted as urine, with the remaining 99% being reabsorbed into the blood.

It has been mentioned that the hypothalamus, the renin-angiotensin-aldosterone system, and the kidney are responsible for maintaining extracellular fluid volume and osmolarity. Actually, the three work in concert because the hypothalamic hormone, antidiuretic hormone (ADH, also called vasopressin), and aldosterone, produced in the adrenal cortex, exert their effects through the kidney.

Antidiuretic hormone is produced in the supraoptic nucleus of the hypothalamus but is stored in and secreted by the posterior pituitary gland. A potent water-conserving hormone, its action is to increase the water permeability of the distal convoluted tubule and the collecting duct, thereby facilitating the reabsorption of water into the peritubular capillaries. The mechanism by which the hormone exerts this effect is not completely understood. However, ADH increases the activity of adenylate cyclase in the tubular epithelial cells, and the resulting elevation in cyclic AMP (cAMP) concentration is believed to result in the recruitment of water transport units that become inserted into the luminal membrane of the cells. Evidence for the involvement of cAMP in the process is found in the fact that exogenously administered cAMP or inhibitors of phosphodiesterase, which prolong cAMP activity, mimic the action of ADH. The release of ADH from the posterior pituitary is triggered by increased extracellular water osmolarity or by decreased intravascular volume. The hypothalamic response to high extracellular fluid osmolarity is attributed to shrinkage of neurons within the gland caused by the movement of water out of the neurons into the higher osmotic interstitial fluid. This shrinkage then acts as the signal to the posterior pituitary to release the hormone.

A decrease in blood volume affects the activity of distention receptors and baroreceptors at various sites throughout the vascular network, and this information is relayed to the hypothalamus. Another hormone, angiotensin II, released indirectly by distention receptor relaxation (reduced blood volume) in renal arterioles, stimulates the hypothalamus directly with the release of more ADH.

Increased extracellular fluid osmolarity or decreased blood volume therefore influences what is known as the water output area of the hypothalamus. The term *water output function* refers to the fact that, because of the resulting increase in ADH, renal tubular reabsorption of water increases and urine output decreases. However, these factors also stimulate the water intake area of the hypothalamus, resulting in the conscious sensation of thirst. A greater intake of water thus follows, resulting in a dilution of extracellular fluid and increased blood volume, which in turn reduces the release of ADH as fluid homeostasis is restored. The release of ADH and the induction of the thirst sensation in response to plasma osmolarity are illustrated graphically in Figure 14.3.

Figure 14.3 Relationship of plasma vasopressin to plasma osmolality. The arrow indicates the plasma osmolality at which the sensation of thirst is stimulated. *Source:* Vokes T. Water homeostasis. Ann Rev Nutr 1987;7:386.

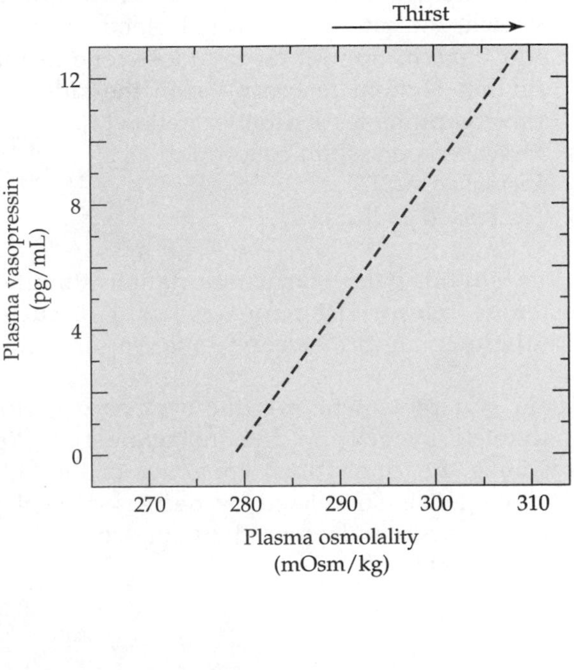

Another hormone that plays an important role in the maintenance of fluid balance is aldosterone, which is produced and secreted by the adrenal cortex and, like ADH, exerts its effect through the kidney. Aldosterone stimulates the active reabsorption of sodium ions in the distal and collecting tubules via a mechanism that involves the transcription and translation of new proteins, which may be Na^+ channels in the luminal membrane, certain mitochondrial enzymes, or Na^+/K^+-ATPase [1]. Evidence that protein induction is indeed a part of the mechanism of aldosterone action is provided by the fact that actinomycin D and puromycin, which are inhibitors of protein synthesis, inhibit electrolyte balance regulation. By stimulating sodium reabsorption, aldosterone increases extracellular fluid osmolarity, thereby promoting fluid retention by the body via the hypothalamus-ADH mechanism already discussed. This is why high-sodium diets are contraindicated for individuals whose fluid "balance" is already upset by excessive retention of water, as with hypertension and edema.

Several different substances influence, according to their plasma concentration, the release of aldosterone. They are listed here and discussed again in the following section on maintenance of electrolyte balance. Listed in decreasing order of their potency in stimulating aldosterone release, they are:

1. Increased angiotensin II. This potent polypeptide hormone is a participant in the renin-angiotensin pathway of aldosterone stimulation. It reacts with receptors on adrenal cell membranes, stimulating the synthesis and release of aldosterone.
2. Decreased atrial natriuretic peptide (ANP). ANP is a peptide hormone synthesized in atrial cells and released in response to increased arteriolar stretch, indicative of elevated blood pressure. It functions in opposition to aldosterone in that it inhibits sodium reabsorption in the kidney and thereby promotes sodium excretion [2].
3. Increased potassium concentration.
4. Increased ACTH.
5. Decreased sodium.

Angiotensin II is particularly important in stimulating aldosterone release. Therefore, we will discuss the renin-angiotensin-aldosterone system in greater detail.

Renin is a proteolytic enzyme synthesized, stored, and secreted by cells in the juxtaglomerular (near or adjoining the glomerulus) apparatus of the kidney. Renin secretion is stimulated by decreased renal perfusion pressure that is sensed by the distention receptors and baroreceptors within the juxtaglomerular apparatus. Renin hydrolyzes angiotensinogen (a freely circulating protein synthesized by the liver) to angiotensin I, an inactive decapeptide. Angiotensin I is then acted on by a second proteolytic enzyme, angiotensin-converting enzyme (ACE), synthesized in vascular endothelial cells (particularly those in the blood vessels of the lung), producing the potent octapeptide angiotensin II. Angiotensin II then interacts with specific receptors on adrenal cortical cells, leading to the release of aldosterone. Along with its sodium-retaining activity, aldosterone promotes the urinary excretion of potassium.

Let's review very briefly the mechanism of action of angiotensin II in increasing the synthesis and release of aldosterone from the adrenal cortex. Stimulatory signals resulting from polypeptide hormone-receptor interactions generally follow one of two major routes. One operates through an accelerated synthesis of cAMP with a consequent increase in protein kinase activity. The second route involves signals mediated by hydrolytic products of phospholipids along with increased intracellular calcium concentrations. It is the second of these mechanisms that applies in the case of angiotensin II action.

A sequential cascade of reactions follows the interaction of angiotensin II with its receptor, involving G proteins, phospholipase C, and inositol triphosphate. Phospholipase C raises intracellular Ca^{2+} concentration by increasing Ca^{2+} conductance through Ca^{2+} channels, and inositol triphosphate releases Ca^{2+} from its storage in the endoplasmic reticulum. The elevated concentration of intracellular Ca^{2+} is stimulatory to appropriate synthetic enzymes, mediated through the Ca^{2+}-binding protein calmodulin [3]. This results in an increase in the synthesis and release of aldosterone. Calmodulin is present in all eukaryotic cells. Figure 11.5 illustrates this type of hormonal mechanism.

The sequence of events that comprise the renin-angiotensin-aldosterone system is illustrated in Figure 14.4. Although not shown in the figure, angiotensin II can be hydrolyzed further to angiotensin III by the hydrolytic removal of an aspartic acid residue by a plasma aminopeptidase. Angiotensin III is also physiologically active. In fact, it has been observed to be more potent than angiotensin II in its aldosterone-stimulating ability. However, the plasma concentration of angiotensin III is significantly less than that of angiotensin II, and therefore its contribution to the maintenance of fluid balance is less dramatic. In addition to its role in the conservation of body water through aldosterone action, angiotensin II is a potent

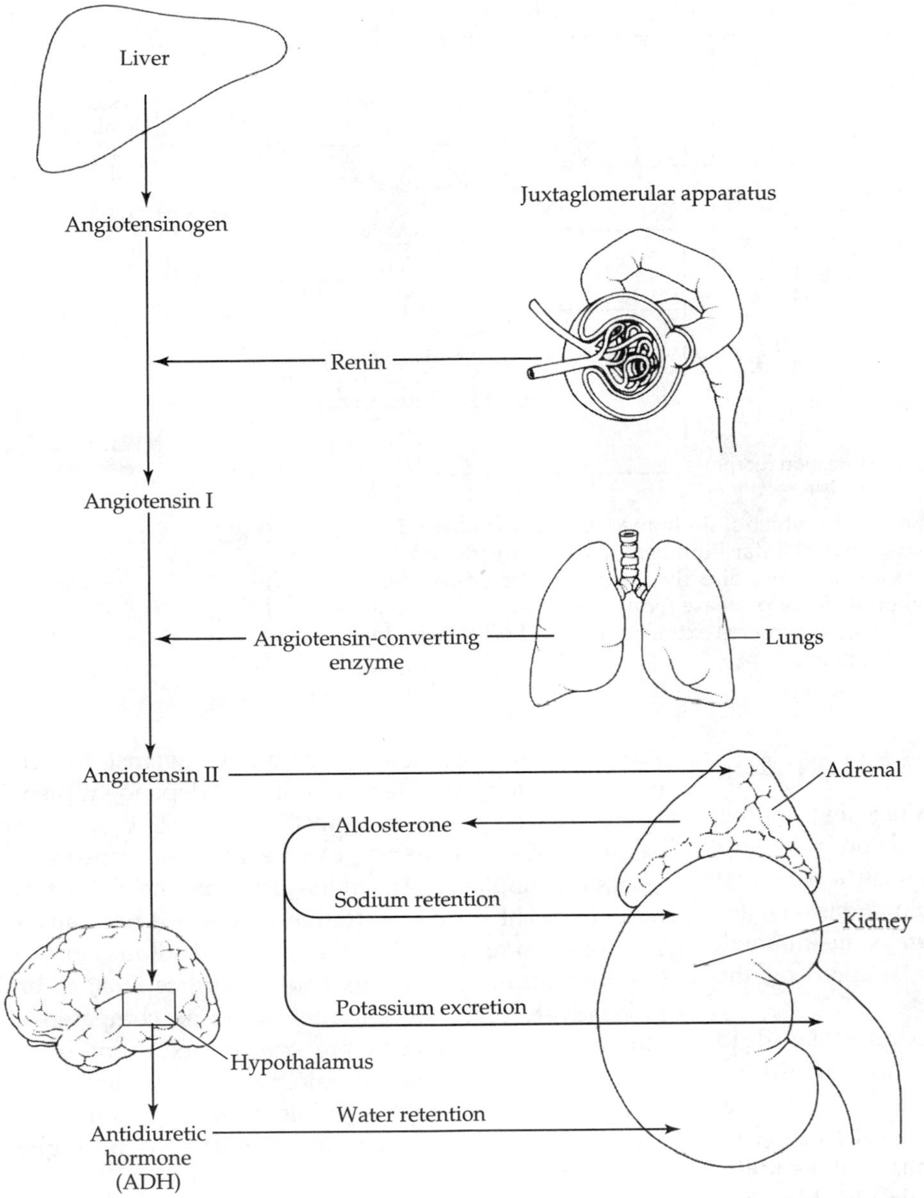

Figure 14.4 The renin-angiotensin-aldosterone system, illustrating the cooperation of kidneys, liver, lungs, adrenals, and hypothalamus in this mechanism of fluid homeostasis.

vasoconstrictor, reducing the glomerular filtration rate and therefore the filtered load of sodium. Also, recall that angiotensin II stimulates the hypothalamic thirst center and the release of ADH, both of which increase body water volume. Figure 14.5 illustrates the central role of the hypothalamus and the action of angiotensin II in the hormonal regulation of fluid homeostasis.

Alterations in food intake can profoundly affect water and electrolyte balance. During the initial days of a period of fasting, for example, there is a marked increase in the renal excretion of sodium, whereas prolonged fasting tends to conserve the ion. Refeeding causes a marked retention of sodium, probably due to the ingestion of carbohydrate. Consequently, a rapid regain of body weight follows, caused by an increase in total body water secondary to the stimulation of vasopressin and thirst by the rise in plasma osmolarity. These alterations in sodium and water balance in subjects as a result of early-phase fasting and refeeding account for the demonstrated weight loss and weight regain to a far greater extent than would be predicted from the changes in caloric balance [4].

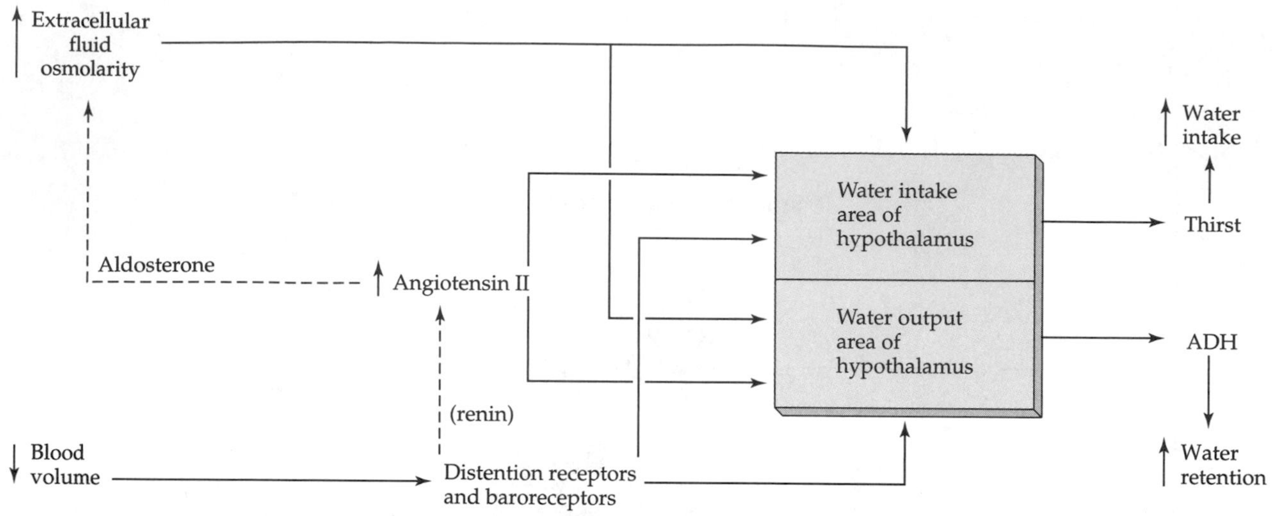

Figure 14.5 A summary of the mechanisms by which fluid homeostasis is maintained. Water depletion stimuli such as increased extracellular fluid osmolarity or decreased blood volume can stimulate the hypothalamus either directly or through the production of angiotensin II, formed by the action of the renal protease renin. The renin-angiotensin-aldosterone system (shown by dashed arrows) increases extracellular fluid osmolarity by promoting renal tubular reabsorption of sodium.

MAINTENANCE OF ELECTROLYTE BALANCE

The term *electrolytes* refers to the anions and cations that are distributed throughout the fluid compartments of the body. They are distributed in such a way that within a given compartment—the blood plasma, for example—electrical neutrality is always maintained, with the anion concentration exactly balanced by the cation concentration.

The cationic electrolytes of the extracellular fluid include sodium, potassium, calcium, and magnesium. These are electrically balanced by the anions chloride, bicarbonate, and protein, along with relatively low concentrations of organic acids, phosphate, and sulfate. The major electrolytes are listed in Table 14.2. Most are categorized nutritionally as macrominerals and, as such, have already been discussed in Chapter 11 from the standpoint of their absorption, function, dietary requirements, and food sources. The maintenance of pH and electrolyte balance, the focus of this chapter, is a responsibility that rests almost exclusively with the kidney.

All filterable substances in plasma—that is, all the plasma solutes except the larger proteins—freely enter the glomerular filtrate from the blood. Some of these substances are metabolic waste products and are excreted in the urine with little or no reabsorption in the tubules. However, most of the materials in the glomerular filtrate must be salvaged by the body. This is accomplished through their tubular reabsorption by either active or passive mechanisms, or both. Active transport allows substances to pass across membranes against concentration gradients by the action of ATP-dependent membrane transport systems (p. 16). Glucose is a prime example of a solute that can be actively transported across the tubular cells from the urine into the blood even though the blood concentration of glucose normally is 20 times that of urine. Another group of solutes, including ammonium, potassium, and phosphate ions, occurs in relatively high concentration in urine compared to blood. These substances are transported from blood into the tubular cells, also against a concentration gradient. Passive transport, the simple diffusion of a material across a membrane from a compartment of higher

Table 14.2 Electrolyte Composition of Body Fluids

	Plasma (mEq/L)	Interstitial Fluid (mEq/L H_2O)	Intracellular Water (mEq/L H_2O)
Cations	153	153	195
Na^+	142	145	10
K^+	4	4	156
Ca^{2+}	5	(2–3)	3.2
Mg^{2+}	2	(1–2)	26
Anions	153	153	195
Cl^-	103	116	2
HCO_3^-	28	31	8
Protein	17	—	55
Others	5	(6)	130
Osmolarity (mosm/L)		294.6	294.6
Theoretic osmotic pressure (mm Hg)		5,685.8	5,685.8

concentration of the material to a compartment of lower concentration, is not energy demanding. This process, too, functions within the renal tubular cells. We will now look at the renal regulation of several major electrolytes.

Sodium

Sodium is freely filtered by the glomerulus. In a healthy individual, nearly all (99.5%) of the sodium is reabsorbed. About 70% of the filtered sodium is reabsorbed by the proximal tubule, 15% by the loop of Henle, 5% by the distal convoluted tubule, and ~10% by the collecting ducts. Sodium is the major cation found in extracellular fluid.

Active reabsorption of sodium ions in the proximal tubule results in the passive reabsorption of chloride ions, bicarbonate ions, and water. The accompanying transfer of the anions chloride and bicarbonate with the cation sodium is required in order to maintain the necessary electrical neutrality of the extracellular fluid, while the water transfer maintains a normal osmotic pressure. Virtually all cells contain a relatively high concentration of potassium and a low concentration of sodium, whereas the blood plasma and most other extracellular fluids have high sodium and low potassium concentrations, as can be seen in Table 14.2. Clearly, energy must be expended to maintain this gradient across the cell membrane; otherwise, each ion would simply diffuse through the membrane until its intracellular and extracellular concentrations were the same. The gradient is maintained by the Na^+/K^+-ATPase pump, which has been discussed in Chapter 1. The Na^+/K^+-ATPase pump is the mechanism by which the renal tubular cells "pump" sodium into the blood in exchange for potassium in such a way as to conserve sodium while allowing a constant loss of potassium in the urine.

Active reabsorption of sodium occurs in the distal convoluted tubule under the influence of aldosterone. The mechanism is highly selective for sodium ion and is accompanied by little water diffusion. This makes it an important system for the regulation of extracellular fluid osmotic pressure. The increased retention of sodium by this mechanism also increases the osmolarity of plasma and therefore is accompanied by water retention. When extracellular fluid osmotic pressure increases, tubular water reabsorption is stimulated through ADH release (Fig. 14.5).

Chloride

The concentration of chloride in the extracellular fluid parallels that of sodium, and chloride generally accompanies sodium in transmembrane passage. However, recall that chloride reabsorption is passive in the proximal tubule. Chloride is probably reabsorbed actively in the ascending limb of the loop of Henle and the distal tubule.

Potassium

Potassium is the chief cation of intracellular fluid, and maintenance of a normal level is essential to the life of the cells. The healthy person maintains potassium balance by the daily excretion in the urine of an amount of the cation equal to the amount ingested minus the small amount excreted in the feces and sweat.

Potassium is freely filtered at the glomerulus, and its active tubular reabsorption occurs throughout the nephron, except for the descending loop of Henle. Only ~10% of the filtered potassium enters the distal tubules, which, along with the collecting ducts, are able to both secrete and reabsorb potassium. The distal tubule is the site at which changes in the amount of potassium excreted are achieved. Several mechanisms are involved in this control.

- The first of these mechanisms is dependent on the cellular potassium content. When a high-potassium diet is consumed, the concentration of potassium rises in cells, including the distal renal tubular cells, providing a concentration gradient that favors the secretion of the cation into the lumen of the tubule. This results in an increase in potassium excretion.
- Another important mechanism in the regulation of potassium balance involves the hormone aldosterone, which, besides stimulating distal tubular reabsorption of sodium, simultaneously enhances potassium secretion at that site. The elevated plasma level of potassium directly stimulates the production and release of aldosterone from the adrenal cortex. Recall that another mechanism for effecting aldosterone release is through decreased renal perfusion pressure and the associated renin-angiotensin-aldosterone pathway.
- A third mechanism of renal conservation of potassium occurs in the collecting duct and involves potassium's active reabsorption coupled with the secretion of protons at that site [5]. The movement of K^+ into the cells of the collecting duct from the urine and the movement of H^+ in the opposite direction are catalyzed by an H^+/K^+-activated adenosine triphosphatase (H^+/K^+-ATPase), functioning similarly to the Na^+/K^+-ATPase pump discussed previously.

Calcium and Magnesium

Tubular reabsorption of calcium is associated with the reabsorption of sodium and phosphate in the proximal tubule, and reabsorption of all three ions, as well as fluid, occurs in parallel. Renal tubular reabsorption of calcium is closely linked to the action of parathyroid hormone (PTH) (p. 348). This hormone exerts parallel inhibition of the reabsorption of calcium, sodium, and phosphate in the proximal tubules. However, stimulation of the reabsorption of calcium in the distal tubules by PTH is markedly disproportionate to that of sodium and phosphate.

The major pathway of calcium excretion is the intestinal tract. Urinary excretion, ~150 mg/day for the average adult, amounts to only ~1% of that filtered by the glomerulus. The remaining 99% is effectively reabsorbed at proximal and distal tubular sites. Calcium balance is achieved largely by control of the intestinal absorption of the ion rather than by regulation of its urinary excretion. The percentage of ingested calcium absorbed decreases as the dietary calcium content increases, so the amount absorbed remains relatively constant. The slight increase in absorption that occurs with a high-calcium diet is reflected in an increased renal excretion of the cation.

The filtration of magnesium at the glomerulus and its subsequent active reabsorption through the tubular cells parallel the filtration and reabsorption of calcium.

Homeostatic regulation of the ions discussed is crucial to many body functions. For example, greatly decreased extracellular potassium (hypokalemia) produces paralysis, whereas elevated potassium levels (hyperkalemia) can result in cardiac arrhythmias. Excessive extracellular sodium (hypernatremia) causes fluid retention, and decreased plasma calcium (hypocalcemia) produces tetany (intermittent spasms of the muscles of the extremities) by increasing the permeability of nerve cell membranes to sodium. Magnesium deficiency is also associated with tetany.

Table 14.2 lists the fluid electrolytes and their approximate normal compartment concentrations. In terms of electrolyte balance only, it is clear that the contribution of sodium to the total cation milliequivalents (mEq) is quite large compared to that of potassium, calcium, and magnesium and that a correspondingly high percentage of anion milliequivalents is contributed by chloride and bicarbonate together. The concentration of these three major ions is used to calculate the so-called anion gap, a clinically useful parameter for establishing metabolic disorders that can alter electrolyte balance. The value is calculated by subtracting the measured anion (chloride + bicarbonate) concentration from the measured cation (sodium) concentration: Measured cations (Na^+) − measured anions ($Cl^- + HCO_3^-$) = Anion gap. Under normal conditions, the value is ~12 mEq/L but may range from 8 to 18 mEq/L. Deviation from a normal anion gap is most commonly associated with increases or decreases in the concentration of certain unmeasured anions such as proteins, organic acids, phosphate, or sulfate. For example, the production of excessive amounts of organic acids, such as would occur in lactic acidosis or ketoacidosis, increases the unmeasured anion concentration at the expense of the measured anion bicarbonate that is neutralized by the acids. Such a condition would therefore cause a greater anion gap.

Considering the effect of plasma osmolarity on water intake and retention, it is logical that should sodium ion accumulate in the body water for any reason, a concomitant rise in blood pressure (essential hypertension) would result. Clinical evidence for this correlation is provided by the hypertension experienced by patients with adrenal adenomas, whose high levels of aldosterone cause excessive retention of sodium. There is also an apparent causal relationship between dietary intake of sodium (as sodium chloride) and the etiology of hypertension, as suggested by studies conducted through one or more of the following designs:

- relating salt consumption to the prevalence of hypertension,
- development of hypertension in animals fed high-salt diets, or
- response of hypertensive patients fed low-salt diets.

An abundance of reported observations deals with the positive correlation of salt intake and hypertension among societies that ingest salt to variable extents. Such observations have led to the generally accepted conclusion that the incidence of hypertension is predictable from average daily sodium intake. Also, convincing animal studies dating back to the 1950s have demonstrated a direct correlation between sodium chloride and hypertension. In spite of these findings, however, there is a lack of evidence of a cause-and-effect relationship among the individuals of a normotensive population. In fact, investigations on the effect on blood pressure of sodium chloride loading among normotensives have revealed no correlation between high salt intake and hypertension. Furthermore, among subjects with borderline essential hypertension, a low-sodium diet is minimally effective in lowering blood pressure. This suggests that plasma sodium concentrations are unalterable if the homeostatic mechanisms controlling it are intact. It has become generally accepted that the differences between those who respond to sodium diet therapy and those who do not have a genetic foundation.

People who are salt-sensitive are called responders, and those showing salt insensitivity are labeled nonresponders. The condition of nonresponders who have essential hypertension does not improve with a low-salt diet. Likewise, normotensive nonresponders can consume as much as 4,600 mg sodium daily (somewhat higher than the sodium intake of the typical Western diet) without risk. Among the genetically disposed (i.e., salt sensitive) individuals, a comparable intake would likely favor the development of hypertension. For people in this population, a restriction of sodium intake to ~1,400 mg or less is recommended.

Although a genetic link to salt sensitivity is generally accepted, biochemical mechanisms of the condition are not clearly understood—though not for lack of relevant research. A literature review of the many investigations designed to explain the biochemical basis of salt sensitivity and nonsensitivity is available [6].

In summary, the implication of sodium in hypertension remains controversial. It is unlikely that it functions alone in the etiology of the disease, and it may be a contributing factor only in the wake of other biochemical disturbances. The involvement of other cations such as calcium, magnesium, potassium, and cadmium cannot be overlooked [6]. Potassium intake has been linked to a reduction in blood pressure, especially in people on high-sodium diets. Although the mechanism remains unknown, potassium may affect natriuresis, baroreflex sensitivity, catecholamine function, or the renin-angiotensin-aldosterone system [7].

ACID-BASE BALANCE: THE CONTROL OF HYDROGEN ION CONCENTRATION

The hydrogen ion concentration in body fluids must be controlled within a narrow range. In fact, its regulation is one of the most important aspects of homeostasis, because merely slight deviations from normal acidity can cause marked alteration in enzyme-catalyzed reaction rates in the cells. Hydrogen ion concentration can also affect both the cellular uptake and regulation of metabolites and minerals and the uptake and release of oxygen from hemoglobin.

The degree of acidity of any fluid is determined by its concentration of protons (H^+). The hydrogen ion concentration in body fluids is generally quite low: it is regulated at approximately 4×10^{-8} mol/L. Concentrations can vary from as low as 1.0×10^{-8} mol/L to as high as 1.0×10^{-7} mol/L, but values outside this range are not compatible with life. From these values, it is apparent that expressing H^+ in terms of its actual concentration is awkward. The concept of pH, which is the negative logarithm of the H^+ concentration, was devised to simplify the expression. It allows concentrations to be expressed as whole numbers rather than as negative exponential values:

$$pH = -\log [H^+]$$

Bracketed values symbolize concentrations. We will use this designation to signify concentrations of other substances besides protons throughout this discussion. The pH of extracellular fluid, in which the H^+ concentration may be assumed to be approximately 4×10^{-8} mol/L, can therefore be calculated as follows:

$$pH = -\log (4 \times 10^{-8})$$

$$\text{or } pH = \log (1/(4 \times 10^{-8}))$$

$$\text{(dividing)} = \log (0.25 \times 10^{8})$$

$$= \log 0.25 + \log 10^{8}$$

$$\text{(taking logs)} = -0.602 + 8$$

$$pH = 7.4$$

As the value of the negative exponent of 10 becomes larger—that is, as the molar concentration of H^+ becomes smaller—the pH correspondingly increases. Low acidity therefore denotes low H^+ concentration and high pH, whereas high acidity is associated with high H^+ concentration and low pH.

An acid, as it relates to fluid acid-base regulation, may be defined as a substance capable of releasing protons (H^+). The metabolism of the major nutrients continuously generates organic acids, which must be neutralized. Chapter 4 explained how lactic acid and pyruvic acid can accumulate in periods of oxygen deprivation, and Chapter 6 described how fatty acids are released from triacylglycerols during lipolysis. Also, the acidic ketone bodies, acetoacetic acid and β-hydroxybutyric acid, can increase significantly during periods of prolonged starvation or low carbohydrate intake. Carbon dioxide, the product of the complete oxidation of energy nutrients, is itself indirectly acidic, because it forms carbonic acid (H_2CO_3) on combination with H_2O. Acidic salts of sulfuric and phosphoric acids are also generated metabolically from sulfur- or phosphorus-containing substances.

The term *acidosis* refers to a rise in extracellular (principally plasma) H^+ concentration (a lower pH) beyond the normal range. Abnormally low H^+ concentration, in contrast (i.e., high plasma pH), results in **alkalosis.** To guard against such fluctuations in pH, three principal regulatory systems are available:

- buffer systems within the fluids that immediately neutralize acidic or basic compounds;
- the respiratory center, which regulates breathing and the rate of exhalation of CO_2; and
- renal regulation, by which either acidic or alkaline urine can be formed to adjust body fluid acidity.

ACID-BASE BUFFERS

A buffer is anything that can reversibly bind protons. In the body, a buffer is a chemical solution designed to resist changes in pH despite the addition of acids or bases. A buffer usually consists of a weak acid, which can be represented as HA, and its conjugate base (A^-). The conjugate base, therefore, is the residual portion of the acid following the release of the proton. The conjugate base of a weak acid is basic, because it tends to attract a proton and to regenerate the acid. Therefore, the dissociation of a weak acid and the reunion of its conjugate base and proton comprise an equilibrium system:

$$HA \leftrightarrow H^+ + A^-$$

The equilibrium expression for this reaction, called the acid dissociation constant (K_a), is represented as

$$K_a = \frac{[H^+][A^-]}{[HA]}$$

The equation can be rearranged to

$$[H^+] = \frac{K_a [HA]}{[A^-]}$$

Taking the negative logarithm of both sides of the equation gives

$$-\log [H^+] = -\log K_a - \log \frac{[HA]}{[A^-]}$$

These values become

$$pH = pK_a + \log \frac{[A^-]}{[HA]}$$

This equation is referred to as the Henderson-Hasselbalch equation. It shows how a buffer system composed of a weak acid and its conjugate base resists changes in pH if strong acid or base is added to the system. For example, if the molar concentrations of the conjugate base and the acid are equal, then the ratio of $[A^-]$ to [HA] is 1.0, and the logarithm of this ratio is 0, making the pH of the system equal to the pK_a of the acid.

The pK_a, which is the negative logarithm of the acid dissociation constant (K_a), of any weak acid is a constant for that particular acid and simply reflects its strength (i.e., its tendency to release a proton). If a strong acid or base is added to this system, the ratio of $[A^-]$ to [HA] changes and therefore the pH changes, but only slightly. Suppose, for example, that both the conjugate base and the free acid are present at 0.1 mol/L concentrations, and suppose also that the pK_a of the acid is 7.0. As shown above, if the ratio is 0.1 : 0.1, the pH is 7.0. The addition of enough hydrochloric acid (a strong acid) to the buffer in the example to make its final concentration 0.05 mol/L will shift the equilibrium to the left (to make HA). The 0.05 mol/L of H^+ (from the fully dissociated HCl) will combine with an equal molar amount of A^- to form HA. The new $[A^-]$ concentration therefore becomes 0.05 mol/L (0.1 − 0.05), and [HA] will be 0.15 mol/L (0.1 + 0.05). The logarithm of this new ratio (0.05 : 0.15, or 0.33) is −0.48. Inserting this value into the Henderson-Hasselbalch equation, we can see that the pH decreases by only 0.48. In other words, the pH decreased from 7.0 to 6.52 by making the system 0.05 mol/L hydrochloric acid. In contrast, this same concentration of HCl in an unbuffered, aqueous solution would produce an acid pH between 1.0 and 2.0.

The physiologically important buffers that maintain the narrow pH range of extracellular fluid at ~7.4 are proteins and the bicarbonate (HCO_3^-)–carbonic acid (H_2CO_3) system. Proteins have the most potent buffering capacity among the physiological buffers, and, because of its high concentration in whole blood, hemoglobin is most important in this respect. The binding of oxygen to hemoglobin is influenced by the pH of the blood. For the proper uptake and release of oxygen in the erythrocyte to occur, it is crucial for the pH regulation to be operating. As **amphoteric** substances (substances that possess both acidic and basic groups on their amino acid side chains), proteins are capable of neutralizing either acids or bases. For instance, the two major buffering groups on a protein are carboxylic acid (R—COOH) and amino (R—NH_3^-) functions, which dissociate as shown:

1. $R{-}COOH \leftrightarrow R{-}COO^- + H^+$
2. $R{-}NH_3^+ \leftrightarrow R{-}NH_2 + H^+$

At physiological pH, the carboxylic acid is largely dissociated into its conjugate base and a proton, so the equilibrium as shown is shifted strongly to the right. At that same pH, however, the amino group, being much weaker as an acid (a stronger base), is only weakly dissociated, and its equilibrium greatly favors the right-to-left direction. If protons, in the form of a strong acid, are added to a protein solution, they are neutralized by reaction 1, because their presence will cause a shift in the equilibrium toward the undissociated acid (right to left). Strong bases, as contributors of hydroxide (OH^-) ions, will likewise be neutralized because, as they react with the protons to form water, the equilibrium of reaction 2 (as illustrated) shifts to the right to restore the protons that were neutralized.

The bicarbonate–carbonic acid buffer system is of particular importance because it is through this system that respiratory and renal pH regulation is exerted. This buffer system is composed of the weak acid carbonic acid (H_2CO_3) and its salt or conjugate base, bicarbonate ion (HCO_3^-). The carbonic acid dissociates reversibly into H^+ and HCO_3^-:

$$H_2CO_3 \leftrightarrow H^+ + HCO_3^-$$

The buffering capacity of this reaction is due to the fact that either added protons or added hydroxide ions will be neutralized by corresponding shifts in the equilibrium, similar to the carboxy-amino group buffering by proteins described earlier. The H_2CO_3 can be formed not only from the acidification of HCO_3^-, as shown in the right-to-left reaction shown above, but also from the reaction of dissolved CO_2 with water. Recall that CO_2 is formed as a result of total oxidation of the energy nutrients as well as various decarboxylation reactions. The gas diffuses from tissue cells into the extracellular fluids and then into erythrocytes, where its reaction with water to form H_2CO_3 is accelerated by the zinc metalloenzyme carbonic anhydrase. The overall reaction involving carbon dioxide, carbonic acid, and bicarbonate ion is as follows:

$$3.\ \underset{(gas)}{CO_2} \leftrightarrow \underset{(dissolved)}{CO_2} \leftrightarrow H_2CO_3 \leftrightarrow H^+ + HCO_3^-$$

In the lungs, these equilibrium reactions are shifted strongly to the left in the circulating erythrocytes because of the release of protons from hemoglobin as hemoglobin acquires oxygen to become oxyhemoglobin. This shift allows the exhalation of carbon dioxide.

Normally, the ratio of the concentration of HCO_3^- to H_2CO_3 in plasma is 20 : 1, and the apparent pK_a value for H_2CO_3 is 6.1. Using the Henderson-Hasselbalch equation, we can show how a normal plasma pH of 7.4 results from these values:

$$pH = pK_a + \log\frac{[HCO_3^-]}{[H_2CO_3]}$$

$$= 6.1 + \log\frac{20}{1}$$

$$= 6.1 + 1.3$$

$$pH = 7.4$$

Alterations in the 20 : 1 ratio of $[HCO_3^-]$ to $[H_2CO_3]$ clearly change the pH. In the next section, we will show how respiratory and renal regulatory systems function to keep this ratio, and therefore the pH, relatively constant.

RESPIRATORY REGULATION OF pH

Should plasma levels of CO_2 rise, perhaps because of accelerated metabolism, more H_2CO_3 will be formed. This, in turn, will cause a fall in pH as it dissociates to release protons (reaction 3). The elevated CO_2 itself, as well as the resulting increase in hydrogen ion concentration, is detected by the respiratory center of the brain, resulting in an increase in the respiratory rate. This hyperventilation significantly increases CO_2 loss through the lungs and therefore decreases the amount of H_2CO_3. This mechanism increases the ratio of HCO_3^- to H_2CO_3 by reducing H_2CO_3, thus elevating the pH to a normal value. Conversely, if plasma pH rises for any reason (because of either an increase in HCO_3^- or a decrease in H_2CO_3), the respiratory center is signaled accordingly and causes a slowing of the respiration rate. As CO_2 then accumulates, the H_2CO_3 concentration rises and the pH decreases.

RENAL REGULATION OF pH

Although the intact respiratory system acts as an immediate (in minutes) regulator of the HCO_3^-/H_2CO_3 system, long-term control (hours or days) is exerted by renal mechanisms. The kidneys regulate pH by controlling the secretion of hydrogen ions, by conserving or producing bicarbonate, and by synthesizing the ammonia from glutamine to form ammonium ions. The secretion of hydrogen ions occurs in conjunction with the tubular reabsorption of sodium ions through the mechanism of countertransport, an active process involving a common Na^+/H^+ carrier protein and energy sufficient to move the protons from the tubular cells into the tubule lumen against a concentration gradient of protons. In subjects on a normal diet, ~50 to 100 mEq of hydrogen ions are generated daily. Renal secretion of the protons is necessary to prevent a progressive metabolic acidosis. The renal tubules are not very permeable to bicarbonate ions because of the charge and the relatively large size of the ions. They therefore are reabsorbed by a special indirect process. The hydrogen ions in the glomerular filtrate convert filtered bicarbonate ions to H_2CO_3, which dissociates into CO_2 and H_2O. The CO_2 diffuses into the tubular cell, where it combines with water, in a reaction catalyzed by carbonic anhydrase, to form H_2CO_3. The relatively high tubular-cell pH allows the dissociation of the H_2CO_3 into HCO_3^- and H^+, after which the bicarbonate reenters the extracellular fluid and the proton is actively returned to the lumen by the Na^+/H^+ carrier. The net result is to excrete an H^+ and to reabsorb a bicarbonate ion, even though it is not the same bicarbonate ion. These events, by which hydrogen ions are secreted against a concentration gradient in exchange for sodium ions and bicarbonate is returned to the plasma from the glomerular filtrate, are summarized in Figure 14.6.

The pH of the urine normally falls within the range of 5.5 to 6.5, despite the active secretion of hydrogen ions throughout the tubules. This is largely due to the partial neutralization of the hydrogen ions by ammonia, which is secreted into the lumen by the tubular cells. Ammonia is produced in large amounts from the metabolic breakdown of amino acids. Although most of the nitrogen is excreted in the form of urea, some is delivered to the kidney cells in the form of glutamine. In the renal tubule cells, ammonia is hydrolytically released from the glutamine by the enzyme glutaminase and is secreted into the urine (Chap. 7). Because it is a basic substance, ammonia immediately combines with protons in the collecting ducts to form ammonium ions (NH_4^+), which are excreted in the urine primarily as their chloride salts.

Should metabolic acidosis occur, such as in starvation or diabetes, an increase in the urinary excretion of ammonia occurs concomitantly to compensate. This is because the diminished intake and use of carbohydrate stimulate gluconeogenesis and therefore an enhanced excretion of ammonia, formed from the higher rate of amino acid catabolism.

Like respiratory regulation, renal regulation of pH is directed at the maintenance of a normal ratio of [HCO_3^-] to [H_2CO_3]. In a situation of alkalosis, for example, in which the plasma ratio of HCO_3^- to H_2CO_3 increases as the pH rises above 7.4, there is a net increase in the excretion of bicarbonate ions. This increase occurs because the high extracellular HCO_3^- concentration increases its filtration, while the relatively low concentration of H_2CO_3 decreases the secretion of H^+. Therefore, the fine balance between HCO_3^- and H^+ that normally exists in the tubules no longer is in effect. Also, because no HCO_3^- ions can be reabsorbed without first reacting with H^+ (Fig. 14.6), all the excess HCO_3^- will pass into the urine, neutralized by sodium ions or other cations. In effect, therefore, HCO_3^- is removed from the extracellular fluid, restoring the normal ratio of HCO_3^- to H_2CO_3 and pH.

In acidosis, the ratio of plasma HCO_3^- to H_2CO_3 decreases, meaning that the rate of H^+ secretion rises to

Figure 14.6 Renal tubular cell reactions illustrating the origin of and the active secretion of hydrogen ions in exchange for sodium ions, as well as the mechanism for tubular reabsorption of bicarbonate. Solid arrows indicate reactions or active transport, while dashed arrows signify diffusion.

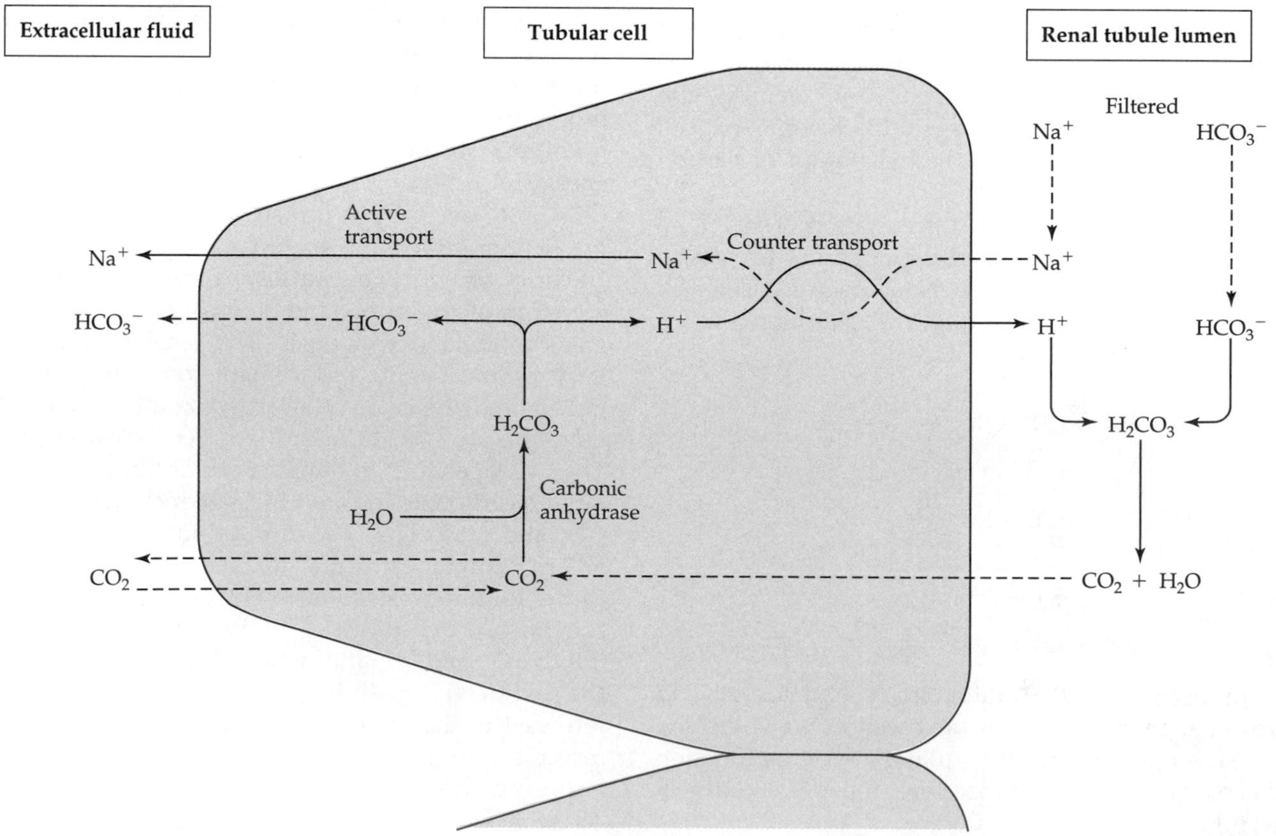

a level far greater than the rate of HCO_3^- filtration into the tubules. As a result, most of the filtered HCO_3^- will be converted to H_2CO_3 and reabsorbed as CO_2 (Fig. 14.6), while the excess H^+ will be excreted in the urine. As a consequence, the extracellular fluid ratio of $[HCO_3^-]$ to $[H_2CO_3]$ increases, as does the pH.

The importance of the kidney in the homeostatic control of body water, as well as in electrolyte and acid-base balance, has been emphasized in this chapter. The material has been presented as a review of the principles involved in such control and of the effect of diet on fluid and electrolyte homeostasis. Although a detailed account of renal physiology is beyond the scope of this text, excellent sources that deal specifically with this subject are available [8,9].

summary

The maintenance of body fluids and electrolytes is of vital importance for sound health and nutrition. Intracellular fluid provides the environment for the myriad of metabolic reactions that take place in cells. The interstitial fluid compartment of the extracellular fluid mass allows the migration of nutrients into cells from the bloodstream and the return to the bloodstream of metabolic waste products from the cells. These fluids contain the electrolytes, dissolved minerals that have important physiological functions. Their concentrations and their intracellular and extracellular distribution must be precisely regulated, and the mechanism for achieving this regulation is exerted largely through the kidney. The homeostatic maintenance of fluid volume is also the responsibility of this organ.

Fluid volume control by the kidney is mostly hormone mediated. ADH, produced in the hypothalamus, stimulates the tubular reabsorption of water from the glomerular filtrate. Aldosterone, a product of the adrenal cortex, increases the reabsorption of sodium ions, which indirectly stimulate ADH release through the resulting rise in extracellular fluid osmotic pressure. Thirst centers in the brain, which respond to fluctuations in blood volume or extracellular fluid osmolarity, are also important regulators of fluid balance by their influence on the amount of fluid intake.

The macrominerals sodium and potassium, and other ions of nutritional importance such as calcium, magnesium, and chloride, are freely filtered by the renal glomerulus but are selectively conserved by tubular reabsorption via active transport systems. Potassium is an example of a mineral that is regulated in part by tubular secretion into the filtrate. Secretion of the ion from the distal tubular cells increases as its concentration in those cells rises because of increased dietary intake. Potassium, like sodium, is regulated by aldosterone. Elevated plasma potassium stimulates the release of aldosterone, which exerts opposing renal effects on the two minerals—enhanced reabsorption of sodium and an increase in potassium excretion. Normal physiological function depends on proper control of the body fluid acid-base balance.

Many metabolic enzymes have a narrow range of pH at which they function adequately, and these catalysts are intolerant of pH swings of more than several tenths of a unit from the average normal value of 7.4 for extracellular fluids. The plasma is well buffered, primarily by proteins and by the bicarbonate–carbonic acid system. However, conditions of acidosis or alkalosis can result in situations such as an overproduction of organic acids, as would occur in diabetes or starvation, or respiratory aberrations that may cause abnormal carbon dioxide ventilation. Therefore, restoration of normal pH may be necessary and is accomplished through compensatory mechanisms of the kidneys and lungs. These organs function to maintain a normal ratio of bicarbonate to carbonic acid. The bicarbonate concentration is under the control of the kidneys, which can either conserve the ion by reabsorbing it to a greater extent or increase its excretion, depending on whether the ratio needs to be decreased or increased to compensate for a pH disturbance. The carbonic acid value is controlled by the respiratory center. Its concentration can be increased or decreased by changes in the respiratory rate. Hyperventilation, for example, lowers the value by "blowing off" carbon dioxide, whereas a slowing of respiration retains carbon dioxide and therefore raises the carbonic acid level. From their effects on the bicarbonate : carbonic acid ratio, it can be reasoned that hyperventilation can raise the pH and respiratory suppression can lower the pH in a compensatory manner.

References Cited

1. Goodman HM. Basic Medical Endocrinology. San Diego: Academic Press, 2003, Chap. 7.

2. Van de Stolpe A, Jamison RL. Micropuncture study of the effect of ANP on the papillary collecting duct in the rat. Am J Physiol 1988; 254:F477–83.

3. Hadley ME. Endocrinology, 5th ed. Englewood Cliffs, NJ: Prentice Hall, 2002, pp. 79–82.

4. Vokes T. Water homeostasis. Ann Rev Nutr 1987;7:383–406.

5. Wingo CS, Cain BD. The renal H-K-ATPase: physiological significance and role in potassium homeostasis. Ann Rev Physiol 1993;55:323–47.

6. Luft FC. Salt and hypertension: recent advances and perspectives. J Lab Clin Med 1989;114:215–21.

7. Suter P. Potassium and hypertension. Nutr Rev 1998;56(#5):151–53.

8. Windhager EE, ed. Handbook of Physiology. Section 8, Renal physiology, vols I, II. New York: Oxford University Press, 1992.

9. Valtin J, Schafer J. Renal Function, 3rd ed., Boston: Little, Brown and Co., 1995.

Suggested Readings

Kleinman LI, Lorenz JM. Physiology and pathophysiology of body water and electrolytes. In: Kaplan LA, Pesce AJ, eds. Clinical Chemistry: Theory, Analysis, and Correlation. St. Louis: Mosby, 1996, Chap. 24.

A clearly written clinical approach to fluid and electrolyte homeostasis, with diagrammatic illustrations of the regulatory mechanisms of fluid and electrolyte control.

Sherwin JE. Acid-base control and acid-base disorders. In: Kaplan LA, Pesce AJ, eds. Clinical Chemistry: Theory, Analysis, and Correlation. St. Louis: Mosby, 1996, Chap. 25.

A brief introduction to the physiological buffer systems and a clinical approach to the regulation of acid-base balance.

Vokes T. Water homeostasis. Ann Rev Nutr 1987;7:383–406.

A discussion of the mechanisms of water balance regulation and the pathology associated with deficiencies in the regulatory system.

Web Sites

www.nih.gov/health/consumer/conicd.htm
National Institutes of Health: Consumer Health Information page
thriveonline.com
@ America Online (AOL)

perspective

Fluid Balance and the Thermal Stress of Exercise

The discussion of sports nutrition in Chapter 8 centered on (1) the selective use of energy-yielding substrates during exercise of varying durations and intensities and (2) how physical performance can be enhanced by maximizing substrate stores via the judicious intake of energy nutrients. Another very important dimension in the demands of sport and exercise is **thermoregulation,** the control of body temperature within a narrow range. A drop in deep body (core) temperature of 10°F and an increase of just 5°F above normal is tolerated, but fluctuation beyond this range can result in death. Strenuous exercise challenges this control because it is markedly thermogenic owing to its stimulation of metabolic rate. Recall that the energy-producing systems are <40% efficient and the remainder of the energy is given off as heat. The fact that there has been an average of three heat-related deaths per year in football since 1995 attests to the seriousness of hyperthermia.

Various mechanisms of thermoregulation are responsible for maintaining thermal balance in the body. Muscular activity is one of the most influential factors contributing to heat gain in body core temperature. Others include hormonal effects, the thermic effect of food, postural changes, and environmental changes. Countering the heat gain factors are mechanisms that protect against hyperthermia by removing heat from the body, including radiation, conduction, convection, and evaporation. In an otherwise normal individual engaged in strenuous exercise, evaporation (of sweat) provides the most important physiological defense against overheating. Evaporation of 1.0 ml of sweat is equivalent to ~0.6 kcal of body heat loss. Therefore, even at maximal exercise—at which 4.0 L O_2/minute are consumed, equivalent to ~20 kcal/minute of heat produced—core temperature would be expected to rise just 1° every 5 to 7 minutes. This is because sweating, assumed to be maximal at 30 mL/minute, would cool the body only to the extent of about 18 kcal/minute.

Approximately 80% of the energy released during exercise is in the form of heat. If this heat is not removed from the body, the heat load due to metabolic activity, combined with environmental heat during strenuous exercise, could lead to a dramatic increase in body temperature. Hyperthermia can result in lethal heat injury. It has already been pointed out that the major mechanism for heat loss is the evaporation of sweat and that nearly 600 kcal are eliminated by the cooling effect of the evaporation of 1 L of sweat. Among the remaining mechanisms for heat removal, radiation is the next most important. In radiation, heat generated in the working muscles is transported by blood flow to the skin, from which it can subsequently be exchanged with the environment. For both of these thermoregulatory mechanisms, body water is clearly the major participant, and there has been considerable interest in assessing various strategies for its replacement during strenuous exercise.

Firm evidence indicates that depletion of body water from sweating beyond 2% of body weight can cause significant impairment of endurance through deficiencies in thermoregulatory and circulatory functions. The most likely explanations for this impairment are as follows:

- A reduced plasma volume and therefore reduced hemodynamic capacity to achieve maximal cardiac output and peripheral circulation. As plasma volume declines, reduced skin blood flow and a fall in stroke volume follow. Heart rate increases to compensate but cannot offset the stroke volume deficit [1].
- Altered sweat gland function, whereby sweating ceases in an autonomic control attempt to conserve body water.

As a result of these reactions, body temperature rises quickly, drastically increasing the chance of cramps, exhaustion, and even heatstroke, the last having a mortality rate of 80%. Sweat losses of 1.5 L/hour are commonly encountered in endurance sports, and under particularly hot conditions sweat rates exceeding 2.5 L/hour have been measured in fit individuals. Marathon runners can lose 6% to 8% of body weight in water during the 26.2-mile event, and plasma volume may fall 13% to 18%. It is not uncommon, therefore, for a 150-lb runner to lose 0.5 lb of water (equivalent to an 8-oz glass of water) per mile in a hot environment.

Dehydration results when fluid loss exceeds intake, with the degree of dehydration directly proportional to the fluid disparity. The primary goal of fluid replacement is to maintain plasma volume so that circulation and sweating can proceed at maximal levels. The maximum rate of sweating is greater than the maximum rate for absorbing water from the intestinal tract, so at maximum effort some dehydration is bound to occur. It is difficult for the endurance athlete to avoid a negative water balance because it is both impractical and distasteful to attempt to replenish the copious amount lost in the course of a marathon. It is distasteful because the necessary intake far exceeds the thirst desire, a stimulus that is delayed behind rapid dehydration. It has been estimated that athletes, when left on their own, replace only about half the water lost during exercise [2]. However, the force-feeding of fluids to exactly balance fluids lost is ideal from the standpoint of athletic performance, although the dramatic effects of lesser amounts of fluid replenishment during exercise are also well documented. The experimental design on which such conclusions are generally based is comparison of the extent of fluid intake with performance and certain physiological parameters such as heart rate and body temperature. Study groups are commonly composed of subjects who, in the course of prolonged exercise, are (1) force-fed fluids beyond the thirst desire, (2) allowed to drink fluid ad libitum (as desired), and (3) deprived of fluid intake. Force-fed subjects display superior performance, lower heart rate, and lower body core temperature than the other groups, and the ad libitum group outperforms the deprived group in these parameters.

An imposing question in sports nutrition that is surrounded by controversy is whether electrolyte replacement is necessary during prolonged exercise. Based on the knowledge that sweat contains electrolytes (sodium, potassium, chloride, and magnesium), it was reasoned that significant losses of these occurred during endurance athletics and that their replacement was necessary to optimize performance. In the 1970s, sports drinks supplemented with electrolytes and sometimes glucose (GE drinks) began to appear on the market and were sold under names such as Gatorade, PowerAde, and All-Sport. Whether such supplementation is necessary depends on the level of intensity of the exercise and therefore on the quantity of sweat lost.

The electrolyte content of sweat in the average individual is very low compared with body fluids. Table 1 compares the electrolyte concentrations of sweat and blood serum. In the case of sodium and chloride ions, dehydration through sweating has the effect of concentrating these electrolytes in extracellular and intracellular water because of their relatively low concentration in sweat. Therefore, in marathon-level exertion, in which a total sweat loss of 5 to 6 L or less is incurred, rehydration with water alone is adequate, because only ~200 mEq of sodium and chloride would be lost from a relatively large body store. Some research suggests that good-tasting electrolyte-glucose solutions encourage the athlete to consume more fluid than would be consumed using only water as a replacement fluid. The enhanced fluid intake therefore is probably beneficial even though the electrolytes might not be needed. Drinking water would have the effect of lowering the osmolality of the blood, which would reduce the thirst reflex.

Table 1 Average Electrolyte Concentrations in Sweat and Blood Serum (mEq/L)

	Na^+	K^+	Cl^-	Mg^{2+}
Sweat	40–45	3.9	39	3.3
Blood serum	140	4.0	110	1.5–2.1

The American Academy of Pediatrics makes recommendations for exercising children, including the use of flavored beverages that contain electrolytes for the reasons stated above [3]. Although some researchers regard potassium losses during exercise in the heat as constituting a potential health problem, this view too is controversial given the relatively small amount of the ion lost. On the basis of the potassium content of sweat (shown in Table 1), it can be estimated that a sweat loss of 5 L would induce a potassium deficit of <20 mEq, or well under 1% of the estimated total body store of 3,000 mEq for a 70-kg man.

Only under severe conditions of prolonged, high-intensity exercise in the heat would electrolyte replacement be indicated. In such a case, electrolyte loss may exceed the amount provided in the daily diet, and some sodium supplementation may be necessary. The quantity provided by adding one-third teaspoon of table salt to a liter of water would be adequate [4]. It is doubtful whether potassium supplementation is called for under similar conditions, for the reasons discussed.

References Cited

1. Sawka M. Physiological consequences of hypohydration: exercise, performance and thermoregulation. Med Sci Sports Exerc 1992;24:657.
2. Noakes T. Fluid replacement during exercise. Exerc Sports Sci Rev 1993;21:297.
3. American Academy of Pediatrics. Pediatrics 2000; 106:158–59.
4. McArdle W, Katch F, Katch V. Exercise Physiology, 4th ed. Baltimore, MD: Williams & Wilkins, 1996, Chap. 25.

Web Site

www.umass.edu/cnshp/index.html

Center for Nutrition in Sport and Human Performance at the University of Massachusetts

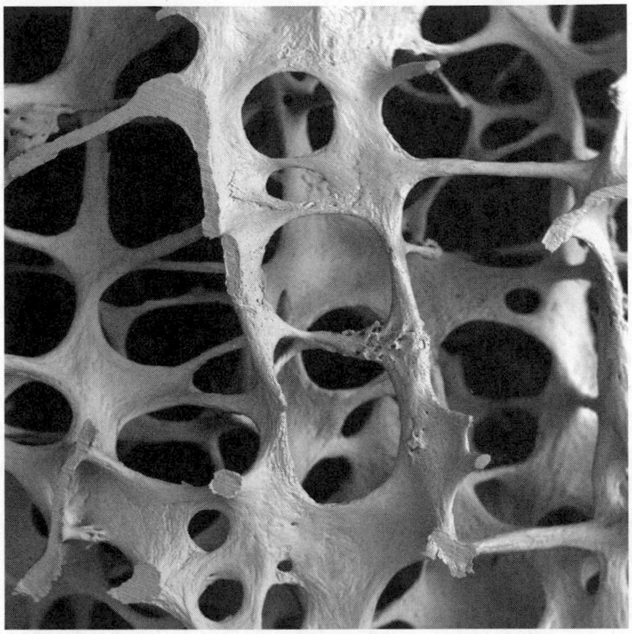

Osteoporosis in an 89-year-old human female

chapter 15 Body Composition and Energy Expenditure

An innate characteristic of maturation and aging is a change in body composition and body weight. These compositional changes occur throughout the life cycle, beginning with the embryo and extending through old age. Rapid growth entails not only an increase in body mass but also a change in the proportions of components making up this mass. Young adulthood is a period of relative homeostasis, but in some people modifications of body composition can occur. Following the more or less homeostatic period of young adulthood is the period of progressive aging, when some undesirable changes in body composition and often weight inevitably occur. Energy expenditure, which influences body weight and composition, is a function of basal metabolic rate, the thermal effect of foods, and physical activity. Nutrition professionals need knowledge of recommended body weight, body composition, and components and assessment of energy expenditure in order to be better prepared to determine nutrient needs and to identify and/or prevent disease.

BODY WEIGHT: WHAT SHOULD WE WEIGH?

Recognition of body weight as an indicator of health status is probably universal and as old as humanity itself. In fact, in 1846 English surgeon John Hutchinson published a height-weight table based on a sample of 30-year-old Englishmen and urged that future census taking include such information, believing it to be valuable in promoting health and detecting disease [1]. Today, scientists and health professionals recognize that the risk of many diseases—including heart disease, stroke, diabetes mellitus, hypertension, osteoarthritis, infertility, and some (endometrial, colon, and kidney) cancers—increases with excess body weight. Furthermore, a low body weight may be indicative of malnutrition or an eating disorder and may pose risks for other diseases, such as osteoporosis. What represents too much weight or too little weight for a given height? Unfortunately, recommendations from health experts vary. We will discuss some of the more currently accepted approaches to weight assessment as well as some older approaches.

Body Mass Index

Body mass index (BMI), first described in the 1860s and known as Quetelet's Index, is at present one of the most accepted approaches to assessing appropriate weight for a given height. The body mass index is considered to be indicative of body adiposity but does not measure body fat. Body mass index is calculated from a person's height and weight as shown in this formula:

$$\text{Body mass index} = \frac{\text{Weight}}{\text{Height}^2}$$

with weight measured in kilograms (kg) and height measured in meters (m) and raised to a power of 2.

Body mass index is considered a good index of total body fat in both men and women and has generally replaced calculations of percent relative body weight (see the section "Height-Weight Tables") and percent ideal body weight (see the section "Formulas") for classifying individuals as underweight or overweight. For adults, classification of weight based on body mass index by the National Institutes of Health is as follows:

- BMI $<$18.5 kg/m^2, underweight (with $<$16 suggesting a possible eating disorder);
- BMI 18.5 to 24.9 kg/m^2, healthy/low health risks;
- BMI $\geq$25 kg/m^2, overweight and associated with increased risk of disease;
- BMI $\geq$30 kg/m^2, obese (class I) and associated with further increased risk of disease;
- BMI $\geq$35 kg/m^2, obese (class II) and associated with higher risk of disease; and
- BMI $\geq$40 kg/m^2, extremely or morbidly obese (class III) [2–4].

Figure 15.1 shows the classification of BMI for various weights and heights.

Using the formula to calculate the BMI of a 5-ft 11-in. (or 71-in.) man weighing 165 lb would involve two conversions before plugging numbers into the body mass index formula. First, to convert weight in pounds (lb) to weight in kilograms (kg), divide by 2.2 because there are 2.2 lb per 1 kg: 165 lb ÷ 2.2 lb/kg = 75 kg. Next, convert height in feet and inches to meters (m). Because there are 39.37 in. per 1 m, divide the man's height of 71 in. by 39.37 in./m to get 1.803 m. With weight in kilograms and height in meters, the formula can be used: BMI = 75 kg ÷ (1.803 m)^2 = 75 kg ÷ 3.25 m^2 = 23.1 kg/m^2.

While the body mass index is a valuable approach to assessing weight, like many other methods it does not determine body composition. Thus, individuals such as athletes may have large amounts of lean body mass and a high body mass index (and thus be considered overweight or obese by classification) but have low body fat.

Height-Weight Tables

Although now typically replaced by the body mass index, height-weight tables were once one of the main methods used to determine an adult's recommended weight. Several different sets of tables have been developed over the years and are reviewed in this section.

The Metropolitan Life Insurance Company has developed height-weight tables for adult men and women based on information obtained from a specific population: individuals interested in obtaining insurance. However, because insurance companies look to insure those individuals likely to live a long life, the data in the tables represent weights for height at a particular age of people who applied and were accepted for insurance over a period of several years [1]. In 1942 and 1943, the Metropolitan Life Insurance Company introduced the concept of "ideal" weights for women and men, respectively. In 1959, these tables were revised as a result of a (build and blood pressure) study by the Society of Actuaries indicating that lower-than-average weight for height, even for young adults, could be associated with longevity. In the revised tables, weights considered appropriate for the various heights and frame sizes were termed "desirable" rather than

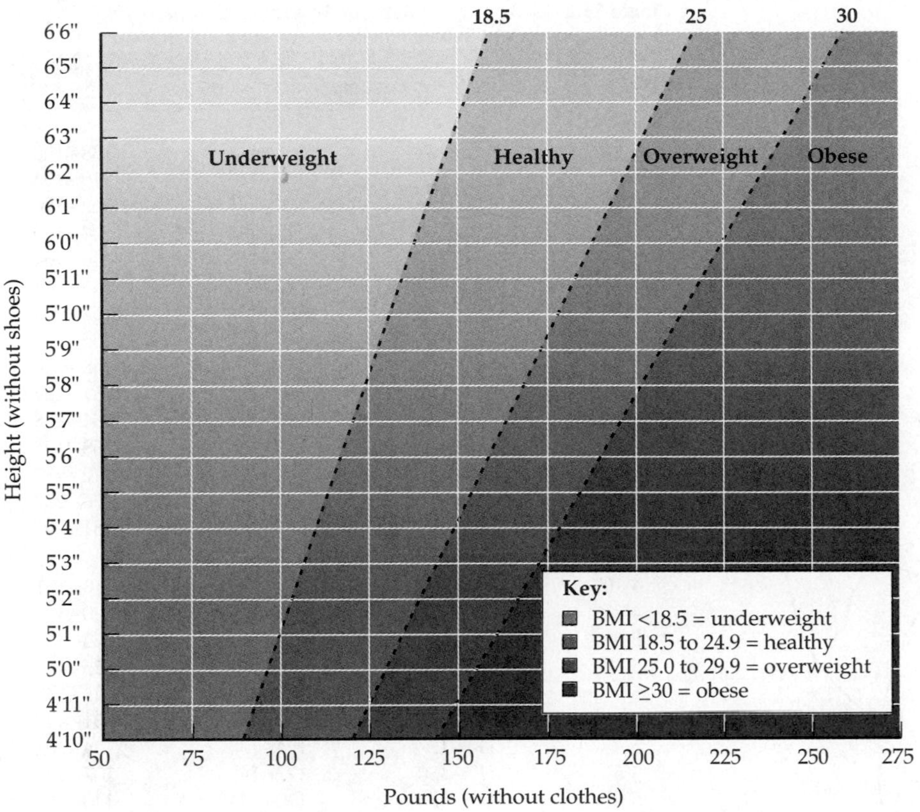

Figure 15.1 BMI values used to assess weight. *Source:* U.S. Department of Agriculture and U.S. Department of Health and Human Services, *Nutrition and Your Health: Dietary Guidelines for Americans.* Washington, DC, 2000, p. 7.

ideal. Yet, the method for determining frame size was omitted.

In 1983, height-weight tables based on the actuary body build study [5] and on direct measurement of frame size as determined from elbow breadth measurements (Fig. 15.2 and Table 15.1) were published by the Metropolitan Life Insurance Company (Table 15.2). Weight-for-height figures were designated "acceptable" rather than ideal or desirable and were somewhat higher than those in the earlier height-weight tables. The increases (~10% in shorter people and ~5% in people of medium height [6]) were a reflection of the mortality data collected in the 1979 actuary build study [5], which showed that insured men and women under 30 years of age tended to be heavier than their counterparts in the 1959 build and blood pressure study. Of particular interest was the reduced mortality found to be associated with mild to moderate overweight in shorter-than-average people.

Dividing a person's actual weight by the midpoint of the weight range for his or her frame size gives the Metropolitan relative weight (MRW) or relative body weight (RBW). This method was used to identify people who might be at risk because of overweight or obesity (or because of underweight) [7]. People at risk included those individuals with weight for height either well below the lowest end of the acceptable range or well above the highest end of the acceptable range. Extremes in either direction more than likely pose some health risks.

In 1990, the U.S. Department of Agriculture published suggested weights for adults age 19 to 34 years and age 35 years and older as part of its *Dietary Guidelines for Americans,* 3rd edition [8]. These weights for heights were given such that the higher weights in the range applied to men and the lower weights in the range applied to women. These suggested weights were slightly higher at the upper end of the ranges than those in the 1983 Metropolitan Life height-weight tables. However, the 1990 suggested weights for adults (as well as the 1983 Metropolitan Life height-weight tables) have been criticized by some as being too liberal [9].

In the 1995 edition of the *Dietary Guidelines for Americans,* recommendations for weight for height for the two age groups, adults 19 to 34 years and adults 35 years and older, were collapsed into one category applicable to all adults (Table 15.3). As with the 1990 publication, the weights for heights in the 1995 publication were given in ranges where the higher and lower weights in the ranges applied to men and women, respectively, with no consideration given to frame size.

With the fifth edition of the *Dietary Guidelines for Americans,* published in 2000 by the U.S. Department

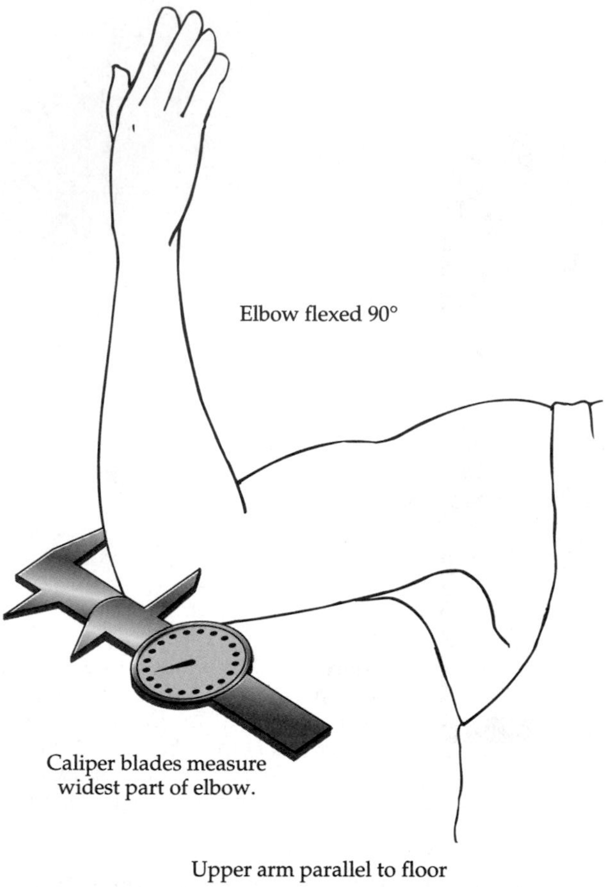

Figure 15.2 Measurement of elbow breadth. Extend your arm and bend the forearm upward at a 90° angle. Keep your fingers straight, and turn the inside of your wrist toward your body. Place the calipers on the two prominent bones on either side of the elbow. Measure the space between the bones with the caliper to the nearest 0.1 cm or 1/8 inch.

Table 15.1 How to Determine Your Body Frame by Elbow Breadth

Height (1-in. heels)	Elbow Breadth (in.)	Height (cm, in 2.5-cm heels)	Elbow Breadth (cm)
Men:			
5′2″–5′3″	$2\frac{1}{8} - 2\frac{7}{8}$	158–161	6.4–7.2
5′4″–5′7″	$2\frac{5}{8} - 2\frac{7}{8}$	162–171	6.7–7.4
5′8″–5′11″	$2\frac{3}{4} - 3$	172–181	6.9–7.6
6′0″–6′3″	$2\frac{3}{4} - 3\frac{1}{8}$	182–191	7.1–7.8
6′4″	$2\frac{7}{8} - 3\frac{1}{4}$	192–193	7.4–8.1
Women:			
4′10″–4′11″	$2\frac{1}{4} - 2\frac{1}{2}$	148–151	5.6–6.4
5′0″–5′3″	$2\frac{1}{4} - 2\frac{1}{2}$	152–161	5.8–6.5
5′4″–5′7″	$2\frac{3}{8} - 2\frac{5}{8}$	162–171	5.9–6.6
5′8″–5′11″	$2\frac{3}{8} - 2\frac{5}{8}$	172–181	6.1–6.8
6′0″	$2\frac{1}{2} - 2\frac{3}{4}$	182–183	6.2–6.9

Note: This table lists the elbow measurements for men and women of medium frame at various heights. Measurements lower than those listed indicate that you have a small frame, while higher measurements indicate a large frame.

Source: Courtesy of Metropolitan Life Insurance Company. Reprinted with permission.

Table 15.2 1983 Metropolitan Life Insurance Company Height and Weight Tables

Height	Weight		
	Small Frame	Medium Frame	Large Frame
Men:*			
5′2″	128–134	131–141	138–150
5′3″	130–136	133–143	140–153
5′4″	132–138	135–145	142–156
5′5″	134–140	137–148	144–160
5′6″	136–142	139–151	146–164
5′7″	138–145	142–154	149–168
5′8″	140–148	145–157	152–172
5′9″	142–151	148–160	155–176
5′10″	144–154	151–163	158–180
5′11″	146–157	154–166	161–184
6′0″	149–160	157–170	164–188
6′1″	152–164	160–174	168–192
6′2″	155–168	164–178	172–197
6′3″	158–172	167–182	176–202
6′4″	162–176	171–187	181–207
Women:†			
4′10″	102–111	109–121	118–131
4′11″	103–113	111–123	120–134
5′0″	104–115	113–126	122–137
5′1″	106–118	115–129	125–140
5′2″	108–121	118–132	128–143
5′3″	111–124	121–135	131–147
5′4″	114–127	124–138	134–151
5′5″	117–130	127–141	137–155
5′6″	120–133	130–144	140–159
5′7″	123–136	133–147	143–163
5′8″	126–139	136–150	146–167
5′9″	129–142	139–153	149–170
5′10″	132–145	142–156	152–173
5′11″	135–148	145–159	155–176
6′0″	138–151	148–162	158–179

*Weights at ages 25–59 years based on lowest mortality.
Weight in pounds according to frame (in indoor clothing weighing 5 lb, shoes with 1-in. heels).

†Weights in pounds at ages 25–59 years based on clothing weighing 3 lb, shoes with 1-in. heels).

Source: Courtesy of Metropolitan Life Insurance Company. Reprinted with permission.

of Agriculture and U.S. Department of Health and Human Services, recommendations for weight are no longer based on height-weight tables but instead are based on the body mass index. The 2000 guidelines are similar to those of the National Institutes of Health (NIH): a healthy weight is defined as a BMI of 18.5 to 25, while a BMI from 25 to 30 indicates overweight and a BMI of 30 or higher indicates obesity [10].

Using the NIH and dietary guidelines BMI classifications, analyses of height and weight data on the U.S. population collected from ongoing surveys such as the National Health and Nutrition Examination Surveys (NHANES) are being undertaken. Evaluation of these data has shown that the prevalence of obesity has continued to increase over the last several decades. Data from 1999 to 2000

Table 15.3 Suggested Weights for Adults, 1995 Dietary Guidelines

Height (without shoes)	Weight (lb, without clothes)
4′10″	91–119
4′11″	94–124
5′0″	97–128
5′1″	101–132
5′2″	104–137
5′3″	107–141
5′4″	111–146
5′5″	114–150
5′6″	118–155
5′7″	121–160
5′8″	125–164
5′9″	129–169
5′10″	132–174
5′11″	136–179
6′0″	140–184
6′1″	144–189
6′2″	148–195
6′3″	152–200
6′4″	156–205
6′5″	160–211
6′6″	164–216

Source: U.S. Department of Agriculture, U.S. Department of Health and Human Services. *Dietary Guidelines for Americans*, 4th ed. Washington, DC: Government Printing Office, 1995.

show that >64% of adults are overweight with a BMI ≥25 and that >30% of adults are obese with a BMI ≥30 [11].

Formulas

In addition to the body mass index and height-weight tables, other formulas are available to calculate ideal body weight (IBW). One of the more popular formulas is that by Devine [12,13]:

$$\text{IBW for men} = 50\text{ kg} + 2.3\text{ kg/in.} > 5\text{ ft}$$

$$\text{IBW for women} = 45\text{ kg} + 2.3\text{ kg/in.} > 5\text{ ft}$$

These formulas have been modified somewhat and converted into the following familiar empirical formulas for those with a medium-size body frame:

$$\text{IBW for men} = 110\text{ lb} + 5\text{ lb/in.} > 5\text{ ft}$$

$$\text{IBW for women} = 100\text{ lb} + 5\text{ lb/in.} > 5\text{ ft}$$

A slightly modified formula for men is also used:

$$\text{IBW for men} = 106\text{ lb} + 6\text{ lb/in.} > 5\text{ ft}$$

A 10% range minus and plus the calculated ideal weight allowing for differences in weight due to a small or a large frame size, respectively, is also usually included in the Devine formula.

Frame size traditionally is assessed using either of two methods based on measurements of wrist or elbow breadth and height. In addition, the frame index 2 considers not only elbow breadth and height but also age and gender. The frame index 2 value is determined by the following formula:

$$\text{Frame index 2 value} = \frac{\text{Elbow breadth}}{\text{Height}} \times 100$$

with elbow breadth measured in millimeters (mm) and height measured in centimeters (cm) [14]. Once calculated, a person's frame index 2 value is compared with age-based values (shown in Table 15.4) to determine small, medium, or large frame size.

Table 15.4 Classification of Frame Size Based on Frame Index 2 Values

	Male			Female		
Age (yrs)	Small	Medium	Large	Small	Medium	Large
18.0–24.9	<38.4	38.4 to 41.6	>41.6	<35.2	35.2 to 38.6	>38.6
25.0–29.9	<38.6	38.6 to 41.8	>41.8	<35.7	35.7 to 38.7	>38.7
30.0–34.9	<38.6	38.6 to 42.1	>42.1	<35.7	35.7 to 39.0	>39.0
35.0–39.9	<39.1	39.1 to 42.4	>42.4	<36.2	36.2 to 39.8	>39.8
40.0–44.9	<39.3	39.3 to 42.5	>42.5	<36.7	36.7 to 40.2	>40.2
45.0–49.9	<39.6	39.6 to 43.0	>43.0	<37.2	37.2 to 40.7	>40.7
50.0–54.9	<39.9	39.9 to 43.3	>43.3	<37.2	37.2 to 41.6	>41.6
55.0–59.9	<40.2	40.2 to 43.8	>43.8	<37.8	37.8 to 41.9	>41.9
60.0–64.9	<40.2	40.2 to 43.6	>43.6	<38.2	38.2 to 41.8	>41.8
65.0–69.9	<40.2	40.2 to 43.6	>43.6	<38.2	38.2 to 41.8	>41.8
70.0–74.9	<40.2	40.2 to 43.6	>43.6	<38.2	38.2 to 41.8	>41.8

Source: Matarese L, Gottschlich M. *Contemporary Nutrition Support Practice.* Philadelphia: Saunders, 2003, p. 37. Adapted from Frisancho AR. *Anthropometric Standards for the Assessment of Growth and Nutritional Status.* Ann Arbor: University of Michigan Press, 1990, p. 28.

Using the formulas, a man who is 5 ft 11 in. tall with a medium frame should weigh either 165 lb (110 + [5 × 11] = 165 lb) or 172 lb (106 + [6 × 11] = 172 lb) depending on which formula is used. If the man has a small frame, ideal body weight would be 10% less than that calculated for a medium frame size (i.e., 165 lb − 16.5 lb = 148.5 lb or 172 lb − 17.2 lb = 154.8 lb, respectively). A female who is 5 ft 6 in. tall and has a large frame has an ideal body weight of 143 lb (100 + [5 × 6] = 130 lb + 13 lb [accounting for the 10% addition for the large frame size] = 143 lb).

Dividing a person's actual body weight by the ideal body weight calculated (from the Devine formula) for his or her estimated frame size gives what is referred to as percentage ideal body weight, as shown:

$$\% \text{ IBW} = \frac{\text{Actual body weight}}{\text{Ideal body weight}} \times 100$$

Although largely replaced by use of the body mass index, calculation of % IBW is another approach used for classification of individuals as overweight, obese, or underweight. For example, individuals whose body weight is 10% or more below the ideal for a given height (i.e., ≤90% IBW) are considered underweight, whereas those whose body weight is 10% or more above the ideal for a given height (i.e., ≥110% IBW) are considered overweight. Individuals with a weight for height 20% or more above the ideal (i.e., ≥120% IBW) are considered obese.

Using the formula, a male with a medium frame who is 6 ft 3 in. tall and weighs 260 lb would have a % IBW of 260 lb/(106 lb + [6 lb/in. × 15 in.]) × 100, or 260 lb/196 lb × 100 or 132.7%. At 132.7% IBW, this male would be considered obese.

Regression equations for estimating IBW also have been developed based on the 1959 Metropolitan Life Insurance Company height-weight tables and the ideal body weight tables used by Grant [15] in nutrition assessment. The equation based on the 1959 Metropolitan Life Insurance Company tables (with indoor clothing and shoes) is [16]

$$\text{IBW (lb)} = -139.17 + 3.86(\text{height}) + 9.52(\text{frame}) + 5.01(\text{sex})$$

Based on Grant's tables, corrected for height and nude weight the equation becomes

$$\text{IBW} = -133.99 + 3.86(\text{height}) + 9.52(\text{frame}) + 3.08(\text{sex})$$

In these two equations, height is in inches. Values used for frame size are 1 for small, 2 for medium, and 3 for large. Values for sex are +1 for male and −1 for female.

Although measuring both height and weight is relatively easy and can serve as a screen for underweight, overweight, or obesity, no method (weight for height from tables, formulas, or body mass index) is always a valid indicator of the degree of body fatness. The inadequacy of weight as a valid measure of fatness became clear in World War II when A. R. Behnke, a Navy physician, was able to demonstrate by hydrostatic weighing that several football players who had been found unfit for military service because of excessive weight actually had less body fat than controls of normal weight [17]. The excessive weight of these athletes was due to hypertrophy of muscles rather than excessive adipose tissue [17]. Behnke's work rekindled interest in studying the composition of the human body, an interest that had lain dormant for about 50 years.

THE COMPOSITION OF THE HUMAN BODY

The chemical composition of the human body was first described in 1859 in a book that dealt with the chemical composition of food [18]. Analytic chemistry was a rapidly growing science at the time, and figures describing the chemical composition of the different body tissues were compared with those of various foods. Additional chemical composition data from whole-body analysis of fetuses, children, and adults collected during the next few decades represent a direct (versus indirect) measure of body composition [18–22].

The concept of the reference man and woman (Table 15.5) was developed in the 1970s [23]. These

Table 15.5 Body Composition of Reference Man and Woman

Reference Man	Reference Woman
Age: 20–24 yr	Age: 20–24 yr
Height: 68.5 in.	Height: 64.5 in.
Weight: 154 lb	Weight: 125 lb
Total fat: 23.1 lb (15.0% body weight)	Total fat: 33.8 lb (27.0% body weight)
Storage fat: 18.5 lb (12.0% body weight)	Storage fat: 18.8 lb (15.0% body weight)
Essential fat: 4.6 lb (3.0% body weight)	Essential fat: 15.0 lb (12.0% body weight)
Muscle: 69 lb (44.8% body weight)	Muscle: 45 lb (36.0% body weight)
Bone: 23 lb (14.9% body weight)	Bone: 15 lb (12.0% body weight)
Remainder: 38.9 lb (25.3% body weight)	Remainder: 31.2 lb (25.0% body weight)
Average body density: 1.070 g/mL	Average body density: 1.040 g/mL

Source: McArdle WD, Katch FI, Katch VL. *Exercise Physiology.* Philadelphia: Lea & Febiger, 1981, p. 369. Adapted from Behnke AR, Wilmore JH. *Evaluation and Regulation of Body Build and Composition.* Englewood Cliffs, NJ: Prentice Hall, 1974.

reference figures provide information on body composition based on average physical dimensions from measurements of thousands of subjects who participated in various anthropometric and nutrition surveys [23]. The reference man and woman data provide a frame of reference for comparisons.

As seen in Table 15.5, the reference man weighs 29 lb more than the woman (nonpregnant) and is 4 in. taller. The man has 15% body fat versus the female's 27%. Of the 15% total body fat in the reference man, only 3% is essential fat versus 12% essential fat in the reference woman's 27% total body fat. Essential fat is fat associated with bone marrow, the central nervous system, viscera (internal organs), and cell membranes. In females, essential fat also includes fat in mammary glands and the pelvic region. Note that in the reference man muscle accounts for 44.8% body weight versus 36.0% body weight in the female. The average body densities of the reference man and woman are 1.070 and 1.040 g/mL, respectively.

Table 15.6 provides information on the average values for body fat in U.S. men and women, while Table 15.7 provides mean body composition values [24,25]. Average body fat values for men and women (untrained individuals) typically range from ~12% to 20% and from ~20% to 30%, respectively. Athletes, however, often have a lower percent body fat. For example, female Olympic athletes (runners, jumpers, swimmers, divers, and gymnasts) often have body fat levels in the 11% to 16% range, while many male athletes have <10% body fat [26].

Body composition is influenced by a variety of factors, including age, gender, race, heredity, and stature [27]. Although stature accounts for only a small portion of the variance in lean body mass, its influence is sufficient to require that stature be taken into account when comparing body composition data among individuals or groups of individuals. Taller children and adults have an advantage in lean body mass over their shorter peers [27].

Table 15.6 Average Percentage of Body Fat for Women and Men from Selected Studies

Study	Age (yr)	Stature (cm)	Mass (kg)	Fat (%)	68% Variation Limits*
Younger women:					
North Carolina, 1962	17–25	165.0	55.5	22.9	17.5–28.5
New York, 1962	16–30	167.5	59.0	28.7	24.6–32.9
California, 1968	19–23	165.9	58.4	21.9	17.0–26.9
California, 1970	17–29	164.9	58.6	25.5	21.0–30.1
Air Force, 1972	17–22	164.1	55.8	28.7	22.3–35.3
New York, 1973	17–26	160.4	59.0	26.2	23.4–33.3
North Carolina, 1975	—	166.1	57.5	24.6	—
Massachusetts, 1993	17–30	165.3	57.7	21.8	16.7–27.2
Older women:					
Minnesota, 1953	31–45	163.3	60.7	28.9	25.1–32.8
Minnesota, 1953	43–68	160.0	60.9	34.2	28.0–40.5
New York, 1963	30–40	164.9	59.6	28.6	22.1–35.3
New York, 1963	40–50	163.1	56.4	34.4	29.5–39.5
North Carolina, 1975	33–50	—	—	29.7	23.1–36.5
Massachusetts, 1993	31–50	165.2	58.9	25.2	19.2–31.2
Younger men:					
Minnesota, 1951	17–26	177.8	69.1	11.8	5.9–11.8
Colorado, 1956	17–25	172.4	68.3	13.5	8.3–18.8
Indiana, 1966	18–23	180.1	75.5	12.6	8.7–16.5
California, 1968	16–31	175.7	74.1	15.2	6.3–24.2
New York, 1973	17–26	176.4	71.4	15.0	8.9–21.1
Texas, 1977	18–24	179.9	74.6	13.4	7.4–19.4
Massachusetts, 1993	17–30	178.2	76.3	12.9	7.8–18.1
Older men:					
Indiana, 1966	24–38	179.0	76.6	17.8	11.3–24.3
Indiana, 1966	40–48	177.0	80.5	22.3	16.3–28.3
North Carolina, 1976	27–50	—	—	23.7	17.9–30.1
Texas, 1977	27–59	180.0	85.3	27.1	23.7–30.5
Massachusetts, 1993	31–50	177.1	77.5	19.9	13.2–26.5

*Indicates the range of values for percentage of body fat that includes one standard deviation or about 68 out of every 100 people measured.

Source: Katch FI, McArdle WD. *Introduction to Nutrition, Exercise, and Health,* 4th ed. Philadelphia: Lea and Febiger, 1993, p. 254.

Table 15.7 Mean Body Composition Values for Healthy Males and Females*

Age (yr)	*n*	Weight (kg)	Protein (kg)	TBW (L)	BA (kg)	BCM (kg)	ECW (L)	ECS (kg)	TBF1 (kg)	TBF2 (kg)
Males:										
20–29	12	80.1	13.1	44.9	3.53	35.7	19.8	6.77	18.6	16.8
30–39	12	73.7	11.2	42.3	3.44	32.5	19.0	6.61	16.8	15.6
40–49	12	84.6	12.4	47.2	3.59	35.1	19.8	6.88	21.4	23.0
50–59	12	82.0	12.1	45.0	3.43	33.3	19.3	6.58	21.5	20.7
60–69	10	78.5	11.8	42.1	3.33	30.7	19.9	6.39	21.3	21.5
70–79	10	80.5	11.1	40.4	3.17	27.6	20.3	6.08	25.8	26.5
Females:										
20–29	17	64.6	9.0	33.3	2.78	23.1	16.1	5.33	19.4	20.0
30–39	10	69.3	9.3	33.6	2.69	22.9	16.5	5.17	23.7	24.7
40–49	11	65.2	8.7	31.4	2.60	21.3	15.9	4.99	22.5	22.9
50–59	9	73.6	8.4	31.7	2.40	20.5	15.9	4.61	29.1	22.6
60–69	13	61.7	7.8	28.6	2.26	18.0	15.4	4.34	23.0	23.9
70–79	9	58.3	7.3	27.6	2.03	17.6	14.5	3.89	21.4	22.3

*Protein = 6.25 × total body nitrogen; BCM (body cell mass) = 0.235 × total body potassium (g); ICW (intracellular water) = TBW (total body water) − ECW (extracellular water); BA (bone ash) = total body calcium (TBCa)/0.34; ECS (extracellular solids) = TBCa (total body calcium)/0.177; TBF (total body fat); TBF1 = body weight − (protein + TBW + BA); TBF2 = body weight × (BCM + ECW + ECS).

Source: Modified from Cohn SH, Vaswani AN, Yasumura S, et al. Improved models for determination of body fat by in vivo neutron activation. Am J Clin Nutr 1984;40:255. Am J Clin Nutr, American Society for Clinical Nutrition. Reprinted with permission.

Evidence suggests that bone density and fat-free weight are significantly affected by heredity. The effect of race is evidenced by the difference between North American whites and blacks. Blacks tend to have slightly larger lean body mass than whites, along with thicker and denser bones and hence a larger amount of total body calcium [28].

The influence of gender on body composition appears to exist from birth but becomes dramatically evident at puberty. The differences in body composition between males and females manifested at sexual maturation continue throughout life. Moreover, an age and gender effect is seen in women at menopause, when the female undergoes a further change in body composition. Accelerated loss of calcium from the bones, due in large part to the decline of estrogen production, causes a more rapid decrease in bone density in the elderly woman compared to the elderly man.

The effect of maturation on body composition from birth to 10 years of age has been estimated through the use of "reference infants and children" (Table 15.8) [29,30]. Table 15.9 describes the components of weight gain occurring during these years. Total body water

Table 15.8 Body Composition of Reference Childrern

	Weight (kg)		Fat (%)		Protein (%)		Water (%)		Ash (%)		Carbohydrate (%)	
Age	Males	Females	Males	Females	Males	Females	Males	Females	Males	Females	Males	Females
Birth	3.545	3.325	13.7	14.9	12.9	12.8	69.6	68.6	3.2	3.2	0.5	0.5
4 mo	7.060	6.300	24.7	25.2	11.9	11.9	60.1	59.6	2.8	2.8	0.4	0.4
6 mo	8.030	7.250	25.4	26.4	12.0	12.0	59.4	58.4	2.8	2.7	0.4	0.4
12 mo	10.15	9.18	22.5	23.7	12.9	12.9	61.2	60.1	2.9	2.8	0.5	0.5
18 mo	11.47	10.78	20.8	21.8	13.5	13.5	62.2	61.3	3.1	3.0	0.5	0.5
24 mo	12.59	11.91	19.5	20.4	14.0	13.9	62.9	62.2	3.2	3.0	0.5	0.5
3 yr	14.675	14.10	17.5	18.5	14.7	14.4	63.9	63.5	3.4	3.1	0.5	0.5
4 yr	16.69	15.96	15.9	17.3	15.3	14.8	64.8	64.3	3.5	3.1	0.5	0.5
5 yr	18.67	17.66	14.6	16.7	15.8	15.0	65.4	64.6	3.7	3.1	0.5	0.5
6 yr	20.69	19.52	13.5	16.4	16.2	15.2	66.0	64.7	3.8	3.2	0.5	0.5
7 yr	22.85	21.84	12.8	16.8	16.5	15.2	66.2	64.4	3.9	3.1	0.5	0.5
8 yr	25.30	24.84	13.0	17.4	16.6	15.2	65.8	63.8	4.0	3.1	0.5	0.5
9 yr	28.13	28.46	13.2	18.3	16.8	15.1	65.4	63.0	4.1	3.1	0.5	0.5
10 yr	31.44	32.55	13.7	19.4	16.8	15.0	64.8	62.0	4.1	3.1	0.5	0.5

Source: Adapted from Foman SJ, Haschke F, Ziegler EE, Nelson SE. Body composition of reference children from birth to age 10 years. Am J Clin Nutr 1982;35:1171.

Table 15.9 Weight Increase and Its Components in Reference Children

Age	Weight Increase (g/d)		Fat (%)		Protein (%)		Minerals (%)	
	Males	Females	Males	Females	Males	Females	Males	Females
0–1 mo	29.3	26.0	20.4	21.4	12.5	12.5	0.9	0.8
3–4 mo	20.8	18.6	39.6	39.3	10.9	11.3	0.5	0.4
5–6 mo	15.2	15.0	27.3	32.4	13.2	12.6	0.4	0.4
9–12 mo	10.7	10.0	9.0	11.9	17.0	16.7	0.4	0.3
12–18 mo	7.2	8.7	7.2	10.7	18.4	17.0	0.3	0.3
18–24 mo	6.1	6.2	6.6	7.8	18.7	17.5	0.3	0.2
2–3 yr	5.7	6.0	5.8	7.9	19.1	17.6	0.2	0.2
3–4 yr	5.5	5.1	4.0	8.1	19.7	17.5	0.3	0.2
4–5 yr	5.4	4.7	3.2	11.3	19.9	17.0	0.3	0.2
5–6 yr	5.5	5.1	3.7	13.9	19.8	16.6	0.3	0.2
6–7 yr	5.9	6.4	6.3	19.6	19.5	15.6	0.3	0.2
7–8 yr	6.7	8.2	14.8	21.9	17.9	15.2	0.3	0.2
8–9 yr	7.8	9.9	15.2	24.5	17.9	14.8	0.4	0.3
9–10 yr	9.1	11.2	18.0	27.2	17.5	14.3	0.4	0.3

Source: Adapted from Foman SJ, Haschke F, Ziegler EE, Nelson SE. Body composition of reference children from birth to age 10 years. Am J Clin Nutr 1982;35:1174. Am. J. Clin. Nutr., American Society for Clinical Nutrition. Reprinted with permission.

decreases during the first year of life, primarily because of a rapid increase in fat. The decrease in total body water during the first year of life is followed by a slight increase from age 12 months to about 6 or 7 years (Table 15.8) [29]. Although total body water gradually declines for the next 3 to 4 years, it still exceeds 60% of total body weight at age 10 years. Accompanying the changes in total body water is a change in the ratio of extracellular fluid (ECF) to intracellular fluid (ICF). ECF exceeds ICF volume in the fetus during gestation, but during infancy and childhood the ECF : ICF ratio progressively falls until ICF occupies the majority position [27]. The change in the ECF : ICF ratio occurs with the growth and maturation of lean body mass. Cell hypertrophy and bone development encroach on the space occupied by ECF, while protein accrual results in an increased incorporation of ICF.

The rapid increase in lean body mass begun in the late fetal period continues for a while after birth and then decelerates. The deceleration is followed by a slower but fairly steady growth during the childhood years. The growth curves (body weight and lean body mass) for boys and girls are given in Figure 15.3. Despite the trend toward maturation of lean body mass during the childhood years, maturation appears to be incomplete until sometime during adolescence [27,31]. The percentage of

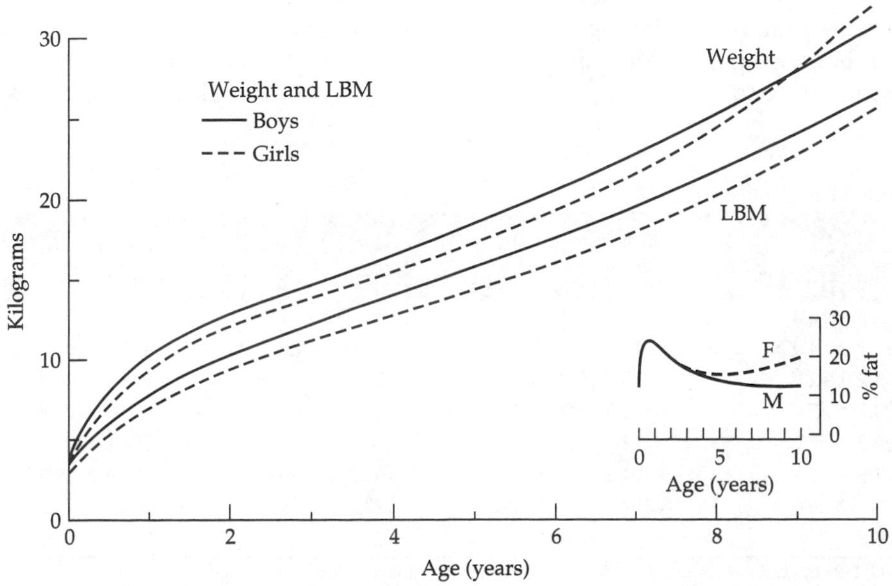

Figure 15.3 Graph of average body weight and lean body mass (LBM) for boys and girls from birth to 10 years. *Source:* Forbes GB. *Human Body Composition.* New york: Springer-Verlag, 1987, p. 154. Reprinted by permission.

water in lean body mass of reference children exceeds that considered average for the adult [31]. In addition, the value for minerals as a percentage of body weight is less than the adult average of 5.2% [18]. These differences in the components of lean body mass in children and adults result in a density of lean body mass in children of <1.10 g/mL, the average density for adults. Studies of children, both male and female, at various stages of maturation have confirmed the increased hydration of lean tissue and its lower density among people who have not yet reached adulthood [31]. As a result of these studies, Lohman [32] has suggested that Siri's [33] equation for determining fatness (p. 531) be replaced by the following equation when body fat composition of prepubescent children is being estimated:

$$\text{Percentage fat} = \frac{5.30}{\text{Body density}} - 4.89 \times 100$$

Although some gender differences are evidenced in the body composition of prepubescent children (Tables 15.8 and 15.9 and Fig. 15.3), they are not of great magnitude. The significant gender differences occur during adolescence and, once established, persist throughout adulthood.

Lean body mass is the body component most significantly affected by gender. In both sexes, serum testosterone levels rise during adolescence. However, the rise is much greater in boys, whose testosterone values approach ten times those of girls. As a result of high testosterone production, boys increase their lean body mass by ~33 to 35 kg between the ages of 10 and 20 years. The increment in girls is only about half as much, ~16 to 18 kg [27,34,35]. The female achieves her maximum lean body mass by about age 18 years, whereas the male continues accretion of lean body mass until about age 20 years [31,36]. By age 15 years the male-to-female ratio of lean body mass is 1.23 : 1, and by 20 years the ratio has increased to 1.45 : 1, well above the ratio for body weight (1.25 : 1) and stature (1.08 : 1). The pronounced gender difference in lean body mass is the primary reason for the gender difference in nutrition requirements [27].

The sharp increase in lean body mass that occurs in boys during the adolescent growth spurt is accompanied by a decrease in the percentage of body fat. The average percentage of body fat in boys age 6 to 8 years is ~13% to 15%; this percentage decreases to 10% to 12% for boys age 14 to 16 years [37]. Although the adolescent female also increases lean body mass during the growth spurt, a higher percentage of the weight gain is due to accretion of essential sex-specific fat. Girls age 6 to 8 years have ~16% to 18% body fat, and by age 14 to 16 years percentage of body fat ranges from 21% to 23% [37].

After 25 years of age, weight gain is usually due to body fat accretion [38]. Although the percentage of body weight due to fat remains lower in males than in females, a slow sustained rise in fat in both sexes occurs throughout adulthood [18,39]. The onset of menarche seems to affect the amount of fat accrued by the female through the early adult years [40]. Earlier sexual maturity in women appears to result in a greater amount of storage fat and a greater risk of obesity. In addition to increased body fat with age, a redistribution of body fat occurs [17,41,42]. Subcutaneous fat decreases with age, while internal or visceral fat increases [43]. The redistribution of body fat to the abdominal cavity is thought to be related in part to decreases in the concentrations of growth hormone and of estrogen or testosterone that occur with aging [44]. Fat placement in the body affects health. For example, fat placement in the abdominal (truncal) region (a so-called apple-shaped person or android obesity) is associated with greater risk of health problems, including heart disease, type 2 diabetes, and some cancers, than fat placement in the hip area (a so-called pear-shaped person or gynoid obesity).

Table 15.10 illustrates the differences between the young and the elderly in the various body components. More marked changes were seen in aging females than in aging males; however, in both males and females,

Table 15.10 Body Composition in Young and Elderly Males and Females

	Males		Females	
Parameters	Young (*n* = 10) (18–23 yr)	Elderly (*n* = 20) (61–89 yr)	Young (*n* = 10) (18–23 yr)	Elderly (*n* = 20) (60–89 yr)
Body weight (kg)	72.60 ± 10.34	61.60 ± 10.40	54.90 ± 2.71	56.10 ± 9.21
Body water (mL/kg)	586.1 ± 64.3	579.9 ± 54.4	531.0 ± 89.9	442.3 ± 57.3
Intracellular volume (mL/kg)	378.2 ± 42.3	375.7 ± 41.8	328.9 ± 64.7	248.3 ± 26.3
Lean body mass (g/kg)	800.7 ± 87.9	790.3 ± 78.1	725.4 ± 112.9	603.6 ± 77.8
Total body fat (g/kg)	199.3 ± 87.9	212.7 ± 66.2	274.6 ± 112.9	396.4 ± 77.8
Extracellular water volume (mL/kg)	207.9 ± 30.8	204.2 ± 37.0	192.1 ± 31.0	192.6 ± 19.4
Interstitial water volume (mL/kg)	167.7 ± 20.8	157.2 ± 19.7	172.5 ± 41.5	148.9 ± 21.2
Plasma volume (mL/kg)	43.2 ± 7.6	47.0 ± 6.2	29.6 ± 5.2	45.1 ± 10.1

Source: Adapted from Fulop T, Worum I, Csongor J, Foris G, Leovey A. Body composition in elderly people. Gerontology 1985;31:6. Karger, Basel.

a decrease in lean body mass (due primarily to a decrease in body cell mass) occurs with aging [39,44,45]. Skeletal muscle loss may be due in part to decreased physical activity and alterations in protein metabolism that might be affected by diminished anabolic hormone concentrations [43]. Decreased lean body mass causes a decrease in total body water. The decrease in total body water is much greater in females than in males. Further examination of body water amounts shows that extracellular fluid volume remains virtually unchanged. However, a redistribution occurs such that interstitial fluid decreases while plasma volume increases [45]. Loss of bone mass and atrophy of organs also occurs with aging.

METHODS FOR THE MEASUREMENT OF BODY COMPOSITION

Division of the body into components is used extensively for in vivo studies of body composition. The body can be categorized atomically in terms of its elements—primarily carbon, oxygen, hydrogen, and nitrogen, which make up ~95% of body mass, along with about another 50 or so elements that make up the remaining 5%. Alternately, the body may be thought of from a nutrient or molecular perspective as consisting of water, protein, fat, carbohydrate, and minerals. Multicompartment models to assess body composition rely on calculations of these different nutrient components.

Densitometry, one standard against which other indirect measurements of body composition are evaluated, separates the body into two components: fat mass and fat-free mass [18,22,46]. According to the two-component model of body composition assessment, fat mass includes essential and nonessential fat (triglycerides, also called triacylglycerols), whereas fat-free mass includes protein, water, carbohydrate (glycogen), and minerals [18,22]. The term *lean body mass* is used synonymously with *fat-free mass* but also includes essential body fat [18,46]. Several methods of body composition assessment are available, some of which are based on the two-component model. Commonly available methods are indirect and provide a means to calculate body components (direct measurement is accomplished only on cadavers). Although different procedures are available, accuracy varies not only with the equipment or method used but also with the technician. Several indirect methods of body composition assessment are reviewed in this section.

Anthropometry

Anthropometry allows for estimation of body composition through measurement at various circumference and skin fold (fat) sites. Skin varies in thickness from 0.5 mm to 2 mm [47]; thus, fat beneath the skin typically represents the major part of the skin fold measurement. The assumption is that a direct relationship exists between total body fat and fat deposited in depots just beneath the skin (i.e., subcutaneous fat). Skin fold measurements can be used in one of two ways:

- scores from the various measurements can be added and the sum used to indicate the relative degree of fatness among subjects, or
- scores can be plugged into various mathematical regression equations developed to predict body density or to calculate percentage of body fat [24,48].

Five sites commonly used for measuring skin fold thickness, shown in Figure 15.4 (labeled A–E), are as follows:

A. Back of the upper arm (triceps)—a vertical fold is measured at the midline of the upper arm halfway between the tip of the shoulder and the tip of the elbow.
B. Subscapula—an oblique fat fold is measured just below the tip (interior angle) of the scapula.
C. Suprailiac—a slightly oblique fold is measured just above the hipbone, with the fold lifted to follow the natural diagonal line at this point.
D. Abdomen—a vertical fold is measured 1 in. to the right of the umbilicus.
E. Thigh—a vertical fold is measured at the midpoint of the thigh, between the kneecap and the hip (inguinal crease) [24,49].

Additional sites often include the pectoral (chest), midaxillary, and calf. The right side of the body is used for most measurements if comparisons are being made to standards derived from data from U.S. surveys that typically measured the right side of subjects. The handedness of the subject affects skin fold measurements taken on the arm such that measurements on the right exceed those on the left by 0.2 to 0.3 standard deviation units [50].

Bias associated with the side of the measurement, however, is less than error due to measurement [50]. All measurements should be repeated at least two or three times, and the average should be used as the skin fold value. Measurement procedures and the use of formulas (see the next paragraph) contribute to procedure error. The precision of skin fold thickness measurements depends on the skill of the anthropometrist; in general, a precision of within 5% can be obtained by a well-trained and experienced anthropometrist [51]. The use of anthropometry for predicting visceral fat content offers limited accuracy [52]. Nevertheless, the method is quite inexpensive compared with the cost of other techniques.

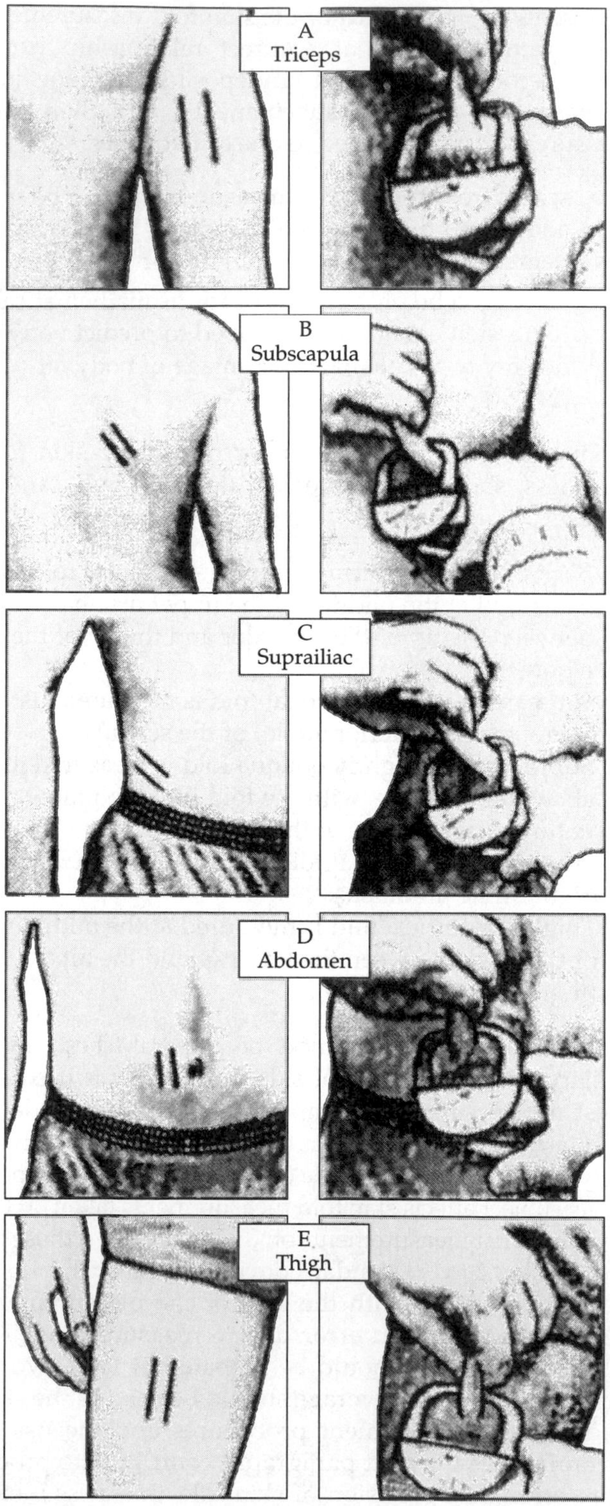

Figure 15.4 Anatomic location of the five fat fold sites: (A) triceps, (B) subscapula, (C) suprailiac, (D) abdomen, (E) thigh.

Several different equations that are population specific have been developed for calculating total body fat from skin fold sites. Equations developed by Katch and McArdle [24] for predicting total body fat in young (age 17–26 years) men and women from the triceps and subscapula skin folds are shown:

$$\text{Young women: \% body fat} = 0.55(A) + 0.31(B) + 6.13$$

$$\text{Young men: \% body fat} = 0.43(A) + 0.58(B) + 1.47$$

where A = triceps fat fold measured in millimeters and B = subscapula fat fold measured in millimeters. Measurements from multiple (at least three) sites are deemed better for overall subcutaneous fat assessment than measurements from only one or two sites [24].

Circumference or girth measurements also may be used to assess body fat. Typical sites of measurement include the abdomen, buttocks, right thigh, and right upper arm. As with skin fold measurements, body fat prediction equations that are age and gender specific have been developed.

Circumference measurements of the waist (abdominal circumference) and hips (gluteal circumference) also provide an index of regional body fat distribution and have been shown to correlate with visceral fat [52]. The ratio of waist to hip circumference is calculated following measurement of the subject's waist and hip. Waist measurements should be made below the rib cage and above the umbilicus in a horizontal plane at the narrow site, or the site of least circumference. Hip circumference should be measured at the site with the greatest circumference around the hips or buttocks. Soft tissue should not be compressed or indented during these measurements, and all measurements should be taken with the subject standing. Reproducibility of circumference measurements is good at 2% [52]. Ratios > 0.8 in women and > 0.95 in men are thought to indicate increased health risk. Waist circumferences > 40 in. (men) and > 35 in. (women), without comparison to hip circumference, also may be used to identify increased abdominal fat and thus increased risk for the development of obesity-associated conditions.

Densitometry/Hydrodensitometry

The principle of hydrostatic weighing on which densitometry or hydrodensitometry is based can be traced to the Greek mathematician Archimedes. He discovered that the volume of an object submerged in water is equal to the volume of water displaced by the object. The specific gravity or density of an object can be calculated by dividing the object's weight (wt) in air by its loss of weight in water. For example, for an individual who weighs 47 kg in air and 2 kg underwater, 45 kg represents the loss of body weight and the weight of the water displaced. Correction for residual air volume in the lungs (RLV) and gas in the gastrointestinal tract (GIGV) must be made.

The calculation of body density is given by the following formula:

$$\text{Body density} = \frac{\text{Wt of body in air}}{\dfrac{\left(\text{Wt of body in air} - \text{Wt of body underwater}\right)}{\text{Density of water}} - \text{RLV} - \text{GIGV}}$$

Residual lung volume is thought to be about 24% of vital lung capacity. The volume of gas in the gastrointestinal tract is estimated to range from 50 to 300 mL. This volume typically is neglected, or a value of 100 mL may be used in calculations. The density or the weight of water is known for a wide range of temperatures and needs to be obtained for the calculation.

Calculating the body density of the human body allows an estimation of body fat. At any known body density, estimating the percentage of body fat in an adult is possible using an equation derived by Siri [33]:

$$\text{Percentage body fat} = \frac{495}{\text{Body density}} - 450 \times 100$$

or an equation derived by Brozek [46]:

$$\text{Percentage body fat} = \frac{457}{\text{Body density}} - 414 \times 100$$

Calculations of body density are derived in part from the knowledge that the density of fat mass is 0.9 g/cm^3 and that the density of fat-free mass is 1.1 g/cm^3 (assuming fat-free mass is composed of ~20.5% protein, 72.4% water, and 7.1% bone mineral). Once the percentage of body fat has been calculated, the weight of the fat and the lean body mass can be estimated as follows [24]:

$$\text{Body weight} \times \text{percentage body fat} = \text{Weight of body fat}$$

$$\text{Body weight} - \text{weight of body fat} = \text{Lean body weight}$$

Various calculations for determining ideal or desirable body weight have been proposed based on information of body composition, such as this formula [53]:

$$\text{Desirable body weight} = \frac{\text{Lean body weight}}{1 - \%\ \text{fat desired}}$$

Calculations would be as follows for a woman who weighs 200 lb, with a measured 40% of this weight as fat:

$$200\ \text{lb} \times 0.40 = 80\ \text{lb (fat weight)}$$

$$200\ \text{lb} - 80\ \text{lb} = 120\ \text{lb (lean body weight)}$$

Because the desirable amount of fat in females ranges from ~20% to 30%, a figure of 25% (0.25) is used in the following equation for the sample woman:

$$\text{Desirable body weight} = \frac{120}{1 - 0.25} = \frac{120}{0.75} = 160\ \text{lb}$$

Underwater weighing is considered a noninvasive and relatively precise method for assessment of body fat. The standard error of estimate of body fat using densitometry has been estimated at 2.7% for adults and ~4.5% for children and adolescents [26]. Limitations of underwater weighing include its relatively high equipment cost, the inability to measure gas volume in the gastrointestinal tract, its impracticality for large numbers of subjects, and the extreme cooperation and time required of subjects, who must be submerged and remain motionless for an extended time period. Thus, the technique is not suitable for young children, older adults, or subjects in poor health. Additional limitations to its use include its assumption that density of lean body mass is relatively constant when in fact bone density typically changes with age [54].

Absorptiometry

Absorptiometry is an imaging technique that involves scanning the entire body or a portion of the body by a photon beam. Single-photon absorptiometry involves scanning the body with photons from ^{125}I (iodine) at a specific energy level. However, this technique does not allow accurate measurement at soft tissue sites. This problem has been eliminated with the development of dual-photon absorptiometry. In dual-photon absorptiometry, the radionuclide source is generally ^{153}Gd (gadolinium), and photons at two different energy levels are emitted. Bone mineral content as well as fat mass and fat-free mass may be estimated from dual-photon absorptiometry.

Dual energy X-ray absorptiometry (abbreviated DEXA or DXA), introduced in the late 1980s, involves scanning subjects with X rays at two different energy levels. The subject lies on a table while a photon source beneath the table and the detector above the table pass across the subject's body. Attenuation of the beam of X rays as it passes over the body is calculated by computer. Percentage of body fat, soft tissue, and bone mineral density (total or specific sites) can be calculated based on the restriction in the flux of the X rays across the fat and the fat-free masses [51,55–57].

Limitations to the use of absorptiometry include the expense of the equipment and the exposure, though minimal, of subjects to radiation. In addition, trained personnel are required to run the instrument and analyze the scans. DXA measurements are highly reproducible and have been shown to correlate with other body composition assessment methods. The technique, however, is not accurate for individuals with metal implants, including, for example, pins or rods. In addition, extremely obese individuals may have difficulty getting on the table, assuming the table can support the weight.

Computerized (Axial) Tomography (CAT or CT)

Computerized or computed (axial) tomography (CT or CAT), another imaging technique involving an X-ray tube and detectors aligned at opposite poles of a circular gantry, allows the taking of visual images and thus the determination of regional body composition such as visceral organ mass; regional muscle mass; subcutaneous and internal fat; and bone density. Subjects lie faceup on a movable platform that passes through the instrument's circular gantry. Cross-sectional images of tissue are constructed by the scanner computer as the X-ray beam rotates around the person being assessed. Differences in X-ray attenuation are related to differences in the physical density of tissues [51]. Calculation of relative surface area or volume occupied by tissues (e.g., bone, adipose, and fat-free tissue) can be done from the images produced by the instrument. Results are highly reproducible [52]. Excessively long exposure of subjects to ionizing radiation and the expense of the equipment are major drawbacks to the use of computerized tomography to assess body composition.

Magnetic Resonance Imaging (MRI)

Magnetic resonance imaging (MRI) is based on the principle that atomic nuclei behave like magnets when an external magnetic field is applied across the body. When an external magnetic field is applied, the nuclei attempt to align with the field. The nuclei also absorb radio frequency waves directed into the body and in turn change their orientation in the magnetic field [51]. Abolishing the radio wave results in the emission of a radio signal by the activated nuclei, and this emitted signal is used to develop a computerized image. Magnetic resonance imaging is used to measure organ size and structure, body fat and fat distribution (subcutaneous, visceral, intra-abdominal), and muscle size, as well as body water contents. The technique is noninvasive and safe; however, the cost is quite high. Reproducibility of visceral fat area measured by magnetic resonance imaging is ~10% to 15% [52]. However, for assessment of adipose tissue distribution, magnetic resonance imaging provided the least variability when compared to skin fold thickness, ^{40}K counting, bioelectrical impedance, total body water assessment with ^{18}O, and hydrostatic weighing [58].

Total Body Electrical Conductivity (TOBEC)

The total body electrical conductivity (TOBEC) technique is based on the change in electrical conductivity when a subject is placed in an electromagnetic field. Subjects lie faceup on a bed, which is rolled into the TOBEC instrument. The instrument then induces an electrical current in the subject. Changes in conductivity, which are proportional to the body's electrolyte content, are measured. Because electrolytes in the body are found associated mostly with lean body mass, TOBEC allows for the estimation of lean body mass and thus fat by difference. Hydration status, electrolyte imbalances, and variations in bone mass may, however, interfere with accuracy. In addition, although the procedure is fast and safe, the equipment is very expensive.

Bioelectrical Impedance Analysis (BIA)

Bioelectrical impedance analysis (BIA), also called bioelectrical impedance (BEI), is similar to TOBEC in that it depends on changes in electrical conductivity. However, in BIA, measurement of electrical conductivity is made on the extremities and not on the whole body. Subjects lie faceup on a bed, with their extremities away from the body. Electrodes are placed on the limbs in specific locations. An instrument generates a current or multiple electrical current frequencies that are passed through the body by means of the electrodes. Opposition to the electric flow current, called impedance, is detected and measured by the instrument. Impedance is the inverse of conductance. The lowest resistance value of an individual is used to calculate conductance and predict lean body mass or fat-free mass. For example, muscle, organs, and blood, which have high water and electrolyte content, are good conductors [43]. Tissues containing little water and electrolytes (such as fat) are poor conductors and have a high resistance to the passage of electrical current [43]. At higher frequencies, estimates of both intracellular and extracellular water can be made, because the current can penetrate cell membranes. At lower frequencies, the flow of the current is blocked, and the measured resistance indicates extracellular water.

Bioelectrical impedance is a safe, noninvasive, and rapid means to assess body composition. The equipment is portable and fairly easy to operate, although it is also relatively expensive. Like TOBEC, bioelectrical impedance readings are affected by hydration and electrolyte imbalances. Thus, the technique is more useful for healthy subjects. Several bioelectrical impedance analysis prediction equations have been developed for various populations.

Ultrasonography or Ultrasound

Ultrasound provides images of tissue configuration or depth readings of changes in tissue density [51]. Electrical energy is converted in a probe to high-frequency ultrasonic energy. The ultrasonic energy is transmitted through the skin and into the body in the form of short pulses or waves. The waves pass through adipose tissue until they reach lean body mass. At the interface between the adipose and lean tissues, part of the ultrasonic energy is reflected back to the receiver in the probe and transformed to electrical energy. The echo is visualized on an oscilloscope. A transmission gel used between the probe and the skin provides acoustic contact. The equipment is portable, and the technique may provide information on the thickness of subcutaneous fat as well as the thickness of muscle mass. Reliability of the technique has improved to >91%, and accuracy is similar to that of skin fold measurements [59].

Infrared Interactance

Infrared interactance is based on the principle that when material is exposed to infrared light, the light is absorbed, reflected, or transmitted depending on the scattering and absorption properties of the material. For assessment of body composition, a probe that acts as an infrared transmitter and detector is placed on the skin. Infrared light of two wavelengths is transmitted by the probe. The signal penetrates the underlying tissue to a depth of 4 cm [51]. Infrared light also is reflected and scattered at the site from the skin and underlying subcutaneous tissues and detected by the probe. Estimates of body composition can be made by analyzing specific characteristics of the reflected light. The method is safe, noninvasive, and rapid; however, overestimates of body fat in lean (<8% body fat) subjects and underestimates of body fat in obese (>30% body fat) subjects have been reported [60]. The accuracy of the technique requires further investigation.

Some methods of body composition assessment use an atomic perspective to quantify one or more components of the body and through various calculations determine the other body components. Measurements of body composition by assessment of total body water, total body potassium, or neutron activation analysis use such an approach.

Total Body Water (TBW)

Quantification of total body water involves the use of isotopes—typically deuterium (D_2O), radioactive tritium (^3H_2O), or oxygen-18 (^{18}O)—and is based on principles of dilution. Water can be labeled with any one of the three isotopes. The water containing a specific amount (concentration) of the isotope is then ingested or injected intravenously. Following ingestion or injection, the isotope distributes itself throughout the body water. Body water occupies ~73.2% of fat-free body mass. After allowing a specified time period (usually 2 to 6 hours) for equilibration, samples of body fluids (usually blood and urine) are taken. Losses of the isotope in the urine must be determined. If ^{18}O is used, breath samples are collected for analysis. Concentrations of the isotope in the breath or body fluids are determined by scintillation counters or other instruments.

The initial concentration (C_1) and volume (V_1) of the isotope given are equal to the final concentration of the isotope in the plasma (C_2) and the volume of total body water (V_2), expressed as $C_1V_1 = C_2V_2$. Thus, total body water (V_2) is equal to C_1V_1 divided by C_2. Once total body water has been determined, the percentage of lean body mass can be calculated. Fat-free mass equals total body water divided by 0.732. Body fat can be obtained by subtracting fat-free mass from body weight. A three-component model (consisting of total body water, body volume, and body weight) has been shown to measure changes in body fat as low as 1.54 kg in individuals [55]. Many studies, however, have shown that the degree of hydration varies considerably in lean body tissue of apparently healthy people. Therefore, implications about total body fat derived from estimation of lean body mass via total body water may be misleading [25,61]. In addition, adipose tissue has been shown to contain as much as 15% water by weight [56]. Thus, measurement of extracellular fluid as well as total body water should be made and subtracted from total body water to give an indication of intracellular water and thus of body cell mass.

Because total body water involves radiation exposure if ^3H is used, the method is not suitable for use with some subjects (such as children and pregnant women). ^{18}O is in itself quite expensive and requires expensive mass spectrometry equipment for its analysis. Deuterated water (D_2O) is relatively inexpensive to purchase but is expensive to measure [43].

Total Body Potassium (TBK)

Total body potassium is also used to assess fat-free mass. Potassium is present within cells but is not associated with stored fat. About 0.012% of potassium occurs as ^{40}K, a naturally occurring isotope that emits a characteristic gamma ray. External counting of gamma rays emitted by ^{40}K provides the amount of total body potassium; however, getting accurate counts of ^{40}K may be difficult because of external or background radiation. After measurement of potassium (^{40}K) radiation from the body, calculation of total body potassium from the data is required. Fat-free mass can be estimated from the total body potassium based on any one of several conversion factors, which vary in men from 2.46 to 3.41 g potassium per kilogram fat-free mass and in women from 2.28 to 3.16 g potassium per kilogram fat-free mass [56]. Total body fat can be calculated by subtracting fat-free mass from body weight. Overestimation of body fat in obese subjects has been reported with total body potassium [60]. The technique should not be used in people with potassium-wasting diseases.

Neutron Activation Analysis

Neutron activation analysis allows for an in vivo estimation of body composition, including total body concentrations of nitrogen (TBN), calcium (TBCa), chloride (TBCl), sodium (TBNa), and phosphorus (TBP), among other elements. A beam of neutrons is delivered to the individual being assessed. The body's atoms (nitrogen, calcium, chloride, sodium, and phosphorus) interact with the beam of neutrons to generate unstable radioactive elements, which emit gamma-ray energy as they revert back to their stable forms. The specific energy levels correspond to specific elements, and the radiation's level of activity indicates the element's abundance [51].

Assessment of many body components may be conducted with neutron activation analysis. For example, measurement of nitrogen allows for lean body mass assessment, and subtracting lean body mass from total body water allows calculation of total body fat [36,38]. Table 15.7 [38] reports body composition information derived from neutron activation for males and females age 20 to 79 years. Neutron activation analysis is noninvasive and provides reliable and reproducible data. However, the equipment is expensive and requires a skilled technologist, and subjects are exposed to significant amounts of radiation.

Overview of Methods

Table 15.11 provides an overview of the methods discussed in this chapter as well as a few additional methods. In brief review, the methods available to assess lean body mass (LBM) or fat-free mass include neutron activation analysis, total body potassium, intracellular water (total body water minus

Table 15.11 Methods for Assessing Body Composition [33,43,49,54]

Method	Description of Method and Comments
Anthropometry	Skin fold thicknesses from a variety of locations, body weight, and limb circumferences can be used to calculate fat, fat-free mass, and muscle size. Measurements can be made in the field but require skilled technicians for accuracy. Skin folds can provide some information about regional subcutaneous fat as well as about total fat. Measurements may not be applicable to all population groups.
Densitometry	Measurement of total body density through determination of body volume by underwater weighing, helium displacement, or combination of water displacement by body and air displacement by head. Measurements can be used to determine body density, which in turn allows calculation of percentage of body fat and fat-free mass. Measurements are precise but must be conducted in laboratory; subject cooperation is necessary for underwater weighing. The method is not suitable for young children or the elderly.
Total body water	Measured by dilution with deuterium (D_2O), tritium (^3H_2O), or oxygen-18 (^{18}O). TBW is used as index of human body composition based on findings that water is not present in stored triglycerides but occupies an approximate average of 73.2% of the fat-free mass. A specified quantity of the isotope is ingested or injected; then, following an equilibration period, a sampling is made of the concentration of the tracer in a selected biological fluid. TBW is calculated from the equation $C_1V_1 = C_2V_2$, where V_2 represents TBW volume, C_1 is the amount of tracer given, and C_2 is the final concentration of tracer in the selected biological fluid. The ECF can be estimated by a variety of methods. Subtracting ECF from TBW allows calculation of fat-free mass. This is a difficult procedure with limited precision, and the cost can be great, particularly when ^{18}O is used as the tracer.
Total body potassium	^{40}K, a naturally occurring isotope, is found in a known amount (0.012%) in intracellular water and is not present in stored triglycerides. These facts allow fat-free mass to be estimated by the external counting of gamma rays emitted by ^{40}K. Instrument for counting ^{40}K is quite expensive and must be properly calibrated for precision. Method is limited to laboratories.
Urinary creatinine excretion	Creatinine is the product resulting from the nonenzymatic hydrolysis of free creatine, which is liberated during the dephosphorylation of creatine phosphate. The preponderance of creatine phosphate is located in the skeletal muscle; therefore, urinary creatinine excretion can be related to muscle mass. Drawbacks to this method include large individual variability of creatinine excretion due to the renal processing of creatinine and the effect of diet. The creatine pool does not seem to be under strict metabolic control and is to some degree independent of body composition. Another technical difficulty is control of accurately timed 24-hour urine collections.
3-methylhistidine excretion	3-methylhistidine has been suggested as a useful predictor of human body composition because this amino acid is located principally in the muscle and cannot be reused after its release from catabolized myofibrillar proteins

Table 15.11 *(continued)*

Method	Description of Method and Comments
	(methylation of specific histidine residues occurs posttranslationally on protein). Some concern exists over the use of 3-methylhistidine as a marker of muscle protein because of the potential influence of nonskeletal muscle protein (skin and gastrointestinal [GI] tract proteins) turnover on its excretory rate. Additional problems with this method are the need for consumption of a relatively controlled meat-free diet and complete and accurate urine collections.
Electrical conductance (a) Total body electrical	Method is based on the change in electrical conductivity when subject is placed in an electromagnetic field. The change is proportional to the electrolyte content of the body, and because fat-free mass contains virtually all the water and conducting electrolytes of the body, conductivity is far greater in the fat-free mass than in the fat mass. From measurement, LBM can be calculated and fat estimated by difference. A primary drawback to this method is the expense of the instrument required; this measurement is a laboratory procedure limited primarily to large clinical facilities.
(b) Bioelectrical impedance analysis	This method is an adaptation of TOBEC; measurement of electrical conductivity is made on extremities rather than the whole body. Determinations of resistance and reactance are made, and the lowest resistance value for an individual is used to calculate conductance and to predict LBM. Equipment is portable and much less expensive than that required for TOBEC, yet precision is comparable.
Absorptiometry (a) Single-photon	Method is used in measurement of local or regional bone. The bone is scanned by a low-energy photon beam and the transmission monitored by a scintillation detector. Changes in transmission as the beam is moved across the bone are a function of bone mineral content (bone density) in that region. Disadvantages of this method are that the bone must be enclosed in a constant thickness of soft tissue and that measurements cannot be used to accurately predict total skeletal mass.
(b) Dual-photon	This method allows estimation of LBM as well as total bone mineral of the whole body. The body is scanned transversely in very small steps over its entire length by radiation from gadolinium-153 (^{153}Gd). This isotope emits two gamma rays of different energies; attenuation measurements at the two discrete photon energies allow quantification of bone mineral and soft tissue. The equipment required for dual-photon absorptiometry is quite expensive, complicated calibration is required, and data collected require complicated mathematical treatment.
(c) Dual X-ray photon	Similar to dual-photon, this method involves scanning subjects at two different energy levels; however, X rays are used instead of a radionuclide source. Radiation exposure to subjects is very low, and the procedure is relatively quick. This method appears to be the best choice for measuring bone mineral density.
Computerized tomography	Method determines regional body composition. An image is generated by computerized processing of X-ray data. Fat, lean tissue, and bone can be identified by their characteristic density-frequency distribution. Information about regional fat distribution can be obtained; it has been used to determine the ratio of intra-abdominal to subcutaneous fat in humans. The size of the liver, spleen, and kidneys can be determined by computerized tomography. Both cost of the equipment and technical difficulties are high. Method is a laboratory procedure presently limited primarily to large medical centers.
Ultrasound	Approach uses instrument in which electrical energy is converted in probe to high-frequency ultrasonic energy. Subsequent transmission of these sound waves through various tissues can be used to calculate tissue thickness. Method is frequently used to determine the thickness of subcutaneous fat layer. Large laboratory instruments and smaller portable equipment are available. Although data suggest a reasonable validity of method, its general use has been limited because the appropriate signal frequency of the probe has not been well defined and the needed constant pressure by the probe to the scan site is difficult to achieve. Changes in pressure by probe application can prejudice ultrasonic determination of adipose tissue thickness.
Infrared interactance	Measurement of body fat is made at various sites on the extremities through use of short wavelengths of infrared light. The amount of fat can be calculated from the absorption spectra and used with a prediction equation to estimate TBF.
Magnetic resonance imaging	Approach is based on fact that atomic nuclei can behave like magnets. When external magnetic field is applied across a part of the body, each nucleus attempts to align with the external magnetic field. If these nuclei are simultaneously activated by a radio frequency wave, once the radio wave is turned off the activated nuclei will emit the signal absorbed; this emitted signal is used to develop image by computer. Method has capability of generating images in response to intrinsic tissue variables and of representing characteristics such as level of hydration and fat content. This method appears to have much potential, but both the cost of equipment and technical difficulties are high.
Neutron activation analysis	This is the only technique currently available for measurement of multielemental composition of the human body. Low radiation doses produce isotopic atoms in tissues; the induced nuclides permit measurement of many elements, including nitrogen, calcium, phosphorus, magnesium, sodium, and chloride. Although precision of measurement is high, so are the technical difficulties and cost of equipment. Method of measuring body composition is limited to a very few laboratories in this country and abroad.

extracellular water), total body electrical conductivity, and bioelectrical impedance analysis. Body fat may be assessed by anthropometry, densitometry, dual-photon or energy X-ray absorptiometry, ultrasound, and infrared interactance. Adipose tissue typically is measured using computerized tomography, magnetic resonance imaging, and ultrasound. Bone mineral density may be assessed using single- or dual-photon absorptiometry as well as via dual energy X-ray absorptiometry.

COMPONENTS OF ENERGY EXPENDITURE

Whether body weight is being maintained, increased, or decreased depends primarily on the extent to which the energy requirements of the body (i.e., total energy expenditure) have been met by energy intake. Total energy expenditure is composed primarily of

- the basal metabolic rate (BMR) or resting energy expenditure (REE),
- the thermic effect of food (TEF), and
- the effect of physical activity or exercise.

A fourth component, thermoregulation, is sometimes included. The average division of energy expenditure among the components, each of which is discussed in the following sections, is shown in Figure 15.5.

Basal Metabolic Rate and Resting Energy Expenditure

Basal metabolic rate (BMR) represents the rate at which the body expends energy to sustain basic life processes such as respiration, heartbeat, renal function, and blood circulation. It also includes the energy needed to remain in an awake state, because the measurements are usually made in individuals shortly after waking. The word *basal*, as it is used in BMR, is often confused with the term *resting*; however, *basal* is more precisely defined than is *resting*. The measurement of oxygen consumed and carbon dioxide produced that is used in calculating energy expenditure is made under closely controlled and standardized conditions. An individual's basal metabolic rate is determined when he or she is in a postabsorptive state (i.e., no food intake for at least 12 hours), is lying down (supine), and is completely relaxed (motionless)—preferably very shortly after awakening from sleep in the morning. In addition, the temperature of the room in which the measurement takes place is made as comfortable as possible (thermoneutral) for the individual. Any factors that could influence the internal work of the individual are minimized as much as possible. For most individuals, BMR is slowest during sleep. BMR is usually converted to units of kcal/24 hours and called *basal energy expenditure* (BEE).

Figure 15.5 Components of energy expenditure and their approximate percentage contribution.

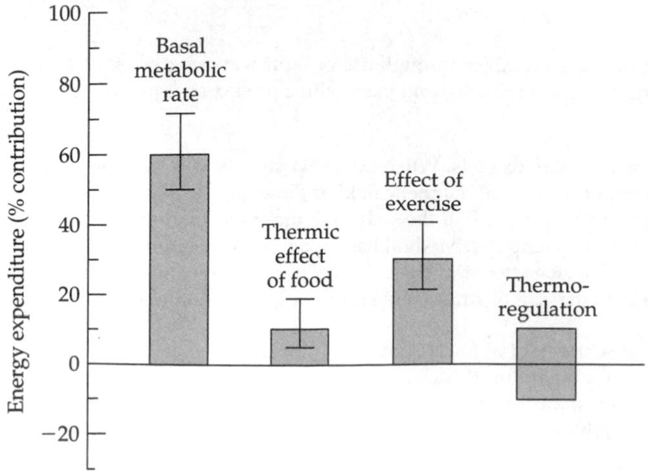

In contrast to BMR, resting metabolic rate (RMR) is measured when the individual is at rest in a comfortable environment, and fasting for 12 hours is not required. Instead, the fast for RMR is usually ~2 to 4 hours. RMR usually is slightly higher (~10%) than BMR because of its less stringent conditions of measurement [62,63]. RMR is thought to account for ~65% to 80% of daily total energy expenditure [62]. BMR accounts for ~50% to 70% of daily total energy expenditure [64]. The term *resting energy expenditure* (REE) is used when RMR is extrapolated to units of kcal/24 hours [65].

Basal metabolism is a result of energy exchanges occurring in all cells of the body. The rate of oxygen consumption, however, is most closely related to the actively metabolizing cells, that is, the body's lean body mass or fat-free mass [66,67]. In aging, for example, fat increases at the expense of fat-free mass, and BMR decreases. With maturation, the proportion of supporting structures (i.e., bone and muscle) increases more rapidly than does total body weight. Bone and muscle, though components of body cell mass, have a much lower metabolic activity than organ tissues but much greater activity than adipose tissue. This difference in the rate of weight accretion between the less active and the more active components of mass means a decrease in the overall metabolic activity of cell mass and a concurrent decrease in BMR per unit of body weight [66]. These changes that occur during maturation explain the lower REE of children as compared to very young infants.

A look at the metabolic activity among the different components of the cell mass in an adult male illustrates its variability. Under normal circumstances, ~5% to 6% of total body weight can be attributed to the weight of the brain, liver, heart, and kidney, whereas ~30% to 40%

of body weight is due to muscle mass [66]. At the same time, the metabolic activity of these organ tissues accounts for ~60% of basal oxygen consumption, whereas muscle mass accounts for only ~25% [66]. Tissues such as bone, glands, intestine, and skin account for 33% of body weight and contribute 15% to 20% of metabolic activity. In contrast, fat usually accounts for at least 20% of body weight but contributes only 5% of metabolic activity. Thus, changes in BMR can occur whenever the proportions of body tissues change in relation to one another [66].

Thermic Effect of Food

A second component of energy expenditure is the thermic effect of food (i.e., the metabolic response to food), also referred to as diet-induced thermogenesis, specific dynamic action, or the specific effect of food. The thermic effect of food represents the increase in energy expenditure associated with the body's processing of food, including the work associated with the digestion, absorption, transport, metabolism, and storage of energy from ingested food. The percentage increase in energy expenditure over BMR due to the thermic effect of food has been estimated to range from ~5% to 30%. Protein in foods has the greatest effect, increasing energy expenditure 20% to 30%. Carbohydrates have an intermediate effect, raising energy expenditure 5% to 10%, while fat increases energy expenditure 0% to 5% [65]. The value most commonly used for the thermic effect of food is 10% of the caloric value of a mixed diet consumed within 24 hours [64,68]. The rise in metabolism following food consumption appears to reach a maximum about 1 hour after eating and is generally, but not always, absent 4 hours postprandial (after eating) [63]. Consequently, the thermic effect of food often is not included in calculations of total energy requirements.

Physical Activity

The effect of physical activity (i.e., voluntary movement, including fidgeting) is the most variable of the components and also the only component that is easily altered. Although on average physical activity accounts for ~20% to 40% of total energy expenditure, it can be considerably less in a truly sedentary person or much more in a very physically active person [64,68]. Factors impinging on energy expenditure during exercise, other than the activity itself, include the intensity, duration, and frequency with which the activity is performed; the body mass of the person; his or her efficiency at performing the activity; and any extraneous movements that may accompany the activity. In addition, oxygen consumption and thus energy expenditure can remain elevated for a short time period after the exercise activity has stopped.

Thermoregulation

An additional component of energy expenditure that is of some importance is thermoregulation, also called adaptive, nonshivering, facultative, or regulatory thermogenesis. Thermoregulation refers to the alteration in metabolism that occurs in the body's maintaining its core temperature. Changes in metabolism occur most often with changes in environmental temperature, especially below the comfort zone (zone of thermoneutrality), but they also occur with overfeeding, trauma, burns, and physical conditioning, among other situations [65]. For example, when temperatures decrease below the comfort zone and a person has not adjusted to the change by altering the thickness of the clothes he or she is wearing, energy expenditure increases to maintain or restore the body temperature to normal. The overall contribution of thermoregulation to energy needs is small, given that most individuals alter clothing as needed to maintain a comfortable body temperature.

ASSESSMENT OF ENERGY EXPENDITURE

In healthy adults, total energy expenditure typically includes basal energy expenditure, energy expended due to the thermic effect of foods, and energy expended due to physical activity. Assessment of energy expenditure can be made through direct or indirect calorimetry or the doubly labeled water method as well as via several calculations using derived formulas. We will discuss each of these methods of assessment.

Direct Calorimetry

Measurement of total energy expenditure can be determined by **direct calorimetry,** which measures the dissipation of heat from the body [69]. Heat dissipation is measured via an isothermal principle, a gradient-layer system, or a water-cooled garment [69,70]. A very simplified version of calorimetry for humans based on the isothermal principle is depicted in Figure 15.6. Total heat loss consists of sensible heat loss and heat of water vaporization. In the isothermal calorimeter (Fig. 15.6), sensible heat loss is determined by the difference in water temperature and in the amount of water flowing in and out of pipes situated within the walls of the chamber where the subject has been placed. Heat removed by the vaporization of water is calculated from the moisture of the air leaving the calorimeter and being absorbed in sulfuric acid. Although the concept of direct calorimetry is relatively simple, direct measurement of body heat loss is expensive, cumbersome, and usually rather unpleasant for the subject or subjects involved [68]. Thus, basal metabolic rate is usually measured indirectly.

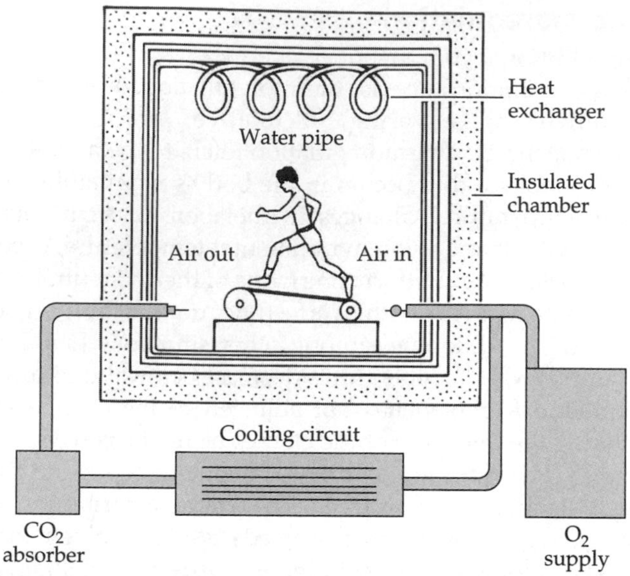

Figure 15.6 A simplified version of the human calorimeter used to measure direct body heat loss (i.e., energy expenditure).

Indirect Calorimetry

Indirect calorimetry measures the consumption of oxygen and the expiration of carbon dioxide. Urinary nitrogen excretion should also be measured, because for every 1 g of nitrogen excreted, ~6 L oxygen is consumed and 4.8 L carbon dioxide is produced [69,71]. Oxygen consumption and carbon dioxide production are measured via portable equipment that may be placed on an individual, enabling collection and analysis of expired air and quantification of inspired air. The exchange of oxygen and carbon dioxide is proportional to metabolism.

The amount of energy expended can be calculated from the ratio of the carbon dioxide expired to the oxygen inhaled. This ratio is known as the respiratory quotient (RQ). Examination of respiratory quotients provides meaningful information with respect to both energy expenditure and overall substrate oxidation. However, with regard to substrate oxidation, no information about metabolism in individual organs and tissues is gained [69]. A brief discussion of the use of the respiratory quotient to assess substrate oxidation is presented next, followed by discussion of the use of the respiratory quotient to determine energy expenditure.

Substrate Oxidation and the Respiratory Quotient

An RQ equal to 1.0 suggests that carbohydrate is being oxidized, because the amount of oxygen required for the combustion of glucose equals the amount of carbon dioxide produced, as shown here:

$$C_6H_{12}O_6 + 6\,O_2 \longrightarrow 6\,CO_2 + 6\,H_2O$$

$$RQ = 6\,CO_2/6\,O_2 = 1.0$$

The RQ for a fat is <1.0 because fat is a much less oxidized fuel source. For example, a fat such as tristearin, as shown in the following reaction, requires 163 mol oxygen for the production of 114 mol carbon dioxide:

$$2\,C_{57}H_{110}O_6 + 163\,O_2 \longrightarrow 114\,CO_2 + 110\,H_2O$$

$$RQ = 114\,CO_2/163\,O_2 = 0.70$$

Calculating the RQ for protein oxidation is more complicated, because metabolic oxidation of amino acids requires removing the nitrogen and some oxygen and carbon as urea, a urinary excretory compound. Urea nitrogen represents a net loss of energy to the body, and only the remaining carbon chain of the amino acid can be oxidized in the body. The following reaction illustrates the oxidation of a small protein molecule into carbon dioxide, water, sulfur trioxide, and urea:

$$C_{72}H_{112}N_{18}O_{22}S + 77\,O_2 \longrightarrow 63\,CO_2 + 38\,H_2O + SO_3 + 9\,CO(NH_2)_2$$

The RQ of this small protein molecule is equal to 0.818.

The average figures 1.0, 0.7, and 0.8 are accepted as the representative RQs for carbohydrate, fat, and protein, respectively. The RQ for an ordinary mixed diet consisting of the three energy-producing nutrients is usually considered to be ~0.85. An RQ of 0.82 represents the metabolism of a mixture of 40% carbohydrate and 60% fat [53]. RQs that are actually computed from gaseous exchange and that come closer to 1.0 or nearer to 0.7 would indicate that more carbohydrate or fat, respectively, was being used for fuel. In clinical practice, an RQ <0.8 suggests that a patient may be underfed and an RQ <0.7 suggests starvation or ingestion of a low-carbohydrate or high-alcohol diet, whereas an RQ >1.0 suggests that lipogenesis is occurring [69].

Energy Expenditure

Once the RQ has been computed from gaseous exchange, the calculation of energy expended is rather simple. Table 15.12 gives the caloric value for 1 L of oxygen and for 1 L of carbon dioxide given various RQs. When the amount of oxygen and/or carbon dioxide in the exchange has been determined, the total caloric value represented by the exchange can be calculated. It is also possible to determine the amount of carbohydrate and fat being oxidized in the production of these calories.

For example, if under standard conditions for the determination of BMR a person consumed 15.7 L oxygen per hour and expired 12.0 L carbon dioxide, the RQ

Table 15.12 Thermal Equivalent of O_2 and CO_2 for Nonprotein RQ

Nonprotein RQ	Caloric Value 1 L O_2	Caloric Value 1 L CO_2	Source of Calories: Carbohydrate (%)	Source of Calories: Fat (%)
0.707	4.686	6.629	0	100
0.71	4.690	6.606	1.10	98.9
0.72	4.702	6.531	4.76	95.2
0.73	4.714	6.458	8.40	91.6
0.74	4.727	6.388	12.0	88.0
0.75	4.739	6.319	15.6	84.4
0.76	4.751	6.253	19.2	80.8
0.77	4.764	6.187	22.8	77.2
0.78	4.776	6.123	26.3	73.7
0.79	4.788	6.062	29.9	70.1
0.80	4.801	6.001	33.4	66.6
0.81	4.813	5.942	36.9	63.1
0.82	4.825	5.884	40.3	59.7
0.83	4.838	5.829	43.8	56.2
0.84	4.850	5.774	47.2	52.8
0.85	4.862	5.721	50.7	49.3
0.86	4.875	5.669	54.1	45.9
0.87	4.887	5.617	57.5	42.5
0.88	4.899	5.568	60.8	39.2
0.89	4.911	5.519	64.2	35.8
0.90	4.924	5.471	67.5	32.5
0.91	4.936	5.424	70.8	29.2
0.92	4.948	5.378	74.1	25.9
0.93	4.961	5.333	77.4	22.6
0.94	4.973	5.290	80.7	19.3
0.95	4.985	5.247	84.0	16.0
0.96	4.998	5.205	87.2	12.8
0.97	5.010	5.165	90.4	9.58
0.98	5.022	5.124	93.6	6.37
0.99	5.035	5.085	96.8	3.18
1.00	5.047	5.047	100	0

Source: Adapted from McArdle W, Katch F, Katch V. *Exercise Physiology*, 2nd ed. Philadelphia: Lea and Febiger, 1986, p. 127.

The original source is Weber. Die Bedeutung de verschiedenen Nährstoffe als Erzeuger der Muskelkraft. Pflgers Archiv zur Physiologie, 1901:83(1):557–71.

would be 12.0/15.7, or 0.7643. From Table 15.12, the caloric equivalent for an RQ of 0.76 is 4.751 for 1 L oxygen or 6.253 for 1 L carbon dioxide. Based on the caloric equivalent for oxygen, calories produced per hour are 15.7 × 4.751, or 74.59. Based on the caloric equivalent for carbon dioxide, calories produced per hour are 12.0 × 6.253, or 75.04. If we then use 75 kcal/h as the caloric expenditure, then under basal conditions the BMR for the day would be ~1,800 kcal (75 kcal/h × 24 h). At this RQ of 0.76, fat is supplying almost 81% of energy expended (Table 15.12).

Because under ordinary circumstances the contribution of protein to energy metabolism is so small, the oxidation of protein is ignored in the determination of the so-called nonprotein RQ. If a truly accurate RQ is required, a correction, though minimal, can be made by measuring the amount of urinary nitrogen over a specified time period. As mentioned earlier, for every 1 g of nitrogen excreted, ~6 L oxygen is consumed and 4.8 L carbon dioxide is produced. The amount of oxygen and carbon dioxide exchanged in the release of energy from protein can then be subtracted from the total amount of measured gaseous exchange.

Measurement of the energy expended in various activities has also been made primarily through indirect calorimetry. The method for measuring gas exchange, however, differs from that used for determining BMR. The subject performing the activity for which energy expenditure is being determined inhales ambient air, which has a constant composition of 20.93% oxygen, 0.03% carbon dioxide, and 78.04% nitrogen. Air exhaled by the subject is collected in a spirometer (a device used to measure respiratory gases) and is analyzed to determine how much less oxygen and how much more carbon dioxide it contains compared with ambient air. The difference in the composition of the inhaled air and the exhaled air reflects the energy release from the body [53]. A lightweight portable spirometer (Fig. 15.7) can be worn during the performance of almost any sort of activity, and thus freedom of movement outside the laboratory is possible. In the laboratory, the Douglas bag is routinely used to collect expired air [53].

Tables are available that list the kilocalories expended per kilogram body weight per minute or hour for a wide variety of activities. Table 15.13, an example of such a table, groups various activities together according to their average level of energy expenditure. Information on the energy needs associated with physical activities, coupled with the information on basal or resting energy needs derived from indirect calorimetry, allows assessment to be made of the total energy needs of an individual. Table 15.14 provides information on the energy expended on various activities and on basal metabolism for individuals of different body weights.

Doubly Labeled Water

The doubly labeled water method also allows for the assessment of total energy expenditure of individuals. In this technique, a stable isotope of water is given to individuals as $H_2{}^{18}O$ and as ^2H_2O, and the disappearance of the $H_2{}^{18}O$ and ^2H_2O is measured in the blood and urine for about 3 weeks. The disappearance of the $H_2{}^{18}O$ is representative of the flux of water (i.e., water turnover) and of the production rate of carbon dioxide. The disappearance of the ^2H_2O represents water

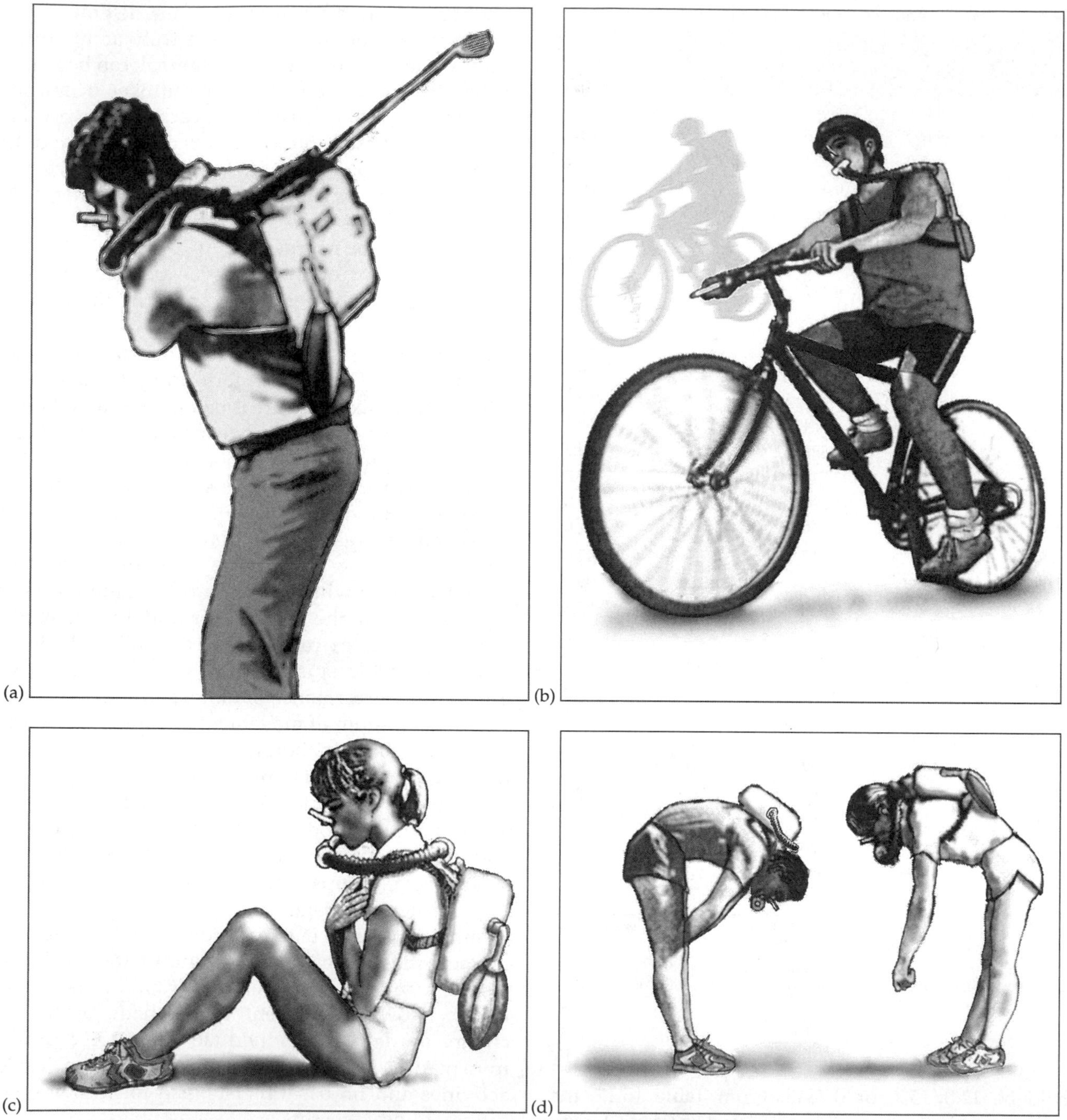

Figure 15.7 Measurement of oxygen consumption by portable spirometer during (a) golf, (b) cycling, (c) sit-ups, and (d) calisthenics.

turnover alone. Thus, the difference between the disappearance rate of $H_2{}^{18}O$ and that of ${}^{2}H_2O$ corresponds to the production rate of carbon dioxide. To assess oxygen consumption, a food quotient (FQ) is calculated from diet records kept by the individuals throughout the time period. In subjects maintaining body weight, the food quotient is equal to the respiratory quotient. Oxygen consumption, and thus energy expenditure, may be calculated from the FQ and carbon dioxide production.

Use of the doubly labeled water method to assess total energy expenditure has been shown to be accurate with good correlation with indirect calorimetry. The main source of error in the technique lies with the use of

Table 15.13 The Energy Cost above Basal Associated with Different Activities

Energy Level	Type of Activity	Energy (kcal/kg/minute*) Woman	Man
a	Sleeping or lying still, relaxed†	0.000	0.000
b	Sitting or standing still (such as sewing, writing, eating)	0.001–0.007	0.003–0.012
c	Very light activity (driving a car, walking slowly on level ground)	0.009–0.016	0.014–0.022
d	Light exercise (sweeping, eating, walking normally, carrying books)	0.018–0.035	0.023–0.040
e	Moderate exercise (fast walking, dancing, bicycling, cleaning vigorously, moving furniture)	0.036–0.053	0.042–0.060
f	Heavy exercise (fast dancing, fast uphill walking, hitting tennis ball, swimming, gymnastics)	0.055	0.062

*Measured in kilocalories per kilogram per minute above basal energy. Where ranges are given, pick the midpoint within the range, unless you have reason to believe you are unusually relaxed or energetic when performing the activity. For example, for "sitting," a man should normally pick 0.007; if he is sitting very relaxed, 0.003; if very tense, 0.012.

†For purposes of this table, these are assumed to be at the basal level of activity.

Source: Modified from Whitney E, Cataldo C. *Understanding Normal and Clinical Nutrition*, St. Paul, MN: West, 1983.

food records, which may not necessarily be accurate, and with the calculation of oxygen consumption from the food quotient [65].

Derived Formulas

In contrast to the doubly labeled water technique, which has been adapted for use in humans only since the 1980s, estimating basal metabolic rate or resting energy expenditure rather than measuring it has been the practice among clinicians since about 1925. Many different methods for estimating energy needs have been used over the years. Estimations have been based on body surface area, body weight, and/or calculations from regression equations that take into account the person's gender, age, weight, and height and have been shown to correlate with measurements from indirect calorimetry or from doubly labeled water.

One estimate of basal metabolic rate for all mammals, including humans, is based on body weight raised to the power of 0.75 [66,72]. The equation BMR (kcal/day) $= 70 \times W^{0.75}$ uses weight (W) measured in kilograms and raised to the power of 0.75 multiplied by 70 for estimating BMR. Table 15.15 provides sample body weights raised to the power of 0.75 to aid the reader in performing calculations.

Because of the relatively narrow range of human body size, calculations from the preceding equation give an estimate that is reasonably close to the BMR value obtained from the formula of 1 kcal/kg/h for men and 0.9 kcal/kg/h for women.

Using the two formulas to estimate the BMR of a 70-kg man illustrates their comparable results:

1. $\text{BMR} = 70 \times 700^{0.75} = 70 \times 24.2 = 1{,}694$ kcal/day
2. $\text{BMR} = 1\ \text{kcal} \times 70\ \text{kg} \times 24\ \text{hours} = 1{,}680$ kcal/day

---

The derived regression equations probably most often used [73] to estimate BMR in the clinical setting are those derived by Harris and Benedict in 1919 based on indirect calorimetry [74], and only slightly modified. Using the Harris-Benedict equations, BMR (kilocalories per day) is predicted in separate equations for men and women based on weight in kilograms (W), height in centimeters (H), and age in years (A):

$$\text{Men: BMR} = 66.5 + (13.7 \times W) + (5.0 \times H) - (6.8 \times A)$$

$$\text{Women: BMR} = 655.1 + (9.56 \times W) + (1.85 \times H) - (4.7 \times A)$$

Other equations, by Mifflin and St. Jeor [75], predict REE (kilocalories per day) for men and women as follows:

$$\text{Men: REE} = (10 \times W) + (6.25 \times H) - (5 \times A) + 5$$

$$\text{Women: REE} = (10 + W) + (6.25 \times H) - (5 \times A) - 161$$

A female who is 35 years old, weighs 125 lb (56.82 kg), and is 5 ft 5 in. tall (165.1 cm) would have a BMR of 1,339 kcal (using the Harris-Benedict equation) and an REE of 1,264 kcal (using the Mifflin–St. Jeor equation).

The various equations used to calculate energy expenditure are reevaluated regularly in scientific literature. Reevaluations have shown that predicted values for BMR are often higher than the actual expenditure and may not be applicable to all individuals, for example, those who are obese [73,76]. Thus, dietitians must be alert to the literature for recent findings and recognize the limitations and implications of the use of the various equations.

Table 15.14 Energy Expended on Various Activities*

Activity	kcal/lb/min†	kcal/min at Different Body Weights				
		110 lb	125 lb	150 lb	175 lb	200 lb
Aerobic dance (vigorous)	0.062	6.8	7.8	9.3	10.9	12.4
Basketball (vigorous, full court)	0.097	10.7	12.1	14.6	17.0	19.4
Bicycling						
13 mph	0.045	5.0	5.6	6.8	7.9	9.0
15 mph	0.049	5.4	6.1	7.4	8.6	9.8
17 mph	0.057	6.3	7.1	8.6	10.0	11.4
19 mph	0.076	8.4	9.5	11.4	13.3	15.2
21 mph	0.090	9.9	11.3	13.5	15.8	18.0
23 mph	0.109	12.0	13.6	16.4	19.0	21.8
25 mph	0.139	15.3	17.4	20.9	24.3	27.8
Canoeing (flat water, moderate pace)	0.045	5.0	5.6	6.8	7.9	9.0
Cross-country skiing						
8 mph	0.104	11.4	13.0	15.6	18.2	20.8
Golf (carrying clubs)	0.045	5.0	5.6	6.8	7.9	9.0
Handball	0.078	8.6	9.8	11.7	13.7	15.6
Horseback riding (trot)	0.052	5.7	6.5	7.8	9.1	10.4
Rowing (vigorous)	0.097	10.7	12.1	14.6	17.0	19.4
Running						
5 mph	0.061	6.7	7.6	9.2	10.7	12.2
6 mph	0.074	8.1	9.2	11.1	13.0	14.8
7.5 mph	0.094	10.3	11.8	14.1	16.4	18.8
9 mph	0.103	11.3	12.9	15.5	18.0	20.6
10 mph	0.114	12.5	14.3	17.1	20.0	22.9
11 mph	0.131	14.4	16.4	19.7	22.9	26.2
Soccer (vigorous)	0.097	10.7	12.1	14.6	17.0	19.4
Studying	0.011	1.2	1.4	1.7	1.9	2.2
Swimming						
20 yd/min	0.032	3.5	4.0	4.8	5.6	6.4
45 yd/min	0.058	6.4	7.3	8.7	10.2	11.6
50 yd/min	0.070	7.7	8.8	10.5	12.3	14.0
Table tennis (skilled)	0.045	5.0	5.6	6.8	7.9	9.0
Tennis (beginner)	0.032	3.5	4.0	4.8	5.6	6.4
Walking (brisk pace)						
3.5 mph	0.035	3.9	4.4	5.2	6.1	7.0
4.5 mph	0.048	5.3	6.0	7.2	8.4	9.6
Wheelchair basketball	0.084	9.2	10.5	12.6	14.7	16.8
Wheeling self in wheelchair	0.030	3.3	3.8	4.5	5.3	6.0

*The values listed in this table reflect both the energy spent in physical activity and the amount used for BMR.
†To calculate kcalories spent per minute of activity for your own body weight, multiply kcal/lb/min by your exact weight and then multiply that number by the number of minutes spent in the activity. For example, if you weigh 142 lb, and you want to know how many kcalories you spent doing 30 min of vigorous aerobic dance: 0.062 × 16 = 8.8 kcal/min, 8.8 × 30 (min.) = 264 kcal spent total.
Source: Whitney EN, Rolfes SR. *Understanding Nutrition*, 9th ed. Belmont, CA: Wadsworth Thompson Learning, 2002, p. 248.

Use of the Harris-Benedict or Mifflin–St. Jeor equations, among other formulas mentioned, provides information on an individual's basal or resting energy needs. To determine total energy needs for an individual, the energy required for physical activity must be added to the energy needed for basal needs. Depending on the type, duration, intensity, and frequency of physical activity, energy needs for physical activity may vary from ~20% to 70% or more of basal metabolism. Activity factors can be multiplied by basal energy calculations to address the energy needs of physical activity.

Using the formulas, for example, a person with basal energy needs of 1,580 kcal who does little activity (i.e., sedentary) may expend only ~20% of kilocalories per day being physically active and thus would require 1,580 kcal basal + (1,580 kcal × 0.20 activity) = 1,580 kcal basal + 316 kcal activity = 1,896 kcal. This calculation also may be written as 1,580 kcal basal × 1.20 activity factor = 1,896 kcal. Energy needed for the thermic effect of food is not included in many equations used to calculate total energy needs,

Table 15.15 Body Weights in Kilograms Raised to the Power of 0.75

Weight (kg)	Weight$^{0.75}$ (kg)	Weight (kg)	Weight$^{0.75}$ (kg)
1	1.0	51	19.1
2	1.68	52	19.4
3	2.28	53	19.6
4	2.83	54	19.9
5	3.34	55	20.2
6	3.83	56	20.5
7	4.30	57	20.8
8	4.75	58	21.0
9	5.19	59	21.3
10	5.62	60	21.6
11	6.04	61	21.8
12	6.44	62	22.1
13	6.84	63	22.4
14	7.24	64	22.6
15	7.62	65	22.9
16	8.00	66	23.2
17	8.38	67	23.4
18	8.75	68	23.7
19	9.10	69	23.9
20	9.46	70	24.2
21	9.8	71	24.4
22	10.2	72	24.7
23	10.5	73	25.0
24	10.8	74	25.2
25	11.2	75	25.5
26	11.5	76	25.8
27	11.8	77	26.0
28	12.2	78	26.2
29	12.5	79	26.5
30	12.8	80	26.7
31	13.1	81	27.0
32	13.5	82	27.2
33	13.8	83	27.5
34	14.1	84	27.7
35	14.4	85	28.0
36	14.7	86	28.2
37	15.0	87	28.5
38	15.3	88	28.7
39	15.6	89	29.0
40	15.9	90	29.2
41	16.2	91	29.4
42	16.5	92	29.7
43	16.8	93	29.9
44	17.1	94	30.2
45	17.4	95	30.4
46	17.7	96	30.7
47	18.0	97	30.9
48	18.2	98	31.1
49	18.5	99	31.4
50	18.8	100	31.6

Source: Adopted from Pike R, Brown M. *Nutrition: An Integrated Approach*, 3rd ed. New York: Macmillan (formerly Wiley), 1984, p. 749.

but when it is used a value of 10% of basal energy needs is usually used. Thus, using the above example and including the thermic effect of foods (TEF) in the calculation, a person with basal energy needs of 1,580 kcal would need another 1,580 kcal basal × 0.10 TEF = 158 kcal for TEF. Total energy needs would be 1,580 kcal + 316 kcal + 158 kcal, or 2,054 kcal.

Based on data on total daily energy expenditure measured by the doubly labeled water method, the Food and Nutrition Board has developed several equations to calculate estimated energy requirements (EER). For an adult, "the estimated energy requirement is defined as the dietary energy intake that is predicted to maintain energy balance in a healthy adult of a defined age, gender, weight, height, and level of physical activity consistent with good health" [65]. Formulas to calculate the estimated energy requirements for adults follow:

Adult men: EER = 662 – (9.53 × age) + PA (15.91 × weight + 539.6 × height)

Adult women: EER = 354 – (6.91 × age) + PA (9.36 × weight + 726 × height)

where age is in years, weight is in kilograms (kg), and height is in meters (m) [65]. PA in the equation refers to physical activity coefficients and varies with the level of activity and with gender. PA values for different physical activity levels are given below. The appropriate PA value should be inserted into the EER equation to calculate total energy expenditure.

PA Values for Different Physical Activity Levels [65]				
Gender	Sedentary	Low active	Active	Very active
Men	1.00	1.11	1.25	1.48
Women	1.00	1.12	1.27	1.45

Adults are individuals 19 years of age or older. These formulas apply to individuals with healthy body weights (BMI of 18.5 to 25 kg/m^2). The formula for women is applicable to women who are not pregnant or lactating.

summary

Although differences in weight for height among individuals have traditionally been used for estimating recommended body weight, height-weight tables and formulas provide limited information about true body composition. Presently, estimations of body composition for the general public are derived from anthropometric measurements. With an accurate measure of height, weight, and skin folds from selected areas of the body, the percentage of body fat can be determined. Then, by difference, lean body mass can be estimated. Certain skin fold or circumference measurements, as well as use of more elaborate equipment such as DEXA and bioelectrical impedance analysis, can also provide some information about distribution of body fat, a factor that may be as important to health as or even more important to health than percentage of total body fat.

Despite the differences in the various body components that have been noted among individuals and population groups, it is clear that the component showing the greatest variability is the one over which we have the most control—total body fat. Although changes in energy balance produce weight changes, the extent of these changes varies from person to person. One of the greatest problems in making predictions of energy needs centers around estimations of energy expenditure. Energy expenditure has three defined components: basal metabolic rate, thermic effect of foods, and the effect of exercise or physical activity, none of which is constant.

References Cited

1. Weigley ES. Average? Ideal? Desirable? A brief review of height-weight tables in the United States. J Am Diet Assoc 1984;84:417–23.

2. National Institutes of Health. Clinical Guidelines on the Identification, Evaluation, and Treatment of Overweight and Obesity in Adults. Bethesda, MD: National Institutes of Health, National Health, Lung, and Blood Institute, 1998.

3. Abernathy R, Black D. Healthy body weights: an alternative perspective. Am J Clin Nutr 1996;64(suppl3):448S–51S.

4. Sandowski S. What is the ideal body weight? Family Practice 2000;17:348–51.

5. Build Study 1979. Chicago: Society of Actuaries and Association of Life Insurance Medical Directors of America, 1980.

6. Callaway CW. Weight standards: their clinical significance. Ann Intern Med 1984;100:296–98.

7. Schulz LO. Obese, overweight, desirable, ideal: where to draw the line in 1986? J Am Diet Assoc 1986;86:1702–4.

8. U.S. Dept. of Agriculture and U.S. Dept. of Health and Human Services. Nutrition and Your Health: Dietary Guidelines for Americans, 3rd ed. Washington, DC: USDA, 1990.

9. Marwick C. Obesity experts still say less weight is still best. JAMA 1993;269:2617–18.

10. www.health.gov/dietaryguidelines

11. Flegal K, Carroll M, Ogden C, Johnson C. Prevalence and trends in obesity among U.S. adults, 1999–2000. JAMA 2002;288:1723–27.

12. Devine BJ. Gentamicin therapy. Drug Intell Clin Pharm 1974; 8:650–55.

13. Robinson J, Lupklewica S, Palenik L, Lopez L, Ariet M. Determination of ideal body weight for drug dosage calculations. Am J Hosp Pharm 1983;40:1016–19.

14. Frisancho AR. Anthropometric standards for the assessment of growth and nutritional status. Ann Arbor, MI: University of Michigan Press, 1990, p. 28.

15. Grant A, DeHoog S. Anthropometry. In: Nutritional Assessment and Support, 3rd ed. Seattle: Grant, 1985, p. 11.

16. Giannini VS, Giudici RA, Nerrukk DL. Determination of ideal body weight. Am J Hosp Pharm 1984;41:883–87.

17. Behnke AR, Feen BG, Welham WC. The specific gravity of healthy men. JAMA 1942;118:495–98.

18. Friis-Hansen B. Body composition in growth. Pediatrics 1971; 47:264–74.

19. Mitchell HH, Hamilton TS, Steggerda FR, Bean HW. The chemical composition of the adult human body and its bearing on the biochemistry of growth. J Biol Chem 1945;158:625–37.

20. Widdowson EM, McCance RA, Spray CM. The chemical composition of the human body. Clin Sci 1951;10:113–25.

21. Forbes RM, Cooper AR, Mitchell HH. The composition of the human body as determined by chemical analysis. J Biol Chem 1953;203:359–66.

22. Clarys JP, Martin AD, Drinkwater DT. Gross tissue weights in the human body by cadaver dissection. Hum Biol 1984;56:459–73.

23. Behnke AR, Wilmore JH. Evaluation and Regulation of Body Build and Composition. Englewood Cliffs, NJ: Prentice Hall, 1974.

24. Katch FI, McArdle WD. Introduction to Nutrition, Exercise, and Health, 4th ed. Philadelphia: Lea and Febiger, 1993, pp. 223–58.

25. McArdle WD, Katch FI, Katch VL. Exercise Physiology, 3rd ed. Philadelphia: Lea and Febiger, 1991.

26. Barr SI, McCargar LJ, Crawford SM. Practical use of body composition analysis in sport. Sports Med 1994;17:277–82.

27. Forbes GB. Human Body Composition—Growth, Aging, Nutrition and Activity. New York: Springer-Verlag, 1987.

28. Moore FD, Olesen KH, McMurrey JD, et al. The body cell mass and its supporting environment: body composition in health and disease. Philadelphia: Saunders, 1963.

29. Foman SJ, Haschke F, Ziegler EE, Nelson SE. Body composition of reference children from birth to age 10 years. Am J Clin Nutr 1982;35:1169–75.

30. Fomon S, Nelson S. Body composition of the male and female reference infant. Ann Rev Nutr 2002;22:1–18.

31. Boileau RA, Lohman TG, Slaughter MH, et al. Hydration of the fat-free body in children during maturation. Hum Biol 1984; 56:651–66.

32. Lohman TG. Research relating to assessment of skeletal status. In: Body Composition Assessment in Youth and Adults. Report of the Sixth Ross Conference on Medical Research. Columbus, OH: Ross Laboratories, 1985, pp. 38–41.

33. Siri WE. Gross composition of the body. In: Lawrence JH, Tobias CA, eds. Advances in Biological and Medical Physics. New York: Academic Press, 1956, pp. 239–80.

34. Tepperman J, Tepperman HM. Metabolic and Endocrine Physiology, 5th ed. Chicago: Year Book Medical, 1987.

35. Baker ER. Body weight and the initiation of puberty. Clin Obstet Gynecol 1985;28:573–79.

36. Cohn SH, Vartsky D, Yasumura S, Vaswani AN, Ellis KJ. Indexes of body cell mass: nitrogen versus potassium. Am J Physiol 1983;244:E305–10.

37. Nieman DC. Fitness and Sports Medicine: An Introduction. Palo Alto: Bull, 1990.

38. Cohn SH, Vaswani AN, Yasumura S, Yuen K, Ellis KJ. Improved models for determination of body fat by in vivo neutron activation. Am J Clin Nutr 1984;40:255–59.

39. Forbes GB, Reina JC. Adult lean body mass declines with age: some longitudinal observations. Metabolism 1970;19:653–63.

40. Garn SM, LaVelle M, Rosenberg KR, Hawthorne VM. Maturational timing as a factor in female fatness and obesity. Am J Clin Nutr 1986;43:879–83.

41. Borken GA, Hults DE, Gerzof SG, et al. Comparison of body composition in middle-aged and elderly males using computed tomography. Am J Phys Anthropol 1985;66:289–95.

42. Komiya S. Aging, total body water and fat mass in males between ages 9 and 77 years. Ann Physiol Anthropol 1984;3:149–51.

43. Heymsfield SB, Matthews D. Body composition: research and clinical advances. JPEN 1994;18:91–103.

44. Seidell J, Visscher T. Body weight and weight change and their health implications for the elderly. Eur J Clin Nutr 2000;54:S33–39.

45. Fulop T, Worum I, Csongor J, Foris G, Leovey A. Body composition in elderly people. Gerontology 1985;31:6–14.

46. Brozek J, Grande F, Anderson JT, Keys A. Densitometric analysis of body composition: revision of some quantitative assumptions. Ann NY Acad Sci 1963;110:113–40.

47. Clarys JP, Martin AD, Drinkwater DT, Marfell-Jones MJ. The skinfold: myth and reality. J Sports Sci 1987;5:3–33.

48. Sinning WE, Dolny DG, Little KD, et al. Validity of "generalized" equations for body composition analysis in male athletes. Med Sci Sports Exerc 1985;17:124–30.

49. Harrison GG, Buskirk ER, Carter JEL, Johnston FE, et al. Skinfold thicknesses and measurement technique. In: Lohman TG, Roche AF, Martorell R. Anthropometric Standardization Reference Manual. Champaign, IL: Human Kinetics Publishers, 1988, pp. 55–80.

50. Martorell R, Mendoza F, Mueller WH, Pawson IG. Which side to measure: right or left. In: Lohman TG, Roche AF, Martorell R. Anthropometric Standardization Reference Manual. Champaign, IL: Human Kinetics Publishers, 1988, pp. 87–91.

51. Lukaski HC. Methods for the assessment of human body composition: traditional and new. Am J Clin Nutr 1987;46:537–56.

52. Van der Kooy K, Seidell JC. Techniques for the measurement of visceral fat: a practical guide. Internl J Obesity 1993;17:187–96.

53. McArdle WD, Katch FI, Katch VL. Exercise Physiology, 2nd ed. Philadelphia: Lea and Febiger, 1986.

54. Pace N, Rathbun EN. Studies on body composition: III. The body water and chemically combined nitrogen content in relation to fat content. J Biol Chem 1945;158:685–91.

55. Jebb AS, Murgatroyd PR, Goldberg GR, Prentice AM, Coward WA. In vivo measurement of changes in body composition: description of methods and their validation against 12-d continuous whole-body calorimetry. Am J Clin Nutr 1993;58:455–62.

56. Jensen MD. Research techniques for body composition assessment. J Am Diet Assoc 1992;92:454–60.

57. Genant H, Engelke K, Fuerst T, Gluer C, Grampp S, Harris S, Jergas M, Lang T, Lu Y, Majumdar S, Mathur A, Takada M. Noninvasive assessment of bone mineral and structure: state of the art. J Bone Min Res 1996;11:707–30.

58. Fuller MF, Fowler PA, McNeill G, Foster MA. Imaging techniques for the assessment of body composition. J Nutr 1994;124:1546S–50S.

59. Fanelli MT, Kuczmarski RJ. Ultrasound as an approach to assessing body composition. Am J Clin Nutr 1984;39:703–9.

60. Garrow JS. New approaches to body composition. Am J Clin Nutr 1992;35:1152–58.

61. Andres R. Mortality and obesity: the rationale for age-specific height-weight tables. In: Andres R, Bierman EL, Hazzard WR, eds. Principles of Geriatric Medicine. New York: McGraw-Hill, 1985, pp. 311–18.

62. Danforth E. Diet and obesity. Am J Clin Nutr 1985;41:1132–45.

63. Food and Nutrition Board, Commission on Life Sciences, National Research Council. Recommended Dietary Allowances, 10th ed. Washington, DC: National Academy Press, 1989, pp. 24–38.

64. Ravussin E, Bogardus C. A brief overview of human energy metabolism and its relationship to essential obesity. Am J Clin Nutr 1992;55:242S–45S.

65. Food and Nutrition Board. Dietary Reference Intakes for Energy, Carbohydrates, Fiber, Fat, Protein, and Amino Acids. Washington, DC: National Academy Press, 2002.

66. Grande F. Body weight, composition and energy balance. In: Olson RE, Broquist HP, Chichester CO, Darby WJ, Kolbye AC, Jr, Stalvey RM, eds. Nutrition Reviews' Present Knowledge in Nutrition, 5th ed. New York: The Nutrition Foundation, 1984, pp. 7–18.

67. Welle S, Nair K. Relationship of resting metabolic rate to body composition and protein turnover. Am J Physiol 1990;258:E990–98.

68. Horton ES. Introduction: an overview of the assessment and regulation of energy balance in humans. Am J Clin Nutr 1983;38:972–77.

69. Jequier E, Acheson K, Schutz Y. Assessment of energy expenditure and fuel utilization in man. Ann Rev Nutr 1987;7:187–208.

70. Webb P. Human Calorimeters. New York: Praeger, 1985.

71. Westerterp KR. Food quotient, respiratory quotient, and energy balance. Am J Clin Nutr 1993;57:759S–65S.

72. Garrow JS. Energy balance in man—an overview. Am J Clin Nutr 1987;45:1114–19.

73. Daly JM, Heymsfield SB, Head CA, Harvey LP, Nixon DW, Katzeff H, Grossman GD. Human energy requirements: overestimation by widely used prediction equation. Am J Clin Nutr 1985; 42:1170–74.

74. Harris J, Benedict F. A Biometric Study of Basal Metabolism in Man. Publication 279. Washington, DC: Carnegie Institution, 1919.

75. Mifflin MD, St Jeor ST, Hill LA, Scott BJ, Daugherty SA, Koh YO. A new predictive equation for resting energy expenditure in healthy individuals. Am J Clin Nutr 1990;51:241–47.

76. Roth-Yousey L, Reeves R, Frankenfield D. Let the evidence speak: indirect calorimetry and weight management guides. Food and Nutrition Conference and Expo, San Antonio, TX, 2003.

perspective

Eating Disorders

Despite its increasing prevalence in our society, obesity is still generally considered unacceptable. Few things can create as large a sensation in the media as a new weight reduction diet guaranteed to remove that unwanted fat. The authors of the sensational new diet are interviewed on television talk shows, newspapers give publicity to the new diet (and its authors), and the book promoting the "new and revolutionary" diet joins its companions on the shelves of all bookstores. The fact that the new diet book has so many companions on the bookshelves attests to the fact that none of these "new and revolutionary" diets is successful in helping people reduce weight and keep it off. Nevertheless, following some sort of weight reduction diet appears to be a way of life among many Americans, particularly women.

The desire by girls and women to be thin has a foundation: the ideal female body image is dictated to a large extent by fashion magazines, *Playboy* centerfolds, and beauty pageant contestants. Society considers thin to be healthy. In fact, the body mass index of the winners of the Miss America pageant since 1922 has significantly declined over time, with recent winners considered undernourished, having body mass indices between 16.9 and 18.5 [1]. Children as young as 9 years of age have been found curtailing their food intake to avoid becoming fat [2]. A female's body size too often impacts her self-worth and self-esteem. Body image distress results when individuals become dissatisfied with their weight, and, if the individuals are of the belief that their weight and shape are central to their self-worth as a person, an eating-disorder mindset often ensues [3]. Eating disorders are particularly prevalent among young females. In fact, 90% to 95% of those affected by anorexia nervosa and bulimia are young, white females from middle- and upper-middle-class families; relatively few cases have been documented in males [4].

The incidence of eating disorders has consistently increased [5]. The prevalence of anorexia nervosa among U.S. adolescent girls and young women is estimated to be between 2% and 3% using the criteria of the American Psychiatric Association [6]. The estimated prevalence of bulimia nervosa is thought to be higher, ranging from 3% to 19% in adolescents and college-age females [7,8]. If the criteria of the American Psychiatric Association were not used, the prevalence of eating disorders or disordered eating likely would be much higher.

Anorexia Nervosa

Being too thin is dangerous, even deadly. Of the many psychiatric disorders, anorexia nervosa possesses the highest mortality rate [9]. If left untreated, ~18% to 20% of individuals with anorexia nervosa die within a 20-year period [10,11]. Given that this condition often affects children before they hit puberty, death may occur in persons only in their 20s or 30s.

Anorexia nervosa, described over 100 years ago as "loss of appetite due to a morbid mental state," is actually misnamed because its victims do not experience loss of appetite unless they have reached a moribund state. Anorectics relentlessly pursue thinness, remaining thin through self-inflicted starvation and excessive amounts of strenuous exercise. Individuals with anorexia nervosa have a distorted body image and fear weight gain. Moreover, women who develop anorexia nervosa tend to be perfectionists. They often have a poor self-image and want to please others because their perceived self-worth is heavily dependent on the words and actions of others (such as teachers, coaches, or instructors).

Diagnostic criteria for anorexia nervosa (Table 1) include refusal to maintain at least 85% of normal weight for height (or a body mass index of at least 17.5 kg/m^2), denial of a low current body weight, fear of gaining weight (failure to show expected weight gain during growth), and **amenorrhea** (absence of at least three consecutive menstrual cycles) [12]. Preoccupation with food and abnormal food consumption patterns are also typical of anorexia nervosa.

Eating patterns of individuals with anorexia nervosa mostly fall into one of two categories: the restricting type or the binge eating–purging type. Anorectics with the restricting type will eat to a limited extent without regularly inducing vomiting or misusing laxatives or diuretics. Individuals with the binge eating–purging type alternate between restricting food intake and bouts of binge eating or purge behavior with laxative and/or diuretic misuse or self-induced vomiting [13,14].

The cause(s) of anorexia nervosa are unknown, but the disease seems to be multifactorial. At least two sets of issues and behaviors are entangled. Issues include those concerning food and body weight and those involving relationships with oneself and with others [15,16]. Conflict regarding maturation and problems with separation, sexuality, self-esteem, and compulsivity

Table 1 Diagnostic Criteria for 307.1 Anorexia Nervosa

A. Refusal to maintain body weight at or above a minimally normal weight for age and height (e.g., weight loss leading to maintenance of body weight less than 85% of that expected; or failure to make expected weight gain during period of growth, leading to body weight less than 85% of that expected).
B. Intense fear of gaining weight or becoming fat, even though underweight.
C. Disturbance in the way in which one's body weight or shape is experienced, undue influence of body weight or shape on self-evaluation, or denial of the seriousness of the current low body weight.
D. In postmenarcheal females, amenorrhea, i.e., the absence of at least three consecutive menstrual cycles. (A woman is considered to have amenorrhea if her periods occur only following hormone, e.g., estrogen, administration.)

Specify type:

Restricting Type: during the current episode of Anorexia Nervosa, the person has not regularly engaged in binge-eating or purging behavior (i.e., self-induced vomiting or the misuse of laxatives, diuretics, or enemas)

Binge-Eating/Purging Type: during the current episode of Anorexia Nervosa, the person has regularly engaged in binge-eating or purging behavior (i.e., self-induced vomiting or the misuse of laxatives, diuretics, or enemas)

Source: Reprinted with permission from the Diagnostic and Statistical Manual of Mental Disorders, Text Revision, Copyright 2000. American Psychiatric Association.

often are associated with the development of anorexia nervosa [15]. A genetic basis for the condition also has been suggested.

The initial weight loss of the anorectic may not always be the result of a deliberate decision to diet; weight loss may occur unintentionally, for example, as the result of the flu or a gastrointestinal disorder [13]. However, following the initial weight loss, whatever its cause, additional diet restriction (often coupled with excessive exercise to induce further weight loss) is deliberate. Weight loss or control of body weight becomes the overriding goal in life, especially during stressful periods when pressures become overwhelming [13]. The anorectic learns the caloric contents of foods and the energy expenditure associated with various activities. Because anorectics have such a disturbed body image and such an intense fear of becoming fat, they may continue starving themselves to emaciation and even death should intervention be delayed too long.

The effects of anorexia nervosa on the body are similar to the effects of starvation (that is, protein-calorie malnutrition or **marasmus**). Growth and development slow. Adipose tissue, lean body mass, and bone mass are lost. Organ mass may be lost, and/or organ function may become impaired. Loss of heart muscle can result in the weakening of the heart and an irregular heartbeat, among other serious complications. The gastrointestinal tract atrophies such that peristalsis is slowed, gastric emptying is delayed, and intestinal transit time is lengthened. The secretion of digestive enzymes as well as digestive juices also is diminished. Constipation often results, along with abdominal distention after eating just small amounts of food. Hormone and nutrient levels in the blood become altered. Skin typically becomes dry, hair loss from the head occurs while **lanugo**-type (soft woolly) hair may appear on the sides of the face and arms, and body temperature drops. Table 2 lists some potential consequences of anorexia nervosa.

Table 2 Some Potential Medical Complications of Anorexia Nervosa

Gastrointestinal	Hematologic
Gastric distention	Anemia
Constipation	
	Skeletal
Cardiovascular	Stress fractures
Heart muscle atrophy	Premature osteoporosis
Bradycardia	
Hypotension	Muscle
Arrhythmias	Depleted muscle mass
Mitral valve prolapse	
Peripheral edema	Brain
	Abnormal electrical activity
Endocrine/metabolic	Confusion
Amenorrhea	
Low body temperature	

Treatment of anorexia nervosa is multidisciplinary (involving physician, dietitian, nurse, psychologist, psychiatrist, and family therapist, among others) and may be accomplished through outpatient and/or inpatient care depending on the severity of the individual's condition. Assessment for inpatient treatment generally includes an evaluation of the individual's mental status, how much the individual is eating, current weight (inpatient if <25%–30% of ideal), speed of weight loss, motivation and compliance, family support, purging behavior, and comorbid complications, especially those affecting the heart [9,16]. Whether the patient is treated as an inpatient or as an outpatient, goals for the patient's health are established, often with a written contract signed by the patient as well as by members of the health care team.

Summaries of treatment outcomes involving thousands of individuals treated for anorexia nervosa show that the majority (~40%–50%) of individuals recover completely, ~30% improve, 20% to 25% continue to experience chronic problems with the condition, and another 10% to 15% die due to medical complications, suicide, or malnutrition [7,17,18]. Mortality typically is highest in individuals who have exhibited severe weight loss, who have had the condition for a prolonged duration, and who developed the condition at an older age [6,7,16].

A long-term consequence of anorexia nervosa is osteoporosis, which occurs much earlier in those who have (or have had) anorexia nervosa than in those who have not suffered from the condition. Osteoporosis is associated with the amenorrhea and weight loss that occurs with anorexia nervosa. Factors associated with anorexia nervosa such as poor energy and nutrient (especially vitamin D and calcium) intakes, low blood estrogen concentrations, high blood cortisol concentrations, and low insulinlike growth factor 1 concentrations contribute to the problem. Adolescents with anorexia nervosa are less likely to reach peak bone mass. Bone formation is impaired and bone resorption increased in adolescents and women with anorexia nervosa, leading to diminished bone mineral density, premature osteoporosis, and increased fracture risk [19,20]. Bone mineral density has been shown to be significantly correlated with the age of onset and the duration of anorexia nervosa [20]. While weight gain and the resumption of normal menstrual function can improve bone mineral density, the bones do not appear to catch up to normal to correct the deficit that occurred during the amenorrhea [21]. Studies investigating the effectiveness of hormone replacement and other drugs for the treatment of osteoporosis associated with anorexia nervosa in young women are ongoing.

Bulimia Nervosa

Bulimia nervosa, another eating disorder, is a condition characterized by recurring binge eating coupled with self-induced vomiting and misuse of laxatives, diuretics, or other medications to prevent weight gain. Binge eating is marked by a sense of lack of control over eating during the binge episode. A binge is defined as eating an amount of food larger than most people would eat during a similar time period and under similar circumstances [12]. Bulimia denotes a ravenous appetite (or "ox hunger") associated with powerlessness to control eating [13]. Criteria [12] for the diagnosis of bulimia nervosa are given in Table 3.

Bulimia occurs primarily in young women, especially college-age women who are of normal weight or slightly overweight. The typical bulimic, rather than being overly concerned with losing weight and becoming very thin (like the individual with

Table 3 Diagnostic Criteria for 307.51 Bulimia Nervosa

A. Recurrent episodes of binge eating. An episode of binge eating is characterized by both of the following:
   (1) eating, in a discrete period of time (e.g., within any 2-hour period), an amount of food that is definitely larger than most people would eat during a similar period of time and under similar circumstances
   (2) a sense of lack of control over eating during the episode (e.g., a feeling that one cannot stop eating or control what or how much one is eating)
B. Recurrent inappropriate compensatory behavior in order to prevent weight gain, such as self-induced vomiting; misuse of laxatives, diuretics, enemas, or other medications; fasting; or excessive exercise.
C. The binge eating and inappropriate compensatory behaviors both occur, on average, at least twice a week for 3 months.
D. Self-evaluation is unduly influenced by body shape and weight.
E. The disturbance does not occur exclusively during episodes of Anorexia Nervosa.

Specify type:

Purging Type: during the current episode of Bulimia Nervosa, the person has regularly engaged in self-induced vomiting or the misuse of laxatives, diuretics, or enemas.

Nonpurging Type: during the current episode of Bulimia Nervosa, the person has used other inappropriate compensatory behaviors, such as fasting or excessive exercise, but has not regularly engaged in self-induced vomiting or the misuse of laxatives, diuretics, or enemas.

Source: Reprinted with permission from the Diagnostic and Statistical Manual of Mental Disorders, Text Revision, Copyright 2000. American Psychiatric Association.

anorexia nervosa), seeks to be able to eat without gaining weight [13]. Other factors associated with the development of bulimia include a history of sexual abuse, psychoactive substance abuse or dependence, and/or a family history of depression or alcoholism [7,22].

Bulimia often starts with dieting attempts in which hunger feelings get out of control. These dieting attempts, usually based on food abstinence or excessive food restriction, lead to binge eating. Once binge eaters discover that they can undo the consequences of their overeating by vomiting the ingested food, they begin to binge not only when they are hungry but also when they are experiencing any distressing emotion [7,13]. Most binge eating is done privately in the afternoon or evening, with an intake of about 3,500 kcal [23,24]. Favorite foods for binging usually are dessert and snack foods very high in carbohydrates. Embarrassment usually prevents the bulimic from revealing his or her food-related behavior even to those closest to him or her [4].

Diagnosis is usually dependent on self-reported symptoms or on treatment for related problems or conditions. Conditions that may develop as the result of bulimia are listed in Table 4. The gastrointestinal tract is greatly affected by repeating vomiting and the use of laxatives. Repeated vomiting also causes other problems, including skin lesions or calluses on the dorsal side of the hands (especially over the joints), severe dental erosion, swollen enlarged neck glands, reddened eyes, headache, and fluid and electrolyte imbalances. Laxative misuse may exacerbate fluid and electrolyte losses and, when coupled with vomiting, may lead to heart arrhythmias and heart failure. The presence of lesions or calluses on the hands, the swollen neck glands, and the frequent trips to the bathroom after meals often are recognized by health professionals and family or friends and facilitate detection and diagnosis of the problem.

Table 4 Some Potential Medical Complications of Bulimia Nervosa

Gastrointestinal	Cardiovascular
Erosion of the teeth	Arrhythmias
Dental caries	
Sore throat	Respiratory and skeletal
Swollen parotid glands	Aspiration pneumonia
Esophageal rupture or tears	Rib fracture
Stomach tear	
Gastroesophageal reflux disease	Endocrine/metabolic
Constipation	Irregular menses or amenorrhea
Cathartic colon	Electrolyte imbalance

The treatment of bulimia, like that of anorexia nervosa, is multidisciplinary. Goals typically focus on the elimination of binge-purge behaviors, normalization of eating habits, weight maintenance, and resumption of normal menses if affected [7]. The patient is most likely to be hospitalized with problems such as electrolyte imbalance, drug (e.g., laxatives, diuretics) dependence, severe depression, or suicidal tendencies [7]. The prognosis of those suffering from bulimia nervosa is similar to those with anorexia nervosa. About 50% of individuals recover, but about half of these continue to have some abnormal eating habits; another 30% continue to have a nonspecified eating disorder [7].

Disordered Eating

Eating disorders (Table 5) [12] other than anorexia nervosa or bulimia nervosa also are present within the U.S. population. The characteristics of disordered eating are similar to those of anorexia nervosa and bulimia and include fear of being fat, restrained eating, binge eating, purge behavior, and distorted body image; however, individuals with disordered eating do not meet the criteria for anorexia nervosa or bulimia nervosa (Tables 1 and 3) [25]. Disordered eating is common among female athletes and often exists as part of what is known as the female athlete triad.

The female athlete triad, defined as the combination of disordered eating, amenorrhea, and osteoporosis, was first described in 1992 [26]. The condition appears most often in women participating in sports in which physique and body image are important and/or extra body weight is undesirable. Women most at risk include long-distance runners, figure skaters, gymnasts, ballet dancers, and swimmers and divers [7,21,27]. However, because of societal pressures to be thin and because of the perfectionist tendencies of many females, all female athletes are at risk for the female athlete triad [28].

Disordered eating among athletes is common, with an estimated prevalence of 15% to 62%. The disordered eating, however, can vary considerably. To lose or maintain body weight, some athletes may restrict food intake mildly to severely while

Table 5 307.50 Eating Disorder Not Otherwise Specified

The Eating Disorder Not Otherwise Specified category is for disorders of eating that do not meet the criteria for any specific Eating Disorder. Examples include

1. For females, all of the criteria for Anorexia Nervosa are met except that the individual has regular menses.
2. All of the criteria for Anorexia Nervosa are met except that, despite significant weight loss, the individual's current weight is in the normal range.
3. All of the criteria for Bulimia Nervosa are met except that the binge eating and inappropriate compensatory mechanisms occur at a frequency of less than twice a week or for a duration of less than 3 months.
4. The regular use of inappropriate compensatory behavior by an individual of normal body weight after eating small amounts of food (e.g., self-induced vomiting after the consumption of two cookies).
5. Repeatedly chewing and spitting out, but not swallowing, large amounts of food.
6. Binge-eating disorder: recurrent episodes of binge eating in the absence of the regular use of inappropriate compensatory behaviors characteristic of Bulimia Nervosa.

Source: Reprinted with permission from the Diagnostic and Statistical Manual of Mental Disorders, Text Revision, Copyright 2000. American Psychiatric Association.

others may also use diet pills, diuretics, and laxatives. Still others may binge and purge.

While amenorrhea occurs in only 2% to 5% of women in the general population, 3% to 66% of female athletes experience amenorrhea [21]. The amenorrhea occurring in athletes may be primary or secondary. Generally, primary amenorrhea is found in females who by about age 14 years have not menstruated. Secondary amenorrhea refers to the absence of three to six menstrual cycles in a year in females who have previously had a regular menstrual cycle or to a 1-year absence of menstrual bleeding in females with previously irregular periods [21,29]. The causes of amenorrhea in athletes, as in women with eating disorders, are not clearly understood. They are thought to relate to synergistic effects of excessive amounts of physical activity and/or training, constant stress or anxiety, low amounts of body fat, weight fluctuations, and poor diet, especially an extreme energy (caloric) deficit [29,30]. The effect of these various factors is to evoke changes in the release of hormones such as follicular stimulating and luteinizing hormones that then lead to alterations in the release of estrogen and progesterone (among other hormones), which in turn can cause amenorrhea. The amenorrhea—more specifically, the diminished serum estrogen concentrations—in turn causes medical problems.

One main complication of an estrogen deficit is its effect on the body's skeletal system. Female athletes with amenorrhea and disordered eating have an increased risk for osteoporosis, which in young athletes has been defined as premature loss of bone, inadequate bone formation, or both with resulting low bone mass, stress fractures, and other orthopedic problems [30,31]. High levels of hormones such as cortisol, common in athletes, as well as extensive training regimens also can contribute to bone loss. While weight-bearing exercises promote bone mineralization to improve bone density, this protection is considerably diminished without estrogen [27]. Young athletes are losing bone during a phase of life when they should be accruing bone, and thus they are compromising the attainment of peak bone mass. Studies have found that over 50% of athletes with amenorrhea have low bone mass or bone densities at least one standard deviation below the mean [7,32,33]. As with others suffering from eating disorders, while resumption of menses helps improve bone mass, recovery from the loss of bone associated with amenorrhea is not thought to be complete [34–36].

The early identification and treatment of eating disorders are crucial if serious complications are to be avoided. Just as obesity is associated with increased risk for a variety of diseases, eating disorders are associated with a multitude of risks, including death. Combating eating disorders is difficult. Not only must the victims be treated, but the images and values of society must also be rehabilitated [37].

References Cited

1. Rubinstein S, Caballero B. Is Miss America an undernourished role model? JAMA 2000;283:1569.
2. Pugliese MT, Lifshitz F, Grad G, Fort P, Marks-Katz M. Fear of obesity. N Engl J Med 1983;309:513–18.
3. Devlin M, Zhu A. Body image in the balance. JAMA 2001;286:2159.
4. Herzog DB, Copeland PM. Eating disorders. N Engl J Med 1985;313:295–303.
5. Engles J, Johnston M, Hunter D. Increasing incidence of anorexia nervosa. Am J Psychiatry 1995; 152:1266–71.
6. Brown J, Mehler P, Harris R. Medical complications occurring in adolescents with anorexia nervosa. West J Med 2000:172:189–93.
7. Walsh J, Wheat M, Freund K. Detection, evaluation, and treatment of eating disorders. J Gen Intern Med 2000;15:577–90.
8. Rome E. Eating disorders. Obstet Gynec Clin N Am 2003;30:353–77.
9. Anzai N, Lindsey-Dudley K, Bidwell R. Inpatient and partial hospital treatment for eating disorders. Child Adoles Psych Clin N Am 2002;11:279–309.
10. Powers P, Santana C. Childhood and adolescent anorexia nervosa. Child Adol Psych Clin 2002; 11: 219–35.
11. Eckert E, Halmi K, Marchi P, Grove W, Crosby R. Ten year follow-up of anorexia nervosa: clinical course and outcomes. Psychol Med 1995;25:143–56.
12. Diagnostic and Statistical Manual of Mental Disorders, 4th ed. Washington, DC: American Psychiatric Association, 1994, pp. 544–45, 549–50.
13. Casper RC. The pathophysiology of anorexia nervosa and bulimia nervosa. Ann Rev Nutr 1986; 6:299–316.
14. Emerson E, Stein D. Anorexia nervosa: empirical basis for the restricting and bulimic subtypes. J Nutr Ed 1993;25: 329–36.
15. Reiff D, Reiff K. Position of the American Dietetic Association: nutrition intervention in the treatment of anorexia nervosa, bulimia nervosa, and binge eating. J Am Diet Assoc 1994;94:902–7.
16. Mehler P. Diagnosis and care of patients with anorexia nervosa in primary care settings. Ann Intern Med 2001;134:1048–59.
17. Treasure J, Schmidt U. Anorexia nervosa. Clin Evid 2002;7:824–33.
18. Steinhausen H. The outcome of anorexia nervosa in the 20th century. Am J Psychiatry 2002;159:1284–93.
19. Lucas A, Melton J, Crowson C, O'Fallon W. Long term risk among women with anorexia nervosa: a population-based cohort study. Mayo Clinic Proc 1999;74:972–77.
20. Katzman D. Osteoporosis in anorexia nervosa: a brittle future. Curr Drugs Targets—CNS & Neurolog Dis 2003;2:11–15.
21. Hobart J, Smucker D. The female athlete triad. Am Fam Physician 2000;61:3357–64,3367.
22. Johnson J, Cohen P, Kasen S, Brook J. Childhood adversities associated with risk for eating disorders or weight problems during adolescence or early adulthood. Am J Psychiatry 2002;159:394–400.
23. Muuss RE. Adolescent eating disorder: bulimia. Adolescence 1986;21:257–67.
24. Mitchell JE, Pyle RL, Eckert ED. Frequency and duration of binge-eating episodes in patients with bulimia. Am J Psychiatry 1981;138:835–36.
25. Mellin LM, Irwin CE, Scully S. Prevalence of disordered eating in girls: a survey of middle-class children. J Am Diet Assoc 1992;92:851–53.
26. Otis C, Drinkwater B, Johnson M, Loucks A, Wilmore J. ACSM Position Statement: The female athlete triad. Med Sci Sports Exerc 1997;29:i–ix.
27. Golden N. A review of the female athlete triad (amenorrhea, osteoporosis and disordered eating). Int J Adolesc Med Health 2002;14:9–17.

28. Smith A. The female athlete triad: causes, diagnosis, and treatment. Physic Sports Med 1996;24:67–76.

29. Sabatini S. The female athlete triad. Am J Med Sci 2001;322:193–95.

30. Kleposki R. The female athlete triad: a terrible trio implications for primary care. J Am Acad Nurs 2002;14:26–31.

31. Sanborn C, Horea M, Siemers B, Dieringer K. Disordered eating and the female athlete triad. Clin Sports Med 2000;19:199–213.

32. Snead D, Stubbs C, Weltman J, Evans W, Veldhuis J, Rogol A, Teates C, Weltman A. Dietary patterns, eating behaviors, and bone mineral density in women runners. Am J Clin Nutr 1992;56:705–11.

33. Rencken M, Chesnut C, Drinkwater B. Bone density at multiple skeletal sites in amenorrheic athletes. JAMA 1996;276:238–40.

34. Drinkwater B, Nilson K, Ott S, Chesnut C. Bone mineral density after resumption of menses in amenorrheic athletes. JAMA 1986;256:380–82.

35. Drinkwater B, Bruemner B, Chesnut C. Menstrual history as a determinant of current bone density in young athletes. JAMA 1990;263:545–48.

36. Keen A, Drinkwater B. Irreversible bone loss in former amenorrheic athletes. Osteoporosis Int 1997;4:311–15.

37. Bulimia among college students. Nutr Rev 1987;45:10–11.

Web Sites

www.anred.com
www.nationaleatingdisorders.org
www.nimh.nih.gov/public/eatingdisorder.cfm
www.questia.com

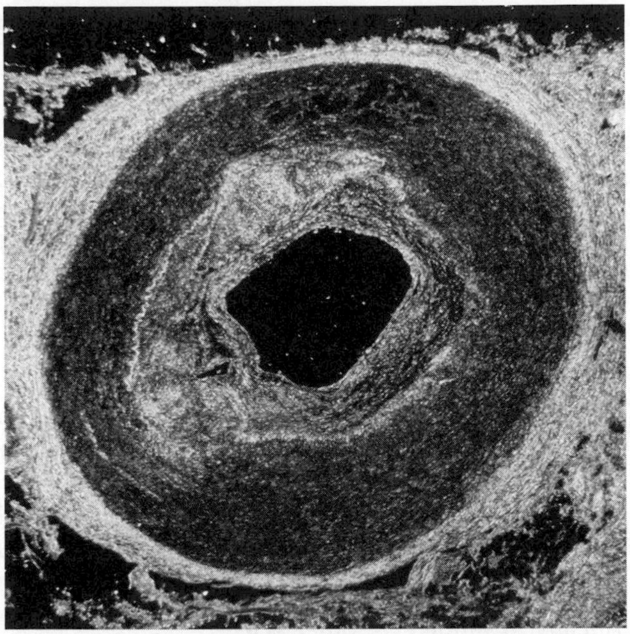

Atherosclerosis, a cross section through an obstructed artery

chapter 16

Experimental Design and Critical Interpretation of Research

RESEARCH IS A PROCESS THAT SEEKS, FINDS, AND TRANSFERS new knowledge. Although many definitions of research have emerged, probably none is more comprehensive and poignant than that taken from *Webster's Dictionary of the English Language:*

> ***Research:*** A studious inquiry or examination, especially a critical and exhaustive investigation or experimentation having for its aim the discovery of new facts and their correct interpretation, the revision of accepted conclusions, theories, or laws in the light of newly discovered facts or the practical application of such conclusions, theories, or laws.

At the core of this definition is that research discovers new facts (if there is no discovery, there was no research) and then correctly interprets those facts.

All of the information contained within this text was derived from research, and the reference list at the end of each chapter allows the reader to examine the source of the information. Publications cited in a bibliography reveal to the reader the premise or justification of the research, the experimental methodology by which it was conducted, and the author's interpretation of the results. Through such publications, findings and facts in the nutrition arena are routed through the appropriate scientific journals to the public. Perhaps more than any other discipline, nutrition furnishes an unrelenting barrage of news through the media, because nutrition touches the lives of all of us by appealing directly to our concept of good health. Unfortunately, along with the profusion of nutrition news comes the probing question as to what is reliable and what is not. It is imperative that the student of nutrition recognize this problem and learn to separate fact (derived from carefully constructed research) from fictional information passed along via anecdotal reports and hearsay.

The refereed or peer-reviewed journals offer the best source of information. The research procedures and results submitted by the investigator to these journals for publication are critically examined by other scientists knowledgeable in that particular area of research. This peer review process screens proposed publications for quality and soundness, ensuring the reliability of research papers that are ultimately published in that journal. Journals that feature nutrition-related investigations that have won the respect of practitioners over the years include *The American Journal of Clinical Nutrition, Nutrition Journal, Nutrition Reviews,* and *Journal of the American Dietetic Association.* Many other excellent journals frequently publish nutrition-related reports. Students who regularly consult the nutrition literature will learn to recognize these and distinguish them from weaker publications. The qualifications of the suppliers of information in other than peer-reviewed journals should be examined carefully and the reliability of the information judged accordingly.

As its title indicates, this chapter seeks to acquaint the reader with the various experimental methodologies (designs) available to the researcher and to offer information that may be helpful in both understanding research terminology and critiquing existing research publications.

THE SCIENTIFIC METHOD

Research uses a process referred to as the scientific method to solve problems or to resolve previously unanswered questions. The scientific method contains the following fundamental components:

1. *The research purpose or problem:* expresses the question to be answered or the problem to be solved
2. *The hypothesis:* a prediction of the outcome of the research that will follow and therefore a solution to the problem or an answer to the question
3. *Experimentation:* the conducting of the research itself using one of the many methodologies available to the researcher
4. *Interpretation or analysis:* interpreting the data collected from the experimentation so as to understand what it means
5. *Conclusion:* answers the originally posed question, and confirms or disproves the hypothesis
6. *Theory formulation:* a statement founded on the conclusion

Research can be thought of as occurring in a cyclic process, with the components of the scientific method arranged as illustrated in Figure 16.1. However, thinking of research in terms of a closed circle may be misleading. Research does not dead-end into finality with the theory statement. To the inquisitive mind of the researcher, a conclusion from one experiment invariably gives rise to new questions and problems. Research is therefore nonending, and its cyclic nature, as illustrated in Figure 16.1, may be more meaningfully represented as a spiral or helix, twisting inexorably upward toward a limitless goal.

Research design, particularly that which lends itself to the physical and biological sciences, must include the components listed. To be considered a fact, the theory formulated must be verified by other investigators who carry out the experiment under the same controlled conditions used in the original research. If the theory is verified, it becomes accepted as fact until further advances in research can disprove it.

Historical Applications

Antoine Lavoisier is credited with being the first to implement the scientific method in his research, which he conducted during the 18th century. Up until that time, inquiry into problems had been only a philosophical exercise. His approach to problem solving is illustrated by the following steps [1,2]:

- Using Priestley's earlier discovery that oxygen is involved in burning, Lavoisier formulated the hypothesis that respiration in animals was a form of combustion.
- Lavoisier carried out experimentation under controlled conditions on animals (guinea pigs). Oxygen consumption, heat production, and

Figure 16.1 The cyclic nature of research from theory to conclusion.

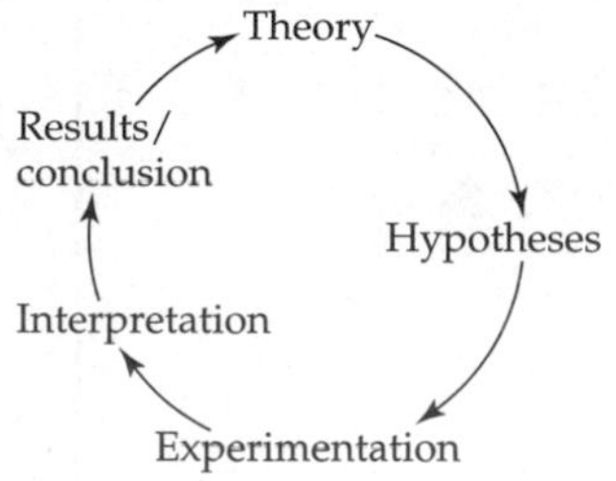

production of carbon dioxide by animals confined in airtight chambers were carefully measured.

- From the measurements (data) collected, Lavoisier interpreted the results: a pattern could be identified between oxygen consumption, carbon dioxide production, and heat emanating from the animal body.

- Based on his interpretation of the data, Lavoisier formulated the theory that consumption of oxygen is related to the amount of carbon burned or heat produced in the animal body. Then, to validate his theory, he performed similar controlled experiments on other animals, including humans.

THE INFLUENCE OF KNOWLEDGE BASE AND TECHNOLOGY ON RESEARCH: A HISTORICAL EXAMPLE

Nutrition research, designed to expand the nutrition knowledge base, began with Lavoisier's revelations about energy metabolism (around 1789) [2] and moved at a rather slow pace until the beginning of the 20th century. At about that time, many important discoveries and technological advances allowed a rapid expansion of the nutrition knowledge base. Nutrition research continued to flourish throughout the 20th century.

The cyclic nature of research makes clear that one prerequisite of productive research is an investigator who is familiar with the existing knowledge base of the subject under study and with how others have investigated the subject. This prerequisite is showcased admirably in the studies of Rose [3] and Young [4], who investigated the dietary essentiality of amino acids. Their studies are described briefly here. Though dated, they provide an example of well-planned research that emphasizes the cyclic nature of the investigative process.

A particularly fertile field in nutrition and biochemical research has been protein composition and metabolism. Scientific inquiry has been directed toward identification of the indispensable amino acids followed by quantitative determination of human requirements for these amino acids and for total protein. Rose, after comparing the work of previous investigators (Osbourne and Mendel, Fischer, and others) on the amino acid composition of proteins with that from his own laboratory, undertook the identification of those amino acids that are indispensable to animals and/or humans. He began his investigations with weanling rats and then extended them to humans (graduate students). The data obtained from rats were used as the starting point for the more difficult and costly studies on human beings. The experimental approach used by Rose was to keep a particular amino acid in the diet as the single independent variable and compare this with maximum weight gain as the criterion for the dependent variable. He found through a series of experiments that only 10 of the 19 to 20 amino acids ordinarily found in proteins are required by the rat: arginine, histidine, isoleucine, leucine, lysine, methionine, phenylalanine, threonine, tryptophan, and valine.

In his follow-up study on humans, Rose continued to use individual amino acids in the diet as the independent variable, but he used nitrogen equilibrium as the criterion for the dependent variable to determine indispensability. Rose's 13-year study on the indispensable amino acids and their requirements in the adult male (1942–1955) resulted in identification of those amino acids that are indispensable (essential) to human beings, their range of requirements, a tentatively proposed minimum requirement, and a definitely safe intake (Table 16.1). One troubling aspect of the study was the increased caloric intake required to maintain nitrogen equilibrium when subjects were fed amino acids rather than protein as their nitrogen source. In the discussion of his studies, Rose cites their limitations, noting particularly the small number of subjects, the artificiality of using diets containing mixtures of amino acids rather than proteins, and the attendant need for increased caloric intake on the part of the subjects. Rose concludes his studies by stating [3]:

> By reference to [Table 16.1], it should be possible to predict with reasonable accuracy how much of a given protein or diet, if its content of amino acids is known, would be required to maintain nitrogen equilibrium, provided the moderate quantity of extra nitrogen needed by the body for synthesis is already present or is added to the food. Such calculations must take account of the availability of the amino acids in the materials under investigation, since the processing and preservation of foods and their preparation for consumption may modify the nutritional usefulness of the component proteins. (p. 644)

Up to the present, these studies by Rose, published in 1957, have been used to a large degree as the basis for the estimation of adults' needs for the indispensable amino acids. They also have provided a basis for development of an amino acid pattern against which the biological value or "completeness" of a protein is measured.

The hypotheses comprising Rose's theory began to be tested by Young in the late 1960s, and those studies continue today. Young's research has contributed to the refinement of methods and procedures in assessing the amino acid needs of humans and is probably leading to a new, increased estimate of adults' amino acid requirements. The modification of the amino acid requirements in adult humans that may result from Young's research does not in any way negate the usefulness of Rose's

Table 16.1 The Daily Amino Acid Requirements of Young Men

Amino Acid	Number of Quantitative Experiments	Range of Requirements Recorded (g)	Minimum Proposed Tentatively (g)	Definitely Safe Intake (g)	Subjects in N Balance on Safe Intake or Less
L-tryptophan	3*	0.15–0.25	0.25	0.50	42
L-phenylalanine	6	0.80–1.10†	1.10	2.20	32
L-lysine	6	0.40–0.80	0.80	1.60	37‡
L-threonine	3§	0.30–0.50	0.50	1.00	29
L-methionine	6	0.80–1.10‖	1.10	2.20	23
L-leucine	5	0.50–1.10	1.10	2.20	18
L-isoleucine	4	0.65–0.70	0.70	1.40	17
L-valine	5	0.40–0.80	0.80	1.60	33

All values were determined with diets containing the eight essential amino acids and sufficient extra nitrogen to permit the synthesis of the nonessential amino acids.

*Fifteen other young men were maintained in nitrogen balance on a daily intake of 0.20 g, though their exact minimum needs were not established. Of the 42 subjects maintained on the *safe* intake or less, 33 had 0.30 g daily or less.

†These values were obtained with diets devoid of tyrosine. In two experiments, the presence of tyrosine was found to spare the phenylalanine requirement to the extent of 70% and 75%.

‡Ten of these subjects had an intake of 0.80 g or less.

§In addition to these 3 subjects, 4 young men had diets containing 0.60 g of L-threonine daily, and 16 others had 0.80 g daily. No attempt was made to determine the exact minimum requirements of these 20 subjects, but all were in positive balance on the amounts shown.

‖These values were obtained with diets devoid of cystine. In three experiments, the presence of cystine was found to spare the methionine requirement to the extent of 80% to 89%.

Source: Rose WC, Wixon RL, Lockhart HB, et al. The amino acid requirements of man, XV. The valine requirement: summary and observations. J Biol Chem 1955;217:992. Reprinted with permission.

theory. The research energy expended in rejecting a theory propels science even further ahead.

During the time of Young's research on amino acid metabolism, many weaknesses in the use of nitrogen balance as the dependent variable for studying protein metabolism have been identified. These weaknesses include the following:

1. Nitrogen equilibrium gives no specifics about protein metabolism in individual tissues or organs.
2. Results using the nitrogen balance technique often overestimate need because losses of nitrogen through the skin are seldom measured.
3. Nitrogen balance is significantly affected by energy intake.
4. Nitrogen balance can be greatly influenced by the length of the experimental period, which makes interpreting a specific nitrogen balance difficult.

As Young became aware of the limitations of nitrogen balance as a criterion for amino acid adequacy and as alternative methods for assessment of protein status became available (through technologic advances), he began a new series of studies on amino acid requirements in adults. An alternative dependent variable that Young used extensively during the late 1960s and early 1970s was the plasma amino acid response curve [5–8]. Subsequently, following the advent of stable isotopes, the tracing of amino acid distribution and use within the body became possible. As a consequence, distribution and use of an amino acid replaced the amino acid response curve as the dependent variable. Concurrently, by combining the isotope tracer technique with the measurement of nitrogen balance, Young collected some convincing evidence to support his hypothesis that adults need more of the indispensable amino acids than had been indicated through the measurement of nitrogen balance alone.

These examples of research efforts illustrate the effects on outcome of (1) a broadening of the knowledge base and (2) advances in technology. Young, unlike Rose, had available to him the knowledge of the positive effect of increased caloric intake on nitrogen balance and of other disadvantages associated with nitrogen balance studies. In addition, Young gained advantage from the advent of isotope tracer techniques and other technological advances.

RESEARCH METHODOLOGIES

Many different types, or classifications, of research exist. One of the broadest classifications of research is according to *application:* is the research basic or applied? Basic research seeks to expand existing knowledge by discovering new knowledge. Applied research, in contrast, seeks to solve problems primarily in a field setting. Other classifications of research may be according to *strategy* (historical, survey), *degree of experimental control* (experimental vs. nonexperimental), *time dimension* (cross-sectional vs. longitudinal), *setting* (laboratory, field), or *purpose* (descriptive or analytical).

Despite the diversity of research classifications, the methods by which research can be carried out are more concisely categorized. Two broad methodological approaches encompass essentially all research: *qualitative methods* and *quantitative methods.* They are distinguished from each other according to the nature of the data collected in the study. All the data emerging from a research study reaches the researcher in the form of either words or numbers. *If the data are verbal, the methodology is qualitative; if the data are expressed in numbers, the methodology is quantitative.* Within these major categories, four discrete subdivisions of methodological approaches can be used in research: historical methods and descriptive survey methods, both of which are qualitative approaches, and analytical survey methods and experimental methods, which are quantitative in nature. We will describe each of these methods, along with illustrative examples taken from the literature. The text by Leedy [9] provides a good review of research methodologies.

Historical Method (Qualitative)

Historical research seeks to explain the cause of past events and to interpret current happenings on the basis of these findings. Sources of information for the historical researcher are primarily documentary, existing in the form of written records and accounts of past events as well as literary productions and critical writings. The researcher relies, if possible, only on primary data, that is, data that are "firsthand" and therefore minimally distorted by the channels of communication. Generally, information gathered by historical research does not need to be analyzed by any form of statistical treatment or data analysis.

Descriptive Survey Method (Qualitative)

A word that distinguishes the descriptive survey method from other research methods is *observation.* The investigator observes, across a defined population group, whatever variable is under study. The variable may be physical (size, shape, color, strength, etc.) or cognitive (achievement, beliefs, attitudes, intelligence). The researcher first observes very closely the population bounded by the parameters that were set for the study and then carefully records what was observed for future interpretation. It is important to note that observation does not involve only visual perception but also (most likely) tests, questionnaires, attitude scales, inventories, and other evaluative measures. In fact, most descriptive surveys use well-designed questionnaires as the instrument of observation.

The keeping of records, which can be thought of as a preservation of facts, is an important feature of the descriptive survey method. Observation and record keeping are exemplified by the case study, which follows the symptomatology, treatment, conclusions, and recommendations as they apply to a patient under study. A case report is a report of observations on one subject, while a case series involves observations on more than one subject. Generally, the subjects being observed have a condition or disease in common. This form of research design is useful in attempts to identify variables or generate hypotheses that may be important in the etiology, care, or outcome of patients with a particular disease or condition.

An example of a case report is the investigation by Sedlet and Ireton-Jones [10]. These researchers studied energy expenditure in a patient who, on initial evaluation at an eating disorder clinic, presented with a semifast-binge eating pattern. Findings of the investigation were documented as a case report study, preliminary to further research. Energy expenditure in the subject was assessed prior to and following nutrition intervention. Basal energy expenditure (BEE) was estimated by the Harris-Benedict equation (Chap. 15). Actual measured energy expenditure (MEE) was determined by indirect calorimetry. The investigators found that the patient's BEE was 53% higher than her MEE when, on initial evaluation, she was in the semifast-binge eating pattern. Modification of her eating pattern to three meals a day, providing a total of ~1,200 kcal/day, was accomplished over a 4- to 6-week period. After the modification, her MEE increased and was essentially the same as her BEE (Table 16.2), whereas her activity level remained the same throughout treatment. The subject seemed more willing to continue the modified eating pattern (three meals per day) when she was able to eat each day and not gain weight.

Findings from this case report helped generate an ongoing research project to determine whether the data presented can be substantiated in a study involving a group of patients with bulimia. There is limited information about actual versus estimated energy

Table 16.2 Energy Intake versus Expenditure of JK (a bulimic patient)

Treatment Period	Intake (kcal/day range)	BEE (kcal/day)	MEE (kcal/day)	BEE/MEE (% difference)
Pretreatment semifast-binge	600–3,800	1,266	829	53
Nutrition counseling follow-up				
2 months	1,000–1,200	1,257	1,203	4
6 months	1,000–1,200	1,252	1,193	5
7 months	1,000–1,200	1,252	1,202	4

Source: Sedlet KL, Ireton-Jones CS. Energy expenditure and the abnormal eating pattern of a bulimic: a case report. J Am Diet Assoc 1989;89:16.

expenditure in bulimia and also about ways acceptable to patients to modify their food intake pattern.

The classic work of Goldberger on pellagra [11], involving observations of groups of children, illustrates a case series study. Goldberger described qualitatively the population and environment at two orphanages in Mississippi in 1914 as a preliminary study in his research on pellagra. By careful, systematic observation, he noted the following:

1. The incidence or absence of pellagra among both the orphan residents and the staff
2. Age groups affected by disease or free of the disease
3. Opportunity for close contact among groups
4. Sanitary conditions
5. Foods eaten by the different groups of residents and staff

In this preliminary inquiry, he found that the disease pellagra was confined almost exclusively to a group of 6- to 12-year-old children. The different diet given to the 6- to 12-year-old groups was the only factor he observed at this point that might explain the occurrence of the disease among these groups. The finding led him to test his hypothesis in later experimental dietary studies, eventually leading to our current knowledge that pellagra is caused by niacin deficiency. The prevalent theory at the time of Goldberger's work was that pellagra was an infectious disease spread by unsanitary conditions. Goldberger's ability as a researcher is demonstrated by his refusal to be constrained by prevailing beliefs.

Data for case series studies are often collected from existing records, and such studies are considered retrospective ("looking back") studies. A disadvantage of the retrospective study is that observations of the different variables of interest may not have been recorded in a standardized way and thus may not be comparable. Alternately, data for case series may be collected concurrently, providing an opportunity to standardize procedures. An advantage of case series studies is that they are relatively easy to perform and are inexpensive. They may provide data to justify the need for future analytic study, especially when the data are concerned with a condition or disease about which information is limited.

Bulimia (Perspective, Chap. 15), a disease requiring nutrition intervention but about which little is known, has been studied by observation. Pyle et al. [12] reported a case series study of 34 subjects with bulimia. Among the characteristics described were frequency of binge eating, fasting, self-induced vomiting, and use of laxatives. An eating pattern of binge eating combined with periods of fasting was common.

Other older but classic examples of descriptive survey studies are the Ten-State Nutrition Survey [13] and the National Health and Nutrition Examination Surveys (NHANES I, II, and III) [14, 15]. These surveys can also be classified as cross-sectional studies; that is, all subjects across the population were studied at approximately the same time, and each subject was studied once, not continuously.

The Ten-State Nutrition Survey was designed to oversample among low-income populations in selected states in the United States. Thus, application of the findings (external validity, to be discussed later) was limited, and results could not be applied to the U.S. population in general. Findings from the Ten-State Nutrition Survey provided some evidence for the need to expand food programs in low-income populations. The NHANES data, in contrast, were collected from a statistically selected sample to represent the 194 million noninstitutionalized civilians age 1 to 74 years in the United States. Data were collected systematically and by standardized methods of measurement from the sample population. The survey used both qualitative and quantitative methods. The NHANES data are considered baseline information for the U.S. population at the time of the survey.

Analytical Survey Method (Quantitative)

The analytical survey method is best described by contrasting it with the descriptive survey method just discussed. While the descriptive survey method involves observations that can be described in words and conclusions drawn from those words, the analytical survey uses a language not of words but of numbers. Because values obtained from an analytical survey are numerical, the data are said to be quantitative.

The quantitative data of an analytical survey are analyzed by statistical tools from which conclusions can be inferred. Statistical analysis of numerical data may include

- measures of central tendency (mean, median, mode),
- measures of dispersion (range, standard deviation, coefficient of variation), or
- measures of correlation (correlation coefficient, regression analysis).

These measurements fall within a category called descriptive statistics. Another category of statistics, called inferential statistics, has two principal functions:

1. To predict or estimate from a random sample a certain parameter in a general population
2. To test null hypotheses based on statistics

The null hypothesis postulates that there is no statistically significant difference between phenomena that occur by pure chance and the statistically evaluated behavior of the data as they have been observed by the researcher. As an illustration of the testing of the null hypothesis, suppose a study is to be conducted on the level of serum iron among vegetarians and nonvegetarian, omnivorous consumers. In keeping with a quantitative study, the data will be numerical, in this case, serum iron concentration expressed in milligrams per deciliter. Before the data are collected, the null hypothesis holds that there is no statistical difference in the criterion serum iron concentration between the two groups. If, in fact, the experimental statistical findings confirm this, the null hypothesis is said to be accepted. However, if it is shown that there is a statistically significant difference in the level of serum iron between the two groups, then the null hypothesis is rejected.

Observational research designs can also be included in the category of analytical surveys. The use of the word *observational* in describing this type of research may at first seem confusing, because observation is also the hallmark of descriptive surveys. Remember, however, that the observational research designs discussed here are examples of an analytical study and, as such, produce numerical, quantitative data that are interpretable by the application of statistics. Descriptive surveys, on the other hand, though based on observation, rely on written data and are qualitative, not quantitative.

Observational designs may take the form of epidemiological or cohort studies, neither of which involves experimentally induced changes in variables. **Epidemiology** has been defined as "the study of the distribution of a disease or condition in the population, and the factors that influence the distribution." A **cohort** is a group of subjects entered into a study at the same time and followed up at intervals over a period of time. A cohort study is also called a prospective ("looking ahead") study.

Three examples of observational nutrition-related studies are the classic Seven Countries Studies reported by Keyes [16], the Framingham Study [17], and the Nurses' Health Study [18]. In the Seven Countries Studies, the outcome of interest was coronary heart disease (CHD). Factors under consideration because of their possible association with CHD included dietary total calories, total fat, animal fat, saturated fat, total protein, animal protein, and sucrose. Data regarding CHD and the dietary factors were collected from population groups in each country by trained teams using systematic, standardized methods of measurement. Data were statistically analyzed for possible association of any of the studied dietary factors. Figure 16.2 shows the relationship of one dietary factor, saturated fat, to the incidence of CHD.

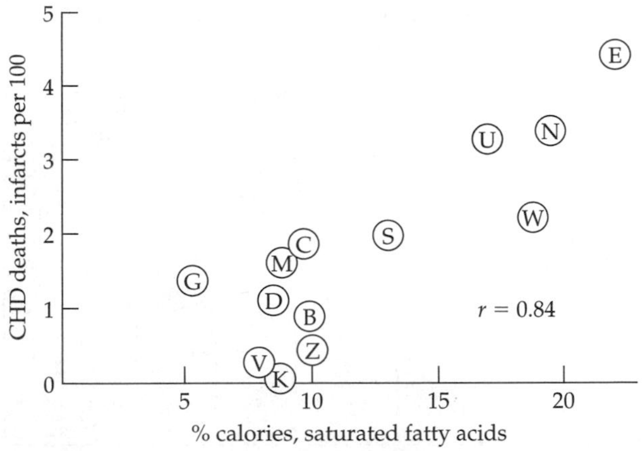

Figure 16.2 Diet-heart associations. B, Belgrade faculty; C, Crevalcore; D, Dalmatia; E, East Finland; G, Corfu; K, Crete; M, Montegiorgio; N, Zutphen; S, Slovonia; U, U.S. railroad; V, Velika Krsna; W, West Finland; Z, Zrenjanin. *Source:* Inter-society Commission for Heart Disease Resources, Atherosclerosis Group. Keys A, ed. Coronary heart disease in seven countries. Circulation 1970(1)42:211. Reprinted with permission.

The Framingham Study was a long-term, longitudinal study initiated in the town of Framingham, Massachusetts, in 1948. The term *longitudinal* refers to a study conducted on a group (cohort) over a certain period of time, a feature of the cohort study. The Framingham Study was designed to investigate the distribution of CHD in the sample population and possible causal factors associated with the disease. The study began with a cohort of 2,336 men and 2,873 women age 29 to 62 years, randomly selected from the population. Data regarding cardiovascular condition and possible causal factors of CHD were systematically collected from subjects at specified time intervals, using standardized methods of measurement. Data from the Framingham Study indentified hypercholesterolemia, hypertension, and cigarette smoking as three major risk factors in CHD. Information from that study was also used to show comparative risk at different levels of blood cholesterol (Fig. 16.3).

The Nurses' Health Study began in 1976 and continues to the present. This very large cohort (initially in excess of 122,000 participants) is composed of married, female registered nurses born between 1921 and 1946. The advantage of this cohort, in addition to its large size, is that the participants are broadly dispersed geographically, having been chosen from the 11 states with the largest number of registered nurses. Several of the studies conducted on this cohort have been based on the effect of diet on various health parameters, including cancer and cardiovascular disease. One such study resulted in the published finding that there appears to be no causal relationship between the intake of dietary total fat or specific major types of fat and breast cancer [19]. The finding was based on food-frequency questionnaires returned by 88,795 participants. It represents a refutation of the previously alleged, though

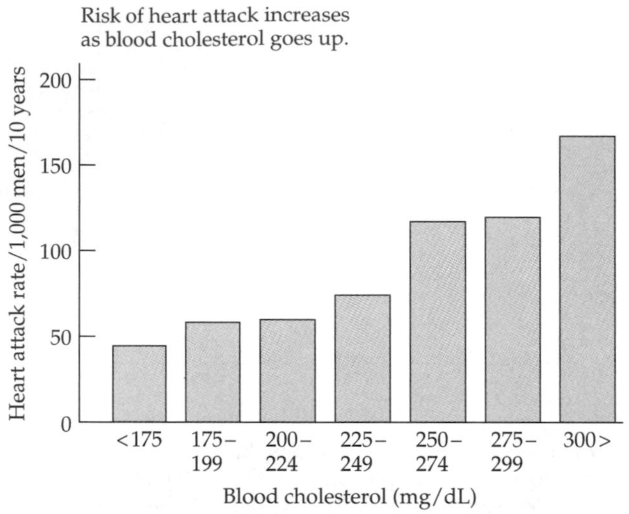

Figure 16.3 Risk of heart attack as related to blood cholesterol. *Source:* Inter-society Commission for Heart Disease Resources, Atherosclerosis Group. Primary prevention of atherosclerotic disease. Circulation Dec 1977;42:A55–95. Reprinted with permission.

not scientifically documented, connection between dietary fat and breast cancer.

The results and conclusions of an experiment, and eventually the establishment of scientific fact, ultimately depend on the statistical treatment of data, a field of considerable scope. This section is intended simply to acquaint the reader with some statistical terms commonly used in the analysis of numerical data. For the interested reader, many comprehensive texts on applied statistics offer a more in-depth treatment of the subject [20,21].

Experimental Method (Quantitative)

Among the research methodologies, the experimental method is the one most commonly encountered in the nutrition literature. The hallmark of the experimental method is control. So basic is control to this method that it is frequently referred to as the control group–experimental group design. Such a study uses two or more population groups with the subjects of each group matched, characteristic by characteristic, as closely as possible to the subjects of the other group(s). One group serves as a control and as such is not exposed to any extraneous change. The experimental group is exposed to the alteration under study, and whatever change is noted in this group relative to the subjects of the control group is presumed to be caused by the extraneous variable(s).

The experimental method can also use just one group, a method sometimes called a pretest-posttest approach. In its simplest form, a group of subjects is first evaluated (pretest) and then subjected to the experimental variable (test) and reevaluated (posttest). So-called crossover studies are also commonly used. In this type of study, a control group is not subjected to a particular experimental variable, while an experimental group is subjected to the variable, and differences in the data are noted. Then the original control group is exposed to the variable, therefore becoming the experimental group, and the original experimental group is not exposed to the variable and thus becomes the control group. This approach corrects for any inherent differences in the two groups that might confound the experimental data.

In short, the experimental method is based on cause and effect. It involves intervention on the part of the researcher, who introduces a variable and records its effect. Experimental research designs allow the investigator to control or manipulate one or more variables in an effort to examine the relationship between the variables. Variables typically are designated as dependent and independent. The independent variable is the variable controlled or manipulated by the investigator. The dependent variable occurs as the result of the influence of the independent variable. In other words, the dependent variable reflects the effects of the independent variable. As in the case of the analytical survey method, many traditional descriptive and inferential statistical tools can be used to analyze the data.

Because experimental methodology is so commonly used in nutrition research, numerous examples can be given to illustrate its use. Following are two classic illustrative examples of research employing the experimental method.

Experimental Atherogenesis

Armstrong et al. [22], using the experimental research design, tested the hypothesis that diet-induced **atheromas** (lipid plaques on the arterial wall) may regress in primates by use of appropriate diet (the independent variable). The investigators conducted their study with 40 adult male rhesus monkeys. To serve as controls, 10 of the monkeys were fed a low-fat, cholesterol-free diet throughout the study. The other 30 were fed the same low-fat, cholesterol-free diet for a control period of 6 weeks and then were fed a high-fat, high-cholesterol diet (an atherogenic diet, i.e., a diet conducive to lipid plaque formation) for 17 months. The composition of the diets is given in Table 16.3. The 30 monkeys were then divided into three groups matched for body weight and **hyperlipidemia** (the presence of excess fat or lipids in the blood).

Group 1, on the atherogenic diet, was autopsied for determination of baseline atherosclerosis. For 40 months, group 2 was fed a low-fat, cholesterol-free diet, and group 3, a linoleate-rich corn oil diet. All diets throughout the study included supplements to make them complete in all essential nutrients. Control and study animals were autopsied at the end of the study to determine the

Table 16.3 Major Characteristics of Diets

	Group 1 Atherogenic	Group 2 Low Fat	Group 3 Corn Oil
Protein	16	19	15
Carbohydrate	43	77	45
Fat	41	4	40
Cholesterol	1.2	0	0

Note: Values for protein, carbohydrate, and fat are percentages of total calories; cholesterol values are percentages by weight.

Source: Armstrong ML, Warner ED, Connor WE. Regression of coronary atheromatosis in rhesus monkeys. Cir Res 1970;27:60. Reprinted with permission.

Table 16.4 Luminal Narrowing (%)

	Main Coronary				
Group	Left	Right	LAD	L c'flex	R dist
1	60 ± 8	56 ± 7	53 ± 18	57 ± 9	65 ± 10
2	17 ± 4	14 ± 3	21 ± 4	22 ± 6	16 ± 5
3	25 ± 5	26 ± 3	30 ± 5	23 ± 6	18 ± 5

Abbreviations of branch arteries: LAD = left anterior descending; L c'flex = left circumflex; R dist = distal continuation of right main coronary artery. Values are means ± SE (standard error).

Source: Armstrong ML, Warner ED, Connor WE. Regression of coronary atheromatosis in rhesus monkeys. Cir Res 1970;27:60. Reprinted with permission.

degree of atheromatosis (the dependent variable). Autopsies showed that the cross-sectional area of the lumen of five major coronary arteries was significantly greater in monkeys fed the regression diets (group 2, low-fat diet; group 3, linoleate-enriched diet) than in the monkeys with baseline atherosclerosis (group 1). Table 16.4 provides a comparison of the groups. The investigators were able to show for the first time regression of atheromatosis in nonhuman primates by modification of diet.

Clinical Trial to Prevent Coronary Heart Disease (CHD)

The randomized clinical trial, an experimental research design, is frequently used in medical research studies involving humans. Clinical trials are usually conducted after preliminary trials have been done with experimental animals, and they typically test the benefits of one or more treatments. Subjects in clinical trials are those who have the condition to be treated and should be representative of the population to which results are to be applied. Subjects are assigned randomly to a treatment group. In some instances, only one treatment is available and a placebo is used for the control group. Subjects who enroll in the study must be informed that they have an equal chance of being assigned either to the treatment group or to the control (placebo) group. Ideally, to avoid bias, a clinical trial should be "double blind," with neither the subject nor the investigator knowing which group is which.

A classic example of a clinical trial is the Lipid Research Clinics Coronary Primary Prevention Trial (LRC-CPPT) [23]. This research project, sponsored by the National Heart, Lung, and Blood Institute of the National Institutes of Health (NIH), illustrates a number of important points that must be considered in the design of a randomized clinical trial.

The LRC-CPPT was undertaken to determine whether reducing blood cholesterol levels lowers the risk of CHD in humans. Earlier studies had shown that elevated blood cholesterol levels were a major risk factor in CHD. Numerous studies had also shown that blood cholesterol levels in animals and in humans could be reduced by diet and drugs. Previous clinical trials had not been considered conclusive because of a number of problems in research design. These previous clinical trials, however, along with findings from earlier studies (e.g., epidemiological studies, clinical investigations, and animal studies), were extremely useful in designing the LRC-CPPT. A particularly helpful aspect of the earlier clinical trials was the identification of pitfalls in experimental design, including absence of double-blind testing, too small sample size, treatment groups that were not identical, and questionable statistical procedures. Typical problems and pitfalls in research are considered later in the chapter.

In the LRC-CPPT, the study population consisted of people known to be at high risk for CHD. Those under consideration for the study, therefore, were men age 35 to 59 years who were asymptomatic for CHD but exhibited primary hypercholesterolemia (a plasma cholesterol ≥265 mg/dL). Subjects were 3,810 men, screened from ~48,000 age-eligible men. Informed consent was received from each subject entered into the trial.

Subjects were randomly selected to receive either the drug cholestyramine (a resin previously tested for safety and effectiveness in reducing total cholesterol and low-density lipoprotein cholesterol) or a placebo. Both subjects and investigators were unaware of the treatment assignment (i.e., it was double blind). A moderate cholesterol-lowering diet, designed to lower cholesterol levels by 3% to 5%, was prescribed to all subjects. Maintaining all the subjects on the same diet throughout the study minimized the opportunity for confounding the study results because of different dietary intakes.

Twelve lipid research clinics (LRCs) participated in the trial. To ensure comparability of data over the entire study period, a common protocol documenting all procedures in detail was adhered to by clinic personnel trained and certified in standardized procedures. All aspects of the study were carefully monitored by the Central Patient Registry and Coordinating Center and by the Program Office.

Table 16.5 Selected Variables before and during Treatment

Variable	Placebo Preentry	Placebo First Year	Placebo Seventh Year	Cholestyramine Resin Preentry	Cholestyramine Resin First Year	Cholestyramine Resin Seventh Year
Mean systolic blood pressure, mm Hg	121	120	122	121	120	122
Mean diastolic blood pressure, mm Hg	80	79	78	80	78	78
Mean Quetelet index, g/cm^2 **	2.6	2.6	2.7	2.6	2.6	2.7
Mean weight, kg	81	81	83	80	80	82
% current smokers	37	35	26	38	36	27
Mean cigarettes/d for current smokers	25	24	25	26	25	26
% regular exercisers	30	*	27	31	*	28
Median alcohol consumption, g/wk	61	58	51	64	57	53

*No assessment of exercise was done in the first year.

**QI = weight in g/(height in cm).

Source: Lipid Research Clinics Program: The Lipid Research Clinics Coronary Primary Prevention Trial Results. I. Reduction in incidence of coronary heart disease to cholesterol lowering, JAMA 1984;251:357.

Table 16.5 illustrates the close similarity of the drug and placebo groups before and during treatment for selected variables that include the major known risk factors for CHD. Any change in risk factors other than cholesterol levels during the treatment period could have posed an alternative explanation for the observed treatment benefit.

The results of the trial showed that the cholestyramine group experienced a 19% reduction in the risk of the primary end point (i.e., definite CHD death and/or definite nonfatal myocardial infarction). The data also showed that a 1% reduction in blood cholesterol level yields approximately a 2% reduction in CHD rates.

Subjects were followed for a minimum of 7 years and for as long as 10 years, with the average follow-up being 7.4 years. Subjects attended clinics every 2 months during the follow-up. At clinic visits, subjects received the drug or the placebo, dietary and drug counseling to encourage adherence, and standardized examinations and evaluations according to the detailed protocol. All subjects who entered the study were followed to the completion of the trial irrespective of their levels of adherence or frequency of visits. At the completion of the trial, contact was made with all men who discontinued visits during the trial. Thus, it was possible to know the vital status of every subject.

Experience in the LRC-CPPT met design goals in several features of the study, as shown in Table 16.6. Twenty-seven percent of subjects did not adhere (nonadherers) to taking cholestyramine for 7 years. This percentage was less than the expected goal of 35%. However, a nonadherer was defined as a subject taking less than half a packet of medication daily, and the prescribed dose was six packets of medication per day. Thus, many subjects considered to be adherers were not taking the total prescribed dose. As a consequence, the goal of 28% reduction in cholesterol levels of men assigned to cholestyramine treatment was not met. Actual reduction in cholesterol levels amounted to 13.9%. In addition, although the 19% reduction in the primary end point (incidence of CHD death) was well below the goal of 36%, the reduction in CHD deaths has been judged to be clinically significant.

Investigators in the LRC-CPPT expressed caution against extrapolating the results of the study to predict results from use of drugs that are not bile acid sequestrants like cholestyramine. In addition, the study was not designed to show whether lowering cholesterol by diet decreased CHD deaths. It is known, however, that cholesterol levels can be reduced by dietary modification, and findings from the LRC-CPPT support the view that lowering cholesterol by diet would be beneficial. That view was later strongly supported by the Consensus

Table 16.6 Comparision of LRC-CPPT* Design Goals and Actual Experience

Design Feature	Goal	Experience
Sample size	3,550	3,808†
Duration of follow-up, year	7	7–10
Lost to follow-up	0	0
Reduction of plasma total cholesterol levels in placebo group	4%	4.8%
Nonadherers‡ at year 7	35%	27%
Reduction of plasma total cholesterol levels in men adhering to cholestyramine resin treatment	28%	13.9%§
Seven-year incidence of primary end point in placebo group	8.7%	8.6%
Reduction in primary end point	36%	19%

*Lipid Research Clinics Coronary Primary Prevention Trial.

†After removal of four type III participants.

‡A nonadherer is someone averaging less than half a packet of cholestyramine resin per day.

§Computed for seventh year.

Source: Lipid Research Clinics Program: The Lipid Research Clinics Coronary Primary Prevention Trial Results. I. Reduction in incidence of coronary heart disease to cholesterol lowering. JAMA 1984;251:360.

Conference on lowering blood cholesterol to prevent heart disease [24]. The LRC-CPPT was a long, complex, expensive clinical trial. Nevertheless, the experimental design method involving randomized clinical trials can also be used for much less expensive studies.

TERMS THAT DESCRIBE RESEARCH QUALITY

Descriptive terms that reflect the effectiveness or quality of a research effort include

- validity,
- accuracy,
- reliability, and
- precision.

The "truth" of research lies within the validity of its collected data. Validity represents the extent to which the process or technique being used is measuring what it is supposed to be measuring. *Validity is concerned with the effectiveness of the measuring instrument.* The term *instrument,* as it applies in research, is broadly defined, with applications ranging from survey questionnaires to pieces of scientific equipment.

There are several types of validity. Face validity relies on the subjective judgment of the researcher and involves asking the following questions: (1) Is the instrument measuring what it is supposed to be measuring? (2) Does the sample being measured adequately represent the behavior or trait being measured? Criterion validity uses as an essential component a reliable and valid criterion (i.e., a standard against which to measure the results of the instrument that is doing the measuring). Validity can also be expressed as internal or external, and both types are very important in research. Internal validity refers to causal relationships, that is, whether an experimental treatment made (caused) a difference. External validity refers to the generalizability of the results of the research to a population group that was not studied.

The terms *accuracy* and *reliability* are related, because both are concerned with how close to the "truth" a measurement is. Accuracy is expressed as the difference between the measured values of an instrument and the true values. The more accurate a measurement, the closer the result is to the true value. Reliability refers to the instrument used in the study and indicates the degree of accuracy that it generates. An instrument may be reliable within a broad range of accuracy. This concept can be illustrated by the use of a sundial as an instrument for telling time. It is a reliable timepiece if one is concerned only with whether the time of day is early afternoon or late afternoon. However, the sundial has poor reliability for more specific timing, such as informing the observer when it is time to turn on the television to see a favorite show or to leave to catch a bus. In both of these cases, the sundial's accuracy—that is, the quantitatively expressed nearness of the measured time to the true time—is poor.

The term *precision* is a very useful expression of the consistency or repeatability of multiple analyses performed on the same sample or subject. Procedures used in research should generate the same data from the same sample with repetition. For example, multiple assays of serum glucose performed on the same serum sample provide an indication of the precision of the instrument used. It is important to understand the difference between precision and accuracy. A method may be highly precise (i.e., replicate values may be very close to one another) yet not be accurate. In contrast, widely disparate replicate values (i.e., poor precision) might yield an accurate average value. However, imprecise measurements are not a property of quality research.

INITIATION OF RESEARCH

The only prerequisite for initiation of research is an inquiring mind. The novice is likely to be intimidated by reports of sophisticated research that has required expensive equipment, extensive personnel, and a generous budget. Not all research needs to be conducted at this level. It can be simple and inexpensive while still serving the purpose of broadening the knowledge base.

Initiation of research requires familiarity with the characteristics of research. These characteristics are shown in Table 16.7. The first characteristic suggests that research begins with a question: Why does something occur, or what causes something? Research demands that the problem be identified and stated clearly. Research requires a plan. It seeks direction through hypotheses. Research deals with data and their meaning. And, as shown in Figure 16.1, research is circular. To be certain that all these characteristics are included in a research project, the following four steps should be followed [25]:

1. *Select the research topic or problem to be solved.* Choosing a topic or problem narrow enough to be manageable often can be difficult. A review of published literature in relation to the selected research topic is necessary in order to have a basis on which to build present research and precisely define the research.

2. *Clearly state the question to be researched.* Components of the question include who/which (i.e., the subjects or units being assessed are identified), what (i.e., the factor of interest is stated specifically), and how assessed (i.e., the outcome to be assessed is stated specifically).

Table 16.7 Checklist for the Evaluation of Research

1. Is the central problem for research (and its subproblems) clearly stated?
2. Does the research evidence plan and organization?
3. Has the researcher stated his or her hypotheses?
4. Are the hypotheses related to the principal problem or the subproblems of the research?
5. Are the assumptions stated? Are these assumptions realistic for the research undertaken?
6. Is the research methodology that has been employed clearly stated?
7. If the research is of experimental design, was it in vivo or in vitro work? If in vivo, were humans or animals used? Was there a control group? What were the sex, number, and age of experimental (and control) subjects? What was the length of the experiment? Was there a sufficient number of subjects and/or sufficient time allowed to warrant meaningful conclusions?
8. Is the statistical treatment of data clearly defined and are statistics presented in a straightforward manner?
9. Are the conclusions that the researcher presents justified by the facts presented?
10. Is there any indication whether the hypotheses are supported or rejected?
11. Are limitations of the study identified?
12. Is there any reference to or discussion of related literature or studies by other investigators?
13. Are specific areas for further research suggested?
14. By whom was the research sponsored? Could results be influenced in any way by the source of funding?

3. *Prepare a research plan/proposal.* The proposal should include

a. a statement of the research question (from step 2);
b. a review of literature (from step 1);
c. the significance of the research; and
d. a description of research design, which should specify the specifics of the investigation (i.e., methods, data analysis, and the appropriate statistical analysis).

Putting the plan in writing forces the researcher to think through all aspects of the investigation and can serve as a clearly defined guide for carrying out the project. The plan becomes a working document that can be converted into the research report. A written plan is more likely to be followed without modification over time.

Depending on the level of the research, the plan may range from a simple outline to a complicated, detailed request for funding from a foundation or government agency. Regardless of the level of investigation, established guidelines must be followed whenever live subjects are used. Review of proposed research projects by committees on ethical standards ensures that procedures are acceptable. These committees operate in academic institutions at the departmental and university level. Funding agencies and organizations are very careful about considering only those proposals that strictly adhere to the guidelines.

4. *Plan for the collection and preparation of data.* Once the method for data collection has been selected (or designed), a pilot study can be conducted to point out any adjustments or modifications that need to be made. The pilot study also may provide a good indication of the value of the data being collected. Improvements in research design often result from a pilot study.

Once the research procedures have been refined, the planning stage is finished and the research study can be conducted. Carrying out the research involves the collection of data, followed by the crucial steps of interpreting the data and reporting the results. The problem that initiated the research finally is addressed, and results of the investigation are interpreted in the framework of existing theory and past research, if such is attainable. Either the problem is solved, or the process must begin again. Many valuable outcomes are possible from even the simplest research projects if they are well planned. An interest in problem solving coupled with diligence in planning an orderly, stepwise progression in problem solution provides the essentials for scientific inquiry.

PROBLEMS AND PITFALLS IN RESEARCH

In general, a clear understanding of the steps or components of the research process provides a good checklist against which to evaluate research presented in publications or to plan one's own research study. Attention to these components also provides a guide to problems and pitfalls that can plague research.

The logical progression of components in the research process was discussed in the previous section and reproduced in checklist form in Table 16.7. A complete plan for this logical progression of the elements of research (including the question, research design, and exact statistical analysis) should be in place before any

Table 16.8 Commonly Encountered Problems in Research

Insoluble problems in studies:
Lack of representative sampling
Vague target population definition with poor selection of subjects
Lack of random allocation of treatments
Lack of proper handling of confounding (nuisance) variables
Lack of appropriate controls
Lack of blinded subjects and evaluators
Lack of objective measurement or assessment of outcome
Possibly soluble problems in studies:
Inadequate assurance of group comparability
Inappropriate choice of sample units
Use of calculated normal limits for skewed distributions; multiple significance testing
Incorrect denominators for rates, risks, or probabilities
Misuse and incorrect presentation of age data
Improper handling of problems arising from incomplete follow-up in longitudinal studies
Spurious associations between diseases or between a disease and apparent risk factors
Ambiguity concerning descriptive statistics used

research activity begins. If this is done, then the research study will in fact be following a predetermined protocol, in a manner similar to a National Aeronautics and Space Administration (NASA) launch.

Despite the best-laid plans, some problems can occur during a research study. As summarized in an editorial by Vaisrub [26], problems that can be considered as either "soluble" or "insoluble" may arise in the course of a research study. Examples of both types of problems are given in Table 16.8.

One of the more difficult and error-prone areas of research is the application of statistics in the analysis of data. Typically, this involves rejection or retention of a null hypothesis. Should the statistics be invalid, the null hypothesis may be rejected when it should have been retained, or it may be retained when it should have been rejected. The most common cause of such errors is insufficient power of the statistical test ("power" refers to the likelihood of falsely rejecting a null hypothesis). In view of the magnitude of the subject, statistical data analysis is not addressed in this chapter. However, excellent pertinent references are available to the interested reader [20,21,27].

EVALUATION OF RESEARCH AND SCIENTIFIC LITERATURE

Although the library "research" paper cannot be considered research because it is not gathering new data or using existing data for a new purpose, it does involve the selection and transfer of existing information and therefore requires careful evaluation of scientific literature. Like initiation of research, evaluation requires familiarity with the characteristics of research. The questions posed in Table 16.7 can serve as a guide in identifying the quality of published research articles. The type of publication in which the research article is published is also important. Publication in a peer-reviewed or refereed journal indicates that the article has been reviewed by some of the researcher's peers to determine its worth for publication. However, while peer review helps enhance the quality of a research publication, it is not a guarantee of a high-quality study.

There is a form of research synthesis that attempts to solve research problems through literature reviews. A popular technique to accomplish this is called meta-analysis. A full discussion of the technique is beyond the scope of this text, but briefly it is a way to quantitatively compare (using statistical measures) treatment effects from studies with similar treatments. Meta-analysis involves additional steps beyond the typical literature research review paper. After the problem to be studied is identified, definitive criteria are reported for the literature analysis. Additionally, the results included from the various studies are converted to a quantitative standard that allows the use of statistical techniques as a means of analysis [28].

Although most quality research articles appear in refereed journals, many excellent invited reviews from prestigious investigators may appear in other journal publications, such as *Nutrition Today, Nutrition in Clinical Practice,* or *Contemporary Nutrition.* These reviews are not original research but are summaries of research in a particular area (subject) and are based on information formerly published in refereed journals. What distinguished these reviews from meta-analysis is the lack of a quantitative standard and statistical analysis of the data from multiple published reports. The information in review articles is secondhand and thus may have become somewhat distorted because of imperfections inherent in communication. Review articles, however, can be extremely helpful in providing an overview of some particular topic. When specifics are important, the original report should always be consulted.

The introduction to this chapter emphasized that because of intense public interest in nutrition and health, the media floods us with nutrition-related information. This information wears two faces: that based on sound scientific research and that which comes from anecdotal reporting, hearsay, or quackery. The well-informed student of nutrition must learn to distinguish these and to critically evaluate the source of a report. This may be easy to do at the extremes of "good" science and quackery, but many times information falls between these extremes and distinguishing between the two becomes more of a challenge. Articles designed to help the nutrition student do this appear frequently in respected literature sources. Two such articles are referenced here [29,30].

NUTRITION RESEARCH ON THE INTERNET

Nutrition is big business on the Internet, just as it is in all other forms of mass communication. Nutrition topics take many popular guises: weight loss diets and healthy heart diets, recipes for lowering cholesterol, tips on how to reduce the risk of cancer or boost sports prowess, and herbal therapies for all of these.

Professional nutrition research on the Internet should follow all the guidelines of good research discussed in this chapter. In addition, users of the medium must recognize some Internet-specific caveats. In seeking out new information on the Internet while at the same time attempting to separate hearsay, anecdotal reporting, and quackery from authentic information, the reader should ask the following questions:

- *What is the source of the Web site?* Most Web sites have owners and/or sponsors who may have a proprietary interest in promoting a product or an agenda. Also, because the Web is worldwide, some Web sites originating in another country may use different guidelines or principles. The source is always posted, sometimes in small print at the bottom of the home page.
- *Who are the contributors?* Nutritionists and health care professionals should be prominently listed as contributors to a Web site. For example, the Web site **onhealth.com** has a page listing the contributing members of its medical advisory board.
- *Is the Web site efficiently managed?* The site should be frequently updated. Generally, the most recent updates are posted. Within the limits of the computer used, moving between pages should be quick and easy. There should also be a "search" component to access all the resource information of the Web site.
- *What links to other Web sites and databases are provided?* There should be links to other reputable professional sources of information such as the National Library of Medicine's MEDLINE, which holds records and abstracts from over 3,500 medical journals and other publications. Databases that are accessed should provide abstracts of the research publications. In some cases, it is possible to order complete articles on-line.

Research on the Internet is novel, convenient, and appealing, but it is important to remember that it is simply a technologically advanced medium designed to disseminate vast amounts of information to, in many cases, unwary users. The information it provides must be evaluated for authenticity at least to the same degree as information accessed through the more traditional library search.

summary

This chapter has identified characteristics of research, noted the process for evaluating scientific literature, and identified problems that can plague a research study. It has also described methodologies used in research, giving examples of nutrition-related research in which various methodologies were used.

Certainly, one chapter cannot provide sufficient depth of information for performing outstanding research. Study and coursework in the various elements of the research process, as well as apprenticeship to a more experienced investigator, are normally required. It is hoped, however, that the material offered in the chapter, together with the supplemental references, has at least armed the reader with new insight into proper research protocol and imparted a higher level of confidence with respect to becoming a critical reviewer of the literature.

Expansion of the nutrition knowledge base depends on ongoing nutrition research at every level. Knowledge about the total human depends on research at the molecular, cellular, organ or tissue, and system levels. Examples of research at the different levels have been given in this chapter and throughout the book.

References Cited

1. Lusk G. The Basics of Nutrition. New Haven, CT: Yale University Press, 1923.

2. McCollum EV. A History of Nutrition. Boston: Houghton Mifflin, 1957.

3. Rose WC. The amino acid requirements of adult man. Nutr Abst Rev 1957;27:631–47.

4. Young VR. 1987 McCollum Award lecture. Kinetics of human amino acid metabolism: nutritional implications and some lessons. Am J Clin Nutr 1987;46:709–25.

5. Young VR, Scrimshaw NS. Endogenous nitrogen metabolism and plasma free amino acids in young adults given a "protein free" diet. Br J Nutr 1968;22:9–20.

6. Young VR, Hussein MA, Murray E, et al. Plasma tryptophan response curve and its relation to tryptophan requirements in young adult men. J Nutr 1971;101:45–60.

7. Ozalp I, Young VR, Nagchaudhuri J, et al. Plasma amino acid response in young men given diets devoid of single essential amino acids. J Nutr 1972;102:1147–58.

8. Young VR, Toutisrin K, Ozalp I, et al. Plasma amino acid response and amino acid requirements in young men: valine and lysine. J Nutr 1972;102:1159–70.

9. Leedy PD. Practical Research Planning and Design, 7th ed. Upper Saddle River, NJ: Merrill Prentice Hall, 2001.

10. Sedlet KL, Ireton-Jones CS. Energy expenditure and the abnormal eating pattern of a bulimic: a case report. J Am Diet Assoc 1989;89:74–77.

11. Terris M, ed. Goldberger on Pellagra. Baton Rouge: Louisiana State University Press, 1964.

12. Pyle RL, Mitchell JE, Eckart ED. Bulimia: a report of 34 cases. J Clin Psych 1981;42:60–64.

13. U.S. Department of Health, Education and Welfare. Ten-State Nutrition Survey, 1968–1970. Washington, DC: U.S. Government Printing Office, 1972.

14. National Center for Health Statistics. Plan and operation of the National Health and Nutrition Examination Survey. Rockville, MD: U.S. Department of Health and Human Services, 1975.

15. National Center For Health Statistics. Plan and Operation of the Third National Health and Examination Survey. Hyattsville, MD: U.S. Department of Health and Human Services, 1994.

16. Keys A, ed. Coronary heart disease in seven countries. Circulation 1970;41(suppl1):1–211.

17. Gordon T, Kannel WB. Premature mortality from coronary heart disease. The Framingham Study. JAMA 1971;215:1617–25.

18. Belanger CF, Hennekens CH, Rosner B, Speizer FE. The Nurses' Health Study. Am J Nurs 1978;78(6):1039–40.

19. Holmes MD, Hunter DJ, Colditz GA, Stampfer MJ, et al. Association of dietary intake of fat and fatty acids with risk of breast cancer. JAMA 1999;238(10):914–20.

20. Stephens LJ. Beginning Statistics (Schaun's Outline Series). New York: McGraw-Hill, 1998.

21. Jaeger RM. Statistics: A Spectator Sport, 2nd ed. Newbury Park, CA: Sage Publications, 1990.

22. Armstrong ML, Warner ED, Connor WE. Regression of coronary atheromatosis in rhesus monkeys. Circ Res 1970;27:59–67.

23. Lipid Research Clinics Program: The Lipid Research Clinics Coronary Primary Prevention Trial Results. I. Reduction in incidence of coronary heart disease to cholesterol lowering, and II. The relationship of reduction in incidence of coronary heart disease to cholesterol lowering. JAMA 1984;251:351–64,365–74.

24. Lowering blood cholesterol to prevent heart disease. Consensus Conference. JAMA,1985;253:2080–86.

25. Touliatos J, Compton N. Research Methods in Human Ecology and Home Economics. Ames, IA: Iowa State University Press, 1988.

26. Vaisrub N. Manuscript review from a statistician's perspective (editorial). JAMA 1985;253:3145–47.

27. Daniel WW. Biostatistics: A Foundation for Analysis in the Health Sciences, 4th ed. New York: Wiley, 1987.

28. Thomas JR, Nelson JK. Research Methods in Physical Activity, 4th ed. Champaign, IL: Human Kinetics, 2001.

29. Ashley JM, Jarvis WT. Position of the American Dietetic Association: food and nutrition misinformation. J Am Diet Assoc 1995;95:705–7.

30. Hansen B. President's address, 1996: a virtual organization for nutrition in the 21st century. Am J Clin Nutr 1996;64:796–99.

Suggested Readings

Monsen ER, Cheney CL. Research methods in nutrition and dietetics: design, data analysis and presentation. J Am Diet Assoc 1988; 88:1047–65.

This extremely useful article can serve as a guide for students who are learning the mechanics of research as well as for practitioners in the field of nutrition. Practical examples of research that could be conducted inexpensively in the work setting are given.

The Surgeon General's Report on Nutrition and Health. DHHS (PHS) publication no. 88-50210. Washington, DC: U.S. Government Printing Office, 1988.

This 725-page report includes extensive evidence for the relationship between nutrition and several chronic diseases. Results of research reported to support evidence of relationship are based on a wide array of studies: dietary studies, experiments with laboratory animals, genetic and metabolic research, and epidemiological studies. Issues of special priority for continuing research are listed after discussion of each disease.

Touliatos J, Compton N. Research Methods in Human Ecology and Home Economics. Ames, IA: Iowa State University Press, 1988.

This is an excellent up-to-date book on the how-to's of applied research.

Web Sites

www.eurekalert.org
EurekAlert; American Association for the Advancement of Science

www.cspinet.org
Center for Science in the Public Interest

www.quackwatch.com
Quackwatch, member of the Consumer Federation of America

www.nlm.nih.gov
National Library of Medicine: MEDLINE

onhealth.com
On Health

www.nejm.org
New England Journal of Medicine

www.ama-assn.org/public/journals/jama/jamahome.htm
Journal of the American Medical Association

www.navigator.tufts.edu
Tufts University Nutrition Navigator

www.ncahf.org
National Council against Health Fraud

www.ilsi.org/pubs.html
Nutrition Reviews

www.faseb.org/ajcn
American Journal of Clinical Nutrition

APPENDIX

Stereoisomerism and Carbohydrates

This appendix provides a more complete discussion of stereoisomerism as it relates to carbohydrates. A more extensive discussion can be obtained from a general biochemistry text. This topic is important because most enzymes and transport mechanisms for carbohydrates, fats, and amino acids are stereospecific. An understanding of the implications and nomenclature therefore aids in the understanding of nutritional biochemistry. Many organic substances, including the carbohydrates, are optically active. This means that if a plane-polarized light is passed through a solution of the substances, the plane of light will be rotated to the right (dextrorotatory) or to the left (levorotatory). The direction and extent of the rotation are characteristic of a particular compound and depend on the substance's concentration and temperature and on the wavelength of the light. The right or left direction of light rotation is expressed as + (dextrorotatory) or − (levorotatory), and the number of angular degrees indicates the extent of rotation. As an example, a solution of glucose is known to have a rotation of +52.7°.

Optical activity is attributed to the presence of one or more asymmetrical or chiral carbon atoms in the molecule. Chiral carbon atoms have four different atoms or groups covalently attached to them. Shown in Figure A is a chiral carbon atom with its bonds directed

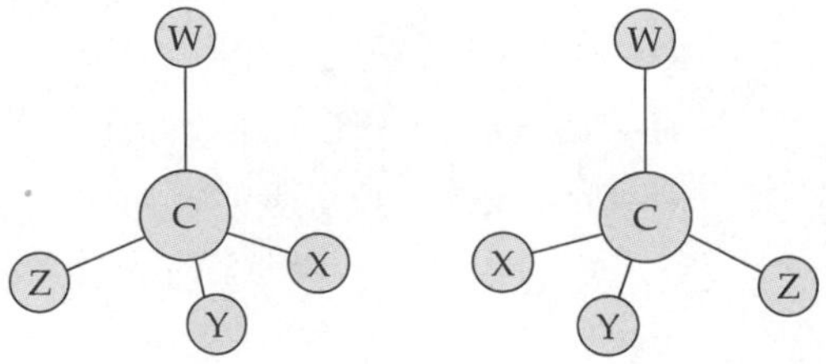

Figure A

D-glyceraldehyde L-glyceraldehyde

Figure B

toward the hypothetical atoms or groups W, X, Y, and Z. The carbon atom can be thought of as being situated in the geometric center of a tetrahedron, with its four bonds directed toward the corners of that tetrahedron. Because the molecule is asymmetrical, it is possible to construct a similar but not identical figure by simply exchanging the positions of any two of the groups. The two models shown bear the same groups and therefore the same molecular formula, but they are not identical, as evidenced by the inability to superimpose them by mental manipulation. In fact, they are mirror images of each other and are said to be enantiomers, a special class within a broader family of compounds called stereoisomers. Stereoisomers are compounds having two or more chiral carbon atoms that have the same four groups attached to them but are not mirror images of each other.

If an asymmetrical substance rotates the plane of polarized light a certain number of degrees to the right, its enantiomer will rotate the light the same number of degrees to the left. Enantiomers exist in D or L orientation. If a compound is structurally D, its enantiomer will be L. The D and L designations do not predict the direction of rotation of plane-polarized light. Instead, the designation is simply a structural analogy to the reference compound glyceraldehyde, whose D and L forms are by convention drawn as shown in Figure B. The distinction between D and L configurations of enantiomers therefore rests with the direction of the –OH bond on the single, chiral carbon of the molecule. Note that in the D configuration it points to the right and in the L configuration to the left. Remember that these forms are not superimposable.

Monosaccharides having more than three carbons will have more than one chiral center. The highest-numbered chiral carbon indicates whether the molecule is of the D or the L configuration. Carbohydrates are numbered from the functional aldehyde or ketone end, so the chiral carbon farthest from that end determines the configuration. The configuration is determined by the right or left direction of the hydroxyl group attached to that carbon atom. Carbon-atom numbering and the D versus L designation are illustrated in Figure C for the aldohexose glucose and the ketohexose fructose. Because the highest-numbered asymmetrical carbon atom in these structures is number 5, this becomes the designator atom for either the D or the L stereoisomer. Notice, however, that in going from the D to the L isomer, the direction of the hydroxyl groups on all asymmetrical carbons is reversed, not only that on the number 5 carbon (see Fig. C). Monosaccharides of the D configuration are much more important nutritionally than their L isomers because they exist as such in dietary carbohydrate and are metabolized specifically in that form. The enzymes involved in carbohydrate digestion and metabolism are stereospecific for D sugars, meaning that they react only with D sugars and are inactive toward the L forms.

The structures in Figure C are shown as open-chain, or Fischer projection, models, in which the carbonyl (aldehyde or ketone) functions are free. The monosaccharides generally do not exist in open-chain form, but they are shown that way here to clarify the D-L concept and to illustrate the so-called anomeric carbon, the carbon atom comprising the carbonyl function. Note that the anomeric carbon is number 1 in the aldose (glucose) and number 2 in the ketose (fructose).

The fact that the monosaccharides do not exist in open-chain form while in solution is evidenced by the fact that they do not undergo reactions characteristic of true aldehydes and ketones. Actually, the molecules cyclize, producing forms called hemiacetals if the sugar is an aldose and hemiketals if the sugar is a ketose. The hemiacetal or hemiketal bonds are formed by the

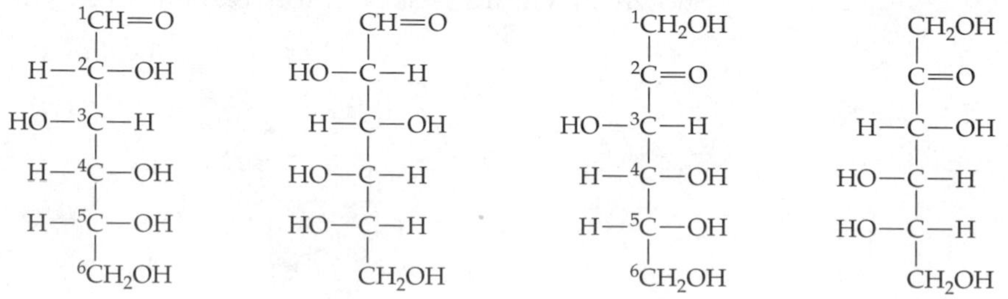

D-glucose L-glucose D-fructose L-fructose

Figure C

reaction of an alcohol group with an aldehyde or ketone group, respectively. Therefore, the participating groups within a monosaccharide are the aldehyde or ketone of the anomeric carbon atom and the alcohol group attached to the highest-numbered chiral carbon atom. This is illustrated using D-glucose and D-fructose in Figure D. The formation of the hemiacetal or hemiketal

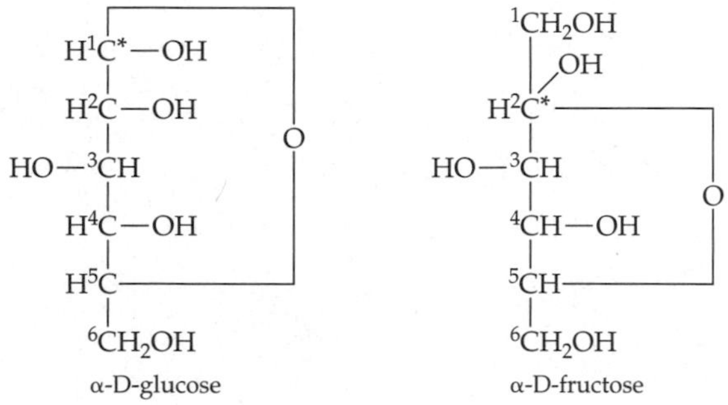

Figure D

produces a new chiral center at the anomeric carbon, designated by an asterisk in the structures in Figure D, and therefore the bond direction of the newly formed hydroxyl becomes significant. In the cyclized structures shown, the anomeric hydroxyls at position 1 for D-glucose and position 2 for D-fructose are arbitrarily directed to the right, resulting in an alpha (α) configuration. Should the anomeric hydroxyl be directed to the left, the structure would be in a beta (β) configuration. Cyclization to the hemiacetal or hemiketal can produce either the α- or β-isomer; however, in aqueous solution, an equilibrium mixture of the isomers exists, with the concentration of the β form being roughly twice that of the α form. If a pure solution of either isomer is prepared, the optical rotation of the solution will change as the equilibrium concentrations of the two forms are approached. This change in optical rotation, called mutarotation, results from the interconversion of the α- and β-isomers. In essence, the α-hemiacetal can change to the open structure and then cyclize again, to either the α or the β configuration.

Glossary

Achlorhydria Lack of hydrochloric acid in gastric juice.

Activation energy Energy introduced into the reactant molecules to activate them to the transition state so that an exothermic reaction can take place.

Acute Having a rapid or sudden onset.

Alkalosis A condition in which the pH of the blood is above 7.45.

Amenorrhea The absence of at least three consecutive menstrual cycles.

Amphibolic pathway A pathway that is involved in both the catabolism and the biosynthesis of carbohydrates, fatty acids, and amino acids.

Amphipathic Refers to a molecule that has a polar region at one location and a nonpolar region at another.

Amphoteric Something that can react as either an acid or a base.

Anomeric carbon The carbon that forms a ring structure with the reducing carbon reacting with the OH group on the highest-numbered chiral carbon of a monosaccharide.

Anticodons Three-base sequences of nucleotides on molecules of a transfer RNA (tRNA).

Antral Pertaining to the antrum, the lower or distal portion of the stomach.

Apolipoprotein The protein component of a lipoprotein.

Apoprotein A protein that bind to ligands (other compounds).

Apoptosis An organized series of events that, once triggered, lead to cell death.

Aromatic compound An organic compound that contains a benzene ring.

Ataxia Impaired muscle coordination, especially when trying to perform voluntary muscular movements.

Atheroma A mass of plaque consisting of degenerated, thickened arterial intima, occurring in atherosclerosis.

Autolysis The digestion of intracellular components (including organelles) by lysosomes.

Autophagy The breakdown or digestion of the body's proteins, such as those found in the blood or within cells.

Beriberi A condition resulting from a thiamin deficiency.

Bile A body fluid made in the liver and stored in the gallbladder that functions in the emulsification of fat and micelle formation for fat absorption.

Buffer A compound that ameliorates a change in pH.

Calpains A calcium-dependent protease involved in protein turnover in the body.

Carboxylation The addition of a carboxyl group to a molecule.

Catabolism The breaking down of organic molecules to produce energy.

Cathepsins A group of enzymes involved with the breakdown or digestion of the body's proteins.

Cells The basic units for all organisms that arise from preexisting cells.

Chaperones Soluble intracellular proteins that bind to and deliver minerals to specific intracellular locations.

Chelators Small organic compounds that form a complex with another compound such as a mineral.

Chemiosmotic theory A process by which there is a movement of protons down an electrochemical gradient and the energy generated is used to phosphorylate ADP to make ATP.

Chiral carbon Carbon atoms with four different atoms or groups covalently attached to them.

Chronic Long and drawn out in duration.

Chylomicron A type of lipoprotein that transports fats and fat-soluble vitamins from the intestine into the lymph and then blood for use by body cells.

Chylomicron remnant What is left over from a chylomicron after the action of blood lipoprotein lipase removes part of the triglycerides.

Chyme Partially digested food.

Cobalophilins A group of proteins, sometimes called R proteins, that are found in digestive juices and bind to vitamin B_{12} to facilitate absorption.

Codon A three-base sequence in a DNA or mRNA molecule that specifies the location of a single amino acid in a polypeptide chain.

Cohort A group of individuals that share common characteristics.

Colloids Substances comprised of very small particles that are suspended uniformly in a medium.

Colorimetric titration A method of measuring the volume of one reagent required to react with a measured volume of another reagent using an indicator that changes color.

Complementary base pairing The pairing of nucleotide bases in two strands of nucleic acids; A pairs with T or U, G pairs with C.

Complete protein A protein that contains all the essential (indispensable) amino acids in the approximate amounts needed by humans.

Connexin A protein involved in the formation of junctions between cells.

Coulometric titration A method for determining the amount of a substance released during electrolysis by measuring the electrical charge. (*Note:* A coulomb is a unit of electrical charge.)

Cytochromes Heme-containing proteins that serve as electron carriers in oxidative phosphorylation.

Cytokines A generic term for non-antibody protein messengers released from a macrophage or lympocyte that is part of an intracellular immune response.

Cytoplasm The continuous aqueous solution of the cell and the organelles contained in it.

Cytoplast A cell from which the nucleus has been removed.

Cytoskeleton Microtubules and microfilaments in the cell providing internal reinforcement and communication.

Deamination The removal of an amino (NH_2) group from an amino acid.

Dehydrogenases Enzymes that catalyze reactions in which hydrogens and electrons are removed from a reactant.

Desaturation The process of converting a saturated compound to an unsaturated one.

Dietary fiber Nondigestible (by human digestive enzymes) carbohydrates and lignin that are intact and intrinsic in plants.

Dipeptidylaminopeptidase A protein-digesting enzyme that breaks apart dipeptides.

Direct calorimetry Measurement of the dissipation of heat from the body.

Disaccharides Sugars formed by combining two monosaccharides through a glycosidic bond between the hydroxyl group of one monosaccharide and the hydroxyl group of another.

Dowager's hump A deformity of the spine characterized by a humpback or being bent forward; also called *kyphosis.*

Eicosanoids Biologically active substances derived from arachidonic acid.

Electron transport chain The sequential transfer of electrons from reduced coenzymes to oxygen that is coupled with ATP formation.

Elongation The extension of the polypeptide chain of the protein product during protein synthesis.

Endocrine system All of the body's hormone-secreting glands.

Endocytosis Uptake of a substance into a cell through the formation of vesicles formed from the plasma membrane.

Endopeptidase An enzyme that hydrolyzes amino acids linked to other amino acids in the interior of a peptide/protein.

Endoplasmic reticulum (ER) A network of membranous channels pervading the cytoplast and providing continuity between the nuclear envelope, the Golgi apparatus, and the plasma membrane.

Endothermic (reaction) A reaction in which the products have more free energy than the reactants, requiring energy.

Enkephalins Peptides that bind to opioid receptors found in the brain and gastrointestinal tract.

Enterocyte An intestinal cell.

Enterohepatic circulation The movement of a substance, such as bile, from the liver to the intestine and then back to the liver.

Enzymes Protein catalysts that increase the rate of a chemical reaction in the body.

Epidemiology The science concerned with the study of those factors that influence the frequency and distribution of disease.

Equivocal Uncertain or ambiguous.

Erythrocyte A red blood cell.

Estimated average requirement The amount of a nutrient thought to meet the nutrient requirements of 50% of healthy individuals in a specified age and gender group.

Eukaryotic cells Cells with a defined nucleus surrounded by a nuclear membrane.

Exocytosis A process by which compounds may be released from cells.

Exons The segments of a gene that code for a sequence of nucleotides in a specific molecule of mRNA.

Exopeptidase An enzyme that hydrolyzes amino acids off the terminal end of a peptide or protein.

Exothermic (reaction) A reaction in which the reactants have more free energy than the products, giving off energy as heat.

Exudate Fluids that have exuded (been forced or pressed) out of a tissue or its capillaries.

Ferment To break down substrates anaerobically to yield reduced products and energy.

Fermentation An anaerobic breakdown of carbohydrates and protein by bacteria.

Fibrotic Pertaining to fibrosis, formation of fibrous tissue as a reactive or repair process.

Free energy The potential energy inherent in the chemical bonds of nutrients.

Free radical An atom or molecule that has one or more unpaired electrons.

Functional fiber Nondigestible carbohydrates that have been isolated, extracted, or manufactured and have been shown to have beneficial physiological effects in humans.

Gap junctions Channels between cells.

Gene A section of chromosomal DNA that codes for a single protein.

Genome The sum of all the chromosomal genes of a cell.

Gluconeogenesis The formation of glucose by the liver or kidney from noncarbohydrate precursors.

Glucose tolerance factor (GTF) A chromium-containing compound whose structure has yet to be characterized but may potentiate the action of insulin in the body.

Glycocalyx The layer of glycoprotein and polysaccharide that surrounds many cells.

Glycogenesis The pathway by which glucose is converted to glycogen.

Glycogenolysis The pathway by which glycogen is enzymatically broken down to glucose.

Glycolysis The pathway by which glucose is converted to pyruvate.

Glycoproteins Proteins covalently bound to a carbohydrate.

Glycosaminoglycan An unbranched polysaccharide consisting of alternate units of two different sugars.

Glycosidases/carbohydrases Digestive enzymes that hydrolyze polysaccharides to their constituent monosaccharide units.

Golgi apparatus The part of the cell responsible for modifying macromolecules synthesized in the endoplasmic reticulum and packaging them to be transported to the cell surface or cytoplasm.

Haptocorrins A group of proteins, sometimes called R proteins, that are found in digestive juices and bind to vitamin B_{12} to facilitate absorption.

Hartnup disease A hereditary disorder in which tryptophan absorption and excretion are abnormal.

Hemochromatosis An inherited disorder characterized by excessive iron absorption and iron overload in the body.

Heterodimers Complexes formed between two or more different receptors.

Hexosemonophosphate shunt The pathway that metabolizes glucose-6-phosphate to pentose phosphate, producing NADPH.

Homeostasis The tendency to stability in the internal environment of an organism.

Homodimers Complexes formed between two of the same receptors.

Hormones Chemical messengers synthesized and secreted by endocrine tissue (glands) and transported in the blood to target tissues or organs.

Hydrolases Enzymes catalyzing cleavage of bonds between carbon atoms and some other kind of atom by the addition of water.

Hydroperoxyl radical HO_2^- or H—O—O$^-$.

Hydroxyapatite A crystal-lattice-like substance with the formula $Ca_{10}(PO_4)_6(OH)_2$ found in bones and teeth.

Hypercalciuria High urinary calcium excretion.

Hyperglycemia A glucose blood level above normal.

Hyperinsulinemia A level of insulin in the blood that is above normal.

Hyperkalemia High concentrations of potassium in the blood.

Hyperlipidemia A general term for an elevated blood level of any lipid.

Hyperphosphatemia High concentrations of phosphorus in the blood.

Hyperplasia Excessive cell proliferation.

Hyperpnea An abnormal increase in the rate and depth of breathing.

Hypertrophied Grown larger or increased in size.

Hypertrophy Enlargement of the size of cells to increase the size of an organ.

Hypocalcemia Low concentrations of calcium in the blood.

Hypochondriasis Abnormal anxiety about one's own health.

Hypoglycemia A blood glucose level that is below normal.

Hypokalemia Low concentrations of potassium in the blood.

Hyponatremia Low concentrations of sodium in the blood.

Immunoproteins Proteins made by plasma cells that help destroy foreign substances in the body; also called *immunoglobulins* or *antibodies.*

Indirect calorimetry Measurement of the consumption of oxygen and the expiration of carbon dioxide by the body used to estimate metabolic rate.

Introns Noncoding regions of a gene.

In vitro In a test tube or culture (outside the body).

In vivo Within the body.

Ion An electrically charged atom or group of atoms; positively charged ions are called *cations,* and negatively charged ions are called *anions.*

Ischemia Deficiency of blood in a tissue.

Isomer Two different chemical compounds that have the same molecular formula.

Isomerases Enzymes catalyzing the interconversion of optical or geometric isomers.

Isoprenoid Refers to the structure of the side chains of vitamins E and K.

Isotope infusion The direct introduction of an isotope (either radioactive or stable) into the bloodstream.

Keratinocytes Cells that produce the protein keratin.

Ketone bodies Compounds (acetoacetate, β-hydroxybutyrate, and acetone) formed during the oxidation of fatty acids in the absence of adequate four-carbon intermediates.

Krebs cycle An aerobic metabolic cycle in the mitochondria that produces ATP; also called the *citric acid cycle.*

Kyphosis A deformity of the spine characterized by a humpback or being bent forward; also called *dowager's hump.*

Lanugo Fine, soft, lightly pigmented hair that usually is found on a fetus toward the end of pregnancy but may appear on malnourished individuals.

Leukotrienes Biologically active compounds derived from arachidonic acid.

Ligands Small molecules that bind to a larger molecule.

Ligases Enzymes that catalyze the formation of bonds between carbon and other atoms.

Limiting amino acid The amino acid with the lowest amino acid or chemical score; it is the amino acid present in a protein in the lowest amount compared with a reference protein.

Lingual Pertaining to the tongue.

Lipophilicity The state of being attracted to lipids and thus repelled by water.

Lipoproteins Complexes of lipids and proteins that play a role in the transport and distribution of lipids.

Lyases Enzymes that catalyze cleavage of carbon-carbon, carbon-sulfur, and certain carbon-nitrogen bonds without hydrolysis or oxidation-reduction.

Lysosomes Cell organelles that contain digestive enzymes.

Macronutrients The dietary nutrients that supply energy, including fats, carbohydrates, and proteins.

Marasmus Malnutrition due to a prolonged intake of a diet deficient in energy (kcal).

Microflora Bacteria adapted to living in a specific environment such as the intestines.

Microvilli Extensions of intestinal epithelial cells designed to present a large surface area for the absorption of dietary nutrients.

Mitochondria Cellular organelles that are the site of energy production by oxidative phosphorylation and the site of the Krebs cycle; they are surrounded by an outer membrane that is very permeable and an inner membrane that is only selectively permeable.

Monosaccharides The simplest form of carbohydrates that cannot be reduced in size to smaller carbohydrate units.

Motility Movement.

Mucins Glycoproteins found in some body secretions such as saliva.

Nervous system The system of nervous tissue made up of neurons and glial cells.

Nuclear envelope A set of two membranes containing nuclear pores and surrounding the nucleus.

Nucleoli Regions of the nucleus containing condensed chromatin and sites for synthesis of ribosomal RNA.

Nucleotides A phosphate ester of the 5′-phosphate of a purine or pyrimidine in N-glycosidic linkage with ribose or deoxyribose, occurring in nucleic acids.

Nystagmus Constant, involuntary movement of the eyeball.

Oligomer Polypeptide chains joined to form a functional protein.

Oligosaccharides Short chains of monosaccharide units joined by covalent bonds.

Oncogenes Genes capable of causing a normal cell to convert to a cancerous cell.

Ophthalmoplegia Paralysis of the ocular muscles.

Oscilloscope An instrument used to visualize echoes as part of an ultrasound examination.

Osmosis The net movement of the solvent (such as water) from a solution of lesser to one of greater concentration when the two solutions are separated by a membrane that selectively prevents passage of solute molecules but is permeable to the solvent.

Osmotic pressure A property of a solution that is proportional to the nondiffusible solute concentration.

Osteoblasts Bone-forming cells.

Osteoclasts Cells that break down or resorb bone.

Osteomalacia A disorder characterized by bone mineralization defects that may occur in adults due to inadequate vitamin D intake.

Oxidation An enzymatic reaction in which there is an addition of oxygen to or the removal of electrons or hydrogen from the reactant.

Oxidative phosphorylation The pathway in the mitochondria that makes ATP from ADP and P_i.

Oxidoreductases Enzymes catalyzing all reactions in which one compound is oxidized and another reduced.

Oxygenation reactions Reactions involving the introduction of or requiring one or more oxygen atoms.

Parenchymal cells The functional cells of an organ such as the liver.

Pellagra A condition resulting from a niacin deficiency.

Peroxisomes Cell organelles containing enzymes that perform oxidative catabolic reactions.

Peroxyl radical O_2^{2-}.

Petechiae Skin discolorations due to ruptured small blood vessels.

Phagocytosis An endocytotic process in which material is engulfed into a cell.

Phospholipids Lipids that belong to a class of complex lipids containing phosphate and one or more fatty-acid residues.

Phosphorolysis The process by which there is sequential release of individual glucose units from glycogen.

Phosphorylation The metabolic process of adding a phosphate group to an organic molecule.

Phytochemical A nonnutritive substance that is biologically active and found in plants.

Phytyl tail Refers to the structure of the side chains of vitamins E and K.

Pinocytosis Uptake of a substance into a cell through the formation of vesicles formed from the plasma membrane.

Plasma membrane The membrane encapsulating the cell.

Polymer A substance with a high molecular weight made up of a chain of repeating units.

Polysaccharides Long chains of monosaccharide units that may number from several into the hundreds or thousands.

Porphyrin The nitrogen- and iron-containing nonprotein portion of hemoglobin.

Postprandial Occurring after a meal.

Potentiometry A method using electrodes that allows for the direct measurement of various anions and cations such as potassium, sodium, and chloride.

Preprandial Occurring before a meal.

Probiotics Products containing specific strains of microorganisms in sufficient numbers to alter the microflora of the gastrointestinal tract, ideally to exert beneficial health effects.

Prokaryotic cells Primitive cells that do not contain a defined nucleus.

Propagation The ongoing generation of free radicals following the initiation stage of free radical formation.

Prophylactic A substance or regime that helps in the prevention of disease or illness.

Prostaglandins Biologically active compounds derived from arachidonic acid.

Proteases Enzymes that digest (break down) proteins.

Protein kinases A family of enzymes that transfers a phosphate group to another protein from ATP.

Proteoglycans Large molecules made up of proteins and glycosaminoglycans.

Proteolytic Refers to the breakdown of protein.

Quenching A process by which electronically excited molecules such as singlet molecular oxygen are inactivated.

Receptors Macromolecules (usually proteins) that bind a signal molecule with a high degree of specificity that triggers intracellular events.

Recommended dietary allowance The average daily dietary intake level of a nutrient that is thought to be sufficient to meet the nutrient requirements of about 97% of healthy individuals.

Reflex An involuntary response to a stimulus.

Reperfusion The resupply of an organ or tissue with oxygen and/or nutrients.

Replication The synthesis of a daughter duplex DNA molecule identical to the parental duplex DNA.

Resin A compound that is usually solid or soft-solid and usually exists as a polymer.

Respiratory quotient (RQ) The ratio of the volume of CO_2 expired to the volume of O_2 consumed.

Rhodopsin A vitamin A–containing protein found in the eye.

Rickets A condition in infants and children resulting from vitamin D deficiency.

Ryanodine receptor A calcium channel in the sarcoplasmic reticulum of muscle that opens to permit the release of calcium.

Sarcoplasmic reticulum The smooth endoplasmic reticulum that is found in muscle cells and is the site of the calcium pump.

Scintillation counter An instrument used to measure concentrations of isotopes in a sample.

Scurvy A condition resulting from vitamin C deficiency.

Seborrheic dermatitis An inflammatory skin condition.

Sense strand The strand of DNA that serves as a template for mRNA.

Short-chain fatty acids Fatty acids typically containing two to four carbons.

Sideroblastic anemia An inherited disorder affecting red blood cell production and function.

Singlet molecular oxygen An electronically excited radical in which one of oxygen's electrons is excited to an orbital above the one it normally occupies.

Sphingolipids Phospholipids containing the amino alcohol sphingosine rather than glycerol.

Splanchnic Pertaining to the internal organs (viscera), especially the intestines.

Standard reduction potential The tendency of a molecule to donate or receive electrons.

Steatorrhea The presence of an excessive amount of fat in the feces.

Stellate cells Storage cells of the liver.

Stereoisomers A group of compounds having the same structure but different configurations.

Sterols A subclass of lipids containing a cyclopentanoperhydrophenanthrene ring system, a hydroxyl group, and a side chain.

Substrate-level phosphorylation The transferring of a phosphate group from one organic molecule to another.

Superoxide radical An oxygen-centered free radical, O_2^-.

Teratogenic Causing birth defects in a fetus.

Tetany A condition resulting from inadequate blood calcium concentrations and characterized by prolonged muscle contraction.

Thalassemia A hereditary form of anemia associated with defective synthesis of hemoglobin.

Thermogenesis The production of heat within the body.

Thermoregulation A regulatory mechanism that keeps heat production and loss about equal.

Thiobarbituric acid reactive substances Compounds such as hexanal, pentanal, or pentane that react with thiobarbituric acid and suggest oxidative damage has occurred.

Thromboxanes Biologically active compounds derived from arachidonic acid.

Tolerable upper intake level The highest daily intake level that is likely to cause no risk of adverse health effects to most individuals in the general population.

Tonic Pertaining to or characterized by tension or contraction.

Transcaltachia Rapid intestinal calcium absorption stimulated by the active form of vitamin D.

Transcription The process by which the genetic information (base sequence) in a single strand of DNA is used to specify a complementary sequence of bases in an mRNA chain.

Transducin A G protein found in the eye that responds to changes in opsin and is involved in the visual cycle.

Transferases Enzymes that catalyze reactions not involving oxidation and reduction in which a functional group is transferred from one substrate to another.

Transition state Energy level at which reactant molecules have been activated and can undergo an exothermic reaction.

Translation The process by which genetic information in an mRNA molecule specifies the sequence of amino acids in the protein product.

Translocation Movement of a compound or agent across a cell membrane, such as the intestinal cell, and into the blood.

Transport proteins Proteins that transport nutrients in blood or into and out of the nucleus of a cell.

Tropical sprue A disease common in tropical regions and characterized by weakness, weight loss, poor nutrient digestion and absorption, and steatorrhea.

Ubiquinol The alcohol form of ubiquinone, a fat-soluble molecule that functions in electron transport and ultimately ATP generation; also called *coenzyme* Q_{10} or CoQ_{10}.

Ubiquitin A protein that attaches to other proteins within cells or tissues to promote the degradation of the protein.

Vascular system The circulatory pathway that delivers blood to and from organs.

VO_2 max The maximal uptake of oxygen as measured during a test with increasing work intensity.

Ward's triangle A region within the pelvis (hip).

Xenobiotics Foreign chemicals such as drugs, carcinogens, pesticides, food additives, pollutants, or other noxious compounds.

Xerophthalmia Dryness of the conjunctiva and keratinization of the epithelium of the eye following inflammation of the conjunctiva associated with vitamin A deficiency.

Zwitterion An amino acid with no amino or carboxyl groups in its side chain.

Zymogen An inactive form of an enzyme, also referred to as a *proenzyme*.

Index

Page numbers in bold indicate definitions;
page numbers with *f* indicate figures;
page numbers with *t* indicate tables.

B

H

M

Q

R

U